Practical Manual of Physical Medicine and Rehabilitation

Commissioning Editor: Dolores Meloni
Project Development Manager: Cecilia Murphy
Project Manager: Anne Dickie
Design Manager: Stewart Larking
Illustration Manager: Mick Ruddy
Illustrator: Martin Woodward
Marketing Managers: Jennie Finn (UK) and Laura Meiskey (US)

Practical Manual of Physical Medicine and Rehabilitation

SECOND EDITION

Jackson C. Tan MD PT PhD CIME
Adjunct Assistant Clinical Professor
Rusk Institute of Rehabilitation Medicine
New York University Medical Center
New York, New York, USA
and
Medical Director
Occupational and Rehabilitation Center
Jacksonville, Florida, USA

Foreword by

Mathew H.M. Lee MD MPH FACP
Howard A. Rusk Professor of Rehabilitation Medicine
and Chairman
Department of Rehabilitation Medicine
Rusk Institute of Rehabilitation Medicine
New York University Medical Center
New York, New York, USA

NON SOLUS
ELSEVIER
MOSBY

ELSEVIER
MOSBY
An affiliate of Elsevier Inc

First edition 1998
Second edition 2006

ISBN 0 3230 3285 0

British Library Cataloguing in Publication Data
A catalogue record for this book is available from the British Library

Library of Congress Cataloging in Publication Data
A catalog record for this book is available from the Library of Congress

Notice
Medical knowledge is constantly changing. Standard safety precautions must be followed, but as new research and clinical experience broaden our knowledge, changes in treatment and drug therapy may become necessary or appropriate. Readers are advised to check the most current product information provided by the manufacturer of each drug to be administered to verify the recommended dose, the method and duration of administration, and contraindications. It is the responsibility of the practitioner, relying on experience and knowledge of the patient, to determine dosages and the best treatment for each individual patient. Neither the Publisher nor the author assume any liability for any injury and/or damage to persons or property arising from this publication.

The Publisher

Printed in China
Last digit is the print number: 9 8 7 6 5 4 3 2 1

The Publisher's policy is to use **paper manufactured from sustainable forests**

Contents

Reviewers

Jung H. Ahn MD
Clinical Professor of Rehabilitation Medicine
Rusk Institute of Rehabilitation Medicine
New York University Medical Center
New York, New York, USA

Chapter 5.7 Voiding dysfunctions

Augusta S. Alba MD
Chief, Department of Rehabilitation Medicine
Coler Goldwater Specialty Hospital and Nursing Facility
Roosevelt Island, New York, USA

Chapter 5.12 Chronic pulmonary problems

Federico Balagué MD
Department of Rheumatology, Physical Medicine and Rehabilitation
Hôpital Cantonal
Bertigny, Fribourg, Switzerland

Chapter 3.1 Differential diagnoses of pain

Matthew N. Bartels MD MPH
Associate Professor of Clinical Rehabilitation Medicine
Columbia University College of Physicians and Surgeons
Director, Cardiac and Pulmonary Rehabilitation/Human Performance Laboratory
New York-Presbyterian Hospital/Columbia University Medical Center
New York, New York, USA

Chapter 2.7 Exercise tolerance testing; Chapter 5.13 Cardiac problems

Nancy Bergstrom PhD
Theodore J. and Mary E. Trumble Professor of Aging Research
Director, Center on Aging
University of Texas School of Nursing
Houston, Texas, USA

Chapter 5.2 Pressure ulcers

Murray E Brandstater MBBS PhD MRCP FRCP(C)
Professor and Chair of Physical Medicine and Rehabilitation
Loma Linda University of Affiliated Hospitals
Loma Linda, California, USA

Chapter 5.3 Venous thromboembolism

Joan E. Edelstein MA PT FISPO
Special Lecturer
Columbia University College of Physicians and Surgeons
New York, New York, USA

Chapter 4.3 Orthoses

Andrew A. Fischer MD PhD
Associate Clinical Professor of Rehabilitation Medicine
Mount Sinai School of Medicine
City University of New York
New York, New York, USA

Chapter 4.11 Trigger point therapy

Matthew D. Flynn CP FAAOP
President, Eastside Orthotics and Prosthetics Inc
Clinical Instructor of Orthopedic Surgery and Rehabilitation Medicine
New York-Presbyterian Hospital/Columbia University Medical Center
New York, New York, USA

Chapter 4.4 Prostheses

Glen Gillen EdD OTR FAOTA
Assistant Professor
Programs in Occupational Therapy

Columbia University College of Physicians and Surgeons
New York, New York, USA

Chapter 4.5 Adaptations for activities of daily living

Ellen A. Goldberg MA CCC-SLP
Manager, Speech–Language Pathology
Department of Rehabilitation Medicine
New York-Presbyterian Hospital/
Columbia University Medical Center
New York, New York, USA

Chapter 5.5 Neurogenic communication disorders

Cornelia N. Golimbu MD
Clinical Professor of Radiology
New York University Medical Center
New York, New York, USA

Chapter 2.2 Noninvasive imaging studies; Chapter 2.3 Invasive imaging studies

Carl V. Granger MD
Director, Uniform Data System for Medical Rehabilitation
Professor and Chairman Emeritus of Rehabilitation Medicine
School of Medicine and Biomedical Science
University at Buffalo, The State University of New York
Buffalo, New York, USA

Chapter 2.8 Functional assessment instruments

Sheila E. Horn DO
Clinical Assistant Professor of Rehabilitation Medicine
Rusk Institute of Rehabilitation Medicine
New York University Medical Center
New York, New York, USA

Chapter 2.1 Laboratory tests; Chapter 2.9 Psychologic tests; Chapter 4.5 Adaptations for activities of daily living; Chapter 5.11 Work-related musculoskeletal problems

Arthur C. Jimenez MD
Clinical Professor of Rehabilitation Medicine
New York University Medical Center
Chairman, Department of Rehabilitation Medicine
Hospital for Joint Diseases – Orthopedic Institute
New York, New York, USA

Chapter 5.10 Acute and chronic pain

Carolyn B. Kisner MS PT
Associate Professor
Department of Physical Therapy
College of Mount St. Joseph
Cincinnati, Ohio, USA

Chapter 4.2 Therapeutic exercises

Ted A. Lennard MD
Clinical Assistant Professor of Physical Medicine and Rehabilitation
University of Arkansas for Medical Sciences
Private Practice, Springfield Neurological and Spine Institute
Springfield, Missouri, USA

Chapter 4.10 Nerve blocks

Jeri A. Logemann PhD CCC-SLP
Professor of Otolaryngology and Maxillofacial Surgery and Neurology
Ralph and Jean Sundin Professor of Communication Sciences and Disorders
Northwestern University
Evanston, Illinois, USA

Chapter 5.6 Dysphagia

Arturo C. Magboo PT MD
Clinical Director of Physical Therapy
Occupational and Rehabilitation Center
Jacksonville, Florida, USA

Chapter 4.1 Physical modalities

Gerald A. Malanga MD
Director, Pain Management, Overlook Hospital
Director, Sports Medicine, Mountainside Hospital
Associate Professor of Physical Medicine and Rehabilitation
UMDNJ-New Jersey Medical School
Newark, New Jersey, USA

Chapter 1.1 Clinical evaluation and documentation

Margareta Nordin DSc PT
Director, Occupational and Industrial Orthopedic Center
Professor of Orthopedic Surgery and Environmental Medicine

New York University Medical Center
New York, New York, USA

Chapter 2.5 Musculoskeletal and work-related tests

John B. Redford MD
Professor Emeritus of Rehabilitation Medicine
Kansas University Medical Center
Kansas City, Kansas, USA

Chapter 4.7 Manual and powered mobility systems

Edwin F. Richter MD
Clinical Associate Professor of Rehabilitation Medicine
Rusk Institute of Rehabilitation Medicine
New York University Medical Center
New York, New York, USA

Chapter 5.4 Spasticity

Gregg L. Ruppel MEd RRT RPFT
Adjunct Professor
Division of Pulmonary, Critical Care, and Occupational Medicine
Director, Pulmonary Function Laboratory
St. Louis University School of Medicine
St. Louis, Missouri, USA

Chapter 2.6 Pulmonary function tests

Francisco H. Santiago MD
Attending Physician
Departments of Neurology and Physical Medicine/Rehabilitation
Bronx-Lebanon Hospital Center
Bronx, New York, USA

Chapter 2.4 Electrodiagnostic tests

Marcalee Sipski MD
Director, VA R&D Center of Excellence in SCI
Project Director, South Florida Model SCI System
Professor of Rehabilitation Medicine
University of Miami School of Medicine
Miami, Florida, USA

Chapter 5.9 Problems in human sexuality

Kevin Sperber MD
Clinical Assistant Professor of Rehabilitation Medicine
Columbia University College of Physicians and Surgeons
New York-Presbyterian Hospital/ Columbia University Medical Center
New York, New York, USA

Chapter 4.9 Joint and soft tissue injections

Michelle A. Stern MD
Assistant Clinical Professor of Rehabilitation Medicine
Columbia University College of Physicians and Surgeons
New York-Presbyterian Hospital/ Columbia University Medical Center
New York, New York, USA

Chapter 3.2 Differential diagnoses of nonpain problems;
Chapter 4.8 Pharmacologic agents;
Chapter 5.1 Deconditioning;
Chapter 5.8 Bowel dysfunction

Charng Shen Wang MA PT AP CMT
President, American Rehab Connection
Orange City, Florida, USA

Chapter 4.6 Gait aids and gait patterns

Foreword

It is with much honor, pride, and delight that I am able to write the foreword to the second edition of Dr. Tan's popular book. This extraordinary book was written when Dr. Tan was a resident at the Rusk Institute of Rehabilitation Medicine. Dr. Tan, who, in addition to his MD degree, also has a BS Physical Therapy and a PhD in Physical Therapy, is more than qualified to write this practical manual in the field of physical medicine and rehabilitation (PM&R).

For this second edition, Dr. Tan has fully revised and updated the contents, based on new research and, when available, the latest published consensus, guidelines, and recommendations from different panels of experts. Dr. Tan's revisions have been peer reviewed and critiqued by a distinguished panel of 29 reviewers. This carefully selected panel includes physiatrists as well as experts in other fields of medicine and allied health professions.

As in the previous edition, this handy and concise book encompasses both the diagnostic and the practical therapeutic tools necessary in the practice of PM&R. It also includes the practical diagnosis and treatment of basic clinical problems commonly seen in PM&R. Physicians who have mastered these basic problems will be able to apply them in the many different clinical scenarios encountered in both in- and out-patient practice in PM&R.

Following the format and style of the first edition, each chapter covers its particular topic comprehensively and is presented in strict outline format, following a logical and sensible classification, to aid easy understanding and retention. The book, which maintains a singular, coherent voice and style, also has extensive cross-referencing. The line drawings from the first edition have been redrawn and updated. The appendices, which include a mini-atlas of normal radiographic and MRI films, have been retained from the first edition.

This user-friendly book will be useful not only for PM&R practitioners, residents, and students, but also for practitioners in other fields of medicine, such as orthopedics, rheumatology, neurology, occupational medicine, pain medicine, family medicine, gerontology, internal medicine, and other PM&R-related specialties. Allied health professionals, such as physical therapists, occupational therapists, speech–language pathologists, respiratory care practitioners, rehabilitation nurses, orthotists, and prosthetists will also find this book very informative.

In the foreword of the first edition, I stated that Dr. Tan represents the next generation of physiatrist, trained here at the Rusk Institute, who will continue the legacy of excellence and achievement left by the late Dr. Howard Rusk. I am glad and proud to have been proven right, as evidenced by this edition and, hopefully, by many more editions to come.

Mathew H.M. Lee

Preface to the second edition

Reading furnishes the mind only with materials of knowledge;
it is thinking that makes what we read ours.
– John Locke

More than 6 years have passed since the publication of the first edition of the *Practical Manual of Physical Medicine and Rehabilitation*. The initial conception of this book during my early years of residency at the Rusk Institute of Rehabilitation Medicine, New York University Medical Center, was even longer than that (at least 12 years). Between then and now, the number of similar types of "pocket" books written specifically for the field of physical medicine and rehabilitation (PM&R) has more than doubled – a good indicator that PM&R is growing and flourishing.

The positive response to the first edition has been overwhelming. Apparently, this book has filled the need for a portable, concise, practical, in-depth, and user-friendly reference manual in the field of PM&R. Through word of mouth, the first edition found a niche, not only among PM&R residents, students, and practitioners, but also among other medical specialists (e.g., neurologists, rheumatologists, internists, gerontologists, family doctors, orthopedic surgeons, pain specialists, and occupational medicine doctors), allied health professionals (e.g., physical therapists, occupational therapists, speech–language pathologists, rehabilitation nurses, respiratory care practitioners, prosthetists, orthotists, rehabilitation psychologists, vocational counselors, and social workers), and non-health practitioners interested in PM&R (e.g., lawyers, case managers, rehabilitation administrators, and insurance adjusters).

In writing the second edition, I first revised, updated, and, when needed, expanded each chapter of the first edition. These revised chapters were then peer reviewed by a panel of 29 reviewers, each selected according to his or her expertise and knowledge of the contents of the chapter. The comments and suggestions of the reviewers were then incorporated into the second edition. However, due to space limitation and the style of the book, some of the reviewers' inputs were not included. One example of this is the recommendation for extensive referencing of the chapter contents. In this case, the reader is referred to the textbooks or articles cited in the bibliography following the chapter.

Although the basic science of PM&R has not changed drastically, there have been numerous changes since the first edition, namely (to mention a few): a new World Health Organization International Classification of Impairments, Ability, and Participation; changes in concepts and terminologies for flexibilities and resistance exercises; new exercise testing protocols for pulmonary patients (e.g., the

National Emphysema Treatment Trial protocol); a revised definition of female sexual dysfunction through the formation of the panel of the International Consensus Development Conference of Female Sexual Dysfunction; new pentad concepts in trigger point injection therapy; new guidelines and recommendations for treatment of neuropathic pain, venous thromboembolisms, cardiac patients, dysphagic patients, and other conditions; newly approved drugs, as well as newly withdrawn drugs, and revised warnings and dosages (e.g., for non-steroidal anti-inflammatory drugs); and new technologies in orthotics, prosthetics, adaptations for activities for daily living, wheelchairs, and different physical modalities. All of these changes have been incorporated into the second edition. Moreover, in the pharmacology section of this book, a new section on drugs used in Parkinson's disease has also been added.

When available, I have deferred to the latest guidelines and recommendations written by panels of experts using evidence-based medicine (e.g., American College of Chest Physicians for the management of venous thromboembolisms and the Consortium for Spinal Cord Medicine for the management of pressure ulcers). However, when none is available, I (with the help of the reviewers) have done my best to determine the most appropriate diagnostic or therapeutic regimens based upon current standards of practice of PM&R and of medicine.

Readers of the first edition will be familiar with the five-part presentation of this edition, encompassing PM&R clinical evaluation, diagnostic tests, differential diagnoses, management tools, and basic problems. At the end of the book, appendices of commonly used reference values, normal anatomy, and a mini-atlas of normal skeletal radiographs and MRIs of the brain and spine are also included. I believe that by mastering these five parts and learning how to manage the basic PM&R problems, one can practically manage most clinical conditions encountered in the practice of adult PM&R.

Each chapter of this book has been written in a user-friendly format and style, following a tight, strict, and practical classification and outline of the topic. When needed, composite tables and figures, as well as extensive cross-referencing to different parts of the book, have been employed for complete understanding and faster retention of the subject matter. For the second edition, all the figures have been redrawn and updated and a two-tone page design added for easier reading. Due to space limitation, the appendix containing addresses and phone numbers of PM&R resources has not been included in this edition as this information can now be easily obtained via the Internet. In keeping with the "practical" aspect of the book, emphasis is placed on practical clinical management, rather than pathophysiology and epidemiology, and on details of PM&R procedures, rather than on surgical procedures.

As with the first edition, this book is intended to be used as a supplement and complement, rather than a substitute, to the bigger (nonportable) but more comprehensive textbooks available in PM&R. The recommendations presented in this book are meant to be used as guidelines, not dogmas. These guidelines are certainly not "recipes" for treatment but should be considered as "menus" or "tools" from which one can judiciously choose in formulating the overall management plan for the patient. In keeping with the dictum of the first edition, I have sought to provide the most relevant and cutting-edge clinical information in a clear, concise, and easy-to-read manner with as much depth as is possible while maintaining practicality and portability. However, because medicine, as a scientific field, is constantly evolving and improving, I would recommend that readers continually update their knowledge through peer-reviewed journals, lectures, conferences, books, and the Internet.

Although every effort has been made to ensure the accuracy of this book, it is always possible that there may be some errors or mistakes. Any such errors or mistakes are all mine, and not the reviewers, as I have had the final say on every word that goes into or out of this book. As with the first edition, I would appreciate feedback on any such errors so that they can be corrected in the subsequent printings and editions.

I sincerely hope that the reader finds this book useful in the daily practice of his or her chosen field, be it PM&R or other related fields.

Jackson C. Tan

Dedication

This book is dedicated to all who continue to seek knowledge and pursue the highest form of excellence in the alleviation of pain and restoration of hope, dignity, and ability.

I also wish to dedicate this book to the loves of my life:

my wife, Darlene,
my two sons, Lance and Liam,
George,
and finally, Yumi, who patiently awaits us at the Rainbow Bridge.

Acknowledgements

Our knowledge is the amassed thought and experience of innumerable minds.
– Ralph Waldo Emerson

As with the first edition, this book would not have been possible without the help and sacrifice of many good and wonderful people. In particular, I am grateful to:

Darlene Tan, a beautiful person in every sense of the word, my soulmate, best friend, better (best!) half, dearest wife, and cherished mother of our two loving boys. Always a source of wise counsel, she not only helped in the editing of the book, but also managed the household and cared for Lance, Liam, and George while I took time off to write.

My two boys, Lawrence (Lance) Everett Tan and Liam Garrett Tan, both precious and precocious, loving and endearing, sweet and funny, wise and innocent, joyful, blissful, blessed, budding beings of the human race – I love them tremendously.

All my reviewers, who, despite their busy practices, found the time to peer review my revisions, in particular, Sheila Horn DO and Michele Stern MD, both of whom reviewed multiple chapters of the book (some even without credit) and cheered me on.

The hard-working staff of Elsevier, in particular Rolla Couchman, the original commissioning editor, who initiated the second edition by visiting me in Florida with a solid proposal backed by an assurance of full commitment from Elsevier, and Gillian Whytock (from Prepress Projects), who guided the book straight through the finish line.

The staffs of: the Borland Health Sciences Library, the University of Florida Health Science Center, Jacksonville, FL; the University of Florida Health Science Center Libraries, Gainesville, FL; and the Thomas G. Carpenter Library, University of North Florida, Jacksonville, FL, for courteous and generous services.

Un Beng and Ah Wan Tan (my parents); Freddie, Emerald, Merry June Grace, and Fred Gerald Tan; Stevenson Tan; Ronald and Marianne Warnke; Dennis, Mellani, and Mishani Denyz Tan, and other relatives and friends in America, Canada, and the Philippines, for moral support.

Annie R. Aquino, who helped take care of our household, our children, and our dog.

Robert and Annemarie Lindsey and Charng Shen and Mein Li Wang, for friendship and moral support.

Dohee Steve Kwak, for computer assistance.

Adolfo and Lourdes DeGuzman, who helped take care of our children during the initial writing stage.

The staff (past and present) of the Occupational and Rehabilitation Center, Jacksonville, FL, in particular, Carlos A. Oteyza MD, Mario Sabban, Arturo Magboo RPT MD, Virginie Balisi RPT, Julie Stevens LMT NMT, David Hall LMT, Angie Casiple LMT BSPT, Jhoanna Javier BSPT, Crystal Shaffer LMT, Lynette and Ruel Villanueva, Leilani Human CMA, Xandra Faircloth, Sheri Fowler, Mary Trader, Nellie Baldwin, Vickie Muller, Sharon Brown, and Gail Fleming-Easter LMT.

Everyone who helped make the first edition possible.

And, last but not least, all my wonderful patients, from whom I continue to learn and grow as a doctor and as a person.

PART I

PHYSICAL MEDICINE AND REHABILITATION: CLINICAL EVALUATION

CHAPTER 1.1
Clinical evaluation and documentation

Physical Medicine and Rehabilitation (PM&R) as a medical specialty was officially sanctioned by the American Board of Medical Specialties in 1947. The shortened name of PM&R is physiatry (from the Greek *physio*, or nature), and its practitioner is called a physiatrist. PM&R encompasses the diagnosis and treatment of physical and functional disorders involving the neuromuscular, musculoskeletal, and cardiopulmonary systems. Unlike other fields of medicine, the primary concern of PM&R is not the identification and cure of disease. Rather, its primary goal is the patient attaining the fullest physical, psychological, social, vocational, avocational, and educational potential consistent with physiologic or anatomic impairment and environmental limitations.

To understand the impact of a disease on the patient's life, the physiatrist must understand the distinctions between impairment, disability, and handicap as defined by the World Health Organization (WHO 1980).

- **Impairment** refers to "any loss or abnormality of psychological, physiological, or anatomical structure or function." It represents the problem at the tissue and organ level. Examples include muscular weakness, limited joint range of motion, pain, and confusion.
- **Disability** refers to "any restriction or lack resulting from an impairment of the ability to perform an activity in the manner or within the range considered normal for a human being." It represents the problem at the whole-person level. Examples include the inability to walk, run, or ski after suffering a stroke. In 1997, the World Health Organization (WHO 1997) suggested that instead of disability, the more positive terminology ability (defined as the nature and extent of functioning at the level of the person) be used instead.
- **Handicap** refers to "a disadvantage for a given individual, resulting from an impairment or a disability, that limits or prevents the fulfillment of a role that is normal (depending on the age, sex, and social and cultural factors) for that individual." It represents the problem at the societal level. Examples include difficulties with social integration, economic self-sufficiency, and negotiation of architectural barriers (e.g., wheelchair inaccessibility). Instead of handicap, the WHO in 1997 suggested that the term handicap should be substituted with participation (defined as the nature and extent of a person's involvement in life situations in relationship to impairments, activities, health conditions, and contextual factors).

The goals of PM&R are achieved by an interdisciplinary team approach consisting of the patient and his or her support system (family or significant others), physiatrist, physical therapist (PT), occupational therapist (OT), psychologist, speech–language pathologist (SLP), rehabilitation nurse, social worker, vocational counselor, recreational therapist (RT), prosthetist–orthotist, nutritionist, and other health professionals involved in the rehabilitation of the patient (e.g., psychiatrist, respiratory care practitioner, kinesiotherapist or corrective therapist, chaplain, maxillofacial prosthetist, dentist, podiatrist, audiologist, bioengineer, hospital-based or special-education teacher, pharmacist, durable medical equipment vendor, child-life specialist, horticultural therapist, music therapist, dance therapist, animal-assisted therapy specialist).

The basic elements of a physiatric evaluation are the same as with other medical specialties. A thorough history-taking and physical examination is important, with emphasis on the assessment of functions and activities of daily living (ADL).

I. History

A. CHIEF COMPLAINT, i.e., reason for seeking physiatric attention. If possible, record in the patient's own words to assess the patient's intellect, perception, and concerns about existing illness and dysfunction. The focus should be on functional loss or the reason for the loss of function (e.g., inability to walk, talk, or eat after suffering from a stroke).

B. SOURCE OF INFORMATION. As much as possible, try to obtain information from the patient. If necessary, the patient's primary caregiver or medical records may corroborate. In patients with communication disorders, such as in a stroke or traumatic brain injury patient, assistance from a family member is needed (if available, a speech therapist would be helpful).

C. HISTORY OF PRESENT ILLNESS, i.e., chronological narrative of the patient's chief complaint. Describe each symptom using the "**O-PP-Q-RR-S-TTT** or **$OP^2QR^2ST^3$**" mnemonic:

- Other associated manifestations
- Provocative (aggravating) factors
- Palliative (relieving) factors
- Quality (character)
- Region (location and extension)
- Radiation to a distant site (if present)
- Severity (intensity)
- Timing (onset, duration, frequency, pattern of involvement, progression)
- Tests results
- Treatments effects

In the history of present illness, record the hand dominance and the functional history (compare current with premorbid functioning). The **functional history** describes how the chief complaint affects the patient's physical and functional independence at home, at work, or at school. The key functions include self-care (feeding, grooming, bathing, dressing, and toileting), sphincter control (bladder and bowel), mobility/transfers (bed, chair, toilet, and shower), locomotion (ambulation on level ground and stairs, with or without gait aids; use of mobility devices such as wheelchair; operation of motor vehicles), social cognition (social interaction, problem solving, and memory), and communication. The degree of independence (or dependence) can be briefly described as full independence, modified independence (i.e., with an assistive device or modification of the environment), requiring close or distant supervision by another person, requiring assistance (minimal, moderate, or maximal assistance), or fully dependent.

D. PAST HISTORY. General state of health, prior hospitalizations (medical, surgical, psychiatric, and rehabilitation), past traumas and accidents, past surgeries, blood transfusions and reactions, vaccinations (flu and pneumococcal), recent travels, past minor and major psychiatric illnesses, and past illnesses (diabetes, hypertension, coronary artery disease, pneumonia, bronchitis, chronic obstructive pulmonary disease, hepatitis, rheumatic fever, cancer). For pediatric patients, include birth history, growth and developmental milestones, significant childhood illnesses, and immunizations.

E. ALLERGIES. Type of allergic reaction to any food, drug, chemicals, or pets.

F. CURRENT MEDICATIONS. All current prescription and nonprescription drugs; record their dose, frequency, and duration.

G. PERSONAL HISTORY provides the clinician with an opportunity to modify the patient's unhealthy behavior through counseling. Knowing the patient's current and premorbid life-style or personality can help in setting realistic rehabilitation goals.

1. Life-style and habits

a. ***Avocational*** (recreational or leisure) interests. Indoor and outdoor sports (note frequency, duration, and intensity to estimate fitness level), intellectual pursuits, social interactions, organizations, and group functions.

b. ***Diet***. Usual dietary habits, special diets, caffeine use, ability to prepare meals and snacks.

c. ***Cigarette smoking***. Quantity in pack years.

d. ***Recreational drug use***. Depressants, stimulants, opiates, cannabis derivatives, and hallucinogens.

e. ***Sexual history***. Sexual preference, sexual promiscuity, most recent sexual experience.

f. ***Alcohol use***. A "yes" response on the CAGE questionnaire (see Table 1.1-1) is suspicious for alcohol abuse and, therefore, warrants further investigation.

2. Religious beliefs relevant to health and rehabilitation.

3. Premorbid personality and emotional response to previous illnesses and family troubles.

H. SOCIAL HISTORY. Knowing the patient's home situation and available support systems can help in discharge planning.

1. Home situation and architectural barriers. Owns or rents home, location of home (urban, suburban, or rural), distance between home and rehabilitation facilities, number of outside and inside steps, accessibility to elevator or ramps, availability of space for entry ramps, and accessibility of the kitchen, bathroom, bedroom, living room, and laundry room. Also ask patient's specific expectations

Table 1.1-1 CAGE questionnaire for screening of alcohol abuse or alcohol dependency

C:	"Have you ever felt you ought to **C**ut down on your drinking?"
A:	"Have people ever **A**nnoyed you by criticizing your drinking?"
G:	"Have you ever felt bad or **G**uilty about your drinking?"
E:	"Have you ever had a drink first thing in the morning (**E**ye-opener) to steady your nerves or get rid of a hangover?"

Note: A "no" answer is scored as 0 and a "yes" answer as 1. A total score of 2 or greater significantly increases the probability of alcoholism, thus warranting additional screening.

From: Ewing JA: Detecting alcoholism: the CAGE questionnaire. JAMA *252:1905–1907, 1984, copyright ©1984, American Medical Association, with permission.*

regarding household chores, such as meal preparation, shopping, home maintenance, cleaning, and child-rearing.

2. **Marriage history and status**
3. **Family, significant others, support system**

I. VOCATIONAL (AND ECONOMIC) HISTORY helps in retraining patients for possible return to the work-force or in assisting patient in securing alternative employment or gainful activities.

1. **Educational and training history**. Educational level, abilities, special skills, licenses, and certifications.
2. **Work and/or military history**. Type and place of work, work environment (include physical barriers at work and use of any special supports or adaptive aids), military service, return-to-work history after previous injury.
3. **Financial situation, insurance, and litigation**. Sources of income, investments, insurance resources, disability classifications, debts, and litigation status.

J. FAMILY HISTORY helps in understanding patient's support structure and for genetic counseling of inheritable disease. Record the age and health status of each immediate family member. If deceased, indicate the age and probable cause of death. Ask for family history of diabetes, heart disease, hypertension, cancer, rheumatic disease (rheumatoid arthritis, osteoarthritis, seronegative spondyloarthropathies, e.g., ankylosing spondylitis), gout, stroke, kidney stones, psychiatric disorders, neuromuscular disorders, or any hereditary conditions.

K. REVIEW OF SYSTEMS. Carefully screen all the systems for clues to disease (not previously identified in history-taking) that may adversely affect the rehabilitation outcome.

1. **General**. Overall state of health, usual weight, recent weight change, sleeping habits, appetite, fever, chills, night sweats, fatigue.
2. **Skin**. Pressure ulcer, rash (with or without sun sensitivity), pruritus, color (or ischemic) changes, pigmentation, nodules.
3. **Lymphatic**. "Swollen glands" or masses in the neck, axilla, groin; lymphedema.
4. **HEENT**

a. ***Head***. Headache, trauma.

b. ***Eyes***. Pain, dryness, conjunctivitis, scotoma.

c. ***Ears***. Earache, ear discharge.

d. ***Nose and sinuses***. Epistaxis, nasal stuffiness or congestion, drainage, sinusitis.

e. ***Mouth and Throat***. Condition of teeth, gums, and tongue; last dental examination; mouth disorders (sores, masses, dryness, tightness); sore throat; change in voice.

5. **Breasts**. Pain, history of lumps, bleeding, symmetry, nipple discharge. In female patients, ask if she performs self-examination and note her last mammogram date.
6. **Respiratory**. Cough, sputum (quantity, color), hemoptysis, wheezing, shortness of breath, pain associated with breathing.
7. **Cardiac**. Chest pain, palpitations, dyspnea, orthopnea, paroxysmal nocturnal dyspnea, edema, heart murmurs, history of high blood pressure, syncope, exercise tolerance.
8. **Peripheral vascular**. Varicose veins, thrombophlebitis, claudication, Raynaud's phenomenon.
9. **Gastrointestinal**. Swallowing problems, reflux symptoms, abdominal pain, nausea, vomiting, increased girth, jaundice, blood from mouth or rectum, change in bowel habits (constipation, diarrhea, incontinence), use of laxatives.
10. **Genitourinary**. Dysuria, frequency, urgency, hesitation, nocturia, pyuria, flank pain, hematuria, renal stones, discharge, venereal disease, bleeding. In patients

with neurogenic bladder, ask about fluid intake, voiding schedules, bladder emptying techniques, incontinence, retention, and incomplete emptying.

a. ***Male sexuality***. Libido, erection, ejaculation, fertility, dyspareunia.

b. ***Female sexuality***. Libido, vaginal and clitoral sensation, orgasm, fertility, dyspareunia.

c. ***Gynecologic/reproductive***. Age at menarche, last menstrual period, frequency and duration of periods, number and complications of pregnancies, live births, miscarriages, age at menopause, contraception.

11. Musculoskeletal. Pain, swelling, stiffness, limitation of range of motion, arthritis, gout, cramps, myalgia, fasciculation, atrophy, hypertrophy, fracture, deformity.

12. Neurologic

a. ***Consciousness level***. Change in level of consciousness, convulsions.

b. ***Cognitive***. Change in memory or thinking.

c. ***Speech and language***. Change in reading, speaking, and writing ability.

d. ***Cranial nerves***

I. Altered sense of smell

II, III, IV, VI. Diplopia, blurred vision, field cuts, glasses

V. Weakness of muscles of mastication

VII. Facial weakness, dysarthria, loss of taste

VIII. Deafness, imbalance, dizziness, vertigo, tinnitus

IX, X, XII. Difficulties in swallowing and speaking

XI. Difficulties in turning head or in shrugging

e. ***Sensory***. Loss or change of sensation (touch, pain, temperature), dysesthesia, hyperpathia.

f. ***Motor***. Weakness, paralysis, tremors, involuntary movements.

g. ***Gait***. Stability, use of assistive or mobility devices, falls, endurance.

13. Psychiatric. Personality changes, extreme mood change, insomnia, anxiety, depression, obsessive and phobic ideas, past major and minor psychiatric care, history of psychotherapy or psychotropic pharmacological intervention, suicidal ideation or prior suicidal attempts.

14. Endocrine. Heat or cold intolerance, polydypsia, polyuria, polyphagia.

15. Hematologic. Easy bruising, transfusion reactions, excessive bleeding, history of anemia.

II. Physical examination

The basic techniques of physiatric physical examination (i.e., inspection, palpation, percussion, and auscultation) are the same as with other medical specialties (see Supplemental references). Emphasis is placed on musculoskeletal, neurological, and functional examinations.

A. VITAL SIGNS. Blood pressure (indicate which arm; measure in supine, sitting, and standing positions to rule out orthostasis), pulse (rate and regularity), respiration (rate and rhythm), temperature, weight, height.

B. GENERAL DESCRIPTION. State of health, general appearance, apparent age, nutritional status, body development, personal hygiene, cooperativeness, hostile or threatening behavior, signs of anxiety or distress.

C. INTEGUMENT.

1. Skin. Color, temperature, turgor, atrophy, lesions.

2. Pressure ulcers. Location (usually over bony prominence), diameter (cm), depth, wound type (e.g., abrasion, scab, blister, ulcer with eschar or slough), appearance, color, drainage (character, volume, or odor), and presence of epithelization and/or granulation tissue, edema, and tunneling or sinus tracts. The periwound area (e.g., erythema, induration, maceration) should also be described. For clinical grading or staging of pressure ulcers, refer to Table 5.2-1 in Chapter 5.2.

3. **Hair**. Distribution, amount, texture, areas of hair loss, facial hairs.
4. **Nail**. Infection, hygiene, long toenails, ingrown toenails.

D. **LYMPH NODES**. Posterior auricular, cervical, supraclavicular, axillary, inguinal areas (if with lymphadenopathy, note size, consistency, mobility, tenderness).

E. **HEENT**

1. **Head**. Size, shape, symmetry, lesions, craniofacial anomalies, neurosurgical procedures, shunt sites, shunt bulb compressibility.
2. **Eyes**. Eye dryness, conjunctival and scleral color, corneal lesions, eyelid nodules, adequacy of lid closure, fundi.
3. **Ears**. Drainage, tympanic membrane.
4. **Nose and sinuses**. Polyps, lesions, drainage, sinus tenderness (frontal and maxillary).
5. **Mouth and throat**. Lesions, ulcers, tooth loss, dentures, hygiene.
6. **Temporomandibular joint**. Crepitation, tenderness, swelling, mouth opening size.

F. **NECK**. Nuchal rigidity, carotid pulsations and bruits, jugular venous distension, thyroid gland, trachea, skin around tracheostomy site (type and size of tracheostomy tube).

G. **THORAX AND DIAPHRAGM**. Chest wall shape, tenderness, deformity, breathing pattern, chest expansion (normal is >6 cm at nipple line), use of accessory muscles, cough force and efficiency, hiccups.

H. **LUNGS**. Quality and intensity of breath sounds, "e" to "a" change, whispered pectoriloquy ("ninety-nine"), wheezes, crackles (rales), rhonchi, or rubs.

I. **HEART**. Thrills, point of maximal impulse, S_1 and S_2 intensity and splitting, murmurs (timing, intensity, pitch, location, radiation, quality), abnormal heart sounds (S_3, S_4, clicks, rubs, snaps, gallops).

J. **BREASTS AND NIPPLES**. Masses, tenderness, rashes, ulceration, discharge.

K. **ABDOMEN**. Obesity, scars, rigidity, distension, ascites, venous pattern, masses (pulsatile and nonpulsatile), tenderness, guarding, bowel sounds, abdominal bruits, hepatosplenomegaly.

L. **RECTAL**. Lesions, inflammation, masses, hemorrhoids, perineal sensation, sphincter tone, fecal occult blood, prostate (size, shape, and consistency), bulbocavernosus reflex.

M. **GENITOURINARY**. Costovertebral angle tenderness, hernia.

1. **Male genitalia**. Circumcision, ulcers, nodules, masses, scars, inflammation, tenderness, discharge, fistulas, hypospadia, testicular descent and symmetry.
2. **Female genitalia**. Nodules, masses, discharge, swelling.

N. **PERIPHERAL VASCULAR SYSTEM**. Peripheral arteries (describe symmetry and grade intensity of brachial, radial, popliteal, femoral, dorsalis pedis, and posterior tibialis pulses), femoral bruits, edema (severity and presence of pitting), distal clubbing, and cyanosis.

O. **MUSCULOSKELETAL SYSTEM**. Note any pain behavior (e.g., marked grimacing, groans, limping) during examination. Refer to Table 1.1-2 for sequence of musculoskeletal examination [for more details, see Hoppenfeld's *Physical Examination of the Spine and Extremities* and Magee's *Orthopedic Physical Assessment* (both listed under Supplemental references)].

1. **Spine**. Surgical scars, spinal posture (cervical lordosis, scoliosis, dorsal kyphosis, lumbar lordosis), shoulder height, pelvic level, trunk tilt [neck range of motion (ROM), back ROM (e.g., Schober's test), neck and trunk strength, spinal and

Table 1.1-2 Sequence of physiatric examination with emphasis on musculoskeletal systems. Testing position and sequence may be modified in patients who cannot assume all positions

Position	Tests
A. Standing	1. Posture and gait analyses; functional lower extremity strength (heel-walk, toe-walk, squatting, transfer in and out of bed or chair) 2. Lower extremity alignment and deformities; position of ankles and feet (e.g., flatfeet, inversion or eversion) 3. Back motion (flexion, extension, lateral bending, Schober's test)
B. Seated	1. Head and neck motion in all planes (include Spurling's test) 2. Temporomandibular joint examination 3. Thoracolumbar rotation with pelvis fixed 4. Routine medical (VS, skin, HEENT, neck, thorax, breasts, lungs, heart, flank) and neurologic examination (mental status, cranial nerves, reflexes, sensory, coordination) 5. Upper extremity: inspect, palpate, measure girth, screen strength (see Table 1.1-4) and functional ROM: a. Shoulder complex (arm elevation from side to 180° above head; internal rotate by reaching dorsum of hand to highest level of spinous process; external rotate by putting hand behind the neck or head) b. Glenohumeral joint (fix scapula, abduct arm, and do internal and external rotations) c. Elbow: flexion and extension d. Wrist and hands (wrist motion; fist; grip and pinch; pronation and supination; thumb distal phalange flexion and extension; opposition) 6. Lower extremity: inspect, palpate, screen strength (see Table 1.1-4) and ROM: a. Hip flexion b. Knee extension and flexion c. Ankle dorsiflexion, plantar flexion, inversion, eversion
C. Supine	1. Routine medical examination (skin, abdomen, genitalia, peripheral vascular systems) and neurologic examinations 2. Low back (abdominal strength; traction maneuvers, e.g., SLR, Gaenslen) 3. Hips: rolling, abduction, adduction, flexion (knee to chest), internal and external rotation with hips flexed to 90°; maneuvers (Thomas's, Ober's) 4. Leg length measurement; girth 5. Knees: patella (patellar click sign; bulge sign); popliteal area (synovial cyst); knee stability (Drawer's, Lachman's, Apley's, medial and lateral stress tests) 6. Ankle and feet: malleoli; dorsiflexion and plantar flexion; subtalar motion inversion and eversion 7. Toes: alignment and deformity
D. Side-lying	1. Hip abduction and adduction 2. Rectal and perineal examinations
E. Prone	1. Inspect and palpate cervical, thoracic, lumbosacral, sacroiliac, gluteal areas 2. Hip extension (knee straight and bent) 3. Head, neck, and trunk extension

paraspinal tenderness, muscle tightness and spasm, compression tests (Spurling's test), traction maneuvers, e.g., straight leg raising (SLR) and Gaenslen's test].

2. **Limbs**. Alignment (e.g., genu varum or valgum), contractures, deformities, limb length discrepancy, limb girth asymmetry, winging (scapular), erythema,

Table 1.1-3 Screening tests of upper and lower extremities used to grossly assess the musculoskeletal system (ROM and MMT) as well as the central and peripheral nervous system

Muscle	Spinal roots*	Peripheral nerve	Test
Upper extremity†:			
Upper trapezius	Cranial nerve XI, C3, C4	Spinal accessory; cervical roots	Shrugging
Deltoid	**C5**, C6	Axillary	Shoulder abduction
Biceps brachii	C5, C6	Musculocutaneous	Elbow flexion of supinated arm
Brachioradialis	C5, **C6**	Radial	Elbow flexion of neutral arm
Triceps brachii	C6, **C7**, C8	Radial	Elbow extension
Extensor pollicis longus	**C7**, C8	Radial	Thumb distal phalange extension
Extensor carpi ulnaris	**C7**, C8	Radial	Wrist extension
Flexor pollicis longus	C7, **C8**	Median	Thumb distal phalange flexion
Opponens pollicis	C8, **T1**	Median	Thumb opposition
Opponens digiti minimi	C8, **T1**	Ulnar	Fifth digit opposition
Lower extremity‡:			
Iliopsoas	**L1**, **L2**, L3	Lumbar plexus	Hip flexion
Adductor longus	**L2**, **L3**, L4	Obturator	Hip adduction
Quadriceps femoris	L2, **L3**, **L4**	Femoral	Knee extension
Gluteus medius	**L4**, **L5**, S1	Superior gluteal	Hip abduction
Gluteus maximus	**L5**, **S1**, S2	Inferior gluteal	Hip extension
Hamstrings	L5, **S1**, S2	Sciatic	Knee flexion
Tibialis anterior	**L4**, L5	Deep peroneal	Ankle dorsiflexion and inversion
Extensor hallucis longus	**L5**, S1	Deep peroneal	Big toe extensor
Peroneus longus	L5, S1	Superficial peroneal	Ankle eversion
Gastrocnemius	S1, S2	Tibial	Ankle plantar flexion

** A **bold** designation indicates the predominant root supply.*
† Pronator drift can be used to screen proximal shoulder and arm weakness.
‡ Heel tapping can be used to screen proximal lower extremity muscle weakness whereas forefoot tapping screens for distal lower extremity muscle weakness.

hematoma, scar, callous, lesions, swelling, masses, crepitation, fasciculation, atrophy, hypertrophy, tenderness, trigger point, tender point, spasm, spasticity, rigidity, tests that provoke symptoms (e.g., Tinel's test, Phalen's wrist flexion test), amputation (note residual limb shape, length, scar, skin integrity, sensation, ROM, strength). See Table 1.1-3 for screening tests of upper and lower limbs used to grossly assess the musculoskeletal system (ROM and strength) as well as the central and peripheral nervous system. The screening tests are used to determine which specific muscle or joint needs further testing. For muscle strength, the numerical or word/letter grading system may be used (see Table 1.1-4).

a. ***Range-of-motion (ROM).*** Measure active and passive ROM; use the 0° to 180° system (i.e., anatomic position is the zero starting point, except for rotation that uses a point midway between normal rotation range as the zero starting point); record the patient's position and starting joint position during testing;

Table 1.1-4 Grading of manual muscle testing using number, word, and letter system

Number grade[1]	Word grade[2]	Letter grade[2]	Definition
0	Zero	0	No observable or palpable muscle contraction
1	Trace	T	Visible or palpable muscle contraction but no joint motion
2−	Poor minus	P−	Joint moves through incomplete ROM in gravity-decreased position
2	Poor	P	Joint moves through complete ROM in gravity-decreased position
2+	Poor plus	P+	Joint moves through incomplete ROM (<50%) against gravity or through complete ROM against slight resistance in gravity-decreased position
3−	Fair minus	F−	Joint moves through incomplete ROM (>50%) against gravity
3	Fair	F	Joint moves through complete ROM against gravity
3+	Fair plus	F+	Joint moves through complete ROM against gravity and slight resistance*
4	Good	G	Joint moves through complete ROM against gravity and moderate resistance†
5	Normal	N	Joint moves through complete ROM against gravity and full resistance†

Adapted from: [1]*Guarantors of Brain:* Aids to the examination of the peripheral nervous system, *London, 1986, Balliere Tindall;* [2]*Daniels L, Worthingham C:* Muscle testing, *ed 5, Philadelphia, 1986, WB Saunders.*

** Resistance for grades 3+ and above are given at the end range of motion (i.e., break test).*

† Grades 4 and 5 have poor interrater reliability and do not need plus or minus designation.

note the stabilization, alignment, and goniometer type used, as well as the factors affecting the ROM, such as pain, swelling, spasm, spasticity, motivation, cooperation, fear, obesity, and contractures. For functional ROM testing, refer to Tables 1.1-2 and 1.1-3. ROM limitations can be estimated by using the percentage system, i.e., 0 limitation = full ROM; minimal limitation = lacks 1–33% to full ROM; moderate limitation = lacks 33–66% to full ROM; maximal limitation = lacks 66–100% to full ROM. Average ROMs for the spine and limbs are summarized in Appendices A-1 and A-2. Further details on ROM testing can be found in Norkin and White's *Measurement of Joint Motion: A Guide to Goniometry* (see Supplemental references) as well as Chapter 2.5, section I.

b. ***Joint stability***. Determine ankylosis, hypo- or hypermobility, instability, subluxation, and dislocation. Perform maneuvers such as Drawer's test, Lachman's test, and pivot–shift test.

c. ***Muscle strength***. Manual muscle testing (MMT) and dynamometry (see Chapter 2.5, section II) are tests of voluntary movement used to assess weakness due to disorders primarily involving the contractile muscle elements, the myoneural junction, and the lower motor neurons. They are inaccurate for disorders of the upper motor neurons (UMN) or the brain (e.g., cerebral palsy, stroke) because of alteration in reflex activity, which brings about abnormal muscle tone and synergy patterns. Screening tests of muscle strength are presented in Table 1.1-3.

I. **Manual muscle testing (MMT)**. Note distribution of muscle weakness (proximal vs. distal, upper vs. lower limbs); document patient's position and stabilization as well as co-contractions and substitution patterns used during testing; and record factors affecting MMT such as pain, swelling, spasm, spasticity, motivation, cooperation, effort, fear, fatigue, contractures, size, physical condition, and conversion reaction of patient. For grading manual muscle strength, see Table 1.1-4. If possible, MMT must be compared with uninvolved side. Further details about MMT procedures can be found in Hislop and Montgomery's Daniels and Worthingham's Muscle Testing and Kendall, McCreary, and Provance's Muscles Testing and Function (see Supplemental references).

II. **Dynamometry**. Hand-held, isometric, isokinetic, isoinertial dynamometers (for specific dynamometers, see Chapter 2.5, section II).

P. NEUROLOGIC.

1. Mental status.

a. Level of consciousness. Classify level of consciousness using the Glasgow "coma" or responsiveness scale (see Table 1.1-5).

b. Cognition. Alertness, orientation (to time, place, and person), attention (digit repetition), recent and immediate memory recall (recall three named objects or numbers within 5, 10, and 15 minutes), general information (appropriate for age and educational/cultural background), calculations (count by sevens), proverbs explanation, describing similarities (e.g., between apple and orange), and judgment (e.g., how to find a friend in an unfamiliar city). The level of cognitive function or recovery can be classified by using the Rancho Los Amigos descriptive scale (Table 1.1-6).

Table 1.1-5 Glasgow "coma" or responsiveness scale (GCS) classifies and scores the patient's eye, motor, and verbal responses to verbal and physical stimuli

Parameter	Patient's response	Score*
Eye opening (**E**)	Spontaneous eye opening	E 4
	Opens eyes in response to speech	E 3
	Opens eyes in response to pain	E 2
	No eye opening	E 1
Best motor response (**M**)	Obeys verbal commands	M 6
	Localizes painful stimulus	M 5
	Flexion withdrawal from painful stimulus	M 4
	Abnormal flexion response to painful stimulus	M 3
	Extensor response to painful stimulus	M 2
	No motor response	M 1
Best verbal response (**V**)	Oriented; able to converse	V 5
	Disoriented; confused conversation	V 4
	Inappropriate words	V 3
	Incomprehensible sounds	V 2
	No verbal response	V 1

Tabulated with permission from Jennett B, Teasdale G: Aspects of coma after severe head injury. Lancet *1:878–881, 1977. Copyright ©1977 The Lancet Ltd.*

** The GCS score is calculated by adding the E, M, and V scores (lowest possible score is 3 and highest is 15). GCS scores can be used to classify head injury (8 or less = severe; 9–12 = moderate; 13–15 = mild).*

Table 1.1-6 Rancho Los Amigos Levels of Cognitive Functioning or Recovery*

Cognitive level	Description of patient
I. No response	Unresponsive to any stimuli
II. Generalized response	Nonspecific, inconsistent, and nonpurposeful response to any stimuli; response may be physiologic changes, gross body movement, and/or vocalization
III. Localized response	Specific but inconsistent response to stimulus; may follow simple commands (e.g., closing eyes, squeezing hands) but in an inconsistent, delayed manner
IV. Confused, agitated	Heightened state of activity; bizarre, incoherent, and nonpurposeful behavior relative to immediate environment; gross attention to environment is brief; no selective attention; lacks short- and long-term recall; unable to cooperate directly with treatment; may confabulate; may be hostile; needs maximum assistance for self-care
V. Confused, inappropriate	Appears alert; consistent response to simple commands but when command is complex or lacks any external structure, responses are nonpurposeful or fragmented; gross attention to the environment but highly distractible; unable to focus on specific task; with structure, may be able to converse on a social automatic level for short period; often confabulatory; memory is severely impaired; unable to learn new information; needs assistance for self-care and supervision for feeding; may wander off either randomly or with vague intention of "going home"
VI. Confused, appropriate	Shows goal-directed behavior but is dependent on external input or direction; responses may be incorrect due to memory problems, but they are appropriate to the situation; follows simple commands consistently with carryover for relearned tasks such as self-care; needs at least supervision for old learning and maximal supervision for new learning with little or no carryover; past memories show more depth and detail than recent memory; no longer wanders and is oriented (inconsistently) to time and space
VII. Automatic, appropriate	Appears appropriate and oriented within the hospital and home setting; goes through daily routine automatically but robot-like; if with structure, able to initiate social or recreational activities; judgment is impaired; independent in self-care but needs supervision in home and community skills for safety; prevocational evaluation and counseling may be indicated
VIII. Purposeful, appropriate	Alert and oriented; able to recall and integrate past and recent events and is aware of and responsive to environment; shows carryover for new learning and needs no supervision once activities are learned; may continue to have decreased abilities relative to premorbid abilities; decreased level of social, emotional, and intellectual capacities but still functional within society; independent in home and community skills (within patient's physical abilities); vocational rehabilitation is indicated

Condensed from: Professional staff association: Rehabilitation of the head injured adult: Comprehensive physical management, *Downey, CA, 1979, Rancho Los Amigos Hospital, pp. 87–88, with permission from the Adult Brain Unit Service, Rancho Los Amigos Medical Center, Downey, CA.*

**Does not address specific cognitive deficits; no reliability data are available; useful for communicating general cognitive and/or behavioral status particularly in patients with traumatic brain injury, where this scale is commonly used.*

c. ***Perception***. Agnosia (identification of common objects or body parts), unilateral environmental neglect, right–left disorientation, safety awareness (i.e., is patient aware of his or her deficit and the environment? does patient take adequate safety precautions?).

2. **Speech and language**. Communicative skills (residual and premorbid), hearing function, aphasia, apraxia, dysarthria.

a. ***Listening***. Ability to follow verbal commands (single- and multisteps).

b. ***Reading***. Ability to follow written commands (single- and multisteps).

c. ***Speaking***. Naming of at least three objects or pictures indicated by the examiner; ability to state his or her own name, address, and phone; ability to read aloud short paragraphs; ability to say a prolonged "aaah" (test for phonation and resonance deficits), "pa-pa-pa" (lip closure test), "ta-ta-ta" (test of tongue function), "ka-ka-ka" (test of speed, regulatory, and posterior pharyngeal function).

d. ***Writing***. Ability to write his or her own name, address, phone, and a brief paragraph.

3. **Cranial nerves (CN)**

I. Sense of smell

II. Visual acuity (near and far, with and without eyewear), visual fields, color

III. Eye adduction (medial rectus muscle), eye depression (inferior rectus muscle), eye elevation (superior rectus and inferior oblique muscles), pupillary constriction (with CN II), upper lid elevation

IV. Eye intortion with depression and adduction (superior oblique muscle)

V. Mastication (masseter, pterygoids), sensory of forehead, face, and jaw

VI. Eye abduction (lateral rectus muscle)

VII. Facial expression, blink or corneal reflex (with CN V), taste in anterior two-thirds of tongue, "ba-ba-ba"

VIII. Hearing (whisper or use ticking watch), Weber, Rinne, nystagmus

IX, X. Sensory and motor functions of pharynx and larynx (gag reflex, position of uvula, swallowing), "ka-ka-ka"

XI. Shrugging of shoulders (trapezius), movement of head (sternocleidomastoid)

XII. Tongue movement, "la-la-la"

4. **Sensory** (see Appendices B-1 and B-2 for dermatomes).

a. ***Superficial sensation***. Pinprick (use disposable sterile safety pin), light touch (use wisp of cotton), temperature (use hot and cold test tubes).

b. ***Deep sensation***. Joint position or proprioception, deep pain (for upper limb hyperextend small finger; for lower limb, firmly compress calf muscle or Achilles tendon), vibration.

c. ***Cortical sensation***. Two-point discrimination, graphesthesia, stereognosis, double simultaneous stimulation (cortical extinction).

5. **Reflexes**.

a. ***Muscle-stretch or deep tendon reflexes (DTR)***. Commonly tested DTRs include (the main segment is in bold type): biceps brachii (**C5**, C6), brachioradialis (C5, **C6**), triceps brachii (**C7**, C8), quadriceps (L2, **L3**), and gastrocnemius-soleus (**S1**, S2). Less frequently tested DTRs include: jaw jerk (cranial nerve V), internal hamstring (L4, L5, S1, S2), and external hamstring (L5, S1, S2). DTRs on both sides must be compared and graded as: 0 = absent, 1+ = hypoactive, 2+ = normal, 3+ = brisker than average, 4+ = hyperactive with clonus and pathologic reflexes.

b. ***Superficial (segmental) reflexes***. Corneal (CN V and VII), gag (CN IX and X), epigastric (T6–9), hypogastric (T11–L1), cremasteric (L1–2), bulbocavernosus (S2–4), and anal (S3–5) reflexes.

c. ***Pathologic reflexes***. Babinski (Chaddock or Oppenheim), Hoffman, Kernig, bite, tongue thrust, chewing, and suck–swallow reflexes.

Table 1.1-7 Functional grading of balance

Balance grade	Definition
Zero	Patient needs maximal assistance to maintain balance
Poor	Patient needs support to maintain balance
Fair	Patient is able to maintain balance without support; cannot tolerate challenge; cannot maintain balance while shifting weight
Good	Patient is able to maintain balance without support; accepts moderate challenge and can shift weight, although limitations are evident
Normal	Patient is able to maintain balance without support; accepts maximal challenge and can shift weight in all directions

From Leahy P: Motor control assessment. In Montgomery P, Connolly B, editors: Motor control and physical therapy: theoretical framework and practical applications. *Hixson, TN, 1991, Chattanooga Group, p. 75, with permission.*

d. ***Developmental or primitive reflexes and reactions***. Asymmetric tonic neck reflex (ATNR), symmetric tonic neck reflex (STNR), tonic labyrinthine reflex (TLR), positive supporting reaction, crossed extension reflex, associated reactions, grasp reflex, righting reactions, equilibrium reactions, protective extension (parachute), sucking, and rooting reflexes.

6. **Motor control**.

a. ***Muscle tone***. Spasticity (for clinical grading, see Table 5.4-1 in Chapter 5.4), flaccidity (e.g., pendulum and drop arm test), rigidity, dystonia.

b. ***Coordination***. Tests for upper limbs include finger-to-nose and knee-pat tests; tests for lower limbs include toe-to-finger and heel-to-shin tests.

c. ***Alternate motion rate***. Rapid alternating hand movements, tongue wiggling, finger wiggling, foot-patting.

d. ***Involuntary movements***. Tremors, chorea, athetosis, ballismus, dystonia, myoclonus, asterixis, tics.

e. ***Motor planning ability***. Dressing apraxia (inability to put on a coat), constructional apraxia (inability to draw the face of a clock).

f. ***Balance/postural reactions***. Romberg test, sway excursion, verticality (perception of body position in space), balance responses to external displacement and during volitional displacements, adaptability to repeated displacements (see Table 1.1-7 for functional grading of balance).

g. ***Flexibility*** (or ROM; see section II.O.2.a under musculoskeletal examination).

h. ***Movement patterns***. Flexion or extension synergy patterns (see Table 1.1-8 for differentiation and Table 1.1-9 for grading of movement patterns), primitive reflexes (see section II.P.5.d).

i. ***Strength*** (see section II.O.2.c under musculoskeletal examination).

7. **Gait**. Document any gait aids used (note hand used, appropriate sequencing, condition of device; see Chapter 4.6). Observe the gait parameters (described in Table 1.1-10) from front, side, and rear, and note type of pathologic gait (e.g., antalgic, short-leg, coxalgic, metatarsalgic gait). Refer to Chapter 2.5, section VI for details about gait analyses.

Q. FUNCTIONAL NEUROMUSCULAR ASSESSMENT for screening of disabilities (see Table 1.1-11).

R. FUNCTIONAL (ADL) SCALES. The most widely used general (global) scale of function is the Functional Independence Measure (FIM) (see Chapter 2.8,

Table 1.1-8 Synergy patterns of the limbs

Limbs	Flexion synergy components	Extension synergy components
Upper	Scapular retraction/elevation or hyperextension Shoulder abduction, external rotation Elbow flexion* Forearm supination Wrist and finger flexion	Scapular protraction Shoulder adduction,* internal rotation Elbow extension Forearm pronation* Wrist and finger flexion
Lower	Hip flexion,* abduction, external rotation Knee flexion Ankle dorsiflexion, inversion Toe dorsiflexion	Hip extension, adduction,* internal rotation Knee extension* Ankle plantar flexion,* inversion Toe plantar flexion

From: O'Sullivan SB: Stroke. In O'Sullivan SB, Schmitz TJ, editors: Physical rehabilitation: assessment and treatment, *ed 4, Philadelphia, 2001, FA Davis Co., p. 532, with permission.*
** The components which are generally the strongest or most prominent.*

Table 1.1-9 Grading system of movement patterns in patients with upper motor neuron disease

Grade	Definition
0	Unable to initiate movement
1	Initiates movement through 25% of range of motion (ROM)
2	Carries movement through 50% of ROM
3	Carries movement through 75% of ROM
4	Carries movement through full range

Adapted from: Sawner K, Lavigne J: Brunnstrom's movement therapy in hemiplegia: a neurophysiological approach, *ed 2, Philadelphia, 1992, JB Lippincott, p. 207.*

section I). The FIM assesses 18 activities of self-care, mobility, locomotion, communication, and social cognition on a seven-point scale from fully independent to fully dependent. Other ADL scales that are more task specific include Barthel Index, PULSES profile, Klein–Bell ADL Scale, Katz index of independence in ADL, and Kenny self-care evaluation (see Chapter 2.8).

III. Summary and problem list

This includes a summary of the history and physical findings and a separate listing of medical and PM&R problems. The problem list must include diagnoses, secondary abnormalities, specific losses in self-care functions, social functions, vocational functions, and psychological functions. Record date of onset and date of resolution of problems.

Table 1.1-10 Clinical gait analysis

Parameters	Observation
A. Standing balance	Steadiness of position; Patient's attempt to regain balance as examiner pushes patient off balance
B. Body part movements during walking	
1. Posture	Fixed or abnormal postures; Inadequate, excessive, or asymmetrical movements of body parts
2. Head and trunk	Listing or tilting
3. Shoulder	Dipping, elevation, depression, protraction, and retraction
4. Arm swing	Protective positioning or posturing
5. Pelvis and hip	Hip hiking, dropping (Trendelenburg), or lateral thrust
6. Knee	Genu varum, valgum, or recurvatum
7. Ankle and foot	Excessive inversion or eversion
C. Gait cycle factors	
1. Cadence	Rate, symmetry, fluidity, and consistency
2. Stride width	Narrow or broad base; Knee and ankle clearance
3. Stride length	Shortened, lengthened, or asymmetrical
4. Stance phase	Normal heel-strike, foot flat, push off; Knee stability during all components of stance; Coordination of knee and ankle movements
5. Swing phase	Adequate and synchronized knee and ankle dorsiflexion during swing; abduction or circumduction

Adapted from: Erickson RP, McPhee MC: Clinical evaluation. In DeLisa JA and Gans BM, editors: Rehabilitation medicine: principles and practice, *ed 3, Philadelphia, 1998, Lippincott-Raven, p. 105.*

Table 1.1-11 Functional neuromuscular assessment for screening of disabilities

Activity	Patient tasks
A. Bed mobility	
1. Rolling to side	Turn from side to side
2. Supine to sit	Sit at edge of bed
B. Sitting	
1. Static balance	Sit at edge of bed unsupported
2. Dynamic balance reactions	Put on shoes or slippers while seated
C. Transfers	
1. Sit to stand	Stand up from seated position
2. Bed to other surface	Transfer from bed to chair or other surface (note standing pivot ability and equipment used, e.g., sliding board)
D. Standing	
1. Static balance	Stand unsupported
2. Dynamic balance reactions	Put on robe or coat while standing
E. Gait*	
1. Level surface	Walk on level surface
2. Stairs	Ascend and descend a flight of stairs
F. Wheelchair mobility†	
1. Level surface	Propel wheelchair on level surface
2. Ramp	Propel wheelchair up and down ramp

** See Table 1.1-10 and Chapter 2.5, section VI for details on gait assessment. Document gait aids and gait patterns (see Chapter 4.6 for details).*
†See Chapter 4.7 for details.

IV. Physiatric orders/referrals

Physiatric orders/referrals include primary and secondary diagnoses with onset; whether evaluation and/or treatment is requested; goals of treatment with expected duration of treatment or hospital stay; intensity, frequency, and initial duration of treatment desired; precautions (weight-bearing status, assistive devices needed, current medications, associated medical diagnosis); and follow-up date.

V. Admission orders

Use the "**ADC-VAAN-DISML**" mnemonic.

- Admit to: Ward or room; attending and resident physicians responsible for the patient
- Diagnosis: Admitting diagnosis, secondary diagnosis pertinent to nursing care
- Condition: Patient's general condition (stable, fair, poor, critical)
- Vital signs: Type, frequency, and parameters for notifying physician
- Allergies: Medications and food products (describe past reactions)
- Activity limitations: Bed rest, out of bed to wheelchair (specify type of assistance, precautions)
- Nursing orders: Wound care, input and output monitoring, weighing of patient, catheter care
- Diet: Regular diet, restricted diet (e.g., 2 g sodium, 2 g potassium, 300 mg/day cholesterol), diabetic diet (e.g., 1800 cal), dysphagia diet (see Chapter 5.6, section V.A.2.b.1)
- Intravenous fluids: Intravenous solutions and rate of infusion
- Sedatives, analgesics, and other prescription medications (gastrointestinal medications, bowel routine medications, antipyretics)
- Medications: Specify dose, route, frequency, duration, and special restrictions
- Laboratory and other diagnostic tests (see Chapter 2.1): Routine laboratory tests [complete blood count (CBC), serum electroytes with glucose (SMAG), prothrombin time (PT) and activated partial thromboplastin time (aPTT), liver function tests (LFT), and urinalysis (UA)], chest radiographs, electrocardiogram (ECG), special tests

VI. Progress notes

Use the "**SOAP**" mnemonic.

- Subjective: Patient complaints/symptoms and personal impressions
- Objective: Physical signs, test data (laboratory tests, radiograph, ECG), and quantified progress.
- Assessment: Analysis of subjective and objective data with tentative diagnosis or impression
- Plan: Diagnostic studies, therapeutic regimen, additional consultations, patient education required

VII. Discharge summary

Use the "**ROTC-DIC**" mnemonic.

- Reason for admission: Chief complaint, admission diagnosis, and brief history of the present illness

- Objective findings: Physical examinations, laboratory, radiograph, special tests (include pertinent negative findings too)
- Treatment given (medical, surgical, PM&R, PT, OT, psychology, etc.) and patient's response to it
- Complications and Consultations
- Diagnosis: Final diagnosis and final secondary diagnoses
- Instructions on continuing care: Medications (specify dose, route, frequency, and duration), diet, physical activity limitations, home exercises, home equipment, referrals (PT, OT, SLP, nursing, home health attendant), and follow-up appointments
- Condition upon discharge: ambulation status, self-care, ability to work

Further reading

Ferri FF, editor: *Practical guide to the care of the medical patient*, ed 6, St Louis, 2004, Mosby.

Gadi RK, Cifu DX: Physical medicine and rehabilitation: philosophy, patient care issues and physiatric evaluation. In Garrison SJ, editor: *Handbook of physical medicine and rehabilitation basics*, ed 2, Philadelphia, 2003, Lippincott, Williams & Wilkins, pp. 1–9.

Ganter BK, Erickson RP, Butters MA, *et al.*: Clinical evaluation. In DeLisa JA, Gans BM, Walsh NE, *et al.*, editors: *Physical medicine and rehabilitation: Principles and practice*, ed 4, Philadelphia, 2005, Lippincott, Williams and Wilkins, pp. 1–48.

Grynbaum BB, Sury R: Evaluation. In Goodgold J, editor: *rehabilitation medicine*, St Louis, 1988, Mosby, pp. 3–23.

McPeak LA: Physiatric history and examination. In Braddom RL, editor: *Physical medicine and rehabilitation*, ed 2, Philadelphia, 2000, WB Saunders, pp. 3–45.

Sinaki M, editor: *Basic clinical rehabilitation medicine*, St Louis, 1994, Mosby.

Stolov WC, Hays RM: Evaluation of the patient. In Kottke FJ, Lehmann JF, editors: *Krusen's handbook of physical medicine and rehabilitation*, ed 4, Philadelphia, 1990, WB Saunders, pp. 1–19.

World Health Organization: *International classification of impairments, disabilities and handicaps: a manual of classification relating to the consequence of disease*, Geneva, 1980, World Health Organization.

World Health Organization: *International classification of impairments, activities and participations*, Geneva, 1997, World Health Organization.

Supplemental references

Bates B: *A guide to physical examination and history taking*, ed 7, Philadelphia, 1998, JB Lippincott-Raven.

DeGowin RL, Brown DD: *DeGowin's diagnostic examination*, ed 7, New York, 1999, McGraw-Hill.

Hislop HJ, Montgomery J: *Daniels and Worthingham's muscle testing: techniques of manual examination*, ed 7, Philadelphia, 2002, WB Saunders.

Hoppenfeld S: *Physical examination of the spine and extremities*, New York, 1976, Prentice-Hall.

Jenkins DB: *Hollingshead's functional anatomy of the limbs and back*, ed 7, Philadelphia, 1998, WB Saunders.

Kendall F, McCreary EK, Provance P: *Muscles testing and function*, ed 4, Baltimore, 1993, Lippincott, Williams & Wilkins.

Magee DJ: *Orthopedic physical assessment*, ed 4, Philadelphia, 2002, WB Saunders.

Norkin CC, White DJ: *Measurement of joint motion: a guide to goniometry*, ed 3, Philadelphia, 2003, FA Davis.

O'Sullivan SB, Schmitz TJ, editors: *Physical rehabilitation: assessment and treatment*, ed 4, Philadelphia, 2001, FA Davis.

Seidel HM, Ball JW, Dains JE, *et al.*: *Mosby's guide to physical examination*, ed 5, St Louis, 2002, Mosby.

Victor M, Ropper AH, Adams RD: *Adam's and Victor's principles of neurology*, ed 7, New York, 2000, McGraw-Hill.

PART II

PHYSICAL MEDICINE AND REHABILITATION: DIAGNOSTIC TESTS

CHAPTER 2.1
Laboratory tests

Understanding the rationale of any test is important in proper patient care. This chapter covers some of the common laboratory tests used in PM&R. Although some of the tests are clearly in the realm of other specialties (e.g., rheumatology), they are commonly ordered for patients undergoing rehabilitation. All laboratory tests must be interpreted in the context of a careful history, thorough physical examination, and other related tests and measures. For normal values of common laboratory tests, refer to Appendix A-3.

I. Routine tests

These are commonly ordered upon hospital admission and include the following tests.

A. LABORATORY. Complete blood count (CBC) with differential count, erythrocyte sedimentation rate (ESR), serum electrolytes with glucose (SMAG), liver function tests (LFT or FLEX), coagulation profile [prothrombin time (PT) and activated partial thromboplastin time (aPTT)], urinalysis.

B. PLAIN RADIOGRAPH. Chest radiograph (described in Chapter 5.13, section III.C.1) to rule out cardiac and pulmonary pathology; postoperative skeletal radiograph.

C. ELECTROCARDIOGRAM (ECG; described in Chapter 5.13, section III.C.2.a). Baseline ECG especially in patients with cardiac history.

II. Special laboratory studies

A. SERUM PROTEIN ELECTROPHORESIS detects monoclonal and polyclonal patterns of serum proteins. The presence of monoclonal proteins in patients with back pain is suggestive of multiple myeloma. Polyclonal proteins are seen in connective tissue (autoimmune) disorders, chronic infection, chronic active hepatitis, and lymphoproliferative disease, but are sometimes found in normal individuals.

B. ACID PHOSPHATASE is used to provide clues of prostatic malignancy in men with metastatic bone tumor.

C. MUSCLE ENZYMES are increased in myopathies, muscle trauma, strenuous physical exertion (marathon running), and after intramuscular injections. Muscle enzymes commonly measured are creatinine kinase (CK), aldolase, lactic dehydrogenase (LDH), and aspartate aminotransferase (AST). CK, specifically the MM isoform of CK (CK-MM), is probably the most reliable indicator of skeletal muscle damage.

D. THYROID FUNCTION TESTS

1. **Serum thyroid-stimulating hormone (TSH)** is the least expensive and most sensitive marker for primary hypothyroidism. TSH is elevated in primary hypothyroidism [even before the thyroxine (T_4) level falls to an abnormal level]; while in secondary hypothyroidism (caused by pituitary or hypothalamic failure), it is decreased.

2. **Serum total T_4** is increased in hyperthyroidism, and decreased in hypothyroidism; however, it is also greatly affected by the level of serum binding protein [most commonly thyroxine-binding globulin (TBG)] because over 99% of T_4 is bound to TBG. An increase in TBG (e.g., pregnancy, use of oral contraceptives, acute hepatitis or chronic active liver disease, use of marijuana or heroin or methadone, fluorouracil use, and acute intermittent porphyria) will decrease total T_4; while decreased TBG (e.g., androgen or glucocorticoid excess, nephrotic syndrome, severe illness, cirrhosis, or intake of such drugs as phenytoin, furosemide, and salicylate) will increase total T_4.
3. **Tri-iodothyronine resin uptake (T_3RU)** is used to circumvent the problem of changes in serum TBG; however, it must be used only in conjunction with simultaneous measures of total T_4. The T_3RU reflects the unsaturated thyroxine binding sites on TBG and is not a measure of circulating T_3. The T_3RU is high in hyperthyroidism and low in hypothyroidism and pregnancy.
4. **Free T_4 and free T_3** are theoretically the ideal tests of thyroid function, but serum concentrations are so low that they are difficult to measure.

E. CEREBROSPINAL FLUID ANALYSIS is used to identify subarachnoid hemorrhage, meningeal inflammation (meningitis) and neoplasia, presence of various abnormal antigens, antibodies, and other abnormal proteins (e.g., syphilis, multiple sclerosis). It is obtained by lumbar puncture, which is a relatively simple procedure. Lumbar puncture contraindications include clinical evidence of increased intracranial pressure, local infection at the puncture site, or poor patient cooperation.

F. DYSTROPIN is a cytoskeletal protein normally found in equal quantities in skeletal and cardiac muscle. Dystropin deficiency is seen in Duchenne and Becker muscular dystrophy.

III. Rheumatologic laboratory tests

A. ACUTE-PHASE REACTANTS

1. **Erythrocyte sedimentation rate (ESR)** is the rate of fall in millimeters per hour of red blood cells (RBCs) in a standard tube (Westergren method). Normal Westergren ESR values are 0–15 mm/h for males and 0–20 mm/h for females. Rates in the range of 30 mm/h are considered normal in people aged 60 years or older. Elevated ESR indicates nonspecific tissue inflammation (e.g., in the presence of infection, anemia, chronic disease, allergic reaction, malignancy, or in patients taking heparin). However, normal ESR tends to exclude active inflammatory disorders such as acute rheumatic fever, systemic lupus erythematosus (SLE), rheumatoid arthritis (RA), temporal arteritis-polymyalgia rheumatica. ESR can be used to follow the course (including therapeutic responses) of chronic inflammatory disorders. Falsely low ESRs may be found in polycythemia, anisocytosis, spherocytosis, sickle cell disease, or heart failure. Falsely high ESR may be seen in prolonged storage of blood to be tested or tilting of the calibrated tube.
2. **C-reactive protein (CRP)** is present in low concentration in normal serum. It has the ability to give a precipitin reaction with pneumococcal C-polysaccharide and can be measured by a latex agglutination test or rocket electrophoresis. CRP rises rapidly in the presence of inflammation, then fall as the inflammation subsides. It is usually used to monitor the progress of osteomyelitis during antibiotic treatment. The major advantage of CRP testing over ESR testing is that it can be performed on freeze-stored serum. However, both are nonspecific tests of inflammation. In the absence of infection in patients with SLE or scleroderma, CRP levels are inappropriately low.

B. RHEUMATOID FACTORS (RF) are autoantibodies against the Fc (i.e., heavy-chain constant fragment) portion of immunoglobulin G (IgG), which are primarily associated with RA but are also found in other rheumatic diseases, such as Sjögren's syndrome, SLE, scleroderma, and mixed connective tissue disease. They have also been associated with acute viral infections (e.g., mononucleosis, hepatitis, influenza, postvaccination), parasitic infections (e.g., malaria, schistosomiasis, filariasis), chronic inflammatory disease (e.g., tuberculosis, leprosy, syphilis, subacute bacterial endocarditis, salmonellosis), and other hyperglobulinemic states (e.g., cryoglobulinemia, sarcoid, chronic liver disease, other chronic pulmonary disease).

C. ANTINUCLEAR ANTIBODIES (ANAs) react to a variety of nuclear and cytoplasmic cellular antigens found in systemic rheumatic disease, such as SLE, progressive systemic sclerosis, mixed connective tissue disease, and RA. ANA studies are usually reported by pattern, intensity of fluorescence (1+ to 4+), or titer. Values of 2+ to 4+ or titers greater than 1:40 are usually considered significant. By determining the reactivity of ANA-positive sera with nuclear constituents [e.g., double-stranded DNA (dsDNA), single-stranded DNA (ssDNA), histones, etc.], greater diagnostic specificity is attained. For example, antibody to dsDNA is highly specific for SLE and particularly corresponds to active renal disease (dsDNA disappears with remission after immunosuppressive or steroid therapy). Although steroid or immunosuppressive therapy may affect the ANA titer, most clinicians do not rely on serial changes in ANA to monitor disease activity. Instead, ANA studies are performed as an initial screening test for autoantibodies.

1. **Antineutrophil cytoplasmic antibody (ANCA)** is a special case of ANA, which binds relatively selectively to cytoplasmic proteins within neutrophils. A granular cytoplasmic staining pattern (C-ANCA) is highly specific for Wegener's granulomatosis (present in approximately 80% of cases), while a perinuclear pattern (P-ANCA) is seen in polyarteritis nodosa and in other forms of glomerulonephritis. ANCA is also useful in confirming the diagnosis of vasculitis in the presence of histopathological diagnosis.
2. **Anticardiolipin antibody** is another form of ANA found in up to 50% of patients with SLE but it also occurs in individuals without SLE. It is associated with recurrent fetal loss, recurrent venous and arterial thrombosis, thrombocytopenia, and labile hypertension. It has also been reported (but unconfirmed) in patients with stroke and early myocardial infarct.

D. IMMUNE COMPLEXES

1. **Cryoglobulins** are special types of immunoglobulins that precipitate from serum in the cold (0–5°C). Testing for cryoglobulins is the simplest way of detecting immune complexes.

a. ***Mixed cryoglobulins*** consist usually of IgM–IgG immunoglobulins and constitute two-thirds of the cryoglobulins seen in the Western world. They are used in identifying the immune complex syndrome called mixed, or essential, cryoglobulinemia. Other diseases associated with mixed cryoglobulin are autoimmune diseases (e.g., SLE, RA, polyarteritis nodosa, Sjögren's syndrome, scleroderma), lymphoproliferative diseases (e.g., chronic lymphocytic leukemia, macroglobulinemia), renal diseases (e.g., proliferative glomerulonephritis), and liver diseases (Laennec's cirrhosis, biliary cirrhosis, chronic hepatitis). It can also be seen (often transiently) in viral, bacterial, or parasitic infections. Mixed cryoglobulin may be difficult to detect because it tends to be present in small amounts (50–500 mg/dL).

b. ***Monoclonal cryoglobulins*** occur in large amounts (1–5 g/dL) and are easily detected as monoclonal components on electrophoresis of whole serum or the isolated cryoprecipitate. They are generally associated with multiple myeloma, macroglobulinemia, angioimmunoblastic lymphadenopathy, chronic lymphocytic leukemia, and other rarer neoplastic proliferations of plasma cells and lymphocytes.

2. **Complement assay** is one method of detecting immune complexes. The complement system consists of at least 20 different plasma and membrane proteins that play a major role in host defense against microbes by either modifying the membranes of the infectious agents (e.g., opsonization for ingestion by phagocytes, membrane damage), or promoting the host inflammatory response (e.g., chemotaxis of neutrophils and monocytes, anaphylatoxic activity). It can be activated in an enzymatic cascade system (similar to the clotting system cascade) through the classical pathway (activated by the presence of antigen–antibody immune complexes) or through the alternative pathway (activated by the complex polysaccharides found in microbes). Both pathways eventually cleave C3 which subsequently leads to the activation of the membrane attack complex (MAC) with involvement of the terminal complement proteins C5–C9. The activated MAC proteins can insert into the membrane of cells and form a transmembrane channel that leads to cell lysis. They can also remove the lipid from viral envelopes, thus rendering the virus noninfectious.

   The irreversible proteolytic reactions in the complement cascade system result in cleaved proteins or complements that are rapidly cleared from the circulation. If there is an ongoing immunologic event that is activating the complement system in vivo (e.g., SLE or cryoglobulinemia), the plasma levels of these complements may be decreased, especially if the body is in a catabolic state (i.e., with low protein synthesis). Thus, low plasma complement (hypocomplementemia) suggests that there is a high level of circulating immune complexes.

   Complements can be measured by functional immunoassays of individual components or by determining the total hemolytic complement (THC) or CH_{50} assay, which measures the ability of the test serum to lyse 50% of a standardized suspension of sheep RBCs coated with rabbit antibody. Because complement proteins are heat-labile, the collected specimen must be adequately frozen (at −20°C) and assayed within 2 weeks, otherwise the results become inaccurate. Interpretation of an isolated static value is often difficult, hence serial testing is generally recommended for monitoring the disease activity (e.g., in patients with SLE or RA). While low values may suggest ongoing disease, normal or high values are less helpful because complement proteins, which are acute-phase reactants, tend to be increased even with minor intercurrent illnesses. Deficiencies of complements C1 to C4 (i.e., complements during the early classical pathway) are associated with SLE-like syndromes and an increased incidence of infection; while deficiencies of complements C5 to C9 are associated with rheumatic syndromes and an increased incidence of infection, particularly by *Neisseria*. A low CH_{50} is often seen in SLE, cryoglobulinemia, and RA vasculitis.

E. **HUMAN LEUKOCYTE ANTIGEN (HLA) TYPING** is used as a marker to identify certain rheumatic diseases.

1. **HLA-B27** is a major histocompatibility antigen and is positive in patients with ankylosing spondylitis (95%), Reiter's syndrome (80%), psoriatic spondylitis (50–70%), and inflammatory bowel disease (75%). It has been shown that 20% of HLA-B27-positive persons experience ankylosing spondylitis or Reiter's syndrome after an infectious episode.
2. **SSA antigen** is associated with Sjögren's syndrome and SLE while SSB antigen is associated with Sjögren's syndrome only.

F. **LYME SEROLOGIC TESTING** detects antibodies or T-cell response to *Borrelia burgdorferi*. It is used to confirm clinical suspicion of Lyme disease but is not definitive because false-negative results (e.g., during first week of infection before antibodies develop) and false-positive results (e.g., because of cross-reactivity to other spirochetes such as *Treponema pallidum,* in patients with RF or ANA) can occur.

1. **Immunofluorescent assay (IFA)** detects antibodies to whole *B. burgdorferi* seen within weeks of the onset of Lyme disease.
2. **Enzyme-linked immunosorbent assay (ELISA)** has better specificity, sensitivity, and reproducibility than IFA. It detects IgM antibodies, which occur 2–4 weeks after the erythema chronicum migrans rash, then peaks after 8 weeks and normalizes by 4–6 months.
3. **Western blotting** is used to confirm a positive IFA or ELISA, especially late in the course of Lyme disease. It is used only when clinical and serologic tests are doubtful.
4. **Cellular immunity testing** detects the T-cell response to *B. burgdorferi* early in the course of Lyme disease, before the production of antibodies. It is difficult, however, to perform and interpret; therefore, it is not routinely used.

G. **URIC ACID (SERUM)** is increased in gout and is primarily used to confirm the diagnosis of gout. However, it is also increased in asymptomatic hyperuricemia, renal failure, rapidly proliferating neoplasms, postchemotherapy or irradiation, hemolytic anemias, toxemia of pregnancy, excessive dietary intake (e.g., kidney or liver food products), lead poisoning, parathyroid disorders, sarcoidosis, and in the intake of certain drugs (e.g., thiazides, loop diuretics, low-dose aspirin).

H. **SYNOVIAL FLUID** obtained via arthrocentesis (see Chapter 4.9 for arthrocentesis techniques) can be classified into normal, noninflammatory (group I), inflammatory (group II), septic (group III), or hemorrhagic (group IV). The problems with such classifications include: the lack of uniform criteria for inclusion into any one group; and their limited usefulness for diagnosis because a single disease may fall into any group [e.g., SLE and scleroderma can either be inflammatory (group I) or noninflammatory (group II); gout, which is classified as inflammatory (group II) may look purulent (group III) during an acute attack; infected fluids (group III) may show inflammatory (group II) fluid during early infection or when partially treated]. In general, the only two conditions that can be diagnosed using synovial fluid analysis alone are crystal-induced synovitis (group II or inflammatory) and septic arthritis (group III or purulent). As long as the clinician is aware of its limitations, the arbitrary classification of synovial fluids (see Table 2.1-1) may be used to distinguish inflammatory from "noninflammatory" arthritis and to alert the clinician about infectious arthritis when the white blood cell is high or when the fluid looks purulent. The following are some of the possible rheumatologic conditions that may be associated with each group of synovial fluid analysis (note that some conditions, e.g., SLE, may be associated with more than one group):

1. **"Noninflammatory" (group I)**: Osteoarthritis, aseptic necrosis, trauma, osteochondritis dessicans, osteochondromatosis, neuropathic arthropathy, pigmented villonodular synovitis, SLE, scleroderma, and subsiding or early inflammation.
2. **Inflammatory (group II)**: Connective tissue diseases (RA, juvenile RA, SLE, acute rheumatic fever, scleroderma, arthritis accompanying ulcerative colitis and regional enteritis), infectious arthritis (e.g., viral), seronegative spondyloarthropathies (Reiter's syndrome, ankylosing spondylitis, psoriatic arthritis), crystal-induced synovitis (gout, pseudogout), leukemia, lymphoma.
3. **Purulent (group III)**: Tuberculosis, acute bacterial infections, fungal infections, and sometimes gout and RA.
4. **Hemorrhagic (group IV)**: Coagulation disorders (e.g., hemophilia, von Willebrand's disease, anticoagulation therapy, thrombocytopenia), trauma with or without fracture, postsurgical, pigmented (hypertrophic) villonodular synovitis, benign or malignant joint or synovial neoplasm, hemangioma, scurvy,

Table 2.1-1 Classification of synovial fluids*

Synovial fluid	Normal	I	II	III	IV
Viscosity	High	High	Low	Variable	High
Color	Colorless to straw-colored	Straw-colored to yellow	Yellow	Variable	Red
Clarity	Transparent	Transparent	Cloudy	Opaque	Opaque
WBC/mm^3	<200	200–2000	2000–100 000 75 ± 000	Often >75	May be <200
% PMN WBC	<25	<25	Often >50	Often >75	May be <25
Mucin clot	Firm	Firm	Friable	Friable	Firm
FBG	Nearly equal (±10%) to blood	Nearly equal (±10%) to blood	<25 mg/dL lower than in blood	>25 mg/dL lower than in blood	Nearly equal (±10%) to blood

*Group I = "noninflammatory"; group II = inflammatory; group III = septic; group IV = hemorrhagic.
WBC = white blood cell; PMN WBC = polymorphonuclear WBC; FBG = fasting blood glucose.
Adapted from: Zvaiffler NJ: Synovial fluid analysis. In Stein J, editor: Internal medicine, *ed 4, St Louis, 1994, Mosby, p. 2358.*

neuropathic arthropathy, Ehlers–Danlos syndrome, pseudoxanthoma elasticum, sickle cell disease.

IV. Biopsy

A. MUSCLE BIOPSY, usually taken from the deltoid or quadriceps, is performed to distinguish myopathic from neurogenic disease. In primary myopathies, the muscle is characterized by fiber size variation and evidence of degeneration (fiber necrosis and phagocytosis, possibly inflammation) and regeneration (basophilia, fiber splitting). In chronic myopathies, there may be extensive connective tissue proliferation and fatty infiltration. In denervating disease there may be evidence of active (small, angulated fibers) and chronic (fiber-typed grouping and grouped atrophy) denervation. Muscle biopsy is of major diagnostic value in inflammatory muscle disease, steroid myopathy, muscular dystrophy, and infectious myositis. It is also valuable in the diagnosis of myopathy associated with various connective tissue diseases, including vasculitis.

B. SYNOVIAL BIOPSY is obtained via open arthrotomy, under direct vision with arthroscopy, or blindly through closed needle biopsy. However, a closed needle biopsy should not be performed unless there is excessive synovial fluid. It is performed when the diagnosis is unclear despite a thorough clinical examination in patients with chronic nontraumatic synovitis limited to a single or few joints. Its greatest value is in providing a more specific diagnosis in patients with monoarticular or oligoarticular arthritis whose diagnosis is not clear. It also has diagnostic values in acute infection (i.e., showing clusters and sheets of neutrophils and bacteria); chronic infection such as tuberculosis, fungal infections (i.e., showing large numbers of lymphocytes, plasma cells, granulomas, and tubercle bacilli or fungi); and infiltrative or deposition disease such as primary and secondary amyloidosis (i.e., showing amyloid infiltrates), ochronosis (i.e., showing brown pigment sheets), hemochromatosis (i.e., showing hemosiderin deposits), tumors (e.g., pigmented villonodular synovitis, benign and malignant tumors), and multicentric disease (e.g., reticular histiocytosis). It may also be helpful in chronic sarcoidosis, multiple synovial chondromatosus, polymyositis, and scleroderma.

C. **SURAL NERVE BIOPSY** is used to confirm vasculitis especially if there are symptoms of intermittent numbness or weakness or if nerve conduction studies show delayed sural nerve conduction.

Further reading

Hicks JE, Sutin J: Rehabilitation in joint and connective tissue diseases. 2. Approach to the diagnosis of rheumatic diseases. *Arch Phys Med Rehabil* Suppl 69:S78–S83, 1988.

Paget S, Gibofsky A, Beary III JF, editors: *Manual of rheumatology and outpatient orthopedic disorders*, ed 4, Philadelphia, 2000, Lippincott, Williams & Wilkins.

Schumacher Jr HR, Klipper JH, Koopman WJ, editors: *Primer on the rheumatic disease*, ed 10, Atlanta, 1993, Arthritis Foundation.

Stein J, editor: *Textbook of internal medicine*, ed 5, Philadelphia, 2000, Elsevier.

Surks MI, *et al.*: American Thyroid Association guidelines for the use of laboratory tests in thyroid disorders. *JAMA* 263:1529–1532, 1990.

CHAPTER 2.2
Noninvasive imaging studies

Chapters 2.2 and 2.3 cover some of the widely used imaging studies in the PM&R setting. They are by no means complete. The classification of invasive vs. noninvasive procedures is at best arbitrary. In this book, noninvasive imaging studies refer to those that do not involve skin puncture. Hence, imaging studies that involve swallowing of ultrasound probes (e.g., transesophageal echocardiography) or of barium (e.g., videofluoroscopic swallowing studies) are discussed under this chapter even though they can be argued to be "invasive". Interpretation of any imaging studies must be closely correlated with clinical findings (as abnormal findings can possibly be found in asymptomatic individuals).

I. Radiographic imaging

A. **CONVENTIONAL RADIOGRAPHY OR PLAIN RADIOGRAPHY (PLAIN X-RAY)** is usually the initial diagnostic imaging method in the evaluation of bone and joint pain because it is readily available and has relatively low cost. For a systematic way of interpreting radiographs of the musculoskeletal system, use the "ABCs" mnemonic. First check the Alignment of the bone, then the Bone itself, followed by Cartilage and Soft tissue.

1. **Limb radiograph** views commonly used are anteroposterior, lateral, oblique, patellar views of the knee, and standing views of the foot, knee, and hip. Plain radiographs are specific for the diagnosis of bony lesions, such as fractures, neoplasms, and osteomyelitis, but are not as sensitive as radionuclide bone scanning and magnetic resonance imaging (MRI) for early detection of these abnormalities. Radiographic evaluation of nonbony structures (e.g., cartilage, muscle, ligaments, tendons, and synovial fluid) is difficult unless fat or calcification is present. Joint space narrowing may indicate cartilage destruction. Displacement of adjacent fat pads in the knee, elbow, and ankle may be the result of synovitis (this cannot be reliably detected in the hip and shoulder).
2. **Spine radiograph** views commonly used are anteroposterior, lateral, oblique, odontoid, and flexion–extension views. Spine radiographs are useful in patients with suspected spinal trauma, scoliosis, congenital anomalies of the spine, back pain (e.g., spondylolisthesis, spondylolysis, ankylosing spondylitis), point tenderness, osteoporosis, and after spinal surgery (e.g., flexion and extension views of the spine can be used to diagnose instability and evaluate the adequacy of spinal fusion). However, studies have shown that there is almost no correlation between clinical findings and the osteophytes and/or neural foraminal stenosis (especially in the cervical region) seen in conventional radiographs. Detection of multilevel degenerative disease is also a poor indicator of the specific source of the pain. Fractures of the pedicles or the neural arch are difficult to identify in conventional radiographs [computed tomographic (CT) scan is recommended instead].
3. **Skull radiographs** have low diagnostic yield and should not be used routinely to screen headache, seizure, and transient or fixed neurologic deficits. In severe intracranial injury, an immediate CT scan is indicated. Most skull radiographs are currently used in the emergency room on patients with relatively mild head trauma and without neurologic findings to detect fractures, to screen patients for CT examination, and on patients with facial injury, lacerations to the head, or

penetrating missile injury. Skull radiographs can also be used in assessing congenital craniofacial abnormalities, palpable lesions in the scalp, and inflammatory conditions of the paranasal sinuses and mastoids.

B. FLUOROSCOPY is used to determine the position during surgical procedures (e.g., internal fixation of fractures and osteotomies) and during invasive radiologic procedures (e.g., myelography, percutaneous needle biopsy, diskography, arthrography, and facet joint injection). Fluoroscopy may be used for the evaluation of motion and to determine spinal stability. Its main disadvantage is excessive radiation exposure, which can be reduced by videotape recording, e.g., **videofluoroscopic swallowing studies** (see Chapter 5.6, section III.C.1.b) and **video-urodynamics** (see Chapter 5.7, section II.C.2.e).

C. COMPUTER-ASSISTED TOMOGRAPHY (CT) is a cross-sectional imaging technique that uses a narrowly collimated X-ray beam of predetermined slice thickness to provide better soft tissue contrast than with plain radiographs. It is useful in evaluating the extent of bony and soft tissue tumors. In a CT scan, air is black, and fat, cerebrospinal fluid, white matter, gray matter, blood and bone are progressively whiter. Its disadvantage is that it exposes the patient to radiation.

1. **Head CT** without contrast is indicated in acute trauma, hydrocephalus (monitoring ventricular size in shunted patients), intracranial hemorrhage, stroke (distinguishing hemorrhagic from bland infarcts), skull base diseases, and complex craniofacial anomalies. Contrast-enhanced head CT has an intravascular component that enhances normal vessels and abnormal vascular structures, such as aneurysms and vascular malformations, and an extravascular component in which contrast material leaks out of vessels into areas of blood–brain barrier disruptions such as brain tumors, cerebral infarction, and a variety of inflammatory processes. With the advent of MRI, the need for contrast head CT has diminished.
2. **Spine and pelvic CT scans** can be used to diagnose intervertebral disk herniation, spinal stenosis (assessment of the extent of hypertrophic bony changes, calcified ligaments, and bony spurs), degenerative disk and vertebral disease, vertebral and paraspinal tumors and inflammatory lesions, vertebral fractures (e.g., fractures through the pedicles or the neural arch, which are difficult to assess on plain radiographs), pelvic and sacral fractures, and congenital abnormalities. Although CT and MRI are equally helpful in diagnosing lumbar disk disease, CT is not as good as MRI in detecting cervical and thoracic disk herniation. In most patients with back pain and sciatica, CT has eliminated the need for myelography. In the diagnosis of intraspinal lesions, however, CT may be combined with myelography to enhance its sensitivity. Although sagittal and coronal CT images can be obtained by reformatting the obtained data, their resolutions are not as good as with the axial images. If after a CT scan, the diagnosis is not established, then MRI should be considered.

II. Magnetic resonance imaging (MRI)

MRI involves the imaging of protons (the positively charged spinning nucleus of hydrogen atoms that are abundant in water, proteins, lipids, and other macromolecules). When placed in a magnetic field, protons align themselves either with or against the direction of the field. Their alignment direction is reversed when radiofrequency (RF) pulses are applied. As the RF pulse is stopped, the protons then return to their original magnetic alignment (relaxation phase). In the process of relaxation, the protons release the energy acquired during the RF pulse, thus producing a voltage that is measured as the magnetic resonance (MR) signal. The relative brightness or darkness of the MR signal depends on the RF pulse sequence, the proton density of the tissue, and other factors such as blood flow and chemical shift.

MRI can be used to evaluate internal derangement of the knee (e.g., meniscal tears, cruciate, and collateral ligament tears, quadriceps mechanism tears, and bone contusion); osteonecrosis; rotator cuff tears and glenohumeral instability; tendon, ligament, and muscle tears of the ankle, wrist, and elbow; diskovertebral instability and disk herniation; brain disorders (especially white matter diseases); spinal cord disorders (syringomyelia, intrinsic lesions such as cysts and tumors, myelopathy, conus medullaris lesions); bone and soft tissue tumors and metastases; occult fractures; vascular malformations; and hemangiomas. It is superior to the CT scan in detecting cervical and thoracic disk herniation. For the diagnosis of lumbar disk disease, however, MRI and CT are equally helpful. When extensive calcification or hypertrophic changes are present (e.g., calcification of the posterior longitudinal ligament or osteophytes), MRI is inferior to CT scan. In patients with sciatica, MRI (instead of myelography) is recommended to detect lesions of the conus medullaris and other intraspinal lesions (e.g., neoplasms), which may mimic sciatica.

MRI has the following advantages over a CT scan:

- MRI does not use ionizing radiation and has no apparent adverse biologic effects;
- MRI is not subject to bone or dental artifact;
- MRI allows coronal and sagittal imaging with ease and with excellent resolution;
- MRI requires contrast enhancement less often than CT; and
- MRI uses contrast agents that are generally safer than the agents used for CT.

The disadvantages of MRI are:

- It is more expensive than CT;
- It has limited use in acutely ill patients on life support because of interactions between the magnetic field and life support equipment;
- It is often unacceptable to claustrophobic patients;
- It cannot be used in patients with ferromagnetic intracranial aneurysm clips, metallic objects anatomically close to vital vascular or neural structures or in or around the eyes, pacemakers, cochlear implants, neurostimulator devices, or some bullet fragments;
- It has limited use when the area of clinical interest is close to ferromagnetic surgical hardware; and
- It is inferior to CT in detecting acute subarachnoid hemorrhage and in evaluating calcified lesions. Most prosthetic heart valves, as well as most orthopedic materials and devices (including stainless steel screws and wires), are considered safe for MRI. However, ferromagnetic metallic implants cause image artifact ("flare" response), which may interfere with image interpretation. Pregnancy (especially in the first trimester) is considered a relative contraindication to MRI although there is no convincing evidence to suggest a risk to the fetus. Children as well as anxious patients may need to be sedated during MRI.

A. SPIN-ECHO MRI TECHNIQUE uses two RF pulses to achieve soft tissue contrast by differential tissue relaxation times. The images obtained with spin-echo MRI can be weighted depending on the RF pulse sequence, repetition time (TR is the interval between repetitions of the pulse sequence), and echo time (TE is the interval between RF excitation and the measurement of the MR signal). T_1-weighted MR images (short TR of <600 ms and short TE of <32 ms) are obtained quickly to show anatomical detail. T_2-weighted MR images (long TR of 2000–3000 ms and long TE of 60–120 ms) have improved contrast but less spatial resolution and take longer to obtain than T_1-weighted images. An intermediate-density-weighted MR image (or proton-density-weighted or spin-density-weighted image) uses TR of 1500–2500 ms and TE of 15–50 ms.

Table 2.2-1 shows the different signal intensities of different tissues on T_1- and T_2-weighted MR images. In general, fatty tissue (e.g., normal fatty bone marrow) exhibits a bright signal intensity on T_1-weighted sequences, with slightly less bright signal on T_2-weighted sequences. Conversely, pathologic processes (infiltrative disease, infection, bone marrow edema) appear as low signal on T_1-weighted sequences. Both cortical bone and fibrous tissue (including normal ligaments and tendons) maintain low signal intensity on all pulse sequences. Fluids (synovial fluid, edema, cysts) exhibit low signal intensity on T_1-weighted sequences, with markedly bright signal intensity with T_2-weighted sequences.

B. **GRADIENT-ECHO MRI TECHNIQUES** provide rapid image acquisition by using a single RF pulse to achieve soft tissue contrast through variation in pulse sequences. Unlike the spin-echo MRI technique, there is no loss of signal associated with the outflow of blood during the interval between RF pulses. Hence, in gradient-echo MR images laminar blood flow appears bright while turbulent flow and thrombus appear dark. This is in direct contrast to spin-echo MR images, in which rapid blood flow appears dark, slow blood flow appears intermediate, and thrombus appears intermediate or bright. Gradient-echo MRI is extremely useful in the evaluation of articular cartilage and in diagnosing subtle cervical disk disease. In general, bone is black and hyaline cartilage (e.g., disk) are white on gradient-echo MRI.

C. **GADOLINIUM-ENHANCED MRI** is technically an invasive procedure but is discussed here for convenience. It uses an MRI contrast agent (gadolinium diethylenetriamine pentaacetic acid or GD-DTPA) that shortens the T_1 relaxation times. Gadolinium-enhanced images appear bright on T_1-weighted images. It is used in spine and brain imaging especially for tumor diagnosis and detection of multiple sclerosis plaques. It is superior to CT in the detection of tumor-associated features such as edema, cysts, vascularity, hemorrhage, and necrosis. It can distinguish early postoperative scars (which are enhanced because of their rich vascularity) from recurrent disk herniation (which is avascular and is not enhanced). However, long after surgery the scar tissue may become progressively fibrotic with less discernible contrast enhancement. Relative contraindications to GD-DTPA administration include patients with hemolytic anemias (may promote extravascular hemolysis) and impaired renal function (GD-DTPA is cleared through glomerular filtration). The most common adverse reaction is mild headache which is reported in less than 10% of patients.

D. **MAGNETIC RESONANCE ANGIOGRAPHY (MRA)** (see Chapter 2.3, section II.A.2.d).

III. Diagnostic ultrasonography

Diagnostic ultrasonography transmits high-frequency (ultrasound) waves to the tissue and measures the amplitude of the reflected waves and the time it has taken the waves to travel from the transmitter to the receiving crystal. It measures tissue density at known depths and so builds a two-dimensional picture of the tissues, which can be presented in tones of gray. This is known as grayscale or B-mode imaging and is the mode commonly used for imaging solid structures. In this mode, the whiteness is inversely proportional to the density.

Table 2.2-1 Summary of signal intensities on magnetic resonance imaging (MRI)

Tissue	T_1-weighted image*	T_2-weighted image†
Fat	Very bright	Intermediate to dark
Cyst		
Simple	Very dark	Very bright
Proteinaceous	Intermediate to bright	Very bright
Brain		
White matter	Bright	Moderately dark
Gray matter	Moderately dark	Moderately bright
Cerebrospinal fluid	Very dark	Very bright
Multiple sclerosis plaque	Intermediate to dark	Bright
Bland infarct	Dark	Bright
Tumor	Dark	Bright
Meningioma	Intermediate	Intermediate
Abscess	Dark	Bright
Edema	Dark	Bright
Calcification	Variable: poorly seen, dark, or bright	Variable: poorly seen, or dark
Bone marrow		
Yellow	Very bright	Intermediate to dark
Red	Intermediate	Moderately dark
Bone metastasis		
Lytic	Dark	Intermediate to bright
Sclerotic	Dark	Dark
Cortical bone	Very dark	Very dark
Cartilage		
Fibrous	Very dark	Very dark
Hyaline	Intermediate	Intermediate
Intervertebral disk		
Normal	Intermediate	Bright
Degenerated	Intermediate to dark	Dark
Tendons and ligaments	Very dark	Very dark
Inflamed tendons	Intermediate	Intermediate
Torn tendons	Intermediate	Bright
Muscle	Dark	Dark
Gadolinium-enhanced tissue		
Low concentration	Very bright	Bright
High concentration	Intermediate to dark	Very dark
Hematoma		
Acute	Intermediate to dark	Dark
Subacute	Bright rim	Bright
Chronic	Dark rim (±bright center)	Dark rim (±bright center)

** T_1-weighted image = short TR (repetition time) of < 600 ms and short TE (echo time) of < 32 ms.*

† T_2-weighted image = long TR of 2000–3000 ms; long TE of 60–120 ms.

Data adapted from: Edelman RR, Warach S: Magnetic resonance imaging, part I. N Engl J Med *328(10):710, 1993, copyright ©1993 Massachusetts Medical Society. All rights reserved, used with permission.*

A. MUSCULOSKELETAL ULTRASONOGRAPHY can be used to evaluate soft tissue masses and characterize them as either cystic or solid. Ultrasound waves are reflected by bone and cannot be used to evaluate the internal bony structures. Tendons are more echogenic than muscle and can be evaluated in some cases for continuity and inflammation. Ultrasonography of joints has been used in the shoulder for evaluation of the rotator cuff tendons but has not been as accurate as MRI or arthrography. Ultrasound may be used for the evaluation of congenital dislocation of the hip in infants to determine the position of the nonossified femoral head with respect to the acetabulum. In contrast to both CT scan and MRI, ultrasonographs can display structures in motion. Its use in delineating musculoskeletal motion (e.g., motion of the spine and the facet joints), however, is still experimental.

B. ECHOCARDIOGRAPHY uses ultrasound to image cardiac structures and function and to determine flow direction and velocities within cardiac chambers and vessels. It can be performed via either transthoracic or transesophageal ultrasound probes. Transesophageal echocardiography can be classified as an invasive procedure because it entails swallowing the probe. (The diagnostic uses of echocardiography are described in Chapter 5.13, section III.C.2.b.)

C. THYROID ULTRASOUND is used to evaluate the size of the thyroid and the number, composition, and dimensions of the thyroid nodules. Although both solid and cystic nodules can be malignant, solid nodules have a higher incidence of malignancy.

D. RENAL ULTRASOUND is used to assess kidney anatomy for detecting hydronephrosis and kidney stones.

E. VASCULAR DOPPLER is commonly used in PM&R to determine severity or location of peripheral vascular disease or carotid stenosis and to rule out deep venous thrombosis (DVT). Vascular spectral Doppler is used to determine flow velocity. It may be combined with the basic B-mode imaging.

1. Continuous-wave Doppler modality emits and receives ultrasound continuously. It can infer the speed that a target (e.g., red blood cell) is traveling, but it cannot determine from what distance the signal returns (i.e., it cannot state the location of the target). Although it is rapid, easy, inexpensive, and reproducible, it cannot localize occlusions nor provide adequate hemodynamic evaluation.

a. ***Arterial continuous-wave Doppler*** is used for the evaluation of peripheral artery occlusive disease via the ankle/brachial index (ABI), which is determined by taking arterial Doppler measurements from the arm and ankle (i.e., ABI = the highest *ankle* Doppler pressure divided by the highest *brachial* Doppler pressure). The normal ABI should be about 1.1 (±0.2). In diabetic patients, false results may be obtained as a result of medial calcinosis of the artery. Thus an ABI higher than 1.1 in diabetic patients indicates calcified vessels and should be referred to a vascular specialist. ABI of 0.8 to 1.1 indicates venous insufficiency and mild arterial disease, and may need compression therapy. ABI of: 0.6 (±0.2) indicates intermittent claudication; 0.3 (±0.1) indicates ischemic rest pain; and 0.1 (±0.1) indicates an impending tissue necrosis or loss. ABI of less than 0.6 or a change of ABI between examinations of more than 0.15 should be referred to a vascular specialist. Compression therapy is contraindicated in patients with ABI of less than 0.6. If ABI is greater than 0.6, tissue healing will likely occur spontaneously; thus, vascular reconstruction (e.g., vascular bypass or graft surgery) is usually not recommended because 30% of reconstructed vessels can become impatent within 5 years. Vascular reconstruction is only indicated for limb-threatening ischemia (i.e., ischemic rest pain or tissue necrosis or loss).

b. ***Venous continuous-wave Doppler*** may be used to detect DVT. However, its inability to localize the occlusion makes it less useful than duplex scanning using pulsed-wave Doppler.

2. Pulsed-wave Doppler modality emits a burst of ultrasound, waits for a period of time, then opens a "window" to catch the returning signal. Its advantage over continuous-wave Doppler is its range resolution, which allows it to localize the source of occlusion. It is used in **duplex ultrasonography scanning (DUS)** in combination with high-resolution real-time B-mode imaging. In DUS, the pulsed-wave Doppler is used to locate the source of the abnormal flow and the B-mode ultrasound is used to provide a morphologic image of the blood vessel. Color Doppler flow mapping (or **color-flow duplex scanning**; CFDS) is commonly used to facilitate duplex examination of the peripheral vessels, as it allows two-dimensional colored "images" of blood flow to be superimposed on the B-mode imaging. DUS is inexpensive and can be performed quickly; however, test interpretation is technician-dependent.

a. **Carotid duplex scanning** is used to determine stenosis primarily at the carotid bifurcation (e.g., atherosclerotic plaques). For clinical purposes, a stenotic lesion that is identified using CFDS is classified as low grade (40–60%); medium grade (61–80%), or high grade (81–90%). It is of limited use for disease above the region of the carotid bifurcations and is subject to errors of interpretation in cases of high-grade stenosis or complete occlusions.

b. **Venous DUS** is used to locate and quantify the severity of deep or superficial venous thrombosis, assess venous incompetence, and map the superficial veins before surgical harvest for bypass operations. In the detection of infrainguinal DVT (see Chapter 5.3, section III.B.1.a), the compressive technique is commonly used, i.e., a Doppler sensor is placed on the proximal part of the vein as the examiner's hand compresses the vein distally. An obstruction (e.g., thrombus) is detected if the Doppler wave is not augmented upon distal vein compression or if the Doppler wave does not fluctuate significantly during respiration or if the vein is noncompressible (i.e., the vein does not collapse under a force sufficient to distort the artery). For morphological identification of the thrombus, either real-time B-mode grayscale imaging or color imaging (CFDS) may be used.

IV. Plethysmography

This assesses limb volume by detecting changes in the electrical impedance between two electrodes wrapped around the calf.

A. **ARTERIAL PLETHYSMOGRAPHY** measures multiple volume changes (pulse volume recording) in segmental cuffs inflated at a preset pressure. Unlike arterial Doppler studies, it is not affected by medial calcinosis in diabetic patients. However, it is inappropriate for patients who are obese, edematous, or with muscle tremors. Qualitative gradings of the pulse volume recording are normal if the wave has a sharp systolic peak followed by a dicrotic notch (caused by relaxation of arterial wall prior to diastole), mildly abnormal if the dicrotic notch is absent with slow downslope, moderately abnormal if the wave shows flattening of the systolic peak, and severely abnormal if the systolic peak is almost as flat as the baseline.

B. **VENOUS PLETHYSMOGRAPHY** (see also Chapter 5.3, section III.B.1.c).

1. **Impedance venous plethysmography** is used to diagnose proximal venous thrombosis. It involves inflation of a proximal thigh cuff to obstruct venous outflow. After allowing distal filling of the venous system, the cuff is deflated. In the normal limb, plethysmography shows that the leg swells during cuff inflation then rapidly (within 3 to 4 seconds) returns to its normal size upon cuff deflation (because of rapid venous outflow). In the presence of proximal obstruction (most likely because of venous thrombosis), response is "blunted" (i.e., the return to baseline is delayed when the cuff is deflated).
2. **Exercise venous plethysmography** documents or screens for lower limb venous incompetence and quantifies its severity before, during, and after exercise. Normally, plethysmography shows a progressive decrease in leg volume during exercise followed by a period when the volume slowly returns to normal.

In venous insufficiency, the exercise-induced decrease in venous volume is less than expected. Moreover, the postexercise return in volume is more rapid than expected when venous incompetence is present.

3. **Phleborheography** uses multiple pneumatic cuffs to monitor changes in leg volume at various sites in the leg and thigh during respiration and leg compression. It is time consuming and interpretation is subjective.

V. Thermography

Thermography is the use of electronic screening devices to detect infrared rays emitted from the skin, which is directly equivalent to the body surface temperature. A pictorial heat map is then constructed, which shows areas of increased vasodilatation ("hot spots") or vasoconstriction ("cold spots") as a result of autonomic responses to disease or trauma in nerve root or peripheral nerves. It is considered a physiological instead of an anatomical test and may be used to help in diagnosis of neuromuscular pain or inflammation (e.g., radiculopathy, carpal tunnel syndrome, "trigger point", complex regional pain syndrome type I: reflex sympathetic dystrophy, or type II: causalgia). Its usefulness as a diagnostic tool remains controversial.

Further reading

Edelman RR, Warach S: Magnetic resonance imaging, part I. *N Engl J Med* 328(10):708–716, 1993.

Edelman RR, Warach S: Magnetic resonance imaging, part II. *N Engl J Med* 328(11):785–791, 1993.

Firooznia HF, Golimbu C, Rafii M, *et al.*: *MRI and CT of the musculoskeletal system*, St Louis, 1992, Mosby.

Lanzer P, Rosch J, editors: *Vascular diagnostics*, New York, 1994, Springer-Verlag.

Merritt JL, Anderson JM, Fisher SV, *et al.*: Rehabilitation of musculoskeletal and soft tissue disorders. Part 6: Diagnostic tests and examination. *Arch Phys Med Rehabil* Suppl 69:S146–S149, 1988.

Paget S, Gibofsky A, Beary III, JF, editors: *Manual of rheumatology and outpatient orthopedic disorders*, ed 4, Philadelphia, 2000, Lippincott, Williams & Wilkins.

Ramsey RG: *Neuroradiology*, ed 3, Philadelphia, 1994, WB Saunders.

Stein J, editor: *Textbook of internal medicine*, ed 5, Philadelphia, 2000, Elsevier.

Sussman C, Bates-Jensen BM: *Wound care: a collaborative practice manual for physical therapists and nurses*, Gaithersburg, MD, 1998, Aspen Publishers.

CHAPTER 2.3
Invasive imaging studies

As stated in Chapter 2.2, any imaging study is useless without close clinical correlation (because abnormal findings can be found even in asymptomatic individuals). The following include some of the commonly used invasive imaging studies in the PM&R setting. The invasive imaging studies discussed in this chapter include only those that involve skin puncture (e.g., for introduction of contrast dye or radionuclide compounds).

I. Nuclear medicine

A. **BONE MINERAL ANALYSES** are used to diagnose osteoporosis and determine fracture risk. Single- and dual-beam photon absorptiometries use radioisotopes and are considered invasive. Dual-energy X-ray absorptiometry and quantitative computed tomography (QCT) scans are noninvasive non-nuclear medicine studies but are included here for convenience. In the diagnosis of osteoporosis, bone trabecular measurements (which can be determined more accurately by QCT scan) are more important because the trabecular bone turnover is eight to nine times that of cortical bone.

1. **Single-beam photon absorptiometry** uses iodine-125 to measure the cortical bones in the forearm, primarily the distal radius. Although it can delineate bone density accurately (with a precision of 2–3%), it does not distinguish trabecular bone from cortical bone. It has limited usefulness because the cortical density of forearm bones does not necessarily correlate with that of weight-bearing bones.
2. **Dual-beam photon absorptiometry (DPA)** uses a multi-energy isotope (gadolinium-135) to analyze the density of both trabecular and cortical weight-bearing bones (i.e., lumbar vertebral body and femoral neck) with a precision of 2–3%. The scanning, however, is time consuming.
3. **Dual-energy X-ray absorptiometry (DEXA)** uses a dual X-ray source to replace the isotope source used in DPA. It measures the same bones as in DPA but has lower radiation exposure and greater precision than DPA and can be performed much more rapidly. The newer DEXA scanner, which scans the vertebral body from the lateral side (instead of posteriorly to anteriorly), is preferred because it eliminates the inclusion of the cortical bone of the posterior vertebral elements in its measurement of bone density (hence a more accurate measurement of the trabecular density of the vertebral body can be made).
4. **QCT scan** detects trabecular bone loss, independent of cortical bone loss, and is the only modality that can detect vertebral trabecular bone loss in its early phases, when treatment is most effective. It can also measure the amount of vertebral body collapse. Although a QCT scan is more expensive than a DEXA scan, the information provided is more accurate.

B. **RADIONUCLIDE BONE SCANNING** uses technetium-99m phosphate complexes (fluorine-18 or strontium-88m were used in the past) to detect physiologic changes in the bone as compared with anatomic changes seen on radiography. Increased uptake of the radionuclide reflects increased bone blood flow and increased osteoblastic activity as a result of new bone formation. However, this is nonspecific and can be caused by infection, tumor, fractures, or synovitis. A **three-phase bone scan**, which includes blood flow and blood pool scans, as well as static images 2–4 hours or more after injection, can be used to evaluate localized bone or joint pain (the early phases may be helpful in diagnosing infection and soft tissue abnormalities). The radiation exposure from a bone scan is similar to that from a radiograph series of the lumbar spine. Bone scan has similar sensitivity to but less specificity than magnetic resonance imaging (MRI) in the early diagnosis of many bone and joint problems. It is less expensive than MRI and can survey the entire skeleton during one examination.

A bone scan is the procedure of choice in the evaluation of skeletal and spinal metastases and has largely replaced radiography for this purpose. It is more sensitive than plain radiographs in revealing metastatic tumors that are only a few millimeters in diameter, as only metastases larger than 1.5 cm in size and with more than 50% demineralization can generally be detected with plain radiographs. Osseous lesions of multiple myeloma are not usually seen in technetium-99m radionuclide bone scans; therefore radiography remains the screening method of choice for this neoplasm. A bone scan is indicated in patients with bone or joint pain whose radiographs are negative or inconclusive. It is useful in diagnosing subtle nondisplaced traumatic fractures (e.g., navicular stress fracture), prosthetic loosening of total joint arthroplasty (especially of the femoral components), joint infections such as early osteomyelitis and disk space infections (increased sensitivity when triple-phase bone scan is performed, or in conjunction with gallium or indium scan), avascular necrosis (in early stage, there is no focal uptake, but in reparative stage, there is increased uptake; however, MRI is the current procedure of choice), and metastatic disease as a cause of undiagnosed pain. Although three- or four-phase bone scans have previously been used to help diagnose complex regional pain syndrome (CRPS type I: reflex sympathetic dystrophy, and CRPS type II: causalgia), the International Association for the Study of Pain (IASP) does not require any laboratory testing in its CRPS diagnostic criteria (see Chapter 3.1, Table 3.1-1).

C. RADIONUCLIDE INFECTION SCANS are not very specific because increased uptake may also occur in noninfectious conditions.

1. **Gallium-67 citrate scans** have high sensitivity for infection in the bones or soft tissues but are nonspecific because increased uptake may be seen in noninfectious conditions such as fractures, tumors, or noninfectious inflammatory conditions (e.g., inflammatory arthritis). When used in conjunction with a bone scan, their specificity for infection may be increased. Infection is likely if the gallium scan shows more intense uptake than the bone scan at the affected site or if the uptake of gallium is not congruent with the uptake on the bone scan. Unfortunately, only one-third or less of bone infections meet these criteria. There are reports of false-negative gallium scans in chronic infections and in patients treated with antibiotics prior to the scan.
2. **Indium-111 or technetium-99m-labeled leukocyte scans** do not collect in areas of neoplasia and are more specific than bone scans or gallium scans in detecting bone or joint infection. However, increased uptake may also be seen in noninfectious conditions. They are useful in the evaluation of acute osteomyelitis, and possibly total joint arthroplasty infections. Unlike gallium, they are also useful in the presence of pseudoarthrosis. When used in conjunction with a bone scan or radiolabeled colloid scans, their specificity for infection may be increased.

D. RADIONUCLIDE VENTILATION–PERFUSION LUNG SCAN (V/Q SCAN) is commonly used to rule out pulmonary embolism. It consists of a perfusion scan and a ventilation scan. The perfusion scan is obtained by gamma camera imaging of the distribution of intravenously injected radionuclide (technetium-99m-labeled macroaggregates of albumin or iodine-labeled fibrinogen), which are trapped in the pulmonary capillary bed and which accumulate in clots. Normal perfusion scans show homogeneous distribution of radioactivity throughout both lungs and thus rule out pulmonary embolism. An abnormal perfusion lung scan, however, is not specific for pulmonary embolism because any process that destroys or constricts pulmonary arterial vessels (e.g., pneumonia, emphysema) can cause perfusion defects. Hence a ventilation lung scan is performed by having the patient breathe a radioactive gas such as xenon-133, which distributes evenly throughout the lungs. In the presence of airway obstruction, the xenon-133 may be trapped in the proximal airway, thus making interpretation difficult. If the ventilation scan is normal or if it does not match the perfusion defect (which is greater than or equal to one pulmonary segment), then there is a high probability of pulmonary embolism. Based on the relative size of the perfusion and ventilation defects and radiographic abnormalities, a low, intermediate, or indeterminate probability may be designated.

E. RADIONUCLIDE VENOGRAPHY for the detection of thrombi in the proximal veins of the lower limbs is still in the developmental stage.

F. QUANTITATIVE RADIONUCLIDE RENAL SCAN is used to monitor renal function and drainage.

1. **Technetium-99m (^{99m}Tc) scan.** ^{99m}Tc-dimercaptosuccinic acid (DMSA) is used for both differential function and evaluation of the functioning areas of the renal cortex. ^{99m}Tc-mercaptoacetyltriglycine (MAG3) is used to assess urinary tract drainage as well as differential function.
2. **Iodine-131 hippuran scan** is used to monitor renal perfusion and determine glomerular filtration rate and excretory renal plasma flow.

G. THYROID RADIOISOTOPE SCINTISCANNING uses iodine-123 for evaluation of thyroid function and the noninvasive assessment of thyroid anatomy. It is used to assess thyroid nodules to define whether they are functional (hot or warm nodules, which are usually benign) or nonfunctional (cold nodules, which are more likely malignant), to permit localization of the thyroid, localization of metastatic deposits of differentiated thyroid cancer or of residual normal thyroid tissue after surgery, to evaluate thyroid anatomy, and to distinguish multinodular goiter from other goitrous enlargements of the thyroid.

H. SINGLE PHOTON EMISSION COMPUTED TOMOGRAPHY (SPECT) uses scintigraphy and computer-assisted tomography (CT) to evaluate overlapping structures in femoral head osteonecrosis, patellofemoral syndrome, and healing spondylotic defects. It may provide increased detail and may be helpful in diagnosing acute traumatic spondylosis or pars stress fracture, determining acute or pre-existing fracture, and detecting photopenic areas in avascular necrosis.

II. Contrast imaging

A. CONTRAST VASCULAR IMAGING

1. **Venography (phlebography)** of the lower limbs involves the injection of diluted contrast medium into a superficial vein of the foot followed by spot radiographs taken at different intervals of contrast injection. Demonstration of an intraluminal filling defect in all films and views is accepted as the final diagnostic test for determining deep vein thrombosis. MRI may be used to image the vein [magnetic resonance venography (MRV)] with high sensitivity and specificity. However, MRV is expensive and has limited availability.
2. **Angiography**

a. ***Conventional or catheter cerebral angiography*** uses X-rays to image iodinated contrast material injected intra-arterially via the femoral artery. The image may be made on a radiograph directly or the radiographic data may be digitized and electronically subtracted from another exposure obtained during contrast injection (called digital subtraction angiography). It is used in the assessment of aneurysms, vascular malformations and fistulas, arterial stenoses, occlusions, and collateral circulation in vascular occlusive diseases including atherosclerosis, trauma, and vasculitis, and in evaluation of vascular intracranial and skull base tumors.

b. ***Spinal angiography*** is used for the diagnosis of and for pre-embolization or presurgical mapping of spinal arteriovenous malformation and occasionally for vascular tumors such as hemangioblastomas.

c. ***Pulmonary angiography*** has been replaced by CT as the choice method of visualizing the pulmonary vasculature and in the diagnosis of pulmonary embolism. Current techniques, however, cannot consistently show obstruction in small subsegmental arterial branches.

d. ***Magnetic resonance angiography (MRA)*** combines MRI with angiography. It uses the flow effects inherent to MRI to image vascular anatomy. Vascular images are generated either by simultaneously suppressing signal from static tissue while maximizing signal in inflowing blood (time-of-flight angiography) or by modifying magnetic field gradients to use information present in radiofrequency phase changes in flowing blood (phase-contrast angiography). MRA is used for screening intracranial cerebrovascular disease (e.g., aneurysms) and extracranial vasculature pathology (e.g., for evaluation of carotid stenosis and suspected vessel thrombosis). It can also be used for study of aorta or cardiac malformations. Although it has less spatial resolution than conventional angiography and is limited by its high cost and sensitivity to patient motion (producing various artifacts), MRA remains the preferred imaging modality because it is less invasive.

B. INTRAVENOUS PYELOGRAPHY (IVP) OR EXCRETORY UROGRAPHY is used to visualize the size, shape, and function of the whole urinary tract (kidney, ureters, and bladder) and to detect hydronephrosis, pyelonephritis, calculi, tumor, and renovascular hypertension. A radio-opaque substance (iodinated solution) is injected intravenously, and a series of radiographs are taken 3, 5, 10, 15, and 20 min after contrast injection. At the end of the test, the patient voids and another radiograph is taken to visualize the residual contrast in the bladder. The major disadvantage of IVP is the potential for allergic reactions to the contrast, radiation exposure, and patient inconvenience (patient needs to be nil-by-mouth and to take laxatives). It could cause contrast nephropathy in patients with insulin-dependent diabetes mellitus or serum creatinine of $\geq$1.5 mg/dL.

C. MYELOGRAPHY is the radiographic examination of the spinal canal and spinal cord by means of contrast medium, which is injected into the subarachnoid space by lumbar (and occasionally cervical) puncture. Low-osmolar, iodinated, nonionic, water-soluble contrast agents are used because they are absorbed into the blood stream and excreted through the kidneys. Myelography is used to detect extradural or intradural abnormalities (herniation of the intervertebral disks, spinal stenosis, nerve root compression from bony spurs, spinal cord tumors), nerve root asymmetries, congenital anomalies of the root sleeves (e.g., conjoined root sleeves or root cysts), arachnoiditis, obstruction to cerebrospinal fluid flow, and cord compression. In patients with sciatica, myelography should only be performed when diagnosis is still in doubt after performing CT scans and MRI. In this case, postmyelography CT scan should always be carried out. The combination of myelography and postmyelography CT is superior to MRI alone in the diagnosis of nerve root compromise by bony or soft tissue structures, facet joint disease, neural foramina and central spinal canal stenosis, extent of cauda equina compression, communication of the thecal sac with adjacent cystic structures, and the presence and extent of certain types of spinal vascular malformations. Although relatively safe, postmyelographic side-effects such as headache, nausea, vomiting, vasovagal episodes, and leg pain may occur. Other complications of myelography include seizures, hypersensitivity reactions, bleeding, aseptic meningitis, infection, and cardiovascular complications.

D. DISKOGRAPHY involves direct injection of contrast material into the intervertebral disk through a needle placed in the disk. Leakage of contrast material out of the nucleus pulposus has been claimed to indicate disk pathology; however, this is vigorously disputed by others. Disk abnormalities, however, may also be found in asymptomatic patients. Provocation testing may be performed during the injection to determine if the pain is similar to the patient's usual pain syndrome. Diskography is currently not recommended for the diagnosis of disorders of the intervertebral disks. It is neither sensitive nor reliable; false positives are frequent; and findings do not necessarily correlate with those of other, more reliable techniques. Moreover, it has the inherent risks of invasive procedures (e.g., disk space infection and allergic reaction to iodinated contrast material).

E. ARTHROGRAPHY involves the intra-articular injection of water-soluble contrast media, with or without air, to evaluate articular structures such as cartilage, synovium, and ligaments. Injection of air alone may be used to detect loose bodies. Rare complications include infection and anaphylactic reactions to contrast material. Vasovagal reaction, which may occur during arthrography, should not be mistaken for an allergic reaction. Arthrography has been largely replaced by MRI but may still be used if MRI is contraindicated or if the patient is unable to tolerate MRI because of claustrophobia.

1. **Shoulder arthrography** can be used to diagnose rotator cuff tears, adhesive capsulitis, labral and capsular deformity that may occur after shoulder dislocation, bicipital tendon abnormalities, articular and synovial pathologies, infection, and impingement syndrome. In patients with subtle injuries of the glenoid labrum, MR arthrography (intra-articular injection of Gd DTPA [gadolinium diethylenetriamine pentaacetic acid] diluted 1/200) has been proven to provide more details of fibrocartilage abnormalities.
2. **Elbow arthrography** can be helpful in detecting loose bodies in the joint and in the diagnosis of articular cartilage defects and osteochondral fractures.
3. **Wrist arthrography** is most useful in demonstrating ligamentous disruption in the post-traumatic wrist. It can also be used to detect tears of the triangular fibrocartilage and abnormal synovial communications within the wrist joint.
4. **Hip arthrography** is used in adults to evaluate painful hip prostheses (for loosening of hardware or for infection), synovial proliferative disease (cartilage destruction and loose bodies), osteochondral fractures, and communicating bursae and abscess cavities. In infants and children it may be used to assess the septic hip (by obtaining aspirate and assessing joint damage) and to evaluate the position of the cartilaginous femoral head with respect to the acetabulum in Legg–Calvé–Perthes disease, congenital dislocation of the hip, and coxa vara deformities.
5. **Knee arthrography** is used mainly to diagnose meniscal injuries, but it may also be used to outline collateral and cruciate ligament tears, articular cartilage alterations, synovial processes, masses, and periarticular synovial cysts (popliteal cysts). Postarthrogram CT scans of the knee are helpful in evaluating the mediopatellar plicae and the patellar cartilage.
6. **Ankle arthrography** is useful in the evaluation of acute ligamentous injuries and in assessing chronic osseous and osteocartilaginous abnormalities (e.g., osteochondritis dissecans).

Further reading

Firooznia HF, Golimbu C, Rafii M, *et al.*: *MRI and CT of the musculoskeletal system,* St Louis, 1992, Mosby.

Merritt JL, Anderson JM, Fisher SV, *et al.*: Rehabilitation of musculoskeletal and soft tissue disorders. Part 6: Diagnostic tests and examination. *Arch Phys Med Rehabil* Suppl 69:S146–S149, 1988.
Nordin BEC, Chatterton BE, Need AG, *et al.*: The definition, diagnosis, and classification of osteoporosis. *Phys Med Rehabil Clin North Am* 6(3):395–414, 1995.
Paget S, Gibofsky A, Beary III, JF, editors: *Manual of rheumatology and outpatient orthopedic disorders*, ed 4, Philadelphia, 2000, Lippincott, Williams & Wilkins.
Stein J, editor: *Textbook of internal medicine*, ed 5, Philadelphia, 2000, Elsevier.

CHAPTER 2.4
Electrodiagnostic tests

Electrodiagnostic (EDX) studies involve the recording and analysis of responses of nerves and muscles to electrical stimulation. They are most useful in distinguishing between neuropathic and myopathic origins of peripheral neuromuscular pathology. They can help in the assessment of peripheral neuropathy and/or radiculopathy and determine which segment of the peripheral nerve and/or which spinal root level is involved. This chapter gives a brief overview of EDX. For specific EDX procedures and interpretation, refer to the textbooks listed in the Further reading section.

I. Nerve conduction studies (NCS) or electroneurography

NCS involve the recording and analysis of nerve impulses (action potentials) that are generated in the peripheral nervous system in response to electrical stimulation. Under standardized conditions, normal ranges of latencies [interval (ms) between the onset of the stimulus and the onset of a response], amplitude [the maximum voltage difference (mV or μV) between two points, usually baseline to peak or peak to peak], total duration (ms) of individual potential waveforms (the interval from the beginning of the first deflection from the baseline to its final return to the baseline), the duration of a recurring action potential (the interval from the beginning to the end of the series), and the *maximum conduction velocity* (loosely referred to as *nerve conduction velocity*) can be determined. For reference values of motor and sensory nerve conduction studies, refer to Appendices A-4 and A-5, respectively.

A. **MAXIMUM CONDUCTION VELOCITY OR NERVE CONDUCTION VELOCITY** is the speed of propagation of an action potential along a nerve (motor, sensory, autonomic, or mixed) or muscle fiber. It is calculated from the latency of the evoked potential at maximal or supramaximal stimulation at two different points. The distance between the two points (conduction distance) is divided by the difference between the corresponding latencies (conduction time). The calculated velocity represents the conduction velocity of the fastest fibers and is expressed as meters per second (m/s).

B. **COMPOUND SENSORY NERVE ACTION POTENTIAL (COMPOUND SNAP OR SENSORY POTENTIAL OR SENSORY RESPONSE)** is evoked from afferent fibers by recording electrical activity only from a sensory nerve or from a sensory branch of a mixed nerve, from electrical stimulus applied only to a sensory nerve or a dorsal nerve root, or from an adequate stimulus applied synchronously to sensory receptors. The *sensory amplitude* is measured from the most positive peak to the most negative peak (maximum peak-to-peak voltage). The *sensory latency* (i.e., *onset latency*) is the interval from the onset of stimulus to the initial deflection. The *peak sensory latency* is measured from the onset of the stimulus to the negative peak. The *total sensory duration* is the interval between the first deflection of the waveform from the baseline and its final return to the baseline.

C. **COMPOUND MOTOR NERVE ACTION POTENTIAL OR COMPOUND MUSCLE ACTION POTENTIAL (CMAP)** is evoked from efferent fibers by recording electrical activity only from a motor nerve or a motor branch of a mixed nerve or from an electrical stimulus applied only to a motor nerve or a ventral nerve root.

1. **M-wave** is a compound muscle action potential evoked from a muscle by a single supramaximal electrical stimulus to its motor nerve. The recording electrodes should be placed so that the initial deflection of the evoked potential is negative. Normally, the configuration of the M-wave (usually biphasic) is quite stable with repeated stimuli at slow rates (1–5 Hz). The *motor latency* is the interval from the onset of the stimulus to the onset of the first phase (positive or negative) of the M-wave. The *amplitude* of the M-wave is measured from the baseline to the peak of the first negative phase. The *duration* of the M-wave is the interval between the deflection of the first negative phase from the baseline and its return to the baseline.
2. **Late responses** are evoked potentials with longer latency than the M-wave. Late responses (F- and H-waves) can be used to evaluate proximal lesions (as the impulse travels to the spinal cord and returns to the distal recording electrode).

a. ***F-wave*** is a compound muscle action potential evoked intermittently from a muscle by a supramaximal electrical stimulus to the nerve. Compared with the maximal amplitude M-wave of the same muscle, the F-wave has a smaller amplitude (1–5% of the M-wave), variable configuration, and a longer, more variable latency. The F-wave can be found in many muscles of the upper and lower extremities, and the latency is longer with more distal sites of stimulation. The F-wave is caused by antidromic activation of motor neurons. Abnormal F-wave studies are seen in patients with hereditary motor sensory neuropathy, acute or chronic demyelinating neuropathy, diabetic neuropathy, uremic neuropathy, alcoholic neuropathy, as well as in entrapment neuropathies, amyotrophic lateral sclerosis, and radiculopathies. Reference values for F-wave studies are shown in Appendix A-6. In general, the minimum F-latency is less than 35 ms for the upper limb and less than 60 ms for the lower limb. The side-to-side differences in the minimum F-latency should be less than 2 ms in the upper limb and 4 ms in the lower limb.

b. ***H-wave*** is a compound muscle action potential with a consistent latency evoked regularly, when present, from a muscle by an electrical stimulus to the nerve. It is regularly found only in a limited group of muscles, particularly the soleus muscle (through stimulation of the tibial nerve). It is also recordable over the flexor carpi radialis muscle (through stimulation of the median nerve), although its onset latency is often obscured by the preceding M-wave. The H-wave is most easily obtained with the cathode positioned proximal to the anode. Compared with the maximum amplitude M-wave of the same muscle, the H-wave has a smaller amplitude, a longer latency, and a lower optimal stimulus intensity. The latency is longer with more distal sites of stimulation. A stimulus intensity sufficient to elicit a maximal amplitude M-wave reduces or abolishes the H-wave, hence a submaximal electrical stimulation must be used. The H-wave is believed to be caused by the H, or Hoffmann, reflex. In the H-reflex, the motor neuron to the muscle is activated through a monosynaptic reflex connection in the spinal cord elicited by the electrical stimulation of the afferent fibers in the mixed nerve supplying the muscle. The H-reflex is similar to the stretch reflex but unlike the stretch reflex, which is stimulated via activation of muscle spindles, the H-reflex bypasses the muscle spindle by using electrical stimulation.

The normal latency of the H-wave in adults is 28–35 ms when measured from the soleus muscle. The measured H-latency should be within 5.5 ms of the predicted value, which can be computed by the Braddom–Johnson formula:

$$\text{Predicted H-latency (ms)} = 9.14 + [0.46 \times \text{leg length (cm)}] + [0.1 \times \text{age (years)}]$$

If the H-latency is prolonged or if there is clinical suspicion of S1 radiculopathy (e.g., absent ankle jerk), then contralateral H-latency should be measured. Assuming equal leg lengths, a difference of >1.0 ms between the two legs may indicate S1 radiculopathy. If the H-wave is recorded from the flexor carpi radialis muscle, a difference of >0.8 ms between the two arms may indicate C6 or C7 radiculopathy. Prolonged H-latency has also been reported in patients with early Guillain–Barré syndrome.

c. ***A-wave*** is a compound muscle action potential evoked consistently from a muscle by submaximal electrical stimuli to the nerve and is frequently abolished by supramaximal stimuli. The amplitude of the A-wave is similar to that of the F-wave, but the latency is more constant. The A-wave usually occurs before the F-wave, but may occur afterwards. The A-wave is caused by normal or pathologic axonal branching and may be elicited in pressure injuries of the peripheral nerve, peripheral neuropathies, amyotrophic lateral sclerosis, and root injuries. A-waves have limited clinical significance as they may also be elicited in normal subjects.

d. ***T-wave*** is a compound muscle action potential evoked from a muscle by rapid stretch of its tendon, as part of the muscle stretch reflex.

II. Electromyography (EMG)

EMG involves the use of intramuscular needle electrodes to evaluate motor units (i.e., the anatomic unit of anterior horn cell, its axon, the neuromuscular junctions, and all of the muscle fibers innervated by the axon). The electrical potential reflecting the electrical activity of a single anatomic motor unit is called the motor unit action potential (MUAP). The following MUAP configuration should be described: peak-to-peak amplitude; total duration (probably the most reliable routine EMG feature to use in distinguishing "neuropathic" from "myopathic" conditions); number of phases [monophasic, biphasic, triphasic, tetraphasic, or polyphasic (i.e., more than five phases)]; sign of each phase (negative, positive); number of turns; variation of shape, if any, with consecutive discharges; presence of satellite (linked) potentials, if any. The recruitment characteristics in relationship to the voluntary muscle exertion should also be described. Limb muscles commonly tested in a routine needle EMG session are shown in Table 2.4-1. Motor innervations of upper and lower limb muscles are shown in Appendices B-3 and B-4, respectively.

Most EMG studies are performed to evaluate denervation, which demonstrates fibrillation potentials (biphasic waves with initial positive deflection, duration of less than 5 ms, and high-pitched "ticks" that sound like "rain on a tin roof") and positive sharp waves (biphasic waves with primarily sharp positive deflection followed by a small prolonged negative potential, duration of 10–100 ms, and a dull thud sound recurring in a uniform regular pattern, usually in response to needle movement). Fibrillation potentials and positive sharp waves represent abnormal spontaneous single muscle fiber discharges caused by increased muscle membrane irritability. They may also be seen in inflammatory myopathies (e.g., polymyositis) and almost any other myopathies (except for, possibly, chronic steroid myopathy or thyroid myopathy), neuromuscular junction disorders (e.g., myasthenia gravis), upper motor neuron lesions (e.g., stroke and spinal cord injury), direct muscle trauma, or intramuscular injection or bleeding.

A summary of typical EMG findings in neuropathic and myopathic conditions is shown in Appendix A-7. In general, the MUAPs in neuropathies (in which partial denervation and reinnervation have occurred) have increased polyphasicity, amplitude, and duration; while in myopathic conditions (in which there is loss or impairment of individual muscle fibers), the MUAPs have increased polyphasicity but

Table 2.4-1 Limb muscles commonly tested in a routine needle electromyographic procedure (listed in sequential order of testing)

Muscle	Spinal roots*	Peripheral nerve	Test maneuver
UPPER LIMB			
Lateral deltoid	**C5**, C6	Axillary	Abduct shoulder
Biceps brachii	C5, **C6**	Musculocutaneous	Flex elbow (with forearm supinated)
Triceps brachii	C6, **C7**	Radial	Extend elbow
Flexor carpi radialis	C6, C7	Median	Flex and radially deviate wrist
Abductor pollicis brevis	C8, **T1**	Median	Abduct thumb (perpendicular to palmar plane)
First dorsal interossei	C8, **T1**	Ulnar	Abduct (or radially deviate) index finger
Extensor indicis propius†	C7, C8	Radial	Extend index finger (with other fingers flexed)
LOWER LIMB			
Tibialis anterior	**L4**, L5	Deep peroneal	Dorsiflex foot
Peroneus longus	L5, S1	Superficial peroneal	Evert plantar flexed foot
Gastrocnemius	**S1**, S2	Tibial	Plantar flex foot (with knee extended)
Vastus medialis	L2, **L3**, **L4**	Femoral	Extend knee
Tensor fascia lata	**L4**, **L5**, S1	Superior gluteal	Abduct thigh (with hip flexed)
Gluteus maximus	**L5**, **S1**, S2	Inferior gluteal	Extend hip (with knee flexed)
Hamstrings (e.g., short head of biceps femoris)†	L5, **S1**, S2	Sciatic	Flex knee

A **bold designation indicates the predominant root supply.*
† Optional.

Electrodiagnostic tests

decreased amplitude and duration. Neuromuscular junction diseases tend to mimic the MUAP changes seen in myopathy.

A. INSERTIONAL ACTIVITIES are electrical activities caused by the insertion or movement of the needle electrode. Their magnitude may be described as normal, reduced, or increased (prolonged), with a description of the waveform and repetitive rate.

B. SPONTANEOUS ACTIVITIES (e.g., fibrillation potentials and positive sharp waves) are recorded from muscle at rest after insertional activities have subsided in the absence of any voluntary contraction or external stimulus.

C. INVOLUNTARY ACTIVITIES are MUAPs that are not under voluntary control. The condition under which they occur should be described (e.g., spontaneous or reflex potentials; or, if elicited by a stimulus, the nature of the stimulus must be described).

D. RECRUITMENT (OR INTERFERENCE) PATTERNS are qualitative or quantitative descriptions of the electrical activities recorded from a muscle using needle electrodes during maximal voluntary effort. The recruitment pattern may be described as *full* (no individual motor unit action can be clearly identified), *reduced* or *intermediate* (some of the individual MUAPs may be identified while other individual MUAPs cannot be identified because of overlap), *discrete* (each of several different MUAPs can be identified), or *single* (a single MUAP is identified, firing at a rapid rate during maximal voluntary effort). The force of contraction associated with the recruitment pattern should be specified.

III. Evoked potential studies

Evoked potential studies involve the recording and analysis of electrical waveforms generated in both the peripheral and central nervous systems in response to electric or physiologic stimuli. There are two systems for naming complex evoked potential waveforms. In the first system, the different components are labeled PI for the initial positive potential and NI for the initial negative potential. The subsequent positive and negative potentials are named PII, NII, PIII, NIII, etc. In the second system, the components are specified by polarity and average peak latency in normal subjects to the nearest millisecond. The first nomenclature principle has been used in an abbreviated form to identify the seven positive components (I–VII) of the normal brainstem auditory evoked potential (BAEP). The second nomenclature principle has been used to identify the positive and negative components of visual evoked potentials (N75, P100) and somatosensory evoked potentials (P9, P11, P13, P14, N20, P23). The problem of the second system is that the latencies of the components of evoked potentials depend upon the length of the pathways in the neural tissues. Thus, the components of a somatosensory evoked potential (SEP) recorded in a child have different average latencies from the same components of a SEP recorded in an adult.

A. SOMATOSENSORY EVOKED POTENTIALS are elicited by electrical stimulation of peripheral sensory fibers (commonly used nerves are median nerve, common peroneal nerve, and posterior tibial nerve). The normal SEP is a complex waveform with several components that are specified by polarity and average peak latency. The polarity and latency of the individual component depend on subject variables (e.g., age and sex), stimulus characteristics (intensity and rate of stimulation), and recording parameters (e.g., placement and combination of recording electrodes and amplifier time constants). **Short-latency somatosensory evoked potentials (SSEPs)** are the portion of a SEP wave normally occurring within 25 ms after stimulation of the median nerve at the wrist, 40 ms after stimulation of the common peroneal nerve at the knee, and 50 ms after stimulation of the posterior tibial nerve at the ankle. The SEPs are used to study brachial plexus injuries and to monitor spinal cord function during spine surgery.

B. VISUAL EVOKED POTENTIALS (VEPS) OR VISUAL EVOKED RESPONSES (VERS) are recorded over the cerebrum and are elicited by light stimuli. The VEPs are classified by stimulus rate as transient or steady-state VEPs. The normal transient VEP to checkerboard pattern reversal or shift has a major positive occipital peak at about 100 ms (P100), often preceded by a negative peak (N75). The precise range of normal values for the latency and amplitude of P100 depends on subject variables (e.g., age, sex, and visual acuity), stimulus characteristics (type of stimulator, full- or half-field stimulator, check size, contrast, and luminescence), and recording parameters (e.g., placement and combination of recording electrodes). Abnormal VEPs are seen in optic neuritis (as a result of multiple sclerosis or other demyelinating disease) with latency prolongation up to 250 ms.

C. BRAINSTEM AUDITORY EVOKED POTENTIALS (BAEPS) OR BRAINSTEM AUDITORY EVOKED RESPONSES (BAERS, BERS) measure auditory evoked potentials originating between the eighth cranial nerve and the inferior colliculus in response to sound stimuli. The normal BAEP consists of a sequence of up to seven waves, named I to VII, which occur during the first 10 ms after the onset of the stimulus and have positive polarity at the vertex of the head. It is the most accurate noninvasive procedure in the diagnosis of acoustic neuromas and has the lowest false-positive rate.

IV. Special EDX studies

A. NEUROMUSCULAR JUNCTION (NMJ) STUDIES are used to confirm the diagnoses of myasthenia gravis (MG), which is caused by antibody destruction or blocking of the postsynaptic acetylcholine receptors, and Lambert–Eaton myasthenic syndrome (LEMS), which is caused by an autoimmune attack against calcium channels in the presynaptic nerve terminal, resulting in impaired release of acetylcholine.

1. **Repetitive nerve stimulation (RNS; formerly known as the Jolly test)** uses a series of supramaximal stimuli given to a specific nerve in rapid succession to fatigue the NMJ. RNS causes depletion of acetylcholine, thus allowing inspection of the resultant CMAPs for consistency of amplitude and duration. Although distal nerves (e.g., ulnar or peroneal nerves) can be tested, the proximal nerves tend to have higher diagnostic yields (i.e., spinal accessory, axillary, musculocutaneous, or facial nerves).

   In MG, the single-stimulation CMAP amplitudes are usually normal. Using 2–5 Hz stimulation, there is a decrease of more than 10% in the amplitude of the fourth or fifth CMAP as compared with that of the first. A maximum isometric contraction for 10–15 seconds or a stimulation of 20 Hz for 10 seconds will usually result in a short-lived (15–30 seconds) increase in the CMAP amplitude (i.e., postactivation facilitation), but no greater than 50% above baseline. The intravenous injection of edrophonium hydrochloride (Tensilon), a short-acting acetylcholinesterase inhibitor, usually reverses the decrement in CMAP amplitude in patients with MG (this may, however, also be seen in some patients with LEMS).

   In LEMS, the single-stimulation CMAP amplitudes are usually low. Using 2–5 Hz stimulation, the first response may be increased or there may be a decremental response. With a maximum isometric contraction for 10–15 seconds or a stimulation of 20 Hz for 10 seconds, there is an increase in the CMAP amplitude that is usually greater than 50%, often 200–400%, above the single-stimulation CMAP.

2. **Single-fiber EMG (SF-EMG)** examines the relationship of two single-muscle fibers within one motor unit by using a specialized needle electrode. Normally, during depolarization of a motor axon, the action potential travels distally and excites all the muscle fibers within that motor unit at more or less the same time. The variation in the time interval between the excitation of the two fibers is known as the jitter (reported as mean value of the difference between consecutive interpotential intervals). Muscles commonly studied are the extensor digitorum communis and the orbicularis oculi. In patients with NMJ disorders, the jitter is usually prolonged even without overt clinical weakness. SF-EMG is the most sensitive test to demonstrate impaired NMJ transmission (abnormal in 95–99% of patients with generalized MG). However, SF-EMG, although quite sensitive, is not specific and is typically abnormal in neuropathic and myopathic disease. Hence, SF-EMG should only be reserved for patients with high suspicion of MG whose RNS is negative or equivocal.

B. BLINK REFLEX OR BLINK RESPONSE is used to evaluate trigeminal and facial nerve function, such as in Bell's palsy, trigeminal neuropathy, and multiple sclerosis. It is obtained by stimulation over the supraorbital branch of the trigeminal nerve (afferent arc), with surface recording over both ipsilateral and contralateral orbicularis oculi (which are supplied by the efferent arc of the facial nerve). Normally, there is an early compound muscle action potential (R1 wave) ipsilateral to the stimulation site with a latency of about 10 ms and a bilateral late compound muscle action potential (R2 wave) with a latency of about 30 ms. In general only the R2 wave is associated with a visible twitch of the orbicularis oculi.

Further reading

American Association of Electrodiagnostic Medicine: Guidelines in electrodiagnostic medicine. *Muscle and Nerve* Suppl S1–S300, 1999.

Braddom RL, Johnson EW: Standardization of H-reflex and diagnostic use in S1 radiculopathy. *Arch Phys Med Rehabil* 55:161–166, 1974.

Dumitru D, Mato AA, Zwarts MJ, Amato AA, editors: *Electrodiagnostic medicine*, ed 2, Philadelphia, 2001, Hanley & Belfus.

Johnson EW, Pease WS, editors: *Practical electromyography*, ed 3, Baltimore, 1997, Williams & Wilkins.

Kimura J: *Electrodiagnosis in diseases of nerve and muscle: principles and practice*, ed 3, New York, 2001, Oxford University Press.

Liveson JA, Ma D: *Laboratory reference for clinical neurophysiology*. Philadelphia, 1992, FA Davis.

Nomenclature Committee of American Association of Electromyography and Electrodiagnosis: AAEE glossary of terms in clinical electromyography, *Muscle and Nerve* Suppl 10(8S):G1–G60, 1987.

CHAPTER 2.5
Musculoskeletal and work-related tests

Most of the musculoskeletal and work-related tests are affected by psychosocial factors (e.g., motivation, pain, fear avoidance, anxiety related to test situation, conscious symptom magnification or malingering, unconscious symptom magnification or illness behavior, psychological stress, depression, cognitive changes, and active legal cases); physical condition of the subject (e.g., fatigue, cardiovascular capability, general fitness, and training effect); environmental conditions (e.g., nature of the external load, metabolic conditions, pH level, temperature, noise, and number of people present in testing room); biophysical state of the muscles [e.g., fiber composition, physiological cross-sectional area of the muscle, muscle length, rate of change of muscle length, and joint range of motion (ROM)]; testing protocol used (e.g., axis placement, posture, feedback, instruction, and test design and sequence); and type of device used (e.g., its attachment and calibration). This chapter gives an overview of the common musculoskeletal and work-related tests used in PM&R.

I. Range of motion (ROM) and flexibility measurements

Measurements of ROM flexibility in the clinical setting use simple, uniplanar, noninvasive techniques. In general, intratester reliability for ROM testing is higher than intertester reliability, hence the same examiner must be used for successive ROM measurements. Examiners should also use consistent, well-defined testing positions and anatomical landmarks to align the arms of the goniometer.

A. VISUAL ESTIMATION can be used to quickly gauge the ROM but it is unreliable and, therefore, not acceptable.

B. GONIOMETRIC TECHNIQUES

1. **Universal goniometer** consists of a protractor (180° or 360° scale) with a stationary arm (aligned parallel to the proximal limb segment), a mobile arm (aligned parallel to the distal limb segment), and an axis (placed as close to the joint axis as possible). The angle between the stationary and mobile arms is the ROM measurement. The universal goniometer can measure any joint ROM (a small version called the *finger goniometer* may be used for measuring metacarpophalangeal and interphalangeal joints). It is inexpensive and easy to obtain, transport, and use. Its reliability is generally good to excellent for measuring limb joint ROM, with the upper limb ROM measurement being more reliable than that for the lower limb. However, for the measurement of spinal ROM, the use of the universal goniometer has lower reliability. The reliability of the universal goniometer for ROM measurements of the cervical spine is better than for measurements of the lumbar spine. In measuring cervical spine ROM, the universal goniometer has good intertester reliability for cervical extension and lateral bending but is difficult to align for neck flexion and extension.
2. **Gravity-dependent goniometers** use gravity's effect on pointers and fluid levels to measure joint position and motion. The device is strapped to the distal

limb segment with the proximal limb segment positioned vertically or horizontally. At the end of ROM, the position of the pointer or bubble on the scale is read as the ROM measurement. The advantage of the gravity-dependent goniometers over the universal goniometers when measuring limb joint ROM is that they do not have to be aligned with bony landmarks (i.e., it is not necessary to align the goniometer with the joint axis), and passive ROM is easily assessed because the examiner does not have to hold the goniometer. For trunk ROM, gravity-dependent goniometers are easier to use and more accurate than universal goniometers. Their disadvantages (compared to universal goniometer, tape measure, and flexible ruler) are that they are bulkier, more expensive, not as readily available, and require additional instruction and practice to use properly. Also, they are difficult to use on small joints and in the presence of soft tissue deformity or edema. Moreover, they are difficult to use when measuring transverse plane motion (i.e., rotation) because of their gravity dependence.

a. ***Inclinometer*** is a pendulum-based goniometer consisting of a 360° scale protractor with a counter-weighted pointer maintained in a constantly vertical position. Electronic versions are also available (Cybex electronic digital inclinometer, Orthoranger). The *AMA: Guides to the Evaluation of Permanent Impairment* recommends the inclinometer (in particular the use of double-inclinometer technique) for measurement of spinal ROM to determine the "true" spinal ROM. In the double-inclinometer technique for lumbar ROM measurement, one inclinometer is positioned at T12 and the other one in the midsacral area. The degree of inclination on the sacral inclinometer represents flexion of the hip while the reading on the T12 inclinometer represents total trunk flexion. Their difference is the "true" lumbar flexion. For the thoracic spine, T1 and T12 landmarks are used. The disadvantages of the double-inclinometer technique are that it is relatively expensive and difficult to manipulate, and it needs a considerable amount of practice time to locate the landmarks for instrument placements. Intratester reliability for the double-inclinometer technique is only moderate, while intertester reliability ranges from poor to high. The double-inclinometer technique does not appear to be superior to the tape measure (e.g., modified Schober's technique) in measuring lumbar flexion and extension.

b. ***Fluid goniometer (bubble goniometer or hydrogoniometer)*** uses a 360° scale in a flat, fluid-filled circular tube, which contains a small air bubble.

3. **Combined compass and gravity-dependent goniometers** have the same advantages and disadvantages listed for gravity-dependent goniometers, except that the addition of the compass makes it easier to measure rotational movements. The OB Myrin goniometer cannot measure the small joints of the hand and foot whereas the Cervical ROM Device is designed specifically for measuring neck ROM. They have acceptable intratester and intertester reliabilities. As with gravity-based goniometers, their intertester reliability is higher than that for the universal goniometer, tape measure, and flexible ruler.

a. ***OB-Myrin goniometer*** consists of a fluid-filled ratable container (with ROM scaled in tenths of degrees) mounted on a plate. The container has a compass needle that reacts to the earth's magnetic field (this is used to measure rotational movements in the transverse plane) and an inclination needle that is influenced by gravity (this is used to measure movements in the frontal and sagittal planes).

b. ***Cervical ROM Device*** is an instrument consisting of two gravity-dependent goniometers and a compass attached to a frame mounted over the bridge of a subject's nose and ears. The two gravity-based goniometers measure flexion, extension, and lateral bending of the neck. Neck rotation is measured by the compass in conjunction with a shoulder-mounted yoke containing magnetic poles pointing north.

4. **Electrogoniometer** uses a potentiometer attached to two arms, which are strapped to the proximal and distal limb segments. Movement of the arms causes the resistance in the potentiometer to vary. Variations in voltage can then be calibrated to represent joint ROM. They are expensive and are used mainly in research and occasionally for gait analysis (see section VI.C.1.b).

C. **TAPE MEASURES** are used to determine spinal ROM through observation of a change in distance from one segment to another. For ROM measurement of the thoracolumbar spine, the tape measure technique is the least expensive and easiest to obtain, transport, and use.

1. **Cervical ROM measurements using tape measure** include neck flexion and extension (the distance between chin and suprasternal notch is measured) and side bending (the distance between mastoid process and acromion process is measured).

2. **Thoracolumbar ROM measurements using tape measure**

a. ***Finger-to-floor (FTF) technique*** measures the distance from the tip of the middle finger to the floor in either trunk flexion or side bending. This method is inaccurate for spinal motion because it does not differentiate hip motion from thoracolumbar motion. Also, it is affected by the flexibility of the fingers, wrist, elbow, and shoulder. Despite these, the FTF method is still being used because of its simplicity.

b. ***Skin distraction technique*** is used for the thoracic and lumbar spine ROM measurement. The most commonly used method is the **modified Schober's technique**. The tape is aligned at two points in the spine (from a point 10 cm above the lumbosacral junction and 5 cm below the lumbosacral junction, a total of 15 cm distance). The subject bends forward or backward and the distance is remeasured and then subtracted from the original 15 cm. Although it conforms to the spinal curvature, the modified Schober's technique does not take into account hip motion, which is the largest component of trunk forward flexion beyond 30° of motion. The modified Schober's technique has good reliability and validity and is easier to use than the double-inclinometer method. It is slightly more difficult to use than the FTF because the lumbosacral junction needs to be located.

D. **FLEXIBLE RULER (FLEXIRULE OR FLEXICURVE)** is a pliable metal band encased in a supple nonelastic plastic covering, which is used for measuring lumbar ROM. It can be contoured onto the lumbar spine to accommodate lordosis in measuring spinal ROM. Flexible rulers demonstrate repeatable measurements but are inaccurate in obese patients because of skinfolds. Their validity is questionable, and they are not generally recommended for clinical use.

E. **PHOTOMETRIC (OR VIDEO-BASED) MOTION ANALYSIS SYSTEMS** use infrared light sources, light-emitting diodes (or reflectors), or laser light attached to the body part to measure relative motions of the segments between each light source. They can use either two-dimensional or three-dimensional optical systems to measure dynamic ROM of the spine and limbs during different tasks (including gait; see also section VI.C.1.a). With the recent advancement of computer and optoelectric technologies, video-based motion analysis (e.g., Computerized Motion Diagnostic Imaging, Motion Analysis Spinetrak, Oxford Metrics VICON System, and Peak Performance Systems) can now be automatically digitized with increasing accuracy to quantify ROM. Although they have good validity and reliability (i.e., when properly calibrated), they are relatively expensive.

II. Strength assessment

Strength can be measured either manually [e.g., manual muscle test (MMT)] or using a dynamometer (i.e., an external apparatus onto which the body exerts force or torque). In PM&R, strength measurement can "potentially" be used for prescribing treatment, monitoring treatment progress, and evaluating physical impairment. In the medico-legal field, it can "potentially" be used to test effort consistency, identify maximal exertion, and assess disability. In industry, its "potential" uses are in providing ergonomic and rehabilitation guidelines, and in screening for job preplacement and return-to-work. However, most of the above mentioned "potential" benefits (in particular for trunk strength assessment) remain unproved by randomized controlled studies.

In using dynamometers for strength measurement, the following guidelines are suggested: the subject must be educated and informed of the purpose of the machine; maximum voluntary effort must be exerted by the subject; the axis of joint motion must be aligned with the axis of rotation of the shaft of the machine; the joint must be properly positioned and stabilized to ensure muscle isolation and reproducibility; the uninvolved limb must be tested first; warm-ups must be carried out before testing; verbal commands should be standardized to ensure test reproducibility; visual feedback, if used at all, must be consistent; angular velocity used for testing should be the same as for rehabilitation; the instrument must be calibrated every 2 weeks to ensure validity; and data generated from one system should not be used on another system.

In general the upper-body strength of women is 40–50% less than that of men, and the lower-body strength is 20–30% less than that of men. This holds true for upper-body strength in women even in relation to lean body mass, but the lower-body strength appears equal to that of men in relation to lean body mass. However, there appear to be no differences between the sexes when strength is measured for cross-sectional area of muscle.

A. **MANUAL MUSCLE TESTING (MMT)** is traditionally used for determining patterns of muscle weakness in neuromuscular diseases. However, it is inaccurate for testing strength greater than fair or 3/5 (see MMT grading in Chapter 1.1, section II.O.2.c). MMT has also been shown to be insensitive to 20–25% changes in strength and to overestimate the normalcy of muscle strength. Hence, MMT is inadequate for determination of functional capacity, especially in patients with strength greater than fair or 3/5.

B. **NONDYNAMOMETRIC DYNAMIC CONSTANT EXTERNAL RESISTANCE (DCER; PREVIOUSLY CALLED "ISOTONIC") STRENGTH TESTING** uses the 10 RM (repetition maximum) value (see Chapter 4.2, section II.B.2.a.1).

C. **HAND STRENGTH MEASUREMENTS**

1. **Grip strength** is measured using a standard Jamar dynamometer, which is recommended because it has extensive normative data (from 6 to 75+ years), and it is superior to other grip dynamometers (e.g., Digital Jamar Dynamometer, Martin Vigorimeter, and My-Gripper). Its absolute accuracy is within 5%. For pre- and post-testing, the same dynamometer must be used because different versions may vary. Normally grip is strongest in the dominant upper extremity by about 5–10 lb (2.3–4.5 kg) and is greater in the midposition of grip, being weaker with either a narrow or wide grip.
2. **Pinch strength** is measured using a B & L Engineering pinch gauge (0–60 lb; 0–27.3 kg), which is recommended because it has an accuracy of ±1%, and it has extensive normative data (from 6 to 75+ years) for tip, key, and palmar pinch. It is superior to the Preston pinch gauge.

D. DYNAMOMETRY FOR LIMB MUSCLE GROUPS

1. **Hand-held dynamometry** provides objective measurement of limb muscle group strength by having the patient exert maximal effort against a portable force-measuring device held by the examiner. Nonelectrical units that use either spring or hydraulic systems, display the force exerted on a dial gauge, and electrical units that use load cells, or strain gauges display the exerted force digitally. The "make test" (in which the hand-held dynamometer is held stationary by the tester while the patient exerts maximum effort against it) is preferred over the "break test" (in which the tester exerts a force against the subject's limb segment until it gives way) because the break test may require higher force beyond the capability of the dynamometer or the strength of the tester. Subjects are measured either seated or supine, preferably in a gravity-reduced position with proper stabilization. The muscle groups to be tested are placed in the middle of their length ranges and the dynamometer is positioned perpendicular to the limb. If the test is carried out properly by an experienced tester on a sincere subject, only one trial is needed. Duration of exertion is usually 4–5 seconds. Obviously, the hand-held dynamometer can only be used if the tester is stronger than the subject. Commercially available hand-held dynamometers include Nicholas Manual Muscle Tester, Newman Myometer, Penny and Giles Transducer Myometer, Hammersmith Dynamometer, Force Evaluation and Testing System, and Spark Hand-held Dynamometer.
2. **Isometric (static) dynamometry** for limb muscle groups measures static muscle strength without limb joint movement. The muscle length is kept constant by either soft constraints (verbal instruction) or hard constraints (stabilization straps). Isometric dynamometers measure peak and average force, reaction time, rate of motor recruitment of motor units, maximal voluntary exertion, and fatigue. The advantages of isometric testing are its relative safety, its low cost, its simplicity, and the ease of interpretation. Effective stabilization is easier to attain than in dynamic testing. It also produces less systemic fatigue than dynamic testing devices, hence more muscles can be tested in a given session. It is preferred in conditions in which joint motion causes pain (e.g., contractures).

   Its main disadvantage is that it does not correlate with real-life dynamic activities such as lifting and manual materials handling. However, isometric testing can be performed at multiple points in the arc of joint range of motion to create a strength curve. Isometric testing should be used with precaution in the presence of acute, active musculoskeletal problems, osteoporosis, significant cardiovascular or respiratory pathology, or structural weakness of the abdominal or thoracic wall (immediate postsurgery; hernia). It is contraindicated in the presence of unsplinted fractures, unhealed torn or sutured tendons, and in uncontrolled hypertension.

   Strain-gauge (fixed-load cell) dynamometers are commonly used for testing the isometric strength of limb muscle groups. They use electroconductive materials that are sensitive to loads, i.e., tension, compression, or shear. When the subject pushes or pulls against the dynamometer, the gauge is deformed leading to a change in its electrical resistance and alteration of the current passing through the gauge. The change in voltage can then be calibrated and converted into torque. Most dynamometers used primarily for dynamic testing of muscle performances contain a strain gauge, which can be used for isometric testing by locking the machine either mechanically or through computer control or both.
3. **Dynamic dynamometry for limb muscle groups**

a. ***Dynamic constant external resistance (DCER; previously called "isotonic") dynamometry for limb muscle groups*** uses constant weights or resistance to measure strength at variable speed. The former term "isotonic" implies constant tension, which is not true because muscle tension changes as the leverage changes. Commercially available DCER dynamometers can also be isokinetic like, i.e., allowing contraction at an accommodating speed and an accommodating resistance (e.g., Ariel Computerized Exercise System, Physio-Tek, and Tru-Kinetics) or they can have variable speed with accommodating resistance (e.g., Hydra-Fitness Gym).

b. ***Isokinetic limb muscle group dynamometer*** measures strength as the joint moves at a constant preselected speed (0–500°/s). Isokinetic machines provide resistance that accommodates the muscle as its length : tension ratio changes and as the muscle leverage changes throughout the ROM; therefore, the muscle contracts at its maximal capability at multiple points throughout the ROM. The joint velocity or rate of shortening or lengthening of the muscle is kept constant, i.e., acceleration and jerk are zero. A more accurate term is probably *isovelocity* or maybe *isokinematics* because it is usually the change in angle at a joint that is set as a constant.

In isokinetic testing, the reported torque is that produced by the machine to keep the limb from accelerating beyond the preset speed of the machine. If the muscle force is less than the preset speed, then the machine does not register any force and the isokinetic torque is reported as zero. This should not be interpreted as absence of muscle tension. Because zero does not mean absence of torque, isokinetic torque measures are considered as interval scale, not true ratio scale. Hence, torque ratios (flexion/extension) should not be computed from isokinetic measures, because they are not ratio scaled.

The advantages of isokinetic mode are that it can test at different speeds and it is safe (i.e., the resistance provided by the machine is equal to the force exerted, and the subject never meets more resistance than he or she can handle). Its disadvantages are its cost, constraints in motion pattern, and the patient's unfamiliarity with the task of moving at a preselected speed. Isokinetic testing cannot accurately measure the full arc of muscle performance because of acceleration artifact at the beginning ROM arc and deceleration artifact at the end ROM arc. Also, it does not simulate real life because human beings do not move at constant velocity.

I. **Passive isokinetic systems** allow isokinetic concentric exertions only, e.g., Cybex and Universal Merac.

II. **Active isokinetic systems** allow both isokinetic eccentric and concentric exertions as well as passive ROM testing, e.g., Biodex and Kin-Com.

E. TRUNK DYNAMOMETRY

1. **Isometric trunk dynamometers** have similar principles, advantages, disadvantages, precautions, and contraindications to limb muscle isometric dynamometers (see II.D.2). Unlike the limb, the trunk has more than one axis of motion, making it more difficult to standardize. For accuracy, the chosen axis of motion (e.g., L3) must be used consistently for within-subject and between-subject testing. Proper stabilization, especially around the pelvis, is also important for accurate testing.

a. ***Cable tensiometers*** consist of a harness connected to a cable that is attached to a fixed object, e.g., a wall or floor. When the harness (strapped around the individual's chest) is pulled, the cable is stretched. The tension in the cable is then measured in calibrated units on a tension-sensitive gauge. Cable tensiometers are best used to determine peak isometric torques rather than the average torque.

b. ***Strain-gauge (fixed-load cell) trunk dynamometers*** use electroconductive materials that are sensitive to loads (see II.D.2). The MedX Lumbar Extension Machine and MedX Rotary-Torso Machine use a computer-monitored strain-gauge dynamometer designed for testing trunk isometric strength in a sitting position. In contrast to the other isometric devices, the MedX machines have better stabilization and are able to test isometric strength at multiple points throughout the full trunk ROM. This allows multipositional isometric training, which has been shown to be effective in increasing lumbar extensor strength. Other dynamometers used primarily for testing dynamic trunk strength usually contain a strain gauge, which can be used for isometric testing by locking the machine either mechanically or through computer control or both.

2. **Dynamic trunk dynamometers**

a. ***Isokinetic trunk dynamometers*** have similar principles, advantages, and disadvantages to limb muscle isokinetic dynamometers (see II.D.3.b). Commercial isokinetic trunk devices include Cybex Flexion/Extension Rehabilitation Unit, Cybex Torso Rotation Rehabilitation Unit, Kin-Com Back Testing Device, and Biodex Back System.

b. ***Isoinertial trunk dynamometers*** measure the torque and velocity of trunk motion as the trunk exerts against a constant inertia or load (isoinertial exertion). The only commercially available isoinertial trunk dynamometer is the Isostation B-200 Triaxial Dynamometer, but this device is no longer manufactured.

F. **CERVICAL DYNAMOMETRY** usually uses the isometric mode of strength measurement at different points in the cervical ROM arc (e.g., MedX Cervical Extension Machine and MedX Cervical Rotation Machine).

G. **WHOLE-BODY DYNAMOMETRY** usually includes isometric and dynamic testing of upper and lower limb strengths as well as trunk strength and lifting strength. They include the ARCON, the Baltimore Therapeutic Equipment, the ERGASYS, and the ERGOS (from Work Recovery Systems).

III. Lifting capacity tests

Lifting capacity tests include measurements of the strength and endurance of muscles of the trunk as well as the upper and lower limbs. Manual two-handed lifting can be analyzed by using the lifting analysis method developed by the National Institute for Occupational Safety and Health (NIOSH) (revised, 1994). The NIOSH lifting analysis includes the documentation (by job evaluation or simulation) of the following job variables:

- **Weight of the load or object lifted** (L) – determined by direct weighing;
- **Position of load with respect to the body** – measured in terms of horizontal (H) coordinates (i.e., location of the center of mass of the object measured horizontally from a point on the floor midway between the ankles); vertical (V) coordinates (i.e., location of the center of mass of the object measured at the beginning or origin of the lift from the floor); and vertical travel distance (D) of the hands from the origin to the destination (i.e., release) of the object. If the load begins and ends outside the sagittal plane, it is considered asymmetric and the angle of asymmetry is determined (i.e., the angle subtended by a line from the center of the load to the center of the ankle, measured relative to the mid-sagittal plane);
- **Frequency (F) of lift**, i.e., average lifts/min for high-frequency lifting;
- **Period or duration**, i.e., total time engaged in lifting (i.e., <1 h; 1–2 h; 2–8 h); and
- **Coupling** (C) or grip capability, classified into good, fair, or poor grip.

The L, H, V, D, F, A, and C values are then used to determine the following two parameters for evaluating potentially hazardous lifting activities. The first parameter is the Recommended Weight Limit (RWL; formerly called the Action Limit or AL) which represents the maximum weight of the object being lifted with minimum risk for 90% of the workers (i.e., lifting within the RWL would be protective of about 90% of workers). In the calculation of RWL, the L value is set to a constant of 23 kg (226 N or 51 lb), which represents the maximum value for RWL. In lifting tasks where the RWL is exceeded, there is a risk of back injury for 1% for men and 25% for women. The second parameter is the Maximal Permissible Limit (MPL). The MPL is three times the lifting index (LI), which is calculated by dividing the weight of the object lifted (L) by the RWL. Therefore, any job with an LI of >1.0 would be protective of most workers, whereas jobs with an LI of >3.0 would be hazardous (with relative risk of back injury being 75% for men and 99% for women). If jobs with LI of >3.0 cannot be redesigned to reduce worker's risk, then "administrative controls" should be put in place, such as careful training, medical monitoring, and job-specific placement testing. For the determination of RWL, LI, and MPL, computerized programs, based on the NIOSH lifting guides, have been developed by the University of Michigan (e.g., Three-Dimensional Static Strength Prediction Program).

Using the 1994 NIOSH lifting guide, an analytical model can be derived that can quantitatively predict when either a biomechanical, physiological, or psychological population norm would be exceeded. Biomechanically, the predicted maximum compressive forces on the L5/S1 disk would not exceed 3400 N (approximately 760 lb or 345 kg). Physiologically, the metabolic energy expenditure rates (kcal/min) would not exceed the following population limits developed by Rodgers *et al.*, (1991), i.e., for lifting duration of <1 h, the limit is 4.7 kcal/min if V is <75 cm or 3.3 kcal/min if V is >75 cm; for lifting duration of 1–2 h, the limit is 3.7 kcal/min if V is <75 cm or 2.7 kcal/min if V is >75 cm; and for lifting duration of 2–8 h, the limit is 3.1 kcal/min if V is <75 cm or 2.2 kcal/min if V is >75 cm. Psychologically, the determined maximum acceptable weight-lifting limits (i.e., the RWL) would accommodate 75% of women and 99% of men (or 90% of a mix of men and women performing manual material-handling jobs).

Limitations of the 1994 NIOSH lifting guide include the facts that it does not reflect the dynamic factors (e.g., the speed or rhythmicity) of lifting, i.e., it does not account for the proportionate increase in the load across the L5–S1 motion segment (which is independent of object weight) when the speed of lifting is increased or when the lifting pattern is dysrhythmic or "jerky"; it does not appear to recognize individual risk assessment (i.e., it sets a limit that protects most workers as a group, not as individuals); and it does not account for one-handed lifting.

A. **STATIC OR ISOMETRIC LIFTING TEST (TRAY-LIFTING STRENGTH)** uses a hand dynamometer attached by a cable and pulley system to the bottom of a metal tray. The subject grasps the tray handholds and pulls directly upward. A potentiometer output is displayed on a digital readout after averaging the force sustained from the beginning of the 2nd second to the end of the 4th second of the pull. Isometric lifting tests are easier to standardize than dynamic tests. However, they do not simulate dynamic lifting, and their ability to predict the subsequent development of industrial back injuries remains controversial. Variations in isometric lifting tests include whole-body isometric testing in various positions (e.g., leg lift–squat, torso lift–bent back, arm lift–upright) to simulate dynamic activity.

B. **DYNAMIC LIFTING CAPACITY TESTS** are more valid from the industrial perspective but are difficult to standardize. The primary problems are load acceleration and muscle length changes. Commercial devices and protocols for evaluating dynamic lifting capacity are available from Blankenship, EPIC Functional Capacity Evaluation System, Isernhagen Work Systems, Key Functional Assessment, and Work Evaluation Systems Technology (WEST). A torso electrogoniometric system can also be used to continuously monitor the bending and twisting kinematics of the torso relative to the pelvis, then combined with an external measurement of the peak load moment during a lifting job, to determine risk for low back pain.

1. **Psychophysical lifting tests** are safe and are essentially patient-controlled submaximal strength tests. They are based on psychophysics, which is a field in psychology that deals with the relationship between sensations and physical stimuli. In psychophysical lifting tests, the person increases the load (mass) in small increments until subjective maximum exertion is reached (i.e., the dependent variable measured is the person's subjective feelings of fatigue or perception of what load can be sustained for several hours – all of which could be affected by the environmental temperature, noise, or light). As the characteristics of the lifting or working environment are varied, the acceptable weight may change. These tests permit a person to evaluate the acceptable workload in dynamic tasks, but the results cannot be extrapolated too far beyond the conditions of the test. What is an acceptable load to lift in a well-designed tray with handholds is not necessarily acceptable if the load is unstable or in a container with rough edges. Studies have shown that although psychophysical lifting tests are not predictive of new cases of low back pain, there is a close association between the perception of workload and the prevalence of low back pain. An example of a psychophysical lifting test is the progressive isoinertial lifting evaluation (PILE) test described below.
2. **Progressive isoinertial lifting evaluation (PILE)** is a standardized lifting test protocol that uses both psychophysical and isoinertial lifting characteristics. The lumbar PILE consists of free-style lifting from floor to waist height (0 to 30 inches; 0 to 75 cm), and the cervical PILE is from waist to shoulder height (30 to 54 inches; 75 to 135 cm). The lifting load for men starts at 13 lb (5.9 kg) and is increased by 10 lb (4.5 kg) every 20 seconds, while for women it starts at 8 lb (3.6 kg) and is increased by 5 lb (2.3 kg) every 20 seconds. For every 20 seconds, the subject should lift at a rate of four lifting cycles (i.e., one lifting cycle for lumbar test is from floor to waist then back to the floor; for cervical test, one lifting cycle is from waist to shoulder and back to waist). The test is ended when the subject reaches any of the following: (a) psychological end-point, e.g., complaints of pain, discomfort, or fatigue, or inability to complete four lifting cycles in 20 seconds; (b) aerobic end-point, i.e., when target heart rate range (THRR) is reached (usually 85% of maximum heart rate or lower for cardiac patients; see Chapter 4.2, section III.A.1 for calculating THRR); or (c) safety end-point, i.e., a predetermined "safe limit" of 55–60% of body weight is lifted.

   After completion of lifting, the parameters computed include the maximum weight lifted, the endurance time to discontinuation of test, the final and target heart rates, total work (TW), and total power (TP) consumption. The TW is computed by adding all the weights lifted and multiplying the total by a total distance of 20 feet (6 m) for the lumbar test or 16 feet (4.8 m) for the cervical test. The 20-foot distance for lumbar PILE is computed by multiplying the distance from the floor-to-waist-to-floor (i.e., 30 in $\times$ 2 = 60 in or 5 feet) by four, which is the number of lifting cycles in a 20-second interval. The 16-foot distance for cervical PILE is computed in a similar fashion by using the waist-to-shoulder distance of 24 inches or 2 feet multiplied by two (i.e., 4 feet) then multiplied by four lifting cycles. A sample calculation for a woman who reached an end-point after completing 100 seconds of lumbar lifting at 5-lb increments every 20 seconds is TW = $[8 + 13 + 18 + 23 + 28] \times 20 = 1800$ lb-ft. The TP is computed by dividing TW by the total time (i.e., 1800 lb-ft/100 s = 18 lb-ft/s).
3. **DCER ("isotonic") lifting tests** are easy and relatively inexpensive. Weighted objects such as trays, boxes, push–pull carts, or other objects can be used as test loads. The subjects attempt to move the test objects the desired direction and distance on a trial and error basis. Weight can be added or removed

from the containers so that an estimate of the maximum load or effort can be established. The 10-repetition maximum (10 RM value) system may be used. While easy to conduct, isotonic lifting tests are not easy to standardize because they are easily confounded by the techniques used and the velocity and acceleration of the dynamic movement, which are influenced by the subject's efforts. Useful databases on dynamic efforts have rarely been established because of the high degree of specificity associated with these types of tests.

4. **Isokinetic lifting tests** use an isokinetic device attached to a tray or other object to simulate a lifting task. The force and velocity signals are recorded. During data analysis, the velocity data are integrated to give the displacement data. Thus, during the simulated lifts, a record of instantaneous force at incremental vertical heights can be obtained. Because the isokinetic device eliminates most acceleration, the force generated at a vertical location depends on the force-generating capacity of the body at that position. In these lifts, very large forces are generated at low heights where the lifting capacity is high and the lifter relies on momentum to assist the lift at higher positions. Because the resistance that must be overcome during lifting is frictional as opposed to gravitational, the isokinetic strength testing system is not restricted to vertical force measurements. The system can also be used to profile pushing, pulling, and oblique lifting capacities. The use of an isokinetic testing approach does not eliminate the need for standardization of testing procedures. Of particular importance is the velocity of testing because the force that can be developed by a group of muscles decreases with increasing velocity. Therefore, simulated isokinetic lifting at high velocities results in maximal strength values that are less than those found in tests performed at slower speeds. Although isokinetic testings appear to be more functional, the use of constant speed is not truly physiologic. Few prospective studies have used these parameters as predictors of low back pain.

IV. Aerobic work capacity tests

These tests measure the maximum amount of work that can be done when there is enough oxygen to supply the muscles.

A. **WHOLE-BODY AEROBIC CAPACITY TESTS** use cardiac and cardiopulmonary graded exercise tolerance testing described in Chapter 2.7, sections I.A. and II.A.

B. **UPPER-BODY AEROBIC CAPACITY TESTS**

1. **Arm ergometry** uses a modified bicycle ergometer or an arm ergometer to measure upper-body work by arm cranking (see Chapter 2.7, section I.A.2.b).
2. **Upper-body lifting test**. The weight of the tray is increased in four stages while it is lifted twice per minute around a series of shelves. This test appears to be limited by the discomfort felt at the wrists when the tray is lifted.

V. Work assessment

Work assessment consists of **functional capacity evaluation (FCE)**, which is a broad term that includes tests of manual material-handling capabilities, aerobic capacity, posture and mobility tolerance, anthropometric measurements, activities of daily living, energy conservation techniques, and need for adaptive methods or technology. The information obtained from FCE can be used to establish maximal permissible limits (MPL; see section III) for nonrepetitive activities and to delineate safe parameters for repetitive activities in a normal population. However, objective data (including validity) for the injured or disabled population are lacking. In return-to-work programs, FCE usually refers to physical capacity evaluation and work capacity evaluation, both of which are described in Chapter 5.11, section V.D.

VI. Gait assessment techniques

Gait assessments can be performed qualitatively by informal visual analysis (see Chapter 1.1, section II.P.7) or quantitatively using the techniques described below. Table 2.5-1 shows the variables and determinants of gait, Table 2.5-2 shows the kinematic and kinetic events in normal gait, and Table 2.5-3 shows abnormal gaits and their probable causes. When analyzing gait, the clinician must be aware of the effect of gait speed on the gait cycle and gait patterns (e.g., slow walking can increase the period of double-limb stance, shorten the swing phase, and increase muscular co-contraction to provide greater stability on the lower limbs). Multiple observations may also be needed (in a natural setting if possible) as the patient's self-consciousness of being observed may also alter the gait pattern.

A. OBSERVATIONAL GAIT ANALYSES are performed visually, with and/or without videotaping. The patient is asked to walk, with and/or without shoes (with and/or without orthotic/prosthetic devices or other gait aids, if applicable), on level ground (or on a treadmill) and/or on different surfaces as well as stairs. The gait parameters (see Table 1.1-10 in Chapter 1.1) are then observed from the front, side, and rear. The overall pattern of walking, as well as kinematic gait parameters, are described and analyzed from the foot and up to the trunk and upper limbs. If a videotape is used, certain aspects of the gait cycle can be viewed repeatedly (in slow motion if needed) for closer analyses.

B. FUNCTIONAL COMMUNITY ANALYSES determine the distances required for independent community ambulation (e.g., going to the post office, bank, doctor's office, supermarket, department store, drug store, as well as in crossing intersections). Typical curb heights and crosswalk times in the patient's neighborhood can also be analyzed. The patient's gait ability, as well as endurance, are then evaluated (ideally by bringing the patient out on a field trip) to determine the feasibility of community ambulation (with or without gait aids or assistance from another person). If needed, the patient may be recommended a manual or powered mobility system (see Chapter 4.7) for community use.

C. DYNAMIC GAIT ANALYSIS SYSTEMS

1. Motion analysis system

a. ***Video-based (photometric) motion analysis systems*** (see section I.E) use high-speed infrared cameras to record the relative motion of reflective markers attached to different body parts during ambulation. The information gathered is then digitized by the computer to generate two- or three-dimensional gait kinematic parameters. The system can generate raw data on segment positions that can easily be coordinated with ground reaction forces to compute joint kinetic information. Video-based systems are commonly used in most gait analysis laboratories but are relatively expensive.

b. ***Electrogoniometers*** (described in section I.B.4) may be used to collect single-axial or multiaxial ROM data during ambulation. They are less expensive than video-based motion analysis systems and are useful for remote data collection protocols (in which the use of a video-based system is impractical). However, they are not commonly used because they are cumbersome to the patient (because of the need for attaching the goniometric arms to the proximal and distal segments of the patient's limbs). Moreover, their data cannot be easily used to compute joint kinetic information (because of difficulty in coordinating goniometric data with ground reaction forces).

Table 2.5-1 Definition of gait variables and determinants

Gait parameters	Definition
1. Gait cycle	Period between ipsilateral foot contacts (i.e., two steps or one stride); the functional unit of gait.
2. Spatial variables	
a. Step length	Distance (cm) between foot strikes of contralateral feet; normal range is 37.5 to 50 cm.
b. Stride length	Distance (cm) between foot strikes of ipsilateral feet; normal range is 75 to 160 cm; 1 stride = 2 successive steps = 1 gait cycle.
c. Stride width or base of support	Distance (cm) between the midline of contralateral foot strikes; normal range is 7.5 to 15 cm.
d. Toe out	Angulation of the long axis of the foot (in degrees) to the line of walking progression; the normal range is up to 15°.
3. Temporal variables	
a. Cycle time	Time (seconds) of one complete gait cycle.
b. Stance time	Time (seconds) that one foot is in contact with the support surface.
c. Single-support time	Time (seconds) that one foot is the sole contact with the support surface during one gait cycle.
d. Double-support time	Total time (seconds) that both feet have contact with the support surface; double support is absent in running.
e. Step duration	Time (seconds) between contralateral foot contacts.
f. Stride duration	Time (seconds) between ipsilateral foot contacts.
g. Cadence	Number of steps per unit time; normal cadence ranges from 70 to 130 steps per minute with an energy cost of 100 cal/miles.
4. Gait velocity	Rate (m/s) of forward body motion; i.e., (stride length × cadence)/2; comfortable walking speed is 80 m/min or 3 mph.
5. Center of gravity (COG)	Located 5 cm anterior to second sacral vertebra; COG is displaced 5 cm vertically and 5 cm horizontally during an average adult male step.
6. Gait determinants	Mechanisms used by the body to reduce and smooth out the path of the center of gravity for a smooth and efficient gait.
a. Pelvic rotation	Right and left pelvic rotation around a vertical axis about 4° in each direction.
b. Pelvic tilt	Slight (4°) downward drop of pelvis on the side of the swing limb.
c. Knee flexion in stance	Knee flexion at foot strike and at heel-off (or terminal stance)
d. Ankle dorsiflexion in stance	Movement of the tibia over the foot during the foot-flat (loading response) to mid-stance, and mid-stance to heel-off phases
e. Coordinated knee, ankle, and foot motion	The knee flexes, the ankle plantar flexes, and the foot pronates from foot strike to mid-stance; the knee extends, the ankle plantar flexes, and the foot supinates from mid-stance to heel-off.
f. Pelvic lateral displacement	The base of support and the tibiofemoral angle (with slight genu valgum) allows the tibia to remain vertical and the feet relatively close together.

Table 2.5-2 Normal gait

	Stance phase (60%)				Swing phase (40%)			
	First double limb support or DLS (0–10%)		**Single limb support (10–50%)**		**Second DLS (50–60%)**	**Limb advancement (60–100%)**		
RLA terms	Initial contact	Loading response	Mid-stance	Terminal stance	Pre-swing	Initial swing	Mid-swing	Terminal swing
Traditional terms	Heel (foot) strike	Foot flat	Mid-stance	Heel-off	Toe-off	Acceleration	Mid-swing	Deceleration
Stage of gait cycle	0–2%	0–10%	10–30%	30–50%	50–60%	60–70%	70–90%	90–100%
KINEMATICS								
Pelvis/femur	Internal rotation		External rotation			Internal rotation		
Hip	30° flexion	20° flexion	Extending to 0°	10° hyper-extension	Neutral	20° flexion	20° to 30° flexion	30° flexion
Knee	0° to 5° flexion	15° flexion	Extending to 5° flexion	0° to 5° flexion	35–40° flexion	60° flexion	30° flexion	0° to 5° flexion
Ankle	0° to 3–5° PF	7–15° PF	From PF to 5° DF	10° DF	20° PF	10° PF	0° to 2° DF	0° to 3–5° PF
Subtalar	Eversion	Eversion	Maximum eversion	Inversion	Maximum inversion	Neutral	Neutral	Neutral

(*Continued*)

Table 2.5-2 *(Continued)*

KINETICS				
Iliopsoas	Inactive	**Concentric action**		
Gluteus maximus	**Eccentric action**	Inactive		
Gluteus medius	**Eccentric action**	Inactive		
Hip adductors	Inactive	**Concentric action**	Inactive	
Hamstrings	**Eccentric action**	Inactive	**Eccentric action**	
Quadriceps	**Eccentric action**	Inactive	**Eccentric action**	Inactive
Pretibial	**Eccentric action**	Inactive	**Concentric action**	
Calf muscles	Inactive	**Eccentric action**	**Concentric action**	Inactive

Abbreviations: RLA = Rancho Los Amigos; DF = dorsiflexion; PF = plantar flexion.
Data adapted from: Perry J: Gait analysis: normal and pathological function, *Thorofare, NJ, 1992; Slack; Pathokinesiology Service and Physical Therapy Department:* Normal and pathological gait syllabus, *Downey, CA, 1989, Professional Staff Association of Rancho Los Amigos Medical Center, p. 11; and Mann RA, Mann JA: Biomechanics of the foot. In Goldberg B, Hsu JD, editors:* American Academy of Orthopedic Surgeons (AAOS) atlas of orthoses and assistive devices, *ed 3, St Louis, 1997, Mosby, pp. 135–152.*

Table 2.5-3	Abnormal gaits and their probable causes
Gait pathology	**Probable causes**
1. Foot strike to foot flat	
a. Foot slap	Moderately weak dorsiflexors
2. Foot strike through mid-stance	
a. Genu recurvatum	Weak, short, or spastic quadriceps; compensated hamstring weakness; Achilles tendon contracture; plantar flexor spasticity
b. Excessive foot supination	Compensated forefoot valgus deformity; pes cavus; short limb; uncompensated external rotation of tibia or femur
c. Excessive trunk extension	Weak hip extensor or flexor; hip pain; decreased knee ROM
d. Excessive trunk flexion	Weak gluteus maximus and quadriceps
3. Foot strike through toe-off	
a. Excessive knee flexion	Hamstring contracture; decreased ankle dorsiflexion; weak plantar flexor; long limb; hip flexion contracture
b. Excessive medial femur rotation	Tight medial hamstrings; anteverted femoral shaft; weakness of opposite muscle group
c. Excessive lateral femur rotation	Tight lateral hamstrings; retroverted femoral shaft; weakness of opposite muscle group
d. Increased base of support	Abductor muscle contracture; instability; genu valgum; leg length discrepancy
e. Decreased base of support	Adductor muscle contracture; genu varum
4. Footflat through heel-off	
a. Excessive trunk lateral flexion (Trendelenberg gait)	Ipsilateral gluteus medius weakness; hip pain
b. Pelvic drop	Contralateral gluteus medius weakness
c. "Waddling" gait	Bilateral gluteus medius weakness
5. Mid-stance through toe-off	
a. Excessive foot pronation	Compensated forefoot or rearfoot varus deformity; uncompensated forefoot valgus deformity; pes planus; decreased ankle dorsiflexion; increased tibial varum; long limb; uncompensated internal rotation of tibia or femur; weak tibialis posterior
b. Bouncing or exaggerated plantar flexion	Achilles tendon contracture; gastrocsoleus spasticity
c. Insufficient push off	Gastrocsoleus weakness; Achilles tendon rupture; metatarsalgia; hallux rigidus
d. Inadequate hip extension	Hip flexor contracture; weak hip extensor
6. Swing phase	
a. Steppage gait	Severely weak dorsiflexors; equinus deformity; plantar flexor spasticity
b. Circumduction	Long limb; abductor muscle shortening or overuse
c. Hip hiking	Long limb; weak hamstring; quadratus lumborum shortening

2. **Foot pressure measurements** can be used as aids in gait analyses and also in helping fabricate foot orthoses (e.g., wedges needed to reduce foot pressure in patients with diminished foot sensation).
   a. ***Force-platform systems*** measure direct pressures at the plantar surface of the foot (under barefoot conditions) as well as forces at the foot–ground interface. They use force plates (either strain gauges or piezoelectric sensors) on a walkway to measure foot pressures and to determine the ground reaction forces (i.e., the vertical, horizontal, and rotatory forces that are transmitted through the lower limb during each step), the ground reaction moments about the platform's vertical and horizontal axes, as well as the center of pressure and shear forces.
   b. ***Foot-based pressure measurement devices*** determine the pressure at the foot–shoe interface. They can consist of either shoe insoles with embedded load sensor arrays, or individual load sensors, which are applied to the specific areas of the foot that need to be studied.
3. **Dynamic electromyography (EMG)** uses surface or fine-wire electrodes to quantify the muscle recruitment patterns (i.e., timing and intensity of muscle activities in relation to different muscles of the same limb as well as the opposite limb) during ambulation. The EMG data from the electrodes can be transmitted through a telemetry system or through a cable (i.e., hard-wired) system. The EMG data can then be used to determine which muscles need attention during rehabilitation.
4. **Stride analyses** involve the determination of stride and step width, length, and duration as well as cadence and velocity. Toe-drag and symmetry of foot pressure can also be assessed. A simple method is to use footprint analysis (e.g., ink and paper method) and use a stopwatch to time the steps. A more expensive method is to use foot switches or a sensored walkway (similar to the foot-pressure measurement devices described earlier).
5. **Gait energy-expenditure determinations** are used to evaluate the function of the cardiopulmonary system during walking and running activities, with or without orthoses or prostheses. Parameters measured (e.g., oxygen cost, heart and respiratory rate, and blood pressure) are similar to those used for a cardiopulmonary graded exercise tolerance testing (see Chapter 2.7, section II.A.1). The energy expenditure of ambulation using prostheses is shown in Table 4.4-1 in Chapter 4.4, and the energy expenditure of ambulation using gait aids is discussed in Chapter 4.6, section I.

Further reading

Amundsen LR, editor: *Muscle strength testing: instrumented and non-instrumented systems*, New York, 1990, Churchill Livingstone.

Casey Kerrigan D, Schaufele M, Wen MN: Gait analysis. In DeLisa JA, Gans BM, editors: *Rehabilitation medicine: principles and practice*, ed 3, Philadelphia, 1998, JB Lippincott-Raven, pp. 167–187.

Chaffin DB, Andersson GBJ, Martin BJ: *Occupational biomechanics*, ed 3, New York, 1999, Wiley-Interscience.

Cocchiarella L, Andersson GBJ, editors: *American Medical Association: Guides to the evaluation of permanent impairment*, ed 5, Chicago, 2000, American Medical Association.

Eastman Kodak Company: *Kodak's ergonomic design for people at work*, Hoboken, NJ, 2004, John Wiley & Sons.

Esquenazi A, Talaty M: Gait analysis: technology and clinical applications. In Braddom RL, editor: *Physical medicine and rehabilitation*, ed 2, Philadelphia, 2000, WB Saunders, pp. 93–108.

Esquenazi A, Talaty M: Normal and pathologic gait analysis. In Grabois M, Garrison SJ, Hart KA, Lehmkuhl LD, editors: *Physical medicine & rehabilitation: the complete approach*, Massachusetts, 2000, Blackwell, pp. 242–262.

Giallonardo LM: Gait. In Myers RS, editor: *Saunders manual of physical therapy practice*, Philadelphia, 1995, WB Saunders, pp. 1105–1119.

Inman VT, Ralston HJ, Todd F: *Human walking*, Baltimore, 1981, Williams and Wilkins.
Jacobs K: Preparing for return to work. In Trombly CA, editor: *Occupational therapy for physical dysfunction*, ed 4, Baltimore, 1995, Williams & Wilkins, pp. 329–349.
Mayer TG, Barnes D, Kishino ND, *et al.*: Progressive isoinertial lifting evaluation: Part I. A standardized protocol and normative database. *Spine* 13(9):993–997, 1988.
Mayer TG, Gatchel R, Barnes D, *et al.*: Progressive isoinertial lifting evaluation: Erratum notice. *Spine* 16(5):5, 1991.
National Institute for Occupational Safety and Health (NIOSH): *Applications manual for the revised NIOSH lifting equation*. DHHS (NIOSH) Publication No. 94-110. Cincinnati, OH, 1994, US Department of Health and Human Services.
Norkin CC, White DJ: *Measurement of joint motion: a guide to goniometry*, ed 3, Philadelphia, 2003, FA Davis.
Perry J: *Gait analysis: normal and pathological function*, Thorofare, NJ, 1992, Slack.
Rodgers SH, Yates JW, Garg A: *The physiological basis for manual guidelines*. National Technical Information Service, Report Number 90-227-30, Springfield, VA, 1991.
Saunders JBCM, Inman VT, Eberhardt HD: The major determinants in normal and pathological gait. *J Bone Joint Surg* 35A:543–548, 1953.
United States Department of Labor: *Dictionary of occupational titles: the classification of jobs according to worker trait factors*, ed 4, Washington, DC, 1991, US Government Printing Press.

CHAPTER 2.6
Pulmonary function tests

Pulmonary function testing (PFT) is used to determine the cause of respiratory symptoms (e.g., dyspnea) when it is not clinically apparent, to determine the presence of a suspected pulmonary disease (in patients with high risk factors for respiratory disease), to determine the pattern of pulmonary disease (i.e., obstructive vs. restrictive or combined obstructive and restrictive patterns), to assess the severity of respiratory impairment in patients with known disease (e.g., exercise tolerance in asthmatics), to follow the progression or regression of respiratory disease (e.g., neuromuscular diseases that tend to get progressively worse), to assess response to treatment (e.g., bronchodilators), to carry out preoperative evaluation in patients with pulmonary disease or risk factors, and to assess impairment and disability owing to pulmonary problems.

In the PM&R setting, the PFT is usually performed with the patient at rest to differentiate between obstructive and restrictive pulmonary disorders and to estimate the severity and progression of disease. The patient is usually seated; however, in patients with chronic alveolar hypoventilation (see Chapter 5.12), supine PFT should also be carried out. The PFT measures lung volume and capacity (see Fig. 2.6-1 and Table 2.6-1), flow rates [forced vital capacity (FVC), forced expiratory volume in 1 second (FEV_1), FEV_1/FVC ratio, peak expiratory flow rate (PEF), peak inspiratory flow rate (PIF), forced expiratory flow rate (FEF), and maximum voluntary ventilation (MVV)]; lung diffusion capacity (lung diffusion capacity using carbon monoxide [D_{LCO}]); and blood gases. Chest wall compliance, maximal inspiratory pressure (MIP), and maximal expiratory pressure (MEP) may be measured in patients with chronic restrictive pulmonary disease (e.g., neuromuscular disorders). PFTs can also be performed as part of an integrated cardiopulmonary exercise tolerance testing (see Chapter 2.7, section II.A). Other special PFTs, such as sleep studies and bronchoprovocation inhalation tests, are beyond the scope of this book.

After PFT, the measured values are compared to the predicted normal values based on age, sex, height, and weight. Normally, the measured PFT values should be at least 80% of the predicted values. A guide to the interpretation of PFTs is given at the end of this chapter in section V.

I. Tests of ventilation (lung volume and flow rate)

A. DIRECT SPIROMETRY measures lung capacity, volume, and flow rates by having the patient inhale and exhale over a specified period of time into a tube connected to the spirometer. Modern spirometers use a microprocessor-driven pneumotachometer to measure air flow directly and then to mathematically derive volume. A spirogram, which is a graphic representation of bulk air movement, is depicted as a volume–time tracing or as a flow–volume tracing. The spirometry values are then compared with predicted values for a particular age, sex, height, and weight.

1. **Static lung volume and capacity** are measured using a bell or electronic spirometer. The subject is told to take regular breaths [tidal volume (TV)],

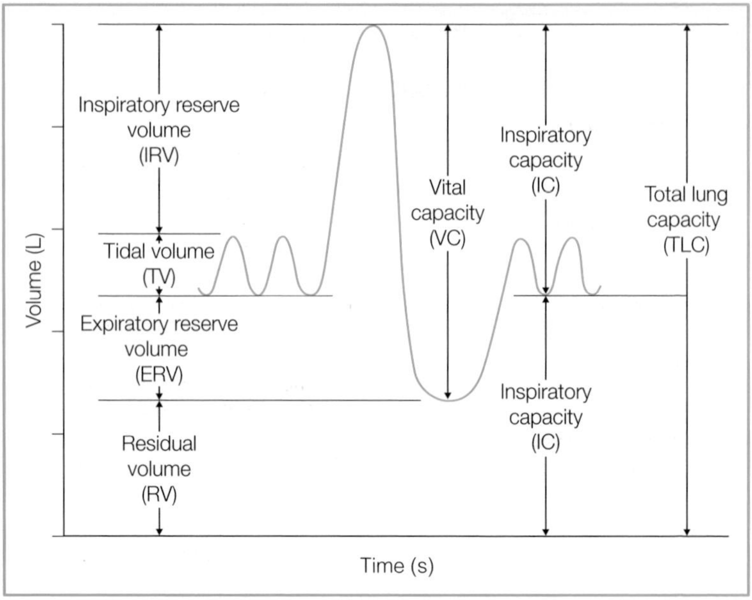

Figure 2.6-1 Spirogram of lung volumes and capacities. *Capacity* refers to two or more volumes. (From Grippi MA, Metzger LF, Sacks AV, *et al.*: Pulmonary function testing. In Fishman AP, editor: *Fishman's manual of pulmonary diseases and disorders*, vol. 1, ed 3, New York, 1998, McGraw-Hill, p. 534, reproduced with permission of the McGraw-Hill Companies.)

then breathe in maximally [inspiratory capacity (IC)] followed by a maximum exhalation [vital capacity (VC)]. The parameters of the measured lung volume and capacity are shown in Fig. 2.6-1 and defined in Table 2.6-1.

a. ***Slow vital capacity (SVC)*** is a subtype of vital capacity [VC = IC + expiratory reserve volume (ERV)]. SVC is the maximum volume of air that can be expired (or inspired) slowly and completely after a full inspiratory (or expiratory) effort. It decreases as restrictive disease increases in severity.

b. ***Inspiratory capacity (IC)*** is the maximal amount of inspired air from end-expiratory tidal volume in normal breathing or from functional residual capacity (FRC). Changes in IC usually parallel changes in SVC and can be used to identify lung or chest wall restriction. Most lung diseases do not affect the IC *per se*, hence in most PFT interpretations the SVC is used instead.

c. ***Expiratory reserve volume (ERV)*** is the maximal amount of air that can be exhaled from end-expiratory tidal volume in normal breathing. It is used to identify lung or chest wall restriction. Decreased ERV indicates a chest wall restriction caused by weak inspiratory muscles or as a result of nonpulmonary causes such as elevated diaphragm (seen in pregnancy, ascites, or obesity), pleural effusion, kyphoscoliosis, thoracoplasty, and massive cardiomegaly.

2. **Dynamic lung volume and flow rate measurements** are used to distinguish between chronic obstructive and restrictive pulmonary diseases. However, a specific diagnosis cannot be made by using these tests exclusively. The obstructive pulmonary pattern (see Table 2.6-2) generally shows normal lung volumes but a reduced FEV_1/FVC ratio because of reduced flow rate on inspiration and expiration; whereas the restrictive pulmonary pattern (see Table 2.6-2) generally shows reduced total lung capacity (TLC) but relatively normal inspiratory and expiratory flow rates.

Table 2.6-1 Definition of static lung volumes and capacity

	Symbol	Definition
Static lung volumes		
Tidal volume	TV*	Amount of air normally inspired or expired with each breath during quiet breathing
Inspiratory reserve volume	IRV	Maximum amount of air inspired from the end-inspiratory level of the TV
Expiratory reserve volume	ERV	Maximum amount of air expired from the end-expiratory level of the TV
Residual volume	RV	RV = FRC − ERV; Amount of air remaining in the lungs at the end of a maximal expiration
Static lung capacities		
Vital capacity	VC	VC = VT + IRV + ERV = IC + ERV; Maximum amount of air that can be inspired from the point of maximum expiration; or the maximum amount of air that can be expired from the point of maximum inspiration; or the maximum amount of air that can be breathed from RV to TLC
Slow vital capacity	SVC	Same as VC but using long, slow breath
Forced vital capacity	FVC	Same as VC but using quick, forceful breath
Inspiratory capacity	IC	IC = TV + IRV; Maximum amount of air inspired from the end-expiratory level of the TV or from FRC
Functional residual capacity	FRC	FRC = RV + ERV; Amount of air remaining in the lungs at the end of a normal exhalation (i.e., at the end-expiratory level of the TV)
Total lung capacity	TLC	TLC = IC + FRC = RV + VC = IRV + TV + ERV + RV; The sum of all air volumes in the entire lungs after maximum inspiration

** The symbol TV is traditionally used for tidal volume to indicate a subdivision of static lung volume; whereas the symbol V_T is used in gas-exchange formulas.*

a. ***Forced expirogram (FVC or time–volume curve)*** is determined by having the subject maximally exhale into a spirometer in which volume is measured against time. It records a maximum rapid exhalation after a maximum inhalation against time (Fig. 2.6-2 demonstrates a normal forced expirogram using a bellows or electronic spirometer).

I. **Forced vital capacity (FVC)** is similar to SVC except that it uses a maximal, forceful expiration. Because forceful expiration prematurely closes the terminal airways (in subjects with airway obstruction), the FVC tends to be lower than the SVC. FVC (in conjunction with FEV_1) can be used to differentiate obstructive from restrictive pulmonary diseases.

Table 2.6-2 Patterns of pulmonary function abnormalities in various pulmonary diseases

Patterns of abnormalities	VC	RV	TLC	FEV_1/FVC	D_{LCO}
A. Obstructive					
1. Asthma	N or ↓	N or ↑	N or ↑	↓	N or ↑
2. Chronic bronchitis	N or ↓	N or ↑	N	↓	N or ↓
3. Emphysema	N or ↓	↑	N or ↑	↓	↓
B. Restrictive					
1. Pulmonary parenchyma	↓	↓	↓	N or ↑	↓
2. Extrapulmonary	↓	↓	↓	N	N
C. Obstructive and restrictive	↓	N or ↓	↓	↓	N or ↓

Abbreviations: VC, vital capacity; RV, residual volume; TLC, total lung capacity; FEV_1, forced expiratory volume in 1 second; FVC, forced vital capacity; D_{LCO}, diffusing capacity of carbon monoxide; N, normal; ↓, decreased; ↑, increased.
Adapted from: Loke JSO: Pulmonary function testing. In Stein J, editor: Internal medicine, *ed 5, St Louis, 1998, Mosby, p. 379, with permission.*

II. **Forced expiratory volume in 1 second (FEV_1)** is the volume of air forcefully expired during the first second after a full breath during the FVC maneuver (see Fig. 2.6-2). It normally comprises over 75% of the vital capacity. In obstructive pulmonary disease, the ratio of FEV_1/FVC is decreased, but in restrictive pulmonary disease, this ratio stays normal (i.e., over 80%) or may be elevated.

b. ***Flow–volume curve*** (***flow–volume loop***; see Fig. 2.6-3) can be generated from successive recording of a forced vital capacity (i.e., expiratory) maneuver and a forced inspiratory vital capacity (FIVC) maneuver using a pneumotachograph, or by calculating it from a forced expirogram.

I. **Peak expiratory flow** (**PEF**; see Fig. 2.6-3) is the highest flow rate achieved at the beginning of the FVC and is reported in liters per second (L/s). The first one-third of the expiratory airflow phase is through the large airways and is dependent on the subject's expiratory effort. But the last two-thirds of the expiratory airflow (i.e., the downslope of the expiratory phase of the flow–volume loop) is dependent on the intrinsic properties of the small airways. The absence of cartilage and decreased elasticity of the small airways predisposes them to collapse (at the same rate) during forced expiration regardless of the patient's effort. Reduced PEF with normal inspiratory airflow is seen in weakness of the expiratory muscles, in poor expiratory effort, and in variable intrathoracic airway obstruction [e.g., chronic obstructive pulmonary disease (COPD), intrathoracic malignancy, and tracheomalacia]. In variable intrathoracic airway obstruction (see Fig. 2.6-4), the trachea widens during inspiration because of the negative pressure created during a maximal forced inspiration (thus, the inspiratory phase remains relatively unaffected); however, during maximal expiration, the abnormal airways are compressed by the markedly positive pleural pressure, thus reducing PEF. The more abnormal and weaker the airways (e.g., terminal bronchioles), the faster is the rate of their collapse during expiration, leading to increased "scooping" of the downslope of the expiratory phase of the flow–volume loop.

II. **Peak inspiratory flow** (**PIF**; see Fig. 2.6-3) is the highest flow rate achieved at the beginning of the FIVC and is reported in L/s. It is dependent on the

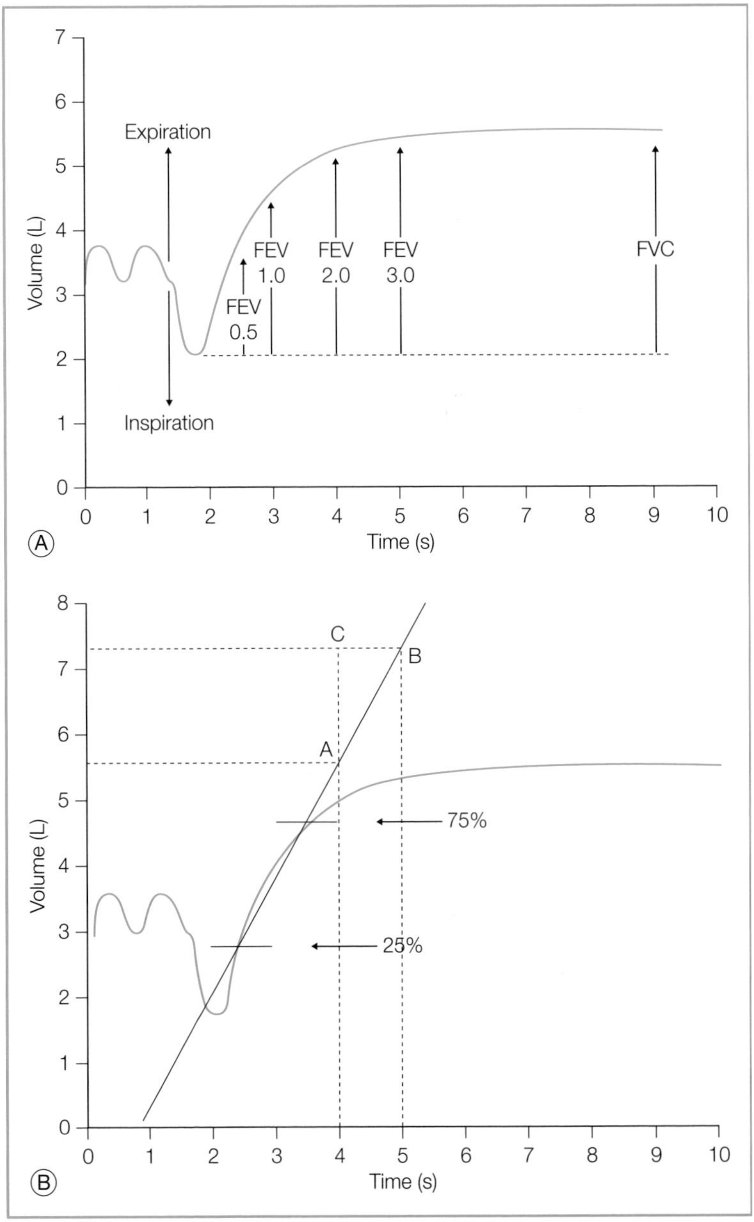

Figure 2.6-2 A normal forced expirogram [forced vital capacity (FVC) or time–volume curve] using a bellows or electronic spirometer. **A**. The subject exhales as forcefully and rapidly as possible to indicate the forced expiratory volume (FEV) at intervals of 0.5, 1, 2, and 3 seconds. The FEV in 1 second (FEV_1) is the most commonly used index of airflow. **B**. The forced expiratory flow rate from 25% to 75% of FVC (*$FEF_{25-75\%}$*) which reflects the average airway flow through large airways (*$FEF_{25\%}$*) and small airways (*$FEF_{75\%}$*). *$FEF_{25\%}$* and *$FEF_{75\%}$* may be determined by multiplying the FVC by 0.25 and 0.75, respectively. (From Ruppel GE: *Manual of pulmonary function testing*, ed 7, St Louis, 1998, Mosby, pp. 32, 34, with permission.)

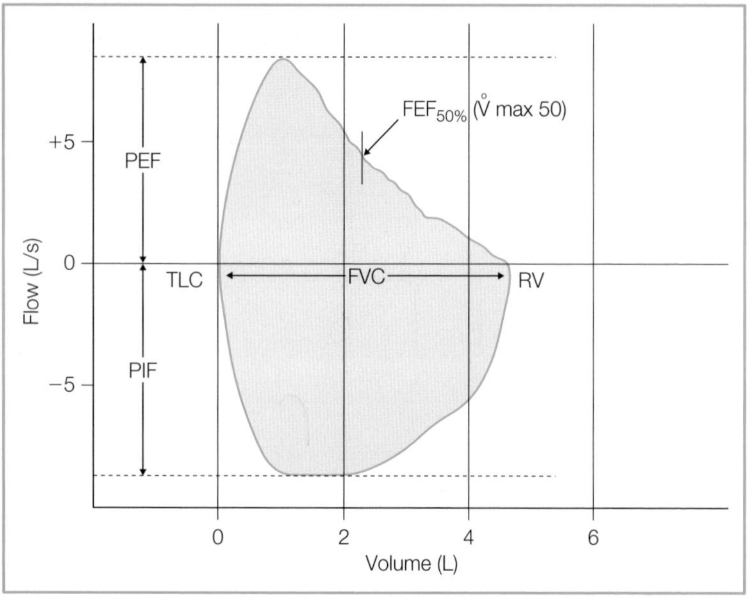

Figure 2.6-3 A normal flow–volume loop generated by successive recording of a forced vital capacity (i.e., expiratory) and a forced inspiratory vital capacity (FIVC) maneuver. In the flow–volume loop, the flow (L/s) is plotted in the vertical axis; whereas the volume (L) is plotted in the horizontal axis. Abbreviations: PEF, peak expiratory flow rate; PIF, peak inspiratory flow; TLC, total lung capacity; FVC, forced vital capacity; RV, residual volume; $FEF_{50\%}$, forced expiratory flow rate at 50% of FVC. (From Ruppel GE: *Manual of pulmonary function testing*, ed 7, St Louis, 1998, Mosby, p. 41, with permission.)

subject's inspiratory effort. Reduced PIF with normal expiratory airflow is seen in weakness of inspiratory muscles (e.g., neuromuscular disease), poor inspiratory effort, and variable extrathoracic airway obstruction (e.g., laryngeal dysfunction). In variable extrathoracic airway obstruction (see Fig. 2.6-4), the trachea narrows during inspiration (thus reducing PIF) because the pressure in the extrathoracic area is less than atmospheric pressure; however, during maximal expiration, the expiratory flow rates remain relatively unaffected because the trachea widens as a consequence of the intratracheal pressure being greater than atmospheric pressure (and thus greater than extrathoracic pressure).

If both inspiratory and expiratory airflows are greatly reduced and have no peaks, the flow–volume loop has a "boxed" appearance. This is indicative of a fixed upper airway obstruction (see Fig. 2.6-4), which can be extrathoracic (e.g., substernal thyroid, tracheal stenosis, tracheal tumor, plugged tracheostomy tube, or foreign body) or intrathoracic (e.g., tumor, rib cage deformity, and sarcoidosis). Although the smaller airways are normal and do not collapse easily, the amount of air getting in and out of the lungs is greatly reduced because of the fixed obstruction.

III. **Forced expiratory flow (FEF)** is the rate of flow at different airway sizes and is thus independent of the subject's effort. It is determined at different percentages of FVC which correspond to different airway sizes.

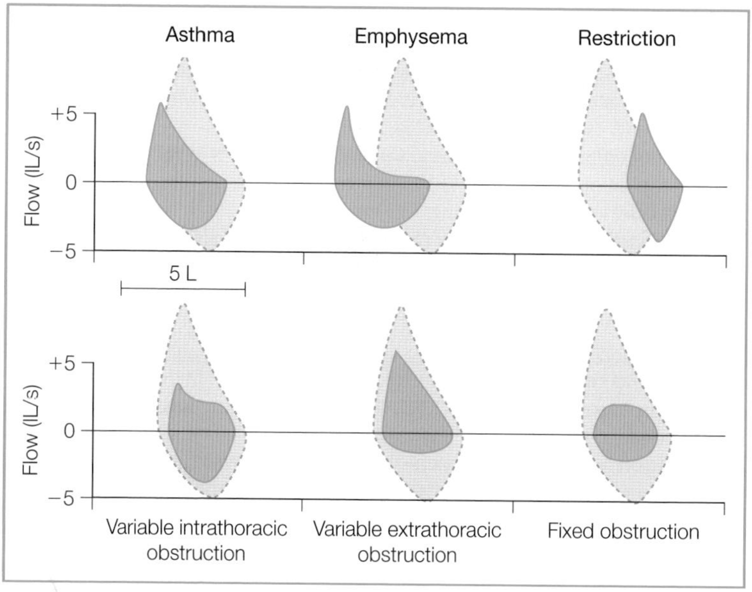

Figure 2.6-4 Flow–volume curve patterns of various chronic obstructive and restrictive pulmonary abnormalities plotted in liters per second against the forced vital capacity. The dotted curve represents the normal flow–volume loop. (From Ruppel GE: *Manual of pulmonary function testing*, ed 7, St Louis, 1998, Mosby, p. 42, with permission.)

It is decreased in obstructive disease and is usually normal in restrictive disease except in severe cases when it can be reduced. By calculating FEF at 25%, 50%, or 75% of FVC, the airway obstruction can be localized. Averaging forced expiratory flow rate from 25 to 75% of FVC ($FEF_{25-75\%}$) reflects average airway flow through small, medium, and large airways (see Fig. 2.6-2).

- **Forced expiratory flow at 25% of FVC ($FEF_{25\%}$)** is decreased in large airway obstruction.
- **Forced expiratory flow at 50% of FVC ($FEF_{50\%}$)** is decreased in medium airway obstruction.
- **Forced expiratory flow at 75% of FVC ($FEF_{75\%}$)** is decreased in small airway obstruction.

3. **Maximum voluntary ventilation (MVV)** is the maximum amount of air a subject can breathe in 12 seconds (expressed in L/min). It is carried out for 12 seconds to prevent hyperventilation and fainting. It reflects thoracic cage compliance, lung compliance, airway resistance, and the available muscle force. It is reduced in obstructive pulmonary disease, poor neuromuscular control, and poor respiratory effort. In emphysema, it is not only reduced but the baseline is also noted to be gradually rising as the ventilation progresses (this is attributed to air trapping). The MVV can be also be estimated by multiplying the FEV_1 by 40.

B. **INDIRECT SPIROMETRIC TECHNIQUES** for determining FRC and derivatives.

1. **Helium dilution or equilibration technique** is a closed-circuit method of measuring residual volume (RV) and FRC. The patient is connected to the

spirometer containing a known concentration of helium, which is virtually insoluble in blood. After some breaths, the helium concentrations in the spirometer and lung equilibrate (i.e., the amount of helium dilution is proportional to the thoracic gas volume). This is measured as the FRC, which is then used to calculate RV (see Table 2.6-1 and Fig. 2.6-1).

a. ***Residual volume (RV)*** is the amount of air that remains in the lungs after maximal expiration (RV = FRC – ERV). An increase in RV is seen in obstructive respiratory diseases with air trapping, e.g., emphysema.

b. ***Functional residual capacity (FRC)*** is the amount of air left in the lungs after tidal or normal respiration (FRC = ERV + RV). Changes in the elastic properties of the lungs are reflected in the FRC. A value below 75% indicates restrictive disease, but a value above 125% suggests air trapping consistent with obstructive airway disease.

c. ***Total lung capacity (TLC)*** is the total amount of air left in the lungs after maximal inspiration (TLC = VC + RV). A decreased TLC is the hallmark of restrictive pulmonary disease.

2. **Nitrogen washout** is an open-circuit method in which the patient exhales into the room. It is assumed that room air as well as the lungs have the same concentration of nitrogen (i.e., 80%). If the patient breathes 100% oxygen, nitrogen is washed out or removed from the lungs. The test begins at FRC and continues until the nitrogen concentration of the exhaled gas is below 1.0%. The volume and the nitrogen concentration of the exhaled gases are measured and a proportion is made to calculate the FRC, which is then used to calculate RV and TLC.

C. **BODY PLETHYSMOGRAPH** can be used to determine FRC. It is a large airtight box, like a telephone booth, in which the subject sits. At the end of a normal expiration, the patient (wearing a nose clip) is asked to make inspiratory efforts against a closed shutter over the mouthpiece (the shutter is closed so that the measured mouth pressure equals alveolar pressure). With each inspiratory effort, mouth pressure falls and lung volume increases. Because the plethysmograph is a closed box, the increase in lung volume produces a corresponding increase in box pressure because its gas volume decreases. The pressure and volume changes within the box as well as the intrathoracic lung volume are recorded. Then Boyle's Law is applied to calculate the FRC.

II. Tests of pulmonary mechanics

A. **BODY PLETHYSMOGRAPH** (see description in section I.C) can also be used to test for airway resistance and static lung compliance.

1. **Airway resistance (RAW)** is the pressure required to produce a given flow. It can be measured with a body plethysmograph or more commonly by inferring it from dynamic lung volumes and expiratory flow rates.

2. **Static lung compliance** is defined as the volume change/unit pressure change and reflects lung elasticity or stiffness.

B. **MANOMETRIC TECHNIQUES** measure the MIP and MEP by having the subject forcibly inhale and exhale through a closed mouthpiece attached to a pressure gauge. Both MIP and MEP reflect the strength of the respiratory muscles. They are reduced in patients with pulmonary diseases caused by neuromuscular disorders (see neuromuscular etiologies in Chapter 5.12, section III.B.1).

III. Measurement of lung diffusion capacity using carbon monoxide (D_{LCO})

Lung diffusion capacity is determined as the subject inspires maximally (from RV) a gas containing a small concentration of carbon monoxide, holds his breath for 10 seconds, then slowly exhales back to RV (**single-breath D_{LCO} technique**). An aliquot of alveolar gas is analyzed for carbon monoxide and the amount absorbed during that breath is then calculated and expressed in mL carbon monoxide absorbed/min/mmHg. It assesses the lung for gas-exchange abnormalities arising from alveolar–capillary pathology (i.e., transfer of gas into the blood). The amount of gas transferred across a tissue is in part directly proportional to the tissue area and inversely proportional to the tissue thickness.

The D_{LCO} is reduced in loss of functioning of the alveolar–capillary bed with decreased lung volume (e.g., lung resection, diffuse interstitial fibrosis, asbestosis, scleroderma, histiocytosis-X, sarcoidosis, and pneumonia), loss of pulmonary capillary bed with relatively normal lung volume (e.g., emphysematous lungs, multiple pulmonary emboli, sarcoidosis, and collagen vascular disease), failure of air to reach alveoli because of poor distribution of ventilation (e.g., severe bronchospasm, pneumonia, foreign body, blocked bronchus, hilar tumor, and pulmonary embolism), and in reduced oxygen binding sites as a result of low numbers of red blood cells (anemia).

Elevated D_{LCO} may be seen in increased pulmonary blood volume (e.g., left-to-right cardiac shunt, left heart failure, alveolar hemorrhage, during exercise, at high altitude, and in the supine position) and in increased red blood cell production (polycythemia).

The D_{LCO} can be used to differentiate different COPD subtypes, e.g., emphysema usually has reduced D_{LCO}, and asthma and chronic bronchitis usually have normal D_{LCO}. Pure restrictive pulmonary diseases with normal pulmonary blood flow and capillary bed (e.g., those caused by neuromuscular disease or chest wall disease) have normal D_{LCO}.

IV. Measurement of blood gases

Blood gas measurements are used to determine the adequacy and the efficiency of gas exchange.

A. ANALYSIS OF ARTERIAL BLOOD GASES (ABG) in room air is used to measure arterial oxygen tension (PaO_2), hemoglobin saturation (SaO_2), arterial carbon dioxide tension ($PaCO_2$), and alveolar–arterial oxygen tension difference or $P_{A-a}O_2$. The PaO_2 is the most sensitive indicator of pulmonary gas-exchange abnormalities of any etiology. A hemoglobin saturation (SaO_2) of less than 90%, which usually corresponds to PaO_2 of less than 60 mmHg, indicates seriously compromised tissue oxygenation. The $PaCO_2$, which is normally kept within the narrow range of 35–45 mmHg, determines the subject's ventilatory status. Hence, hypocapnia ($PaCO_2 < 35$) indicates hyperventilation, while hypercapnia ($PaCO_2 > 45$) indicates hypoventilation. If hypercapnia is persistent, especially when the patient is asleep, positive-pressure airway mechanical ventilators (see Chapter 5.12, section IV.A.4.a) should be considered during sleep. The $P_{A-a}O_2$, i.e., the A–a gradient, is another way of measuring pulmonary gas-exchange. $P_{A-a}O_2$ is the difference between the calculated alveolar oxygen tension (P_AO_2) and measured PaO_2. Normally the $P_{A-a}O_2$ is less than 10–15 mmHg. It remains normal when the decreased PaO_2 is solely due to alveolar hypoventilation, a low inspired oxygen tension, or a decrease in respiration. If $P_{A-a}O_2$ is increased, it is indicative of impaired diffusion, ventilation–perfusion mismatching, or intrapulmonary shunting.

B. TRANSCUTANEOUS OXIMETRY (PULSE OXIMETRY) can be used to monitor arterial oxygen saturation at rest, during exercise, during activities of daily living, and during sleep. It closely correlates with oxygen saturation obtained by ABGs except during severe peripheral hypoperfusion, during carbon monoxide poisoning, when skin pigmentation is extremely dark, or when saturation is below 70%. As with ABGs, a pulse oximeter reading of oxygen saturation of less than 90%, which usually corresponds to a PaO_2 below 60 mmHg, indicates seriously compromised tissue oxygenation. This is explained by the oxygen–hemoglobin dissociation curve, which shows a steep decline in SaO_2 if PaO_2 is below 60 mmHg or if the measured oxygen saturation (e.g., by pulse oximeter) is below 90%.

V. Interpretation of PFTs

Interpretation of test results is contingent upon the quality of the testing session. The subject should be able to follow instructions for the test and should have given his or her best effort. Although PFTs cannot diagnose a specific disease, they can differentiate between obstructive and restrictive patterns of pulmonary disease. Patterns of pulmonary abnormalities in various pulmonary disease states are shown in Table 2.6-2 and Fig. 2.6-4. The degree of severity of the pulmonary disease is determined by the percentage of the measured value compared to the predicted value (i.e., normal if >80%, mild if 65–79%, moderate if 50–64%, and severe if <50% of predicted values). The PFTs for the very young (<20 years old) or very old (>75 years old) subjects should be interpreted with caution because of the lack of normative data in these age groups. All PFTs should be correlated with clinical findings.

A. OBSTRUCTIVE PULMONARY DISEASE (see Table 2.6-2) features reduced inspiratory and expiratory flows but generally normal lung volumes. Because it is an airflow disease, the hallmark is a reduced FEV_1/FVC ratio (i.e., <70%). Also, there is scooping of the downslope of the expiratory phase of the flow–volume loop because of increased airway resistance. The TLC, FRC, and RV may be increased. The major cause of reversible obstructive pulmonary disease is asthma. For COPD, the major risk factor is tobacco. A normal FEV_1/FVC ratio excludes obstructive pulmonary disease. A low FEV_1/FVC ratio in the setting of increased FEV_1 and FVC, however, can be a variant of normal (seen in athletes). If the FEV_1/FVC ratio is low in the presence of elevated FRC (>125%) or elevated RV, it is indicative of emphysema and is the result of air trapping and lung hyperinflation. If the FEV_1/FVC ratio and the $FEF_{75\%}$ are both low, it is indicative of small airway obstructive disease (e.g., because of bronchospasm in asthma). All patients with obstructive patterns should be tested for reversibility with bronchodilators, i.e., improvement in FVC or FEV_1 of more than 12% and more than 200 mL within 15 minutes of bronchodilator treatment. Lack of PFT improvement after a single bronchodilator treatment should be interpreted with caution because it reflects one particular bronchodilator agent given at that particular time of testing. The agent may not have been administered properly or the patient may have responded only to long-term therapy. In determining bronchodilator responsiveness, the FEV_1/FVC ratio should not be used.

B. RESTRICTIVE PULMONARY DISEASE (see Table 2.6-2) features reduced lung volumes but normal flow rates on inspiration and expiration. Because it is a lung-volume disease, its hallmark is reduced TLC (<80% of predicted TLC) with normal or elevated FEV_1/FVC ratio. Restrictive pulmonary diseases caused by abnormalities of the pulmonary interstitium (e.g., interstitial pulmonary fibrosis, lobectomy, and massive pneumonia) have abnormal D_{LCO}, but those caused by chest wall restriction (e.g., kyphoscoliosis; elevated diaphragm because of obesity, ascites, or pregnancy; massive cardiomegaly; pleural effusion; and neuromuscular disease) may have normal D_{LCO}. In general, a normal TLC precludes restrictive pulmonary diseases.

C. **COMBINED OBSTRUCTIVE AND RESTRICTIVE PULMONARY DISEASE** (see Table 2.6-2) has features of both obstructive and restrictive pulmonary diseases, e.g., low FEV_1/FVC ratio with low TLC.

Further reading

Beliveau WJ: Use and interpretation of pulmonary function tests. In Ferri FF, editor: *Practical guide to the care of the medical patient*, ed 5, St Louis, 2001, Mosby, pp. 665–670.

Grippi MA, Metzger LF, Sacks AV *et al.*: Pulmonary function testing. In Fishman AP, editor: *Fishman's manual of pulmonary diseases and disorders*, vol. 1, ed 3, New York, 1998, McGraw-Hill, pp. 533–573.

Irvin CG, Corbridge T: Physiologic evaluation of patients for pulmonary rehabilitation. *Seminars in Respiratory Medicine*, 14(6):417–429, 1993.

Loke JSO: Pulmonary function testing. In Stein J, editor: *Textbook of internal medicine*, ed 4, St Louis, 2000, Elsevier, pp. 1590–1596.

Ruppel GL: *Manual of pulmonary function testing*, ed 7, St Louis, 1998, Mosby.

West JB: *Pulmonary pathophysiology: the essentials*, ed 6, Baltimore, 2003, Williams & Wilkins.

CHAPTER 2.7
Exercise tolerance testing

Exercise tolerance testing (ETT; also called exercise stress testing) can be used for diagnostic, prognostic, and functional purposes. In the PM&R setting, ETT is mainly used to determine the functional work capacity, which in turn can be used to determine disability as well as guide the cardiac and/or pulmonary rehabilitation (e.g., to determine the intensity of the prescribed exercise or activity). In patients with predominantly cardiovascular diseases (e.g., coronary artery disease or after uncomplicated myocardial infarcts), ETT is primarily used to measure cardiac parameters [e.g., electrocardiogram (ECG), blood pressure (BP), heart rate (HR)]. In patients with predominantly pulmonary diseases (e.g., chronic obstructive pulmonary diseases), ETT measures cardiopulmonary parameters (e.g., breathed gas concentrations of O_2 and CO_2; blood gases) in addition to cardiac parameters. This chapter gives an overview of ETT as used in the PM&R setting for determining functional work capacity. Exercise tolerance testing for diagnostic purposes is beyond the scope of this book.

I. Cardiovascular ETTs

Cardiovascular (CV) ETTs (i.e., ECG exercise tests) for determining functional work capacity as well as for determining prognosis (i.e., risk stratification) are justified only in patients with coronary heart disease and with uncomplicated myocardial infarcts (according to the general consensus of the American College of Cardiology/ American Heart Association). Their usefulness for determining functional work capacity in the following conditions remains controversial: (a) apparently healthy men over age 40 who are sedentary and plan to enter a vigorous exercise program, (b) patients with valvular heart disease, and (c) patients with hypertension or cardiac pacemakers who wish to engage in static or dynamic exercise training. The absolute and relative contraindications to ETT in general are listed in Table 2.7-1, and the end-points for exercise termination are listed in Table 2.7-2.

Prior to ETT, the patient is advised not to drink caffeinated beverages for at least 24 hours and not to eat for at least 3 hours. Patients are also told to wear comfortable, loose-fitting clothes and comfortable walking shoes for the ETT session. Most of the CV-ETT protocols use continuous incremental workloads (i.e., the exercise is uninterrupted and the workload is increased in stages) and are referred to as graded ETT or GXTT. Although some CV-ETT protocols make no allowance for warm-up or cool-down because of the extra time required, it is always prudent to include a warm-up and cool-down period, especially in the PM&R setting in which the CV-ETT is primarily used for determining functional work capacity. The benefits of proper (low-load) warm-up include gradual adjustment of the heart to the increased work demand, reduced incidence of ST-T segment depression during exercise, and reduced incidence of muscular injuries and patient anxiety. The cool-down or recovery period, which should be at least 3 minutes, can help prevent pooling of the peripheral circulation and possible fainting.

A. CV GRADED-ETTs (CV-GXTTs) use continuous incremental workloads, which begin at a low workload and progress to higher workloads until either subjective or objective "maximal" end-points (see Table 2.7-2) preclude further exercise or a predetermined "submaximal" end-point is reached [e.g., target heart rate

Table 2.7-1	Absolute and relative contraindications to exercise tolerance testing

Absolute contraindications

A. Unstable or severe CV disorders
1. Acute (e.g., ≤2 days) myocardial infarction (MI); or recent complicated MI
2. Unstable angina
3. ECG parameters: recent (within 4 weeks) changes in resting ECG suggesting MI or acute cardiac events; serious cardiac dysrhythmias (e.g., rapid ventricular or atrial arrhythmias)
4. Severe (>70%) left main coronary obstruction
5. Severe valvular (e.g., aortic) stenosis
6. Severe symptomatic left ventricular dysfunctions or obstructions (e.g. severe hypertrophic obstructive cardiomyopathy)
7. Dissecting aortic aneurysm
8. Acute congestive heart failure (decompensated)
9. Resting blood pressure ≥200/≥120 mmHg
10. Acute myo-, endo-, or pericarditis
11. Acute deep venous thrombosis, thrombophlebitis, or cardiac thrombi

B. Pulmonary conditions
1. Blood gas shows: $PaO_2 < 40$ mmHg in room air; $PaCO_2 > 70$ mmHg
2. $FEV_1 < 30\%$ of predicted value
3. Asthma attack
4. Acute pulmonary emboli or infarct

C. Noncardiopulmonary conditions
1. Any acute or serious systemic disorders (e.g., fever, infections, severe anemia, renal failure, thyrotoxicosis)
2. Acute psychosis
3. Neurologic or musculoskeletal conditions precluding adequate exercise
4. Drug or alcohol intoxication
5. Inability to give consent
6. Inappropriate pretesting documentation or medical indication

Relative contraindications

A. Stable or less serious CV disorders
1. ECG parameters: severe S-T segment depression at rest; frequent or complex ventricular ectopy; tachy- or bradycardic dysrhythmias; second- or third-degree atrioventricular block; atrial fibrillation with uncontrolled ventricular rate
2. Suspected or <70% left main coronary obstruction or its equivalent
3. Moderate stenotic valvular heart disease
4. Less severe hypertrophic cardiomyopathy (e.g., asymmetric septal hypertrophy)
5. Ventricular aneurysm
6. Chronic congestive heart failure
7. Severe arterial hypertension (systolic BP > 200 mmHg and diastolic BP > 110 mmHg)
8. Significant pulmonary hypertension
9. Fixed-rate pacemaker (rarely used)

B. Noncardiopulmonary conditions
1. Uncontrolled metabolic disorders (diabetes mellitus or myxedema)
2. Chronic systemic diseases (e.g., hepatitis, AIDS, mononucleosis, malnutrition)
3. Known electrolyte abnormalities (e.g., hypokalemia; hypomagnesemia)
4. Drug effect
5. Neurologic or musculoskeletal conditions that can be exacerbated by exercise
6. Advanced or complicated pregnancy
7. Nonpsychotic psychiatric illnesses
8. Inability to cooperate or lack of motivation

Partly adapted from American Association of Cardiovascular and Pulmonary Rehabilitation (AACVPR). Guidelines for cardiac rehabilitation and secondary prevention programs, *ed 4, Champaign, IL, 2004, Human Kinetics Publishers, p. 73.*

Table 2.7-2	End-points for exercise tolerance testing
Determinant	**Specific end-points**
Subjective	1. Subject wants to stop 2. Significant and progressive angina 3. Marked fatigue 4. Severe dyspnea 5. Other limiting symptoms (e.g., light-headedness or dizziness, near syncope, headache, blurred vision, ataxia, confusion, nausea, vomiting, leg claudication, cramps, severe joint pains, etc.)
Objective	**A. ECG changes** 1. Ischemic changes: >2-mm horizontal or downsloping S-T depression or elevation; T-wave inversion; or Q-wave 2. Accelerated rhythms: supraventricular tachyarrhythmias; ventricular tachycardia or fibrillation; premature ventricular complexes (increasing frequency; multifocal; in couplets; runs of ≥4; R-on-T); atrial tachycardia, fibrillation, or flutter 3. Bradycardias: unexplained inappropriate bradycardia (i.e., pulse rise slower than 2 standard deviations below age-adjusted normal values); onset of second- or third-degree atrioventricular block 4. Intraventricular conduction abnormalities: onset of bundle branch block **B. Blood pressure (BP) and heart rate (HR) parameters** 1. Systolic BP: >250 mmHg; drops >10–20 mmHg; or falls below standing systolic BP 2. Diastolic BP: >120 mmHg; or increases >20 mmHg 3. HR or systolic BP drops progressively or fails to rise despite an increase in exercise load after the initial adjustment period **C. Blood gas parameters** 1. PaO_2: <55 mmHg; or fall of >20 mmHg 2. $PaCO_2$: >65 mmHg; or rise of >10 mmHg **D. Clinical signs of poor perfusion (pallor or cyanosis)**
Others	1. Attainment of predicted (i.e., maximal) or targeted (i.e., submaximal) values [e.g., HR or METS (see specific parameters in Chapter 5.13, section IV.A.2.b) or ventilation] 2. Technical or equipment failure (e.g., dislodged ECG leads; difficulty monitoring systolic BP)

(see Chapter 4.2, section III.A.1 for formula) or target workload as specified by the test protocol]. The incremental work should last for a reasonable period of time, i.e., a minimum of 8 minutes and a maximum of 18 minutes. During CV-GXTT, there is no rest period at all, thus the patient's peak capacity or end-point is reached earlier. The graded-exercise protocol is practical and is most commonly used in CV-ETT protocols.

1. Measured parameters

a. ***Blood pressure (BP)*** of the brachial artery can be determined by using a sphygmomanometer. The predicted rise in BP for sedentary middle-aged men is >205/>95 mmHg. In general, the systolic BP should increase in proportion with the workload, but should not be greater than 250 mmHg. Likewise, the diastolic BP should not exceed 120 mmHg or increase by more than 20 mmHg.

b. ***Electrocardiogram (ECG) pattern and heart rate (HR)*** can be determined by using a 12-lead ECG telemetric monitor. The ECG is taken before the start of the test (in supine and erect positions to ensure that there are no changes in the

Table 2.7-3 Conversion of treadmill workload at different speeds and % grade incline into approximate metabolic equivalents (METs)
MET* level for treadmill speed (mph) at different % grade inclination

% Grade	1.7 mph	2.0 mph	2.5 mph	3.0 mph	3.4 mph	3.75 mph
0	2.3	2.5	2.9	3.3	3.6	3.9
2.5	2.9	3.2	3.8	4.3	4.8	5.2
5.0	3.5	3.9	4.6	5.4	5.9	6.5
7.5	4.1	4.6	5.5	6.4	7.1	7.8
10.0	4.6	5.3	6.3	7.4	8.3	9.1
12.5	5.2	6.0	7.2	8.5	9.5	10.4
15.0	5.8	6.6	8.1	9.5	10.6	11.7
17.5	6.4	7.3	8.9	10.5	11.8	12.9
20.0	7.0	8.0	9.8	11.6	13.0	14.2
22.5	7.6	8.7	10.6	12.6	14.2	15.5
25.0	8.2	9.4	11.5	13.6	15.3	16.8

**1 MET = 3.5 mL of O_2 consumption/kg/min during rest.*
Note: Actual measurement of VO_2 (described under section II.A) should be used if clinically feasible or available, as it is more accurate than estimating VO_2 using the MET equivalent.
Adapted from: American College of Sports Medicine: ACSM's guidelines for exercise testing and prescription, *ed 6, Philadelphia, 2000, Lippincott, Williams & Wilkins, p. 307.*

ECG based solely on position changes), at each stage of the test, and during the recovery period. During GXTT, the following are suggestive but not diagnostic of myocardial ischemia: development of downsloping ST segment depression, development or increase in the number of premature ventricular contractions, and a significant atrial arrhythmia.

c. ***Workload*** can be determined by using a treadmill or a cycle ergometer in accordance with a CV-GXTT protocol (see below). There is a linear relationship between workload and HR up to an age-determined maximum, i.e., the nominal age-adjusted maximum HR of 220 – age in years.

2. **Calculated parameters**

a. ***Rate–pressure product (RPP; or double product)*** is calculated by multiplying HR by systolic BP. The RPP, which is usually a five-digit number, is then converted into a three-digit number by dropping the last two digits. The RPP (see Chapter 4.2, section III.A) has a good correlation with myocardial oxygen consumption and is an excellent indicator of aerobic conditioning (i.e., a high RPP indicates poor physical conditioning and vice versa).

b. ***Metabolic equivalent (MET)*** is an estimation of the metabolic or energy demands of a given activity [i.e., the volume of O_2 consumed (VO_2), see description in section II.A]. One MET is the amount of oxygen consumed by a seated individual at rest (VO_2 rest) and is equal to approximately 3.5 mL oxygen/kg/min. Although actual measurement of VO_2 using ventilatory gas exchange techniques (described under section II.a) is more accurate, it is not always feasible or available in the clinics, hence the less accurate MET equivalent may be used to estimate VO_2 and help determine functional work capacity. To estimate the "maximal" metabolic demand (i.e., "maximal" MET level) from CV-GXTT, the workload must be known. By using Tables 2.7-3 and 2.7-4, the respective "maximal" workloads attained from treadmill and bicycle-ergometer protocols (see below) can be converted into "maximal" MET levels. For example, if the Bruce protocol (discussed in section I.A.2) is used, and the "maximal" exercise

Table 2.7-4 Conversion of bicycle (leg cycle) ergometry workload into approximate metabolic equivalents (METs) for different body weights MET* level for workloads in watts† (W) for different body weight

Weight	50 W‡	75 W	100 W	125 W	150 W	175 W	200 W‡
50 kg	5.1	6.6	8.2	9.7	11.3	12.8	14.3
60 kg	4.6	5.9	7.1	8.4	9.7	11.0	12.3
70 kg	4.2	5.3	6.4	7.5	8.6	9.7	10.8
80 kg	3.9	4.9	5.9	6.8	7.8	8.8	9.7
90 kg	3.7	4.6	5.4	6.3	7.1	8.0	8.9
100 kg	3.5	4.3	5.1	5.9	6.6	7.4	8.2

**1 MET = 3.5 mL of O_2 consumption/kg/min during rest.*
†1 watt = 6 kg-m/min; thus 50 W = 300 kg-m/min = 1.0 kilopond-meter/min.
‡The MET or VO_2 consumption for workloads <50 and >200 W cannot be accurately estimated.
Note: Actual measurement of VO_2 (described under section II.A) should be used if clinically feasible or available, as it is more accurate than estimating VO_2 using the MET equivalent.
Adapted from: American College of Sports Medicine: ACSM's Guidelines for exercise testing and prescription, *ed 6, Philadelphia, 2000, Lippincott, Williams & Wilkins, p. 308.*

level is reached at the treadmill setting of 2.5 mph and 12% grade incline, then the estimated "maximum" MET level is 7 (see Table 2.7-3), i.e., the person is consuming 24.5 mL oxygen/kg/min or seven times the resting rate of 3.5 mL oxygen/kg/min.

The drawbacks in using the relative MET equivalent from the table of activities include (a) the MET level tables tend to overestimate the MET level for patients with cardiopulmonary problems because most of the data used in constructing the table were derived from normal healthy subjects, (b) the maximal MET level obtained during GXTT using lower-limb protocols (e.g., treadmill) may not correlate well with the MET level of predominantly upper-limb activities (e.g., carpentry), and (c) the MET level tables do not take into account the concomitant emotional or physiological stresses that may add to metabolic demands during performance of an activity in real-life settings. Hence, MET tables should be used with great caution and an awareness of their physiologic limitations.

3. **Interpretation guidelines** The CV-GXTT performed in the PM&R setting is usually used to determine the "maximal" functional work capability of the patient (e.g., for exercise prescription). A CV-GXTT is considered "maximal" only if the limiting signs or symptoms are reflective of the person's functional capacity, e.g., if the test were stopped because of the onset of angina or significant changes in ECG, BP, or HR parameters; however, if the patient requests the test to be stopped (e.g., because of some localized muscle fatigue), the test is considered "maximal-volitional". The HR achieved at the end-point of a "maximal" or "maximal-volitional" CV-GXTT test is considered the "maximal heart rate" (MHR), or more accurately the "peak HR", for the purpose of exercise prescription (see Chapter 4.2, section III.A.1 on how to use MHR to compute the target heart rate range used for guiding aerobic exercise intensity). The "maximal" workload attained during the CV-GXTT can also be converted into its "maximum" MET level to estimate the workload's metabolic demand or the VO_2max. The use of MET levels in prescribing aerobic exercise intensity is described in Chapter 4.2, section III.A.2. If a "submaximal" protocol is used, the MHR may need to be adjusted because estimates of VO_2max derived from submaximal performance on a GXTT may vary by 10–15% from the actual or measured VO_2max. Another use of the CV-GXTT is to help classify a patient according to

Table 2.7-5 Correlation of metabolic equivalent (MET) levels to the functional and therapeutic classification of cardiac or cardiopulmonary impairment/disability and to the US Department of Labor classification of work

MET* level	1	2	3	4	5	6	7	8	9	10	11	12	13	14	15	16
Clinical status	← Symptomatic →															
Clinical status		← Limited →														
Clinical status				← Sedentary Healthy →												
Clinical status							← Physically Active →									
Functional class†‡	IV		III		II			← I and Normal →								
Work classification (see Table 5.11-1 in Chapter 5.11 for details)	Sed§		Light		Medium			Heavy to very heavy								

*1 MET (metabolic equivalent) = 3.5 mL of O_2 consumption/kg/min at rest.

† ***New York Heart Association (NYHA) classification***

- ***Class I*** *patients have no limitations as they can perform ordinary physical activity without undue fatigue or symptoms.*
- ***Class II and III*** *patients may experience fatigue or symptoms (e.g., dyspnea, anginal pain) with ordinary activity (Class II) or lighter than ordinary activity (Class III).*
- ***Class IV*** *patients have symptoms at rest and cannot perform any physical activity without discomfort.*

‡ ***Canadian Cardiovascular Society classification***

- ***Class I*** *(Ordinary physical activity, such as walking and climbing stairs, does not cause angina. Angina with strenuous or rapid or prolonged exertion at work or recreation).*
- ***Class II*** *(Slight limitation of ordinary activity; Walking or climbing stairs rapidly, walking uphill, walking or stair-climbing after meals, in cold, in wind, or when under emotional stress, or only during the few hours after awakening; Walking more than two blocks on the level and climbing more than one flight of ordinary stairs at a normal pace and in normal conditions).*
- ***Class III*** *(Marked limitation of ordinary physical activity; Walking one or two blocks on the level and climbing one flight of stairs in normal conditions).*
- ***Class IV*** *(Inability to carry on any physical activity without discomfort; Anginal syndrome may be present at rest).*

§ *Sed, sedentary.*

Adapted from: Dolgin M, editor: The Criteria Committee of the New York Heart Association. Nomenclature and criteria for diagnosis of diseases of the heart and great vessels, *ed 9, Boston, 1994, Little, Brown, and Co, p. 254; Campeau L: Letter to the editor.* Circulation *54:522, 1976; and US Department of Labor Employment and Training Administration:* Dictionary of Occupational Titles, *vol. II, ed 4, revised, Washington, DC, 1991, US Government Printing Press, p. 1013.*

functional capacity (see Table 2.7-5) and to use this functional classification in the determination of maintenance levels for cardiac exercise therapy, in advising patients about recreational and occupational activities (see Chapter 4.2, section III.A.2), and in predicting subsequent cardiac events and prognosis for survival.

a. ***Treadmill CV-GXTTs,*** which use a motor-driven treadmill, are the most commonly used protocols for CV-GXTT in the United States.

I. **Advantages**. The advantages of using a treadmill over a bicycle ergometer include (a) a treadmill permits higher peak cardiopulmonary workload and is a more accurate predictor of VO_2max, (b) walking is familiar to most people, thus less skill is needed, and there is less local fatigue of the leg muscles, (c) treadmill protocols are quite flexible because the speed and grade of treadmill walking can be varied independently to change the workload, and (d) treadmill workloads can be better administered because the patient is forced to keep up with the preset treadmill speed.

II. **Disadvantages**. Treadmills are more expensive, occupy more space, are relatively noisier, and not as convenient for recording the patient's BP, HR, and ECG than bicycle ergometry. During TM test, the patient should not grip the handrail as isometric loading of hand gripping can increase myocardial VO_2 and diastolic blood pressure, leading to increased cardiac risk.

III. **Test protocols**. Treadmill protocols for CV-GXTT vary in terms of percentage grade (i.e., treadmill incline), speed, duration of stages, and size of increments between stages. Although there are variations in the rate of workload increment, most protocols accomplish about the same effect. In general, smaller and more gradual uniform workload increments are preferred for cardiac patients because large, rapid, unequal workload increments tend to result in an overestimation of exercise capacity.

Among the many validated treadmill protocols available (see description of common treadmill protocols in Table 2.7-6), the most widely used is the Bruce protocol because of its ease of administration and economy of time (i.e., it takes a relatively short duration for most subjects to reach maximal effort). However, for most cardiac or cardiopulmonary patients, the standard Bruce protocol is too strenuous. Hence, a less strenuous protocol using 2- to 3-minute stages with low speed and one MET increments (e.g., modified Naughton, modified Balke, and modified Bruce protocols; see Table 2.7-6) should be used. The modified Naughton has also been used to extensively classify cardiac patients into high-risk and low-risk categories (i.e., risk stratification; see Table 5.13-5 in Chapter 5.13). The major disadvantage of using a less strenuous protocol is the longer duration of exercise required to achieve maximal effort (hence they are not practical for healthy subjects). The clinician should carefully evaluate the patient's cardiopulmonary status and decide which particular protocol to use (ideally, one that brings the patient to "maximal" effort in 8–12 minutes) rather than use one protocol for all patients. The patient's "maximal" workload on the treadmill can be converted into METs using Table 2.7-3, and the MET level can then be used to determine the patient's functional classification (Table 2.7-5). In general, one MET represents an increment on the treadmill of roughly 1 mph or 2.5% grade.

b. ***Cycle-ergometer CV-GXTTs***

I. **Upright bicycle ergometer CV-GXTTs** offer a useful alternative for patients who have difficulty with treadmill walking because of ambulatory instability or orthopedic limitations. Upright bicycling is preferred because supine bicycling does not significantly change stroke volume and end-diastolic volumes. The peak values for heart rate during upright cycle ergometry have been shown to be similar to treadmill exercise, although the maximum

Table 2.7-6 Common treadmill protocols for cardiovascular graded-exercise tolerance testing arranged in approximate order of increasing strenuousness

Treadmill§	Protocol
Modified	Set speed q 2 min to: 2.0, 2.0, 2.0, 2.0, 2.0, 2.0, 3.0, 3.0 mph*
Naughton	Set % grade q 2 min to: 0, 3.5, 7.0, 10.5, 14.0, 17.5, 12.5, 15 mph; Corresponding MET† level q 2 min is 2, 3, 4, 5, 6, 7, 8, 9 METs
Cornell	Set speed q 2 min to: 1.7, 1.7, 1.7, 2.1, 2.5, 3.0, 3.4, 3.8, 4.2 mph; Set % grade q 2 min to: 0, 5, 10, then increase by 1%; Corresponding MET level q 2 min is 2, 3, 4, 5.5, 7, 8.5, 10, 11.5, 13 METs
Modified Balke	Set speed q 3 min to: 2.0, 2.0, 2.0, 2.0, 2.0, 2.0, then 3.0 mph thereafter; Set % grade q 3 min to: 0, 3.5, 7.0, 10.5, 14, 17.5, 12.5, 15, 17.5, 20, 22.5 mph; Corresponding MET level q 3 min is 2.5 with 1 MET increase thereafter
Modified Bruce	Set speed q 3 min to: 1.7, 1.7, 1.7, 2.5, 3.4, 4.2, 5.0, 5.5, 6.0 mph; Set % grade q 3 min to: 0, 5, 10, 12, 14, 16, 18, 20, 22%; Corresponding MET level q 3 min is 2, 3, 5, 7, 10, 13, 16, 19, 22 METs
Naughton–Balke	Set and maintain speed q 2 min to: 3.0 mph; Set % grade q 2 min to 2.5, then increase by 2.5%; Corresponding MET level q 2 min is 4, 5, 6, 7, 8, 9.5, 10.5, 11.6, 12.6 METs
USAFSAM‡	Set and maintain speed q 3 min to: 3.3 mph; Set % grade q 3 min to 0, then increase by 5% Corresponding MET level q 3 min is 4, 6, 8, 10, 13, 15 METs
Standard Bruce	Set speed q 3 min to: 1.7, 2.5, 3.4, 4.2, 5.0, 5.5, 6.0 mph; Set % grade q 3 min to 10% then increase by 2%; Corresponding MET level q 3 min is 5, 7, 10, 13, 17, 20, 24 METs

**mph = miles per hour.*
† 1 MET (metabolic equivalent) = 3.5 mL of O_2 consumption/kg/min at rest.
‡ USAFSAM = US Air Force School of Aerospace Medicine.
§ To increase accuracy, the treadmill (TM) should be calibrated properly and used appropriately, i.e., no rail-holding during TM exercise, subject familiarized with the TM, and protocols gradual and individualized.

myocardial VO_2 may be approximately 10% less than for treadmill exercise. The workloads of bicycle ergometers are expressed in units of absolute mechanical power, i.e., watts (W), kg-m/min, or kilopond-m/min (kp-m/min). These can then be converted into MET levels (using Table 2.7-4), which in turn can be used to determine the patient's functional classification (see Table 2.7-5). In general, one MET represents an increment on the bicycle ergometer of roughly 20W (120kg-m/min) for a 70-kg person.

- **Advantages**. The advantages of upright bicycle ergometry compared to treadmill protocols include use of nonweight-bearing exercise and more convenient monitoring of ECG, HR, and BP because of less interference from chest and arm motions. Moreover, bicycle ergometers are cheaper, take up less space, have easy-to-control workload gradations, make less noise than a treadmill, and allow the patient to voluntarily discontinue the test at any time.
- **Disadvantages**. The disadvantages of bicycle ergometry include a VO_2 6–25% less than in treadmill exercise, greater cardiac stress (i.e., BP and RPP

tend to be higher) with added risk of cardiac complications, some patients being unfamiliar with cycling and not learning to use the machine (e.g., because of incoordination), and a greater tendency of the patient to discontinue the test earlier (i.e., submaximally) because of local fatigue of the muscles recruited for the unfamiliar task of bicycling. During bicycle ergometry, the patient should not grip the handlebars tightly because the additional isometric loading of hand gripping can cause exaggerated cardiac response, thus leading to overestimation of the functional capacity by as much as 20% and increased cardiac risk.

- **Test protocols**. The protocol for upright bicycle ergometry CV-GXTT, like treadmill protocols, should bring the patient to "maximal" effort in 8–12 minutes (hence it entails careful assessment of the patient's cardiopulmonary status). The seat height of the bicycle ergometer is first adjusted so that there is only minimal (5°) knee flexion when the foot is at its lowest position on the pedal. The patient is then instructed to warm up for 2–3 minutes by free-wheeling (i.e., cycling with "no resistance") at a rate of 50–60 rpm. This is followed by an initial workload of 10 or 25 W and subsequent progressive workload increases of 25–50 W (150–300 kg-m/min) every 2–3 minutes while the pedaling rate is maintained. Patients with severe deconditioning may use even smaller workload increments of 10–25 W every 1–2 minutes. During the test, HR and BP are measured every 1–2 minutes, and an ECG tracing is taken at the end of each 2- or 3-minute stage. Unlike treadmill protocols, cycle ergometry has no horizontal component because the cycle is stationary. When the end-point is reached (see Table 2.7-2), the resistance is reduced to zero and the patient cycles at the same rate for at least 3 minutes to cool down.

II. **Arm or upper-limb crank ergometer CV-GXTTs** can be used for patients who are unable to use their lower limbs because of neurological, orthopedic, or vascular impairment of lower limbs or for patients for whom arm exercise is necessary in their occupations or avocations. One major disadvantage of arm ergometry is the difficulty in monitoring the blood pressure during exercise. Peak oxygen uptake (or VO_2max) achieved with upper-limb ergometry is between 60 and 80% of that maximally achieved by the lower-limb exercise, depending on the strength of the arm and the shoulder muscles. Hence, upper-limb exercise capacity is a poor predictor of lower-limb exercise capacity and vice versa. The maximum cardiac output for upper-limb exercise is lower than for lower-limb exercise, but the attained peak or maximal HR is similar or slightly less in upper- than lower-limb exercise. In upper-limb exercise, the RPP is also more elevated mostly because of the greater increase in the systolic BP than the HR. The increased systolic BP has been attributed to increased peripheral vascular tone in the nonexercising vascular beds. For a given VO_2, there is a higher myocardial VO_2 during arm ergometry compared to leg ergometry.

Arm crank ergometry testing can be performed while seated or standing. The standing position generally permits a greater use of trunk and postural muscle groups to achieve higher peak cardiopulmonary workload. After 2–3 minutes of "no-load" cranking for warm-up, the workload is initially set to 25–50 W and increased in 2- or 3-minute stages by 10–25 W. The typical peak value achieved by 50–65 year-old men is approximately 100 W (600 kg-m/min). BP may periodically be measured in one arm while the other arm cranks at submaximal intensities, or it may be measured immediately after cessation of a 2-minute stage. However, because of the rapid decline of BP immediately after termination of upright arm-cranking exercise, the immediate postexercise BP values are most likely lower than the peak exercise BP.

Most patients are unable to tolerate a continuous protocol, hence needing an intermittent testing protocol (see below).

B. CV INTERMITTENT-LOAD ETTs include rest periods (which vary from 30 seconds to 2 minutes or longer) between a series of constant workloads, which are repeated at progressively higher intensities. Muscle strength can be restored during rest and greater total stress can subsequently be applied. The ECG and BP can also be recorded with less motion artifact during rest. This approach, however, takes a longer period of time to complete and is not practical for most routine testing in the clinical setting. It is used for arm crank ergometry ETT (e.g., increments of 25 W for 2 minutes separated by 1 or 2 minutes of rest) to improve patient tolerance of the arm exercise and to permit more frequent measurement of immediate postexercise BP. The intermittent method is also occasionally used for lower-limb exercise testing, in more severely impaired patients who can only perform a constant workload such as unloaded pedaling or walking at a slow pace.

C. CV SINGLE-LOAD ETTs

1. **Master's test ("two-step test")** is a crude method of determining physical fitness. It has declined in popularity and has been replaced by the CV-GXTT protocols described above in section I.A.
2. **Bench-stepping test (or sitting-chair step-test)** may be used as a form of CV single-load ETT in patients who are unable to do a formal CV-GXTT (e.g., elderly patients). The following protocol is by Smith and Gilligan (1983). The patient sits with both feet flat on the floor in a straight-backed chair facing a step (e.g., a bench or a pile of books). The distance of the step to the patient is equal to the length of the patient's extended leg. At the count of one (a metronome set at 120 may be used), the arch of the right foot is brought up to touch the edge of the step; on the count of two, the same foot is returned to the floor. On the next count of three, the arch of the left foot touches the step edge and, on four, returns to the floor. This alternating foot process is continued for a 2- and a 5-minute duration, at a rate of 60 steps/min, using a 6-inch-high (15-cm-high) step (stage 1; O_2 cost is 2.3 METs), a 12-inch-high step (stage 2; O_2 cost is 2.9 METs), and an 18-inch-high step (stage 3; O_2 cost is 3.5 METs). Stage 4 (O_2 cost is 3.9 METs) is similar to stage 3 with the addition of the following arm exercises. The right arm is raised (at the same time the arch of the right foot touches the step) and then extended over the leg; as the right foot returns to the floor, the right arm is lowered so that the hand rests on the knee. This process is alternately repeated on the left and right side for 5 minutes. For each stage, the heart rate is recorded after 2 minutes to determine if the patient should proceed to the 5-minute test. The HR is again recorded after the 5-minute test, and if it is still below 75% of age-adjusted maximum HR (i.e., 220 – age), then the patient proceeds to the next stage.

II. Pulmonary ETTs

Pulmonary ETTs are actually integrated cardiopulmonary (CP) ETTs because the pulmonary system is tightly linked to the cardiovascular system. They directly measure cardiac and pulmonary responses while indirectly assessing peripheral gas exchange. In the PM&R setting, they are primarily used to determine functional work capacity in patients with an established pulmonary diagnosis (e.g., for disability evaluation), to evaluate the need for supplemental oxygen during exercise, and to determine the appropriate intensity of prescribed exercise or activity. They may also help provide an objective assessment of complaints of limited exercise capacity and clarify the nature of any limiting factors (e.g., cardiac vs. pulmonary factors in patients in whom history, physical examination, and pulmonary function tests are equivocal). Except for the above reasons, CP–ETT are generally not used for diagnostic purposes because they are time consuming, expensive, and lack specificity (the few conditions in which they have high specificity include psychogenic dyspnea, exercise-induced asthma, deconditioning, myocardial ischemia, and peripheral vascular disease). Their absolute and relative contraindications as well as end-points for exercise termination are similar to those for CV-ETT (see Tables 2.7-1 and 2.7-2).

A. CARDIOPULMONARY GRADED-ETTs (CP-GXTTs) use continuous incremental workload for 6–14 minutes. They can be performed using stationary cycle ergometers or treadmills (see section I.A.1 and I.A.2 for description), allowing the subject to reach the maximal attainable work while measuring the exhaled gas (volume and O_2 and CO_2 concentrations), ventilatory parameters, blood gases, ECG, HR, and BP. Their purpose is to differentiate whether the impairment is the result of cardiac disease or of pulmonary disease (e.g., exercise-induced bronchospasm, ventilatory inefficiency due to ventilation–perfusion [V/Q] mismatch). They can determine the reasons for exercise-related symptoms and can be used to document the patient's progress during rehabilitation by showing changes in symptom-limited oxygen consumption and other physiologic parameters. Protocols used for CP-GXTT in patients with pulmonary disease are shown in Table 2.7-7. They can also help determine cardiopulmonary changes during medical management (e.g., the addition of prostacycline in patients with pulmonary hypertension).

Table 2.7-7 Graded exercise tolerance testing protocols for patients with pulmonary disease

Testing mode	Protocol
I. Treadmill†	
Massachusetts Respiratory Hospital	Set constant speed at 1.5 mph with 0 grade; If FEV_1 is >1 L/s: increase by 4% grade every 2 min, or if FEV_1 is <1 L/s: increase by 2% grade every 2 min.
Naughton	Set constant speed at 2.0 mph with 0 grade; increase 3.5% grade every 3 min.
Balke and Ware	Set constant speed at 3.3 mph with 0 grade; increase 3.5% grade every 2 min.
II. Cycle*†	
Massachusetts Respiratory Hospital	Begin at 25 W; increase 10 W every 20 s; or 5 W every 20 s when FEV_1 is <1 L/s.
Jones	Begin with 17 W, increase 17 W every min.
Berman and Sutton	Begin with 17 W, increase 17 W every min or 8 W every min when FEV_1 is <1 L/s.
Jones and Campbell	Begin with 25 W, increase by 15 W every min.
National Emphysema Treatment Trial (NETT) protocol	With the patient breathing 30% FiO_2, after 5 min rest, begin warm-up by pedaling 3 min with 0 W load, then increase by 5 W per min for MVV < 40 or 10 W per min for MVV ≥ 40, followed by 3 min cool-down at 0 W load.

** Cycle speed is constant at 50 rpm.*
Note: mph, miles per hour; FEV_1, forced expiratory volume at 1.0 s; L/s, liters per second; W, watt; 1 W = 6 kg-m/min; 25 Watts = 150 kg-m/min = 0.5 kilopond-meter/min; MVV, maximum voluntary ventilation.
Adapted from: Brannon FJ, Foley MW, Starr JA, et al.: Cardiopulmonary rehabilitation: basic theory and application, *ed 3, Philadelphia, 1998, FA Davis, p. 299; and National Emphysema Treatment Trial Research Group: A randomized trial comparing lung volume reduction surgery with medical therapy for severe emphysema.* N Engl J Med *2003;* **348**: *2059–2073.*
† To increase accuracy of treadmill (TM) and cycle protocols, machines should be calibrated properly and used appropriately, i.e., no rail-holding during TM exercise, subject familiarized with the TM or ergometer, and protocols gradual and individualized.

1. **Measured parameters.** Measured parameters include the cardiovascular parameters (see section I.A) such as BP, HR, 12-lead telemetric ECG, and the workload provided by the treadmill or cycle ergometer. In addition, they also include the following pulmonary parameters:

a. ***Breathed gas concentrations of oxygen and carbon dioxide,*** i.e., a breath-by-breath determination of the volumes of oxygen uptake (VO_2) and carbon dioxide output (VCO_2), as well as the actual peak oxygen uptake (peak VO_2) or maximum oxygen consumption (VO_2max). The VO_2, VCO_2, and peak VO_2 or VO_2max can be determined by using a headgear with a mouthpiece and a nose clip to collect the necessary gas samples, which are then quantified by a gas analyzer. In modern laboratories, breath-by-breath ventilation can be measured directly at the mouth using a light-weight, disposable flowmeter (which obviates the need for the cumbersome headgear, valve apparatus, and collection tubes) and a pneumotachometer. Although the term VO_2max is usually used interchangeably with the term peak VO_2 (i.e., peak O_2 uptake), they are not exactly the same. Strictly speaking, a true VO_2max can only be established if the patient keeps on exercising at a near maximal exercise level so that there is a VO_2 plateau. Because most patients are unable to maintain a maximal VO_2 plateau, the peak VO_2 (which is the point of highest O_2 uptake during the exercise testing) is used instead of VO_2max. The VO_2max or peak VO_2, which are expressed in L/min or mL/min/kg, are dependent not only on the circulatory system but also on the number of muscles involved in the task being performed (i.e., the more muscles involved, the higher the possible VO_2max; for example, cross-country skiing, which involves the arms and legs, permits the person to reach a higher peak VO_2 or VO_2max than arm cycling).

The predicted VO_2max is highly variable as it depends on several factors such as age, height, genetic body type, physical training, and familiarity with the testing protocol. In general, it is above 2.1 L/min for men and above 1.4 L/min for women. One way of computing for the predicted VO_2max value (mL/min) for sedentary middle-aged men is estimated by calculating [height (cm) – age (years)] $\times$ 21. It has been reported that a normal person is capable of performing a task for up to 8 hours if the maximal workload of that task needs less than 40% of the worker's peak VO_2 or VO_2max. If the actual VO_2max measurement is not feasible, the metabolic equivalent (i.e., METs; see description below and also in section I.A above) for the "maximum" workload may be used to estimate the VO_2max.

b. ***Tidal volume (TV), ventilatory frequency (f), and maximum exercise ventilation (VE_{max})*** can be determined using a pneumotachometer (see Chapter 2.6) before and after the CP-GXTT. Initially, as the exercise begins, there is increasing TV. As the work increases, f also increases. Ventilation is likely to become a limiting factor in CP-GXTT if (a) the VE_{max} approaches within 10–15 L/min of the maximal voluntary ventilation (MVV) measured prior to exercise, (b) the exercise TV approaches to within 10% of the resting inspiratory capacity, or (c) the f is more than 50/min. If early during recovery there is a prompt decrease in HR but no normal prompt decrease in ventilation, it is suggestive of a ventilatory limitation.

c. ***Blood gases*** including arterial oxygen pressure (PaO_2), arterial carbon dioxide pressure ($PaCO_2$), and oxygen saturation (SaO_2) can be determined by sampling the arterial blood gas (see Chapter 2.6, section IV.A). The noninvasive pulse oximetry (see Chapter 2.6, section IV.B) may also be used to measure SaO_2. During heavy exercise, there is a rise in $PaCO_2$, which in turn stimulates ventilation and causes the $PaCO_2$ to decline, thus minimizing the respiratory acidosis. In patients who are limited in their ventilatory ability (e.g., because of severe obstructive or, less commonly, restrictive pulmonary disease), a respiratory acidosis is sometimes seen. The PaO_2 should remain at about 90 mmHg throughout the CP-GXTT. In severe pulmonary disease, shunts or diffusion limitation can lead to decreased PaO_2.

2. **Calculated parameters**

a. ***Rate–pressure product or double product,*** i.e., RPP = HR × systolic BP (see discussion of RPP in section I.A), which is well correlated with myocardial oxygen consumption, indicates aerobic conditioning (i.e., the higher the RPP at a given load, the poorer the aerobic conditioning).

b. ***Metabolic (MET) equivalent*** is fully described in section I.A. Because one MET is equivalent to the resting VO_2 (i.e., VO_2rest = 3.5 mL of O_2 consumption/kg/min), a given MET value can be determined by dividing the measured peak VO_2 or VO_2max by 3.5 (i.e., the resting VO_2). MET equivalents (i.e., METs; see description below and also in section I.A above) for the 'maximum' workload may be used in PM&R clinics to estimate VO_2 if actual measurement of VO_2max or peak VO_2 is impractical or not available. These MET equivalent tables (see Tables 4.2-3 and 4.2-4 in Chapter 4.2) were constructed from actual measurements of VO_2max in normal subjects during different activities or exercises. The limitations and disadvantages of using the MET equivalent tables for CP-GXTT interpretation and for exercise prescription are discussed in section I.A and in Chapter 4.2, section III.A.2.

c. ***Peak O_2 pulse*** can be calculated either by dividing peak VO_2 or VO_2max by the peak heart rate (i.e., mL O_2/heartbeat) or by multiplying the effective ventricular stroke volume with the difference between the arterial and mixed-venous oxygen contents. Peak O_2 pulse can estimate cardiac stroke volume only in the absence of anemia, hypoxemia, or shunt. In general, the peak O_2 pulse at maximum exercise is greater than 12 mL O_2/heartbeat in men and greater than 8 mL O_2/heartbeat in women. During the CP-GXTT, the peak oxygen pulse normally increases in a curvilinear fashion from rest to exhaustion. A smaller than appropriate increase of the peak O_2 pulse indicates dysfunction in oxygen transport and an inefficient cardiopulmonary system. The peak O_2 pulse is reduced if the maximal stroke volume is decreased (e.g., valvular heart disease, coronary artery disease, cardiomyopathy, pulmonary vascular disease, or peripheral vascular disease), the arterial oxygen content is decreased (e.g., anemia, hypoxemia, or carboxyhemoglobinemia), or the mixed-venous oxygen content is increased (e.g., poor peripheral O_2 extraction or inability to increase exercise to higher levels because of the presence of other systemic diseases).

d. ***Ventilatory or anaerobic threshold (VT or AT) and respiratory exchange ratio (RER or R) or respiratory quotient (RQ).*** During aerobic metabolism, as the workload increases there is a linear increase in ventilation, heart rate, oxygen consumption, and carbon dioxide production. However, during anaerobic metabolism (which is used to supplement energy production when O_2 demand surpasses its supply), this increase becomes nonlinear. The VO_2 point at which this nonlinear response occurs (i.e., when the *rate of* VCO_2 increase exceeds the *rate of* VO_2 increase) is called the ventilatory threshold (VT). It is also called gas-exchange anaerobic threshold (AT) and is also referred to as lactate threshold (LT) because the concentration of lactic acid suddenly rises and the concentration of bicarbonate decreases in the arterial blood. In the average young person, VT or AT occurs at a VO_2 value that is approximately 45 to 60% of the predicted VO_2max. A VT or AT that is less than 40% of the predicted (not the measured) peak VO_2 or VO_2max is abnormal regardless of age, gender, or body size. Causes of low VT or AT include heart failure, anaemia, hypoxemia, low circulatory flow from pulmonary hypertension, and marked deconditioning. Severely low VT or AT (<30% of predicted peak VO_2 or VO_2max) is usually only seen in severe cardiopulmonary disease, and is not due to deconditioning alone.

The AT (or LT) is measured directly by repeated measurement of blood lactate levels; however, this is invasive and inconvenient. Noninvasive, indirect, and more convenient methods using continuous measurement of respiratory gases can be done to determine VT (or AT) by using the V-slope technique or by calculating the respiratory exchange ratio (RER or R). In the V-slope technique (Beaver *et al.*, 1986), the VCO_2 vs. VO_2 curve is divided into two regions, each of which is fitted by linear regression, and the intersection between the two regression lines is regarded as the V-slope VT (or AT).

In the clinic, RER is often used because it is easier to calculate than the V-slope. It has been shown that VT (or AT) corresponds to the point at which the RQ or RER rises above the resting value of 0.7 to 0.85, i.e., when the value approaches the value 0.85 to 0.95 (some clinicians refer to this value as 1.0). Although RER and RQ had been used interchangeably, they are, strictly speaking, not interchangeable because RER and RQ are only equal in steady state condition. Moreover, RQ is defined as the ratio of the CO_2 produced to the O_2 consumed (i.e., VCO_2/VO_2) occurring at the cellular level of metabolism; whereas RER is the equivalent VCO_2/VO_2 at the lung level (i.e., the ratio of CO_2 output to O_2 uptake by the lungs). RQ, which is calculated at the cellular level, is difficult to determine; whereas RER, which is calculated using respiratory gases, is easier to determine in the clinic. RQ always falls between 0.7 and 1.0; whereas RER may exceed 1.0 during heavy non-steady-state or "maximal" exercise due to hyperventilation (which increases CO_2 production by the lungs) and buffering the lactic acid in the blood (which provides a nonmetabolic source of CO_2).

RQ or RER varies depending on the substrate metabolized. Carbohydrate (glucose or glycogen) produces a RQ of 1.0 ($VCO_2/VO_2 = 6CO_2/6O_2$, i.e., one molecule of glucose yields 6 molecules of CO_2 for 6 molecules of O_2 consumed) whereas dietary fat produces a RQ of 0.7 (i.e., $16CO_2/23O_2$). Protein, which has a RQ of 0.8, is not as important as it plays a very small part in energy metabolism. The average RQ during light or moderate exercise is about 0.8 because a mixture of fat and carbohydrate is used for energy. Likewise, RER at rest is about 0.8 (range of 0.70 to 0.85) because, measured VCO_2 produced at rest is about 20 mL/min STPD (at standard temperature of 0°C, barometric pressure of 101.3 kPa, and dry gas) and measured VO_2 consumed at rest is about 250 mL/min STPD (i.e., roughly 70 to 85% of O_2 consumed is converted to CO_2). As more CO_2 is being produced than O_2 consumed is about 0.85 to 0.95, at which point VT or AT is estimated to have been reached, indicating anaerobic metabolism.

The VT or AT can be used to determine the intensity of an activity or exercise (i.e., activities requiring VO_2 above the VT or AT [i.e., RER exceeding 1.0] are considered as heavy or intense (or "maximal" effort), and activities requiring VO_2 below the VT or AT [i.e., RER of less than 0.85–0.95] are considered as mild or moderate). When exercise is done beyond the VT or AT, endurance time is greatly diminished and fatigue (with cramps caused by lactic acid accumulation) usually occurs unless the person is trained to tolerate fatigue and pain. With physical training, both the VT or AT and the peak VO_2 or VO_2max generally increase. Also, the VT (or AT)/peak VO_2 ratio increases to as high as 0.85 in some highly trained endurance athletes.

e. ***Ventilatory equivalents (V_E)*** denote the efficiency of ventilation related to metabolism. Normally, the resting V_E values for oxygen (i.e., V_EO_2) and for carbon dioxide (i.e., V_ECO_2) are 35–60. During exercise near the AT, the V_EO_2 decreases to 23–27, while the V_ECO_2 decreases to 28–30. If the V_EO_2 and V_ECO_2 do not decline appropriately, it is most likely the result of a high dead space volume/tidal volume ratio (VD/TV, see below). When exercising at or above the AT, the resulting metabolic acidosis stimulates further ventilation, thus both V_EO_2

and V_ECO_2 become significantly elevated. Increased V_EO_2 and V_ECO_2 is also caused by inefficient ventilation seen in patients with pulmonary hypertension and restrictive (i.e., interstitial) lung disease. Another cause for elevated V_E is unusually low $PaCO_2$ (e.g., in acute hyperventilation, chronic respiratory alkalosis, or chronic metabolic acidosis), thus arterial blood gases need to be checked to rule this out.

f. ***Dead space volume/tidal volume (VD/TV)*** is calculated from the measured mixed expired carbon dioxide, $PaCO_2$, TV, and the dead space of the breathing valve and mouthpiece or face mask. During exercise, as the TV increases and the airspaces are increasingly perfused with highly carbon dioxide-laden blood, the VD/TV normally decreases. In normal, sedentary middle-aged men, the VD/TV falls to 0.30 or less at maximal exercise, while in younger men the decrease is even greater. If there is primary or secondary pulmonary vascular disease or severe maldistribution of ventilation to perfusion, the VD/TV does not decline appropriately but may be increased at rest and markedly increased with exercise. Increased VD/VT is also seen in both restrictive lung disease (due to low TV) and obstructive lung diseases (due to inability to expire fixed TV).

3. **Test interpretation**. The use of CP-GXTT for exercise prescription is similar to that for CP-GXTT described above. For specifics on how to use it for prescribing aerobic exercise intensity, see Chapter 4.2, section III.A. The CP-GXTT can also be used to determine the need for supplemental oxygen during exercise (see Chapter 5.12, section IV.A.3 for parameters on the prescription of O_2 supplementation).

a. ***Treadmill CP-GXTTs*** provide a more accurate functional assessment of the patient with mild to moderate pulmonary disease than does a bicycle ergometer test. For a full discussion on the advantages and disadvantages of treadmill testing, refer to section I.A.1. Some of the commonly used treadmill protocols for CP-GXTT in pulmonary patients are shown in Table 2.7-7. These protocols are extremely low levels (i.e., low speed, low increment, and low MET levels). For less impaired patients in whom these protocols may be too slow, the modified treadmill protocols for cardiac patients may be used (see Table 2.7-6). In general, the Bruce protocol is rarely indicated in pulmonary patients because of its high workload. To convert the patient's "maximal" workload on the treadmill into METs, refer to Table 2.7-3.

b. ***Bicycle ergometer CP-GXTTs*** have the same indications, advantages, and disadvantages as those used for CV-GXTT (see section I.A.2). Some of the low-level bicycle protocols commonly used for CP-GXTT in pulmonary patients are shown in Table 2.7-7. To convert the patient's "maximal" workload on the bicycle ergometer into METs, refer to Table 2.7-4. The bicycle ergometer test is preferred by most pulmonary patients. In patients with severe pulmonary disease, the bicycle ergometer test is better than the TM test because exercise effort is less, supplemental O_2 can be used, and metabolic measures are easier to calculate.

B. **CONSTANT WORKLOAD CP-ETTs** use a series of constant workloads, which can be repeated at progressively higher intensities with rest periods in between. They may take one or more days to complete. Patients using constant workloads can achieve a peak VO_2 or VO_2max for a given task similar to that when using the more practical continuous incremental workload. Constant workload CP-ETTs may be used for evaluating the efficacy of oxygen breathing or drug therapy in relieving symptoms or for an accurate measurement of the AT (see AT description in section II.A above).

C. **TIMED WALKING TEST** is easy and inexpensive and can be used as an objective way of measuring exercise performance before and after a therapeutic intervention. The patient is asked to walk as far as possible in 6 minutes (this may be modified to 12 minutes, or, in patients with severe pulmonary conditions, to as low as 2 or 3 minutes). The HR, BP, and walking time and distance are then measured. The results of the test, as described by Kenneth Cooper, have been shown to positively correlate with FVC and VO_2max as determined by CP-GXTT (i.e., incremental treadmill or bicycle ergometry test). Additional parameters that may be measured during the timed walking test are oxygen saturation, ECG, and perceived exertion.

Further reading

American College of Sports Medicine: *ACSM's guidelines for exercise testing and prescription*, ed 6, Philadelphia, 2000, Lippincott, Williams & Wilkins.

Beaver WL, Wasserman K, Whipp BJ: A new method for detecting anaerobic threshold by gas exchange. *J Applied Physiol* 60:2020–2027, 1986.

Brannon FJ, Foley MW, Starr JA, *et al.*: *Cardiopulmonary rehabilitation: basic theory and application*, ed 3, Philadelphia, 1998, FA Davis.

Ellestad MH: *Stress testing: principles and practice*, ed 5, New York, 2003, Oxford Press.

Fardy PS, Yanowitz FG, Wilson PK: *Cardiac rehabilitation, adult fitness, and exercise testing*, ed 3, Philadelphia, 1996, Lippincott, Williams & Wilkins.

Flores AM, Zohman LR: Rehabilitation of the cardiac patient. In DeLisa JA, Gans BM, editors: *Rehabilitation medicine: principles and practice*, ed 3, Philadelphia, 1998, Lippincott-Raven, pp. 1337–1357.

Froelicher VF, Myers JN: *Exercise and the heart*, ed 4, Philadelphia, 2000, WB Saunders.

Gibbons RJ, Balady GJ, Bricker JT, *et al.*: ACC/AHA 2002 guideline update for exercise testing: summary article: a report of the American College of Cardiology/American Heart Association Task Force on Practice Guidelines (Committee to Update the 1997 Exercise Testing Guidelines). *Circulation* 106(14):1883–1892, 2002.

Hansen JE, Wasserman K: The integrated cardiopulmonary exercise stress test. In Demeter SL, Andersson GBJ, editors: *American Medical Association: disability evaluation*, ed 2, St Louis, 2003, Mosby, pp. 342–360.

Myers JN, Froelicher VF: Exercise testing and prescription. *Phys Med Rehabil Clin North Am* 6(1):117–151, 1995.

Salazar-Schicchi J, Haas F, Reggiani JL: Exercise stress testing. In Haas F, Axen K, editors: *Pulmonary therapy and rehabilitation. Principles and practice*, ed 2, Baltimore, 1991, Williams & Wilkins, pp. 121–131.

Smith EL and Gilligan C: Physical activity prescription for the older adult. *Phys Sportsmed* 11:91–101, 1983.

Solberg G, Robstad B, Skjønsberg OH, *et al.*: Respiratory gas exchange indices for estimating the anaerobic threshold. *J Sports Sci Med* 4, 29–36, 2005.

Stein J, editor: *Textbook of internal medicine*, ed 4, St Louis, 2000, Elsevier.

Subcommittee on Exercise Testing: Guidelines for exercise testing: A report of the American College of Cardiology American Heart Association Task Force on Assessment of Cardiovascular Procedures. *J Am Coll Cardiol* 8:725–738, 1986.

Wasserman K, Hansen JE, Sue DY, *et al.*: *Principles of exercise testing and interpretation: including pathophysiology and clinical applications*, ed 4, Philadelphia, 2004, Lippincott, Williams & Wilkins.

CHAPTER 2.8
Functional assessment instruments

Functional assessment instruments (FAIs) are standardized tests used to quantify change in function over time as a result of rehabilitation intervention (i.e., functional outcome). They are used not only for the management of individual patients (e.g., for planning treatment, determining effective and efficient treatment, maintaining continuity of care) but also for developing and improving treatment resources (e.g., performing program evaluation, quality assurance, and medical care audit studies to detect deficiencies in care and then to improve care). FAIs can be used in different health-care settings (inpatient, outpatient, and long-term facilities) to detect functional, cognitive, affective, and continence dysfunction not usually recognized on clinical examination. The following are some of the more popular FAIs used in PM&R.

I. FAIs measuring basic activity of daily living (B-ADL)

These are earlier forms of FAIs, which typically measure B-ADL skills, i.e., mobility and self-maintenance skills (e.g., feeding, dressing, grooming, bathing, personal hygiene, and toileting activities); see Chapter 4.5, section II.A.

A. BARTHEL INDEX measures 10 items: bowel control, bladder control, feeding, personal grooming and hygiene, dressing, bathing, toilet use, transfer, mobility, and stair negotiation. Items are scored according to a weighted numerical system with total scores ranging from 0 (totally dependent) to 20 (totally independent). By multiplying each item score by 5, an equivalent score of 0 to 100 may be obtained. Its inter-rater reliability is >0.95 and its test–retest reliability is 0.89. It was widely used in the United States to assess disability and rehabilitation outcome in patients with stroke or spinal cord injury. A maximum Barthel score does not necessarily signify independence in all ADL because it does not measure cognition or higher levels of functions (e.g., instrumental activities of daily living or IADLs such as cooking, housekeeping, and socialization are not assessed).

B. PULSES PROFILE measures the following: Physical condition or basic health/illness status, Upper limb functions, Lower limb functions and mobility, Sensory components (sight and communication), Excretory function (bowel and bladder control), Support factors (psychosocial, emotional, family, social, financial support). Each section is graded from 1 (no abnormalities) to 4 (severe abnormalities limiting independence) with scores ranging from 6 to 24. Its scoring system and rating criteria were modified in 1975. Its inter-rater reliability is >0.95 and its test–retest reliability is 0.87. It is currently used to detect functional change before discharge among various patient populations, especially in patients with stroke or spinal cord injury in whom substantial functional improvement is likely to occur. Its limitation is that it lacks subscore detail in discrete ADL variables.

C. KATZ INDEX OF INDEPENDENCE IN ADL evaluates the patient's functional independence in bathing, dressing, going to the toilet, transfers, continence, and feeding. Through observation, the rater determines which assistance is needed, that is, active personal assistance, directive assistance, or supervision.

Using specific rating criteria, the patient's level of independence is ranked ordinally as A, B, C, D, E, F, G, or "other". An A signifies independence in all six functions, while G signifies dependence in all rated functions. "Other" signifies dependence in at least two functions but not classifiable as C, D, E, or F. Its coefficient of scalability is 0.89. It is used to study the results of treatment and prognosis in the elderly and chronically ill (e.g., recovery in stroke and the need for care among patients with rheumatoid arthritis). Its limitations are that it is mainly descriptive and the hierarchy of items signifying dependence is deterministic. Also, it does not assess walking or stain-climbing ability.

D. **KENNY SELF-CARE EVALUATION** measures 17 items in the following six categories: bed mobility, transfers, locomotion, dressing, personal hygiene, and feeding. The scoring ranges from 0 (completely dependent) to 4 (independent), the highest score being 24, which indicates maximum independence on the ADL skills assessed. Although it is sensitive to changes in overall function of the patient and can be used to document rehabilitation progress, it is not as widely used as the other scales. No formal reliability coefficients have been reported.

II. FAIs measuring B-ADL plus functional communication and social cognition

A. **FUNCTIONAL INDEPENDENCE MEASURES (FIM)** (see Fig. 2.8-1) is the most widely used functional assessment instrument in medical rehabilitation. It measures 18 items in six categories: self-care, sphincter control, mobility, locomotion, communication, and social cognition. Each item is scored on a seven-point ordinal scale (where 1 is total assistance; 7 is complete independence) with the total score ranging from 18 to 126. The score is a direct observational measure and may be based on information provided by a reliable observer, usually a trained clinician. Sometimes the information may be gathered from the patient or a family member, such as by telephone interview conducted by a trained clinician. Its interrater reliability is 0.95. The strength of the FIM instrument is that it measures social cognition and functional communication as well as mobility and activities of daily living (ADL), and it uses a seven-point scale, which is more sensitive for classification purposes and for detecting change compared with other scales. Contrary to the proclamations of some authors that it has "ceiling" and "floor" effects at the upper and lower ends of function, the main use of the FIM instrument is to validate the need for assistance from another person (burden of care) in personal care tasks as a measure of disability. FIM data are stored by the **Uniform Data System for Medical Rehabilitation** (UDS_{MR}) in databases collected from the United States and other countries to be used for program evaluation and outcome comparisons in rehabilitation. Item transformation through Rasch analysis has established two equal-interval measures of motor (13 items) and cognitive (5 items) functioning. Assessment ratings are based upon probabilistic relationships among FIM instrument items in an expected hierarchy from easy to difficult items. In general, it is expected that of the motor items, eating would be the easiest and that stair climbing would be the hardest. Of the cognitive items, expression and comprehension would be easiest and problem-solving would be the hardest. Since January 2002, the Medicare prospective payment system for inpatient rehabilitation facilities in the US requires collection of FIM instrument data in a modified form through the IRF–PAI (Inpatient Rehabilitation Facility–Patient Assessment Instrument). Prospective payment is determined through CMGs (case-mix groups that are based upon the relative severity of disability at admission.

UDS$_{MR}$^{SM} FIM^{SM} Instrument

Self-care	Admission*	Discharge*	Goal
A. Eating			
B. Grooming			
C. Bathing			
D. Dressing – upper			
E. Dressing – lower			
F. Toileting			
Sphincter control			
G. Bladder			
H. Bowel			
Transfers			
I. Bed, chair, wheelchair			
J. Toilet			
K. Tub, shower			
Locomotion (W-walk, C-wheelchair, B-both)			
L. Walk/wheelchair			
M. Stairs			
Communication (A-auditory, V-visual, B-both; V-vocal, N-nonvocal, B-both)			
N. Comprehension			
O. Expression			
Social cognition			
P. Social interaction			
Q. Problem solving			
R. Memory			

* Leave no blanks. Enter 1 if not testable due to risk

FIM levels

No helper

7 Complete independence (timely, safely)
6 Modified independence (device)

Helper – modified dependence

5 Supervision (subject = 100%)
4 Minimal assistance (subject = 75% or more)
3 Moderate assistance (subject = 50% or more)

Helper – complete dependence

2 Maximal assistance (subject = 25% or more)
1 Total assistance or not testable (subject less than 25%)

Figure 2.8-1 The Functional Independence Measure (FIM™) instrument rating form. (Reprinted with permission from the Uniform Data System for Medical Rehabilitation, a division of UB Foundation Activities, Inc. (UDS$_{MR}$^{SM}). Copyright 1997. *Guide for the Uniform Data Set for Medical Rehabilitation [including the FIM™ instrument], version 5.1.*, Buffalo, NY, 1997, State University of New York at Buffalo.)

B. **PATIENT EVALUATION AND CONFERENCE SYSTEM (PECS)** uses a seven-point ordinal scale ranging from 1 (dependent) to 7 (fully independent) to measure 115 items divided into 16 different disciplinary sections (i.e., medical, nursing, physical mobility, ADL, communication, medications, assistive device utilization, psychology, neuropsychology, social issues, vocational and educational activity, therapeutic recreation, pain, nutrition, pulmonary rehabilitation, and pastoral care). Each section is completed by the discipline primarily responsible for the specific aspect of care. Analyses of PECS have shown that it has four underlying unidimensional interval subscales (i.e., impairment severity, applied self-care, knowledge of medication, and cognition subscales). The inter-rater reliability for different sections of the PECS ranges from 0.68 to 0.80. PECS focuses on long-term needs and program evaluation. It measures rehabilitation team goals and provides feedback on the patient's frequency of goal achievement. It can be used to predict the level of care needed after discharge from a treatment facility.

C. **LEVEL OF REHABILITATION SCALE III (LORS III)** uses a five-point scale from 0 (unable to perform activity) to 4 (able to perform) to measure five interval subscales assessing ADL, mobility, communications, cognitive ability, and memory. Its ADL subscale, however, does not measure bladder or bowel incontinence. Similar to the UDS_{MR} using the FIM instrument, it uses a national database, i.e., the **LORS-III American Data System (LADS)**, for program evaluation and outcome comparisons in rehabilitation.

III. FAIs measuring instrumental ADL (I-ADL)

FAIs measuring I-ADLs (see Chapter 4.5, section II.B) include more advanced problem-solving skills, and more complex environmental interactions, such as home management (e.g., cleaning, bed-making, laundry, meal preparation), community living skills (e.g., using a telephone, shopping, driving, managing of money), and occupational activities (e.g., leisure, work).

A. **OLDER AMERICANS RESOURCES AND SERVICES (OARS) MULTIDIMENSIONAL FUNCTIONAL QUESTIONNAIRE (MFAQ)** is a multidimensional assessment tool containing more than 100 questions in five domains: social resources, economic resources, mental health, physical health, and ability to carry out ADLs. It uses a six-point scale ranging from 1 (excellent level of functioning) to 6 (totally impaired level of functioning). It was specifically designed to determine the impact of services and of alternative service programs on the functional status of older people. It can be used as individual clinical assessment of personal functional status, surveys of the status of adult populations, assessment of service utilization and service requirements, longitudinal investigations in community, clinic, and long-term care settings, and training of service providers. Its initial and later ratings correlated from 0.47 to 1.00, the majority being over 0.85.

B. **PHILADELPHIA GERIATRIC CENTER (PGC) I-ADL** uses the Guttman scale (i.e., a cumulative scale) to measure the broad base of information necessary for independent living at home and in the community, including questions on use of telephone, walking, shopping, food preparation, housekeeping, laundry, public transportation, and medicine.

IV. FAIs measuring quality of life (QoL)

FAIs measuring QoL entail a multidimensional quantification of the patients' appraisal of and satisfaction with their current level of functioning as compared to what they perceive to be possible or ideal. QoL scales are not criterion referenced because they generally ask the subject to compare himself or herself to his or her prior healthy state. They encompass not only physical functions, but also social and emotional functions. Components of QoL generally include social roles and interactions, functional performance, intellectual functioning, perception of health status, and general satisfaction with life. QoL scales can be useful in helping to indicate the success of rehabilitation.

A. MEDICAL OUTCOMES STUDY (MOS) 36-ITEM SHORT FORM HEALTH SURVEY uses a generic, well-standardized health status scale, **Short Form 36 (SF-36)**, to assess a person's perception of wellness. The SF-36 comprises 36 items that measure health concepts in eight domains: physical limitations because of health problems; limitations in social activities because of physical or emotional problems; limitations in usual role activities because of physical health problems; bodily pain; general mental health (psychological distress and well-being); limitations in usual role activities because of emotional problems; vitality (energy and fatigue); and general health perceptions. It has a possible "floor" effect in seriously ill patients (especially for physical functioning), thus its use may need to be supplemented by an ADL scale. Although widely used in the clinics and in the community, its ability to follow people with disability is not known.

B. SICKNESS IMPACT PROFILE (SIP) is a generic instrument used to provide a descriptive profile of changes in a person's behavior as a result of sickness. It evaluates observable behavior rather than subjective health perceptions. It comprises 136 items related to 12 domains: mobility, ambulation, domestic affairs, social interaction, behavior, communications, recreation, eating, work, sleep, emotions, and self-care. Its scores (range 0–100%) discriminate between psychosocial and physical dysfunction. It has satisfactory internal consistency, good test–retest reliability, and construct validity. Although clinically comprehensive, it is lacking in questions on well-being, happiness, and satisfaction. Because of its broad range of items, the "floor" or "ceiling" effects of SIP are reduced. SIP is commonly used in the research setting, but it is not as widely used as the SF-36 in the clinics because of its length. Like SF-36, the usefulness of SIP for following persons with disability is not known.

C. THE LIFEware^{SM} SYSTEM is an online functional assessment and outcomes tracking system designed for persons with musculoskeletal and neurological disabilities or chronic health conditions. Most frequently it is used to measure functional outcomes in patients after they receive rehabilitation services in an outpatient setting. The LIFEware^{SM} System is applicable for outpatient rehabilitation clinics and ambulatory care settings, as well as private therapy and medical practices. The system consists of over 50 quality of daily living scales and measures (including the FIM™ instrument). These are grouped under seven core domains: physical functioning, cognitive functioning, emotional effect, experience with pain, degree of social interaction and degree of role participation, plus satisfaction with the treatment experience. Assessment forms appropriate for the types of patients being seen are created from various combinations of these scales and measures. Both standard and custom assessment forms are available.

An initial assessment is made prior to a patient receiving therapy services, interim assessments may optionally be performed, and a final assessment is made when treatment is completed. If desired, patient follow-up assessments may also be completed 80–180 days post discharge to document further change or else stability in functional status. For most assessments, patients self-report on the various measures. For some, clinician/therapist input is required, for example, joint specific measures of the knee, shoulder, ankle, etc. Patient data are entered directly into the LIFEware^{SM} system via the Internet or indirectly via fax.

The LIFEware^{SM} system automatically analyzes pre- and post-assessment ratings to create objectified patient reports of functional status and any change following treatment. It also furnishes national benchmark reports whereby a facility or therapist may compare their patient outcomes with those of similar patients across the country. Unique features of the LIFEware^{SM} system include its ability to track the functional status of patients over an indefinite period of time and its ability to alert the clinician to the status of specific items within a measure that fall below a predetermined expected value.

Further reading

Baker JG, Granger CV: Application of Rasch analysis in the development of the Medical Rehabilitation Follow-Along Measure (MRFA). *Am J Phys Med Rehabil* 11:305–313, 1997.

Baker JG, Granger CV, Ottenbacher KJ: Validity of a brief outpatient functional outcome assessment measure. *Am J Phys Med Rehabil* 75:356–363, 1996.

Bergner M, Bobbitt RA, Carter WB, *et al.*: The Sickness Impact Profile: development and final revision of a health status measure. *Med Care* 19:787–805, 1981.

Carey RG, Posavac EJ. Program evaluation of a physical medicine and rehabilitation unit: a new approach. *Arch Phys Med Rehabil* 59(7):330–337, 1978.

Christiansen CH: Functional evaluation and management of self-care and other activities of daily living. In DeLisa JA, Gans BM, Walsh NE, *et al.*, editors: *Physical medicine and rehabilitation: principles and practice*, ed 4, Philadelphia, 2005, Lippincott, Williams & Wilkins, pp. 975–1004.

Clark GS, Granger CV: Functional evaluation and outcome measurement. In Grabois M, Garrison SJ, Hart KA, *et al.*, editors: *Physical medicine and rehabilitation: the complete approach*, Malden, MA, 2000, Blackwell Science, pp. 225–241.

Duke University Center for the Study of Aging and Human Development: *Multidimensional functional assessment: the OARS methodology*. Durham, NC, 1978, Duke University.

Granger CV: The LIFEware system^{SM}. *J Rehabil Outcomes Meas* 3:63–69, 1999.

Granger CV, Ottenbacher KJ, Baker JG, *et al.*: Reliability of a brief outpatient functional outcome assessment measure. *Am J Phys Med Rehabil* 74:469–475, 1995.

Granger CV, Lackner JM, Kulas M, Russell, CF: Outpatients with low back pain: an analysis of the rate per day of pain improvement that may be expected and factors affecting improvement. *Am J Phys Med Rehabil* 82:253–260, 2003.

Granger CV, Hamilton BB, Sherwin FS: *Guide for use of the uniform data set for medical rehabilitation*, Buffalo, 1986, Uniform Data System for Medical Rehabilitation.

Guccione AA: Functional assessment. In O'Sullivan SB, Schmitz TJ, editors: *Physical rehabilitation: assessment and treatment*, ed 4, Philadelphia, 2001, FA Davis, pp. 309–332.

Harvey RF, Jellinek HM: Functional performance assessment: a program approach. *Arch Phys Med Rehabil* 62:456–460, 1981.

Katz S, Ford AB, Moskowitz RW: Studies of illness in the aged. The index of ADL: a standardized measure of biological and psychosocial function. *J Am Med Assoc* 185:914–919, 1963.

Lawton MP: The functional assessment of elderly people. *J Am Geriatr Soc* 19:465–481, 1971.

Linn RT, Granger CV, Disler PB, *et al.*: Applications of functional assessment to musculoskeletal disability evaluation. *Phys Med Rehabil Clin N Am* 12(3):529–541, 2001.

Mahoney FI, Barthel DW: Functional evaluation: the Barthel index. *Maryland State Med J* 14(2):61–65, 1965.

Moskowitz E, McCann CB: Classification of disability in the chronically ill and aging. *J Chronic Dis* 5:342–346, 1957.

Schoening HA, Anderegg L, Bergstrom D, *et al.*: Numerical scoring of self-care status of patients. *Arch Phys Med Rehabil* 46:689–697, 1965.

Uniform Data System for Medical Rehabilitation. *The LIFEware System^{SM} Clinical Guide*. Buffalo, NY, UDSMR, 2002.

Uniform Data System for Medical Rehabilitation. *The LIFEware^{SM} System Standard Quarterly Report Explanation Guide*. Version 1.0. Buffalo, NY, UDSMR, 2004.

Ware JE, Sherbourne CD: The MOS 36-Item Short Form Survey (SF-36): conceptual framework and item selection. *Med Care* 30:473–483, 1992.

CHAPTER 2.9
Psychologic tests

This chapter gives an overview of the common psychologic tests used in PM&R. They are typically administered by a psychologist or a neuropsychologist. Tests used specifically for determining psychological aspects of pain are discussed in Chapter 5.10, section IV.

I. Personality tests

Personality tests provide information about an individual's emotional stability, motivation, interpersonal relations, interests, and attitudes. They usually involve completion of a self-administered questionnaire.

A. MINNESOTA MULTIPHASIC PERSONALITY INVENTORY (MMPI; revised in 1989 as **MMPI-2**) is the most widely used and extensively researched objective test of personality. In PM&R it is commonly used to help determine the presence of conversion disorders in patients with chronic pain. Specific scales on the test have been reported to correlate with chronic pain treatment outcome, with particular emphasis on scales 1 (hypochondriasis), 2 (depression), and 3 (hysteria). Chronic pain patients may also have elevated scale 6 (paranoia) and 8 (schizophrenia) because of sensory disturbances, confusion because of medications, or bizarre interpretation of their symptoms. There are also extensive MMPI data on specific disability groups such as patients with spinal cord injury and multiple sclerosis.

The MMPI contains 556 true–false questions describing one's thoughts, feelings, ideas, attitudes, behaviors, physical and emotional symptoms, and life experiences. Items are grouped into 10 clinical scales on the basis of their ability to distinguish between a criterion group, having certain defined characteristics or displaying certain distinctive behaviors, and the general population. These clinical scales are interpreted with the help of four validity scales that are effective in identifying attempts at malingering and provide a sensitive indicator of unconscious or other subtle distortions of responses. The MMPI provides information on the patient's response style by evaluating various areas, such as literacy, cooperation, tendency toward malingering, comprehension, and use of denial or defensiveness. A score of 70 or greater (98th percentile on general population norms) is traditionally considered suggestive of a pathologic level of the trait in question.

The MMPI requires a sixth-grade reading level and is appropriate for age 15 and above. It needs 1.5–2 hours to complete. A variety of factors, such as race, socioeconomic status, unique family circumstances, and ethnic background, may distort its profile. New norms include larger samples subdivided by gender and age and exclude individuals with a history of major medical or psychiatric illness. They have been shown to validate the original norms. The new MMPI-2 provides larger, nationally represented norms and updated item content with 567 true–false questions; however, it requires an eighth-grade reading level (compared to sixth grade for the original MMPI) and is to be used only with adults aged 18 years or older.

B. MILLON CLINICAL MULTIAXIAL INVENTORY III (MCMI-III) is intended for screening patients suspected of significant personality disorders and is inappropriate for the general patient population. It consists of 175 true–false items written at an eighth-grade reading level and is appropriate for patients aged

18 years or older. It takes 25 minutes to complete. The questions are divided into categories that reflect enduring personality characteristics (i.e., Axis II), clinical syndromes (Axis I), and levels of pathologic severity. The MCMI-III is the only clinically oriented personality inventory reflective of Diagnostic and Statistical Manual of Mental Disorders (DSM-IV) diagnostic categories. However, its orientation toward the detection of pathologic personalities might produce an overly pathologic view of rehabilitation patients. To date, there are no existing normative data that can help guide the use of the MCMI in the rehabilitation setting.

C. **MILLON BEHAVIORAL HEALTH INVENTORY (MBHI)** is a self-report inventory consisting of 150 true–false items based on 20 clinical scales that measure personality styles, physical concerns, and behavioral reactions to disease or illness. Eight of these scales measure basic coping styles (e.g., introversive, inhibitive, cooperative, sociable, confident, forceful, respectful, and sensitive), which are suggestive of patients' styles of relating to their providers. Six of these scales assess psychosocial attitudes, such as chronic tension, recent stress, premorbid pessimism, future despair, social alienation, and somatic anxiety. Three of these scales depict probable responses to illness, including allergic inclination, gastrointestinal susceptibility, and cardiovascular tendency. The three final scales attempt to predict response to pain–treatment, life-threat reactivity, and emotional vulnerability. The test takes 30–45 minutes to complete. Its reliability is good, but its validity remains unproven. It can be used in the PM&R setting to measure patients' attitudes toward their own health and health-care providers.

D. **THE NEUROTICISM, EXTROVERSION, AND OPENNESS PERSONALITY INVENTORY-REVISED (NEO-PI-R)** provides a detailed systematic assessment of normal personality. It measures the five major domains of personality [Neuroticism (vs. Stability), Extraversion (vs. Introversion), Openness to experience, Agreeableness/Antagonism, and Conscientiousness/Undirectedness], as well as the six traits that define each domain, to summarize a person's emotional, interpersonal, experiential, attitudinal, and motivational styles. It is designed for individuals who are at least 17 years old with a sixth-grade reading level. It has both a self-report and an observer rating form. It takes 35–45 minutes to complete and uses a five-point rating scale (from strongly disagree to strongly agree) on 240 items and three validity items. These items do not have references to physical abilities or sensation that might distort the responses of a physically disabled person. Test–retest reliability falls between 0.66 and 0.92. It is limited by its assumption of honesty from the respondent, as well as its lack of subtle items or validity scales. It is also unclear how much the person's current mood (state) may affect his or her response to test items describing long-standing personality characteristics (trait).

E. **STRONG INTEREST INVENTORY (SII)** is the most recent version of the Strong Vocational Interest Blank (SVIB), which is traditionally used to measure vocational interests but can also be used as a valid nonpathology-oriented measure of personality. It asks the respondent to indicate liking, indifference, or dislike for occupations, school subjects, activities, amusements, and types of people. Two subsections ask for preferences between two occupational activities and the self-rated possession of 13 personal characteristics. The test contains 325 items, requires 45–50 minutes to complete, and is written at an eighth-grade reading level.

II. Intellectual ability tests

Tests of intellectual ability are used to measure general intellectual ability to help the physiatrist set appropriate expectations about the rate and complexity of learning that can be legitimately expected from the patient. They can also be used to determine the presence of organic brain dysfunction and provide guidance for post-discharge vocational and educational planning.

A. **STANFORD–BINET INTELLIGENCE TEST, FIFTH EDITION (SB5)** provides a complete assessment of individual intelligence by comprehensively measuring five factors – fluid reasoning, knowledge, quantitative reasoning, visual–spatial processing, and working memory. It includes a wide variety of nonverbal items, hence it is ideal for assessing individuals with limited English, deafness, or communication disorders. It can compare verbal and nonverbal performance – useful in evaluating learning disabilities. Responses are scored according to established procedures to yield mental age and an intelligence quotient (IQ). This is then reported in percentiles. The IQs measured in SB5 include Full-Scale IQ, Verbal and Nonverbal IQ, and Composite Indices spanning five dimensions with a standard score mean of 100, standard deviation (SD) 15. SB5 has enhanced memory tasks that provide a comprehensive assessment for adults and the elderly. It has very high reliabilities (ranging from 0.84 to 0.98). It is appropriate for individuals from 2 to 90+ years old. It includes many untimed tasks with an average testing time of 45–60 minutes.

B. **WECHSLER ADULT INTELLIGENCE SCALE, III (WAIS-III)** comprises 14 subtests (six for verbal IQ; five for performance IQ; one for symbol search; one for matrix reasoning; and one for letter–number sequencing) for individuals ≥16 years old. It takes 75–90 minutes to complete. Raw scores are converted into scale scores and reported in percentiles. It yields a Full Scale IQ, Verbal IQ, Performance IQ, and four indices: Verbal Comprehension, Perceptual Organizational, Working Memory, and Processing Speed. Compared to its older editions, the WAIS-III has: updated norms; culturally up-to-date items; more really easy items and really hard items (to decrease the "floor" and "ceiling" effect); measures for fluid reasoning, or on-the-spot reasoning processes; and computations based on age groups (i.e., if you are 37, you are compared to other 35–44 year olds, rather than a standard age sample of 20–44). It is commonly used in rehabilitation (e.g., as part of neuropsychologic evaluation in patients with traumatic brain injury). Test–retest reliability for the IQs and indices ranges from 0.88 to 0.96.

III. Academic achievement tests

These provide insight into the patient's current level of academic achievement and are used to determine the patient's educational and vocational needs, especially after discharge from the hospital. Those with low achievement levels for reading and math may need special education.

A. **WIDE-RANGE ACHIEVEMENT TEST 3 (WRAT-3)** assesses three types of academic achievement: reading, spelling, and arithmetic. It can be used for individuals from 5 through 75 years old. The test can be completed in 20–30 minutes. Although the WRAT-3 is reliable, the reading subtest does not measure reading comprehension. Instead it requires the subject to recognize and name letters and correctly pronounce individual words. Hence, its critics feel that the reading subtest is limited in testing reading comprehension.

B. **WOODCOCK–JOHNSON III PSYCHO-EDUCATIONAL BATTERY (WJ-III) TESTS OF ACHIEVEMENT** include three tests of academic fluency (i.e., Reading, Math, and Writing) and five oral language tests (Story Recall, Understanding Directions, Picture Vocabulary, Oral Comprehension, and Story Recall-Delayed). It has strong reliability (0.80 and higher) and can be used for individuals from 2 through 95 years old to provide three types of ability/achievement discrepancies: general intellectual ability to achievement, predicted achievement to achievement, and oral language to achievement. The oral language to achievement discrepancy (a new measure offered only in the WJ-III) allows comparison of oral language to academic performance to get an ability/achievement discrepancy evaluation. Hence, the individual's oral language ability becomes the predictor of his or her academic achievement. Unlike WRAT-III, the WJ-III reading score reflects diverse aspects of reading, not just correct word pronunciation. The administration time varies (about 5 minutes per test) and can reach up to 2 hours.

C. PEABODY INDIVIDUAL ACHIEVEMENT TEST-REVISED (PIAT-R) is an individually administered, norm-referenced measure of academic achievement. It is untimed and it scores in six content areas: general information, reading recognition, reading comprehension, mathematics, spelling, and written expression. It is not as comprehensive as the WJ-III, but is better suited for patients with low verbal abilities. The inter-rater reliabilities range from the 0.80s to mid-0.90s and the internal consistency reliability (composites) is in the upper 0.90s.

IV. Neuropsychologic battery tests

Neuropsychologic battery tests are standardized scales designed to test relatively pure cognitive skills and, thus, allow assessment of the presence and site of organic neurologic disease. They are commonly requested in the assessment of mental status after brain injury (e.g., traumatic brain injury, stroke); early diagnosis, assessment of severity, follow-up observation, and counseling in patients with suspected dementia; differentiation of the relative part played by functional and organic components in disease states; detection and evaluation of cognitive deficits in cases of learning disability, mental retardation, etc.; and counseling of patients and their families about management of acquired cognitive deficits.

A. HALSTEAD–REITAN NEUROPSYCHOLOGIC BATTERY (HRNB) consists of five tests of seven variables selected for their ability to distinguish frontal lobe dysfunction. The result is presented as the Halstead impairment index, a summary of values computed by dividing the number of test scores in the impaired range by seven. It should be placed in the context of other test data analyzed by inferential methods including level of performance, pattern of performance, and specific behavioral deficits or pathognomonic signs, and by comparison of performance of the right and left sides of the body. Although HRNB can diagnose the presence and type of brain dysfunction, it does not consistently localize lesions and discriminate psychiatric from organically impaired patients.

B. LURIA–NEBRASKA NEUROPSYCHOLOGICAL BATTERY (LNNB) has 269 items divided into 14 clinical scales. Performance on each item is scored from 0 (no impairment) to 2 (severe impairment). Total administration time is a maximum of 2.5 hours. The LNNB systematically assesses qualitative aspects of the patient's behavior, especially integrated motor performance. Criticisms involve issues of diagnostic unreliability, confounding of scale content, insufficient scale length, and difficulty in examining gradations of impairment.

C. BOSTON PROCESS APPROACH (BPA) combines quantitative and qualitative approaches to neuropsychological assessment. It uses tests with proven validity to identify patients with cognitive deficits. Once identified, these patients are systematically observed and tested (using a core set of frequently used and validated tests to assess intellectual and conceptual function; memory; language; visual–perceptual function; academic achievement; self-control and motor control) to determine their problem-solving strategies. Although the standardized instructions of the core set of tests are adhered to, the BPA also uses modifications to test the limits of the patients, e.g., adding new components to the established tests or asking the patient to respond to test items beyond the standard cut-off scores or time limits for test discontinuation. The BPA does not only concentrate on the test norms and patterns of scores, but also focuses on the manner in which the patient produced the response. Hence, the BPA claims it can potentially provide insight about the most effective cognitive rehabilitation methods to use in the remediation of patients with cognitive deficits.

V. Aptitude tests, vocational interest tests, and achievement or skill tests

These tests all measure global skills or interests in an effort to clarify an individual's vocational potential. They are generally used in the rehabilitation of work-related musculoskeletal problems (Examples are listed in Chapter 5.11, section V.D.2.c.).

VI. Value or attitude tests

Value or attitude tests are used by counselors as a focus for discussion of personal matters, and to assist their clients in gaining better self-understanding. Although they enhance communication in counseling and facilitate progress in vocational planning, the information they yield relates more to personality and life-style than to vocational choices or to questions of vocational success.

VII. Mood assessment tests

Mood assessment tests are used to measure depression and anxiety.

A. THE BECK DEPRESSION INVENTORY (BDI) consists of 21 items with a cumulative scoring system based on questions common in depression, such as sleep disturbance, weight change, fatigue factors, sexual dysfunction, and cognitive components of depressive illness. The patient selects one of four or five statements ranked in order of severity for each item. Scores range from 0 to 63 with high scores indicating greater depression. It requires only 5 minutes to complete. The BDI is commonly used throughout a treatment program for the chronic pain patient as a measure of improvement. It has good validity and reliability.

B. ZUNG SELF-RATING DEPRESSION SCALE is a 20-item, self-report measure yielding a numerical estimate of depression severity. Patients rank each item on a four-point scale indicating frequency of occurrence of symptom. The higher the score, the more severe is the depression. Data on retest reliability and on validity with nonpsychiatric patients are lacking.

C. SPIELBERGER STATE–TRAIT ANXIETY INVENTORY (STAI) is a 40-item, multiple choice, self-report questionnaire designed to measure trait anxiety (TA, i.e., a stable personality characteristic that describes a person's overall tendency to respond in a rather anxious manner, independent of the specific stimulus) and state anxiety [SA, i.e., anxiety (specifically feelings of apprehension, tension, nervousness, and worry) temporarily experienced in response to specific conditions]. TA scores are generally high in psychoneurotic and depressed patients. SA scores increase in response to physical danger and psychological stress, and decrease as a result of relaxation training. The STAI has good reliability and validity.

Further reading

Aronoff GM, editor: *Evaluation and treatment of chronic pain*, Baltimore, 1992, Williams & Wilkins.

Beck AT: *Beck depression inventory: manual,* San Antonio, 1987, Psychological Corporation.

Butcher JN, Spielberger CD, editors: *Advances in personality assessment*, vol. 2. Hillside, NJ, 1983, Lawrence Erlbaum Associates.

Butcher JN, Dahlstrom WG, Graham JR, *et al.*: *MMPI-2: manual for administration and scoring,* Minneapolis, 1989, University of Minnesota Press.

Costa PT Jr, McCrae RR: *NEO-PI-R professional manual*, Odessa, FL, 1992, Psychological Assessment Resources.

Dahlstrom WG, Welsh GS, Dahlstrom WG, editors: *An MMPI handbook, vol. I: clinical interpretation*, revised ed, Minneapolis, 1972, University of Minnesota Press.

Golden CJ, Hammeke TA, Purisch AD: *The Luria–Nebraska battery manual*, Los Angeles, 1980, Western Psychological Services.

Hansen JC, Campbell DP: *Manual for the strong interest inventory*, ed 4, Palo Alto, CA, 1985, Consulting Psychologists Press.

Kaufman AS, Lichtenberger EO: *Essentials of WAIS-III assessment*, New York, 1999, John Wiley & Sons.

Markwardt FC: *Peabody individual achievement test – Revised*, Circle Pines, MN, 1989, American Guidance Service.

Mather N, Jaffe LE: *Woodcock–Johnson III: reports, recommendations, and strategies*, ed 2, New York, 2002, John Wiley & Sons.

Millburg WP, Hebben N, Kaplan E: The Boston Process Approach to neuropsychological assessment. In Grant I, Adams K, editors: *Neuropsychological assessment of neuropsychiatric disorders*, New York, 1986, Oxford University Press, pp. 65–86.

Millon T: *Millon Clinical Multiaxial Inventory III manual*, Minneapolis, 1994, National Computer System.

Millon T, Green CJ, Meagher RB: A new psychodiagnostic tool for clients in rehabilitation settings: The MBHI. *Rehab Psychol* 27(1):23–35, 1982.

Ranlett G, Bleiberg J: Psychological assessment in the rehabilitation setting. In Grabois M, Garrison SJ, Hart KA, *et al.*, editors: *Physical medicine and rehabilitation: the complete approach*, Malden, MA, 2000, Blackwell Science, pp. 303–310.

Reitan RM, Wolfson D: *The Halstead–Reitan neuropsychological test battery: theory and clinical interpretation*, Tucson, AZ, 1985, Neuropsychological Press.

Rohe DE: Psychological aspects of rehabilitation. In DeLisa JA, Gans BM, Walsh NE, *et al.*, editors: *Physical medicine and rehabilitation: principles and practice*, ed 4, Philadelphia, 2005, Lippincott, Williams & Wilkins, pp. 1005–1024.

Roid G: *Stanford-Binet intelligence scales,* ed 5, Illinois, 2003, Riverside.

Wilkinson GS: *Wide-Range achievement test administration manual*, Wilmington, DE, 1993, Wide Range, Inc.

Zung WWK: A self-rating depression scale. *Arch Gen Psychiatr* 12:63–77, 1965.

PART III

PHYSICAL MEDICINE AND REHABILITATION: DIFFERENTIAL DIAGNOSES

CHAPTER 3.1
Differential diagnoses of pain

As with other fields of medicine, the majority of complaints in PM&R are pain related. This chapter deals with the differential diagnoses of acute and chronic pain problems commonly encountered by the physiatrist in both in- and outpatient settings. These differential diagnoses are to be used as a guide in the diagnostic and therapeutic process of pain problems. Other details on acute and chronic pain (i.e., their neurophysiology, psychosocial factors, assessment, and management) are discussed in Chapter 5.10.

Pain problems may be related to either the neuromusculoskeletal systems or the non-neuromusculoskeletal systems. In making the differential diagnosis of pain, general sources of pain must be determined based on the patient's pain description. *Cutaneous pain* from skin and subcutaneous tissues is usually well localized. *Deep somatic pain* from bone, nerve, muscle, tendon, ligaments, periosteum, arteries, and joints is poorly localized and may be referred to the body surface (as cutaneous pain). *Visceral pain* from body organs in the trunk or abdomen usually corresponds to the dermatomes from which the affected organs receive their innervation. As a result of multisegmental innervation, visceral pain is not well localized and is usually referred to the back (generally from organs of the abdomen and pelvis) or shoulder (generally from intrathoracic organs and from the gallbladder). *Referred pain* (from either cutaneous, deep somatic, or visceral structures) is usually well localized but occurs in remote areas supplied by the same (shared) central afferent neurosegment supplying the affected organ. The usual musculoskeletal sites of referred pain are the shoulder, scapula, chest, thoracic spine, lumbar spine, groin, sacroiliac joint, and hip.

I. Neuromusculoskeletal pain problems

Joint pain because of nonsystemic joint dysfunction is sudden, sharp, occurring after some unguarded joint movement, and is associated with warmth or swelling. It is usually limited to one joint, aggravated by movement, and is reduced by rest. *Joint pain of systemic joint disease* can be deep, aching, throbbing, and may be reduced by pressure; it can be sharp or dull, or either constant or occurring in waves. Joint pain of systemic joint disease generally occurs with systemic signs and symptoms (e.g., skin rash, jaundice, fatigue, low-grade fever, and weight loss). *Pain as a result of musculoskeletal neoplasm* is usually constant, not relieved by changing positions or rest, and awakens the patient at night.

Muscular (or soft tissue) pain is induced by movement of musculoskeletal parts (bones, joints, bursae, tendons) or by mechanical forces (pressure or stretch) and is usually relieved by rest. Muscular pain may occur from accumulation of metabolites (e.g., from anaerobic exercise) or from ischemia (e.g., intermittent claudication). *Fibromyalgia pain,* usually seen in females, is insidious, diffuse, generalized, and occurs symmetrically in muscular and bony areas. *Myofascial pain* occurs with equal frequency in both sexes, is associated with acute muscle strain or chronic muscle overuse, is limited to muscles, and occurs asymmetrically in isolated or regional muscles. Both fibromyalgia and myofascial pain are associated with stress, poor sleep pattern, fatigue, depression, and negative laboratory and neurologic results.

Radicular pain is felt in a dermatome and myotome and is caused by the direct irritation or involvement of the root of a spinal nerve. If nerve root irritation is caused by compression, the pain may be relieved by decompression, either nonsurgically (e.g., sitting and bending forward may relieve the pain of spinal stenosis) or surgically. If the pain does not occur in a radicular pattern that conforms to a dermatome or myotome, then other diagnoses should be considered, such as diabetic neuropathy, toxic neuropathy, and psychiatric disorders (e.g., hysterical or conversion reactions). Patients with nonanatomic patterns of radicular pain (e.g., glove and stocking pattern or pain in entire leg) in the absence of any objective findings should be considered for further psychological assessment to rule out nonorganic causes, especially in the presence of inappropriate or exaggerated illness behaviors.

"Nonorganic" neuromusculoskeletal pain, which is usually seen in patients with chronic pain, includes psychosomatic musculoskeletal pain (e.g., tension syndrome or fibrositis), psychogenic musculoskeletal pain, psychogenic modification of organic musculoskeletal pain, and situational spinal pain (e.g., litigation reaction and exaggeration reaction). The usual symptoms of "nonorganic" pain are multifocal pain, nonmechanical pain (present at rest), involvement of entire limb, limb "gives way" (i.e., complaints of knee buckling, which patient is able to catch at the last minute), poor response to treatment (e.g., no response to any treatment, "allergic" to treatment, and refusal of treatment), multiple crises, multiple hospital admissions or consultations, and multiple doctors. Signs of "nonorganic" pain (see Chapter 5.11, section V.B.3) include superficial tenderness (over skin), nonanatomic pain, positive simulated movement tests, positive distraction tests, weakness or numbness of the entire arm or leg, and an "award-winning" performance. A recent study by Giesecke *et al.* (2004) on idiopathic chronic low back pain patients suggests that evidence of augmented central pain processing might offer some organic basis to "nonorganic" pain.

The following differential diagnoses of neuromusculoskeletal pain problems are classified by syndromes and inferred pathophysiology, by specific body region, and by pattern and distribution of musculoskeletal pain.

A. DIFFERENTIAL DIAGNOSIS OF PAIN CLASSIFIED BY SYNDROMES AND INFERRED PATHOPHYSIOLOGY [based on the classification by Portenoy (see Further reading section); excluding headache and facial pain which are classified under systemic pain problems].

1. Neuropathic pain is any acute or chronic pain syndrome in which the sustaining mechanism for the pain is inferred to involve aberrant somatosensory processing in the peripheral or central nervous system (CNS). The following classification is based on inferred predominant pathophysiology rather than on the site of the inciting lesion or on the basis of diagnosis. It classifies whether neuropathic pain is primarily sustained by processes in the CNS or by processes in the peripheral nervous system.

a. Predominating "central" pain generator

I. **Deafferentation pain (anesthesia dolorosa)** is a descriptive term for pain because of injury of the central or peripheral nervous system. The term does not refer to any specific set of known mechanisms, although the pain is inferred to be predominantly the result of a sustaining central mechanism that is independent of activity in the sympathetic nervous system. There is "central sensitization", which is a denervation hypersensitivity of neurons and ectopic foci of spontaneous neuronal activity that develops in the dorsal horn of the spinal cord, thalamus, and, perhaps, cerebral cortex following an injury to afferent pathways. "Central desensitization" may involve changes in the central neurons that may be structural (e.g., transynaptic and transganglionic degeneration or collateral sprouting) or functional (e.g., lowered threshold for activation, exaggerated activation, ectopic discharges, enlarging receptive fields, and loss of normal inhibition).

- **Phantom pain.** Phantom limb pain, phantom pain following amputations of nonlimb structures (e.g., breast, tooth), and phantom body pain [i.e., pain in regions of the body that are totally denervated but not amputated, such as that which occurs after spinal cord transection or peripheral nerve injury; instead of using the confusing term *phantom body pain,* it is better to call it *central pain* (see below) or nonspecifically as *deafferentation pain*].
- **Avulsion of plexus.** Brachial plexus avulsion or lumbosacral plexus avulsion.
- **Postherpetic neuralgia**
- **Central pain syndrome** includes deafferentation pain syndromes that can occur following injury to the CNS. Some have been named by the location of the lesion (e.g., thalamic pain) or by the inciting injury (e.g., poststroke pain). Most however, do not conform to a named syndrome (e.g., pain associated with syringobulbia), hence it is better to use the term *central pain syndrome.*
  - ***Spinal cord lesions.*** Trauma, focal demyelination, infection, vascular lesions, neoplasms, syringomyelia.
  - ***Brainstem lesions.*** Vascular lesions, trauma, infection, neoplasms, syrinx, focal demyelination.
  - ***Cerebral lesions.*** Vascular lesions, trauma (including surgical), neoplasms, and lesions associated with seizures.
- **Others.** Complex regional pain syndrome (CRPS type I: reflex sympathetic dystrophy and CRPS type II: causalgia – described below) and miscellaneous labels for deafferentation pain (e.g., postsurgical pain syndrome and post-thoracotomy pain), which are merely descriptive and do not imply pathophysiology.

II. **Sympathetically maintained pain (SMP)** (Roberts, 1986; see Further reading section) is any pain that is sustained, at least in part, by sympathetic efferent activity. It is usually caused by a partial peripheral nerve lesion [unlike complex regional pain syndrome type I (reflex sympathetic dystrophy or RSD) which can be caused by any type of lesion]. It is hypothesized that SMP is caused by a vicious cycle of nerve injury, which results in sensitization (i.e., lowering of pain threshold) of central projection neurons (e.g., wide-dynamic-range neurons in the spinal cord) leading to their enhanced response to low-threshold mechanoreceptors and an increase in adrenergic receptors in the periphery, which may then be activated further by norepinephrine release from sympathetic fibers.

SMP occurs less commonly than CRPS type I (RSD). The cardinal symptoms of SMP are spontaneous pain (mostly burning; predominantly superficial; no orthostatic component, i.e., intensity is not dependent on the position of the limb), mechanical allodynia (i.e., pain produced by a normally nonpainful stimulus such as light touch, wind, and mild temperature changes), and local hyperalgesia (to cold stimulus). Other symptoms of SMP are autonomic dysregulation (e.g., edema, vasomotor disturbances), involuntary motor response, and trophic changes. The sensory, motor, and autonomic symptoms of SMP are mostly localized to the territory of the affected peripheral or spinal nerve [unlike CRPS type I (RSD) symptoms which occur independently from the site of the preceding lesion]. SMP can usually be alleviated by sympathetic blockade. Unequivocal (and at least temporary) relief of spontaneous and evoked pain after sympathetic blockade confirms the presence of SMP. Examples of neuropathic pain that may have SMP components include CRPS (see section I.A.1.c), phantom pain, avulsion of nerve plexus, postherpetic neuralgia, and metabolic neuropathies.

b. ***Predominating "peripheral" pain generator*** includes "nerve sheath pain", i.e., activation of "normal" nociceptors (e.g., sensitization of C and A-delta nociceptors following injury, "backfiring" of C-fiber with release of pain mediators, unmodulated pain input because of large-fiber loss, and activation of nociceptive nervi nervorum), and dysesthetic pain, i.e., aberrant activity from injured nerves (e.g., neuroma formation from severed nerve, focal demyelination, or formation of nociceptor ephapses or abnormal connections).

I. **Painful polyneuropathies**

- **Metabolic disorders.** Diabetic neuropathy, neuropathy associated with insulinoma, nutritional deficiency (e.g., alcohol-nutritional neuropathy, thiamine deficiency, niacin deficiency, pyridoxine deficiency, and Strachan's syndrome or Jamaican neuropathy, which may be associated with beriberi or pellagra), hypothyroid neuropathy, uremic neuropathy, amyloid neuropathy, and neuropathy associated with Fabry's disease.
- **Drugs or toxins.** Isoniazid, hydralazine, nitrofurantoin, metronidazole, phenytoin, disulfiram, gold, vincristine, cisplatin, alcohol, arsenic, cyanide, lead, and thallium.
- **Neoplasm.** Subacute sensory neuropathy (a subtype of paraneoplastic neuropathy most commonly associated with small cell carcinoma and other carcinomas and lymphomas), nonspecific paraneoplastic sensorimotor neuropathy associated with carcinoma, and sensorimotor neuropathy associated with dysproteinemia (e.g., multiple myeloma, Waldenström's macroglobulinemia, cryoglobulinemia, solitary plasmacytoma, and osteosclerotic plasmacytoma).
- **Connective tissue diseases.** Polyarteritis nodosa, rheumatoid arthritis (RA), systemic lupus erythematosus, and Churg–Strauss disease.
- **Other causes.** Hereditary neuropathy (e.g., hereditary sensory neuropathy type I), painful polyneuropathy associated with Guillain–Barré syndrome, acute intermittent porphyria, sarcoidosis, AIDS.

II. **Painful mononeuropathies** refer to a diverse group of pain syndromes, all of which are inferred to be associated with a known peripheral nerve injury, and are experienced, at least partly, in the territory of the affected nerve. The pain may follow the injury immediately and then persist, or it may occur days, weeks, months, or, rarely, years after nerve injury. The injury may be the result of:

- **Nerve inflammation.** Acute herpetic neuropathy, acute brachial plexus neuropathy (brachial plexitis), lumbosacral plexus neuropathy, and sensory perineuritis.
- **Nerve trauma** from transection (e.g., surgical), stretch, inflammation, or compression of the nerve. The most common types are those caused by neuroma (e.g., residual limb pain) or compression (e.g., low back pain because of spinal nerve compression by herniated nucleus pulposus and nerve entrapment such as carpal tunnel syndrome).
- **Nerve vascular lesion.** Diabetic mononeuropathy (femoral neuropathy, diabetic amyotrophy, lumbar radiculoplexopathy), cranial neuropathy (e.g., oculomotor neuropathy), thoracoabdominal neuropathies, mononeuritis or mononeuritis multiplex due to vasculitis (e.g., polyarteritis nodosa, RA), Sjögren's syndrome, and Churg–Strauss syndrome).
- **Nerve neoplasm** from benign tumors (neurofibroma) or malignant tumors.
- **Lancinating neuralgia** is related to nerve injury and is characterized by brief paroxysmal pain (similar to trigeminal neuralgia).

– ***Cranial neuralgias.*** Trigeminal neuralgia (the most common), glossopharyngeal neuralgia, occipital neuralgia, geniculate (nervus intermedius) neuralgia, supraorbital neuralgia, superior (or vagal) neuralgia. See also headache classification in I.A.4 and I.B.1.

– ***Neuralgia of other sites.*** Intercostal neuralgia, ilioinguinal neuralgia, genitofemoral neuralgia.

c. ***Complex regional pain syndrome (CRPS type I: RSD and CRPS type II: causalgia)*** has been ascribed to both central and peripheral processes. Peripheral processes include activity in nociceptive visceral afferents, which travel with sympathetic efferent fibers; processes unrelated to the sympathetic nervous system that increase activity in somatic nociceptors (e.g., sensitization following injury, C-fiber "backfiring" with release of pain mediators, and ectopic electrical activity from neuroma or areas of focal demyelination); and processes involving a sympathetic–somatic link (e.g., sympathetic hyperactivity that changes peripheral tissues to activate nociceptors in a "vicious cycle"; increased sensitivity of damaged nociceptors to catecholamines released by sympathetic nerves; nociceptor sensitization by prostaglandins released by sympathetic nerve; or formation of sympathetic nociceptor ephapses or abnormal connections). However, recent evidence favors a central mechanism as the fundamental process; the most compelling evidence being that the complete isolation of the painful part from the CNS, for example, by neurectomy or rhizotomy, did not reliably eradicate the pain. Other evidence of a central mechanism of CRPS type I (RSD) includes the occurrence of classic CRPS type I (RSD) following damage to the CNS or viscera.

CRPS type I (RSD) is known by many other names, such as shoulder–hand syndrome, post-traumatic syndrome, symphathalgia, and Sudeck's atrophy. According to the International Association for the Study of Pain (IASP) consensus (Janig *et al.*, 1991; see Further reading section), CRPS type I (RSD) is a "complex disorder or group of disorders that may develop as a consequence of trauma affecting the limbs, with or without an obvious nerve lesion. CRPS type I (RSD) may also develop after visceral diseases, and central nervous system lesions, or, rarely, without an obvious antecedent event. It consists of pain and related sensory abnormalities, abnormal blood flow and sweating, abnormalities in the motor system and changes in structure of both superficial and deep tissues ('trophic' changes). It is not necessary that all components are present. It is agreed that the name 'reflex sympathetic dystrophy' is used in a descriptive sense and does not imply specific underlying mechanisms." CRPS type II (causalgia) typically refers to the same syndrome as CRPS type I (RSD) but produced by peripheral nerve injury. The IASP criteria for CRPS type I and type II are shown in Table 3.1-1.

The underlying central mechanism of CRPS can be either sympathetically maintained or caused by deafferentation. CRPS is distinguished from SMP (see section I.A.1.a.2) in that CRPS is common, develops in the distal region of the affected limb irrespective of the type and the site of the preceding lesion [e.g., minor trauma, partial nerve lesion, bone fracture, and other lesions such as shoulder trauma, myocardial infarction (MI), or even a contralateral cerebrovascular lesion], is usually distally generalized (e.g., glove-like distribution), has common (but not obligatory) spontaneous pain (which has variable character, mostly deep and diffuse, with an orthostatic component, i.e., pain is alleviated by elevating the limb and aggravated by lowering it), and has less common incidence of mechanical allodynia than in SMP. The subtype of CRPS with SMP features responds favorably to sympathetic blockade.

In general, the symptoms of CRPS can be classified into: (a) sensory symptoms, i.e., deep spontaneous pain, hypo- or hyperalgesia, hypo- or hyperesthesia, movement-related pain, diffuse mechanical allodynia (seen in late cases), and hyperpathia (i.e., pain produced by painful stimuli that appears with a delay, outlasts the stimulus, and spreads beyond the site of the stimulus); (b) autonomic symptoms, i.e., distally generalized swelling, warm or cold

Table 3.1-1 The International Association for the Study of Pain (IASP) diagnostic criteria for complex regional pain syndrome (CRPS) type I (reflex sympathetic dystrophy or RSD) and type II (causalgia)

CRPS type I (RSD)	CRPS type II (causalgia)
1. Presence of an initiating noxious event.	1. Presence of more regionally confined presentation about a joint or area, associated with a nerve injury.
2. Spontaneous pain and/or allodynia and hyperalgesia occurring beyond the territory of a single peripheral nerve(s), and is disproportionate to the inciting event.	2. Spontaneous pain and/or allodynia and hyperalgesia are usually limited to the area involved, but may spread variably distal or proximal to the area, not in the territory of a dermatomal or peripheral nerve distribution.
3. There is, or has been, evidence of edema, skin blood flow abnormality (e.g., skin color changes, skin temperature changes more than 1.1°C difference from the homologous body part), or abnormal sudomotor activity in the region of pain since the inciting event.	3. Intermittent and variable edema, skin blood flow change (skin color changes, skin temperature changes more than 1.1°C difference from the homologous body part), or abnormal sudomotor activity, and motor dysfunction, disproportionate to the inciting event, are present about the area involved.
4. The diagnosis is excluded by the *presence* of identifiable major nerve lesion (CRPS type II) or the existence of conditions that would otherwise account for the degree of pain and dysfunction.	4. Diagnosis is excluded by the *absence* of identifiable major nerve lesion (CRPS type I) or the existence of conditions that would otherwise account for the degree of pain and dysfunction.

Note that laboratory testing is not *required for either CRPS type I or II diagnostic criteria. The CRPS criteria are being revised to address such issues as the necessity of the presence of an initiating noxious event; and the minimal number of symptoms or signs needed for diagnosis.*
Adapted and tabulated from Merskey H, Bogduk N: Classification of chronic pain, *Seattle, 1994, IASP Press; and Boas RA: Complex regional pain syndromes: symptoms, signs, and differential diagnosis. In Janig W, Stanton-Hicks M, editors:* Reflex sympathetic dystrophy: a reappraisal. Progress in pain research and management, *vol. 6, Seattle, 1996, IASP Press, p. 82.*

affected limb, marbled, reddish, or cyanotic skin, and hypo- or hyperhydrosis; and (c) motor symptoms, i.e., weakness, tremor (postural or action-related), difficulty in initiating movement, spasm, dystonia, and increased reflexes and tone.

In chronic cases of CRPS, there are trophic changes (e.g., disturbed nail growth, increased hair growth, palmar or plantar fibrosis, thin glossy skin, and hyperkeratosis) and changes in bone (e.g., diffuse distal osteoporosis). The staging of untreated CRPS into acute, dystrophic, and atrophic stages does not always conform to the clinical course, and is, thus, not very useful. It is probably more practical to grade the symptoms of CRPS according to their intensity (i.e., mild, moderate, or severe).

Prior to the IASP diagnostic criteria (see Table 3.1-1), the diagnostic criteria described by Kozin (1986) were used. These were: (a) definite RSD, indicated by pain in association with vasomotor instability, edema, and dystrophic skin and nail changes; (b) probable RSD, indicated by pain, vasomotor instability, and edema; (c) possible RSD, indicated by pain, and vasomotor instability or edema; and (d) doubtful RSD, indicated by pain alone. Although this simple diagnostic classification may be helpful in the clinics, empirical evidence is lacking. The treatment of CRPS is discussed in Chapter 5.10, section VI, and summarized in Table 5.10-2.

2. **Musculoskeletal pain**
a. ***Inflammatory arthropathies.*** Rheumatoid arthritis, seronegative spondyloarthropathies (e.g., ankylosing spondylitis, reactive arthritis, psoriatic arthritis, gut-associated arthritis), infections (e.g., bacterial, postviral).
b. ***Degenerative arthropathies.*** Osteoarthritis, aseptic necrosis, neuropathic ("Charcot") joints.
c. ***Crystal-associated arthropathies.*** Gout, calcium pyrophosphate deposition disease (or pseudogout).
d. ***Soft tissue rheumatic problems.*** Enthesopathies, injury, diffuse (fibromyalgia) and regional (myofascial pain) syndromes (either of which may be superimposed on other pain syndromes).
e. ***Systemic connective tissue diseases.*** Systemic lupus erythematosus (SLE), vasculitides, systemic sclerosis.
f. ***Metabolic bone disease.*** Osteoporosis, osteonecrosis, osteomalacia, Paget's disease.
3. **Low back pain** [based on the classification by Kanner (see Further reading section)].
a. ***Acute low back pain*** (see also section I.B.3.b)
   I. **Acute pain originating in the bony elements.** Vertebral metastases, osteoporosis, vertebral osteomyelitis, traumatic fractures.
   II. **Acute pain originating in the muscles, aponeuroses, and nerves.** Low back strain, locked back syndrome (i.e., slippage of an articular facet with encroachment on the pain-sensitive joint capsule), pain originating in neural structures, radicular pain without spinal pathology, herniated lumbar intervertebral disks.
b. ***Chronic low back pain***
   I. **Somatic nociceptive pain.** Degenerative spine or disk disease, facet disease, spondylolisthesis, fibromyalgia/myofascial pain syndrome.
   II. **Visceral nociceptive pain.** Referred from pelvic organ, the retroperitoneal space, the gallbladder, and the pancreas.
   III. **Neuropathic pain.** Lateral recess syndrome, spinal stenosis, lumbar arachnoiditis, neoplasm (e.g., neoplasm of the cauda equina, filum terminale, or lumbar dura).
   IV. **Psychogenic pain**, which may be associated with malingering, "hysterical features", delusional pain, depression, secondary gain (e.g., monetary compensation), and somatization.
c. ***Failed low back syndrome*** is broadly defined as persistent low back pain, despite usually efficacious therapy, occurring in a heterogeneous and difficult group of patients. In its most limited meaning, it refers to pain after surgery to correct the presumed cause of the pain. It could be the result of incorrect patient selection, incorrect surgery, or complications of surgery.
d. ***Noncancer chronic back pain syndrome*** is pain and disability disproportionate to any recognizable organic cause and is associated with abnormal pain behavior.
4. **Headache and facial pain** (see also section I.B.1)
a. ***Acute headache***
   I. **Focal headache**
   - **Vascular headache.** Complex migraine headache, cluster headache.
   - **Headache caused by meningeal inflammation.** Meningitis, encephalitis.
   - **"Traction headache" associated with increased intracranial pressure (ICP).** Tumor, subdural hemorrhage, intracranial bleeding, acute hydrocephalus, cerebral edema, brain abscess, subdural empyema, benign intracranial hypertension (or pseudotumor cerebri).

II. **Nonfocal headache**

- **Vascular headache.** New-onset migraine headache, reactive vasodilatation headache (e.g., fever, drug-induced, postictal, hypoglycemia, hypoxia, hypercarbia, hyperthyroidism), arterial hypertension (diastolic blood pressure above 120 mmHg), paroxysmal severe hypertension (e.g., pheochromocytoma, coital headache), giant cell ("temporal") arteritis.
- **Headache caused by meningeal inflammation**. Subarachnoid hemorrhage, meningitis, encephalitis.
- **Headache and head pain caused by cranial neuralgias**. Trigeminal neuralgia or "tic douloureux", glossopharyngeal neuralgia, occipital neuralgia, supraorbital neuralgia, geniculate (or nervus intermedius) neuralgia, superior (or vagal) neuralgia.
- **"Traction headache" associated with increased ICP**. Bilateral subdural hemorrhage, dural venous sinus thrombosis.
- **"Traction headache" associated with decreased ICP**. Postlumbar puncture headache.
- **Headache and head pains caused by diseases of eyes, ears, nose, sinuses, teeth, or skull** (e.g., sinusitis, glaucoma, extracranial infections).
- **Headache and facial pain without demonstrable physical findings.** Headache of uncertain cause (tension headache, post-traumatic headache).

b. Chronic/intermittent headache

I. **Headache with demonstrable muscle spasm**. Posturally induced (prolonged computer work, driving), paralesional muscle spasm (cervical spondylosis, cervical disk herniation), psychophysiologic muscular contraction (stress related), "muscle contraction headache", myofascial pain syndrome, temporomandibular syndrome, musculoskeletal headache.

II. **Headache and facial pain without demonstrable physical findings**. Headache of uncertain cause (tension headache), psychogenic headache (hypochondriacal, conversional, delusional, malingering), facial pain of uncertain cause ("atypical facial pain").

III. **Combined tension–migraine headache**. Episodic migraine superimposed on chronic tension headache, chronic daily headache ("rebound HA" associated with analgesic and/or ergotamine use).

IV. **Vascular headache.** Arteriovenous malformation.

V. **"Traction headache" associated with increased ICP**. Chronic hydrocephalus.

5. Pain syndromes associated with cancer

a. Tumor involvement

I. **Intracranial tumors causing headache** (see section I.A.4 for headache classification).

II. **Cranial neuralgias**. Painful trigeminal neuropathy, referred facial pain syndrome (e.g., from lung tumor), painful glossopharyngeal neuropathy.

III. **Bony infiltration of the skull**. Orbital syndrome, parasellar syndrome, middle fossa syndrome, jugular foramen syndrome, clivus metastases, sphenoid sinus metastases, odontoid fracture, jaw metastases.

IV. **Infiltration of peripheral nerve, nerve root, plexus, meninges, and spinal cord.**

V. **Infiltration of hollow viscus, i.e., intestine, biliary tract, and ureters.**

b. Cancer-therapy related

I. **Postsurgical**. Pain after radical neck dissection, pain after mastectomy, pain after thoracotomy, phantom pain, residual limb pain, pain after nephrectomy, postsurgical pelvic floor myalgia.

II. **Postchemotherapy**. Painful chemotherapy-related toxicities, painful polyneuropathy, painful plexopathy from intra-arterial chemotherapy, corticosteroid-associated pain syndrome (e.g., perineal pain, steroid pseudorheumatism, and aseptic necrosis of the femoral and humeral head), postherpetic neuralgia (e.g., as a result of immunosuppressive therapies).

III. **Postradiation therapy**. Radiation injury to the brachial plexus (radiation fibrosis, reversible or transient radiation injury, acute ischemic brachial plexopathy), radiation fibrosis of the lumbosacral plexus, radiation myelopathy, radiation-induced peripheral nerve tumors.

B. COMMON DIFFERENTIAL DIAGNOSES OF ACUTE PAIN BY SPECIFIC BODY REGION

1. **Headache and facial pain** (see also section I.A.4) can be associated with cranial bone; neck (e.g., cervical spine and retropharyngeal tendinitis); eyes (e.g., acute glaucoma, refractive errors, and heterotropia); ears; nose and sinuses (e.g., acute sinus headache); temporomandibular joint; mouth; teeth; or other facial or cranial structures.

2. **Neck pain**

a. ***Acute anterior neck pain.*** Trauma (anterior whiplash injury, blunt laryngotracheal trauma), myofascial pain disorder, thyroid or parathyroid disease, esophageal pathology, lymphadenitis, infection, abscess, internal carotid artery dissection, referred pain (e.g., MI and coronary insufficiency).

b. ***Acute lateral neck pain.*** Myofascial syndromes of the trapezius muscles, sternocleidomastoid muscle trauma or pseudotumor, parotid disorder (e.g., viral parotitis), salivary duct stone, cervical lymphadenitis, referred pain (e.g., pleuritis involving the diaphragm), infections, cysts.

c. ***Acute posterior neck pain.*** Cervical disk degeneration; cervical disk herniation and radiculopathy; disorders mimicking cervical disk herniation [e.g., cervical osteomyelitis and fracture, transverse myelitis, Lyme disease and radiculitis, myofascial syndrome and referred arm pain, osteoarthritis (OA) of the cervical spine with foraminal narrowing]; arthritis-related cervical subluxation, especially of the atlantoaxial joint [e.g., RA, ankylosing spondylitis (AS), and juvenile rheumatoid arthritis (JRA)]; trauma (e.g., whiplash injury, cervical spine fracture, or dislocation); myositis of the posterior neck muscles; occipital migraine/neuralgia; bacterial and viral meningitis; meningismus; coital neck- and head-pain; acute torticollis; and infection.

3. **Back, buttock, and pubic pain**

a. ***Acute midline thoracolumbar pain.*** Pathological vertebral fracture (because of osteoporosis, metastatic carcinoma, multiple myeloma, and pyogenic or tuberculous osteomyelitis), myofascial pain, fractures and soft tissue injuries, acute transverse myelitis, anterior cord ischemia, epidural abscess, herpes zoster virus infection, referred visceral pain (duodenal ulcer, pancreatitis), pneumothorax.

b. ***Acute lumbosacral pain*** (see also section I.A.3.a.). Lumbosacral strain and sprain, disk degeneration (with or without herniation or protrusion), lateral recess stenosis with nerve root compression, spinal stenosis, spondylolysis, spondylolisthesis, facet syndrome (posterior joint syndrome), locked-back syndrome, trauma (e.g., fractures and subluxations, hyperextension injury), pathologic vertebral fractures (as a result of osteoporosis, metastatic carcinoma, multiple myeloma, Paget's disease, primary spine tumor, or pyogenic or tuberculous osteomyelitis), vertebral osteomyelitis, myofascial pain syndrome (gluteus maximus syndrome, quadratus lumborum syndrome, pyriformis syndrome), referred visceral pain (e.g., diverticulitis of the colon and acute pelvic inflammatory disease), acute sacroiliitis (because of Reiter's syndrome), anterior cord ischemia, intraspinal synovial cysts, cauda equina syndrome (because of central disk herniation), infarction of the conus medullaris, acute epidural abscess, acute nontraumatic epidural hematoma.

c. ***Acute buttock pain***. Spondylolisthesis, disk degeneration, myofascial syndrome (gluteus maximus syndrome, quadratus lumborum syndrome), facet syndrome (posterior joint syndrome), hamstring strain or tear, buttock trauma, trochanteric bursitis, nodular fasciitis (episacroiliac lipomas), acute sacroiliitis (e.g., Reiter's syndrome), sacral neuralgia (e.g., genital herpes), furuncle, abscess (injection-related, epidural, anorectal abscess), nontraumatic epidural hematoma, levator ani spasm.

d. ***Acute pubic pain***. Pubic fracture, pathologic fracture of the pubic bone (disease-associated), stress fracture of the pubic bone (athletic activity-associated), Paget's disease, osteitis pubis, osteomyelitis of the pubic bone, pyogenic arthritis of the pubic symphysis, pubic osteolysis, postpartum symphyseal pubic pain.

4. **Scapular and upper limb pain**

a. ***Acute interscapular and scapular pain***. Myofascial pain, pathological fracture of the spine (because of osteoporosis, metastatic carcinoma, multiple myeloma, and pyogenic or tuberculous osteomyelitis), trauma, cervical radiculopathy (because of disk herniation), transverse myelitis, acute epidural abscess, herpes zoster infection, viscerogenic (MI, dissecting aortic aneurysm, common bile duct stone, pyelonephritis, pleuritis, pancreatitis).

b. ***Acute axillary pain***. Fracture of the proximal humerus, anterior costochondritis with axillary pain radiation, axillary myalgic pain, radicular pain involving T1 root, postaxillary dissection pain, breast disorders in women, axillary abscess, hidradenitis suppurativa, axillary–subclavian venous thrombosis, pleuropulmonary disease, pneumothorax, gaseous gastric distension.

c. ***Acute shoulder and upper arm pain***. Calcific tendinitis, subdeltoid bursitis, trauma (proximal humeral fracture, humeral shaft fracture, pathologic fracture of the humerus, anterior or posterior glenohumeral joint dislocation, acromioclavicular separation, clavicular fracture), cervical radiculopathy (C5, C6), neuralgic amyotrophy (brachial neuropathy), acute arthritis (gout or pseudogout of the glenohumeral joint, Reiter's syndrome, Lyme arthritis, septic arthritis, acute rheumatic fever, hepatitis B-associated arthritis), osteonecrosis of the humeral head, bicipital rupture or tendinitis, pectoralis major tendinitis, acute osteomyelitis of the shoulder, acute hemarthrosis of the glenohumeral joint (as a result of anticoagulant therapy or hemophilia), referred pain.

d. ***Acute upper and lower arm pain***. Acute cervical (C6–T1) radiculopathy (as a result of disk herniation, spondylosis, nerve root avulsion, ligamentous or muscular injuries, fracture or dislocation of the lower cervical spine, osteomyelitis, epidural abscess), brachial plexopathy (acute thoracic outlet syndrome, acute brachial neuropathy or neuralgic amyotrophy, blunt or penetrating trauma), myofascial pain, carpal tunnel syndrome, acute arthritis (acute RA, acute gout and pseudogout, Reiter's syndrome, Lyme arthritis, septic arthritis, acute rheumatic fever, hepatitis B-associated arthritis), cellulitis, vascular pain, referred pain (e.g., acute MI or acute coronary insufficiency and chest wall pain).

e. ***Acute elbow and forearm pain***

I. **Diffuse or generalized elbow and forearm pain**. Simple dislocation of the elbow, forearm muscle strain, fractures (supracondylar fracture of the humerus, transcondylar fracture of the humerus, medial epicondylar fracture of the humerus, intercondylar fracture of the humerus, olecranon fracture, radial head fractures, Monteggia's fracture-dislocation of proximal third of ulna, radial head fracture with acute distal radioulnar dislocation), acute C8 radiculopathy, impending Volkmann's ischemic contracture (anterior compartment syndrome of the forearm), acute monoarticular arthritis (septic arthritis, disseminated gonococcal infection, gout, pseudogout, hemophilic hemarthrosis), acute polyarthritis with elbow involvement (rubella arthritis, rubella vaccine-induced arthritis, acute rheumatic fever, acute hepatitis B arthritis, Reiter's syndrome, Lyme disease arthritis), arterial occlusion pain, referred pain (e.g., acute MI or acute coronary insufficiency).

II. **Anterior elbow pain**. Brachialis muscle tear, rupture of the distal biceps muscle tendon, biceps muscle tear, anterior capsular tear, disruption of the annular ligament and anterior radial head dislocation, acute thrombophlebitis.

III. **Posterior elbow pain**. Triceps tendinitis, triceps rupture, valgus extension overload syndrome, stress fracture of the olecranon, olecranon bursitis (septic bursitis, gouty bursitis, traumatic bursitis).

IV. **Medial elbow pain**. Medial epicondylitis ("golfer's" elbow), rupture of the flexor forearm, rupture or injury of the medial collateral ligament, medial epicondylar fracture, little-leaguer's elbow (partial separation of medial epicondyle apophysis), acute ulnar neuropathy, epitrochlear lymphadenitis.

V. **Lateral elbow pain**. Lateral epicondylitis ("tennis" elbow), rupture of the lateral extensor muscle origin, disruption of the annular ligament and anterior radial head dislocation, entrapment of the musculocutaneous or lateral antebrachial cutaneous nerve, osteochondral fracture of the radial head–capitellum articulation.

f. ***Acute wrist pain***

I. **Diffuse or generalized wrist pain**. Neurogenic wrist pain (acute carpal tunnel syndrome, acute ulnar tunnel syndrome), traumatic ulnar translocation of the carpus, acute arthritis of the wrist (septic arthritis, pseudogout, gout, avascular necrosis of lunate, hemophilic arthropathy, idiopathic arthritis), wrist instability radiographic patterns (volar intercalated segment instability, dorsal intercalated segment instability).

II. **Radial wrist pain**. Distal radius fracture (Colles' fracture, Smith's fracture, articular margin fracture of the distal radius and carpal dislocation), scaphoid fracture, trapezium fracture, scapholunate interosseous ligament sprain, radial collateral ligament sprain, noninfectious tenosynovitis (de Quervain's disease, tenosynovitis of the extensor pollicis longus, flexor carpi radialis tendinitis, intersection syndrome, extensor indicis proprius syndrome), infectious tenosynovitis (suppurative flexor pollicis longus tenosynovitis, gonococcal tenosynovitis).

III. **Mid-dorsal wrist pain**. Fractures (capitate fracture, lunate fracture), perilunate sprains and dislocations, volar lunate dislocation.

IV. **Ulnar wrist pain**. Distal radioulnar joint disorders (fracture of the distal ulna or radial sigmoid fossa, fracture of the triquetrum or lunate, triquetrum avulsion fracture, dislocation of the distal ulna, dislocation of the lunate or triquetrum, triangular fibrocartilage complex injury, extensor carpi ulnaris subluxation and/or tendinitis, extensor digiti minimi tendinitis), hamate fracture, pisiform fracture, triquetrolunate sprain, tendinitis (flexor carpi ulnaris tendinitis, digital flexor tendinitis), pisotriquetral arthritis, midcarpal instability.

g. ***Acute hand and finger pain***

I. **Diffuse or generalized hand and finger pain**. Entrapment neuropathies (carpal tunnel syndrome, ulnar tunnel syndrome, proximal causes of neuropathic hand and finger pain, double-crush syndrome), CRPS type I (RSD), acute polyarthritis with wrist and hand involvement (hepatitis B arthritis, rubella-associated arthritis, rubella immunization-associated arthritis, acute RA, SLE arthritis, acute rheumatic fever, acute traumatic arthritis, arthritis–dermatitis syndrome caused by *Neisseria gonorrhoeae*, acute gout, pseudogout, arthritis associated with inflammatory bowel disease, psoriatic arthritis, septic arthritis), mononeuritis multiplex, vascular hand and finger pain (acute arterial embolism), secondary Raynaud's phenomenon (acute arterial occlusive disease, drug therapy), cutaneous disorders of the hand, infections, bites.

II. **Carpometacarpal and metacarpophalangeal pain**. Carpometacarpal dislocation, metacarpal shaft fractures, metacarpophalangeal joint dislocation and ligament injuries (volar plate disruption, collateral ligament sprain, dorsal capsule injuries, fractures of the metacarpal neck and head).

III. **Proximal phalanx and proximal interphalangeal (PIP) pain**. Fractures of the proximal phalanx, PIP joint area (ligament sprains, volar plate injuries, intra-articular fracture-dislocation, collateral ligament tears, volar dislocations, PIP joint deformities, boutonniere deformity).

IV. **Middle phalanx pain**. Fracture, sprain.

V. **Distal interphalangeal pain**. Extensor tendon disruption (mallet finger), flexor tendon disruption from distal phalanx, fracture of the distal phalanx, subungual hematoma, dislocation of the distal interphalangeal joint.

h. Acute thumb pain

I. **Trapeziometacarpal pain**. De Quervain's disease, abductor pollicis longus tendinitis, fractures (Bennett's fracture at the base of first metacarpal, Rolando's fracture at the carpometacarpal joint of the thumb), dislocation.

II. **Metacarpophalangeal joint pain**. Volar plate injury, ulnar collateral ligament injury, radial collateral ligament injury.

III. **Proximal phalanx pain**. Neuropathy of a digital nerve (bowler's thumb), fractures of the proximal phalanx.

IV. **Interphalangeal joint pain**. Dislocation, fracture of the distal phalanx, extensor tendon disruption (mallet thumb).

5. Lower limb pain

a. Acute thigh and leg pain

I. **Diffuse or generalized thigh and leg pain**. Myalgic pain (e.g., after exercise or associated with fever), iliofemoral thrombophlebitis, iliofemoral arterial embolism or thrombosis, polyarthritis, mononeuritis multiplex, acute spondylolisthesis, sacroiliitis, genital herpes.

II. **Anterior and anteromedial thigh and leg pain**. Radiculopathy of L2, L3, or L4 (from disk herniation, facet joint arthritis, previous L5–S1 fusion operation), lumbar plexopathy (L2–L4), femoral neuropathy (with or without iliacus syndrome).

III. **Posterior and/or posterolateral thigh and leg pain**. Sacral plexopathy (L5–S1), panplexopathy (L2–S1), radicular or "sciatic" pain (acute lateral herniation of L4–L5 or L5–S1 disk, nerve root irritation in a stenotic lateral recess or foramen, or due to OA or spondylolisthesis), epidural abscess, cauda equina syndrome, epidural hematoma, midline disk herniation, conus medullaris infarction.

IV. **Lateral thigh and leg pain**. Trochanteric bursitis, meralgia paresthetica.

b. Acute thigh pain

I. **Diffuse or generalized thigh pain**. Muscle strain because of overuse, femoral shaft fracture (traumatic or stress), lumbosacral plexus injury, fever-related myalgias, iliofemoral venous thrombosis, idiopathic dermatomyositis or polymyositis, complex anterior and posterior compartment syndromes, pathologic fracture as a result of bone tumor or cyst, soft tissue sarcoma, infectious polymyositis, rhabdomyolysis and myoglobinuria, thigh infection, sickle cell pain crisis.

II. **Anteromedial thigh and inguinal pain**. Traumatic fractures of the hip and pelvis (femoral neck fracture, intertrochanteric fracture, greater trochanteric fracture, lesser trochanteric fracture, subtrochanteric fracture, central acetabular fracture and fracture-dislocation, fractures at or near the pubic symphysis, impacted fracture of the femoral neck), dislocation and fracture-dislocation of the hip (posterior, anterior), pathologic fracture of the hip (femoral neck, intertrochanteric and femoral shaft), stress fracture of the hip and pelvis, acute arthritis of the hip in adults (septic arthritis, acute gout, acute pseudogout, acute rheumatic fever, acute RA of the hips, chronic RA with acute noninfectious arthritis of the hip, osteoid osteoma, Reiter's syndrome), acute synovitis of the hip in children and adolescents (transient synovitis of the hip, JRA of the hip, Legg–Calvé–Perthes disease, slipped capital femoral epiphysis, pubic osteomyelitis), osteonecrosis of the femoral head, iliopsoas muscle disorders (iliopsoas bursitis, iliopsoas tendinitis, iliopsoas abscess), femoral neuropathy, iliofemoral venous thrombosis, inguinal or femoral hernia, inguinal or femoral lymphadenitis, cellulitis, sexually transmitted disease (e.g., syphilis, gonococcal urethritis, genital herpes, chancroid).

III. **Anterior thigh pain**. Femoral shaft fracture (traumatic), quadriceps injury (muscle strain, contusion, or tendon rupture), radicular pain (L2–L4 spinal roots), femoral neuropathy, femoral shaft stress fracture in athletes, sartorius muscle strain of the thigh, anterior compartment syndrome of the thigh, myositis ossificans traumatica, obturator hernia, referred pain, herpes simplex neuritis.

IV. **Posterior thigh pain**. Radicular pain (disk protrusion, spinal epidural abscess, spinal epidural or subdural hematoma, conus medullaris infarction), hamstring muscle injury (strain, ischial apophysis avulsion), myofascial pain, pyriformis syndrome, hamstring syndrome (gluteal sciatica), ischial bursitis, lumbar facet joint disease, sacroiliitis (Reiter's syndrome or reactive arthritis, septic arthritis), sacroiliac sprain, posterior femoral cutaneous neuropathy, posterior compartment syndrome of the thigh.

V. **Medial thigh pain**. Adductor muscle strain, iliopsoas muscle strain or avulsion fracture of the lesser trochanter, pubic bone disorders (e.g., osteitis pubis), greater saphenous vein phlebitis.

VI. **Lateral thigh and trochanteric pain**. Traumatic fracture of the femoral shaft, trochanteric bursitis, snapping hip syndrome, meralgia paresthetica, acute arthritis of the hip, osteonecrosis of the hip, hip pointer (iliac crest contusion), fracture of the iliac crest apophysis.

c. ***Knee***

I. **Diffuse or generalized knee pain**. Trauma (supracondylar fractures of the femur, patellar fractures, fractures of the proximal tibia, fractures of the tibial spines or intercondylar eminence), knee dislocation (anterior, posterior, medial, or lateral), patellar dislocation, intra-articular ligament injury (anterior cruciate ligament tear, posterior cruciate ligament tear, multiple ligament and meniscus injuries, "dashboard knee"), reflex sympathetic dystrophy of the knee, mimics of septic monoarthritis (pseudogout, gout, traumatic synovitis, foreign body synovitis, acute leukemic arthritis, acute hemarthrosis due to coagulopathy, JRA, acute rheumatic fever, idiopathic monoarthritis, Lyme arthritis, acute RA of the knee), acute septic monoarthritis of the knee (gonococcal or nongonococcal), acute polyarthritis involving the knee (gonococcal or nongonococcal), septic arthritis involving the knee, reactive arthritis, acute rheumatic fever, crystal-induced polyarthritis, hepatitis B-associated arthritis, acute Lyme arthritis, acute RA, rubella arthritis, rubella vaccine-associated arthritis, varicella arthritis, acute JRA, referred pain from the hip (e.g., acute synovitis).

II. **Anterior knee pain**. Patellar tendon injury, patellofemoral pain syndrome, patellofemoral tracking disorders, patellar tendinitis ("jumper's knee"), prepatellar bursitis ("housemaid's or miner's knee"), retropatellar bursitis, infrapatellar bursitis, infrapatellar fat-pad injury, Hoffa's disease (hypertrophy and inflammation of the infrapatellar fat pad), osteochondritis dissecans of the patella, osteochondral fracture of the patella, quadriceps tendon rupture, Osgood–Schlatter disease (tibial tubercle avulsion fracture), synovial plica, meniscal disorders.

III. **Posterior knee pain**. Gastrocnemius muscle strain, hamstring muscle strain, hamstring tendinitis, muscle spasms (cramps), posterior cruciate ligament and/or posterior capsule tear, plantaris muscle strain or rupture.

IV. **Medial knee pain**. Medial meniscus tear (traumatic or degenerative), pes anserine bursitis, tibial collateral ligament bursitis, tibial collateral ligament injury (sprain, rupture), pes anserine-gastrocnemius-related tendinitis, semimembranosus tendinitis, Hoffa's disease (hypertrophy and inflammation of the infrapatellar fat pad), osteonecrosis of the medial femoral condyle, osteonecrosis of the proximal tibia, extra-articular displacement of the medial meniscus.

V. **Lateral knee pain**. Iliotibial band friction syndrome, lateral meniscus tear, biceps femoris tendinitis, tibiofibular joint disorder, osteochondral fracture of the lateral femoral condyle, lateral (fibular) collateral ligament injury, popliteus tenosynovitis, popliteus tendon rupture.

d. Leg

I. **Diffuse or generalized leg pain**. Fractures of the tibial shaft or fibula (traumatic or pathologic), delayed muscle soreness caused by exercise, acute occlusion of the superficial femoral or popliteal artery, cellulitis, sickle cell crisis pain.

II. **Anteromedial leg pain**. Stress fracture of the tibia, stress microfractures of the tibia, medial tibial stress syndrome (periostalgia), soleus syndrome, distal deep posterior compartment syndrome, greater saphenous vein thrombophlebitis, saphenous neuritis, osteomyelitis of the tibia, shin splints related to systemic disease (e.g., Paget's disease of tibia).

III. **Anterolateral leg pain**. Muscle strain or hematoma in the anterior compartment, anterior compartment syndrome, lateral compartment syndrome, compression of the superficial peroneal nerve, fibular fracture, anterior tibial vein thrombosis, pyomyositis.

IV. **Posterior leg (calf) pain**. Deep vein thrombosis, mimics of calf vein thrombosis (complications of a baker's cyst, gastrocnemius muscle strain, soleus muscle strain, hematoma of the calf, acute rhabdomyolysis, rupture of the Achilles tendon, acute posterior compartment syndrome, pyomyositis), benign calf muscle cramps (e.g., after exercise, during pregnancy, at night in elderly persons), muscle cramps as a result of underlying disease (peripheral neuropathy root or plexus lesion, drug-related, metabolic causes).

e. Acute ankle pain

I. **Diffuse or generalized ankle pain**. Acute injuries of the ankle (fracture of the medial or lateral malleolus, disruptions of the medial or lateral ligament of the ankles, fracture of the neck of the talus, fracture of the body of the talus, anterior or posterior ankle dislocation), acute monoarthritis of the ankle [septic arthritis, acute gout, acute pseudogout, RA, CRPS type I (RSD), hemophilic arthropathy, acute hemarthrosis], ankle arthritis associated with acute polyarthritis (polyarticular septic arthritis, acute rheumatic fever, Lyme arthritis, hepatitis B-associated arthritis, rubella and rubella vaccine-associated arthritis, arthritis associated with inflammatory bowel disease, acute polyarticular gout, pseudogout, Reiter's syndrome, RA), osteochondritis dissecans of the talus, acute osteomyelitis, transient migratory osteoporosis.

II. **Anterior ankle pain**. Peritendinitis of the extensor tendons of the foot and toes, cruciate crural ligament (retinaculum) sprain, sprain or rupture of the anterior tibiofibular ligament, fracture of the anterior lip of the distal tibial articular surface.

III. **Posterior ankle pain**. Achilles tendinitis, subcutaneous Achilles bursitis, retrocalcaneal bursitis, partial rupture of the Achilles tendon, complete rupture of the Achilles tendon, fracture of the calcaneal tuberosity.

IV. **Medial ankle pain**. Fracture of the medial malleolus, shin splints (stress fracture of tibia, periostitis, and musculotendinous pain), fracture of the sustentaculum tali, deltoid ligament sprain, tibialis posterior tendinitis, tendinitis of the flexor hallucis longus and flexor digitorum communis.

V. **Lateral ankle pain**. Lateral collateral ligament injuries (anterior talofibular, calcaneofibular, and posterior talofibular ligaments), mimics of anterior talofibular ligament sprain [anterior tibiofibular ligament sprain, fracture of the lateral malleolus, fracture of the lateral process of the talus, fracture of the lateral tubercle of the posterior process of the talus, peroneal tendinitis, traumatic dislocation of the peroneal tendons, ganglion cyst, stress fracture of the fibula, calcaneofibular ligament sprain (isolated)].

f. *Acute foot pain*

I. **Generalized foot pain**. Nerve and root compression syndrome (L5–S1 root compression, superficial or deep peroneal nerve entrapment, sural nerve entrapment, tarsal tunnel syndrome), arthritis (RA, AS, Reiter's syndrome, psoriatic arthritis, gout, pseudogout, acute rheumatic fever, SLE, hepatitis B-associated arthritis, rubella-associated arthritis), sickle cell crisis pain, vascular pain (acute arterial occlusion), nocturnal rest pain, ulcers and gangrene (e.g., due to arteriosclerosis obliterans, progressive ischemia, vasculitis), CRPS type I (RSD), foot cramps, peripheral polyneuropathy (see section I.A.1.b), trauma (crush injury, compartment syndrome, amputation), infection (cellulitis, necrotizing fasciitis, abscess, osteomyelitis), cold injury (frostbite, chilblains), bites, cutaneous disorders (e.g., shoe dermatitis, tinea pedis).

II. **Forefoot pain**. Morton's neuroma (plantar interdigital nerve hypertrophy), inflammatory arthritis of the metatarsophalangeal joint, arterial insufficiency, traumatic metatarsal fractures, forefoot sprain, metatarsalgia caused by high-heeled shoes, metatarsalgia as a result of equinus foot or cavus foot, metatarsalgia as a result of central-ray overload syndrome, metatarsalgia as a result of first-ray insufficiency syndrome or Morton's syndrome (acute march fractures and chronic first-ray insufficiency), Freiberg's disease (osteonecrosis of second and third metatarsal head), second metatarsal space syndrome, idiopathic synovitis of the second metatarsophalangeal joint, bursitis (submetatarsal and interdigital), submetatarsal cysts.

III. **Great toe and medial forefoot pain**. Radicular pain (L5 root), first metatarsophalangeal joint injury (sprain, dislocation or sesamoid fracture, "turf" toe), fracture of the great toe, crush injury of the distal toe (soft tissue injury), dislocation of the interphalangeal joint, hallux valgus, bunion of the great toe, hallux limitus or rigidus, first metatarsophalangeal joint arthritis (septic arthritis and osteomyelitis, podagra as a result of gout or pseudogout), shoe vamp ulcer and bursitis, gangrene or ulceration of the great toe, subungual hematoma, plantar cutaneous lesions (corns, warts, calluses), nail lesions and infection of the hallux, Joplin's neuroma (of plantar digital nerve of great toe), first-ray overload syndrome, calcific tendinitis of the flexor hallucis tendons, tumors.

IV. **Small toe pain**. Dorsal interphalangeal joint area pain and inflammation, trauma (contusions and fractures), arthritis of the small toes, ulcerations of the toes (ischemic, neuropathic), hammer toe deformity, mallet toe deformity, gout tophus, tailor's bunion (bunionette of the fifth toe), Raynaud's disease and phenomenon, plantar cutaneous lesions (corns, warts), tinea pedis, candidiasis, Osler's nodes, subungual tumors.

V. **Midfoot pain**. Plantar fascial pain (plantar fasciitis, heel pain syndrome), longitudinal arch strain, subtalar osteochondral fracture, stress fracture of one or more metatarsal or tarsal bones, OA (first metatarsocuneiform joint, cuboideometatarsal joint), tarsometatarsal joint trauma (sprain or dislocation or fracture-dislocation), midtarsal trauma (Chopart's or the transverse tarsal joint), navicular fractures (traumatic or stress fractures), fracture of the fifth metatarsal (avulsion fractures, diaphyseal or true Jones fractures), aseptic necrosis of the navicular bone, tendinitis (flexor hallucis longus tendinitis, peroneal tendinitis), interosseous myositis or strain, osteomyelitis, acquired flatfoot (rupture of the tibialis posterior tendon, ligamentous or bone failure), plantar abscess.

VI. **Dorsal foot pain**. Acute gout or pseudogout, peripheral polyneuropathy, trauma (metatarsal, tarsal), stress fracture of the metatarsal, OA of the tarsometatarsal joint, tendinitis (extensor hallucis longus muscle, extensor digitorum longus muscle, tibialis anterior muscle), cruciate crural ligament injury, cellulitis, CRPS type I (RSD), peroneal nerve entrapment (superficial or deep), subtalar arthritis or osteochondral fracture, aseptic necrosis of the navicular bone, interosseous muscle strain, acquired pes planus, shoe dermatitis, foot abscess, osteomyelitis, septic arthritis, herpes zoster.

VII. **Diffuse or generalized hindfoot pain**. Intra-articular calcaneal fractures, extra-articular calcaneal fractures (fracture of the medial calcaneal process, fracture of the superior portion of the calcaneal tuberosity, fracture of the sustentaculum tali), ischemic necrosis of the heel.

VIII. **Plantar hindfoot pain**. Heel pain syndrome because of overuse ("plantar fasciitis") or as a result of systemic disorders (e.g., RA, seronegative arthritis, spondyloarthropathies), fat-pad disorders (atrophy, inflammation, fat-pad separation from the calcaneus), stress fracture of the calcaneus, rupture of the plantar fascia, entrapment neuropathy of the first branch of the lateral plantar nerve to abductor digiti quinti muscle, flexor tendinitis (flexor hallucis longus tendinitis, flexor digitorum longus tendinitis).

IX. **Posterior hindfoot pain**. Achilles tendinitis, retrocalcaneal bursitis, superficial Achilles bursitis ("pump bump"), Achilles tendon rupture, calcaneal periostitis and osteitis, fracture of the posterosuperior calcaneal tuberosity, calcaneal osteomyelitis.

X. **Medial hindfoot pain**. Tarsal tunnel syndrome, tibialis posterior tendinitis, flexor hallucis longus tendinitis, calcaneal fractures (medial calcaneal process or sustentaculum tali), calcaneal branch neurodynia.

XI. **Lateral hindfoot pain**. Lateral ankle sprain, peroneal muscle strain, peroneal tendinitis, fracture of the lateral process of the talus, osteochondral fracture of the talar dome, stress fracture of the lateral malleolus, sural nerve entrapment.

C. DIFFERENTIAL DIAGNOSIS OF MUSCULOSKELETAL PAIN BY ITS DISTRIBUTION PATTERN

1. **Acute generalized musculoskeletal pain**. Postexertional in normal individuals, fibromyalgia, viral infection [influenza A virus, Epstein–Barr virus, coxsackievirus, herpes simplex virus, human immunodeficiency virus (HIV)], therapeutic drugs (lovastatin, clofibrate), postimmunization, electrolyte and mineral deficiencies (hyponatremia, hypokalemia, hypocalcemia, hypomagnesemia, hypophosphatemia), alcohol abuse, drug abuse (amphetamines, cocaine, heroin or its contaminants), endocrine disorders (diabetes mellitus, hypo- or

hyperthyroidism, hypoadrenalism, panhypopituitarism, hypoparathyroidism), metabolic muscular disorders, eosinophilia myalgia syndrome, mimics of the eosinophilia myalgia syndrome (e.g., polymyositis, eosinophilic fasciitis, sarcoidosis, dermatomyositis), polymyalgia rheumatica, seronegative RA.

2. **Acute generalized joint pain.** Reactive arthritis (Reiter's syndrome), rubella-associated arthritis, HIV-associated arthritis, acute seropositive RA, crystal-induced polyarthritis due to gout or pseudogout.
3. **Monoarticular joint pain**

a. ***Acute monoarthritis.*** Infectious arthritis (bacterial, Lyme disease), crystal-induced disease such as gout and pseudogout (or calcium pyrophosphate deposition disease), hemarthrosis, which can be due to nontraumatic causes (anticoagulant therapy, dialysis) or trauma, noninfectious inflammatory conditions such as JRA and seronegative spondyloarthropathies (e.g., psoriatic arthritis, Reiter's syndrome), periarticular syndrome (e.g., erythema nodosum, inflammatory bowel disease, acute sarcoidosis), monoarticular presentation of a polyarticular disease (e.g., RA).

b. ***Chronic monoarthritis.*** Infectious arthritis (e.g., pyogenic bacteria, fungal, Lyme, tuberculous), noninfectious inflammatory conditions such as RA, pauciarticular JRA, sarcoid arthropathy and seronegative spondyloarthropathies (e.g., psoriatic arthritis, Reiter's disease), noninflammatory conditions such as OA, avascular necrosis of bone (osteonecrosis), neoplasia (pigmented villonodular synovitis, synovial chondromatosis), neuropathic ("Charcot") joint.

4. **Polyarticular joint pain**

a. ***Acute migratory polyarthritis.*** Neisserial infection (e.g., gonorrhea), reactive or postinfectious arthritis (e.g., acute rheumatic fever, Reiter's syndrome, poststreptococcal arthritis), early stage of Lyme disease, viral infection (e.g., rubella, mumps, Epstein–Barr virus), serum sickness (occasionally), acute leukemia, inflammatory bowel disease, familial hypercholesterolemia.

b. ***Acute nonmigratory polyarthritis.*** RA, serum sickness, SLE, polyarticular JRA, acute phase of seronegative spondyloarthropathies (e.g., psoriatic arthritis, Reiter's syndrome, AS, enteropathic arthritis), crystal-induced disease (acute polyarticular gout and pseudogout), sarcoidosis, vasculitis, hematologic disorders (e.g., leukemia, sickle cell disease, lymphoma), serum sickness, viral arthritis (e.g., HIV, Epstein–Barr virus).

c. ***Chronic polyarthritis.*** RA, SLE, polyarticular JRA, sarcoid arthritis, connective tissue disease (e.g., scleroderma, polymyositis) and overlap syndromes, chronic phase of seronegative spondyloarthropathies (e.g., psoriatic arthritis, Reiter's syndrome, AS), OA, crystal-induced disease (chronic polyarticular gout and pseudogout).

II. Non-neuromusculoskeletal pain-related problems

Cardiac pain develops as a result of ischemia induced by increase cardiac workload resulting from exertion, cold, or emotion. It may subside with rest and relaxation. *Mediastinal pain* is induced by activities of the esophagus (swallowing), musculoskeletal movement, or aorta (increased systolic thrust). *Pleural and tracheal pain* is associated with respiratory movements. *Arterial pain*, usually throbbing, is seen in arteritis, migraine, and vascular headaches and is aggravated by increased systolic pressure (e.g., exercise, fever, bending over). *Gastrointestinal tract pain* is increased with peristaltic activity (especially if there is obstruction, e.g., impacted stool) and is aggravated by eating and may be relieved with fasting or by vomiting or bowel movement. *Pain induced by gastric juice* is related to food intake and may be relieved by food or antacids. *Visceral pain* from abdominal organs (e.g., kidneys, liver, spleen, and pancreas) is intensified by body positions or movements that increase intra-abdominal pressure.

Further reading

Asbury AK, Fields HL: Pain due to peripheral nerve damage: an hypothesis. *Neurology* 34:1587–1590, 1984.

Braunwald E, Kasper DL, Fauci AS, *et al.*, editors: *Harrison's principles of internal medicine*, ed 16, New York, 2004, McGraw-Hill.

England JD, Asbury AK: Peripheral neuropathy. *The Lancet* 363:2151–2161, 2004.

Galer BS, Schwartz L, Allen RJ: Complex regional pain syndromes – type I: reflex sympathetic dystrophy, and type II: causalgia. In Loeser JD, editor: *Bonica's management of pain*, ed 3, Philadelphia, 2001, Lippincott, Williams & Wilkins, pp. 388–411.

Giesecke T, Gracely RH, Grant MA, *et al.*: Evidence of augmented central pain processing in idiopathic chronic low back pain. *Arthritis Rheum* 50(2):613–623, 2004.

Goldman L, Ausiello D, editors: *Cecil textbook of medicine*, ed 22, Philadelphia, 2003, WB Saunders.

Goodman CC, Snyder TEK: *Differential diagnosis in physical therapy*, ed 3, Philadelphia, 2000, WB Saunders.

Headache Classification Committee of the International Headache Society: Classification and diagnostic criteria for headache disorders, cranial neuralgias, and facial pain. *Cephalalgia* 8 (suppl. 7):1–96, 1988.

Healey P, Jacobson EJ: *Common medical diagnoses: an algorithmic approach*, ed 3, Philadelphia, 2000, WB Saunders.

Janig W, Blumberg H, Boas RA, *et al.*: The reflex sympathetic dystrophy syndrome: consensus statement and general recommendations for diagnosis and clinical research. In Bond MR, Charlton JE, Woolf CJ, editors: *Pain research and clinical management: Proceedings of the VIth World Congress on Pain*, vol. 3, Amsterdam, 1991, Elsevier, pp. 372–375.

Kanner RM: Low back pain. In Portenoy RK, Kanner RM, editors: *Pain management: theory and practice*, Philadelphia, 1996, FA Davis, pp. 126–144.

Kozin F: Reflex sympathetic dystrophy syndrome. *Bull Rheum Dis* 36:1–8, 1986.

Macnab I, McCulloch J: *Neck ache and shoulder pain*, Baltimore, 1994, Williams & Wilkins.

Paget S, Gibofsky A, Beary III JF, editors: *Manual of rheumatology and outpatient orthopedic disorders*, ed 4, Philadelphia, 2000, Lippincott, Williams & Wilkins.

Portenoy RK: Neuropathic pain. In Portenoy RK, Kanner RM, editors: *Pain management: theory and practice*, Philadelphia, 1996, FA Davis, pp. 83–125.

Roberts WJ: A hypothesis on the physiological basis for causalgia and related pains. *Pain* 24:297–311, 1986.

Stein J, editor: *Textbook of internal medicine*, ed 5, Philadelphia, 2000, Elsevier.

Wiener SL: *Differential diagnosis of acute pain by body region*, New York, 1993, McGraw-Hill.

Wall PD, Melzack R, editors: *Textbook of pain*, ed 4, Philadelphia, 1999, WB Saunders.

CHAPTER 3.2
Differential diagnoses of nonpain problems

This chapter deals with the differential diagnosis of common PM&R problems that do not have pain as the primary feature although pain may play a secondary role in some of them. They are encountered in either the in- or outpatient setting of a PM&R practice. The diagnosis and treatment of many of these problems may not fall within the realm of physiatric practice *per se*; however, recognizing the potential diagnosis and knowing when to refer them to another specialist is important for good patient care. As in the previous chapter, these problems are divided into the neuromusculoskeletal system and non-neuromusculoskeletal system. The following list is by no means exhaustive.

I. Neuromusculoskeletal nonpain-related problems

A. WEAKNESS (SEE FIG. 3.2-1)

1. Neurogenic causes

a. ***Upper motor neuron and cortical disorders***. Vascular (e.g., stroke, intracranial hemorrhage, and cerebral palsy), demyelinating (e.g., multiple sclerosis); infectious (e.g., encephalitis, meningitis, Creutzfeldt–Jakob disease, and AIDS), structural (e.g., neoplasm, Arnold–Chiari malformation, syringomyelia, and syringobulbia), exogenous (e.g., traumatic brain injury, cervical spinal cord injuries, and drug-induced causes), degenerative (primary lateral sclerosis [PLS]).

b. ***Combined upper and lower motor neuron disorders***. Amyotrophic lateral sclerosis, progressive bulbar palsy, cervical myelopathy with radiculopathy, syringomyelia, spinal cord tumor or arteriovenous malformation, Lyme disease, human immunodeficiency virus (HIV)-associated motor neuron disease.

c. ***Lower motor neuron disorders***

I. **Motor neurons**. Spinal muscular atrophy, poliomyelitis, postpolio syndrome, progressive muscular atrophy (PMA).

II. **Peripheral nervous system**. Guillain–Barré syndrome, plexopathies, radiculopathies, compressive neuropathies, acute intermittent porphyria (AIP), Charcot–Marie–Tooth (CMT) disease, chronic inflammatory demyelinating polyradiculoneuropathy (CIDP), multifocal motor neuropathy (MNN).

III. **Neuromuscular junction**. Myasthenia gravis, Lambert–Eaton myasthenic syndrome, botulism.

2. Myopathic causes (usually presents with proximal weakness).

a. ***Muscular dystrophy***. Duchenne muscular dystrophy, Becker-type muscular dystrophy, fascioscapulohumeral dystrophy, limb-girdle dystrophy, myotonic dystrophy, oculopharyngeal dystrophy, congenital myopathies.

b. ***Rheumatologic disorders***. Primary amyloidosis, sarcoid myopathy, dermatomyositis, polymyositis, rheumatoid arthritis, polyarteritis nodosa, systemic lupus erythematosus, polymyalgia rheumatica, fibromyalgia, cervical and lumbar spondylosis, Paget's disease of bone, scleroderma, Sjogren's syndrome.

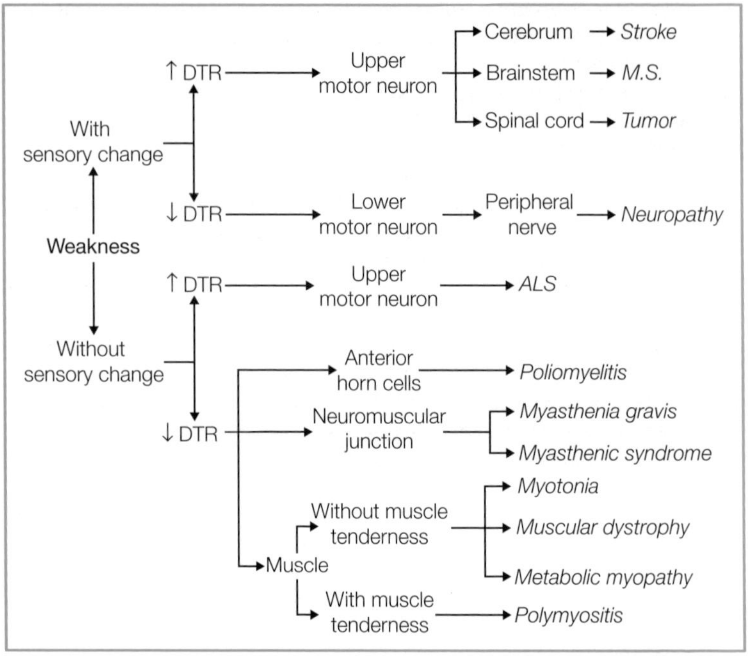

Figure 3.2-1 Algorithm of differential diagnosis of weakness. Patients without sensory disturbances may still have nervous system disease, especially if the weakness is associated with hyper-reflexia, as in amyotrophic lateral sclerosis. Most patients, however, exhibit hyporeflexia, as seen in anterior horn cell lesions, diseases of the neuromuscular junction, or primary muscle disorders. DTR, deep tendon reflexes; MS, multiple sclerosis; ALS, amyotrophic lateral sclerosis. (From Kimura J: *Electrodiagnosis in diseases of nerve and muscle: principles and practice*, ed 3, New York, 2001, Oxford University Press, reproduced with permission of the Oxford University Press.)

c. ***Toxin- and drug-induced myopathies***. Steroid myopathy, hypokalemic myopathy, alcoholic myopathy, drug-induced myopathy (D-penicillamine, colchicine, chloroquine, clofibrate, cimetidine), drug-induced rhabdomyolysis and myoglobinuria.

d. ***Metabolic myopathies***. Familial periodic paralysis, electrolyte imbalance (hypo- or hyperkalemia, hypercalcemia, hypermagnesemia, hypophophatemia), vitamin D deficiency, renal tubular acidosis, mitochondrial myopathy, McArdle's syndrome, familial myoglobinuria, acid maltase deficiency, carnitine 6 deficiency, other metabolic storage disease.

e. ***Endocrine myopathies***. Hypothyroid myopathy, thyrotoxic myopathy, acromegalic myopathy, hyperparathyroidism, Cushing's syndrome, diabetes mellitus (DM).

f. ***Infectious myopathy (with myositis)***. Viral (poliomyelitis, rabies, coxsackie, influenza, rubella, Epstein–Barr viruses and HIV), bacterial (staphylococcal, streptococcal, salmonella, clostridial, *Mycobacterium leprae, Mycoplasma pneumoniae*), parasitic (trichinosis, toxoplasmosis, *Trypanosoma cruzi, Echinococcus alveolaris*), fungal (*Candida tropicalis*).

g. ***Congenital myopathy***. Central core disease, nemaline myopathy, myotubular or centronuclear myopathy, congenital fiber type disproportion, cytoplasmic body myopathy.

h. ***Others***. Endogenous depressive psychosis.

B. PARAPLEGIA OR TETRAPLEGIA

1. Neurogenic causes

a. ***Upper motor neuron and cortical disorders***

I. **Brain**. Vascular (e.g., bilateral cerebral infarction, ventral pontine infarction, bilateral medullary pyramid infarction, and cerebral palsy), neoplastic [frontal lobe tumor, brainstem glioma, parasagittal tumor (paraplegia)], demyelinating (e.g., multiple sclerosis), hydrocephalus (e.g., Arnold–Chiari malformation), degenerative (e.g., PLS).

II. **Spinal cord**. Trauma (spinal cord injury), vascular (e.g., anterior spinal artery thrombosis, spinal arteriovenous malformation, epidural hematoma, hematomyelia, and arteritis), neoplasm [primary intramedullary (ependymoma, astrocytoma) or extramedullary (neurofibroma, meningioma), secondary extradural metastasis], inflammatory (idiopathic transverse myelitis, multiple sclerosis), degenerative [cervical spondylotic myelopathy, intervertebral disk prolapse, vertebral disease with myelopathy, atlantoaxial subluxation (e.g., in rheumatoid arthritis)], congenital (spina bifida, syringomyelia), infectious [herpes zoster or simplex myelitis, HIV myelopathy, tuberculosis (Pott's disease), spinal epidural abscess, syphilitic meningomyelitis], nutritional (subacute combined degeneration due to vitamin B_{12} deficiency), granulomatous (sarcoidosis), others (decompression myelopathy in divers, myelopathy of systemic disease, toxin-induced).

b. ***Combined upper and lower motor neuron disorders,*** e.g., amyotrophic lateral sclerosis.

c. ***Lower motor neuron disorders***

I. **Motor neurons**. Spinal muscular atrophy, poliomyelitis, PMA.

II. **Peripheral nervous system**. Guillain–Barré syndrome, acute intermittent porphyria, neoplasm, heavy metal poisoning.

III. **Neuromuscular junction**. Myasthenia gravis, botulism.

2. Myopathic causes. Polymyositis, rhabdomyolysis, familial periodic paralysis, electrolyte imbalance (hypo- or hyperkalemia, hypercalcemia, hypermagnesemia, hypophosphatemia).

C. HEMIPLEGIA OR HEMIPARESIS

1. Vascular. Stroke, transient ischemic attacks, reversible ischemic neurologic deficit, cerebral palsy, vasculitis.

2. Trauma. Traumatic brain injury (brain contusion, subdural hematoma, epidural hematoma).

3. Brain tumor. Primary or metastatic.

4. Demyelinating disease. Demyelinating disease (multiple sclerosis, acute necrotizing myelitis).

5. Infections. Brain abscess, encephalitis, subdural empyema, meningitis.

6. Other. Hypoglycemia, migraine syndrome, Todd's paralysis, nonketotic hyperosmolar coma, leukodystrophies.

D. GAIT DISORDERS

1. Wide-based unsteady gait (ataxia)

a. ***Cerebellar ataxia***. Wernicke's encephalopathy, alcoholic cerebellar degeneration, multiple sclerosis, vertebrobasilar artery ischemia, neoplasms, hemorrhage, abscess, infarct, following hyperthermia, hypoxic encephalopathy, non-Wilsonian hepatocerebral degeneration (posthepatic coma), hypoparathyroidism, congenital, hereditary (ataxic telangiectasia).

b. ***Sensory ataxia*** (loss of postural or proprioceptive sense). Polyneuropathy (diabetic), tabes dorsalis, multiple sclerosis, subacute combined degeneration of the spinal cord, vitamin B_{12} deficiency, spinal cord tumor, hereditary (Friedreich's ataxia).

c. ***Others***. Frontal lobe lesions (tumors, thrombosis of anterior cerebral artery, hydrocephalus), labyrinthine destruction (neoplasm, injury, inflammation, compression), parainfectious (Guillain–Barré syndrome, acute ataxia of childhood and young adults), hydrocephalus (normal pressure), paraneoplastic syndromes, hypothyroidism, myopathy, toxins (phenytoin, alcohol, sedatives, organophosphates), Wilson's disease (hepatolenticular degeneration), meningomyelopathy, Creutzfeldt–Jakob disease, hysteria, AIDS, disequilibrium (see section II.B.5).

2. **Hemiparetic gait**. Cerebral palsy (CP), stroke, Parkinson's disease.
3. **Gluteus medius insufficiency gait (Trendelenberg gait)**. Poliomyelitis, myelodysplasia.
4. **Gluteus maximus or lurch gait**. Muscular dystrophy.
5. **Back knee (quadriceps paralysis) gait**. Poliomyelitis.
6. **Drop foot gait (steppage gait)**.

a. ***With sensory deficit.*** L5 radiculopathy, lumbar plexopathy, sciatic nerve palsy, peroneal neuropathy (compression or injury at fibular head, diabetes), early GBS, hereditary motor and sensory neuropathy (e.g., Charcot–Marie–Tooth disease).

b. ***Without sensory deficit***. ALS, scapuloperoneal variety of fascioscapulohumeral muscular dystrophy.

7. **Calcaneus gait or triceps gait pattern**. Clubfoot surgery.
8. **Spasticity-related gait abnormality (equinovarus foot, valgus foot, striatal toe, stiff [extended] knee, flexed knee [crouch gait], adducted thighs [scissoring gait], flexed hip, persistent great toe hyperextension [hitchhiker toe])**. SCI, MS, stroke, TBI, CP.

E. INVOLUNTARY MOVEMENT DISORDERS, including tics (Tourette's syndrome), athetosis (e.g., in cerebral palsy), and the following:

1. **Dystonia** (sustained abnormal fixed posture).

a. ***Primary generalized dystonia***. Idiopathic torsion dystonia (hereditary or sporadic).

b. ***Secondary dystonia***. Acquired [e.g., cerebral palsy, poststroke, head trauma, drug induced (neuroleptic, anti-Parkinson), vascular malformation, multiple sclerosis, brain tumor, encephalitis, peripheral trauma], degenerative disorders (e.g., Parkinson's disease, progressive supranuclear palsy, rigid Huntington's disease, olivopontocerebellar degeneration), neurologic disorder with identifiable metabolic defect (e.g., Wilson's disease) or suspected metabolic defect (e.g., ataxia telangiectasia).

c. ***Focal dystonia***. Blepharospasm, torticollis, spastic dysphonia, writer's cramp.

d. ***Stiff-man syndrome***. Associated with diabetes, vitiligo, and thyroiditis.

2. **Tremor** (oscillating involuntary movement of the joint).

a. ***Tremor at rest (pill-rolling)***. Parkinsonian tremor.

b. ***Action tremor***

- I. **Postural tremor**. Essential tremor, enhanced physiologic tremor, neuropathic tremor.
- II. **Intention tremor**. Cerebellar intention tremor.
- III. **Task-specific tremor**. Primary writing tremor.

c. ***Medication-induced tremor***. Thyroid extract (synthroid), epinephrine, amphetamine, phenylephrine, and other sympathomimetics, caffeine, theophylline and other xanthines; nicotine; lithium; phenothiazines; methyl bromide; monosodium glutamate; corticosteroids (in high doses); insulin and oral hypoglycemic agents; alcohol withdrawal; metal intoxication (lead, arsenic, bismuth, mercury, manganese); tricyclic antidepressants.

3. **Chorea** (irregular, brief movements of the limbs and trunk accompanied by facial grimacing, head movements, and a peculiar dancing gait).
a. ***Huntington's disease***
b. ***Non-Huntington's disease.*** Acute rheumatic chorea (Sydenham's disease), chorea gravidarum, systemic lupus erythematosus, chorea acanthocytosis, glutaric acidemia, methylmalonic aciduria, familial calcification of the basal ganglia, acute vascular hemichorea, senile chorea.
4. **Dyskinesia (drug-induced)**
a. ***Acute.*** Levodopa, bromocriptine, anticholinergics, dopaminergic agonists, antihistamines, oral contraceptives.
b. ***Chronic tardive dyskinesia.*** Neuroleptic drugs.
5. **Myoclonus** (brief muscle jerk, which can be spontaneous, or evoked by voluntary movement or sensory stimuli).
a. ***Physiologic.*** Sleep jerks, hiccups.
b. ***Essential.*** Familial essential myoclonus, sporadic essential myoclonus, startle syndrome.
c. ***Epileptic myoclonus***
d. ***Symptomatic myoclonus.*** Toxic or metabolic encephalopathy, viral encephalitis, spinocerebellar degeneration, basal ganglia degeneration, Alzheimer's disease, Creutzfeldt–Jakob disease, storage disease with progressive myoclonus epilepsy, posthypoxic, focal CNS damage.

G. PARESTHESIA

1. **Peripheral neuropathy.** CMT, CIDP, GBS, AIP, Denny–Brown syndrome.
2. **Peripheral nerve entrapment, compression, or trauma.** Intervertebral disk herniation with radiculopathy, thoracic outlet syndrome, carpal tunnel syndrome, plexopathies.
3. **Arteriosclerotic peripheral vascular disease**
4. **Spinal cord disease.** Spinal cord or nerve root compression, tabes dorsalis, subacute combined degeneration of the spinal cord.
5. **Motor neuron disease.** ALS.
6. **Brain disease.** Vascular (e.g., stroke), demyelinating (e.g., MS), structural (e.g., neoplasm, syringomyelia, syringobulbia), exogenous (e.g., TBI).
7. **Connective tissue disease.** SLE, polyarteritis nodosa, Sjögren's syndrome.
8. **Toxins.** Heavy metals (metallic elements such as arsenic, lead, and mercury), antibiotics and chemotherapy, Vitamin B_6 overdose, alcoholism.
9. **Infections.** Lyme disease, HIV, leprosy.
10. **Metabolic imbalance.** Hyperkalemia, hypophosphatemia, hypocalcemia, respiratory alkalosis, hypothyroidism, diabetes, malnutrition, vitamin B_{12} deficiency.

II. Systemic (non-neuromusculoskeletal) nonpain-related problems

The following are differential diagnoses of common PM&R problems that do not have pain as a primary feature although pain may play a secondary role in some of them:

A. GENERAL PROBLEMS

1. **Chronic fatigue**
a. ***Psychogenic origin*** (80% of cases). Anxiety states, depression, "chronic fatigue syndrome".
b. ***Fatigue of physical origin*** (20% of cases). Infectious disease (febrile states, tuberculosis), metabolic disorders (diabetes mellitus, hypothyroidism, hyperparathyroidism, hypopituitarism, Addison's disease), blood dyscrasias (anemia, lymphoma, leukemia), renal disease (acute renal failure, chronic renal failure),

liver disease (acute hepatitis, chronic hepatitis, and cirrhosis), chronic pulmonary disease, chronic cardiovascular disease, neoplastic disease, neuromuscular disease with weakness.

2. Fever acquired in the hospital (nosocomial)

a. ***Infectious***. Sepsis associated with intravascular therapy, urinary catheter-associated bacteriuria, lower respiratory infection (pneumonia), surgical wound infection (deep wound abscess), cardiac bypass (postperfusion syndrome caused by cytomegalovirus or Epstein–Barr virus), upper respiratory infection (sinusitis, pharyngitis, colds), pacemaker and prosthesis infections, skin and soft tissue infections, infections incubating at the time of hospital admission, bacteremia without an apparent source (may be the result of endocarditis, osteomyelitis, pressure ulcers).

b. ***Noninfectious***. Reactions to therapeutic agents (medications, contrast dyes), surgical procedures, intravascular catheter-induced inflammation without concurrent infection, transfusion of blood products, thrombophlebitis, pulmonary embolism, instrumentation (e.g., angiography, colonoscopy, bronchoscopy, and cystoscopy), therapeutic devices (e.g., nasotracheal intubation), noninfectious illnesses (e.g., arthritis, gout, malignancy, hepatitis, appendicitis, and intracerebral bleeding, etc.), hematomas, factitious (self-induced) fever.

3. Anxiety

a. ***Psychiatric disorder***. Anxiety disorders, depressive illness, schizophrenia.

b. ***Disease of the CNS***. Postconcussion syndrome, vascular disease, degenerative disorders, seizures.

c. ***Endocrine and metabolic disorders***. Hyperthyroidism and hypothyroidism, hyperparathyroidism, hyperadrenocorticism, hypoglycemia, pheochromocytoma.

d. ***Drug effects***. Sympathomimetic agents, corticosteroids, alcohol.

e. ***Drug withdrawal syndromes***. Alcohol, barbiturates.

f. ***Miscellaneous***. Menopause, mitral valve prolapse, porphyria.

B. NEUROLOGIC PROBLEMS

1. Acute confusional states

a. ***Metabolic dysfunction***. Electrolyte imbalance (hyper/hypoglycemia, hyper/hyponatremia, hyper/hypomagnesemia, hyper/hypocalcemia), hyper/hypothermia, hepatic failure, renal failure, hypoxia, hyper/hypocarbia, endocrinopathies (thyroid storm, myxedema, adrenal dysfunctions), acidosis, alkalosis, porphyria, vitamin deficiencies.

b. ***Drugs and toxins***. Psychoactive medications, alcohol, toxic ingestions, drug and alcohol withdrawal, carbon monoxide poisoning.

c. ***Infections***. Systemic infections, CNS infections (meningitis, encephalitis).

d. ***Seizures***. Complex partial seizures, psychomotor and absence seizures, status epilepticus, postictal states.

e. ***Brain disease***. Focal brain lesions (right parietal lobe, medial occipital lobes, right frontal lobe), generalized brain lesions (head trauma, concussion, skull fractures, hypertensive encephalopathy, subdural hematoma, intracranial bleed, space-occupying masses, herniation, vasculitis, petechial hemorrhages, brainstem lesions).

f. ***Others***. Psychiatric illness, arrhythmia.

2. Dementia

a. ***Focal neurologic***. Trauma (cerebral contusion), tumor, chronic subdural hematoma, multiple sclerosis, vascular dementia (multiple cerebral infarcts, single cerebral infarcts, lacunar infarcts), Huntington's chorea, Pick's disease, normal-pressure hydrocephalus, Parkinson's disease, progressive supranuclear palsy, olivopontocerebellar degeneration.

b. ***Nonfocal neurologic.*** Lupus cerebritis, brain abscess, progressive multifocal leukoencephalopathy, acute and chronic meningitis, limbic encephalitis, carcinomatosis, Creutzfeldt–Jakob disease, Whipple's disease, postconcussion syndrome, Alzheimer's disease, senile dementia, Wernicke's encephalopathy, paraneoplastic syndromes.

c. ***Metabolic and endocrine abnormalities.*** Pernicious anemia (vitamin B_{12} or cyanocobalamin deficiency), pellagra (niacin deficiency), Wernicke–Korsakoff syndrome (thiamine deficiency), hyper/hypocalcemia, hyper/hypomagnesemia, hyper/hypothyroidism, hypoparathyroidism, chronic hypoglycemia, chronic hypoxemia, hepatic encephalopathy, Cushing's disease, Addison's disease, chronic renal disease (uremia), chronic dehydration.

d. ***Others.*** Depression (pseudodementia), schizophrenia (dementia praecox), syphilis, AIDS encephalopathy, heavy metal intoxication (mercury, lead, aluminum), drug induced (chronic drug toxicity).

3. **Seizure** must be differentiated from syncope, transient ischemic attacks, migraine, hypoglycemia, paroxysmal vertigo, narcolepsy, and psychogenic spells. The usual causes of seizure include:

a. ***Metabolic.*** Hyper/hypoglycemia, hyper/hypomagnesemia, hyper/hyponatremia, hypocalcemia, hypoxia, acid–base disturbance, organ failure (renal, hepatic), drug withdrawal (alcohol, sedatives), drug intoxication (aminophylline, lidocaine, cocaine, amphetamine).

b. ***Focal cortex lesion.*** Infarction, contusion, concussion, tumor, abscess, meningitis, encephalitis, cerebritis, subdural hematoma, intracranial bleed, postoperative scar.

c. ***Cardiovascular.*** Hypertension, heart block, myocardial infarction, brady- or tachyarrhythmia.

d. ***Congenital (hereditary or acquired).*** Idiopathic, perinatal injury, maldevelopment, degenerations.

4. **Ill-defined dizziness** other than vertigo (see section II.B.6), syncope, or disequilibrium (see section II.B.5). Consider psychiatric disorders, such as hyperventilation syndrome, anxiety neurosis, hysterical neurosis, and affective disorders (depression).

5. **Disequilibrium** (feeling of unsteadiness without rotation).

a. ***Multiple sensory deficits*** (diminished proprioception with concomitant visual loss, extrapyramidal dysfunction, orthostatic hypotension, or vestibular disturbances).

b. ***Cerebellar dysfunction.*** Alcoholic cerebellar dysfunction, tumors, infarcts.

c. ***Extrapyramidal diseases.*** Parkinson's disease, progressive supranuclear palsy.

d. ***Schwannomas and other cerebellopontine angle tumors.*** Schwannoma, meningioma, epidermoid tumors, other posterior fossa tumors.

e. ***Nonfunctioning labyrinths***

f. ***Drug-induced disequilibrium.*** Anticonvulsants (e.g., barbiturates, phenytoin, ethosuximide, carbamazepine), alcohol (ethanol, methanol) intoxication, salicylates, cinchona alkaloids (e.g., quinine and quinidine), tranquilizers (e.g., diazepam, lorazepam, and flurazepam), aminoglycoside antibiotics (e.g., tobramycin, amikacin, and gentamicin).

6. **Vertigo and nystagmus** (vertigo is the illusion of motion usually accompanied by nausea, vomiting, nystagmus, and disequilibrium).

a. ***Peripheral or labyrinthine.*** Otitis media, acute labyrinthitis (bacterial, viral, syphilitic), vestibular neuronitis, benign positional vertigo, barotrauma, posttraumatic vertigo (labyrinthine concussion, perilymph fistula), Ménière's disease, cerebellopontine angle tumor (acoustic schwannoma), lesions of the eighth nerve (acoustic neuroma, meningioma, mononeuropathy, metastatic carcinoma), mastoiditis, Cogan's syndrome, ototoxic drugs (alcohol, quinine, salicylates, aminoglycoside antibiotics, such as streptomycin and gentamicin), "physiologic" (motion sickness, vision-induced vertigo, vertigo at heights), temporomandibular joint syndrome.

b. ***CNS or central***. Vertebrobasilar artery insufficiency, posterior fossa tumor or other brain tumors (meningioma, hemangioma), infarction/hemorrhage (cerebral cortex, cerebellum, or brainstem), cerebral vasculitis, arteriovenous malformation, intracranial aneurysm, basilar migraine, multiple sclerosis, CNS infections (viral, bacterial), granulomatous meningitis, herpes zoster oticus (Ramsay–Hunt syndrome), temporal lobe epilepsy (vestibular epilepsy, seizure aura), Arnold–Chiari malformation, syringobulbia, migraine headache, persistent vestibular dysfunction, diplopia.

c. ***Others***. Drugs (tranquilizers, antihypertensives, antidepressants), metabolic (hypoxia, anemia, fever), hypotension, severe hypertension, cardiac arrhythmia, functional disorder, psychogenic (hyperventilation, hysteria).

Further reading

Bradley WG, Daroff RB, Fenichel GM, *et al.*, editors: *Neurology in clinical practice: principles of diagnosis and management*, ed 4, Boston, 2003, Butterworth-Heinemann.

Healey P, Jacobson EJ: *Common medical diagnoses: an algorithmic approach*, ed 3, Philadelphia, 2000, WB Saunders.

Kasper DL, Braunwald E, Fauci AS, *et al.*, editors: *Harrison's principles of internal medicine*, ed 16, New York, 2004, McGraw-Hill.

Paget S, Gibofsky A, Beary III JF, editors: *Manual of rheumatology and outpatient orthopedic disorders*, ed 4, Philadelphia, 2000, Lippincott, Williams & Wilkins.

Samuels M, editor: *Manual of neurologic therapeutics*, ed 6, Philadelphia, 1999, Lippincott, Williams & Wilkins.

Samuels MA, Feske S, editors: *Office practice of neurology*, ed 2, New York, 2003, Churchill Livingstone.

Stein J, editor: *Internal medicine*, ed 5, St Louis, 1998, Mosby.

PART IV

PHYSICAL MEDICINE AND REHABILITATION: MANAGEMENT TOOLS

CHAPTER 4.1
Physical modalities

Modalities that use physical energy for their therapeutic effect (called physical modalities) are commonly prescribed in PM&R. They include thermotherapy (heat and cold), hydrotherapy, electrotherapy (including biofeedback), light therapy (ultraviolet radiation, laser), manipulation and mobilization, traction, massage, acupuncture, magnetotherapy, and extracorporeal shock-wave therapy. Because of the passive nature of most of these modalities, they should not be prescribed indiscriminately. They should only be given for a short period as an adjunct, not as a substitute, to active modalities such as exercise and education.

I. Therapeutic heat

The physiologic response of tissue to heat depends on the intensity of heat applied (therapeutic range is 40–45.5°C or 104–113.9°F), the length of time of heat exposure (therapeutic range is 3–30 min), the size/volume of area to be heated, and the rate of temperature rise in the tissues (i.e., if heat rise is faster than heat dissipation, overheating may occur). Therapeutic heat causes vasodilation, which can either be local or consensual (i.e., distal vasodilation via a reflex mechanism). In the subacute and chronic stages, vasodilation can help in resolving inflammatory infiltrates and exudates, and in promoting tissue healing (by increasing nutrient supply to the heated area). Other therapeutic effects of heat include an increase in nerve pain threshold, an increase in metabolic rate, a decrease in the firing rate of muscle spindles, and an increase in the plastic elongation of collagen fibers in connective tissues (i.e., when heat is combined with stretching).

General applications of heat include relief of pain and muscle spasm, reduction of joint stiffness, and increase in joint range of motion. General contraindications and precautions include acute inflammation, trauma, or hemorrhage; bleeding disorders (e.g., hemophilia); insensate skin (e.g., complete spinal cord injury); inability to communicate or respond to pain (e.g., coma or dementia); poor thermal regulation (e.g., from neuroleptics); sites of malignancy; areas of ischemia (e.g., arterial insufficiency); atrophic skin (e.g., patients on prolonged steroid regimens); immature scar tissue; edema; and open wounds and infected skin lesions. Use of any form of heat must be supervised, especially in the elderly and the very young, because excessive heat may cause skin burn.

Methods of heat transfer include conduction (via physical contact between two surfaces), convection (through current movements in liquid or gases), and conversion (through absorption of electromagnetic energy, e.g., radiant heat, ultrasound, microwave, and short waves). Therapeutic heating agents can either be superficial or deep.

A. SUPERFICIAL HEATING AGENTS are used to heat joints with relatively little soft tissue covering (e.g., hand and foot) or to cause a deeper effect (e.g., relief of muscular spasm) through reflex mechanisms. They achieve maximum tissue temperatures in skin and subcutaneous fat.

1. Conductive heat agents

a. ***Hot moist packs (hydrocollator packs)*** are canvas bags filled with hydrophilic silicate and stored on racks in 70–80°C (158–176°F) water. The pack is wrapped in six to eight layers of towels and can be applied for 20–30 minutes.

For home treatment, patients may use an electrically controlled, moist heating pack (e.g., Thermophore) or a microwavable gel pack.

b. ***Paraffin*** is a mixture of one part mineral oil to seven parts paraffin wax heated to 52–54°C (125.6–129.2°F). The mineral oil lowers the melting point of the paraffin and the combination has a low specific heat, which allows the paraffin to be tolerable even at 47–54.4°C (118–130°F). Paraffin is most commonly used on irregular surfaces such as the distal extremities of patients with rheumatoid arthritis, hand contractures, and scleroderma. It may be applied by dipping the extremity 8 to 10 times followed by wrapping in wax paper or a plastic bag then covering with a towel to retain heat or by continuous immersion of the extremity in the paraffin bath. Application time is 20–30 minutes.

2. Convective heating agents

a. ***Fluidotherapy*** uses a device that blows hot air through a container holding fine cellulose particles (made of beads or corn husks) to produce a dry, warm, air–fluid mixture with properties similar to those of a liquid. Temperature ranges from 38.8–47.8°C (102–118°F). The limb may be immersed for 20–30 minutes.

b. ***Hydrotherapy*** (see section III below for details).

c. ***Dry hydrotherapy*** (see section IX.B.6 below for details).

3. Radiant heating agent (infrared lamp). Infrared radiant energy is absorbed by the skin and converted to dry, superficial heat. Unlike hot packs, there is no discomfort from the weight of an object; however, only one body surface at a time can be heated. Distance from lamp to skin is usually 45–60 cm (18–24 in). Application time is 20–30 minutes.

B. DEEP HEATING AGENTS can increase tissue temperature to a depth of 3–5 cm or more without overheating the skin and subcutaneous tissue. They are used to heat deeper structures such as the hip joint or the belly of the trapezius muscle. Deep heat is produced from the conversion of energy into heat as it penetrates the skin into the ligaments, muscles, bones, and joint capsules. The forms of energy used are high-frequency sound waves (ultrasound), high-frequency currents (short-wave diathermy), and electromagnetic radiation (microwave diathermy). Ultrasound is convenient and is commonly used, but both short-wave and microwave diathermies are cumbersome and are seldom used.

1. Ultrasound. Ceramic and quartz piezoelectric crystals are used to convert electric signals to ultrasonic sound waves (with high frequency of 0.8–1.0 MHz), which are propagated through and absorbed by the tissues and converted to heat. Ultrasound is absorbed and attenuated most in bone followed by, in decreasing order, tendon, skin, muscle, and fat. It is markedly attenuated by air and is totally reflected at the air–tissue interface. At the interface of bone and soft tissue there is a further increase in temperature because of the change in level of absorption and attenuation. Ultrasound, as a thermal agent, is used as an adjunct in the management of soft tissue dysfunctions including joint contracture, scar tissue (keloids), tendinitis, bursitis (calcific bursitis), myositis ossificans, skeletal muscle spasm, musculoskeletal pain, and postherpetic neuralgic pain. It produces temperatures of up to 46°C (114.8°F) in deep tissue (e.g., bone and muscle interface).

The nonthermal effects of ultrasound include cavitation (gas bubble production in a sound field because of turbulence), acoustic streaming (unidirectional movement of compressible material or medium as a result of pressure asymmetries caused by the traveling ultrasonic waves), and standing waves (superposition of high- and low-pressure waves at a half-wavelength interval). Acoustic streaming and stable cavitation are believed to cause wound contraction and protein synthesis. Both thermal and nonthermal effects of ultrasound may facilitate tissue healing in dermal ulcers, incision wounds, tendon surgery, bone fractures, and nerve compression injury. The nonthermal effects of ultrasound are used in extracorporeal shock-wave therapy (see section XII below).

Ultrasound waves can be delivered continuously or in pulses. The usual dosage range is from 0.5 to 2.0 watts/cm^2 for 5–10 minutes, applied daily or every other day. It may be applied directly to regular surface skin by stroking in linear or circular sweeps using a coupling medium (e.g., a water-soluble gel) or, rarely, by a stationary method. In areas with an irregular surface (e.g., hand and ankle), both the ultrasound transducer and the area to be treated are placed under water with a distance of 1 cm between skin and transducer. The ultrasound transducer must be moved constantly to avoid hot spots, unstable cavitation (gas bubbles that continue to grow in size and then collapse), blood cell stasis, or blood vessel (endothelial cell) damage.

In addition to the general contraindications of heat, ultrasound should not be applied over fluid-filled cavities (e.g., eyes, testes, and pregnant uterus), the heart, cardiac pacemakers, brain, cervical and stellate ganglia, laminectomized spine, thrombophlebitic sites, growing epiphyses, infected bone, and malignant tumor. Its use in metal implants is controversial. Although studies have shown that metal implants do not concentrate heat energy, ultrasound must be used with caution in the presence of metal implants (e.g., screws, plates, or uncemented prostheses). When methylmethacrylate cement is used in joint replacements, however, ultrasound should not be used because of the possibility of loosening via unstable cavitation in the cement.

A form of ultrasound in which topical medications (mixed with the ultrasound coupling medium) are driven through the skin is called **phonophoresis (sonophoresis)**. Phonophoresis probably induces transdermal migration by increasing cell permeability through the thermal effects of ultrasound. Commonly used topical medications include corticosteroids (e.g., 1% or 10% hydrocortisone and dexamethasone) or local anesthetics [e.g., 1% lidocaine (Xylocaine)]. Its main indications include tendinitis (e.g., of Achilles, patellar, or bicipital tendons), tenosynovitis, epicondylitis (e.g., tennis elbow), chronic suprahumeral impingement of shoulder, osteoarthritis, bursitis, capsulitis, strains, fasciitis, contracture, scar tissues, neuromas, and adhesions. Common ultrasound parameters include 1 or 2 MHz of continuous (or pulsed) ultrasound with an intensity of 1–3 W/cm^2 for 5–7 minutes per site. It may be given once per day for 3 or 4 consecutive days for a total of 10 days. Prolonged use should be avoided as it may cause tissue (e.g., tendon) weakening. Phonophoresis should not be confused with iontophoresis, which uses a direct current to drive medications through the skin (see section V.A.1.a).

2. **Short-wave diathermy** uses radio waves (usually 27.12 MHz in the United States; other frequencies are 13.56 and 40.68 MHz) to heat the tissue by conversion. These radio waves, delivered either continuously or in pulses by a short-wave diathermy machine, are transmitted through the area to be treated via a circuit element (i.e., a capacitor or inductor) and tuned as if the patient and the machine were components of a radio transmitter. It raises the temperature up to 15°C in the subcutaneous fat and 4–6°C in the muscle. It is applied for 15–30 minutes. Clinical indications include muscle spasm, muscle and joint contractures, and tendinitis or bursitis. In addition to the aforementioned contraindications of general heating, it should not be used in the presence of jewelry, pacemakers, transcutaneous nerve or muscle stimulators, electrophrenic pacers, cerebellar stimulators, urinary bladder stimulators, surgical implants, contact lenses, metallic intrauterine devices, and the menstruating or pregnant uterus. Moist wound dressings, moist clothing, and perspiration can focus the heat and lead to overheating.
3. **Microwave diathermy** uses electromagnetic radiation at frequencies of 915 and 2450 MHz to heat the tissue by conversion. Like short-wave diathermy, it raises the temperature in the subcutaneous fat (up to 10–12°C) more than muscle (3–4°C). It is applied for 15–30 minutes and is used to heat relatively

superficial muscles and joints. It is also used to help resolve hematoma and to produce local hyperthermia in cancer treatment. It has the same contraindications as short-wave diathermy.

II. Therapeutic cold

The physiologic effects of cold include local vasoconstriction, distal vasoconstriction (via a reflex mechanism), a decrease in metabolic rate and in the release of vasoactive agents (e.g., histamine), an increase in nerve pain threshold, a decrease in motor and sensory nerve conduction, a decrease in the sensitivity of muscle spindle to stretch (controversial), an increase in tissue viscosity with decreased tissue elasticity (this may increase joint stiffness), and a transient increase in systolic and diastolic blood pressure. Methods of cold transfer include conduction (e.g., using an ice pack) and evaporation (i.e., the use of volatile liquids, such as fluorimethane, which evaporates upon contact with the skin producing a cool steam, which extracts heat from the skin surface). Although therapeutic cold is restricted to superficial application, the physiologic effect lasts longer than that of heat.

General applications of cold include relief of pain and muscle spasm, reduction of spasticity and clonus, and control of inflammation and edema in the acute (within 24–48 h) post-traumatic stage. General contraindications and precautions include symptoms of cold sensitivity (e.g., Raynaud's phenomenon, cold urticaria, cryoglobinemia, paroxysmal cold hemoglobinurias, and cold intolerance), areas with compromised circulation (e.g., ischemic areas in patients with peripheral vascular disease affecting the arterial system), the initial 2–3 weeks of wound healing, insensate skin (if cold is used, skin must be closely monitored for burns), severe hypertension (if cold is used, blood pressure must be monitored closely), and patients who are unable to communicate or respond to pain (e.g., comatose or demented patients). Use of cold must be closely supervised, especially in the elderly and the very young, because excessive cold may cause skin burn.

Depending on the size of the area to be cooled, as well as its accessibility to cold application, one of the following methods of cold application can be used.

A. **COLD PACKS** are vinyl bags filled with silica gel or a sand slurry mixture stored in a refrigeration unit at –5°C (23°F). The pack is wrapped in moist towels and can be applied for 20–30 minutes. For home treatment, patients may use commercial gel packs (stored in a household freezer) or cold packs that are chemically activated by squeezing or hitting them against a hard surface.

B. **ICE MASSAGE** consists of rubbing a piece of ice onto the skin in overlapping strokes. The ice may be frozen in paper cups or onto a tongue depressor, i.e., ice "lollipops". Ice massage is indicated for cooling a small area (e.g., muscle belly, tendon, or trigger point) before deep-pressure massage. Analgesia can be attained in 7–10 minutes.

C. **ICE TOWELS** are terrycloth towels soaked in a bucket of crushed ice or in ice–slush mixture, wrung out, and wrapped around a joint. The towel must be changed after 4–5 minutes to retain its coldness. This method is impractical.

D. **COLD BATHS** are water-filled containers (e.g., iced whirlpool) with temperatures of 13–18°C (55.4–64.4°F) into which the distal limb is immersed for cooling. Treatment time is from 20 to 30 minutes.

E. **VAPOCOOLANT SPRAYS** use volatile liquids such as ethyl chloride or fluorimethane for inhibiting spasms [in combination with "spray and stretch" exercise (see Chapter 4.11, section II.A.1.b), "spray and limber" exercise (see Chapter 4.11, section II.A.1.a)] and for local skin anesthesia. Fluorimethane is less volatile and less flammable than ethyl chloride.

F. **CONTROLLED COLD COMPRESSION UNITS** use sleeves containing circulating cold water (with adjustable temperature) into which the edematous limb is placed. This sleeve is then attached to an intermittent pump unit.

III. Hydrotherapy (aquatic therapy)

Hydrotherapy is the external use of water for treating physical dysfunctions. This effect is achieved through the physical properties of water (i.e., buoyancy, pressure, relative density, and viscosity), temperature, and agitation. Because of buoyancy, the percentage of weight bearing is reduced to 50% when immersion is up to the anterior superior iliac spine, 33% when immersion is up to the xiphoid process, and 10% when immersion is up to the C7 spine. Buoyancy also provides assistive exercise (when motion occurs toward the water surface) and resistive exercise (when motion occurs away from the water surface). Hydrostatic pressure helps in circulation and decreases the tendency of blood to pool in the lower part of the body. Relative density (measured in specific gravity) provides support for the body or limb, thus reducing stress on the weight-bearing joint. The viscosity of water is low, so providing little friction with low-speed movements. As speed increases, there is also an increase in turbulence (positive pressure) and drag (negative pressure), hence there is greater friction, making movements more difficult. The thermal effects of hydrotherapy are the same as in local heat or cold application except that there is a greater systemic effect because of the immersion of the larger body surface. Cold can decrease heart rate and increase blood pressure by peripheral vasoconstriction. Heat increases heart rate and causes an initial increase in blood pressure, followed by a drop in blood pressure as a result of vasodilation. Respiratory rate increases in both heat and cold hydrotherapy but less markedly with heat. The methods of heat or cold transfer are by conduction and convection.

The nonthermal (mechanical) effect of hydrotherapy is achieved through water pumps or turbines, which agitate the water and provide massage and debridement. The physiologic effects of water agitation include relief of pain and muscle spasm (through mechanical stimulation of skin receptors, which may act as a counterirritant or as a stimulation to large sensory afferents, thus blocking pain input), mechanical debridement, and facilitation of exercise. If only a mechanical effect is desired, water at neutral temperature (33–36°C or 91.4–96.8°F) is well tolerated.

Indications for hydrotherapy include wound and burn treatment, joint mobilization after cast removal, rheumatoid arthritis, and muscle spasm. Aside from having the same general contraindications and precautions as therapeutic heat and cold, it is also contraindicated in patients with urinary incontinence (unless catheterized), bowel incontinence, colostomy, open wounds (unless the wounds are small and covered with waterproof dressing; or unless the individual tank is sterilized), danger of bleeding or hemorrhage; severe kidney disease (because of the inability to adjust to fluid loss during immersion); intravenous lines (unless they are properly clamped and fixated), uncontrolled seizures, uncontrolled autonomic dysreflexia or blood pressure, acute fever >100°F within the past 24 h, tracheostomy (unless covered with a waterproof dressing), water and airborne infections or diseases (e.g., influenza, gastrointestinal infections, typhoid, tuberculosis, or cholera), skin infections (e.g., tinea pedis or ringworm), vital capacity of less than 1 liter, unstable angina, atrial fibrillation, incipient cardiac failure, severe peripheral vascular disease, or severe mental disorder.

Hydrotherapy may be used in patients infected with human immunodeficiency virus or hepatitis virus as long as universal precautions are observed. It may be applied on open and infected wounds as long as the individual tanks are sterilized (commonly used whirlpool disinfecting additives include povidone-iodine solution, sodium hypochlorite, household bleach, and chloramine-T). It may be used in menstruating women with an internal collection device. Patients with indwelling, external, or suprapubic catheters may use leg bags, sport bags, or bed bags in the water (the bag should be emptied before hydrotherapy and as frequently as needed). Patients with orthotic stabilization devices (e.g., soft collars, Philadelphia collars) may participate in hydrotherapy as long as the devices are dried after used or an extra dry set of the device or their pads are used after treatment. It must be used with caution in patients with fear of water; controlled seizures; stable angina and controlled blood pressure. Hydrotherapy using heat can cause fatigue and should be used with caution in patients with deconditioning, multiple sclerosis, and Guillain–Barré syndrome.

A. **WHIRLPOOLS** are tanks used for partial body immersion. The "limb" tank is used for immersion of one or both upper limbs or the distal lower limb. The "lowboy" and "highboy" tanks are used for lower limb immersion or immersion of the trunk up to the mid-thoracic level. In the lowboy tank the patient is in the long sitting position and can perform full range-of-motion (ROM) exercises with both knees. In the highboy tank, the patient is seated in chest-high water with flexed hips and knees. The usual temperature is 37.8–38.9°C (100–102°F) for the lower limbs and 37.8–40.6°C (100–105°F) for the upper limbs. Temperatures of 43°C (109.4°F) to as high as 45 or 46°C (113 or 114.8°F) may be applied for 5–20 minutes.

B. **HUBBARD TANKS** are used for whole body immersion. The shape and design of the tank allow for motion of all four limbs and accessibility of the patient to the therapist. Temperatures should be less than 39°C (102.2°F) to avoid systemic problems. For mild heating, 36.7–37.2°C (98–98.9°F) may be used, while for more vigorous heating, 37.8–38.3°C (100–100.9°F) may be used. Duration of treatment is 10–20 minutes depending on cardiopulmonary tolerance.

C. **POOL THERAPY** (see Chapter 4.2, section V for discussion of aquatic exercise) is used to promote patient relaxation, improve circulation, restore mobility, strengthen muscles, provide gait training with reduced stress on weight-bearing joints, provide endurance training, and improve psychological and emotional outlook (because patients are usually able to ambulate better in water by using water's buoyancy). Specific clinical indications include rheumatoid arthritis, orthopedic patients with musculoskeletal disorders (e.g., chronic back pain) or surgery (e.g., joint replacements, arthroscopic knee surgery), patients with neurologic disorders (e.g., multiple sclerosis in nonheated pools and incomplete paraplegia), or those with partial peripheral lesions (e.g., poliomyelitis, polyneuritis), and in mild cases of spastic cerebral palsy (e.g., postrhizotomy). Unlike whirlpool therapy, pool patients must not have open or discharging wounds (however, a small open wound with a waterproof dressing may be allowed in the pool). For patients with spasticity or for those requiring immersion for up to 20–45 minutes, lower temperatures of 30–34.5°C (86–94°F) are used. Patients with multiple sclerosis require temperatures of 29°C (84°F) or less. Arthritic patients may be immersed for 10–20 minutes at higher temperatures of 36–37°C (96.8–98.6°F). For recommendations on water temperatures used for aquatic exercises, refer to Chapter 4.2, section V).

D. **CONTRAST BATH** is a special technique of treating the distal limb using the whirlpool tank. It alternates exposure of the limb to heat (38–44°C or 100.4–111°F) and cold (10–18°C or 50–64.4°F) to produce reflex hyperemia. Typical treatment begins with an initial soaking of the limb in the warm whirlpool for 10 minutes, followed by four cycles of alternate 1- to 4-minute cold soaks (in a basin of water) and 4- to 6-minute warm soaks (in the whirlpool tank). It is used for rheumatoid arthritis, reflex sympathetic dystrophy, joint sprains, muscular strains, mild peripheral vascular diseases, and to toughen amputation stumps. Aside from the general contraindication to heat and cold, it should not be used when patients have small vessel disease caused by diabetes, arteriosclerotic endarteritis, or Burger's disease.

E. SITZ BATH is the immersion of the pelvis in a hot, cold, or contrasting (hot/cold) bath. It may be used for the relief of postpartum perineal pain, hemorrhoidal pain, and anorectal pain. It has the same general contraindication as the use of heat or cold.

F. PULSED LAVAGE is the use of an electrically powered device to generate pressure (from 4 to 15 lb/in^2 or psi) in a system that delivers a pulsating stream of irrigation solution (usually normal saline) to loosen and clean wound debris and increase tissue perfusion, thus providing a clean wound bed for granulation formation. It may be used concurrently with a suction device to remove wound debris and the irrigating fluid. It can be used for wound cleaning in patients who need to remain in their room (e.g., for medical isolation), or in patients with tracheostomies or ventilators, or in the patient's home. It is contraindicated near areas with exposed blood vessels, eyes, and dura.

G. SHOWER CART uses overhead retractable shower heads (each with independently adjustable water temperature and pressure) to provide gentle spray or shower hydrotherapy during mechanical debridement of large surface area burns and other wounds under relatively sterile conditions. It was developed to reduce the risk of autocontamination and cross-contamination with conventional whirlpool baths or Hubbard tanks. Compared to the Hubbard tank, it uses significantly less water, less space, and needs less maintenance.

IV. Light therapy

A. ULTRAVIOLET RADIATION (UVR) has a wavelength of 200–400 nm (bactericidal wavelength is 253.7 nm) and can be produced by a small, handheld, low-pressure mercury or "cold quartz" lamp. Ultraviolet radiation interacts with tissue and bacteria, causing nonthermal photochemical reactions and alterations in DNA and cell proteins. Its physiologic effects include a bactericidal effect on motile bacteria, an increase in vascularization at wound margins, hyperplasia and exfoliation (peeling), tanning, increased vitamin D production, and excitation of the calcium metabolism. The major clinical indication for UVR today is the treatment of wounds (aseptic or septic) and dermatologic conditions such as psoriasis (using Goeckerman technique, i.e., application of coal tar ointment to skin prior to UVR), acne, and folliculitis.

Dosages are determined by the exposure time required to produce erythema on the volar aspect of the forearm. Minimal erythemal dose (MED), also called first-degree erythema, is the exposure time necessary to produce a faint erythema within a few hours in average Caucasian skin. The MED subsides within 24 hours. A 2.5-MED exposure produces second-degree erythema in 4–6 hours with pain and subsides in 2–4 days, followed by desquamation. A 5-MED exposure produces third-degree erythema in 2–4 hours with pain and local edema followed by marked desquamation. A 10-MED exposure produces fourth-degree erythema with superficial blister. Usual UVR prescription doses begin with 1 or 2 MED and are kept to less than 5 MED. Treatment is given two to three times per week.

Ultraviolet radiation must be used with caution in people using photosensitizing drugs or cosmetics; in patients with fair complexion, scars, or atrophic skin; or in the presence of acute renal and hepatic failure, severe diabetes, hyperthyroidism, generalized dermatitis, advanced arteriosclerosis, and active, progressive pulmonary tuberculosis. To prevent conjunctivitis and photokeratosis, the eyes of both patient and therapist must be shielded (using UV goggles or cotton pledgets). Contraindications include porphyrias, pellagra, sarcoidosis, and the acute onset of psoriasis, lupus erythematosus, eczema, herpes simplex, and xeroderma pigmentosum.

B. LOW-POWER COLD LASER or **LOW-LEVEL LASER THERAPY**. LASER is the acronym for Light Amplification by Stimulated Emission of Radiation. Lasers emit photons (energy particles of light), which can interact with biological molecules to produce light-induced thermal or chemical reactions in the body. Laser devices can either be thermal (hot) or nonthermal (i.e., cold, low-power, or soft). In PM&R, low-power cold lasers produced by helium–neon gas (He-Ne lasers) or by gallium–arsenide semiconductors (Ga-As lasers) are commonly used to produce nonthermal or photochemical reactions in the cells, also referred to as photobiology or biostimulation. He-Ne lasers deliver a red beam with a wavelength of 632.8 nm in a continuous wave and have direct effects in the first 2–5 mm of soft tissue and indirect effects up to a depth of 10–15 mm. Ga-As lasers are invisible, with a wavelength of 904 nm delivered in pulse mode, and have direct penetration of 1–2 cm and indirect penetration of up to 5 cm.

The physiologic effects of cold lasers include facilitation of wound and ulcer healing by stimulating fibroblasts; increasing the tensile strength of a laser-treated wound; increasing phagocytosis by leukocytes with bactericidal effects; increasing T- and B-lymphocyte activities; reduction of edema by decreasing prostaglandin E_2; reducing scar tissue formation by promoting epithelization with less exudative material and with more regular alignment of collagen; pain reduction by reducing action potential amplitude and decreasing sensory conduction velocity; and promotion of bone healing by bone and articular cartilage remodeling.

Clinical uses include wound and ulcer healing, burns, sprain, strain, tendinitis, contusions, pain (e.g., acute and chronic musculoskeletal pain, arthritic pain, headache, orofacial pain, and neuropathic pain), and fracture nonunion. For pain treatment, the laser may be applied over acupuncture points or at painful nerve sites or by combining with electrical stimulation.

Contraindications include cancerous tissue, areas of hemorrhage, direct stimulation into the eyes (may cause retinal burns), and the first trimester of pregnancy. A temporary increase in pain or syncopal feeling may be experienced during treatment, but these are generally self-limited.

The usual dose is 0.05–0.5 joules/cm^2 for acute conditions and 0.5–3.0 joules/cm^2 for more chronic conditions for three to six treatments. Treatment time is in s/cm^2 and varies with the prescribed joules/cm^2. The effectiveness of low-level laser therapy is controversial.

V. Electrotherapy

Electrotherapy is the therapeutic use of electricity to transcutaneously stimulate the nerve or the muscle or both using surface electrodes. Its physiologic effects include muscle group contraction, which can increase joint ROM, re-educate muscles, retard muscle atrophy, and increase muscle strength; increase in circulation with the relief of pain and muscle spasm via a muscle pumping effect, and the release of polypeptides and neurotransmitters (e.g., β-endorphins, dopamine, enkephalins, vasoactive intestinal polypeptides, and serotonin); inhibition of pain fibers via stimulation of large peripheral type A nerve fibers (e.g., gate-control theory and central-biasing theory); wound healing and osteogenesis (via tissue regeneration and remodeling); and for driving medicated ions through the skin (iontophoresis).

Clinical indications include pain management (acute and chronic musculoskeletal pain, chronic neurogenic pain, general systemic pain), joint effusion or interstitial edema (acute and chronic); protective muscle spasm; muscle disuse atrophy; dermal ulcers and wounds; and circulatory disorders (venous insufficiency, neurovascular disorder).

General contraindications include circulatory impairment (e.g., arterial or venous thrombosis and thrombophlebitis), stimulation over the carotid sinus, stimulation across the heart (especially in patients with demand pacemakers), pregnancy, seizure disorders, fresh fractures, active hemorrhage, and malignancy. Direct current can cause electrochemical burns and should not be used on skin with decreased sensation.

Treatment time per session is variable; it can be 1–5 minutes per trigger point in the monopolar treatment of chronic musculoskeletal pain; 10–30 minutes for acute pain and circulatory disorders; 30–60 minutes for skin ulcers and wounds; 2–4 hours for edema control; and there can be from a few to many repetitions for muscle strengthening. It can be once or twice daily or three times per week for a few weeks. For treatment time using transcutaneous electrical nerve stimulators (TENS), see section V.B.2.

In PM&R, transcutaneous electrical stimulators (TES) can be classified by the type of current as direct current (DC), alternating current (AC), or pulsed current. They can also be classified by their stimulation effect as subliminal (nonperceived) current, TENS, and neuromuscular electrical stimulator (NMES). Technically speaking, all pulsed and most AC currents (except when used for subliminal or subthreshold stimulation) are TENS because they work transcutaneously and excite the peripheral nerves. However, in common usage, TENS refers to the small, portable, battery-operated TES unit used for pain relief. The TES used for neuromuscular stimulation of innervated muscles are called NMES.

A. TES CLASSIFICATION BY TYPE OF THERAPEUTIC CURRENT

1. **Direct current (DC)** is an electrical current that flows in one direction for at least 1 second.

a. ***Continuous or uninterrupted low-voltage DC (galvanic current)*** is used to promote healing of superficial skin ulcers (mainly by changing skin pH and causing reflex vasodilation) and to facilitate union of fracture. It is the current used to drive ions through the skin in **iontophoresis**. Indications for iontophoresis include administration of local anesthetics (e.g., 1% lidocaine) in neuritis or bursitis; reduction of edema in acute and chronic musculoskeletal inflammatory conditions (e.g., bursitis, tendinitis, and ligamentous sprain) using topical corticosteroids (e.g., 1% or 10% hydrocortisone and dexamethasone), sodium salicylate, or hyaluronidase (Wydase); promoting muscle relaxation and vasodilation using magnesium sulfate (Epsom salts); softening scars and adhesions using sodium chloride; and reducing calcium deposits in calcific tendinitis using acetic acid (acetate). Iontophoresis can also be used for the treatment of skin conditions like idiopathic hyperhydrosis using tap water, small (<1 cm) open ischemic ulcers using zinc oxide, and fungus infections (*Tinea pedis*) using copper sulfate.

It is contraindicated in people with previous allergic reaction to the iontophoresis agent and in insensate skin. The intensity of iontophoresis currently ranges from microamperes (more comfortable but takes longer to apply) to 5 mA (or even up to 30 mA). Although transdermal penetration of drugs via iontophoresis or phonoresis has been reported in animal studies, this has not been clearly substantiated in humans. Except for occasional superficial skin blisters caused by iontophoresis, both iontophoresis and phonophoresis are safe, noninvasive, and generally not associated with the systemic side-effects of the medication.

b. ***Modulated DC*** can either be reversed, interrupted, or surged (ramped). It is not commonly used because it is uncomfortable and can potentially cause skin burns. It has been used to directly stimulate denervated muscle fibers and to retard atrophy. However, recent studies have shown that electrical stimulation of denervated muscles may be deleterious possibly because of muscle fiber degeneration (with or without associated fibrosis) and retardation of reinnervation.

2. **Alternating current (AC)** is an electrical current that changes the direction of flow (i.e., with reference to the zero baseline) at least once every second.

a. ***Continuous or uninterrupted AC*** is a bidirectional current, with no interval between pulses and no modulation. This current is often referred to simply as AC and is the household electrical current used in North America (i.e., 60 Hz AC).

b. ***Modulated AC***

I. **Time-modulated** AC in burst mode is referred to as "**Russian**" **current**. It has been used for muscle re-education. However, it has a fixed-phase duration, uses unnecessarily high total current, is not indicated for strong contraction of small muscles, and is less versatile and less comfortable than symmetric biphasic pulsed current. Studies have shown that pulsed current (i.e., pulsed high-volt monophasic or biphasic currents) is just as effective as "Russian" current for muscle re-education during motor stimulation.

II. **Amplitude-modulated** AC can be produced by mixing two AC sources with different frequency to generate **interferential current (IFC)**, also known as a **beat pulse** or **alternating modulation frequency**. One of the two currents is usually held at 4000 Hz, whereas the other is held constant or varied over a range of 4001 to 4100 Hz. IFC can reportedly stimulate sensory, motor, and pain fibers. Because of its frequency, the interferential wave is claimed to meet low impedance when crossing the skin to enter the underlying tissue. This deep tissue penetration can then be adjusted to stimulate parasympathetic nerve fibers for increased blood flow. IFC has been used for the relief of acute superficial pain or chronic deep aching pain from various tissue origins, for vascular conditions (e.g., Raynaud's disease, venous insufficiency, and orthostatic hypotension), and for urogenital dysfunction (e.g., urinary stress incontinence). However, its effectiveness over other forms of current (e.g., pulsed current) remains controversial. Like the "Russian" current, IFC has a fixed-phase duration, uses unnecessarily high total current, and is less versatile and less comfortable than symmetric biphasic pulsed current during motor stimulation.

IFC systems (e.g., IF-400) typically use four electrodes near pain sites, but a recent device called the **Dynatron STS** uses eight electrodes applied bilaterally to the lower legs, feet, arms, and hands to form four intersecting stimulation channels that follow the peripheral nerves across the spine. This is supposed to normalize the sympathetic nervous system, thus reducing pain systematically rather than locally in chronic pain conditions associated with the sympathetic nervous system. The effectiveness of Dynatron STS in treating chronic pain is controversial.

3. **Pulsed current** is an electrical current conducted as a signal of short duration with each pulse lasting only a few milliseconds or microseconds followed by an interpulse interval. Pulsed current is classified by its waveform as either monophasic (one phase to each pulse) or biphasic (two opposing phases in each pulse).

a. Monophasic pulsed current

I. **Low-voltage monophasic pulsed current (diadynamic current)** usually has a sinusoidal wave and provides direct excitatory responses. It is very uncomfortable and is obsolete.

II. **High-voltage monophasic pulsed current** (HVPC) is used for wound healing (e.g., pressure ulcer and postsurgical wounds), pain modulation (e.g., before debriding burns and in hand injuries), edema and muscle spasm reduction (e.g., sprains and strains), muscle re-education and maintenance of muscle integrity (e.g., disuse atrophy), and prevention of postoperative deep vein thrombosis. Like the modulated AC, HVPC has a fixed-phase duration, uses unnecessarily high total current, is not indicated for strong contraction of large muscles, and is less versatile and less comfortable than symmetric biphasic pulsed current during motor stimulation.

b. Biphasic pulsed current

I. **Asymmetric biphasic pulsed current (Faradic current)** used to be mistaken as a form of AC. This low-voltage current is not very comfortable and has limited clinical use because of the limited current modulation.

II. **Symmetric biphasic pulsed current with interphase** (also termed **intrapulse**) **interval** is an optimally designed current, which is comfortable and can be used for stimulating peripheral nerves and for connective tissue regeneration and osteogenesis.

B. TES CLASSIFICATION BY STIMULATION EFFECT

1. **Subliminal or nonperceived current or low-intensity stimulators (LIS),** also called microcurrent electrical neuromuscular stimulation (MENS) or microcurrent electrical stimulator (MES), and marketed under various names (e.g., Microcurent, MENS Therapy, Electro-Acuscope, Myopulse, Myomatic, MENS-O-MATIC, Alfastim, Pain Suppressor, Biopulse, etc.) use a low-frequency, low-intensity current (i.e., 1000 mA) given below the threshold of nerve stimulation ("subliminal"). It has been used in alcohol and drug addiction, acute and chronic pain, protective muscle spasm, inflammation, and in promoting regeneration of tissue (connective tissues, bones, nerves) for fracture healing, wound healing, ligament healing, and tendon healing. Its efficacy, however, remains controversial.

2. **Transcutaneous electrical nerve stimulation (TENS)** is the transmission of electrical current to stimulate nerve fibers for the symptomatic relief of pain. Its proposed mechanism of pain control is based on the gate-control theory of Melzack and Wall (i.e., stimulation of large A fibers modulates pain-input transmission of small-diameter A-delta and C fibers at the dorsal horn), the "central-biasing" or "central control trigger" theory (a modification of the gate-control theory wherein large fiber activates central inhibitory mechanisms that descend to modulate pain transmission neurons within the dorsal horns), and the endogenous opiate pain-control theory (e.g., β-endorphin).

The TENS unit is a portable, battery-powered device the size of a cigarette pack. It transmits current impulses through lead wires and electrodes attached to the patient's skin. Some units offer monophasic pulses, while others offer symmetrical or asymmetrical biphasic pulses; few offer burst or amplitude-modulated AC pulses. Some bigger, nonportable TES units, for example IFC units and HVPC units, can also be used as a TENS system. Short-wave diathermy can be pulsed at a high-frequency (27 MHz) electromagnetic radiation and can be used as a TENS alternative instead of a deep heating device.

Most TENS units have three stimulation parameters: pulse rate, pulse duration, and amplitude (or intensity). The pulse rate and duration are usually preset, but the intensity is adjustable. The four common modes of TENS stimulation as described by Mannheimer are listed in Table 4.1-1. In the conventional mode, the onset of relief is within 1–20 minutes with post-TENS analgesia equal

Table 4.1-1 Types of TENS stimulation. The frequency and duration are usually preset. The amplitude or intensity is adjusted until the desired level of paresthesia (P) or contraction (C) is reached

Stimulation modes*	Frequency (pps or Hz)	Duration (μs)	Amplitude (mA)
1. Conventional†	high 50–100 Hz	narrow 30–75 μs	P = mild C = none 10–30 mA
2. Strong low rate‡ (acupuncture-like)	low 1–4 Hz	wide 150–200 μs	P = highest tolerable C = rhythmic 30–80 mA
3. Pulse burst or pulse train:			
a. Low-intensity	2 bursts/second 70–100 Hz/burst	narrow 40–75 μs	P = mild C = none 30–60 mA
b. High-intensity	2 bursts/second 70–100 Hz/burst	wide 150–200 μs	P = mild C = rhythmic 30–60 mA
4. Brief intense§	high 100–150 Hz	wide 150–200 μs	P = highest tolerable C = nonrhythmic or tetanic 30–80 mA

* *Usual patient preference: conventional > modulated > pulse-burst > strong low rate > brief intense.*
† *Conventional mode: onset of relief is within 1–20 minutes with post-TENS analgesia equal to that of stimulation duration or even lasting 1–3 hours or longer; used for all types of pain (especially musculoskeletal pain).*
‡ *Strong low rate mode, the onset of relief is within 20–30 minutes with post-TENS analgesia lasting 2–6 hours; used in chronic neuropathic pain (e.g., reflex sympathetic dystrophy), deep structural pain, fibrositis/myofascial pain syndrome.*
§ *Brief intense mode is seldom used except as an adjunct to joint mobilization.*
Adapted from Mannheimer JS, Lampe GN: Electrode placement techniques. In Mannheimer JS, Lampe GN, editors: Clinical transcutaneous electrical nerve stimulation, *Philadelphia, FA Davis, 1984, p. 338, with permission.*

to that of stimulation duration or even lasting 1–3 hours or longer; however, in the strong low-rate mode, the onset of relief is within 20–30 minutes with post-TENS analgesia lasting 2–6 hours. The prolonged effects could probably be the result of the release of endorphins.

In the newer TENS units, the current may be modulated, i.e., one or more parameters (rate, duration, or intensity) can be set automatically to fluctuate according to a preset level, usually within a range of 40–100% from the starting level, once or twice each second. The aim of TENS modulation is to improve patient tolerance and prevent nerve accommodation. Among the TENS stimulation modes, patient preference is usually conventional > modulated > pulse-burst > strong low rate > brief intense. The brief intense mode is seldom used except as an adjunct to joint mobilization.

Another TENS mode, called hyperstimulation or noninvasive electroacupuncture, uses a very small probe-type stimulating electrode (with tip diameter of 1–3 mm) to generate high current density and produce very noxious cutaneous stimulation that is sharp and burning, without resultant muscle contraction. Its pulse duration is very long (e.g., 500 μs). Although its pulsed frequency can exceed 100 Hz, it usually ranges from 1 to 4 Hz. Its required current amplitude usually does not exceed 50 μA. Hyperstimulation has received limited but promising assessment because of its noxious nature.

A TENS unit called **Codetron** uses random stimulations every 10 seconds at the six electrode sites. It is believed that frequency changes in stimulation sites will avoid the occurrence of habituation and accommodation from repetitive signals. Its effectiveness remains controversial.

TENS has been shown to be highly effective in alleviating pain and reducing analgesic medications following Cesarian section, orthopedic and thoracic operations as well as mixed surgical procedures. It is also beneficial in acute musculoskeletal pain, but its effectiveness in chronic pain remains controversial. Treatment duration of TENS is usually 30 minutes to 1 hour per session, with a maximum of 2 hours per session, for a total of 8 hours per day. This is continued for 3 weeks and then gradually reduced in the next 8 to 12 weeks.

3. **Percutaneous electrical nerve stimulation (PENS) or percutaneous neuromodulation therapy (PNT)** is the application of acupuncture-like needles inserted through the skin into soft tissue or muscle at dermatomal levels corresponding to local pathology. When applied at various acupuncture sites, it is called **electroacupuncture** (see acupuncture description in section X). It usually uses a 5-Hz frequency with a pulse width of 0.5 ms. Its frequency may be lowered to 1 Hz if relief is not attained within 15 minutes. Unlike TENS, it is claimed to bypass the local skin resistance and deliver electrical stimuli at the precisely desired level in close proximity to the nerve endings located in soft tissue, muscle, or periosteum of the involved dermatomes. It has been used to reduce pain, improve function, and reduce the use of opioid analgesia in patients with lower back pain and postherpetic neuralgia. Its efficacy is controversial.
4. **Neuromuscular electrical stimulators (NMES)** are TES units used for the stimulation of muscles with intact peripheral nervous system or muscles that are decentralized (i.e., following central nervous system or spinal cord injury). Their use in denervated muscles is controversial due to reports of deleterious effects such as retardation of reinnervation and degeneration of muscle fibers. The NMES is more powerful than the TENS unit and is usually modulated to provide interrupted current for stronger motor excitation.

   The NMES is used to strengthen or maintain muscle mass (i.e., retard atrophy) or both during or following periods of immobilization. (The NMES has been shown to increase muscle strength even without voluntary effort by the subject. It can also convert type II fast muscle fibers into type I slow fibers, although this change is reversible after cessation of NMES.) It can maintain or gain joint ROM (in soft tissue joint contractures), enhance voluntary motor control (through facilitation technique or muscle re-education program), temporarily reduce the effects of spasticity, and act as semipermanent replacement of conventional bracing (e.g., to gain normal shoulder alignment of subluxed shoulders in hemiparetic patients and to assist dorsiflexion in stroke patients with foot drop or in spinal cord injury patients).

   In patients with paralysis as a result of decentralization, NMES can be used for conditioning and strengthening exercises (e.g., computerized NMES to induce coordinated knee flexion and extension so the patient can pedal a bicycle ergometer or exercise using an isokinetic knee dynamometer). When NMES is used to activate multiple muscles in a coordinated sequential manner to attain specific functional goals (e.g., functional ambulation in paraplegics and hand grasp and standing transfers in tetraplegics), it is called **functional electrical stimulation (FES)** or **functional neuromuscular stimulation (FNS)**.
5. **H-wave muscle stimulation** uses a bipolar, exponential decaying waveform to emulate the H waveform found in nerve signals (i.e., Hoffman or H-reflex; this is not the same as the H-wave in electromyography, which is described in Chapter 2.4, section I.C.2.b) and to enable greater and deeper penetration of a low-frequency current, while using significantly less power than other TES. It is

claimed to be much safer, less painful, and more effective than other TES. It has a low-frequency setting, which is used for muscle contractions, and a high-frequency setting, which is used for pain relief (i.e., "TENS" effect). Both low and high frequencies can be applied to the same patient simultaneously. It has been approved by the Food and Drugs Administration (FDA) for relaxation of muscle spasm, prevention of retardation of disuse atrophy, edema control, muscle re-education, prevention of postoperative venous thrombosis, and in maintaining or improving range of motion. It may be effective in reducing pain caused by chronic diabetic peripheral neuropathy, but has not been shown to be effective in treating chronic pain as a result of ischemia. It is usually applied for 10–30 minutes.

6. **Transcranial electrical stimulation (TCES)** is the application of surface electrodes on two opposing sides of the head. It is claimed to provide direct and/or indirect effects on the central nervous system to modulate neural activity, alter nerve excitation, and affect the quantities of neurotransmitters, neuromodulators, and/or neurohormones. TCES have been used to treat migraine and tension headaches; control anxiety and insomnia; improve mood in traumatic brain injury patients; and treat children with cerebral palsy and delayed motor development. TCES remains experimental and needs further investigation before it is widely accepted.
7. **Electroceutical therapy**, also known as **bioelectric nerve block**, uses special step-down transformers to alter high-frequency current (ranging from 1 to 20 000 Hz compared to the 0.5 to 100 Hz used in TENS) into bioelectric impulses, which are designed to mimic the human bioelectric system. There are two distinctive electroceutical classifications: stimulatory class in which repetitive action potentials are induced in excitable cells (depolarization and repolarization activity), and multi-facilitatory class that produces biophysical effects without repetitive action potential propagation. Electroceutical therapy is claimed to block axonal transmissions in the management of neuropathic pain (nonmalignant pain) as well as pain associated with cancer (malignant pain). However, scientific evidence is lacking.

VI. Biofeedback

Biofeedback is the process of monitoring internal physiological events using equipment (usually electronics) that can display these otherwise involuntary or unfelt events in the form of visual and auditory signals. These signals are then fed back to the patients so they learn how to manipulate them and thus regulate their own internal physiological events. It is used in psychotherapy, for relaxation in patients with chronic pain (e.g., tension headache, vascular headache, and chronic neck and back pain), Raynaud's disease, urinary and fecal incontinence, sports medicine, and psychoimmunology. Specific PM&R conditions that might benefit from biofeedback include stroke, spinal cord injury, cerebral palsy, traumatic brain injury, multiple sclerosis, dystonias and dyskinesias, peripheral nerve denervation, and orthopedic disorders. Biofeedback has no specific medical contraindication; however, it should only be prescribed if patients have potential for voluntary control, are well-motivated and cooperative, and are able to follow commands (e.g., no receptive aphasia). In general, biofeedback training is given two or three times per week with each session lasting about 30–45 minutes. Between training sessions the patient is given detailed instructions to carry out a program of repetitive, daily, self-administered exercises at home. The length of biofeedback training varies from 3 months to 2 years. Biofeedback treatment programs must be regularly monitored by the physiatrist to ensure that the patients are benefiting from them.

A. MYOELECTRIC OR ELECTROMYOGRAPHIC BIOFEEDBACK is the most widely used form of biofeedback in PM&R. It transduces muscle potentials into auditory or visual cues to help the patient learn how to increase or decrease voluntary muscular activities. It is used for muscle recruitment in patients with peripheral nerve injury, muscle weakness as a result of immobilization, joint surgery, deconditioning, pain, antagonists to spastic muscles, muscle–tendon transfers, re-education of weak or flaccid muscle, and recovery of shoulder control poststroke. It can also be used to help relax patients with stress-related hyperarousal, pain, spasticity, rigidity, and torticollis.

B. POSITION BIOFEEDBACK is used to help patients regulate position and movement so they can develop appropriate timing and coordination. It can be used to train for head position control; coordination and control of hand movements in ataxia and following hand surgery; and knee joint position in children with cerebral palsy, adults with hemiplegia, and prosthesis wearers. It can also be used to train muscles that are difficult to isolate (e.g., pronation and supination of forearm) in stroke patients.

C. PRESSURE OR FORCE BIOFEEDBACK is used to determine the amount of force being transmitted through a body segment or assistive device, for example, training of symmetrical standing gait in hemiplegics, use of a feedback cane to determine the amount of force borne by the cane, and gait analysis.

D. BLOOD PRESSURE BIOFEEDBACK uses regular plethysmography to train patients how to relax. This is usually used in conjunction with EMG biofeedback and biofeedback for temperature control of limbs.

E. PERINEAL EMG BIOFEEDBACK uses pressure transducers in the anal canal or vagina, for sphincteral control training in patients with incontinence.

F. RESPIRATORY BIOFEEDBACK is used for training breathing functions in patients with respiratory problems, for example, asthma and high-level spinal cord injury.

G. TEMPERATURE AND PERIPHERAL BLOOD FLOW BIOFEEDBACK is used by clinical psychologists usually for relaxation. It is also used for Raynaud's disease.

H. ELECTROENCEPHALOGRAPHIC (EEG) BIOFEEDBACK is used mainly for relaxation training.

VII. Spinal traction

Spinal traction is a pulling force applied to the cervical or lumbar spine for the following physiological effects: vertebral joint distraction; prevention and loosening of adhesions within the dural sleeves, nerve roots, and adjacent capsular structures; reduction of compression and irritation of the nerve root and disk; improvement of the circulation within the epidural spaces of nerve root canals; and reduction of pain, inflammation, and muscle spasm.

The most common clinical indication of spinal traction is to relieve pain from disk herniation, with or without concomitant nerve root compression. In acute lumbar disk herniation, lumbar mechanical traction has been used to keep the patient immobile in bed.

The main reason for spinal traction failure is inadequate pull because of insufficient weight and improper neck or body positioning or both. Hence spinal traction must never be used by anyone with inadequate training. Cervical and lumbar traction are contraindicated in spondylotic myelopathy, malignancy (e.g., lytic lesions), osteopenia, spinal infection (e.g., diskitis and tuberculosis), acute soft tissue injury, congenital spinal deformity, hypertension, or cardiovascular disease, and in anxious patients who are unable to relax. Additional contraindications for cervical traction are cervical ligamentous instability (e.g., in rheumatoid arthritis, Down's syndrome, or patients with hypermobile joints), atlantoaxial subluxation with spinal cord compromise, vertebrobasilar arterial insufficiency, atherosclerosis of the carotid or vertebral arteries, and acute whiplash injury. Most of these conditions are commonly seen during old age, thus spinal traction must be used with caution in the elderly. In lumbar traction, additional contraindications (as a result of the use of chest and abdominal harness) include pregnancy, cauda equina compression, aortic aneurysm, active peptic ulcers, hiatal or other hernia, and restrictive lung disease or other breathing disorder.

Prescription of spinal traction depends more on the practitioner's empirical observation than on objective data. The parameters to be considered are positioning, weight to be used, duration, and sustained (static) vs. intermittent application. Most importantly, the patient must be comfortable and the traction must not cause or aggravate pain.

Spinal traction is usually used in conjunction with other modalities for relaxation, such as heat and massage. Patients receiving traction must be given exercises and postural re-education to maintain the effect of traction. Ideally, mechanical spinal traction should only be started if active modalities or manual traction have not achieved the desired goal. If the symptoms have worsened or if there is no improvement after six to eight sessions, traction should be discontinued.

A. CERVICAL TRACTION

1. **Manual cervical traction** is a type of spinal manipulation used as a trial before application of mechanical (motorized or home) traction. The patient is positioned in a supine position with the head supported on the therapist's hand so that the patient's neck is flexed to about 20–25°. A traction force is then applied by the therapist to the patient's occiput (not to the mandible).
2. **Mechanical cervical traction** uses free weights and pulley systems to pull the cervical spine. Depending on the patient's size, neurologic symptoms, specific lesions, and comfort, the weight used ranges from 10 to 50 lb (4.5–22.7 kg) applied for 15–20 minutes (a 10-lb minimum is necessary to counterbalance the weight of the head) with the patient's neck flexed 20–30° in either a seated or supine position. The greater the traction force, the shorter the traction time needed. Treatment is provided three to four times per week for 10 to 15 sessions (or 3–4 weeks).

a. ***Intermittent mechanical cervical traction*** is a motorized traction with adjustable rest periods (in seconds) in between traction pulls. Compared to sustained (static) traction, it is more comfortable and patients can tolerate a greater weight. It must be monitored by a physical therapist during treatment, which is both an advantage (because the amount of weight and neck position are monitored) and a disadvantage (because the patient must come to the physical therapy office for treatment).

b. ***Sustained (static) mechanical cervical traction***

I. **Motorized static mechanical cervical traction** applies a constant level of traction to induce fatigue in the paraspinal muscles so that more pull can theoretically be transmitted to the cervical spine. Compared to intermittent traction, it is less comfortable and most patients can only tolerate a small amount of weight.

II. **Nonmotorized static mechanical cervical traction** can be used at home. Patient compliance is paramount for the success of home cervical traction. The newer home cervical traction units (i.e., Saunders Cervical HomeTrac and Glacier Cross' Pronex cervical traction), applied in the supine position without a chin strap, do not strain the temporomandibular joint. They are easier to set up and use and are more comfortable to use than the traditional "over-the-door" cervical traction unit.

- **The traditional "over-the-door" cervical traction unit** consists of a head harness (with chin strap), rope and pulley system, and a counterweight [usually a bag filled with 20 lb (9 kg) or more of water or sand]. They can be applied in a seated position (by attaching the pulley system over the door or onto the wall) or in supine position (by attaching the pulley system to the bed). They can put strain on the temporomandibular joint (TMJ) and are usually ineffective, probably because of incorrect use (inadequate amount of weight, improper head and neck position). Hence, a physical therapist must regularly monitor the patient's technique of application by having the patient demonstrate it.
- The **Glacier Cross' Pronex cervical traction unit** cradles the supine head and neck on two soft foam cushions (one cushion supporting the occiput and the other resting against the upper trapezius). It uses an air-inflated bellows between the cushions to provide up to 20 lb (9 kg) of continuous traction. The amount of traction applied is controlled by the patient by squeezing an inflator bulb (to increase pressure) or releasing a knob (to reduce pressure).
- The **Saunders Cervical HomeTrac cervical traction unit** can provide up to 50 lb (23 kg) of traction and can position the supine head at angles ranging from 15 to 25° by using a forehead strap and self-adjusting neck wedges. It provides traction by using a specially designed pneumatic pump, which is controlled by the patient using a hand-held pump.

B. LUMBAR TRACTION needs a large amount of force to attain lumbar distraction (usually between 65 and 200 lb [30–91 kg] or 40–50% the patient's body weight).

1. **Manual lumbar traction** is a type of spinal manipulation used as a trial before the application of mechanical lumbar traction. Because of the tremendous amount of force needed to separate the lumbar vertebrae, a split table (with a fixed and a mobile segment) is usually needed to decrease frictional forces between the body and the table surface. The patient is either positioned side-lying to provide manual traction to a specific vertebral level or supine for a unilateral leg-pull manual traction.
2. **Mechanical lumbar traction** uses a split table, a nonslip traction harness, and either a pulley system or a friction-free surface system. The patient is positioned in a neutral spinal position either supine with hips flexed to about 90° or prone. A harness is attached around the patient's pelvis (to deliver a caudal pull), while his or her upper body is stabilized with a thoracic harness. The pelvic harness is then connected to the pulley system (or friction-free surface system), which provides traction by weights or by a motorized or hand-pump device. In some women, the thoracic harness may cause discomfort to their breast.

a. ***Intermittent mechanical lumbar traction*** uses a motorized pulley system, which provides rest periods (e.g., 5–15 seconds) between each traction pull [progressive force of up to 50 lb (23 kg) applied for 7–60 seconds]. The treatment protocol can either be pre-programmed or patient-controlled. Treatment duration is usually between 20 and 30 minutes. It is better tolerated than sustained mechanical lumbar traction.

b. ***Sustained (static) mechanical lumbar traction***

I. **Motorized static mechanical lumbar traction** uses a motorized pulley system that provides a steady amount of moderate weight (less than that of intermittent lumbar traction but greater than that of continuous lumbar traction) for 10–30 minutes (or up to 1 hour). It is not as well tolerated as intermittent traction.

II. **Nonmotorized static mechanical lumbar traction** can be used at home. As with home cervical traction, patient compliance is important for its success. To date, only the **Saunders STx** and **Saunders Lumbar HomeTrac** units have split treatment surfaces that are friction free and can be actively moved to apply up to 200 lb of traction to the lower back. The patient is supine with the lumbar curve in neutral or any degree of flexion or extension position. The patient's thorax and pelvis are secured to the traction unit using non-slip surface harnesses. A hand-held pump with gauge is used to apply the prescribed lumbar traction force that can be sustained and released (immediately, if needed) by the patient.

c. ***Continuous mechanical lumbar traction*** uses a motorized pulley system that provides light weights for several hours (up to 20–40 hours). It is not effective in distracting the lumbar vertebrae, and its sole use is to enforce bedrest during acute disk herniation.

3. **Autotraction** uses a specially designed table on which the patient administers sliding tractive force by pulling with the hands on the grasp bar at the head of the table while a traction belt restrains the pelvis to the table. This active form of traction seems to provide more symptomatic relief than the passive forms of lumbar traction and has the advantage of having the patient regulate the traction force. Treatment is usually applied every 2–3 days for 6 to 10 treatments.
4. **Powered autotraction devices (e.g., VAX-D; DRS System; Spina System; DRX 2000, 3000, and 5000; and Lordex Traction Unit)** are air-powered auto-traction tables, split down the middle to apply cycles of tension axially to the lumbar vertebral column. They can provide static, intermittent, and cycling distraction forces to relieve pressures on structures that may be causing low back pain (e.g., herniated disks, degenerative disk disease, posterior facet syndrome, and sciatica). The patient lies prone on the table and fixes the upper body by grasping adjustable handgrips, designed to eliminate the use of a chest harness. A pelvic harness applies distraction forces (ranging from 20–100 lb) primarily to the lateral pelvic crests along the natural anatomical lines of the spinal column with minimal anterior–posterior pressures. Treatment consists of a series of 10 to 20 decompression–relaxation cycles administered five times per week for a total of 20 treatments, with each session lasting 30–45 minutes. The procedure is generally safe as the patient can release the handgrip at any time to end the session. To date, they have not been shown to be more effective than other forms of lumbar traction.
5. **Gravity or inversion traction** is a positional traction that uses the weight of the body hanging upside down from a bar to distract the lumbar vertebrae. This is often accompanied by numerous musculoskeletal and other complaints and is contraindicated in patients with hypertension, bleeding disorders, and glaucoma. It should be prescribed with caution, or not at all.

VIII. Manipulation

Manipulation as done in PM&R by either a physiatrist or physical therapist is a skilled passive, mechanical movement applied to a specific joint or to a joint segment to restore its motion or extensibility and to reduce pain. It must be differentiated from massage (applied to soft tissue), mechanical traction (nonspecific), and active exercise. While manipulation may be used alone, it is usually helpful to add short-term nonsteroidal anti-inflammatory drugs (see Chapter 4.8, section I.A.3) or other analgesics and to diminish the postmanipulation tissue inflammatory reaction. In acute cases, a brace might be necessary to immobilize the spine. Active modalities, such as exercise and education, must be provided to maintain the effects of manipulation and prevent recurrence.

Various hypotheses for pain relief achieved with manipulation include mechanical or reflex relaxation of soft tissues as a result of the restoration of the vertebral range of motion, normalization of a bulging disk by the suction forces created or by stretching the posterior longitudinal ligament, which pushes the disk material anteriorly, away from pain-sensitive structures, and alteration of proprioceptive input to the spinal cord causing the "gate" to close.

A. SPINAL MANIPULATION is the application of passive maneuvers (anterior–posterior glide, lateral flexion tilt, forward flexion tilt, extension tilt, rotation, and distraction) to the spine to restore its normal motion and to reduce pain caused by altered biomechanics. It is indicated in mechanical musculoskeletal pain problems of the back, pelvis, and neck in which loss of vertebral function or localized tenderness on induced motion may be a contributing factor.

Spinal manipulation should only be carried out by a skilled practitioner. Depending on its velocity, manipulation can be classified as thrust (using high velocity and low amplitude) or nonthrust (usually using low velocity and high amplitude). In general, the higher the velocity used in manipulation, the more contraindications arise. In the nonthrust technique, contraindications include vertebral malignancy, infection or inflammation, cauda equina syndrome, myelopathy, spondylosis, multiple adjacent radiculopathies, vertebral bone disease, vertebral bony joint instability (e.g., fracture or dislocation), and rheumatic disease in the cervical region.

Aside from the above, additional contraindications for thrust manipulation include fixed spinal deformities and anomalies, systemic anticoagulation (disease-related or pharmacologic), severe diabetes, atherosclerosis, severe degenerative joint disease, vertigo, or signs and symptoms of vertebrobasilar arterial disease or insufficiency, spondyloarthropathies, inactive rheumatologic disease, ligamentous joint instability, or congenital joint laxity and syndromes (e.g., Marfan and Ehlers–Danlos), aseptic necrosis, local aneurysm, osteomalacia, osteoporosis, osteopenia, objective radicular signs, hypermobility, obsessional fixation on pain, absence of any pain-free direction of vertebral motion. In clearly defined root pain without objective signs of radiculopathy, use of manipulation remains controversial.

In many of the aforementioned conditions, and even in pregnancy, gentle nonthrust techniques can be used. In muscle energy, some of the absolute contraindications are only relative contraindications (e.g., osteoporosis, diabetes, noncervical rheumatoid disease, degenerative joint disease, joint laxity). One specific contraindication for muscle energy is concurrent myositis (because of the patient's active contraction).

Manipulation must only be used on a short-term basis in conjunction with other active modalities such as exercises and patient education. Duration is determined on an individual basis. Thrusting usually has an immediate effect with improvement within 1 week postmanipulation. The muscle energy effect may take longer. Lack of improvement in objective findings after 2–4 weeks suggests the need for re-evaluation.

1. Thrust spinal manipulation (chiropractic "adjustment") uses high-velocity and low-amplitude maneuvers, delivered at the end of the pathologic spinal ROM ("barrier") either directly (in the direction of the barrier) or indirectly (in the opposite direction of the barrier) with the purpose of increasing passive ROM. The facets of the involved vertebral segments are first "locked" by positioning the patient. The involved vertebral segment is then passively moved to its barrier so that all slack motion is removed. A brief (10–100 ms), controlled thrust is applied by the manipulator to increase the passive ROM. This may be associated with an audible "pop" or "click". If the thrust is applied over a spinous or transverse process, it is called short-lever technique. If applied distant from the vertebra through the locked vertebral column, it is called long-lever technique. Although extremely rare, accidents and even death have been reported with the use of thrust manipulation in the neck.

2. **Nonthrust spinal manipulation** consists of gentle, persuasive pressure performed at the end of the pathologic spinal ROM or within its available ROM. Unlike thrust manipulation, it uses relatively slow and controlled movements; hence, there is immediate sensory feedback to the therapist by the patient during the time of application.

a. ***Articulatory technique ("spinal mobilization")*** uses maneuvers with high amplitude but low velocity.

   I. **Graded oscillation technique** uses alternate (on and off) oscillatory pressure at different parts of the available ROM. The oscillation amplitude is graded on a scale of 1 to 4. Its vibratory nature activates the sensory mechanoreceptors to reduce pain and improve proprioception.

   II. **Progressive stretch mobilization** uses a successive series of short-amplitude, spring-type pressures or a series of short-amplitude stretch movements to overcome mechanical or soft tissue restrictions. It is given at progressive increments and is also graded on a 1 to 4 scale.

   III. **Continuous stretch** is the application of a sustained, gradually increasing stretch or a pressure without interruption for immediate tissue feedback; it is used to improve mobility in soft tissue contractures.

b. ***Muscle energy ("isometrics")*** is the most common nonthrust form of spinal manipulation. It requires muscle contraction on the part of the patient from a precisely determined position in a specific direction against a distinct counterforce. Its force direction can be direct (in the direction of the barrier) or indirect (in the opposite direction of the barrier). It has three phases (contraction, relaxation, and stretch) that are comparable to the contract–relax form of active inhibition exercise (see Chapter 4.2, section I.C.1). As in thrust manipulation, slack motion is first removed. Then the patient exerts moderate forces against the operator (force direction can be direct or indirect) for 5–10 seconds, followed by relaxation. The original barrier to movement is then reassessed (there should be less barrier and greater ROM) and the procedure is repeated two or three times. To maintain the gains in ROM, active flexibility exercise must be prescribed.

c. ***Functional technique*** uses active-assistive positioning of a joint away from the motion barrier of restriction (i.e., indirect technique) and into a position of ease to inhibit reflex muscle guarding. The patient is asked to relax by breathing in and out. When muscle relaxation is sensed by the practitioner during expiratory phase, the patient's joint is repositioned into a new position of ease.

d. ***Counterstrain (Jones technique)*** involves application of pressure into the sensitive myofascial trigger point while the muscle and related joint are maintained in the position of maximal relaxation to inhibit reflex muscle guarding and spasm. This pressure is applied for at least 90 seconds and is followed by a slow passive return to neutral so that muscle guarding and spasm do not recur.

e. ***Craniosacral therapy*** assumes that an innate cranial rhythmic impulse can be palpated on the body by an experienced practitioner. Part of the cranial rhythmic impulse causes an ebb and flow of the cerebrospinal fluid, which can presumably be palpated and manipulated by the practitioner using various techniques (e.g., compression of the fourth ventricle by laying of hands on the occipital condyle). Because the parasympathetic nervous system is situated in the cranial and sacral portions of the nervous system, the therapeutic effects are often attributed to the effects on the autonomous nervous system. Craniosacral therapy is highly controversial.

B. PERIPHERAL JOINT MANIPULATION AND MOBILIZATION is the application of passive maneuvers (anterior–posterior glide, lateral glide, distraction, flexion tilt, extension tilt, and rotation) to a limb joint to increase its passive ROM. Clinical indications include painful limb joints with reflex muscle guarding and muscle spasm, reversible joint hypomobility, and joints with progressive limitation and functional immobility. They are contraindicated in joints with hypermobility, effusion, or acute inflammation. Extra caution must be observed in the presence of malignancy (e.g., lytic lesions), osteoporosis, unhealed fracture, excessive pain, or total joint replacement. In patients with inadequate knee flexion after total knee arthroplasty, joint manipulation under anesthesia may be performed (usually by an orthopedic surgeon).

1. **Thrust manipulation of peripheral joint** uses high-velocity, short-amplitude maneuvers at the end of the pathologic limit of the limb joint to alter its positional relationships, to break adhesions, or to stimulate joint receptors. It is indicated in a peripheral limb joint with loss of ROM because of immobilization resulting from trauma or adhesive capsulitis. Its capability to realign intrasynovial structures, such as a displaced meniscus, is highly controversial.
2. **Nonthrust manipulation of peripheral joint**

a. ***Peripheral joint mobilization*** uses slow and controlled movements which are applied at a speed slow enough that the patient can stop the movement. Depending on the patient's response, a rhythmic oscillation (graded oscillation technique) or a sustained distraction (sustained translatory joint-play technique) may be used. In general, oscillation techniques are used for pain management and sustained techniques are used for loss of joint play with decreased functional range.

b. ***Muscle energy ("isometrics")*** can also be performed in the peripheral joint (see section VIII.A.2.b).

c. ***Functional technique*** can also be performed in the peripheral joint (see section VIII.A.2.c).

d. ***Counterstrain*** can also be carried out in the peripheral joint (see section VIII.A.2.d).

IX. Massage

Massage is the systematic, mechanical stimulation of the soft tissues of the body by means of rhythmically applied pressure and stretching for therapeutic purposes. Physiological effects of massage can either be mechanical (i.e., increase in venous return and lymphatic drainage, breaking of adhesion and softening of scars, loosening of secretions) or reflexive (i.e., increase in circulation via reflex vasodilation, general relaxation and sedative effects, increased perspiration and secretion of sebaceous glands, and decreased pain probably caused by gate control or release of endogenous opiates or neurotransmitters). The "laying of hands" also has psychological effects and can promote a sense of general well-being.

Massage is used to reduce excessive fluids in interstitial spaces or joints (e.g., lymphedema), increase circulation to paralyzed muscles, restore tight muscles to normal length, mobilize tissues that are abnormally adhered to surrounding structures, increase tolerance of tissues to pressure, relieve pain and muscle spasm, loosen secretions (e.g., in chronic obstructive pulmonary disease), promote specific and general relaxation, and enhance psychological well-being. Massage does not alter the general metabolism and has no effect on obesity, muscle mass, muscle strength, muscle recovery rate, or the rate of atrophy of denervated muscle.

Contraindications include any acute inflammatory conditions of the skin, soft tissues, or joints as a result of bacterial action (phlebitis, cellulitis, synovitis, abscesses, septic arthritis), open wounds, burns, nerve entrapments (e.g., carpal tunnel syndrome), bursitis, rheumatoid and gouty arthritis, rheumatic fibrositis, panniculitis (subcutaneous fat inflammation), arteriosclerosis, venous thrombosis or embolism, severe varicose veins, clotting disorders (or during anticoagulation), fractures, and malignancies.

Treatment time depends on the size of the area to be treated. It usually takes 15–30 minutes for trunk massage (abdomen, back, or neck) and 5–15 minutes for limb massage. Generally, limb massage is performed from distal to proximal (centripetally); however, if there is swelling (e.g., lymphedema), the proximal part must be massaged before the distal part ("uncorking effect"). Massage should always be used in conjunction with other forms of treatment, preferably active modalities such as exercises. If possible, the patient should be taught self-massage.

A. MASSAGE USING THE HANDS is more effective than massage using mechanical devices because the hand can assess (through palpation) as well as treat.

1. Western massage

a. Classical massage is the blending of the following strokes (a popular form is the Swedish massage, which involves percussion, petrissage, and deep tissue massage):

I. **Effleurage**: Light gliding strokes over skin without moving deep muscle masses used for muscle relaxation.

II. **Petrissage**: Kneading manipulations that intermittently lift, press, and roll the muscles under the fingers or hands, used for increasing circulation and reducing edema.

III. **Percussion (tapotement)**: Series of brisk alternating blows (e.g., hacking, slapping, beating, pinching, tapping with fingertips, cupping, or clapping) used to stimulate circulation, desensitize operated sites (e.g., amputee stump), and dislodge secretions (in chest physical therapy).

IV. **Vibration**: Fine tremulous movement made by hand or finger to cause the part to vibrate. It can be soothing when applied gently or stimulating when done more vigorously. It can be used in conjunction with percussion to loosen secretions.

V. **Friction**: Circular motions of the fingertips with pressure applied so that the therapist's fingers and the patient's skin move as one. It is used to loosen or break up underlying adhesions of healed scar tissue.

b. Cross-fiber friction massage is a deep friction massage applied parallel or perpendicular to the muscle, tendon, or ligament fibers to loosen any adherent fibrous tissue. It can also aid in absorption of local edema or effusions and in reducing local muscle spasm. When done over trigger points, it can have reflex effects.

c. Connective tissue massage (CTM) or Bindegewebsmassage is a series of pulling strokes carried out in the layers of the connective tissue on the body surface to stimulate cutaneovisceral reflex (via autonomic nervous system) and affect visceral organs whose innervation corresponds to cutaneous dermatomes. This claim, however, remains controversial. A variation of CTM, called Rolfing, involves vigorous, pounding massage of the deep connective tissue.

d. Soft tissue mobilization is a forceful form of passive stretching of the muscular and fascial system element through its restrictive direction in a manner and at a speed that are within the ability of the patient to control the movement. It incorporates movement and joint position with the basic application of CTM techniques. It places the fascia and muscle in an elongated rather than a shortened or relaxed position thus exposing the tissue to be treated, stretching the connective tissue, and changing the resting length of the muscle.

e. ***Myofascial release*** is the application of prolonged light pressure in specific directions into the fascia system to release soft tissues from the abnormal grip of tight fascia. It is a gentle form of passive stretching.

2. **Eastern massage** closely resembles CTM in its claim to affect visceral organs via peripheral manipulation of the nervous system (cutaneovisceral reflex). Like CTM, it remains controversial.

a. ***Acupressure*** is a Chinese form of massage that uses finger pressure over acupuncture points or over trigger points to decrease pain. It can supposedly increase endogenous opiates after 1–5 minutes of pressure at a single point. Other specific forms of acupressure are reflexology/zone therapy (which uses the sole of the foot) and auriculotherapy (which uses the ear).

b. ***Shiatsu*** is the Japanese form of acupressure.

B. MASSAGE USING MECHANICAL DEVICES loses the "laying of hands" effect and is often not as effective as manual massage.

1. **Hand-held or hand-strapped devices** usually provide percussion (percussor), vibration (vibrator), and suction (e.g., massage suction-roller). Vibrators with frequencies of 100–200 Hz and an amplitude of 1.5 mm are commonly used for muscle facilitation and muscle re-education in patients with upper motor neuron lesions and for temporary relief of musculoskeletal pain.
2. **Stationary massage devices** are not moved during their use. The body part to be massaged is placed upon the stationary device that vibrates (e.g., vibrating pads, vibrating belts or strap, massage roller pad).
3. **Alternating pressure mattresses and pads** (see Chapter 5.2, section VI.B.3.b) use massage-like actions for the treatment and prevention of pressure sores (by emptying and refilling superficial blood vessels).
4. **Intermittent compression devices** use a hollow cuff, sleeve, or boot that is worn around a limb or part of it and then intermittently filled with air or water to provide centripetal rhythmic compression for the relief of lymphedema. The best known is the Jobst pneumatic intermittent compression unit, which is mostly used for postmastectomy lymphedema of the upper limb.
5. **Devices for hydromassage** provide massage by pressure and movement of water, e.g., shower massage, underwater jet massage, whirlpool baths, and Jacuzzi.
6. **Dry hydrotherapy** (e.g., AquaMED; AquaMassage) uses a waterbed-like device that contains interior jets, which rotate and pulsate while releasing streams of pressurized heated water along the patient's body. This heated hydrotherapy is delivered in a dry environment with the patient either lying or sitting.

X. Acupuncture

Acupuncture is a neurostimulatory technique that induces analgesia and other neurophysiologic effects by the insertion of small 28–36 gauge, 1.25–5.0 cm long, solid needles into acupuncture points found on the skin at varying depths, typically penetrating the underlying musculature. Many of the acupuncture points that are distributed along meridians (hypothetical lines through which the life force, i.e., *Chi* or *Qi*, flows) on the surface of the body were found to correspond to motor points. The enhanced sensitivity and reactivity of the acupuncture points may be the result of their greater concentration of pain fibers and vascular structures. On the trunk, the points are found at segmental innervation levels where nerves and blood and lymphatic vessels penetrate the muscle fascia. On the face and head, they are found near the cranial nerves and blood and lymphatic vessels. On the ear, there appears to be a relationship between the acupuncture points and the cranial nerves and blood vessels, although the traditional postulate is that the body is represented in the ear in the shape of an inverted homunculus. Recent studies show that acupuncture stimulation need not be applied at the points indicated by the traditional acupuncture charts, and it is believed that intense stimulation rather than inserting the needle at the precise site is more crucial to its effectiveness.

Acupuncture has been used as an adjunctive treatment in the management of mild-to-moderate acute and chronic pain syndromes including musculoskeletal pain (e.g., epicondylitis, back and neck pain, fractured ribs, temporomandibular pain, foot pain, osteoarthritis, and headache), neuropathic pain (e.g., postherpetic neuralgia, trigeminal neuralgia, and phantom limb pain), cancer pain, and other pain syndromes; asthma; gastrointestinal disorders; menstrual problems; chronic stress; obesity; depression; insomnia; withdrawal for addictive substances; and immune dysfunctions.

The mechanism of action of acupuncture remains controversial. Popular Western theories include neuropharmacological theory (e.g., involving the opioid system, such as the release of endorphins and enkephalins, or the nonopioid system, such as the serotonergic system), neurophysiologic theory (as shown by its effectiveness in increasing heart rate and blood pressure as well as altering gastrointestinal function, blood chemistry, and immunologic reactions), hyperstimulation theory (i.e., central nervous system hyperstimulation "drowns out" pain messages), gate-control theory (i.e., stimulation of large- or medium-sized afferent nerve fibers in muscles blocks out the small-fiber input), autonomic nervous system theory, and distraction and counterirritation theory. The placebo effect theory has been proposed but is weakened by studies showing partial analgesia in animals such as monkeys, rats, and mice.

Acupuncture is an invasive therapy and is contraindicated in patients who are anticoagulated, have infection at the site of needle insertion, or have active, blood-borne infection. Potential complications include needle-related complications (e.g., breaking a needle; causing bleeding; creating local infection; transmitting disease, such as hepatitis B, human immunodeficiency virus, or cytomegalovirus; and invading nontargeted tissues causing pneumothorax, paresthesias, or nerve damage) and technique-related problems (e.g., vasovagal reactions and fainting, lack of therapeutic effect, and delay in providing more conventional therapy).

The number of acupuncture points used and the number of treatments provided depend on the practitioner's preference, type of pain, and chronicity and seriousness of the problem. Because acupuncture tends to be cumulative, an average course of treatment before significant results occur may be 2 or 3 times per week for 3–6 weeks. The average length of each treatment varies from 20 to 30 minutes. After insertion of the acupuncture needle, the patient should feel a sensation of warmth, heaviness, soreness, or local fullness. The needle can be left untouched, twirled, or connected to a low-volt current. Studies show that 50–80% of patients may exhibit a short-term benefit from acupuncture, especially when it is used as a component of a comprehensive treatment program. To date, there are few controlled studies on the clinical efficacy of acupuncture. One of the problems in performing a controlled study on acupuncture is the difficulty in doing an adequate controlled double-blind study (e.g., in the use of sham acupuncture, inserting the needle at an incorrect point may have some pain reduction effect; also, because the acupuncturist is aware of the difference, he or she might transmit his or her expectations to the patient). Recent meta-analyses produced mixed and inconclusive results and did not specify which types of pain problems acupuncture can or cannot alleviate.

The consensus statement of the 1997 National Institutes of Health (NIH) consensus panel on acupuncture stated that "promising results have emerged showing the efficacy of acupuncture in postoperative and chemotherapy nausea and vomiting, nausea of pregnancy, and postoperative dental pain". The panel also concluded that acupuncture may be effective as an adjunct therapy, an acceptable alternative, or as part of a comprehensive treatment program for conditions including addiction, stroke rehabilitation, headache, menstrual cramps, tennis elbow, fibromyalgia, low back pain, carpal tunnel syndrome, and asthma.

XI. Magnetic therapy (magnetotherapy)

Magnetotherapy is the therapeutic use of magnets (or magnetic energy fields) to transcutaneously affect the nerve or the muscle or both. Magnetic field strength is measured in gauss or teslas (10 000 gauss = 1 tesla). It is claimed to help regenerate nerves and reduce pain in patients with musculoskeletal pain (neck pain, mechanical low back pain, fibromyalgia, muscle soreness, rheumatoid arthritis, osteoarthritis), postpolio syndrome pain, multiple sclerosis, diabetic neuropathic pain, fracture, and neurogenic bowel. It is contraindicated in patients with hemorrhage, pregnancy, and pacemakers. The claim that it increases circulation has not been demonstrated. The efficacy of magnetic therapy is controversial and further studies are needed.

A. **PERMANENT STATIC MAGNETIC FIELD THERAPY** uses iron oxide (Fe_3O_4), neodymium, and/or boron, which are combined as a ceramic (rigid) or neoprene (flexible) substance. It can be either **unipolar** [i.e., several discrete magnets are aligned with the same pole (negative pole or biomagnetic north pole) facing the patient's skin] or **bipolar** [i.e., different shaped magnets (triangles, squares, strips, concentric circles) are aligned in alternating patterns so that both north (or negative) and south (or positive) poles face the patient's skin either in a concentric pattern of circles or a checkerboard pattern]. Static magnetic field magnets are commercially available as pads, disks, wraps, bands, inserts, belts, necklaces, earrings, and bracelets applied as close as possible to the area of concern. Static magnetic field strength ranges from 100 to 500 gauss and is claimed to penetrate up to 20 mm of epidermis and dermis. To date, there is no scientific evidence to support the claim that static magnets can relieve pain or influence the course of any disease.

B. **PULSED ELECTROMAGNETIC FIELD (PEMF) THERAPY** uses an electric device in the form of a pulse generator connected to coils. The magnetic field is produced by the waveform generator that drives a current through electromagnetic coils. In the transformer mechanism, current passes through coils adjacent to tissue, causing current flow in the tissue. PEMFs induce electric fields, therefore the effect is based on the effects of induced electrical fields. Unlike static magnets, PEMFs move electrical charges or induce an electric current and have been FDA approved for treating slow-healing fractures and also for incontinence. PEMF promotes various healing mechanisms, and has been found to promote bone tissue regeneration (even where bone nonunion exists), connective tissue regeneration, wound tissue regeneration (even where chronic wounds exist), nerve tissue regeneration with no reported expected or unexpected adverse reactions. Its effectiveness is controversial.

XII. Extracorporeal shock-wave therapy (ESWT)

This technique uses electrohydraulic, electromagnetic, or piezoelectric generators to produce low- or high-energy acoustical shock waves to initiate structural changes on tissue, stimulate bone growth, stimulate the regenerative process in tissue, or cause structural changes in calcium deposits followed by reabsorption of the calcium by the body. It is theorized to facilitate the neovascularization process, cause a hyperstimulation analgesic effect, or stimulate osteoblast activation. Musculoskeletal disorders in which ESWT has been used include plantar fasciitis, lateral epicondylitis, calcific tendonitis, avascular necrosis, and fractures (stress fractures, delayed union, and nonunion). However, further studies are needed to determine its effectiveness.

Further reading

Alon G: Evaluation of clinical electrical stimulators. *Physical Therapy Practice* 1(2):7–19, 1992.

Basford JR: Electrical therapy. In Kottke FJ, Lehmann JF, editors: *Krusen's handbook of physical medicine and rehabilitation*, ed 4, Philadelphia, 1990, WB Saunders, pp. 375–401.

Basford JR: Therapeutic physical agents. In DeLisa JA, Gans BM, Walsh NE, *et al.*, editors: *Physical medicine and rehabilitation: principles and practice*, ed 4, Philadelphia, 2005, Lippincott, Williams & Wilkins, pp. 251–270.

Basmajian JV, editor: *Manipulation, traction and massage*, ed 3, Baltimore, 1985, Williams & Wilkins.

Basmajian JV: Biofeedback in physical medicine and rehabilitation. In DeLisa JA, Gans BM, Walsh NE, *et al.*, editors: *Physical medicine and rehabilitation: principles and practice*, ed 4, Philadelphia, 2005, Lippincott, Williams & Wilkins, pp. 271–283.

Cameron MH: *Physical agents in rehabilitation: from research to practice*, ed 2, St Louis, 2003, Saunders.

Han JS, Terenius L: Neurochemical basis of acupuncture analgesia. *Ann Rev Pharmacol Toxicol* 22:193–220, 1982.

Kitchen S, editor: *Electrotherapy: evidence-based practice*, ed 11, Edinburgh, 2002, Churchill Livingstone.

Lee MHM, Liao SJ: Acupuncture for pain management. In Lennard TA, editor: *Physiatric procedures in clinical practice*, Philadelphia, 1995, Hanley & Belfus, pp. 49–56.

Lehmann JF, de Lateur BJ: Diathermy and superficial heat, laser, and cold therapy. In Kottke FJ, Lehmann JF, editors: *Krusen's handbook of physical medicine and rehabilitation*, ed 4, Philadelphia, 1990, WB Saunders, pp. 283–367.

Mannheimer JS, Lampe GN: Electrode placement sites and their relationships. In Mannheimer JS, Lampe GN, editors: *Clinical transcutaneous electrical nerve stimulation*, Philadelphia, 1984, FA Davis, pp. 249–329.

McLean B, Fives HE: Stimulation-induced analgesia. In Warfield CA, Bajwa ZH, editors: *Principles and practice of pain management*, ed 2, New York, 2003, McGraw-Hill, pp. 413–425.

Melzack R: Folk medicine and the sensory modulation of pain. In Wall PD, Melzack R, editors: *Textbook of pain*, ed 4, Philadelphia, 1999, WB Saunders, pp. 1209–1217.

Michlovitz SL, editor: *Thermal agents in rehabilitation*, ed 3, Philadelphia, 1996, FA Davis.

National Institute of Health (NIH) Consensus Panel: Consensus statement 107: Acupuncture. *NIH Consensus Statement* 15(5):1–34, Nov 3–5, 1997.

Nelson RM, Hayes KW, Currier DP, editors: *Clinical electrotherapy*, ed 3, Stanford, CT, 1999, Appleton & Lange.

Prentice WE, editor: *Therapeutic modalities for sports medicine and athletic training*, ed 5, New York, 2003, McGraw-Hill.

Ramos G, Martin W: Effects of vertebral axial decompression on intradiscal pressure. *J Neurosurg* 81:350–353, 1994.

Rowlingson JC, Kessler RS, Dane JR, *et al.*: Adjunctive therapy for pain. In Hamill RJ, Rowlingson JC, editors: *Handbook of critical care pain management*, New York, 1994, McGraw-Hill, pp. 229–249.

Shankar K, Randall, KD: *Therapeutic physical modalities*, Philadelphia, 2002, Hanley & Belfus.

Sverdlik SS: Principles of physical medicine. In Goodgold J, editor: *Rehabilitation medicine*, St Louis, 1988, CV Mosby, pp. 773–786.

Tan JC: Massage as a form of complementary and alternative healing modality for physical manipulation. In Wainapel SF, Fast A, editors: *Alternative medicine and rehabilitation: a guide for practitioners*, New York, 2003, Demos, pp. 77–97.

Washington State Department of Labor and Industries: *Technology Assessment*. Available at: *http://www.lni.wa.gov/ClaimsInsurance/Providers/TreatmentGuidelines/TechAssess/default.asp*. Accessed July 17, 2004.

Weber DC, Brown AW: Physical agent modalities. In Braddom RL, editor: *Physical medicine and rehabilitation*, ed 2, Philadelphia, 2000, WB Saunders, pp. 440–458.

Wientraub MI: Clinical applications of magnetic therapy for neuropathic pain. In Wainapel SF, Fast A, editors: *Alternative medicine and rehabilitation: a guide for practitioners*, New York, 2003, Demos, pp. 373–377.

Weiting JM, Andary AT, Holmes TG, *et al.*, editors: *Physical medicine and rehabilitation: principles and practice*, ed 4, Philadelphia 2005, Lippincott, Williams & Wilkins, pp. 285–309.

CHAPTER 4.2
Therapeutic exercises

Therapeutic exercise is defined by the American Physical Therapy Association (2001) as "the systematic performance or execution of planned physical movements, postures, or activities intended to enable the patient to (1) remediate or prevent impairments, (2) enhance function, (3) reduce risk, (4) optimize overall health, and (5) enhance fitness and well-being." It involves the positive and progressive application and adjustment of forces of the appropriate type and amount to the body system to ultimately improve the overall function of the individual and to help meet the demands of daily living. Therapeutic exercise may include mobility exercises; muscle performance exercises (including strength, power, and endurance); aerobic capacity/endurance conditioning and reconditioning; balance; coordination training; agility training; body mechanics and postural stabilization; neuromotor development activities training; neuromuscular education or re-education; gait and locomotion training; and relaxation exercises.

The systemic effects of active rhythmic therapeutic exercise (i.e., excluding relaxation exercise) generally include increased blood flow to the muscle because of increased demands for oxygen; increased heart rate (HR), probably through neural influence; increased arterial pressure with heavy exercise (because of increased stroke volume, increased cardiac output, increased HR, and increased peripheral resistance to blood flow); increased oxygen demand and consumption; and increased rate and depth of respiration. Its effects on the hormonal and catecholamine secretions of the body include decreased insulin secretion with increased glucagon secretion to maintain blood glucose level, and increased secretion of catecholamines and other hormones when the exercise is sustained for at least 20 minutes for a minimum of 3 days per week (Fig. 4.2-1).

As active rhythmic therapeutic exercise continues at a constant rate, the HR, blood pressure, and cardiac output reach a steady state. When this type of exercise is terminated, there is an initial rapid decrease in HR and then a slower return to normal. Abrupt cessation of active rhythmic exercise may cause a sudden drop in blood pressure, hence, a cool-down period is recommended. Likewise, sudden vigorous exercise may cause electrocardiogram (ECG) abnormalities with syncopal episodes, hence, a warm-up period is recommended. If active rhythmic exercise continues beyond the body's ability to maintain it, fatigue and muscle soreness ensue. Muscle soreness usually peaks 48 hours after active rhythmic exercise (known as delayed-onset muscle soreness) and lasts 5–7 days (up to 2 weeks) probably because of tissue damage as well as subsequent structural changes in the muscle fibers to improve their metabolic capacity. This muscle soreness is greater following eccentric (lengthening) exercises than in concentric (shortening) exercises. The long-term (adaptive) cardiovascular changes that occur in the rhythmic endurance and strengthening exercises are discussed in their respective sections below.

In prescribing therapeutic exercises, the factors to be considered are type of exercise, objectives of exercise [e.g., to increase range of motion (ROM), strength, endurance, coordination, or to promote relaxation]; details of exercise instructions (e.g., frequency, duration, repetitions, types and amount of resistance, sequence of progression, exercise equipment,

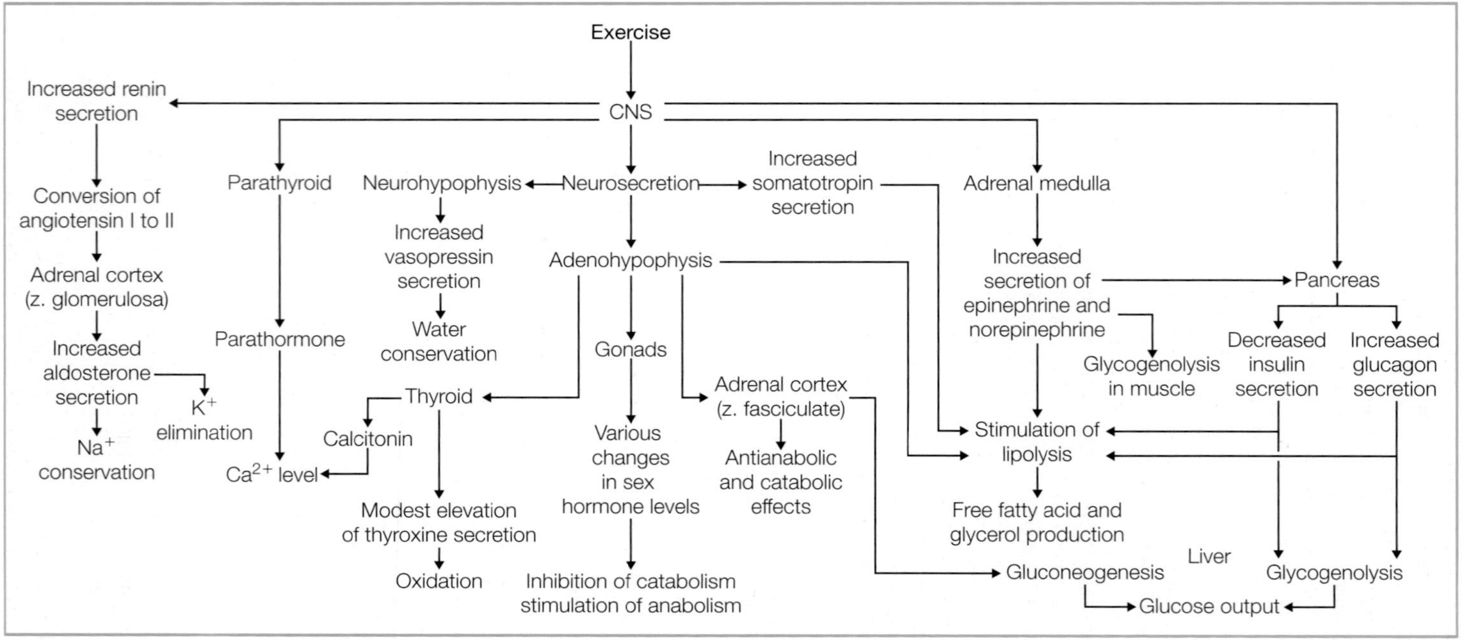

Figure 4.2-1 Effects of active rhythmic exercise on hormonal and catecholamine secretions for the control of body metabolism, i.e., mobilization of energy and protein resources. (Redrawn from Torg JS, Shephard RJ: *Current therapy in sports medicine*, ed 3, St Louis, 1995, Mosby Year Book, p. 504, with permission.)

preferred time of day for exercise, environment, and warm-up and cool-down periods), and other general concerns (e.g., time or schedule, pain, medical problems, general contraindications, cost, and motivation). To increase patient compliance, exercises should be simple and enjoyable and have meaning for the patient. They should not be burdensome, and they should not drastically change one's life-style. The therapist should explain to the patient what to expect during and after the exercise program. Muscle soreness that is labeled "good pain" should be distinguished from "bad pain", such as sharp or radiating pain. Patients must be supervised closely to make sure the exercise goals are achieved. This should be reinforced with a home program by using either an exercise booklet or customized written or computer-generated instructions and drawings, accompanied by an explanation of the purpose of each exercise. Training by using a quota system and by providing positive reinforcement are effective, especially in patients with chronic problems.

This chapter gives an overview of therapeutic exercises, except gait and locomotion training (discussed in Chapter 4.6). For details on how to design specific exercise programs for different disease process (rheumatic disease, scoliosis, stroke, multiple sclerosis, spinal cord injury, chronic obstructive pulmonary disease, peripheral vascular disease, amputation, cancer, total joint replacement, coronary artery disease, etc.], refer to Kisner and Colby's *Therapeutic Exercise: Foundations and Techniques* and Basmajian and Wolf's *Therapeutic Exercise* (see Further reading section).

I. Mobility exercises

Mobility exercises are used to maintain or restore the mobility of soft tissues (e.g., muscle, connective tissue, and skin) and joints so the patient has the ROM to perform normal functional movements.

A. RANGE OF MOTION (ROM) EXERCISES are not synonymous with stretching (see section I.B). ROM exercises *maintain* ROM *within* the available range while stretching *increases* ROM by lengthening the shortened structures, such as connective tissues, including joint capsules, muscles, and tendons *beyond* the available range. Types of ROM exercises include: active (AROM; performed by the patient without assistance), active-assistive (A-AROM; performed by the patient with assistance by another person or a mechanical device), and passive (PROM; performed for the patient by another person or by a mechanical device). ROM exercises can be performed actively with absent or minimal active muscle contraction such as in Codman's pendular exercise (prescribed for impingement syndromes, adhesive capsulitis or frozen shoulder) in which the pendular shoulder movement is mainly propelled by gravity rather than muscle contraction. Both AROM and A-AROM exercises will neither maintain nor increase strength (if muscles are very strong to begin with), and they will not develop skill or coordination (except in the movement patterns used). PROM exercises will *not* prevent muscle atrophy, increase strength or endurance, or assist circulation to the extent that active muscle contraction will.

Historically, ROM exercises are contraindicated when motion is disruptive to the healing process (e.g., immediately after acute tears, fractures, and surgery). Based on recent evidence, carefully controlled motion within the limits of pain-free motion can be performed during the early phases of healing to promote early recovery. ROM exercises should, however, be discontinued if the patient shows signs of increased inflammation (i.e., increased pain, swelling, heat, or redness). Another contraindication of ROM exercises is when patient response or the condition is life-threatening. However, after myocardial infarction, coronary artery bypass surgery, or percutaneous transluminal coronary angioplasty, AROM of the upper extremities and limited walking near the bed may be tolerated as long as there is careful monitoring of symptoms, perceived exertion, and blood pressure. Moreover, PROM may be carefully initiated to the major joints and AROM to the ankles and feet to minimize the risk of deep venous thrombosis.

Each ROM exercise (done actively if possible) should be repeated three to five times and performed once or twice daily for at least 2–3 days per week. Patterns in ROM exercises can be done through the anatomic planes of motion, combined patterns of motion [diagonal patterns similar to proprioceptive neuromuscular facilitation (PNF) patterns], or functional patterns (e.g., patterns used in teaching activities of daily living and in instructing the blind in functional activities). ROM exercises performed slowly within full ROM with minimal effort are also called **limbering exercises**. In limbering exercises, elimination of gravity by positioning helps (e.g., performing hip flexion and extension in a side-lying position). The ROM exercises may be combined with stretching by following the slow dynamic movement with a static stretch held for 10–30 seconds, and they can be performed using manual assistance, mechanical assistance, or self-assistance from the patient. The following are commonly used equipment in ROM exercises:

1. Equipment used in self-assisted ROM (S-AROM)

a. ***Wand, cane, wooden stick, T-bar, or dowel rod*** may be used in any condition where there is weakness in one upper extremity, including hemiparetic patients with some voluntary muscle control in the involved upper limb, but requires guidance or assistance to complete the ROM at the shoulder or elbow. The normal limb is used to move the involved extremity through the ROM.

b. ***Finger ladder (wall climbing) device*** can motivate the patient to do shoulder ROM by providing objective reinforcement. Patients should not be allowed to substitute shoulder ROM with trunk side-bending, toe-raising, or scapular elevation.

c. ***Shoulder wheel***, which is permanently attached to a wall, can be adjusted to various heights and arm length to motivate the patient to do active shoulder ROM. Resistance can be added to the wheel for strengthening exercises.

d. ***Overhead pulleys*** are used to assist an involved limb in performing ROM. Two pulleys are attached to an overhead bar or to the ceiling about shoulder-width apart. A rope is passed over both pulleys, and a handle is attached to each end of the rope.

e. ***Suspension*** is used to free a body part from the resistance of friction while it is moving. The involved part is suspended in a sling attached to a rope that is fixed to an appropriate point above the body segment. In a vertical fixation, the point of attachment of the rope is over the center of gravity of the moving segment. The part can then move like a pendulum, describing an arc. Because of its small ROM, this type of suspension is primarily used for support. In an axial fixation, the point of attachment of all ropes supporting the part is above the axis of the point to be moved. The part moves on a flat plane, parallel to the floor. This allows for maximum movement of a joint (vertical and axial fixation).

f. ***Skate or powder board*** is a device placed under the involved upper or lower limb to help increase ROM by reducing the effect of friction and gravity on the moving limb.

g. ***Reciprocal exercise unit ("restorator")*** is used to provide some hip and knee flexion/extension to an involved lower limb by using the strength of the normal lower limb. The device is mobile in that it can be attached to a patient's bed, wheelchair, or standard chair. It can be used for reciprocal patterning, endurance training, and initiating a strengthening program.

2. **Continuous passive movement (CPM) machine** is a mechanical device that passively moves a desired joint continuously through a controlled ROM without patient effort for as long as 24 hours a day. It is effective in lessening the negative effects of joint immobilization following limb surgery. It can prevent development of adhesions, decrease contracture formation, decrease postoperative pain, increase synovial fluid lubrication of the joint, decrease joint effusion and wound edema thus improving wound healing, increase the rate of intra-articular cartilage healing and regeneration, and provide a quicker return of ROM. Its effectiveness in increasing lower-limb circulation and preventing deep vein thromboses remains controversial. It should be used only as an adjunct to other exercise programs because it serves only to maintain ROM without the strengthening component.

B. STRETCHING refers to any therapeutic maneuver used to increase the mobility of soft tissues and subsequently improve ROM by lengthening structures that have adaptively shortened and have become hypomobile over time. Stretching is indicated when ROM is limited as the result of adhesions, contractures, and scar tissue formation, causing functional limitations or disabilities; when restricted motion may lead to structural deformities that are otherwise preventable; when there is muscle weakness and shortening of opposing tissue; as part of a total fitness program designed to prevent musculoskeletal injuries; and prior to and after vigorous exercise to potentially minimize postexercise muscle soreness. It is contraindicated when a bony block limits joint motion; after a recent fracture before bony union is complete; when there is an acute inflammatory or infectious process (i.e., heat and swelling) or when soft tissue healing could be disrupted in the tight tissues and surrounding region; whenever there is sharp, acute pain with joint movement or muscle elongation; when a tissue trauma (e.g., hematoma or effusion) is observed; when hypermobility already exists; or when contractures or shortened soft tissues are needed to provide increased joint stability (in lieu of normal structural stability or neuromuscular control) or increased functional abilities (particularly in patients with paralysis or severe muscle weakness).

Prior to stretching, the following may be used to elongate both contractile and noncontractile tissues: general relaxation (e.g., Jacobson's progressive relaxation described in section VI.A.2), heat (see Chapter 4.1, section I), cold (e.g., ethyl chloride spray; see Chapter 4.1, section II.E), massage (see Chapter 4.1, section IX), biofeedback (see Chapter 4.1, section VI), warm-up exercise, and joint traction or oscillation. During stretching, proper alignment or positioning of the patient and the specific muscles and joints to be stretched is necessary for patient comfort and stability. For an effective stretch, it is important to stabilize (or fixate) either the proximal or distal attachment site of the muscle–tendon unit being stretched.

Stretching should be applied gently at a low intensity by means of a low load to help inhibit the stretch reflex and to encourage connective tissue creep (i.e., increase in strain with time under constant load). In **static stretching** (also called **sustained, maintained, or prolonged stretching**), the soft tissues are lengthened just past the point of tissue resistance and then held in the lengthened position for an extended period of time with sustained stretch force. Its duration ranges from 15 seconds to several minutes when manual stretch or self-stretches are done, but can last for an hour to several days or weeks when a mechanical device is used. In **static progressive stretching**, the shortened soft tissues are held in a comfortable lengthened position until a degree of relaxation is felt by the patient or therapist. Then the shortened tissues are incrementally lengthened even further and again held in the new end-range position for an additional duration of time. In **cyclic (intermittent) stretching**, a relatively short-duration (between 5 and 10 seconds) stretch force is repeatedly but gradually applied (in a controlled manner at a relatively low intensity), released, and then reapplied in multiple repetitions in a single treatment session. Cyclic stretching should not be confused with **ballistic stretching**, which uses a rapid, forceful intermittent stretch (i.e., a high-speed and high-intensity stretch with very short duration). Except in young healthy subjects who participate in a conditioning program, ballistic stretching must be avoided because it facilitates the stretch reflex (increasing the tension in the muscle being lengthened), and it can also cause microtrauma in the muscle. Ballistic stretching is contraindicated in elderly or sedentary patients with musculoskeletal pathology or chronic contractures.

1. **Manual stretching** is the application of external force (by a therapist or caregiver) to move the involved body segment *slightly beyond* the point of tissue resistance and available ROM to increase the ROM (this is in contrast to ROM exercises, which stay within the limits of tissue extensibility to maintain the available length of tissues). The intensity and duration of the stretch, which are controlled by the therapist, are dependent on the patient's tolerance and the therapist's strength and endurance. In general, it uses a gentle, controlled, end-range, static, and progressive stretch held for about 30–60 seconds and then repeated for several more cycles. It is indicated in the early stages of a stretching program to provide optimal stabilization and to help the therapist determine how a patient responds to varying intensities or durations of stretch. Manual stretches can be carried out passively (called **passive stretching**) in patients with no neuromuscular control of the body segment to be stretched. When done passively, extreme caution must be observed in patients with known or suspected osteoporosis, prolonged immobilization, bone malignancy, excessive pain, hypermobility of associated joints, and total joint replacements. Manual stretching can also be performed with assistance from the patient (using the agonist contraction technique described below in section I.C.2) particularly if the patient is apprehensive and is having difficulty relaxing.
2. **Active stretching** (also called **self-stretching** or **flexibility exercises**) is carried out independently by the patient after careful instruction and supervised practice. It is usually integrated into the home exercise program and may be combined with active inhibition techniques (described below in section I.C) and can be carried out by the patient using body weight as the stretch force.
3. **Mechanical stretching** uses a device to provide either a constant load with variable displacement or constant displacement with variable loads. It applies a very-low-intensity stretch force (low-load) over a prolonged period of time to elongate tissues.

a. ***Prolonged mechanical (or positional passive) stretching*** is the application of a low-intensity external force (5–15 lb; 2.3–6.8 kg) using a mechanical device for 15–30 minutes or as long as 8–10 hours at a time, depending on the type of device used, the severity of the impairment, and the patient's tolerance. A weighted traction and pulley system, a dynamic splint or brace (e.g., **Dynasplin®**; **ERMI Flexionater®** or **Extensionater®**, **Joint Active Systems®**) or serial casts may be used. In noncontractile tissues, plastic deformation occurs; whereas, in muscles, sarcomeres are added in series.

b. ***Cyclic (intermittent) mechanical stretching*** is similar in intensity and duration to manual passive stretching. Instead of using an external manual force, however, it uses mechanical equipment in a cyclic mode. The intensity of the stretch, the length of each stretch cycle, and the number of stretches per minute are adjustable.

C. ACTIVE INHIBITION is a technique in which the patient reflexively relaxes the muscle to be elongated prior to the stretching. The muscles to be inhibited should be innervated and under the patient's control.

1. **Hold–relax (or contract–relax)** is also called "**muscle energy**" (see Chapter 4.1, section VIII.A.2.b) by manual therapists. The patient performs an isometric contraction of the tight muscle for 5–10 seconds against resistance (the contraction may be maximal or submaximal). The patient then relaxes the muscle and the therapist passively lengthens the tight muscle through the gained range. The prestretch contraction of the tight muscle causes that same muscle to relax as a result of autogenic inhibition.
2. **Agonist contraction** involves the patient's active contraction of the "agonist" (muscle opposite the tight muscle) against resistance to cause a reciprocal inhibition of the tight muscle (called the antagonist) so that the tight muscle can lengthen more readily as it is stretched. This is effective in tight muscles that are painful (because of muscle spasm) or in the early stages of healing. It is least effective when the ROM is close to normal.
3. **Hold–relax with agonist contraction** (also called **contract–relax–contract** or **hold–relax–contract**) combines the autogenic inhibition and reciprocal inhibition techniques. The patient performs a contraction and relaxation on the tight muscle (as in contract–relax technique) followed by a concentric contraction of the muscle opposite the tight muscle. Then the patient actively moves his or her own limb through the gained range.

D. PERIPHERAL JOINT MOBILIZATION AND MANIPULATION (SEE CHAPTER 4.1 SECTION VIII).

II. Resistance exercises

Resistance exercises refer to any active exercise in which a dynamic or static muscle contraction is resisted by an outside force (applied either manually or mechanically) to enhance muscle performance (i.e., the capacity of a muscle or a group of muscles to generate strength, power, and endurance).

- **Muscle strength** refers to the ability of contractile tissue to produce tension and a resultant force (i.e., motor output such as torque or work) based on the demands placed upon the muscle. It is the greatest measurable force that can be exerted by a muscle or muscle group to overcome resistance during a single, maximum effort. **Strengthening exercise (strength training)** is defined as the systematic procedure of a muscle or muscle group lifting, lowering, or controlling heavy loads (resistance) for a relatively short time. It is used primarily to increase muscle strength, although it may also increase local muscle endurance. To effectively increase muscle strength, active muscle activation is recommended, although studies seem to suggest that neuromuscular electrical stimulation, a passive modality, can also increase muscle strength as long as the muscle is not denervated (e.g., normally innervated muscles or decentralized muscles; see Chapter 4.1, section V.B.3). General guidelines in prescribing strengthening exercise include starting at submaximal resistance (e.g., 50% of maximum voluntary exertion capability) with gradual increment toward maximal voluntary exertion capability; using low repetitions, which can be increased up to 12–15 times per set for one to three sets; training 2–3 days per week; exercising large muscle groups before smaller groups; exercising in an even manner; and avoiding overfatigue and substitution of motion.
- **Muscle power** is related to strength and speed of movement and is defined as the work (force × distance) produced by a muscle per unit of time (force × distance/time). In short, it is the rate of performing work. Power can be expressed by either a single burst of high-intensity activity (called **anaerobic power**, e.g., lifting a heavy box onto a ledge) or by repeated bursts of less intense muscle activity (called **aerobic power**; e.g., climbing a flight of stairs).

- **Muscle endurance**, also called **local endurance**, is the local ability of a specific muscle to contract repeatedly against a load (resistance), generate and sustain tension, and resist fatigue over an extended period of time. This is in contrast to generalized cardiopulmonary endurance, which is produced by total body endurance exercises as described in section III. **Endurance exercise (endurance training)** is characterized by having a muscle contract and lift or lower a light load for many repetitions or sustain a muscle contraction for an extended period of time, i.e., low-intensity, high repetitions, and prolonged period of time.

The foundation of resistance exercise is based on three principles: (a) **Hellebrandt's "overload" principle**, i.e., increase in muscle performance occurs only if the load that is greater than what the tissue is accustomed to is applied to the point of fatigue; (b) **The SAID principle (Specific Adaptation to Imposed Demand)**, which is the basis for the principle of **specificity of training** (also referred to as **specificity of exercise**), i.e., improvement of strength, power, and endurance is highly specific to the training method used; and (c) **Reversibility principle**, i.e., increase in muscle performance in response to resistance exercise program is transient unless training-induced improvements are regularly used for functional activities or unless an individual participates in a maintenance program of resistance exercises.

In the normal skeletal muscle, factors that influence the capacity of muscles to generate tension include:

- Cross-section and size of the muscle (i.e., the larger the diameter, the greater the tension-producing capacity);
- Fiber arrangement and fiber length (i.e., short fibers with pinnate and multipinnate design produce high force, such as quadriceps; whereas a long parallel fiber design produces a high rate of shortening but less force, such as the sartorius muscle);
- Fiber type distribution of muscle (i.e., high percentage of the tonic, slow-twitch type I fibers results in low force production and slow rate of maximum force development, but greater resistance to fatigue; whereas a high percentage of the phasic, fast-twitch type IIA and IIB fibers results in rapid high force production and rapid fatigue);
- Length–tension relationship of muscle at time of contraction (i.e., muscle produces greatest tension when it is near or at the physiological resting position at the time of contraction);
- Recruitment of motor units (i.e., the greater the number and synchronization of motor units firing, the greater the force production);
- Frequency of firing of motor units (i.e., the higher the frequency of firing, the greater the tension);
- Type of muscle contraction (i.e., force output of eccentric > isometric > concentric muscle contraction); speed of muscle contraction or force velocity relationship (i.e., for concentric contraction, increased speed leads to decreased tension; whereas for eccentric contraction, increased speed leads to increased tension); and
- Other factors (including energy stores available to the muscle; the influence of fatigue and recovery from exercise; age; gender; and psychological factors, i.e., attention, motivation, and feedback).

For the first 4–8 weeks of resistance training, the initial, rapid gain in the tension-generating capacity of skeletal muscle is almost totally the result of neural adaptation attributed to motor learning and improved coordination, with increased recruitment in the number of motor units firing and an increased rate and synchronization of firing. Subsequently, there are adaptive changes in the muscle itself, e.g., hypertrophy of the muscle and tendon, and possibly muscle hyperplasia. For specific physiologic adaptation to strength training and endurance training, refer to Table 4.2-1.

Table 4.2-1 Physiologic adaptations (i.e., chronic physiologic responses) to strength and endurance training

Variable	Strength training adaptations	Endurance training adaptations
Skeletal muscle structure	• Hypertrophy of muscle fibers: greater in type II fibers • Hyperplasia (possibly) of muscle fibers • Fiber type composition: – Remodeling of type IIB to type IIA (thus, more fatigue resistance); – No change in type I to type II distribution (i.e., no conversion) • Capillary bed density: ↓ or no change (because of increase in number of myofilaments per fiber) • Mitochondrial density and volume: ↓ (thus, reduced oxidative capacity)	• Hypertrophy: minimal or no change • Capillary bed density: ↑ • Mitochondrial density and volume: ↑
Neural system	• Motor unit recruitment: ↑ number of motor units firing • Rate of firing: ↑ (↓ twitch contraction time) • Synchronization of firing: ↑	
Metabolic system	• ATP and CP storage: ↑ • Myoglobin storage: ↑ • Stored triglycerides: Not known	• ATP and CP storage: ↑ • Myoglobin storage: ↑ • Stored triglycerides: ↑
Enzymes	• Creatine phosphokinase: ↑ • Myokinase: ↑	• Creatine phosphokinase: ↑ • Myokinase: ↑
Body composition	• Lean body (fat-free) mass: ↑ • % body fat: ↓	• Lean body (fat-free) mass: no change • % body fat: ↓
Connective tissue	• Tensile strength of tendons, ligaments, and connective tissue in muscle: ↑ • Bone: ↑ bone mineral density; no change or possible ↑ in bone mass	• Tensile strength of tendons, ligaments, and connective tissue in muscle: ↑ • Bone: ↑ mineralization with weight-bearing activities

ATP = adenosine triphosphate; CP = creatine phosphokinase.
Adapted from: Kisner C, Colby LA: Therapeutic exercise foundations and techniques, *ed 4, Philadelphia, 2002, FA Davis, p. 69, with permission.*

Resistance exercises (unlike cardiopulmonary endurance exercises in section III) have few long-term cardiovascular effects. There is little or no change in resting heart rate (HR), resting blood pressure (BP), resting stroke volume, resting myocardial oxygen consumption, and arteriovenous oxygen difference. Likewise, there is little change in left ventricular wall thickness and mass because the increments of BP are maintained for only a few seconds at a time. However, there is decreased exercise HR, better sustained exercise stroke volume, slower rate of rise of exercise BP, and reduced myocardial oxygen consumption during exercise. Hemoglobin level may sometimes be increased in hypertrophied muscles.

Among the modes of resistance exercises, isometric (i.e., static increase in muscle tension without joint movement; see section II.A) and isokinetic (i.e., dynamic resistance exercise with constant velocity; see section II.B.1.c) resistance exercises produce the greatest rise in exercise BP. Moreover, isometric resistance exercises can decrease local blood flow to the contracting muscle leading to complete blood vessel occlusion when performing 70% of maximum voluntary exertion capability.

In the presence of muscle or joint inflammation and pain (e.g., acute rheumatoid arthritis and polymyositis), dynamic resistance exercises (performed using concentric or eccentric contractions, or both) are contraindicated, but static (isometric) exercises may be performed gently. In severe cardiac or respiratory diseases or disorders associated with acute symptoms (e.g., within the first 12 weeks of myocardial infarction or coronary artery bypass graft surgery; severe coronary artery disease, carditis, or cardiac myopathy; uncontrolled hypertension), resistance training is also contraindicated. During resistance training, precautions should be taken to avoid: Valsalva phenomenon (especially in cardiac patients because it causes a temporary fall in stroke volume; and in patients with abdominal surgery or abdominal wall hernia); substitution of motions (especially when muscles are weak because of fatigue, paralysis, or pain); overtraining and overwork (especially in patients with easy fatigability, e.g., multiple sclerosis, peripheral vascular disease, cardiac disease, and pulmonary disease); exercise-induced muscle soreness (i.e., acute muscle soreness, which develops during or directly after strenuous exercise; and delayed-onset muscle soreness, which begins 12–48 hours after exercise and peaks at 48–72 hours); and pathologic fracture (in osteoporotic patients and in patients with malignancy and radiation therapy).

A. ISOMETRIC (STATIC) RESISTANCE EXERCISE occurs when tension is generated in the muscle without visible joint movement or appreciable change in total muscle length. It is most efficient when the exertion occurs at the resting length of the muscle. Its main advantage is that it is easy to perform and requires little time and set-up. It is used to prevent or minimize muscle atrophy when the joint cannot be moved because of external immobilization (e.g., splints, casts, skeletal traction); to activate muscles to begin re-establishing neuromuscular control but protect healing tissues when joint movement is not advisable after surgery or soft tissue injury; to develop postural or joint stability; to improve muscle strength when the use of dynamic resistance exercise could compromise joint integrity or cause joint pain or inflammation; and to develop static muscle strength at particular points in the ROM consistent with specific task-related needs.

The limitation of isometric exercise is that strength is improved only at or closely adjacent to the training angle, with little or no carryover to the dynamic exercise of coordination training. It also does not cause hypertrophy and is not as effective as resisted dynamic exercises for developing muscle endurance. It must be used with caution in patients with cardiovascular problems, because it can cause ventricular arrhythmias and significantly increase blood pressure during exercise. General guidelines in prescribing isometric exercise include: use of exercise load of 60–80% of maximum voluntary exertion capability, which is held for 6–10 seconds per contraction, and repeated 8–12 times per set for one to three sets (with rest intervals between sets). The resistance must be progressively increased to continue to overload the muscle as it becomes stronger. Rhythmic breathing must also be emphasized to prevent Valsalva phenomenom.

1. **Types of isometric exercises**

a. ***Muscle-setting exercises*** are low-intensity isometric exercises performed against little to no resistance, which are used primarily to promote muscle relaxation and circulation and to decrease muscle pain and spasm during acute stages of healing. Although they can help retard muscle atrophy, they do not improve strength, except in very weak muscles. Examples are quadriceps-setting and gluteal-setting exercises.

b. ***Stabilization exercises*** are used to develop a submaximal but sustained level of co-contraction to reduce instability and enhance joint or postural stability by means of midrange isometric contractions against resistance in antigravity positions and in weight-bearing postures if weight bearing is permissible. Variations include rhythmic stabilization (used as a progression of alternating isometrics and is designed to promote stability through co-contraction of the proximal stabilizing musculature of the trunk as well as shoulder and pelvic girdle; typically performed in weight-bearing positions), alternating isometrics (manual resistance is applied in a single place on one side of a body segment and then on the other; the patient is instructed to "hold" his or her position as resistance is alternated from one direction to the opposite direction), and dynamic stabilization.

c. ***Multiple angle isometric exercise regimen*** uses resistance at least every 20° through the ROM. The "rule of tens" by Davies uses 10 sets of 10 repetitions of 10-second contractions every 10° in the range of motion. It is used to improve strength throughout the ROM when joint motion is permissible but dynamic resistance exercise is painful or inadvisable.

2. **Isometric exercise regimen**

a. ***Brief maximal isometric exercise regimen (Hettinger and Muller)*** uses a single isometric contraction against fixed resistance, held for 5–6 seconds, once per day, five or six times per week. This protocol has been shown to be ineffective for increasing muscle strength.

b. ***Brief repetitive isometric exercise (BRIME) regimen (Liberson and Asa)*** uses 5 to 10 brief but maximum isometric contractions (each bout held for 6–15 seconds) performed against resistance 5 days per week. It is more effective than the single brief maximal isometric exercise.

3. **Isometric exercise load**

a. ***Manual isometric exercise*** uses resistance force applied by the therapist or caregiver. It is carried out in the anatomic planes of motion or in diagonal patterns known as PNF patterns. A specific muscle may also be strengthened by resisting the action of that muscle as described in manual muscle testing procedures. The direction of resistance is directly opposite to the desired motion. Resistance is usually applied to the distal end of the segment where the muscle to be strengthened is attached to generate the greatest amount of external torque with the least amount of effort from the therapist. In older patients prone to osteoporotic fractures, however, a more proximal lever arm (i.e., resistance applied closer to the joint) must be used. Proper stabilization must be provided to avoid substitution of motion. The resistance is appropriate if maximum pain-free effort is done smoothly. Usually 8 to 10 repetitions per set of a specific action are adequate (as they induce fatigue). The exercise set may be repeated two or three times per session after an adequate period of rest.

b. ***Mechanical isometric exercise*** usually uses the same equipment as that used for dynamic exercises or testing (see section II.B.3.b). The joint is kept from moving by the use of either soft constraints (verbal instructions) or hard constraints (use of stabilization straps or mechanically locking the equipment).

B. DYNAMIC RESISTANCE EXERCISE involves muscle contraction that causes joint movement and excursion of a body segment as the muscle contracts and shortens (i.e., **concentric** contraction; which accelerates body segments, e.g., lifting a load) or lengthens under tension (i.e., **eccentric** contraction; which decelerates body segments, e.g., lowering a load). Both concentric and eccentric contractions are necessary for functional abilities in daily life, e.g., ascending and descending stairs; standing up from seated position and sitting back down). Cross-training or cross-exercise effect (i.e., a slight increase in strength in the same muscle group of the opposite, unexercised extremity) has been shown to occur during concentric and eccentric training. Concentric contraction has less mechanical efficiency than eccentric contraction, i.e., a maximum concentric contraction produces less force than a maximum eccentric contraction under the same conditions (thus, greater load can be lowered than lifted). Because eccentric contractions act as muscular shock absorbers, eccentric training is needed to prevent injury or reinjury during activities that involve high-intensity deceleration and quick changes of direction. The use of eccentric activities (e.g., running downhill) may also improve muscular endurance more efficiently than concentric contraction because muscle fatigue occurs less quickly with eccentric exercise. Eccentric exercise puts greater stress on the cardiovascular system than concentric exercise, thus rhythmic breathing must be emphasized to prevent Valsalva phenomenon. The incidence of exercise-induced delayed-onset muscle soreness is greater with high-intensity, rapidly progressed eccentric exercise, more so than concentric exercise.

Dynamic exercises can be performed in an open-chain or closed-chain. **Open-chain exercises** (e.g., biceps or hamstring curls) involve motions in which the distal segment (hand or foot) is free to move in space, without necessarily causing simultaneous motions at adjacent joints. Limb movement only occurs distal to the moving joint, where the resistance is applied. They use external rotary loading, usually require external stabilization (manually or with equipment), and are typically performed in nonweight-bearing positions. **Closed-chain exercises** (e.g., prone push-ups; squats) involve motions in which the body moves on a distal segment that is fixed or stabilized on a support surface. The joint movements are interdependent with relatively predictable movement patterns in adjacent joints. Movement of body segments may occur distal and/or proximal to the moving point, with resistance applied simultaneously to multiple moving segments. They use axial loading, usually require internal stabilization (by means of muscle action, joint compression and congruency, and postural control), and are typically performed in weight-bearing positions.

1. Types of dynamic exercises

a. Dynamic constant external resistance (DCER) exercise (formerly called **isotonic exercise**) is a dynamic exercise where a limb moves through a ROM against a constant load or weight with uncontrolled (variable) speed of movement. The term DCER is preferred to the term isotonic exercise because *isotonic* falsely assumes that the muscle exerts the same force throughout the range of motion, when in fact, as the muscle lengthens and shortens, the lever arm changes and consequently the forces in the muscle change. During DCER exercise, the contracting muscle is only challenged maximally at one point in the ROM where the maximum torque of the resistance matches the maximum torque output of the muscles. Despite this limitation, DCER continues to be the mainstay of the resistance exercise program.

b. Dynamic variable resistance (DVR) exercise uses specially designed resistance equipment to impose varying levels of resistance on the contracting muscles to load the muscle more effectively (than DCER) at multiple points in the ROM. DVR systems, such as the Nautilus®, Eagle®, and Universal® DVR systems use a camshaft device in the weight-cable system to provide maximal load at multiple points rather than at just one point in the ROM as the muscle exerts concentrically and eccentrically. Other variable resistance units (e.g., Keiser Cam II® system) use pressurized pneumatic resistance. These machines occupy a great amount of space because multiple units are usually needed to strengthen different muscle groups.

c. ***Isokinetic exercise*** is a dynamic exercise performed with constant angular joint velocity, i.e., the muscle shortens or lengthens at a constant rate. However, the load or force exerted may be variable. As a result of the specificity of exercise, the strength gain is greatest at the speed trained. To increase strength, isokinetic training at slow speed is more effective. Isokinetic resistance is controlled through a dynamometer, which can provide either passive (allowing only concentric actions) or active (allowing both concentric and eccentric actions) modes. The isokinetic machine is quite safe and can provide a computerized record of the torque for analysis; however, it is costly, does not accommodate all muscle groups, and can greatly increase blood pressure during exercise. Patients must be advised to move maximally, because if they move at a speed lower than the preset speed, there is no torque generated and strengthening exercise is not attained. Isokinetic exercise is usually carried out with five to seven repetitions in three sets. Isokinetic exercise equipment includes Cybex® (most common), Biodex®, Kincom®, Lido®, Merac®, Orthotron II®, and Upper Body Exerciser®.

2. **Dynamic exercise regimen is** designed to provide the most effective and efficient method to improve muscular performance and functional abilities.

a. ***Progressive resistive exercise (PRE)*** is a system of dynamic resistance training in which a constant external load is applied to the contracting muscle by some mechanical means (usually a free weight or weight machine) and incrementally progressed. The application of progressive loading in PRE, which is in accordance with Hellerandt's overload principle (see above explanation in section II), is more effective in improving muscle performance than the application of regressive loading (i.e., diminish resistance as muscle fatigue develops) used in **regressive resistive exercise** or **Zinovieff's Oxford technique**. In PREs, repetition maximum or RM (defined as the greatest amount of weight a muscle can move through the ROM a specific number of times) is used as the basis for determining and progressing the resistance.

I. **DeLorme PRE regimen** starts with the determination of 10 RM (i.e., greatest amount of weight that can be lifted, pulled, or pushed 10 times through full ROM). The patient then performs one set of 10 repetitions at 50% of the 10 RM, a second set of 10 repetitions at 75% of the 10 RM, and a final set of 10 repetitions at the full 10 RM. All three sets are performed at each session with a brief rest period in between sets. Every week, a new 10 RM is determined as strength increases. The above protocol has been modified by DeLateur by adding a few pounds daily to the initial 10 RM in addition to the weekly determination of the new 10 RM. Another modification by McMorris and Elkins uses 10 repetitions at 25%, 50%, 75%, and 100% of the 10 RM.

II. **Daily adjustable progressive resistance exercise (DAPRE) regimen (Knight technique)** was developed to objectively determine when and how much to increase resistance in an isotonic strengthening exercise program. First, an initial working weight (e.g., 6 RM) is determined. The patient then performs 10 repetitions of 50% of working weight (set no. 1), six repetitions of 75% of the working weight (set no. 2), as many repetitions as possible of the full working weight (set no. 3), then as many repetitions as possible of the adjusted working weight (set no. 4). The adjusted working weight is

Table 4.2-2 Guidelines for the daily adjustable progressive resistance exercise or DAPRE (Knight technique)

Number of repetitions performed during set #3	Adjustment to working weight for set #4	Adjustment to working weight for next day
0–2	Decrease 5–10 lb and repeat set	Decrease 5–10 lb
3–4	Decrease 0–5 lb	Same weight
5–6	Keep weight the same	Increase 5–10 lb
7–10	Increase 5–10 lb	Increase 5–15 lb
11	Increase 10–15 lb	Increase 10–20 lb

10 lb = 4.5 kg.
From: Knight KL: Knee rehabilitation by the daily adjustable progressive resistive exercise technique. Am J Sports Med *7:337, 1979, with permission.*

based on the number of repetitions of the full working weight performed during set no. 3. The number of repetitions done in set no. 4 is used to determine the working weight for the next day. Guidelines for the adjustment of the working weight are in Table 4.2-2. The ideal maximum number of repetitions when the patient is asked to perform as many repetitions as possible is five to seven. The DAPRE system eliminates the arbitrary determination of how much weight should be added in a strengthening exercise program on a day-to-day basis. This system can be used with free weights or with weight machines.

b. ***Circuit weight training*** or ***CWT*** (see also Chapter 5.13, section IV.C.2.b) is a system of mechanical resistance training with pre-established sequence (circuit) of continuous exercises performed in succession at individual exercise stations that target a variety of major muscle groups (usually 8–12) as an aspect of total body conditioning. It is designed in specific *exercise order* to minimize muscle fatigue by allowing one part of the body to recover from exercise while exercising another area. It is progressed by increasing the number of sets or repetitions, the resistance, the number of exercise stations, and the number of circuit revolutions. It requires the participant to exercise in short bouts, using light to moderate workloads with frequent repetitions, interspersed with short rest periods. Exercises can be carried out using free weights or weight training units such as the Universal®, Nautilus®, or Eagle® system. CWT exercises could include two or three sets of 8–12 repetitions of 100% 10 RMs or 10–20 repetitions of 40–50% 1 RM, with minimum amount of rest (at least 15–30 seconds up to 1 minute) between sets and stations. A circuit might include the following exercise order: bench press, leg press or squats, sit-ups, upright rowing, hamstring curls, trunk extension, shoulder press, heel raises, push-ups, and leg lifts or lowering. When the use of successive exercise encompasses flexibility exercises and aerobic activities (e.g., calisthenics) as well as weight training, it is called **circuit training**.

c. ***Plyometric training (plyometrics) or stretch-shortening drills*** uses high-velocity eccentric to concentric muscle loading (to develop muscular power and coordination), reflexive reactions (to improve the reactivity of the neuromuscular system), and functional movement patterns (to help patients return to high-demand occupational, recreational, or sports-related activities). It is used in the later stages of rehabilitation of active patients who have at least 80–85% level of strength and 90–95% ROM. Examples of plyometric activities for the upper extremities include dribbling a ball on the floor or against a wall; clap push-ups; stretch-shortening drills with elastic tubing using anatomic and diagonal motions; whereas for the lower extremities, they include hopping and jumping activities.

d. ***Isokinetic regimen*** uses isokinetic machines to provide constant angular joint velocity (see section II.B.1.c). To have the most benefit on function, the velocity used (usually medium velocities, i.e., 60 or 90–180°/second to fast velocities, i.e., 180–360°/second) should closely match the expected velocities of movement associated with specific functional tasks. Because of limited physiological overflow of training effects from one training speed to another, a regimen called **velocity spectrum rehabilitation (VSR)** was developed, which performs isokinetic exercise across a wide range of velocities. One commonly used VSR protocol involves one or two sets of 8–10 (up to 20) repetitions of concentric contractions of antagonist muscle groups (reciprocal training) at multiple velocities, with 15–20 seconds of rest between sets and a 60-second rest between exercise speeds, performed a maximum of three times per week.

3. Dynamic exercise load

a. ***Manual dynamic exercise*** uses resistance force applied by the therapist or caregiver (as in manual isometric exercise; see section II.A.3.a). The therapist may provide variable resistance by adjusting the manual resistance applied to the contracting muscle through the ROM, based on the patient's response so the muscle is loaded maximally at all portions of the range. They are most effective in the early stages of rehabilitation when muscle strength is four-fifths or less. However, the exercise load is subjective and is limited to the strength of the therapist. Also, the speed of movement is slow to moderate (which may not carry over to most functional activities). It is time- and labor-intensive for the therapist and is impractical for improving muscle endurance.

b. ***Mechanical dynamic exercise*** (also called **load-resisting exercise** or **weight training**) is any form of dynamic exercise in which resistance is applied by mechanical equipment. It is most appropriate during intermediate and advanced phases of rehabilitation when muscle strength is four-fifths or greater or when the strength of the patient exceeds that of the therapist. Increases in level of resistance can be incrementally and quantitatively documented. It is practical for improving muscular endurance. It is expensive to purchase and maintain.

I. **Free weights** are graduated weights that are hand-held or applied to the upper or lower limbs. They include barbells, dumbbells, cuff-weights with Velcro closures, sandbags, and weighted boots. Improvised weights may be made from household items, such as the plastic 1-gallon milk jug whose weight can be readily adjusted by varying the amount of water or sand it contains.

II. **Simple weight-pulley systems** use weights or springs for upper- or lower-limb strengthening. They include the pulley-weight systems (free-standing or wall-mounted) and the Elgin exercise unit. The Elgin unit uses a series of interconnected cables and independent weights and pulleys that make it possible for a patient to perform dynamic (or isometric) exercises.

III. **Elastic resistance** devices include TheraBand® and Rehabilitation Xercise® tubing, which are cut at different lengths and set up on bed rails or walls so that the upper or lower limbs or trunk can be strengthened. The resistance provided can be increased by using thicker elastics.

IV. **Dynamic constant external resistance (DCER) units**, such as the N-K Exercise Unit, provide constant external resistance through either a hydraulic force plate friction mechanism or an interchangeable weight resistance system. They are usually designed for the knee but can be adapted for the hip and shoulders.

V. **Dynamic variable resistance (DVR) systems** are described in section II.B.1.b. These machines occupy a great amount of space because multiple units are usually needed to strengthen different muscle groups.

VI. **Equipment for closed-chain training** is used in weight-bearing postures to develop strength, endurance, and stability across multiple joints.

- **Multipurpose exercise units** (e.g., **The Total Gym® System**) use a glide-board to allow performance of a closed-chain exercise in a variety of positions (ranging from partially reclining to standing) to strengthen many different muscle groups in the upper or lower extremities and the trunk.
- **Balance boards** (e.g., **Biomechanical Ankle Platform System** or **BAPS**) are used for proprioceptive training in the upper or lower extremities. They can be used standing, seated, or in the quadruped position.
- **Slide boards** (e.g., **ProFitter®**) consist of a moving platform that slides from side to side across an elliptical surface against adjustable resistance. It can be used for upper and lower extremity closed-chain resisted movements and for trunk stability.
- **Stepping machines** (e.g., **StairMaster®**) allow the patient to perform reciprocal pushing movements against adjustable resistance to make the closed-chain activity more difficult. They provide non-impact, closed-chain strengthening for both upper and lower extremities.
- **Elliptical trainers** and **cross-country ski machine** provide nonimpact, reciprocal resistance to the lower extremities (and also upper extremities) in an upright weight-bearing position. Resistance can be further adjusted by changing the incline.
- **Mini-trampolines** enable the patient to begin gentle, bilateral or unilateral bouncing activities (jog, jump, or hop in place) on a resilient surface (to decrease joint impact).

VII. **Reciprocal exercise equipment** uses repetitive reciprocal exercises to improve lower or upper limb endurance, strength, or reciprocal coordination as well as cardiovascular fitness. They include stepping machines and cross-country ski machines described above, as well as the following.

- **Cycle ergometers** or **stationary bicycles** use a friction device to increase resistance and are used to increase lower limb strength and endurance.
- **Portable resistive reciprocal exercise units** can be wall-mounted and adapted for upper limb exercise or they can be attached to a sturdy straightback chair or a wheelchair as an alternative for patients who cannot use a stationary bicycle.
- **Upper extremity ergometer** (e.g., **Upper Body Exerciser®** or **UBE**) provides resistance exclusively for the upper extremities. They are typically used in a seated position but may also be used in a standing position.

VIII. **Equipment for dynamic stabilization training** (e.g., **Bodyblade®**) consists of an oscillating blade, which provides instability in three planes of motion. The patient drives the blade using rapid alternating contractions of agonist and antagonist muscle groups in an attempt to maintain it in various positions in space, thus producing dynamic stability. Its goal is to develop proximal stability as a foundation of controlled movement.

IX. **Isokinetic testing and training equipment** is described in section II.B.1.c.

III. Cardiopulmonary endurance exercises

These are also known as **conditioning** or **total body endurance exercises** and refer to low-intensity, high-repetition exercises of large groups of muscles to enhance the overall cardiopulmonary fitness of an individual (this is in contrast to the resistance training referred to in section II, which improves only local muscular endurance). Cardiopulmonary endurance exercises increase one's ability to perform repeated motor tasks in daily living and to carry on a sustained level of functional activity, such as walking or climbing stairs.

Long-term cardiovascular effects of cardiopulmonary endurance training include:

- Decreased heart rate (HR) at rest and submaximal effort (thus the HR reserve is increased although the peak HR remains unchanged or is slightly decreased);
- Small (5–10 mmHg) clinically useful decrease in BP at rest and submaximal effort, but increased peak BP during "maximal" exercise (or "peak" exercise because it is difficult to determine if the effort is indeed "maximal" especially if the patient voluntarily terminates the exercise session);
- A 20- to 30-mL increase in peak stroke volume (SV) during "maximal" exercise (probably as a result of increased cardiac preloading caused by plasma volume expansion and decreased afterloading caused by increased ventricular contractility and increased muscle strength);
- Little effect on resting cardiac output with a small decrease in cardiac output during submaximal exercise and an equivalent of 10–20% increase in peak cardiac output during "maximal" exercise [as a result of training-induced increment in peak SV despite absent or slightly reduced peak HR (because cardiac output = SV × HR)]; and
- Reduced myocardial oxygen consumption at rest and submaximal effort, but a small increase in peak myocardial oxygen consumption during "maximal" exercise (as reflected by the unchanged peak HR and the potential increase in peak systolic BP).

Cardiopulmonary endurance training can also decrease the exercise recovery time (i.e., more rapid return of the above changes to resting levels after exertion), increase coronary blood flow (probably because of longer diastolic phase allowing a longer period of coronary perfusion), increase the wall thickness and muscle mass (up to 30%) of the left ventricle (thus increasing end-diastolic volume and ejection fraction), increase aerobic enzymatic activity, increase arteriovenous oxygen difference, and increase maximum ventilatory ability. The hemoglobin concentration remains unchanged or may be slightly decreased because of an expansion of plasma volume. Overall, there is an increase in the oxidative (aerobic) capacity of the muscle.

Another systemic effect of cardiopulmonary endurance exercise is an increased blood cortisol level (Fig. 4.2-1), which in turn promotes protein catabolism (especially in less active muscle) and suppresses protein synthesis. This catabolic effect (occurring during the exercise session) increases the pool of free amino acids, which, after the exercise session, are eventually used as "building materials" for the adaptive synthesis of structural and enzymatic proteins, probably through the mediation of thyroid hormone, growth hormone, insulin, and/or testosterone. There is also improved thermal regulation capability (i.e., increased sweating begins at lower temperatures with less salt content); increased lipolysis (Fig. 4.2-1), which leads to increased free fatty acid and glycerol production; and decreased serum triglycerides (TG) and low-density lipoproteins (LDL) with increased high-density lipoproteins (HDL). The alteration in serum lipid, which lasts for 1–2 days after the exercise session, helps reduce the risk of coronary artery diseases in trained individuals.

The lowered TG and LDL, increased HDL, and increased caloric expenditure during aerobic exercises can all help to reduce the patient's weight. These effects are dependent on the intensity and frequency of the aerobic exercise. To control excess body fat, the aerobic activity should use about 300 kcal per exercise session and be performed for at least 20 minutes for a minimum of 3 days per week. Aerobic exercise for longer durations and at lower intensities, performed for 4 or 5 days per week, may be prescribed to maximize the weight-controlling effect. In addition to aerobic exercises, the overweight or obese patients should lower caloric intake [generally not <1200 kcal/day to allow for a gradual weight loss of about 2 lb (900 g)/week]; gradually reduce fat intake and increase complex carbohydrate and fiber intake; incorporate behavioral techniques to help manage eating and exercise behavior; and participate in peer social support groups. These patients may find regular counseling from behavioral therapists (for about 6 months) as well as periodic physician follow-up helpful.

For a given workload, the increase in blood pressure, heart rate, cardiac output, and oxygen uptake during maximal exercise is greater in cardiopulmonary endurance exercises involving the upper limbs than in those involving the lower limbs. The increase in cardiac output in upper limb exercises is caused by the increased heart rate, not stroke volume. As in strengthening exercises, the overload principle applies to cardiopulmonary endurance exercises, i.e., the body must work close to the point of fatigue (or mitochondrial exhaustion) to increase its metabolic or aerobic capacities.

A. **AEROBIC ENDURANCE EXERCISE** encompasses strengthening and cardiopulmonary endurance exercise. It uses large groups of muscles to increase the oxygen consumption gradually. A combination of arm and leg aerobic exercise is the most effective way of producing cardiopulmonary fitness. Depending on the patient's preference and physical condition, the following low-impact aerobics may be recommended: stationary bicycling, cycling, race-walking, calisthenics, low-impact aerobic exercises, swimming, aquatic exercises, rowing, hiking, and cross-country skiing. All aerobic endurance exercises should be controlled and progressive. They must be performed using correct technique (i.e., knowledge of the basic rules of the sport), proper equipment, and appropriate protective measures (e.g., wearing appropriate shoes; exercising on nonconcrete surfaces; stretching, warming up, and cooling down). Unless the patient is physically well-conditioned and has good musculoskeletal conditions, the following should be avoided: contact sports (e.g., basketball, football, soccer); sports that involve trunk twisting (e.g., tennis, racquetball, squash, golf); and other high-impact activities (e.g., jogging, running, volleyball, hopping, jumping, rope-skipping, high-impact forms of aerobic dancing, downhill skiing).

Each aerobic endurance exercise session should consist of a 5- to 10-minute warm-up period; followed by 20–30 minutes of aerobic training at 40–60% (low-intensity training), or 60–70% (moderate-intensity training), or 70–85% (heavy-intensity training) of their maximal functional capacity (see below for methods of determining exercise intensity); ending with a 5- to 10-minute cool-down period. In patients whose functional capacities are below 3 metabolic equivalents (MET) (see below) short sessions of about 5 minutes should be performed several times a day. Patients with functional capacities above 5 MET should exercise three to five times per week.

There are four methods of aerobic training. (a) *Continuous training* involves the use of submaximal energy throughout the training period (usually for 20–60 minutes), with overload accomplished by increasing exercise duration. It is the most effective way of improving endurance in healthy individuals. (b) *Interval training* involves the use of a properly prescribed relief interval following work or exercise. The relief interval can either be a rest relief (passive recovery) or work relief (active recovery, wherein exercise is continued but at a reduced level from the work period). Interval training tends to improve strength and power more than endurance. (c) *Circuit training* involves the use of successive exercise activities that encompass flexibility exercises and aerobic activities (e.g., calisthenics) as well as weight training. At the end of the last activity, the individual starts from the beginning and again moves through the series; the series of activities is then repeated several times. Circuit training can improve strength and endurance by stressing both aerobic and anaerobic systems. (d) *Circuit–interval training* is a combination of circuit training and interval training.

Depending on such factors as age, functional capacity, health status, and compliance, the rate of exercise progression generally follows three stages: (a) the initial *conditioning stage,* which involves low-intensity exercise for 10–15 minutes (this stage lasts for 4–6 weeks); (b) the *improvement stage,* which involves performing the exercise at the appropriate training intensity (discussed below) with gradual increment in duration until the patient can exercise for at least 20–30 minutes (this stage lasts 4–5 months); and (c) the *maintenance stage,* which involves regular continuation of the routine acquired in the improvement stage (this stage is usually attained after about 6 months of training).

During aerobic exercise, HR must be monitored to ensure that the maximal safe exercise limit is not exceeded, especially in situations that naturally increase HR (e.g., hot, humid weather). In addition to HR, the rate–pressure product (RPP) (also called the double product) should be monitored. The RPP (i.e., RPP = HR × systolic BP; see Chapter 2.7, section I.A) decreases for a given workload as the patient becomes more conditioned during training. The following are techniques commonly used to prescribe and monitor aerobic endurance exercise intensity:

1. **Target heart-rate range (THRR) methods**. The THRR can be used to guide aerobic exercise intensity as follows: if the pulse or heart rate exceeds the upper limit of THRR, then the exercise intensity should be slowed down, but if the pulse or heart rate is less than the lower limit of the THRR, then the exercise intensity should be increased. For a training effect to occur, the exercise intensity must be such that the pulse or heart rate is within the THRR for at least 20–30 minutes.

a. ***Karvonen formula*** uses the heart-rate reserve, which is computed by subtracting the resting HR from the maximal HR. The "maximal" heart rate (MHR) is obtained from an exercise tolerance test (e.g., cardiovascular or cardiopulmonary graded exercise tolerance test described in Chapter 2.7, sections I.A and II.A respectively); while the resting heart rate is obtained with the subject in a seated position. The THRR using the Karvonen formula can then be computed, **(maximal HR – resting HR) (40–85%) + resting HR = THRR.** The low range (40%) and the high range (85%) of the THRR may be lowered for patients with more impaired cardiopulmonary functions or in the initial phase of cardiac rehabilitation (see Chapter 5.13, section IV.A).

b. ***Age-adjusted maximal HR (AAMHR) formula***, which is less accurate, can be used to estimate the THRR in healthy subjects who have not undergone formal graded exercise tolerance testing. The AAMHR is estimated by subtracting the patient's age in years from 220. The THRR using the AAMHR can thus be computed as **(220 – age) (65–85%) = THRR.** Although this method is easier to calculate, it is not generally recommended because it yields significantly lower THRR values. If used at all, the THRR should be adjusted by adding 10–15%.

2. **Metabolic equivalents (MET) method**. The use of MET (see description in Chapter 2.7, section I.A) for prescribing aerobic exercise intensity in patients with cardiopulmonary disease is probably the least accurate and must, therefore, be used with great caution and an awareness of its physiologic limitations. This is partly because most of the experiments used in constructing the table showing the MET equivalent for different activities (see Tables 4.2-3 and 4.2-4) derived their data from normal subjects (e.g., healthy, young men), hence their values tend to be overestimated for patients with cardiopulmonary problems. Moreover, MET levels estimated from an exercise tolerance test using the lower

Table 4.2-3 Classification of self-care or home activities and occupational activities by MET* units

METs	Self-care or home	Occupational
1.5–3 (Very light)	Self-care (washing, shaving, dressing); Light house work (washing dishes, polishing furniture, washing clothes); Writing at desk	Sitting (desk work, clerical, assembly, computer work, driving car/truck, operating crane, radio and television repair, light woodworking, riding lawn mower); Standing (bartending, standing as a store clerk, janitorial work)
3–5 (Light)	House work (mopping or scrubbing floors, cleaning windows, slowly waxing floors, vacuuming); Yard work (raking leaves, hoeing, weeding, pushing light-power mower); Carrying objects (15–30 lb)	Auto repair, machine assembly, stocking shelves (light objects), paperhanging, light carpentry, masonry (plastering, brick laying, pushing wheelbarrow with 100-lb or 45-kg load); welding (moderate load), painting, energetic musician, trailer-truck in traffic
5–7 (Moderate)	Yard work (easy digging in garden, level hand-lawn mowing); Climbing stairs (slowly); Carrying objects (30–60 lb) Shoveling 10 times/min (4.5 kg or 10 lb)	Carpentry (exterior home building), using pneumatic tools, splitting wood
7–9 (Heavy)	Stair climbing (moderate speed); Carrying objects (60–90 lb); Shoveling 10 times/min (5.5 kg or 14 lb)	Digging ditches, sawing hardwood, tending furnace, pick and shovel
>9 (Very heavy)	Climbing stairs (quickly), carrying load upstairs, carrying objects (>90 lb); Shoveling 10 times/min (7.5 kg or 16 lb)	Lumberjack; heavy laborer

10 lb = 4.5 kg.
** One MET (metabolic equivalent) = 3.5 mL O_2 consumption/kg/min at rest.*
Adapted from: Fox SM, III, Naughton JP, Gorman PA: Physical activity and cardiovascular health: Part III. The exercise prescription: Frequency and type of activity. Mod Concepts Cardiovasc Dis *41(6):27–28, 1972; and Haskell WL: Design and implementation of cardiac conditioning programs. In Wenger NK, Hellerstein HK, editors:* Rehabilitation of the coronary patient. *New York, 1978, John Wiley, pp. 214–215.*

limbs (e.g., treadmill or bicycling test) do not determine the exact MET level that might be achieved during upper-limb exercise, nor does it account for the emotional or physiologic stress that may increase the metabolic demand during actual performance of activities.

When the MET equivalent is used for exercise prescription, it is advisable to begin the exercise program with an initial target range of 50–60% of the "maximal" MET level, which is estimated from the cardiovascular or cardiopulmonary graded exercise tolerance test (see Chapter 2.7, section I.A and II.A). For some patients (e.g., the elderly or those with severe cardiopulmonary disease), the initial training intensity may be as low as 40% of the "maximum" MET level. As training effects are achieved, the target range can be increased up to 70–85% of the "maximum" MET level. Using the table of various activities with corresponding MET equivalents (Tables 4.2-3 and 4.2-4), the individual may select activities for training that are known to require energy expenditures within the target MET range. Likewise, if the MET equivalent table is used for advising patients about recreational and occupational activities, the recommended activity should

Table 4.2-4 Classification of recreational and physical conditioning activities by METs for a 70-kg person (see also Table 2.7-3 for determining MET units during treadmill exercise)

METs	Recreational	Physical conditioning
1.5–2	Card playing, flying, knitting, motorcycling, sewing	Standing, walking (1 mph), bed exercise (arm movement, supine or sitting)
2–3	Billiards, bowling, canoeing, golfing with power cart, horseback riding at a walk, powerboat driving, skeet shooting, shuffleboard	Walking (2 mph), level bicycling (5 mph), TM (2 mph, 0% grade = 2.5 MET), very light calisthenics
3–4	Archery, badminton (social doubles), dancing (moderate), fly fishing (standing in waders), golf (pulling cart), horseback riding (trotting), pitching horse shoes, sailing (handling) small boat, softball (excluding pitcher), volleyball (six-person; noncompetitive)	Walking (3 mph), bicycling (6 mph), TM (2 mph, 2.5% grade = 3.2 MET; or 3 mph, 0% grade = 3.3 MET), light calisthenics
4–5	Badminton (singles), ballet, dancing (foxtrot; vigorous), golf (carrying clubs), ping pong, tennis (doubles), rowing (noncompetitive)	Walking (3.5 mph), bicycling (8 mph), TM (2.5 mph, 5% grade = 4.6 MET or 3 mph, 2.5% grade = 4.3 MET), many calisthenics (in general)
5–6	Canoeing (4 mph), horseback riding ("posting" to trotting), skating (9 mph; ice or roller), stream fishing (walking in light current in waders)	Walking (4 mph), bicycling (10 mph), TM (2 mph, 10% grade = 5.3 MET or 3 mph, 5% grade = 5.4 MET)
6–7	Badminton (competitive), dancing (folk; square), skiing (light downhill; touring at 2.5 mph), tennis (singles), water-skiing	Walking (5 mph), bicycling (11 mph), TM (3 mph, 7.5% grade = 6.4 MET), swim (20 yards/min)
7–8	Basketball, canoeing (5 mph), football (touch), hiking (mountain, no backpack), horseback riding (gallop), ice hockey, paddleball, skiing (vigorous, downhill)	Jogging (5 mph), bicycling (12 mph), TM (3 mph, 10% grade = 7.4 METs)
8–9	Basketball (vigorous), fencing, handball (social), rope skipping, ski touring (4 mph), squash (social)	Running (5.5 mph), bicycling (13 mph), TM (3.4 mph, 10% grade = 8.3 MET); swim (30 yards/min)
10+	Handball (competitive), rowing (11 mph = 13.5 METs), ski touring (5 mph), squash (competitive)	Running (6 mph = 10 MET; 7 mph = 11.5 MET; 8 mph = 13.5 MET; 9 mph = 15 MET; 10 mph = 17 MET); TM (3.4 mph, 14% grade = 10 MET); TM (3.4 mph, 18% grade = 12 MET); swim (>40 yds/min)

1 mph = 1.6 kmph, 5 mph = 8 kmph; 1 yard = 0.9 m.
One MET (metabolic equivalent) = 3.5 mL O_2 consumption/kg/min at rest;
TM = treadmill; mph = miles per hour.
Adapted from: Fox SM, III, Naughton JP, Gorman PA: Physical activity and cardiovascular health: Part III. The exercise prescription: Frequency and type of activity. Mod Concepts Cardiovasc Dis *41(6):27–28, 1972, the American Heart Association.*

correspond to a MET level that is 50–80% lower than the "maximum" MET level obtained during exercise tolerance testing. For example, if the "maximum" workload corresponds to a "maximum" MET level of 12 to 13, then an activity corresponding to a level of 8 MET is recommended, i.e., bicycling at 13 mph (20 kmph) or walking at 3.4 mph (5.4 kmph) with 10% grade (Table 4.2-4).

3. **Borg's rate of perceived exertion (RPE) scale method.** Borg's RPE scale (Table 4.2-5) is used by the patient to rate the intensity of exercise. It provides a subjective means of monitoring exercise intensity as patients become more familiar with the "feeling" associated with exercising at the appropriate THRR. A rating of 12 to 13 (somewhat hard) on the 20-point category scale corresponds to about 60% of maximum HR, but a rating of 15 (hard or heavy) corresponds to about 85%. If the category-ratio scale is used (Table 4.2-5), these ratings would be between 4 and 5. Denial of perceived exertion (in competitive individuals) limits the practical application of Borg's RPE scale. Borg's RPE scale is probably more psychological than physiological. Its use allows an individual to concentrate

Table 4.2-5 Category and category-ratio scales for borg's ratings of perceived exertion (RPE)

Category scale for Borg's RPE*†		Category-ratio scale for Borg's RPE†	
6	No exertion at all	0	Nothing at all ("no intensity")
7	Extremely light	0.3	
8		0.5	Extremely weak (just noticeable)
9	Very light	0.7	
10		1	Very weak
11	Light	1.5	
12		2	Weak (light)
13	Somewhat hard	2.5	
14		3	Moderate
15	Hard (heavy)	4	
16		5	Strong (heavy)
17	Very hard	6	
18		7	Very strong
19	Extremely hard	8	
20	Maximal exertion	9	Extremely strong ("maximum intensity")
		•	Absolute maximum ‡ (highest possible)

Note: The RPE scale is commonly used for rating perceived exercise intensity in exercise tolerance testing and in exercise prescription. The scale values of 6 to 20 were chosen to approximate the linear increase in heart rate from 60 to 200 beats per minute as exercise intensity increases. The category-ratio scale is commonly used for intensity evaluation and has been used to rate angina, aches in the working muscles, and pain from loaded passive joint structures.

From: **Borg G: Perceived exertion as an indicator of somatic stress.* Scand J Rehabil Med *2(2–3):92–98, 1970, and* † *Borg G:* Borg's perceived exertion and pain scales, *Champaign, IL, 1998, Human Kinetics. Copyright © Gunnar Borg, 1970, 1985, 1994, 1998, with permission.*

‡ *If the intensity rating is greater than 10, the person can choose any large number in proportion to 10 that describes the proportionate increase in intensity, i.e., if it feels 30% more than at the rating of 10, the RPE would be 13.*

more on how a particular intensity of exercise feels and still have some assurance that he or she is within the THRR. This ability to use the RPE makes it easier for patients to be independent in their own activities and to wean patients off external monitoring devices. In patients with cardiac transplant (see Chapter 5.13, section IV.A.2.a), the RPE is recommended because of denervation of the heart (which decreases the reliability of other parameters such as heart rate).

B. ANAEROBIC ENDURANCE EXERCISES are performed to deplete the glycolytic system, which functions in the first 1–2 minutes of exercise. High-resistance, short-duration exercises at 80% of maximum exertion capacity are needed. Interval training with intense short-duration activity of 1 or 2 minutes has been recommended (e.g., for sprinters).

IV. Motor coordination and skill exercises

These increase one's ability to regulate muscles simultaneously or in sequence to perform apparently simple or complex activities. Motor coordination is controlled by the conscious activation of an individual muscle or the conscious initiation of a preprogrammed engram. General principles of coordination exercises include constant repetition of a few motor activities, use of sensory cues (tactile, visual, proprioceptive) to enhance motor performance, and increase in the speed of the activity over time.

A. FRENKEL EXERCISES are a series of exercises of increasing difficulty to improve proprioceptive control in the lower limbs. They begin with simple movements with gravity eliminated, then gradually progress to more complicated movement patterns using simultaneous hip and knee motions carried against gravity. They are useful for coordination retraining for proprioceptive or cerebellar dysfunction.

B. TRADITIONAL APPROACHES FOR IMPROVING MOTOR CONTROL AND COORDINATION emphasize the need for repetition of specific movement for learning, the importance of sensation to the control of movement, and the need to develop basic movements and postures, with the assumption that when movement is "normalized" then skilled movement would occur automatically (based on the hierarchical theory of motor control wherein development progresses sequentially from lower to higher levels of control). These approaches are aimed at permanently reorganizing the central nervous system (CNS). The four traditional systems presented below differ in whether abnormal spinal and brainstem reflexes should (Brunnstrom) or should not (Bobath) be used to elicit movement when the patient cannot otherwise move, whether redevelopment of motor control should be sought in an ontogenetic sequence (PNF and Rood) or in a proximodistal sequence (Bobath and Brunnstrom), and whether conscious attention should be directed toward the movement itself (Brunnstrom and PNF) or only toward the goal of the movement (Rood and Bobath). None of the traditional systems addresses methods of developing skilled movement. They are used in a variety of neuromotor impairments (e.g., spasticity in spinal cord injury, cerebrovascular accident, traumatic brain injury, and cerebral palsy patients and multiple sclerosis patients with ataxia). Their clinical effectiveness, however, remains to be proved in randomized controlled studies.

1. **Proprioceptive neuromuscular facilitation (PNF) (Kabat and Voss approach)** uses spiral and diagonal components of movement rather than the traditional movements in cardinal planes of motion with the goal of facilitating movement patterns that will have more functional relevance than the traditional techniques of strengthening individual muscle groups. The movement patterns are developmentally sequenced but do not emphasize the inhibition of abnormal reflex activities. It uses resistance during the spiral and diagonal

movement patterns with the goal of facilitating "irradiation" of impulses to other parts of the body associated with the primary movement.

2. **Movement therapy (Brunnstrom approach)** is based on the theoretical concept that damaged CNS has undergone an evolution in reverse and has regressed to phylogenetically older patterns of movement (e.g., limb synergies and primitive reflexes). Thus, synergies, reflexes, and other abnormal movement patterns are seen as a normal part of the recovery process before normal movement is attained. Patients are taught to voluntarily control the motor patterns available to them at that point in their recovery process (e.g., limb synergies). These are subsequently modified into simple to complex movement combination patterns. (For details, refer to Brunnstrom's: *Movement Therapy in Hemiplegia*, New York, 1970, Harper & Row).
3. **Neurodevelopmental technique (NDT) (Bobath approach)** is based on the theoretical concept that pathologic movement patterns (e.g., limb synergies and primitive reflexes) must not be used for training because repeated use of the pathologic efferent pathways may make them too readily available for use at the expense of normal pathways. This approach is opposite to the Brunnstrom and PNF approaches, in which abnormal reflex activity is reinforced rather than inhibited. The goal of NDT is to normalize tone, to inhibit primitive or "abnormal" reflex patterns, and to facilitate automatic reactions and subsequent normal movement patterns. Patients are taught to use patterns of movement that are opposite to abnormal patterns (so called "reflex inhibiting patterns") and are guided by the therapist from "key points of control" to inhibit abnormal motor activity and facilitate more normal motor activity. "Key points of control" refer to points on the body, usually proximal such as shoulder and pelvic girdles, which, when handled by the therapist in a specific manner, can be used to influence or reduce abnormal/spastic movements. (For details, refer to Bobath B: *Adult hemiplegia: evaluation and treatment*, London, 1978, W Heinemann.)
4. **Sensorimotor approach (Rood approach)** uses sensorimotor stimuli to normalize tone and activate purposeful movement and postural responses starting at the patient's current level of development and progressing sequentially to higher levels of control. These sensorimotor stimuli include quick stretch, icing, fast brushing, slow stroking, tendon tapping, vibration, and joint compression to promote co-contraction of proximal muscles.

C. **CONTEMPORARY APPROACHES FOR IMPROVING MOTOR CONTROL AND COORDINATION** are influenced by contemporary skill acquisition and motor development theories. They emphasize motor performance using functional tasks and consider factors other than CNS damage that may affect performance, include remediation of performance components and modification of the environment to improve task performance, stress practice that fits the nature of the task, and reject the assumption of the hierarchical model of motor control and the traditional developmental theories. These approaches are new and need further research.

1. **Motor relearning program (MRP) for stroke patients (Carr and Shepherd approach)** draws heavily from cognitive motor learning theory and is influenced by Bobath's NDT. The patient is considered an active participant whose major goal is to relearn how to move functionally and how to problem solve during attempts at novel tasks. The MRP provides guidelines for evaluating and improving motor control in seven categories of functional daily activities: upper-limb function, orofacial function, sitting up over the side of the bed, balanced sitting, standing up and sitting down, balanced standing, and walking. Instead of providing a specific sequence for intervention, MRP recommends an analysis of the task, practice of the missing component, practice of the task, and transference of training. The five strategies used are: verbal instruction;

visual demonstration; manual guidance; accurate, timely feedback about the quality of performance; and consistency of practice.

Unlike traditional approaches that emphasize repetitive performance of a specific movement for improving skill, MRP teaches general strategies for solving motor problems. In MRP, activities like rolling are not given emphasis as in the traditional approach because MRP does not believe in the hierarchical theory of motor control. Instead of the proximodistal sequence, MRP therapists encourage any active movement in wrist and finger muscles. If possible, hand function is practiced simultaneously with shoulder girdle control and postural adjustments within the context of functional reaching tasks. The therapist's role is to guide the individual in this process and to prevent or remove obstacles that may lead to the use of inefficient compensatory strategies. When the patient can perform activities effectively and automatically in a variety of environmental contexts, then task learning is considered successful.

2. **Contemporary task-oriented approach** uses purposeful activity as the primary treatment modality with the assumption that functional tasks help to organize motor behavior. It assumes that after CNS damage or other changes in personal or environmental systems, the patient's behavioral changes reflect attempts to compensate to achieve functional goals, and that occupational performance emerges from the interaction of multiple systems that represent the unique characteristics of the person and the performance context. Another assumption is that personal and environmental systems are heterarchically organized (i.e., no automatic or inherent ordering of the system in terms of their importance or influence on the motor behavior), and that a person needs to practice and experiment with varied strategies to find the optimal solution for motor problems and to develop skill in performance. Treatment goals are to help the patient develop the optimal movement patterns for performing a task, to achieve flexibility in task performance by providing practice opportunities in varying contexts, to maximize use of personal characteristics and environmental factors that make efficient and effective task performance possible, and to facilitate problem solving by the patient so he can identify his own solutions to motor problems in the home and community environments.

V. Aquatic exercises

Aquatic exercises refer to the use of multidepth immersion pools or tanks (see also Chapter 4.1, section III.C) to facilitate the application of different established therapeutic interventions, including:

- **Aquatic stretching exercises**, which are performed in waist-deep water and are either provided manually by the therapist or independently by the patient (i.e., self-stretching) using aquatic equipment. Aquatic stretching may be better tolerated than land stretching because of the effects of relaxation, soft-tissue warming, and ease of positioning. However, because of its buoyancy, water can be inherently less stable than land.
- **Aquatic strengthening exercises**, which are performed in waist-deep water (to help reduce joint compression, provide three-dimensional resistance, and dampen perceived pain), and are either provided manually by the therapist (typically in a concentric, closed-chain fashion) or independently by the patient with or without equipment. Equipment-assisted aquatic strengthening exercise can be: (a) **buoyancy assisted**, i.e., movement, which may be performed with buoyant equipment, applied vertically directly parallel to vertical forces of buoyancy; (b) **buoyancy supported**, i.e., movement, which may be performed with

buoyant equipment applied horizontally with vertical forces of buoyancy eliminating or minimizing the need to support an extremity against gravity; (c) **buoyancy resisted**, i.e., movement, performed without equipment, directed against or perpendicular to vertical forces of buoyancy creating drag, i.e., negative pressure; or (d) **buoyancy super resisted**, i.e., movement using equipment to generate resistance by increasing the total surface area moving through the water, thus creating greater drag.

- **Aquatic aerobic conditioning**, which is performed in the vertical position in deep-water pools with feet not touching the pool bottom or, alternatively, in 4–6 ft (1.2–1.8 m) water depth. Techniques include deep-water walking/running using a flotation belt (positioned posteriorly), vests, flotation dumbbells, or noodles, running with patient tethered to the edge of the pool or against resistance jets, midwater jogging/running using specially designed socks to prevent skin breakdown, running in immersed treadmill or against forced current or while tethered with elastic tubing for resistance, exercises with immersed equipment such as immersed cycling or upper-body ergometer, and swimming.
- **Aquatic balance and gait training**, can initially be performed in waist deep water, but if there is pain, the patient is moved to chest deep water. If pain persists, a flotation belt is used around the waist to offload the body's weight. Gait training sequence consists of walking or marching forward, backward, and sideways. Water provides an environment in which patients can practice balance and walking tasks without fear of the consequences of falling which are often present with land-based balance and gait training.

The contraindications of aquatic exercises include patients with incipient cardiac failure and unstable angina; respiratory dysfunctions (i.e., vital capacity <1 litre); severe peripheral vascular disease; danger of bleeding or hemorrhage; severe kidney disease (because of the inability to adjust to fluid loss during immersion); open or discharging wounds; colostomy; skin infections (e.g., tinea pedis and ringworm); bowel incontinence; bladder incontinence (unless catheterized); water- and airborne infections or diseases (e.g., influenza, gastrointestinal infections, typhoid, tuberculosis, and cholera); and uncontrolled seizures.

Aquatic exercises must be used with caution in patients with: fear of water; neurologic disorders [e.g., multiple sclerosis patients, whose preferred temperatures are 29°C (84°F) or less, may easily fatigue in water temperatures greater than 33°C (91.4°F)]; controlled seizures; cardiac dysfunction (e.g., angina and abnormal blood pressure); small, open wounds and tracheotomies (which may be covered with waterproof dressings); and intravenous lines, Hickman lines, and other open lines (which may need to be properly clamped and fixated).

With immersion, the body's capability to dissipate heat through normal sweating mechanisms is diminished because there is less skin exposed to the air. Hence, cooler water temperatures are generally used for higher intensity exercise, and warmer temperatures for mobility exercise and for muscle relaxation. The ambient air temperature should be 3°C (5.4°F) higher than water temperature.

For cardiovascular training and aerobic exercise, water temperatures should be between 26°C (78.8°F) and 28°C (82.4°F) to maximize exercise efficiency, increase stroke volume, and decrease heart rate. Intense aerobic training performed above 80% of a patient's maximum heart rate needs water temperature of 22°C (71.6°F) to 26°C (78.8°F) to minimize risk of heat illness.

For aquatic exercises including mobility, strengthening, gait training, and relaxation, water temperatures between 26°C (78.8°F) and 33°C (91.4°F) are used. For patients with acute painful musculoskeletal injuries, aquatic exercise performed at 33°C (91.4°F) may be beneficial. At temperatures greater than 37°C (98.6°F), exercise may be harmful if prolonged or maintained at high intensities, because of the significant increase in cardiac output.

Special equipment for aquatic exercise includes the following.

A. COLLARS, RINGS, BELTS, AND VESTS provide buoyancy assistance to assist with patient positioning. They can be applied to the neck, extremities, or trunk. For neck support and to maintain the head out of the water, inflatable cervical collars are used. Flotation rings are used to support the extremities (e.g., wrists and ankles) in any immersed position. Belts and vests are used to position patients supine, prone, or vertically for shallow- and deep-water exercises.

B. SWIM BARS are buoyant dumbbells used for supporting the upper body or trunk in upright positions and the lower extremities in the supine or prone positions. In deep water, patients can balance in a seated or standing position on long swim bars for balance, proprioception, and trunk strength training.

C. WEBBED GLOVES, HAND PADDLES, AND HYDRO-TONE® BELLS are non-buoyant devices, which only resist motion in the direction of movement. Hydro-tone® Bells, which are large, slotted plastic devices that increase drag during upper extremity motions, generate more resistance than gloves or hand paddles.

D. FINS AND HYDRO-TONE® BOOTS are applied to the feet during lower extremity motions to generate resistance by increasing the surface area moving through the water. Fins are used to provide resistance for the hips, knees, and ankles. Hydro-tone® Boots are used during deep-water walking and running.

E. KICKBOARDS, which come in different shapes and styles, may be used to provide buoyancy in the prone or supine positions, held vertically to create resistance to walking patterns in shallow water, or used to challenge seated, kneeling, or standing balance in the deep water.

VI. Relaxation exercises

Relaxation exercises are performed consciously with active mental and physical participation from the patient to induce a "relaxation response", which is a psychophysiologic state of low arousal characterized by generalized decrease in sympathetic nervous system activity and concomitant decreases in respiratory rate, oxygen consumption, heart rate, blood pressure, arterial blood lactate levels, and muscle tension, as well as increases in skin resistance, skeletal muscle blood flow, and electroencephalographic (EEG) activity. This "relaxation response" has been demonstrated using biofeedback tools (see Chapter 4.1, section VI) in conjunction with relaxation techniques. They are beneficial to most PM&R patients, for example to help reduce pain perception in patients with acute or chronic pain (see Chapter 5.10, section VI.F.3.b) and to reduce cardiopulmonary stress in patients with cardiac and/or pulmonary problems (see Chapters 5.12 and 5.13). For the relaxation technique to be effective, it must be congenial to the patient, help restore the patient's sense of control, be easy to apply in different settings (i.e., portable), offer relatively immediate reduction of pain, promote other pain-related benefits (e.g., reduced intake of pain medication and increased activity), and be cost-effective.

Relaxation exercises can be performed singly or incorporated into the other exercise sessions, such as part of the warm-up or, more commonly, the cool-down session of aerobic exercise and before or after limbering or stretching exercises. At the beginning of training, relaxation exercises should be carried out in a quiet semi-darkened room with the patient in a comfortable supine or semi-reclining position. Constricting garments should be loosened, and small pillows may be used under the head or under the knees to promote muscle relaxation. Biofeedback machines (see

Chapter 4.1, section VI) may be used during the training period. Eventually, the patient must learn how to apply relaxation techniques in more upright postures such as sitting or standing and during other activities. Patients are encouraged to schedule relaxation sessions at home and at work, and to perform them during stressful periods. The following relaxation exercise techniques can be used singly or in combination with controlled-breathing exercises, followed by progressive muscle relaxation, and then dissociative visualization while breathing is maintained in a rhythmic relaxing pattern throughout the session:

A. PHYSIOLOGIC RELAXATION STRATEGIES

1. **Controlled-breathing relaxation exercise** involves slow breathing patterns to promote parasympathetic activity and counteract sympathetic activity. Usually, the pattern of breathing used is a diaphragmatic breathing (see also Chapter 5.12, section IV.B.2.a.1) in which the abdomen swells out during inspiration so that the lower part of the chest and, finally, the upper chest expands and slightly lifts; then the breath is held momentarily and released slowly as the abdomen is drawn in, the diaphragm is lifted, and the chest relaxes.

a. ***"One" breathing technique,*** which is a form of meditation, involves the passive focusing of awareness on the diaphragmatic breathing cycle while silently repeating the word "one" with each exhalation. The patient is instructed to maintain a passive attitude and permit (rather than force) relaxation to occur at its own pace. It can be performed for 10–20 minutes, once or twice daily.

b. ***Eye-movement breathing technique*** involves looking up to the eyebrows without head movement during the inspiratory phase of diaphragmatic breathing, then holding the breath for 2 seconds followed by looking down to the chin without head movement while breathing out very slowly and completely as a "sissing" sound is produced between the teeth and as the abdomen is drawn in as in diaphragmatic breathing. To promote relaxation, the expiratory phase can be prolonged. The cycle is repeated at least four to five times and is usually used before or after other exercises such as limbering or stretching exercises (see Chapter 4.11, section I.C.3.b and II.A.) or in synchrony with muscle stretching of the trunk, neck, or shoulders.

2. **Progressive muscle relaxation exercise (Jacobson)** consists of systematically learning to tense muscle groups (for about 10 seconds) followed by active relaxation and releasing of tension for 10–15 seconds. Usually, about 14 to 16 major muscle groups are sequentially tensed and relaxed. During the tensing and relaxation of each muscle group, the patient is asked to be consciously aware of different feelings associated with tension and with relaxation. To be effective, the patient must be able to recognize or discriminate relaxation from tension, and to voluntarily induce the state of relaxation.

B. COGNITIVE RELAXATION STRATEGIES involve the use of "mental" strategies to induce the "relaxation response". They can be performed singly or usually in conjunction with physiologic relaxation strategies such as controlled breathing.

1. **Dissociative visualization** involves passive focusing on some personally meaningful, pleasing, relaxing, and absorbing memory or image. The technique of focusing may be attending to sensory information such as the colors and sounds of the imagery. Practice sessions usually last 15–20 minutes.

2. **Autogenic relaxation training**, which is a form of self-hypnosis, relies on a series of self-directed formulae to induce the relaxation response through alterations of proprioception and sensation. The patient is instructed to assume a relaxed position, to close the eyes, and to passively concentrate on a series of six standard autogenic formulae such as "my left arm is heavy". Standard formula one focuses on promoting the feeling of heaviness in the limbs, and formula two focuses on promoting the sensation of warmth in the limbs. Formulae three and

four focus on cardiac and respiratory regulation respectively. Formula five focuses on promoting the sensation of warmth in the abdomen, and formula six focuses on the feeling of coolness in the forehead. The patient is instructed to practice these formulae daily until such time as a voluntary shift to a state of wakeful low arousal is readily attained. In addition to the six standard formulae that focus on the psychophysiologic aspects of the relaxation response, there are a series of organ-specific formulae, intentional formulae, and meditative formulae.

3. **Other cognitive techniques** include the use of audiotapes or videotapes with instructions or music for relaxation, guided imagery, hypnosis (see Chapter 5.10, section IV.F.3.e), and meditation such as transcendental meditation.

C. **NONTRADITIONAL (ALTERNATIVE) "PSYCHOPHYSICAL" TECHNIQUES** incorporate physiologic and cognitive relaxation strategies as well as postural re-education techniques. They include the Feldenkrais Method, Alexander Technique, Trager Psychophysical Integration, Tai Chi Chuan, and Hatha Yoga. Although most of the nontraditional techniques are able to induce a "relaxation response", their effectiveness over the more traditional and more cost-effective techniques (e.g., controlled breathing, progressive muscle relaxation, and dissociative visualization) remain controversial and are at best anecdotal.

Further reading

American Physical Therapy Association: Guide to physical therapist practice, ed 2, *Phys Ther* 81(1): S104–S105, 2001.

Basmajian JV, Wolf SL, editors: *Therapeutic exercise*, ed 5, Baltimore, 1990, Williams & Wilkins.

Brannon FJ, Foley MW, Starr JA, *et al.*: *Cardiopulmonary rehabilitation: basic theory and application*, ed 3, Philadelphia, 1998, FA Davis.

Ciccone CD, Alexander J: Physiology and therapeutics of exercise. In Goodgold J, editor: *Rehabilitation medicine*, St Louis, 1988, Mosby-Year Book, pp. 759–772.

DeLateur B: Therapeutic exercise to develop strength and endurance. In Kottke FJ, Lehmann JF, editors: *Krusen's handbook of physical medicine and rehabilitation*, ed 4, Philadelphia, 1990, WB Saunders, pp. 427–464.

Gaupp LA, Flinn DE, Weddige RL: Adjunctive treatment techniques. In Tollison CD, Satterthwaite JR, Tollison JW, editors: *Practical pain management*, ed 3, Philadelphia, 2002, Lippincott, Williams & Wilkins, pp. 108–135.

Hamill RJ, Rowlingson JC: *Handbook of critical care pain management*, New York, 1994, McGraw-Hill.

Hoffman MD, Sheldahl LM, Kraemer WJ: Therapeutic exercise. In DeLisa JA, Gans BM, Walsh NE, *et al.*, editors: *Physical medicine and rehabilitation: principles and practice*, ed 4, Philadelphia, 2005, Lippincott, Williams & Wilkins, pp. 389–433.

Kisner C, Colby LA: *Therapeutic exercise: Foundations and techniques*, ed 4, Philadelphia, 2002, FA Davis.

Pollock ML, Wilmore JH: *Exercise in health and disease*, ed 2, Philadelphia, 1990, WB Saunders.

Simmons V, Hansen PD. Effectiveness of water exercise on postural mobility in the well elderly: an experimental study on balance enhancement. *J Gerontol* 51A(5): 233–238, 1996.

Torg JS, Shephard RJ: *Current therapy in sports medicine*, ed 3, St Louis, 1995, Mosby-Year Book.

Trombly CA, editor: *Occupational therapy for physical dysfunction*, ed 4, Baltimore, 1995, Williams & Wilkins.

CHAPTER 4.3
Orthoses

An orthosis (or brace) is an external device applied to body parts to provide support or stabilization, improve function by restricting or assisting motion, correct flexible deformities, prevent progression of fixed deformities, or reduce pressure and pain by transferring load from one area to another. A temporary orthosis is referred to as a splint. In general, orthoses should be lightweight with reasonable durability, acceptable appearance, easy to maintain and clean, easy to don and doff correctly, and adjustable to accommodate changes in body contour. Most importantly, patients must be motivated to wear it. In patients with fluctuating edema, orthoses are generally not recommended unless the orthosis is adjustable. In the presence of fluctuating muscle tone, different splints or orthoses may be prescribed to meet different demands (e.g., a resting splint at night and a wrist cock-up orthosis during the day while the patient is undergoing rehabilitation activities that may improve muscle tone). If feasible, active exercises and functional activities should be prescribed together with the orthoses.

Orthoses can be constructed from metal, plastic, leather, fabrics (natural or synthetic), wood, rubber, adhesives, or any combination of these basic materials. Metal orthoses are usually adjustable but are heavy and generally are not cosmetically pleasing. Commonly used metals include stainless steel, aluminum alloys, and titanium. Steel is widely used in orthotic joints, springs and bearings, and less commonly in uprights and bands. It is relatively inexpensive, easy to shape, and fatigue-resistant (i.e., high strength); however, it is heavy and needs expensive alloys to prevent corrosion. Aluminum alloys are less corrosion-resistant than steel and have high strength-to-weight ratio. They are commonly used in upper-limb orthoses because of their light weight. Unfortunately, although its static loading strength is good, aluminum has a lower endurance limit (i.e., is unable to withstand repetitive stress without failure) compared to steel. Thus, if loading conditions are great and highly repetitive (e.g., adult lower-limb orthoses), steel is generally superior to aluminum (unless the aluminum is larger than the steel alternative). Titanium is very lightweight and resistant to corrosion, making it desirable for orthotic joints. However, it is not used often because it is more expensive than steel or aluminum.

Plastics are synthetic organic materials, which are used in orthoses because they are lighter (per unit volume) and can provide a closer fit (i.e., it can be molded, extruded, laminated, or hardened into any desired form). Moreover, they are unaffected by fluids (e.g., water, urine, and oils) and are radiolucent. However, they are not adjustable in length and are not as durable as metal (hence they are not commonly used as joints). Plastics used for orthoses can be classified into thermosetting and thermoforming (or thermoplastic) materials.

Thermosetting plastics develop a permanent shape when heat and pressure are applied; therefore, they cannot be softened when reheated and then reshaped. They resist higher temperatures and provide greater dimensional stability than do most thermoplastics, but are more difficult to form than thermoplastics and are more apt to cause allergic reaction (although the risk is lessened when the patient wears a fabric interface between the skin and orthosis). Polyester-resin thermoset plastics are especially useful for laminating purposes in orthotics. Epoxy-resin thermoset plastics, which are also formulated for laminating, are used for their high tensile, compressive, and flexural strength; high-impact resistance; and superior bonding strength. They have good chemical resistance.

Thermoplastics soften and become moldable when heated and harden when cooled. They can be divided into direct-forming and nondirect-forming thermoplastics. Direct-forming thermoplastics (Orthoplast, Aquaplast, Bioplastics, Glassona, Hexcelite, Kay-splint, Lightcast, Polysar, Warm-N-Form) can be molded at temperatures just above body temperature (<80°C or <180°F), hence they may be shaped directly to the body without the need for a cast. Closed-cell foam polyethylene materials, such as Plastazote, require higher temperature (110–140°C) for molding, but air convection cools their surface so rapidly that they can be formed safely on the skin. Direct-forming thermoplastics can be fabricated easily and rapidly (requiring only a supply of hot water, scissors, and a source of hot air, such as a heat gun or an oven) and are mainly used in upper-limb orthotics in which low-stress activity is anticipated.

Nondirect-forming thermoplastics [acrylic, polyethylene, polypropylene, polycarbonate, acrylonitrile-butadiene-styrene and the group of vinyl polymers and copolymers that includes polyvinyl chloride, polyvinyl alcohol, and polyvinyl acetate) require up to 150–160°C (300–350°F) to become moldable, hence they must be shaped over a plaster replica of the body part. They are creep-resistant (i.e., they do not easily change in shape with continued stress and heat) and are ideal for long-term or permanent use, especially when high stress is anticipated (e.g., in lower-limb orthoses and with spastic limbs).

The leathers most commonly used in orthotics are cattle hides that have been vegetable tanned for texture and for prevention of skin irritation. Cattle hides are recommended for shoe construction because they conduct heat well, absorb fluid from the moist air surrounding the foot, draw perspiration away from points of heavy sweating, and stretch as the shoe becomes moist, so preventing constriction of hot or sweaty feet. Cattle hides, however, are relatively expensive.

Fabrics used in orthoses can be natural (e.g., cotton, wool) or synthetic (e.g., polyester, nylon). Cotton canvas is desirable for making a sturdy abdominal front on a trunk orthosis or for use as porous material for the athletic shoe's upper. It is strong, hypoallergenic, and easily absorbs fluid (e.g., perspiration). Cotton flannel is used as padding material. Knitted cotton, which readily conforms to the bodily contour, is often used as a liner under trunk or leg orthoses. Cotton may be combined with polyester to make a relatively inexpensive fabric that is strong and dries easily. However, a corset made of cotton and polyester does not absorb perspiration as much as one made of pure cotton. Nylon is used in hook-and-pile fasteners, which are easier to use than buckles, snaps, buttons, or laces. Fabrics can be interwoven with rubber to make elastic materials, which can be used in straps and other portions of orthoses (e.g., in trunk orthoses) requiring yield during movement. Fabrics are also used in pressure garments to control edema, prevent hypertrophic scarring, and provide some joint stability.

The wood most commonly used in orthoses (e.g., for shoe lifts and arch supports) is cork because of its light weight and shock absorbency. Cork may be combined with rubber (cushion cork) or with thermoplastics (e.g., Thermocork or Birko Cork). Balsa is another wood used in orthoses especially to make shoe elevations.

Rubber (natural or synthetic) is used in orthoses because of its elasticity, shock absorbency, and toughness. It makes good padding and provides excellent traction on shoe soles. A commonly used synthetic rubber is neoprene which is relatively inexpensive and is corrosion resistant. Nitrogen gas can be introduced to neoprene to make it into a closed-cell expanded rubber (e.g., Spenco), which has excellent shock absorbency. Sodium bicarbonate may be introduced into rubber to create an open-cell sponge rubber (e.g., Lynco, Kemblo), which is softer and more porous than other rubbers. Another open-cell rubber is latex foam, which is washable, soft, and very resilient. However, the cells compress permanently after a short period of use. Polyurethane foam (Poron, Sorbothane, Ovafit) is used primarily for covers and pads for orthoses. It can be bonded to other plastics, metal, and wood.

Adhesives, rather than mechanical means (e.g., rivets or thread), are used in orthoses (e.g., in foot orthoses) to attach materials to one another. Synthetic resin adhesives are commonly used in thermoplastic or thermosetting plastics (e.g., to join a strap to the shell of a wrist–hand orthosis) because they can bond to different surfaces. Rubber-based adhesives are used (e.g., in foot orthoses) to provide resistance to impact loads.

This chapter covers only orthoses primarily used for adults. In general, orthotic prescription should include medical diagnosis (e.g., compressive peroneal nerve palsy), current impairment and resulting disability (e.g., flaccid foot drop), type of orthosis [e.g., plastic ankle–foot orthosis (AFO) with flexible ankle held in neutral position], and orthotic goals (e.g., toe clearance during swing-through and prevention of foot slap during early stance).

I. Shoes and lower-limb orthoses

Shoes and lower-limb orthoses are generally used to assist gait, reduce pain, decrease weight bearing, control movement, and minimize worsening of a deformity. The orthosis should fit properly. Any discomfort should be addressed because it will lead to decreased use of orthosis and subsequent loss of function. In patients with decreased sensation or impaired circulation, the skin must be checked regularly for redness, trophic changes, abrasions, and dermatitis. Skin redness should disappear 10 minutes after orthosis removal. The orthosis must be functionally, as well as cosmetically, acceptable to the patient. The patient must be able to easily don and doff it so the patient can rest the desired segment or stand, sit, and perform the prescribed movement comfortably (throughout all phases of gait) when wearing the orthosis.

A. SHOES are an integral part of lower-limb orthoses. They are worn to protect the feet from the external environment and to transfer body weight to the

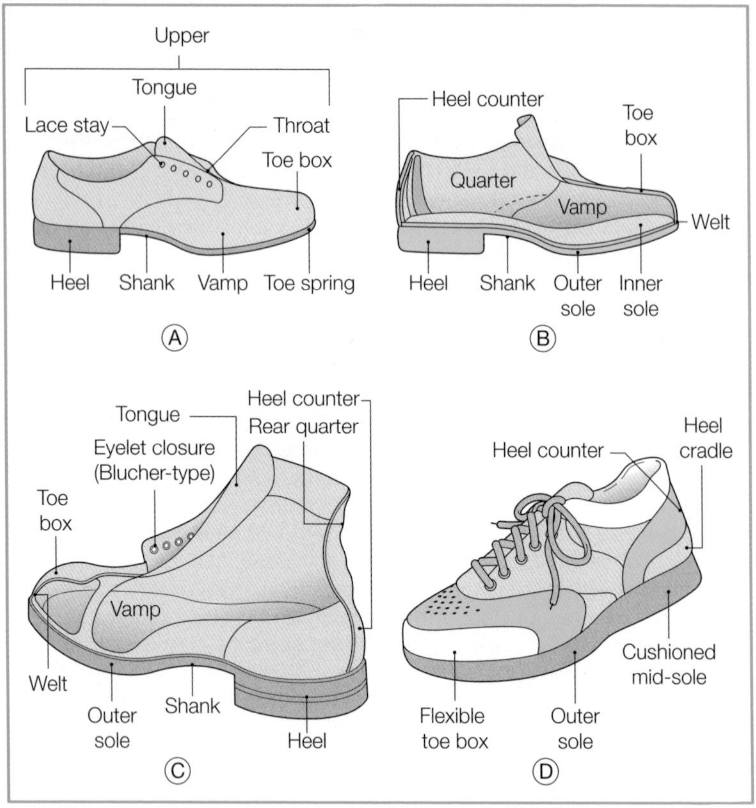

Figure 4.3-1 Parts of three basic shoe types: 1. Low-upper or low-quarter shoe (**A**, external view and **B**, cut view); 2. High-upper or high-quarter shoe (**C**); and 3. Athletic shoe (**D**). The portion of the shoe that covers the dorsal aspect of the foot and encases the heel is called the upper (the anterior component is called the vamp and the posterior part is called the quarter).

ground while walking. In people with orthopedic problems, shoes can be modified to reduce pressure on sensitive or deformed structures by redistributing weight toward pain-free areas. Shoes also serve as the foundation of lower-limb orthoses. Parts of three basic shoe types are shown in Fig. 4.3-1. Different types and styles of shoes used in PM&R are shown in Fig. 4.3-2. A properly fitted shoe should have adequate room for the foot to expand upon bearing weight. The shoe should be at least 1 cm longer than the longest toe and the widest part of the shoe should corres-pond to the foot's widest part. It should be snug from the heel to the ball (i.e., metatarsophalangeal joints) of the foot and should fit closely around the anatomic heel. For adults with foot disorders, the most versatile shoe has an extra-depth (i.e., depth of two insoles to allow the use of shoe inserts; Fig. 4.3-2.D), Blucher-type upper (i.e., no distal attachment of lace stays to leave more room for the entering foot; Fig. 4.3.2.B) with a laced or hook-and-pile closure and a low heel. An accommodative shoe with a spacious toe box is prescribed for patients with hammer-toe, claw-toe or mallet-toe, or bunion.

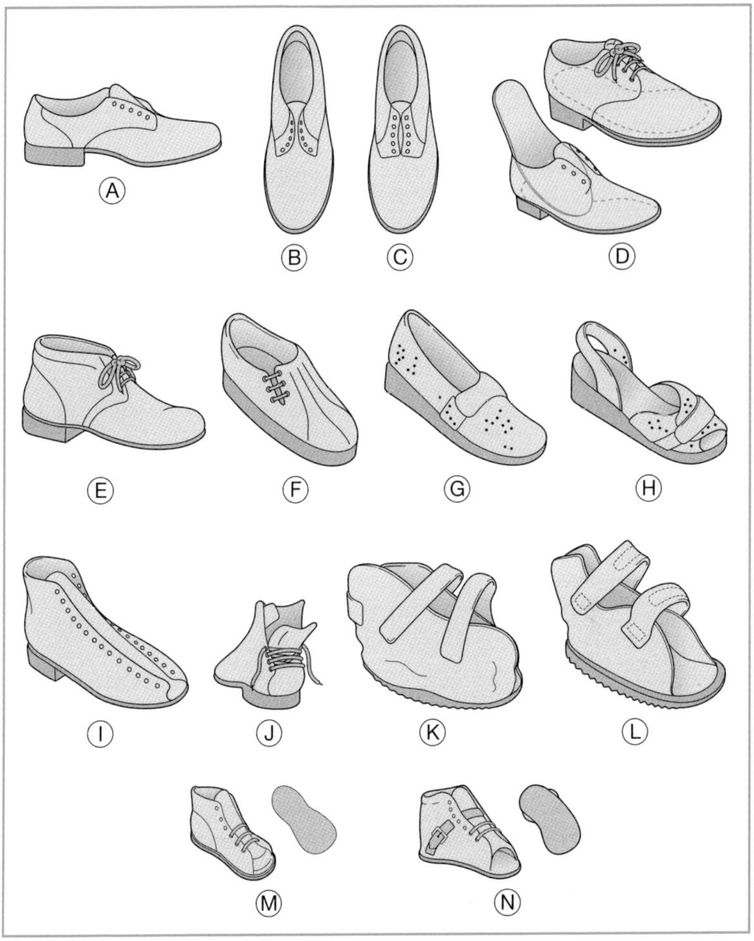

Figure 4.3-2 Different types and styles of shoes used in PM&R. **A**, Low-quarter Oxford-type shoe with lacing. **B**, Low-quarter Oxford-type shoe with Blucher-type lacing (i.e., the lace stays are not stitched to the vamp and remain loose and fully open, thus leaving more room for the entering foot). **C**, Low-quarter Oxford-type shoe with Bal- or Balmoral-type lacing (i.e., the lace stays meet in front and are stitched to the vamp). **D**, Extra-depth shoe (accommodates severe foot deformities such as hammer-toe deformities and allows for shoe insert). **E**, High-quarter (chukka) shoe with lacing. **F**, Custom-molded shoe (for gross deformities of feet such as diabetic neuropathy). **G**, Plastazote shoe. **H**, Plastazote sandal. **I**, Convalescent shoe with anterior lacing. **J**, Convalescent shoe with posterior lacing. **K**, Orthopedic cast boot (closed toes). **L**, Orthopedic cast boot (open toes). **M**, Pediatric prewalker (for mild residual metatarsus varus or for holding the foot in the desired position after casting). **N**, Pediatric clubfoot shoe (for residual or mild to moderate metatarsus varus or when it is necessary to hold a postsurgically corrected clubfoot).

Shoe modifications for common foot problems are shown in Table 4.3-1. Most current lower-limb orthoses (e.g., plastic leaf spring-type AFOs) are made of thermoplastic that can fit inside the shoe. The shoe serves to hold the orthosis in place. For this purpose, individuals may use commercially available shoes with

Table 4.3-1 Suggested shoe modifications for common foot problems in adults

Foot problems (modification goals)	Suggested shoe modifications
Limb shortening (to equalize leg length; improve posture and gait)	Heel elevation (if <½ inch = internal; if >½ inch = external); Heel and sole elevation (if >1 inch); Rocker bar; High-quarter shoe
Arthritis, fusion, or instability of ankle and subtalar joints (to support and limit joint motion; improve gait; accommodate deformities)	High-quarter shoe; Reinforced counters; Long steel shank; Rocker bar; SACH heel
Pes plano-valgo (to reduce eversion; support longitudinal arch)	Thomas heel with medial high wedge; Medial longitudinal arch support with cookie or scaphoid pad
Fixed pes equinus (to provide heel strike; contain foot in shoe; reduce MT head pressure; improve ease of putting on shoe; equalize leg length)	High-quarter shoe; Heel elevation; Heel and sole elevation on other shoe; Modified lace stay for wide opening; Medial longitudinal arch support; Rocker bar, occasionally
Pes varus (to realign flexible deformity; accommodate a fixed deformity; increase medial and posterior weight bearing on foot)	High-quarter shoe; Long lateral counter; Reverse Thomas heel; Lateral shoe and heel wedges for flexible deformity; Medial wedges for fixed deformity; Lateral sole and heel flanges; Medial longitudinal arch support
Pes cavus (to distribute weight over entire foot; restore AP foot balance; and reduce pressure on MT heads)	High-quarter shoe; High toe box; Lateral heel and sole wedges; Metatarsal pads or bars; Molded inner sole; Medial and lateral longitudinal arch support
Calcaneal spurs (to decrease pain)	Heel cushion; Inner relief in heel and fill with soft sponge
Metatarsalgia (to reduce pressure on MT heads; support transverse arch)	Metatarsal or sesamoid pad; Metatarsal or rocker bar; Inner sole relief
Hallux valgus (to reduce pressure on 1st MTP and big toe; prevent forward foot slide; immobilize first MTP; shift weight laterally)	Soft vamp with broad ball and toe; Relief in vamp with cut-out or balloon patch; Low heel; Metatarsal or sesamoid pad; Medial longitudinal arch support
Hallux rigidus (to reduce pressure and motion on first MTP; improve push-off)	Soft vamp; Long steel spring in sole; Sesamoid pad; Metatarsal or rocker bar; Medial longitudinal arch support
Hammer-toes (to relieve pressure on painful areas; support transverse arch; improve push-off)	Soft vamp, extra-depth shoe with high toe box or balloon patch; Metatarsal pad
Unilateral foot shortening (to fit shoe to foot)	Extra inner sole and padded tongue for difference of <1 size; Shoes of split sizes or custom-made
Foot fractures (to immobilize fractured part)	Long steel shank; Longitudinal arch support; Metatarsal pad; Metatarsal or rocker bar

Abbreviations: MT, metatarsal; MTP, metatarsophalangeal joint; SACH, solid ankle cushion heel; AP, anteroposterior.
1 inch = 2.54 cm.
Modified from Ragnarsson KT: Lower extremity orthotics, shoes, and gait aids. In DeLisa JA, Gans BM, Walsh NE, et al., editors: Physical medicine and rehabilitation: principles and practice, *ed 4, Philadelphia, 2005, Lippincott, Williams & Wilkins, p. 1384, with permission.*

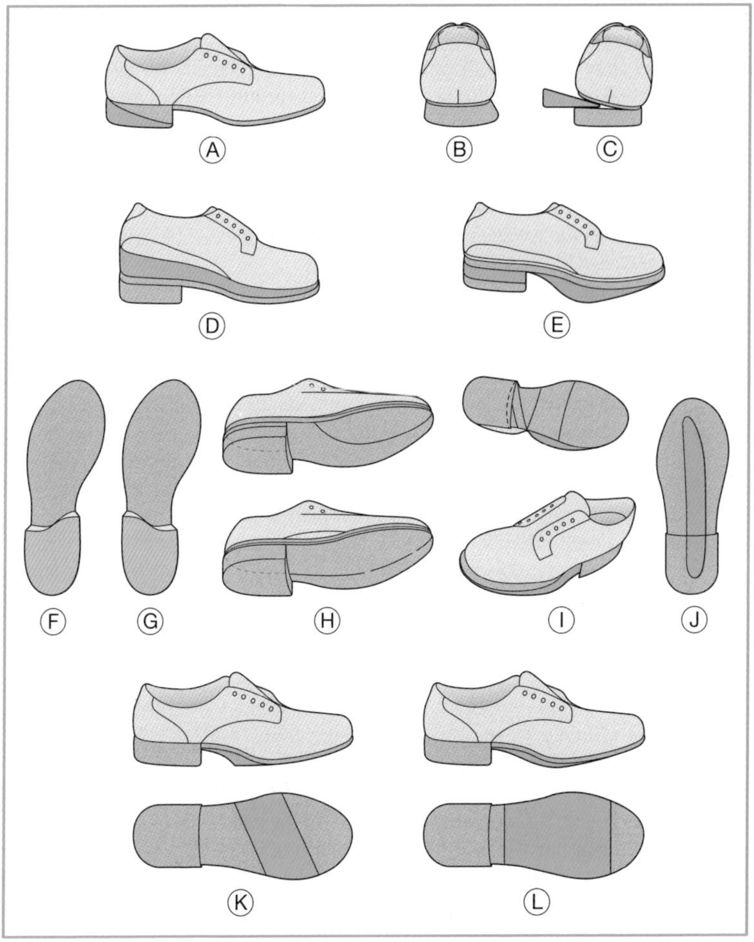

Figure 4.3-3 Types of external shoe modifications (see text for description). **A**, Cushioned heel. **B**, Heel flare. **C**, External heel wedge. **D**, Combination external sandwich-elevation of the heel and sole. **E**, External heel sandwich-elevation (heel lift), with rocker bar at the sole. **F**, Thomas heel (with medial heel extension). **G**, Reverse Thomas heel (with lateral heel extension). **H**, Combination medial sole wedge and external heel wedge (top shows sandwiching in two sections; bottom shows an overlay unit extending the full length of the sole and foot). **I**, Lateral sole flare. **J**, Steel bar. **K**, Metatarsal bar. **L**, Rocker bar sole.

sturdy counters (reinforcement in the posterior portion of the shoe upper) rather than custom-made shoes.

1. **External shoe modifications** (Fig. 4.3-3), unlike internal shoe modification, do not reduce shoe volume. However, they erode as the patient walks and can be conspicuous. The patient is also limited to wearing the shoe that has been modified.

a. ***Heel modifications***

I. **Cushioned heel** (Fig. 4.3-3.A) is a wedge of compressible material inserted into the heel to absorb shock at heel strike. It reduces the knee flexion moment by allowing more rapid ankle plantarflexion and is indicated when the patient wears an orthosis with a rigid ankle or has anatomic ankle limitation.

II. **Heel flare** (Fig. 4.3-3.B) can be applied either medially (to resist hindfoot eversion) or laterally (to resist hindfoot inversion). Medial and lateral heel flares may be used together to provide greater heel stability.

III. **External heel wedge** (Fig. 4.3-3.C, H) can be applied either medially (to rotate hindfoot into inversion) or laterally (to rotate hindfoot into eversion). The shoe must have a counter strong enough to resist the hindfoot from sliding on the wedge incline. External heel wedge can be combined with a sole wedge (described in section I.A.1.b.3).

IV. **Extended heel** can project anteriorly either on the medial side (Thomas, orthopedic, S-shaped, or keystone heel; Fig. 4.3-3.F) or on the lateral side (reverse Thomas or reverse orthopedic or reverse extended heel; Fig. 4.3-3.G). The Thomas heel provides additional support to the medial longitudinal arch, while the reverse Thomas heel supports the lateral longitudinal arch.

V. **Heel elevation (heel lift** or **shoe lift)** (Fig. 4.3-3.D, E) is used to compensate for fixed pes equinus, to help reduce traction and promote healing of Achilles tendonitis, Achilles rupture, or Achilles repair, and, when used with a scaphoid pad, to help reduce pain in plantar fasciitis. A heel elevation or a combination external elevation of the heel and sole can be used to compensate for a leg-length discrepancy of more than 1 cm (½ inch). A leg-length discrepancy of less than 1 cm is usually left uncorrected to aid the swing phase.

*b. **External sole modifications***

I. **Rocker bar** (Fig. 4.3-3.E, L) is a convex rigid strip placed across the sole just posterior to the metatarsal heads. It assists rollover by shifting the rollover point posterior to the metatarsal heads. It also relieves pressure from the metatarsal heads by transferring load to the metatarsal shafts, e.g., to manage ulcers over the metatarsal head in diabetic patients with peripheral vascular disease. It also decreases demand on the plantar flexors.

II. **Metatarsal bar** (Fig. 4.3-3.K) is a flat strip of leather placed across the sole just posterior to the metatarsal heads. It relieves pressure from the metatarsal heads by transferring load to the metatarsal shaft during late stance, for example in metatarsalgia. Because of its flat surface, it does not assist with rollover.

III. **Sole wedge** (Fig. 4.3-3.H) alters mediolateral metatarsal alignment. A lateral wedge tends to pronate the forefoot, while a medial wedge promotes forefoot supination. Sole wedge can be combined with an external heel wedge (described in section I.A.1.a.3).

IV. **Sole flare** (Fig. 4.3-3.I) increases stability. A medial flare resists eversion, while a lateral flare resists inversion of the foot.

V. **Steel bar** (Fig. 4.3-3.J) is inserted between inner and outer soles to prevent motion of the anterior sole and thus reduce stress at the phalanges and metatarsals, particularly in the presence of metatarsal fracture. It is commonly used with the rocker bar to assist rollover.

2. **Internal shoe modifications** (Fig. 4.3-4) are inconspicuous. However, they reduce shoe volume, requiring adequate space for comfortable fit.

*a. **Internal heel modifications***

I. **Heel excavation** or **heel cushion-relief** (Fig. 4.3-4.A) is a soft pad with an excavation under the painful part of the heel (e.g., a calcaneal spur). The excavation is usually filled with a compressible material (e.g., soft Plastazote).

II. **Internal heel wedge** can be applied medially (Fig. 4.3-4.B) to rotate the hindfoot into inversion (e.g., in flexible pes valgus) or laterally (Fig. 4.3-4.C)

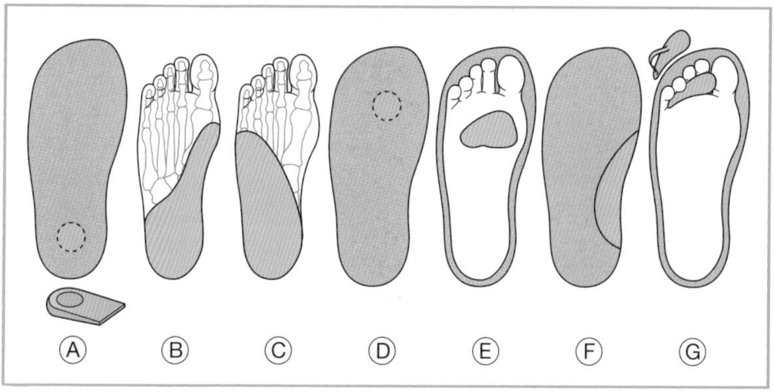

Figure 4.3-4 Types of internal heel and sole modification (see text for description). **A**, Heel excavation. **B**, Medial internal heel wedge. **C**, Lateral internal heel wedge (extended to fifth metatarsal head). **D**, Inner sole excavation. **E**, Metatarsal pad. **F**, Scaphoid pad (navicular pad, cookie insole). **G**, Toe crest.

to evert the hindfoot and relieve pressure on the cuboid (e.g., in flexible pes varus). It also increases the bearing area and can be used in fixed pes varus.

b. ***Internal sole modifications***

I. **Inner sole excavation** (Fig. 4.3-4.D) is a soft pad with an excavation under one or more painful metatarsal heads. The excavation is usually filled with compressible material.

II. **Metatarsal pad** (Fig. 4.3-4.E) is a domed pad glued to the inner sole with its apex under the metatarsal shafts. It reduces stress on the metatarsal heads by transferring load to the metatarsal shafts, for example in metatarsalgia.

III. **Scaphoid pad (navicular pad; cookie)** (see Fig. 4.3-4.F) is a rubber, cork, or plastic foam wedge used to provide medial longitudinal arch support to prevent depression of the subtalar joint. The pad extends from a point 1 cm (½ inch) posterior to the first metatarsal head to the anterior tubercle of the calcaneus. Its apex is between the talonavicular joint and the navicular tuberosity. A semi-rigid scaphoid pad can be used to realign flexible pes valgus. With a heel elevation, the pad can be used in plantar fasciitis to reduce tension on the plantar fascia. It can also be used in the presence of forefoot amputation to support the medial longitudinal arch.

IV. **Toe crest** (Fig. 4.3-4.G) is a crescent-shaped pad placed behind the second through fourth toes. It reduces the stress from the toes by filling the void under each proximal phalanx.

B. INSERTS (INLAYS; Fig. 4.3-5) are foot orthoses that are not glued to the shoe. They usually extend from the posterior border of the foot to a point just posterior to the metatarsal heads. Inserts are generally custom-molded and can be transferred from shoe to shoe. Like internal shoe modifications, inserts usually accommodate the abnormal foot to help restore lower-limb biomechanics.

1. **University of California Biomechanics Laboratory (UCBL) insert** (Fig. 4.3-5.A) is used to realign flexible flat foot (pes valgus), especially in runners. It is made of rigid plastic, custom-fabricated over a plaster mold of the foot held in maximum manual correction. It encompasses the heel and midfoot and has rigid medial, lateral, and posterior walls. It provides a very effective longitudinal arch support.

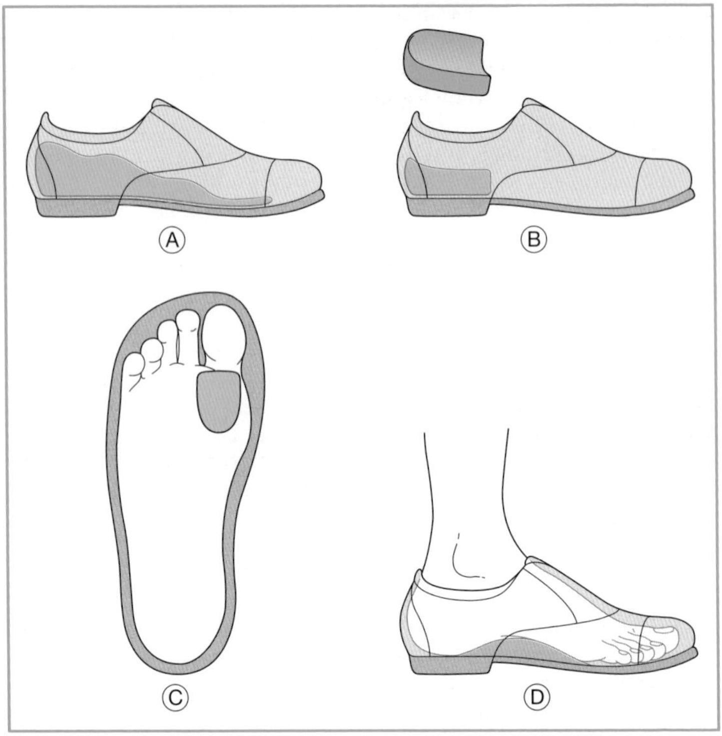

Figure 4.3-5 Types of inserts or inlays (see text for description). **A**, UCBL (University of California Biomechanics Laboratory) insert. **B**, Heel cup. **C**, Sesamoid insert. **D**, Medial longitudinal arch insert.

2. **Heel cup** (Fig. 4.3-5.B) is a prefabricated rigid plastic insert that covers the plantar surface of the heel and extends posteriorly, medially, and laterally up the sides of the heel. It is designed to prevent lateral calcaneal shift (calcaneal valgus) in the flexible flat foot. It can also relieve calcaneal spur.
3. **Sesamoid insert** (Fig. 4.3-5.C) is a three-quarter-length insert with an extension under the hallux to transfer pressure off the first metatarsal head and onto its shaft.
4. **Longitudinal arch insert** can be applied medially (see Fig. 4.3-5.D) to support the medial longitudinal arch or laterally to support the lateral longitudinal arch.

C. **ANKLE–FOOT ORTHOSES (AFOs)** (formerly called **short leg braces** or **below-knee orthoses**) encompass the foot and terminate below the knee. They consist of a foundation (i.e., a shoe and an insert foot plate or a steel stirrup riveted to the shoe), an ankle control component (with the joint usually centered over the tip of the medial malleolus) to assist in dorsiflexion or limit dorsiflexion and plantar flexion, a foot control component to restrict mediolateral motion, and a superstructure including the plastic shell or metal uprights and the proximal band. AFOs are usually prescribed to improve gait and ensure safe ambulation in patients with weak or paralyzed ankle dorsiflexors, plantar flexors, invertors, and/or evertors. They can also be used to prevent or correct deformities, reduce hypertonicity, as well as to stabilize and reduce weight bearing in the foot and ankle. The position of the ankle affects the stability of the knee. When the ankle is plantar flexed, a knee extension moment is created. Conversely, positioning the ankle in dorsiflexion provides a knee flexion force, which can help control genu recurvatum.

AFOs have been shown to reduce the energy cost of ambulation in patients with spastic diplegia (cerebral palsy), lower motor neuron weakness (poliomyelitis), and spastic hemiplegia (stroke). In patients with hemiplegia, AFOs reduce energy expenditure and increase the speed of ambulation. Whether wearing AFOs improves the ability of these patients to ascend and descend stairs remains controversial. Some studies show that metal and plastic AFOs have similar efficiency, but other studies show that plastic spiral and hemispiral AFOs are slightly more efficient than metal AFOs (e.g., for foot drop as a result of lower motor neuron lesion). Other conditions in which AFOs may be recommended are peripheral neuropathy (especially peroneal neuropathy), lumbar radiculopathy, multiple sclerosis, and traumatic brain injury. Guidelines for AFO prescription are shown in Table 4.3-2.

1. **Thermoplastic AFOs** (Fig. 4.3-6.A to H) consist of three sections: a shoe insert, a calf shell, and a proximal calf strap. They are available mass produced or can be custom fitted. Their rigidity depends on the thickness and composition of the plastic and also on the trimlines and shape. They are worn inside the shoe. They are contraindicated in the presence of fluctuating edema or inadequate hip and knee strength.

a. ***Posterior leaf spring*** (Fig. 4.3-6.A) is the most common AFO. It has a narrow calf shell and a narrow ankle with the trimline behind the malleoli. During early stance, the narrow junction between the calf shell and shoe insert bends backward slightly. As the patient enters into the swing phase, the plastic recoils to lift the foot into the neutral position. The posterior leaf spring resists plantar flexion at heel strike and during swing phase (thus preventing foot slapping and toe dragging respectively). Because of its low ankle trimline, it provides minimal mediolateral control. It is indicated for weakness of ankle dorsiflexors, and for moderate to severe spasticity. It is inappropriate for weak plantar flexors.

b. ***Solid AFO*** (Fig. 4.3-6.C) has a wider calf shelf with trimlines in the ankle area extending anterior to the malleoli. It holds the foot in a predetermined position, prevents dorsiflexion and plantar flexion, and resists any varus or valgus deviation of the hindfoot and ankle. It is indicated in structural collapse of foot–ankle, pain because of ankle movement, and severe spasticity with sustained clonus. A solid AFO (Fig. 4.3-6.E) is used to provide maximum mediolateral stability. The anterior band (Fig. 4.3-6.F) is used to prevent knee buckling during the early stance phase. It should not be used if there is significant ankle movement. Modifications are the semi-solid AFO (Fig. 4.3-6.B), which covers part of the malleoli and provides less mediolateral support than the solid AFO, and the hinged solid AFO (Fig. 4.3-6.E; described below).

c. ***AFO with flange*** (Fig. 4.3-6.D) has an extension (flange) that projects from the calf shell medially for maximum valgus control and laterally for maximum varus control of the foot and ankle.

d. ***Hinged AFOs*** (Fig. 4.3-6.E, F) have a pair of ankle hinges, most of which can be set to the desired range of dorsi- or plantar flexion.

e. ***Spiral AFO*** (Fig. 4.3-6.G) is a design in which the single upright spirals from the medial aspect of the shoe insert, passes diagonally around the leg posteriorly, then passes anteriorly to terminate proximomedially where the calf band is attached. This design allows limited rotation in the transverse plane while controlling dorsiflexion/plantar flexion and eversion/inversion. Spiral AFOs are indicated in the presence of weak ankle dorsiflexors or plantar flexors with moderate mediolateral instability and mild weakness of the knee extensors.

Table 4.3-2 Guidelines for prescription of ankle–foot orthoses (AFOs)

Patient group	Suggested AFOs
GROUP I	
• Weakness/absence of dorsiflexors without severe plantar flexor weakness • Good mediolateral stability during stance • Passive ankle dorsiflexion to 90° • Absent to moderate spasticity • Adequate knee stability and strength • Adequate hip strength • Reduced position sense at the ankle	1. Posterior leaf spring AFO 2. Double metal upright AFO with dorsiflexion assist (and plantar flexion assist if needed) 3. Shoe clasp (VAPC) or wire spring AFO
GROUP II	
• Weakness/absence of dorsiflexors and plantar flexors • Tendency to varus/valgus in stance or mediolateral instability in swing • Absent to moderate spasticity • Adequate knee and hip strength (but may be less than in Group I) • Reduced position sense at ankle	1. Double metal upright AFO with dorsiflexion stop at 90° (in the absence of plantar flexors the ankle tends to hyperdorsiflex, creating a knee flexion moment, dorsiflexion must be stopped at 90° to prevent knee buckling). For increased mediolateral stability, the uprights can be attached to an insert molded to realign the foot, or a T-strap can be used 2. Spiral AFO prevents foot drop, resists dorsiflexion during stance (thus assisting push-off) to provide a knee extension moment. It also counteracts a valgus tendency because the spiral starts on the medial side of the foot 3. Hemispiral AFO will counteract a varus tendency as the spiral starts on the lateral side
GROUP III	
• Weak/absent dorsiflexors and plantar flexors • Severe spasticity with equinovarus in swing and stance • Knee and hip strength adequate for weight bearing • Severe position sensory loss associated with spasticity (may be adequate criteria even without weakness) • Pain on ankle movement (may be single criterion)	1. Solid ankle AFO 2. Double upright metal AFO with no ankle movement and correction strap or shoe insert

Tabulated from: Sarno, JE: Below knee orthoses: A system for prescription. Arch Phys Med Rehabil *54:548–552,1973, with permission of WB Saunders Company.*

Spiral AFOs are contraindicated in pronounced imbalance of forces acting on the ankle–foot complex, moderate to severe spasticity, severe mediolateral ankle instability, and fixed ankle deformity.

f. ***Hemispiral AFO*** (Fig. 4.3-6.H) is a design in which the upright starts on the lateral side of the shoe insert and passes diagonally up the posterior leg, terminating proximomedially where the calf band is attached. It makes only half a turn around the leg (whereas the spiral AFO makes a full turn) and provides better

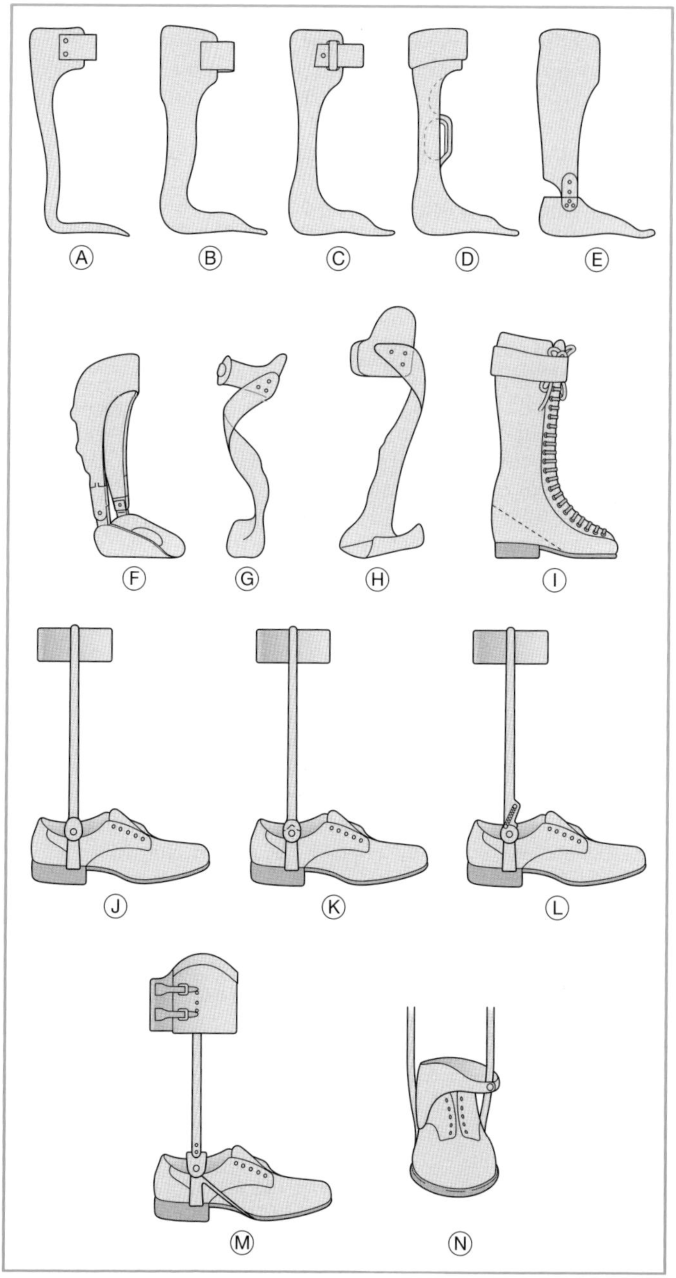

Figure 4.3-6 Types of plastic (**A** to **H**) ankle–foot orthoses (AFOs) and metal (**J** to **O**) AFOs (see text for description). **A**, Posterior leaf spring. **B**, Semi-solid ankle foot orthoses. **C**, Solid AFO. **D**, Solid AFO with flange. **E**, Solid AFO with adjustable hinge. **F**, AFO with adjustable hinge and anterior band. **G**, Spiral AFO. **H**, Hemispiral AFO. **I**, Vannini–Rizzoli stabilizing boot. **J**, AFO with free-motion ankle joint. **K**, AFO with limited motion ankle-joint stop. **L**, AFO with dorsiflexion-assist ankle joint (Klenzak joint). **M**, AFO with weight-relieving brim. **N**, T-strap for varus correction.

control of equinovarus than does the spiral design. It is indicated in weakness of ankle dorsiflexors and evertors with moderate to severe lateral instability or a strong tendency toward equinovarus, internal rotation of the foot, and moderate spasticity. It is contraindicated in severe spasticity with sustained clonus, valgus, and fixed ankle deformity.

g. ***Tone-reducing AFO*** is an orthosis with a broad foot plate to support the foot, extending distally to the toes and over the foot medially and laterally to maintain subtalar alignment. It is designed to inhibit spasticity by maintaining the neutral foot position and hyperextending the toes. It has pads that apply constant pressure to the plantar flexors and invertors. Tone-reducing AFOs are indicated for patients with moderate spasticity (e.g., spastic hemiplegia) with varus instability but whose deformity is not fixed.

2. **Metal–plastic and metal–leather AFOs** (Fig. 4.3-6.J to O) usually consist of two metal uprights (medial and lateral) connected proximally to a calf band (made of plastic or leather-covered metal) and distally to the ankle-joint mechanism, which is anchored to the shoe or foot attachment. The calf band, which provides a reaction point for force application, must be sufficiently wide to distribute forces without exceeding tissue tolerance. A calf band and a plantar flexion stop ankle joint can be used to control knee hyperextension in genu recurvatum. The calf band provides anteriorly directed force on the knee during early stance, while the plantar flexion stop promotes knee flexion during stance phase. Most AFOs have two uprights; however, some have only a posterior upright (e.g., Veterans Administration Prosthetics Center design) or a single medial or lateral upright. In mild dorsiflexor weakness, a single upright may be adequate. The metal uprights are attached to a sturdy shoe by means of a steel stirrup or a caliper (a round tube placed in the shoe heel to allow easy interchangeability of shoes). An alternative is to attach the stirrups to a molded insert, which is fitted into the shoe. The mechanical ankle joints prevent mediolateral instability and either control or assist dorsiflexion or limit plantar flexion by means of stops or assists (springs). The following are variations in the ankle joint and weight-bearing brim of metal–plastic and metal–leather AFOs:

a. ***Free-motion ankle joint*** (Fig. 4.3-6.J) is a stirrup or caliper that does not restrict ankle motion and provides only mediolateral control.

b. ***Ankle-joint stops*** are used to limit motion. They can be used in Achilles tendinitis to limit mediolateral foot motion and prevent instability caused by painful tendinitis. They are also prescribed with a shoe with a rocker-bar sole for patients with plantar flexor paralysis.

   I. **Plantar flexion (posterior) ankle-joint stop** has a posterior angulation at the top of the stirrup or caliper that restricts plantar flexion but allows unlimited dorsiflexion and affects the knee by promoting knee flexion during early stance. It is used for patients with weak dorsiflexors (foot drop) and flexible pes equinus.

   II. **Dorsiflexion (anterior) ankle-joint stop** has an anterior angulation at the top of the stirrup or caliper that restricts dorsiflexion but allows full plantar flexion and affects the knee by promoting knee extension during early stance. It is used by patients with weak plantar flexors to improve late stance.

   III. **Limited-motion ankle-joint stop** (Fig. 4.3-6.K) has anterior and posterior angulations at the top of the stirrup or caliper that limit dorsiflexion and plantar flexion respectively. The angulation of the cut determines the amount of motion. It is recommended in the presence of ankle weakness.

c. ***Ankle-joint assists*** use springs, spring wire, or resilient uprights to assist ankle motion. During the swing phase, dorsiflexion assists prevent toe drag. Dorsiflexion assists are used by patients with flexible pes equinus and weak dorsiflexors. They are contraindicated in patients with severe spasticity or joint instability.

I. **Dorsiflexion-assist spring joint** (**Klenzak joint**; Fig. 4.3-6.L) uses a coil spring located posteriorly that is compressed following heel strike when the spring yields slightly to permit plantar flexion and help prevent inadvertent knee flexion. During the swing phase, the spring rebounds to aid dorsiflexion.

II. **Spring-wire dorsiflexion-assist joint** uses light, flexible, easily adjustable spring-wire uprights attached to the shoe. Because of its flexibility, it does not provide any mediolateral stability.

III. **Veterans Administration Prosthetics Center (VAPC) clasp orthosis** provides dorsiflexion assist by means of a single, resilient, posterior metal upright that clamps onto the shoe counter.

IV. **Bichannel adjustable ankle lock (BICAAL) joint** has posterior and anterior receptacles with springs that can be adjusted to the desired angle. The springs can be replaced by pins to alter the alignment of the joint and thus convert it into adjustable stops.

d. ***Weight-relieving brim*** (Fig. 4.3-6.M) is used to reduce load on the leg and foot for patients requiring limited weight bearing.

e. ***Varus or valgus correction straps (T-straps)*** are leather straps that prevent the foot from deviating in the frontal plane within the shoe. If greater forces are required to correct the varus or valgus, a molded plastic insert with a rigid medial or lateral extension to which an ankle strap is attached can be used. Instead of using T-straps, a solid AFO is generally preferred for optimum varus or valgus control because it has broader area and is easier to don.

I. **T-strap for varus correction** (Fig. 4.3-6.N) attaches to the shoe laterally, encircles the ankle, and buckles on the outside of the medial upright to realign flexible pes varus.

II. **T-strap for valgus correction** attaches to the shoe medially, encircles the ankle, and buckles on the outside of the lateral upright to realign flexible pes valgus.

3. **Vannini–Rizzoli stabilizing boot** (Fig. 4.3-6.I) is an AFO with an inner rigid, calf shell continuous with a footplate angled at about 15° of plantar flexion, thus shifting the center of gravity anterior to the ankle and knee. It immobilizes the leg, ankle, and foot and stabilizes the knee in extension. It is used for patients with spinal cord injury (SCI) to achieve standing balance and ambulation. The patient shifts the center of gravity of the trunk and hips while using parallel bars, a walker, or crutches.

D. **KNEE–ANKLE–FOOT ORTHOSES (KAFO)** (formerly called **long leg brace** or **above-knee orthosis**) consist of an AFO with proximal extension on the thigh to control knee motion and alignment and to maintain knee stability for weight bearing in patients with paralysis or instability occurring at both the knee and the ankle. If weight bearing needs to be relieved at the knee or ankle, forces can be redistributed to as high as the ischial tuberosity and soft tissues of the proximal thigh. The KAFO can be used to stabilize or support the knee in quadriceps paralysis or weakness (e.g., KAFO with knee lock and anterior leg band); control flexible genu valgum or varum (e.g., KAFO with plastic calf shell extended proximally on the medial side for genu valgum control or on the lateral side for genu varum control); and limit weight bearing of thigh, leg, and foot [e.g., KAFO with quadrilateral brim on which patient can sit, with a locked knee, limited motion ankle joints, a patten-bottom (Fig. 4.3-10.D), and a contralateral shoe lift to equalize leg length]. In patients with hemiplegia or head trauma (with marked quadriceps weakness or hamstring spasticity), an AFO is preferred over a KAFO because KAFOs are difficult to don and doff and hamper functional ambulation. To control genu recurvatum, an AFO (with the ankle positioned in dorsiflexion) or a knee orthosis (e.g., Swedish knee cage) is preferred over a KAFO. The orthotic knee joint of a KAFO is usually centered slightly above the medial femoral condyle.

1. Metal–leather and metal–plastic KAFO

a. Double-upright metal KAFO (Fig. 4.3-7.A) has components similar to those of the AFO with the addition of two metal uprights connected to a pair of

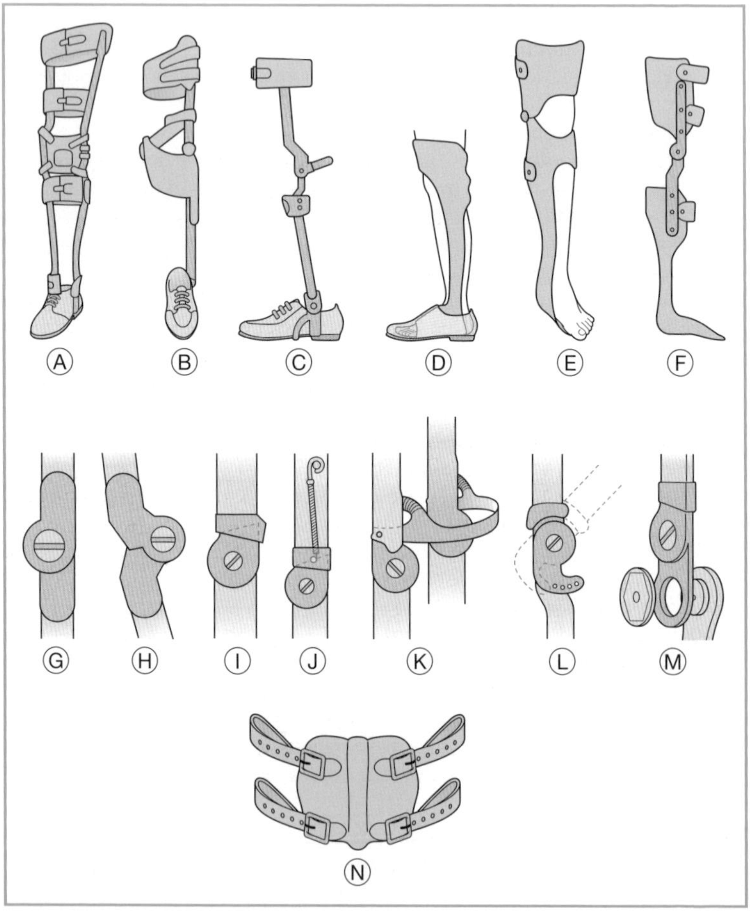

Figure 4.3-7 Types of knee–ankle–foot orthoses (KAFOs) (**A** to **F**) and KAFO locks (**G** to **M**) (see text for description). **A**, Metal KAFO with two uprights and two thigh bands (the distal components are similar to those of AFOs). **B**, Single lateral upright metal orthosis. **C**, Scott–Craig orthosis (double uprights, knee joint with pawl locks and bail control, one posterior thigh band, a hinged pretibial band, an ankle joint with anterior and posterior adjustable pin stops, a cushion heel, and a T-shaped foot plate). **D**, Supracondylar plastic KAFO. **E**, Supracondylar KAFO with conventional metal knee joints and uprights. **F**, KAFO with plastic thigh shell and metal upright. **G**, Free-motion knee joint. **H**, Offset knee joint. **I**, Drop-ring lock. **J**, Spring-loaded pull rod. **K**, Pawl lock. **L**, Adjustable fan lock. **M**, Serrated adjustable knee joint. **N**, Knee cap. (Adapted from New York University Prosthetics and Orthotics Staff: *Lower-limb orthotics*, New York, 1993, Prosthetic-Orthotic Publications, pp. 140–144, with permission.)

mechanical knee joints. The uprights extend up the thigh and are encompassed by two thigh bands. A knee cap (corrective or anterior pads and straps; Fig. 4.3-7.N) may be placed in front of the knee to prevent knee flexion within the KAFO. For genu varum or valgum, the knee cap may include a lateral or medial strap respectively (these buckle around the opposite upright).

The mechanical knee joint may either be single-axis or polycentric. Because most patients needing KAFOs require knee stabilization (rather than increased knee mobility), a single-axis knee joint is used more commonly. Polycentric knee joints follow the natural motion of the knee joint more accurately and are indicated if knee motion is required during walking and the anatomic knee is very unstable. The following are common types of single-axis knee joints:

I. **Free-motion knee joint** (Fig. 4.3-7.G) has unlimited flexion and usually has a stop to prevent hyperextension. It is indicated for patients with a tendency toward genu recurvatum and mediolateral instability but with enough strength to control the knee during weight bearing and ambulation.

II. **Offset knee joint** (Fig. 4.3-7.H) is a hinge with its pivot placed posterior to the anatomic knee axis so that the patient's weight line falls anterior to the offset joint, thus stabilizing the knee during early stance on level surfaces. It allows the knee to flex freely during the swing phase and also allows sitting without the need to manipulate a lock. It should not be used by patients with knee or hip flexion contracture, or with a plantar flexion stop at the ankle. The patient must be careful when ascending a steep ramp as the knee may flex inadvertently.

III. **Locked knee joints** are used to prevent knee flexion during standing and walking. To lock the knee joint, the patient must fully extend the knee, either passively or actively. Hence, locking joints are contraindicated in patients with knee contracture who must use an adjustable knee lock instead. Although locked knee joints provide maximal knee stability, the gait is awkward because of lack of knee flexion.

- **Drop-ring lock** (Fig. 4.3-7.I) consists of a ring that can be dropped over the knee joint (by gravity or with manual assistance) while the proximal and distal uprights are fully extended, thus preventing the uprights from bending. For a KAFO with bilateral uprights, both medial and lateral joints should be locked for greatest stability. A spring-loaded retention button allows the patient or therapist to unlock one upright, then attend to the other one without having the first lock drop. The retention button also prevents inadvertent locking of knee joint in patients who can walk with an unlocked knee but wish to lock the knee joint occasionally. As the patient sits, the retention button can be used to unlock one knee so the person can grasp the chair with one hand for stability, and use the other hand to unlock the other upright. For a KAFO with unilateral lateral upright, a spring-loaded pull rod (Fig. 4.3-7.J) extending to mid-thigh may be added to the drop ring so the patient need not bend to unlock or lock the joint. The spring is used to drive the ring lock down and assist gravity in locking the knee. Drop rings are the most commonly used knee locks to control knee flexion.
- **Pawl lock with bail release** (Fig. 4.3-7.K) consists of a pair of projections (pawls) that fit into matching recesses when the knee is fully extended thus providing simultaneous locking of both uprights. It also has a semi-circular lever (bail) attached posteriorly, which easily unlocks both joints with an upward pull on the bail (either manually or by backing up to a chair). Either the pawls are spring-loaded or an elastic webbing strap is attached to the bail and calf band. The bail is bulky and can be accidentally released if it hits a rigid object.

IV. **Adjustable knee joint** has a proximal component consisting of a drop-ring lock and a distal adjustable knee lock, which can be a fan lock (Fig. 4.3-7.L), a serrated disk (Fig. 4.3-7.M), a dial lock, or a ratchet (step-up) lock. The drop ring, which maintains the desired knee position in standing and walking, can be unlocked to permit full knee flexion when sitting. The adjustable knee joint permits locking in the selected degree of flexion. Adjustable knee joints are used to provide stability in patients with knee flexion contractures. They can also be used for those in whom improvement is anticipated with gradual stretching.

b. ***Single lateral-upright metal KAFO*** (Fig. 4.3-7.B) has a lateral upright only, with thigh and pretibial cuffs made of molded plastic or leather. All the other components are the same as in the double-upright metal KAFO.

c. ***Scott–Craig metal KAFOs*** (Fig. 4.3-7.C) are intended for adults with paraplegia. Each KAFO consists of bilateral uprights, a pawl lock with bail release, a posterior thigh band, and a hinged pretibial band. The distal component is either a plastic solid ankle or a bichannel adjustable ankle lock (BiCAAL) joint (with anterior and posterior adjustable pin stops), and a shoe with a cushion heel and embedded with a longitudinal and transverse (T-shaped) foot plate. The longitudinal plate extends from the heel to the metatarsal heads to provide a rigid platform, while the transverse plate located at the metatarsal head region provides mediolateral stability. The BiCAAL joint is set in about 10° dorsiflexion so the orthosis and patient's limb lean forward slightly. To attain standing balance without crutches, the patient hyperextends the hips to bring the line of gravity behind the hip joints, thus preventing untoward hip or trunk flexion. With the aid of crutches or a walker, the patient is able to ambulate with a swing-to or swing-through gait. Some patients use a two- or four-point gait by shifting the trunk laterally enough to allow the leg to swing forward in a pendular manner. Scott–Craig KAFOs provide orthotic stabilization of the knee, ankles, and foot, and ligamentous stabilization of the hip without recourse to orthotic components at or above the hip.

d. ***Webbing hip rotation control strap*** may be used with a pair of KAFOs if the patient requires control of hip rotation (e.g., toe-in gait). To reduce internal rotation, the patient wears a webbing waist belt to which a pair of straps are secured in the posterior center. Each strap is secured to a D-ring on the lateral upright. To reduce external rotation, a strap passes anteriorly at the groin and connects the uprights of the KAFOs.

2. **Plastic and plastic–metal KAFOs** use thermoplastic materials which are lighter, more cosmetically acceptable, and can be heated for better contour. Unlike leather, plastic does not absorb perspiration. Plastic and plastic–metal KAFOs are indicated for closer fit and more precise control of pressure and for maximum control of the foot, but retain heat in warm, humid weather.

a. ***Supracondylar plastic KAFO*** (Fig. 4.3-7.D) is a plastic orthosis extending from the foot to the lower thigh to resist hypertension force at the knee without hindering flexion and to provide mediolateral stability. In patients with knee extensor weakness, the ankle and foot component holds the ankle in slight plantar flexion, enough to produce a knee extension moment and eliminate the need for a mechanical knee lock. Its disadvantage is that when the patient sits, the suprapatellar portion protrudes. Also, it cannot be used bilaterally because positioning both ankles in plantar flexion would interfere with the patient's anteroposterior stability.

b. ***Supracondylar plastic–metal KAFO*** (Fig. 4.3-7.E) has the same function and design as the supracondylar plastic KAFO except that it has metal knee joints and uprights to allow the orthosis to flex while the patient is seated, thus decreasing protrusion above the knee.

c. ***Plastic shells and metal uprights KAFO*** (Fig. 4.3-7.F) are essentially a posterior leaf spring AFO with double metal uprights extending up to a plastic thigh shell with an intervening knee joint (see section I.D.1.a for different types of knee joints). The proximal contours of the thigh shells are usually quadrilateral in shape to help control rotation and may incorporate an ischial seat for weight bearing.

E. **KNEE ORTHOSES (KOs)** control the knee but not the foot and ankle. As with KAFOs, the orthotic knee joint is usually centered slightly above the medial femoral condyle.

1. **Knee orthoses for patellofemoral disorders** control tracking of the patella as the knee flexes and extends.

a. ***Infrapatellar (Cho-Pat®) strap KO*** (Fig. 4.3-8.A) is a foam-padded strap that encircles the knee immediately below the patella. It is worn during periods of vigorous activity.

b. ***Palumbo KO®*** (Fig. 4.3-8.B) is an elastic sleeve with a patellar cutout, two circumferential rubber straps that apply tension to a crescent-shaped patellar pad (placed laterally), and an elastic counterforce strap, which maintains the position of the pad and prevents axial rotation of the orthosis. It applies medially directed force to the lateral border of the patella and maintains constant pressure during flexion, extension, and rotation of the knee.

2. **Knee orthoses for control in the sagittal plane** control genu recurvatum with minimal mediolateral stabilization. They allow almost complete knee flexion.

a. ***Swedish knee cage*** (Fig. 4.3-8.C) is a prefabricated brace which restricts hyperextension with two anterior straps and one posterior strap held in position by a metal frame medially and laterally. It tends to protrude when the patient sits.

b. ***Three-way knee stabilizer*** (Fig. 4.3-8.D) is similar to the Swedish knee cage, but it has pivotable attachments of the straps, which do not protrude as much in sitting. It has lateral and medial uprights, which provide limited mediolateral stability.

3. **Knee orthoses for control in the frontal plane** consist of thigh and calf cuffs joined by bilateral side bars with mechanical knee joints. In addition to protecting the knee against mediolateral forces (using a pair of three-point force systems), they also provide flexion–extension control by including a hyperextension stop in the mechanical knee joints or by adding a drop lock. The knee joint is usually polycentric to closely approximate anatomic knee motion and contribute better stabilization of the orthosis on the patient's limb.

a. ***Metal–leather KO*** (Fig. 4.3-8.E) has leather thigh and calf cuffs and metal side bars. A pressure pad may be used to apply medial or lateral force to the knee, for genu valgum or genu varum respectively.

b. ***Miami KO®*** has side bars and polycentric joints incorporated into polypropylene calf and thigh shells which cover the anterior limb. A wedge over the medial femoral condyle prevents downward slippage.

c. ***Canadian Arthritis and Rheumatism Society–University of British Columbia (CARS-UBC) KO®*** (Fig. 4.3-8.F) consists of calf and thigh plastic cuffs connected by a telescoping rod, which permits knee flexion. For genu varum, the rod is placed medially with a lateral pad; while for genu valgum, the rod is placed laterally with a medial pad. The three-point pressure system resists varus/valgus forces when the knee is fully extended. It is difficult to don, interferes with clothing, and controls axial rotation minimally.

d. ***Supracondylar KO*** (Fig. 4.3-8.G) is similar to a supracondylar KAFO (section I.D.2.a.) except that it does have an ankle or foot extension (hence it cannot hold the ankle in plantar flexion position to produce a knee extension moment during stance in patients with knee extensor weakness). It controls genu recurvatum

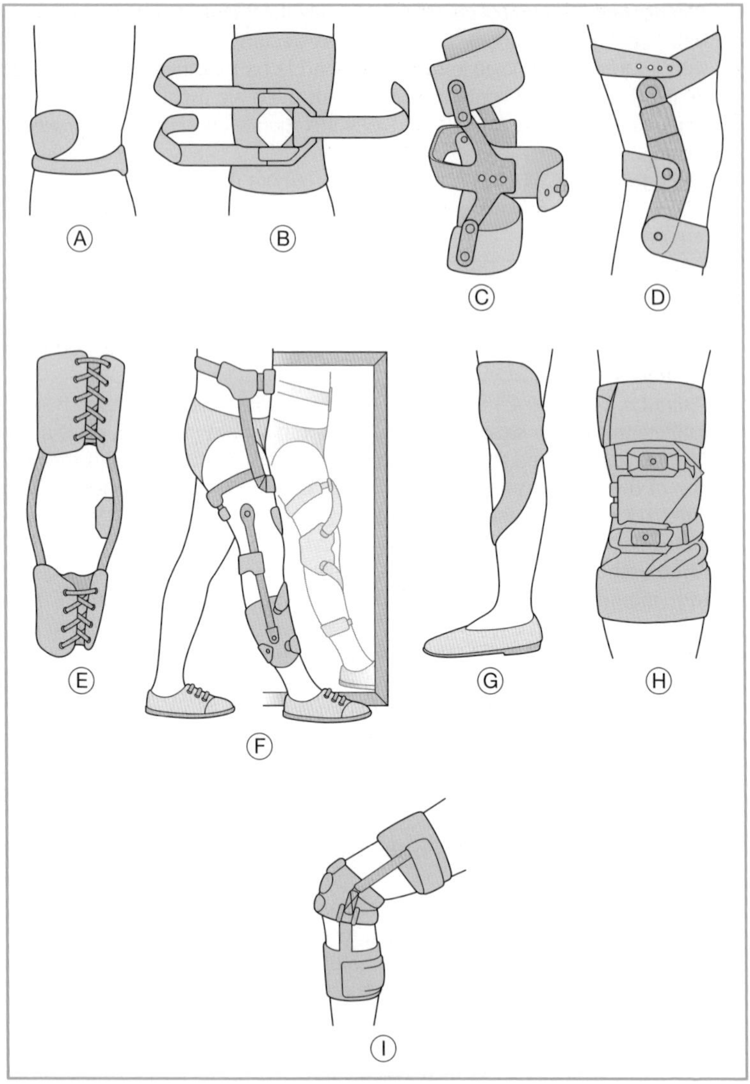

Figure 4.3-8 Types of knee orthoses (KO) (see text for description). **A**, Infrapatellar strap KO. **B**, Palumbo KO. **C**, Swedish knee cage. **D**, Three-way knee stabilizer. **E**, Traditional metal–leather KO with leather thigh and calf cuffs and metal side bars. **F**, Canadian Arthritis and Rheumatism Society–University of British Columbia (CARS-UBC) KO with knee stabilization against genu valgum. **G**, Supracondylar KO. **H**, Lenox–Hill derotation orthosis. **I**, Lerman multiligamentous knee control orthosis. (Adapted from New York University Prosthetics and Orthotics Staff: *Lower-limb orthotics*, New York, 1993, Prosthetic-Orthotic Publications, pp. 150–154, with permission.)

and provides mediolateral knee stabilization. The suprapatellar portion protrudes when the patient is seated.

4. **KO for axial rotation control** also provides angular control in the sagittal (flexion–extension) and frontal (mediolateral) planes. It is used to prevent and

manage sports injuries of the knee, especially in patients with anterior cruciate ligament injury.

a. ***Lenox–Hill derotation orthosis®*** (Fig. 4.3-8.H) uses cuffs or elastic straps that encircle the thigh and leg and oblique bands.

b. ***Lerman multiligamentous knee control orthosis®*** (Fig. 4.3-8.I) is similar to the Lenox–Hill derotation orthosis with the addition of supracondylar pads for additional control of patellar tracking.

F. **HIP–KNEE–ANKLE–FOOT ORTHOSIS (HKAFO)** consists of a pair of KAFOs with the addition of a pelvic band and bilateral hip joints. It is used to reduce gait deviation caused by faulty control of hip abduction, adduction, and rotation (e.g., in paraplegia caused by spina bifida or SCI). It is much more difficult to don than a pair of KAFOs. If the hip joints are locked, the orthosis restricts gait to the swing-to or swing-through pattern. Each orthotic hip joint is positioned slightly above and anterior to the greater trochanter so that the patient can sit upright at 90°.

1. **Pelvic band** surrounds the lower trunk and attaches to the upper part of the hip joint. It is likely to be uncomfortable when the patient sits.

a. ***Bilateral pelvic band*** is more commonly used than a unilateral pelvic band because most conditions requiring a HKAFO have bilateral involvement. It is made of upholstered metal, which curves posteriorly and downward to contact the most prominent portion of each buttock and continues slightly upward to overlie the sacrum. Its ends are located just anterior to the lateral midlines of the pelvis and are connected by a flexible belt.

b. ***Pelvic girdle*** made of molded thermoplastic provides maximum control in patients with bilateral involvement. It is similar to the pelvic part of the molded plastic thoracolumbosacral orthosis used for scoliosis.

c. ***Silesian belt or band*** attaches to the proximal end of the lateral upright and encircles the pelvis. It has no metal joint or rigid band and cannot control motion in the sagittal plane. It offers mild resistance to abduction and rotational forces at the hip. It is rarely used.

2. **Hip joints and locks** consist of metal hinges that connect the lateral uprights of each KAFO to the pelvic band. The hip joints also prevent abduction and adduction, as well as hip rotation.

a. ***Single-axis hip joint with lock*** is most commonly used. It permits flexion and extension and may include an adjustable stop to limit hyperextension. The flexion–extension range can be restricted by a pawl or drop-ring lock similar to that used at the knee joint. The drop-ring lock is useful if hip flexion control is needed, especially in patients with a crouched gait.

b. ***Two-position lock hip joint*** can be locked at full hip extension (for standing and walking) and at 90° of flexion (for sitting). It is indicated in patients whose hip spasticity causes difficulty in maintaining a seated position.

c. ***Double axis (flexion–abduction) hip joint*** has a flexion–extension axis, which may be locked or unlocked, and an abduction–adduction axis, which includes adjustable stops to place limits on these motions as needed.

G. **TRUNK–HIP–KNEE–ANKLE–FOOT ORTHOSES (THKAFO)** incorporate a spinal orthosis attached to a HKAFO to control trunk motion, maintain or modify spinal alignment, and reduce loads on the spine by elevating intra-abdominal pressure. The pelvic band of the spinal orthosis serves as the pelvic band used on the spinal orthosis. It is indicated for paraplegic patients (e.g., because of SCI, poliomyelitis, spina bifida, or muscular dystrophy) but is seldom worn after discharge from the rehabilitation program because it is heavy, cumbersome, and very difficult to don. As with HKAFO, the orthotic knee joint is usually centered slightly above the medial femoral condyle; the orthotic hip joint is positioned so that the patient can sit upright at 90°.

Alternative designs of THKAFO available for paraplegic patients are as follows:

1. **Reciprocating gait orthosis (RGO)** (Fig. 4.3-9) is a THKAFO consisting of a pelvic girdle with a thoracic extension and bilateral hip joints which are connected by one or two metal cables or rods. Both knees are stabilized with knee locks, posteriorly offset knee joints, or pretibial bands and the feet are encased in solid ankle–foot orthoses. For walking, the hip joints can be locked at 180° or set to flex through a range of about 25°. As the patient extends one hip, the coupling mechanism induces hip flexion on the opposite leg or vice versa

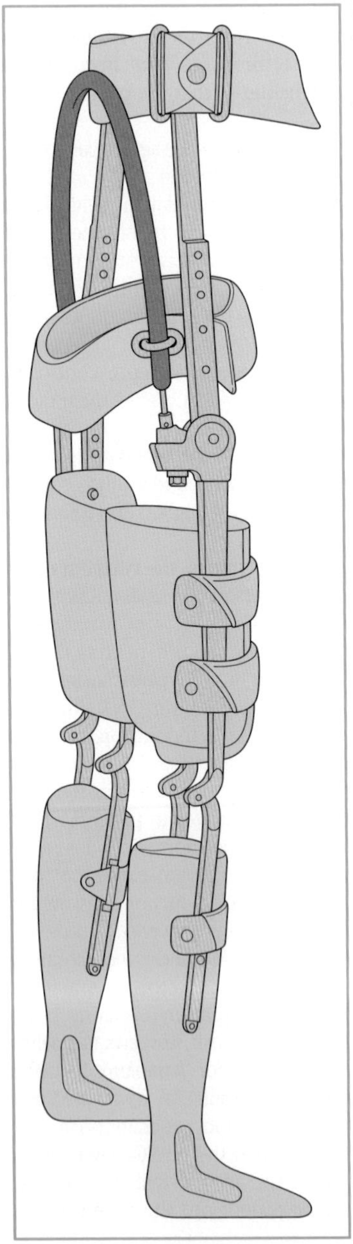

Figure 4.3-9 Reciprocal gait orthosis (RGO). (Redrawn from Lehmann JF: Lower limb orthotics. In Redford JB, editor: *Orthotics etcetera*, ed 3, Baltimore, 1986, Williams & Wilkins, p. 320.)

(i.e., hip extension on one side causes opposite hip flexion). This produces a reciprocal walking pattern not otherwise possible with standard KAFOs or HKAFOs. Using two crutches or a walker, the patient can slowly ambulate with a stable four-point gait with one foot always on the floor. For sitting, the cable can be released to enable both hips to flex. An RGO in combination with functional electrical stimulation can be used for greater aerobic training in paraplegic and possibly tetraplegic (C8) patients.

2. **Hip-guidance orthosis or HGO (Para Walker)** is a THKAFO consisting of ball-bearing hip joints, a shoulder orthosis, and shoes that fit into loops on flat foot plates. The sturdy hip joints guide hip motion in the sagittal plane by using stops that limit hip flexion. Hip extension may be free or may also be limited by a stop. Ambulation occurs through trunk motion transmitted to the lower limbs through the brace. As the patient shifts weight from side to side, the hip joints resist hip abduction and adduction and rotation. The gait maneuver is similar to that used with the RGO.
3. **Prefabricated pediatric THKAFOs,** which include standing frame, swivel base, and parapodium, are beyond the scope of this book.

H. HIP ORTHOSES (HOs) consist of a pair of hip joints and a pelvic band (described in I.F as part of HKAFOs) with the lower bar of the hip joint terminating on a thigh cuff. The thigh cuff may be extended to the medial femoral condyle to provide additional resistance to adduction as well as internal rotation. HOs are most commonly used to resist spastic hip adductors in patients with cerebral palsy. They may also be used after hip arthroplasty to prevent hip dislocation by limiting adduction and flexion of the hip joint (e.g., a postoperative hip-abduction orthosis). The orthotic hip joint is positioned so that the patient can sit upright at 90°.

I. SPECIAL-PURPOSE LOWER-LIMB ORTHOSES

1. **Weight-bearing orthoses** reduce or eliminate weight bearing through the lower limb. The skin and peripheral circulation on the weight-bearing area must be able to tolerate pressure.

a. ***Patellar-tendon-bearing (PTB) AFO*** (Fig. 4.3-10.A) has a proximal design similar to the socket used in a transtibial prosthesis (Chapter 4.4, section I.C.3.a). It supports weight on the patellar ligament and tibial flares with the load being transmitted to the shoe via metal uprights. It is indicated for unloading the mid- or distal tibia, ankle, or foot (e.g., healing os calcis fracture, postoperative ankle fusion, heel with refractory pain, delayed union or nonunion of fractures or fusion, avascular necrosis of the talar body, degenerative arthritis of the subtalar or ankle joint, osteomyelitis of os calcis, and diabetic ulceration). Because little or no ankle motion is allowed, a cushion heel and a rocker bottom are needed to provide smoother gait.

b. ***Ischial weight-bearing KAFO*** (Fig. 4.3-10.B) uses a quadrilateral brim (similar to the quadrilateral socket used in a transfemoral prosthesis; Chapter 4.4, section I.D.2.a) or an ischial (Thomas) ring (Fig. 4.3-10.C) to relieve weight from the femur, knee, or foot. The ischial ring is simpler to fabricate but is less comfortable and less effective in relieving weight because forces are distributed over a smaller area. A patten-bottom shoe (Fig. 4.3-10.D) is used.

c. ***Patten-bottom orthosis*** (Fig. 4.3-10.D) uses uprights (with no ankle joint) that terminate in a floor pad distal to the shoe so the shoe is freely suspended in midair. It is used in conjunction with an ischial weight-bearing orthosis so the weight is transmitted directly to the floor pad. A shoe lift on the opposite side is needed to equalize leg length.

2. **Fracture orthoses** stabilize the fracture site and help promote callus formation. They allow weight bearing and joint movement after an initial rest period when pain and edema subside. They also minimize joint stiffness and reduce

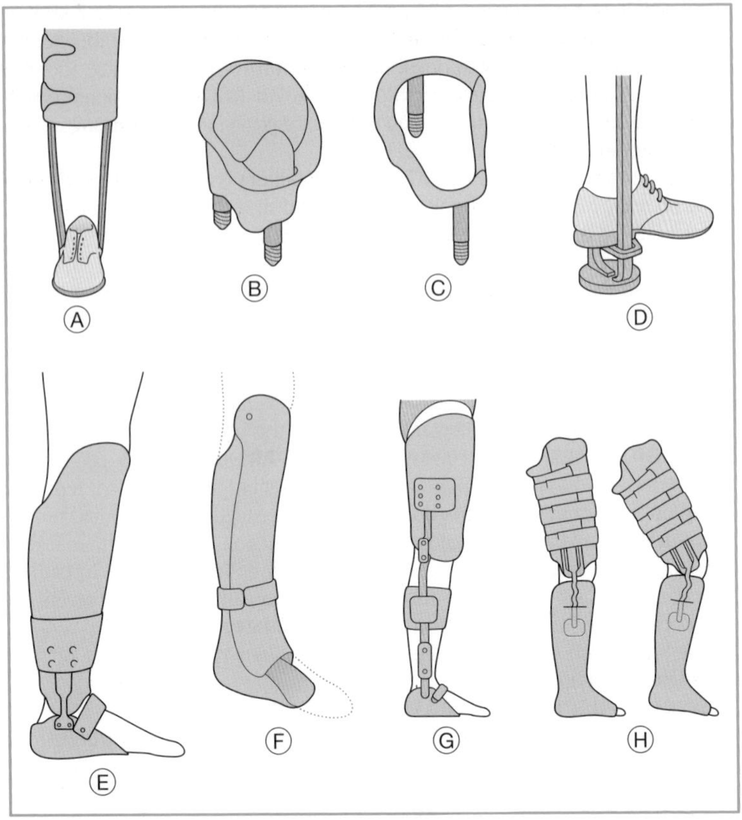

Figure 4.3-10 Types of weight-bearing and fracture lower-limb orthoses (see text for description). **A**, Patellar-tendon-bearing (PTB) orthosis. **B**, Ischial weight bearing orthosis. **C**, Ischial (Thomas) ring. **D**, Patten-bottom orthosis. **E**, Tibial fracture orthosis with plastic cable ankle joint. **F**, Tibial fracture orthosis with Velcro straps. **G**, Femoral fracture orthosis with polycentric metal knee joint. **H**, Femoral fracture orthosis with flexible plastic knee joint. (Adapted from New York University Prosthetics and Orthotics Staff: *Lower-limb orthotics,* New York, 1993, Prosthetic-Orthotic Publications, pp. 155–158, with permission.)

complications such as nonunions. Circumferential compression of the soft tissue can be used to prevent undue bony motion at the fracture site.

a. ***Tibial fracture orthosis*** (Fig. 4.3-10.F) consists of anterior and posterior thermoplastic shells fitted snugly over the leg with hook and pile straps (Velcro®) to ensure compression. Ankle motion is controlled by the distal trimlines, or an ankle joint may be included and may have a stop in either plantar flexion or dorsiflexion. It is used after the tibial and tibial–fibular fractures have been immobilized for about 4 weeks (2 weeks in a long leg cast followed by an additional 2 weeks in a below-knee cast). A design variation uses plastic cable ankle joints (Fig. 4.3-10.E) connected to a plastic heel insert to permit ankle and foot motion while preventing downward displacement of the orthosis. In a tibial plateau fracture, stability may be increased by using a plastic thigh section connected via polycentric knee joints to the distal segment.

b. ***Femoral fracture orthosis*** consists of a thermoplastic thigh and calf component connected via freely moving metal (Fig. 4.3-10.G) or plastic (Fig. 4.3-10.H) knee joints. The thigh component is quadrilateral (for rotational stability) with an ischial seat proximally and is similar to the quadrilateral prosthetic socket. The calf component is attached to the footplate by ankle joints. It is used in fractures of the middle or distal third of the femur when there is callus formation and relatively little pain, usually after immobilization for more than 4–6 weeks. It is contraindicated in proximal femoral fractures because of difficulty in controlling varus angulation.

3. **Pediatric orthoses** include those used for angular and rotational deformities of the leg or foot (e.g., Denis Browne splint, A-frame orthosis, torsion-shaft orthosis, and hip rotation control straps), those that hold the hips in flexion and abduction in congenital hip dislocations (e.g., Pavlik harness, Ilfeld splint, and Von Rosen splint), and those for maintaining the hip in abduction in Legg–Calvé–Perthes disease [e.g., Scottish Rite orthosis, trilateral socket hip abduction orthosis (Tachdjian), Toronto hip abduction orthosis or its variation, and the Newington ambulatory abduction orthosis]. They are, however, beyond the scope of this book.

II. Upper-limb orthoses

Orthoses for the upper limbs are generally used to restore upper-limb function by assisting or supporting weak muscles, substituting for paralyzed muscles, protecting painful or deformed parts, correcting (or minimizing) existing deformities, permitting controlled directional movement, and allowing attachment of assistive devices (e.g., utensil holders; see section II.A.1.c). The orthosis should be fitted so the patient can easily don and doff it and either rest the desired segment or perform the prescribed movement comfortably when wearing the orthosis. Also, the orthosis must be functionally as well as cosmetically acceptable to the patient. When removed, the skin should be unblemished 10 minutes afterwards. Some orthoses for common hand deformities because of neuropathy are shown in Table 4.3-3. Most wrist and hand orthoses can be held in place with a strap, while others need to be suspended from the torso for ambulatory patients (e.g., shoulder or arm slings described in section II.C.1.d) or suspended from the wheelchair for patients using a wheelchair (e.g., balanced forearm orthosis described in section II.C.3.b). Suspension systems commonly used include hoops, shoulder caps, and harnesses.

Traditionally, upper-limb orthoses are classified into *static* (i.e., rigid; gives support without allowing movement) and *dynamic* (also called *functional*; i.e., allows a certain degree of movement). Dynamic orthoses improve functions through the use of joints, levers, pulleys, and external power sources (including rubber bands, springs, and batteries). The traditional classification, however, can be confusing because static orthoses are often used to create movement, and dynamic splints may have components that restrict motion to create movement at another joint. Another way of classifying upper-limb orthoses is by the anatomical joint covered by the orthosis, for example FO (finger orthosis), TO (thumb orthosis), HFO (hand–finger orthosis), WHFO (wrist–hand–finger orthosis), WO (wrist orthosis), WHO (wrist–hand orthosis), EWHO (elbow–wrist–hand orthosis), EO (elbow orthosis), SEWHO (shoulder–elbow–wrist–hand orthosis), SEO (shoulder–elbow orthosis), and SO (shoulder orthosis). This anatomical classification, however, does not indicate function. The following classification, therefore, is used to combine both function and anatomy (based on the classification of upper-limb orthoses of the New York University Prosthetic and Orthotics Faculty published in Bunch WH, Keagy RD, Kritter AS, *et al.*: *American Academy of Orthopedic Surgeons (AAOS) atlas of orthotics: biomechanical principles and application*, ed 2, St Louis, 1985, Mosby-Year Book).

Orthoses

Table 4.3-3 Some upper-extremity (UE) orthoses for common hand deformities due to neuropathy

Nerve injury	Hand deformity	Suggested orthoses
Radial	Wrist drop and drop finger	• Volar wrist-flexion control orthoses (cock-up splint) • MCP extension mobilization orthoses • Wrist mobilization orthoses
Median (distal)	Ape hand*	• Opponens orthoses (C-bar) • Thumb post static orthoses • Dynamic thumb orthoses
Median (proximal)	Active papal sign†	• Buddy splints (taping the index and middle fingers together).
Median and ulnar	Clawhand (also called intrinsic minus hand‡)	• Opponens orthoses with MCP block (lumbrical bar) • MCP flexion mobilization orthoses
Ulnar	Ulnar clawing of the fourth and fifth digits (also called benediction hand or static papal sign)	• Opponens orthoses with MCP block (lumbrical bar) to fourth and fifth digits • MCP flexion mobilization orthoses

MCP, metacarpophalangeal; DIP, distal phalangeal joint.
** Wasting of the thenar eminence and loss of palmar abduction and opposition of the thumb.*
† Loss of DIP flexion of the index and middle fingers as a result of proximal median nerve lesion, thus the index finger remains extended when the patient makes a fist.
‡ Unopposed hyperextension at the MCP joints with secondary flexion at the IP joints as a result of loss of hand intrinsic muscles.

A. WRIST, HAND, AND FINGER ORTHOSES

1. **Assistive and substitutive orthoses** are primarily used to enhance hand function in patients with residual strength (i.e., using assistive orthoses) or no strength (i.e., using substitutive orthoses). They are usually worn throughout the day.

*a. **Positional orthoses***

I. **Opponens orthoses and their variations.** Opponens orthoses are primarily used to position the weak thumb in opposition to other fingers to improve hand function by facilitating three-jaw chuck pinch [e.g., in patients with median/ulnar neuropathy, Guillain–Barré syndrome (GBS); upper motor neuron lesions such as in SCI, stroke, traumatic brain injury (TBI), cerebral palsy]. They can also be used to immobilize the thumb to promote tissue healing [e.g., carpometacarpal (CMC) or metacarpophalangeal (MCP) arthritis/synovitis; late phase of fracture (e.g., scaphoid/thumb); dislocation, subluxation, or collateral ligament injury of the thumb (e.g., CMC/MCP collateral ligament injury or gamekeeper's thumb); cumulative trauma disorders (CTD), (e.g., deQuervain's tenosynovitis and thenar tendinitis); post-surgical thumb (e.g., open reduction internal fixation (ORIF), CMC/MCP fusion, arthroplasty, reconstruction, tendon transfer, tendon/ligament repair, nerve repair, and trapeziumectomy)]; to restrict thumb motion and protect it from harmful internal or external stresses during activities (e.g., arthritis, CTD, and in athletes and performing artists).

- **Basic opponens orthoses** (Fig. 4.3-11.A; also known as short opponens splints, C-bar splints, Engen opponens splints, Rancho opponens splints,

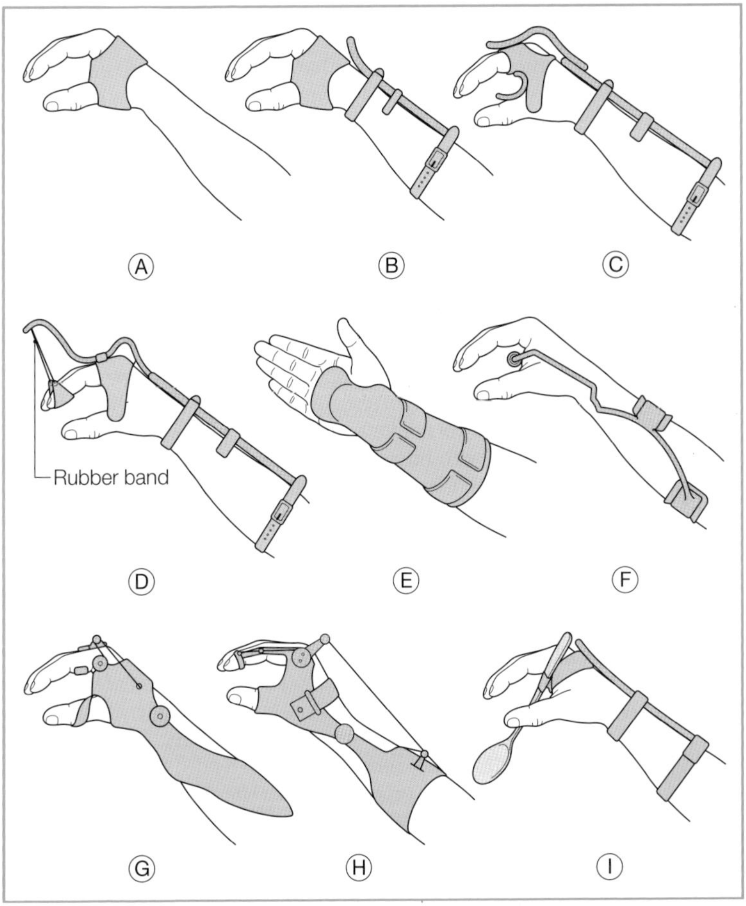

Figure 4.3-11 Assistive and substitutive wrist, hand, and finger orthoses (**A** to **F**, Positional orthoses; **G** to **I**, prehension orthoses). **A**, Basic or C-bar or short opponens orthoses. **B**, Opponens orthoses with wrist control attachments (long opponens orthoses). **C**, Opponens orthoses with lumbrical bar. **D**, Opponens orthoses with finger extension assist assembly (using rubber bands). **E**, Volar wrist-flexion control orthoses (cock-up splint). **F**, Wire wrist-extension assist orthoses (Oppenheimer splint). **G**, Finger-driven hand prehension orthoses. **H**, Wrist-driven prehension orthoses (tenodesis orthoses). **I**, Utensil holders (universal splints, activities of daily living splint).

cone splints, hand-based opponens splints, and static thumb splints) are HFOs that consist of a dorsal and a palmar bar that encircle the mid-palm, with a thumb abduction bar projecting from the palmar bar, and a thumb opponens bar on the first metacarpal.

- **Opponens orthoses with wrist control attachments** (Fig. 4.3-11.B; long opponens splints and thumb spica splints) are WHFOs that have a forearm bar and proximal and distal crossbars for wrist control. In addition to the benefits provided by the opponens orthoses (listed above), (a) the forearm bar maintains the wrist in extension (usually 20°), and prevents wrist dorsi- and volarflexion contractures and (b) the crossbars help prevent ulnar or radial deviation deformities (e.g., in rheumatoid arthritis and systemic lupus erythematosus).

- **Opponens orthoses with lumbrical bar** (Fig. 4.3-11.C; Opponens splints with MCP extension stop assembly, anticlaw splints, hand-based intrinsic-plus splints, clam diggers, and ulnar palsy splints) are HFOs that prevent MCP hyperextension but allow full MCP flexion. In addition to the benefits provided by the opponens orthoses (listed above), they (a) prevent claw-hand deformity (by preventing MCP hyperextension thus preventing proximal interphalangeal (PIP) flexion, which could lead to clawhand deformity) in patients with ulnar or combined median and ulnar neuropathy or in patients with some upper motor neuron lesions (e.g., stroke and TBI), (b) allow active extension of the PIP and distal interphalangeal (DIP) joints in patients with paralyzed or weak intrinsic hand function (e.g., brachial plexus lesion and GBS), and (c) immobilize the MCP to promote tissue healing and to reduce inflammation (e.g., in trigger finger, i.e., digital stenosing tenosynovitis of the flexor tendon).
- **Opponens orthoses with finger extension assist assembly** (Fig. 4.3-11.D) are HFOs that assist PIP and DIP extension [e.g., in patients with interphalangeal (IP) flexion contracture, boutonnière deformity, or postsurgical release of Dupuytren's contracture]. In addition, they also provide the benefits of the basic opponens orthosis (see above).
- **Opponens orthoses with thumb abduction–extension assist assembly** are HFOs that assist thumb extension and/or abduction, in addition to providing the benefits of the basic opponens orthosis.

II. **Wrist control orthoses** are used to promote slight extension of the wrist or to prevent wrist flexion, thus assisting weak grasp (i.e., via tenodesis effect).

- **Volar wrist-flexion control orthoses** (**cock-up splints**; Fig. 4.3-11.E) are plastic WHOs in which the palmar section is extended (usually 20°). They are used to tighten finger flexors (via tenodesis effect) and prevent wrist flexion contracture in patients with radial neuropathy.
- **Wire wrist-extension assist orthoses** (**Oppenheimer splints**; Fig. 4.3-11.F) are WHOs prefabricated from spring steel wire and padded steel bands to assist wrist extension by tensing the steel wire, thus aiding finger flexion through a tenodesis effect.

b. ***Prehension orthoses*** are used to stabilize the thumb, and index and middle fingers while substituting muscle strength from other parts of the body or from an external power source to provide grasping, holding, and releasing functions. They are used for patients with severe paralysis of the upper limb (e.g., SCI and poliomyelitis). The prehension pattern may be a three-jaw chuck or a lateral grasp.

I. **Hand prehension orthoses (or finger-driven hand prehension orthoses)** (Fig. 4.3-11.G) are HFOs that provide prehension through transmission of active flexion of the ring or little finger or both. Active MCP or IP flexion must be present in at least one finger of the hand.

II. **Wrist–hand prehension orthoses** can be classified as WHFOs.

- **Wrist-driven prehension orthoses** (Fig. 4.3-11.H; tenodesis orthoses; flexor hinge splints) are used by patients with C6 complete tetraplegia to provide prehension through tenodesis action and maintain flexibility of the hand and wrist. They may interfere with manual wheelchair propulsion. They are rarely accepted by patients with C7 and C8 tetraplegia who prefer to use their residual motor power or utensil holders.
- **Passive prehension orthoses** have the same design as the finger-driven WHO with the addition of a ratchet assembly (a notched ratchet bar, spring-operated lever, and push lever), thus converting it into a passively operated

orthosis to provide grasp. The term *passive* is used here to describe a mechanism that moves the stabilized fingers by gross motion of the opposite hand or by pushing a lever against a table or similar surface.

- **Electrically driven prehension orthoses**, using a cable, switch, motor, and battery, can be controlled by slight bodily movement (light pressure; often shoulder elevation). They are indicated for patients with tetraplegia (e.g., C5 and higher lesion).

c. ***Utensil holders*** (Fig. 4.3-11.I; universal splints; activities of daily living splints), consist of a handcuff with a palmar pocket into which various utensils can be inserted (see Chapter 4.5, section II.A.3.a.6). Most people with tetraplegia prefer them to complex orthoses because they are inconspicuous, durable, require no daily maintenance, and are inexpensive.

2. **Protective orthoses** are used to protect the wrist, hand, and fingers from potential deformity or damage and pain by restricting active function (e.g., to promote tissue healing) while maintaining a desired position. Most may be worn throughout the day and night to rest the body part.

a. ***Digital stabilizers***

I. **Finger stabilizers**

- **Distal interphalangeal stabilizers (static DIP splints, stax or stack splints, and DIP gutter splints)** are FOs covering the tip of the finger to just distal to the PIP volar crease to immobilize the DIP and allow unrestricted PIP movement, e.g., for patients with DIP fracture. When used by patients with distal extensor tendon repair, the DIP should be positioned in slight DIP hyperextension to take tension off the repaired tissue.
- **Interphalangeal (PIP/DIP) stabilizers** (Fig. 4.3-12.A; static finger splints, eggshell finger casts, and finger gutter splints) are FOs usually used to restrict motions at the PIP and DIP. In general, the IPs are maintained in full extension to keep the collateral ligaments stretched and to prevent IP flexion contractures (unless the condition dictates otherwise). They are used to immobilize and promote healing (e.g., phalanx fracture, PIP/DIP dislocation, PIP/DIP collateral ligament injury, and PIP volar plate injury) and to provide prolonged finger stretch (e.g., burns and contractures).
- **Ring stabilizers**
  - **Swan neck ring (PIP extension-stop digital stabilizers**; see Fig. 4.3-12.B) are FOs that prevent hyperextension of the PIP joint (via a three-point pressure system) while they permit flexion of all joints. They are used by arthritic patients with swan neck deformity or in PIP/DIP volar plate injury.
  - **Boutonnière ring (PIP flexion-stop digital stabilizers**; Fig. 4.3-12.C) are FOs that immobilize the PIP in extension through a three-point pressure system. They should be removed several times a day for ROM exercise. They are used by arthritic patients with boutonnière deformity.
- **Proximal interphalangeal hinged or articulated splints** are FOs used to provide mediolateral stability in patients with PIP strains or sprains, PIP volar plate injury (using PIP hinged joint with extension block), or post-PIP surgery.
- **Metacarpophalangeal ulnar-deviation restriction orthoses** are FOs used to limit ulnar deviation of the MCP with unrestricted (if possible) MCP flexion/extension by arthritic patients with ulnar deviation of the MCPs. Most patients find these orthoses cumbersome and may choose MCP arthroplasty instead.
- **Finger web-space stabilizers (finger web spacers**; Fig. 4.3-12.D) are FOs held firmly in the finger web spaces to increase or maintain the space between digits to prevent finger web-space contractures (e.g., burns, postreconstruction of syndactyly, and postrevision of scar).

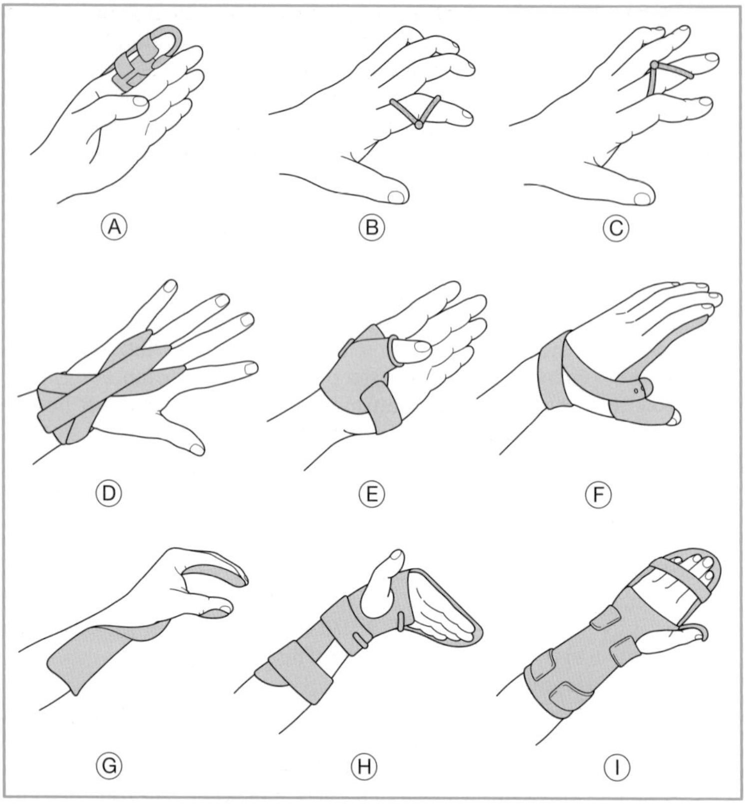

Figure 4.3-12 Protective wrist, hand, and finger orthoses. **A**, IP stabilizer (static finger splints, finger gutter splint). **B**, Swan neck ring (PIP or DIP extension-stop digital stabilizer). **C**, Boutonnière ring (PIP flexion-stop digital stabilizer). **D**, Finger web-space stabilizers (finger web spacers). **E**, Thumb carpometacarpal stabilizers (thumb posts). **F**, Thumb web-space stabilizer (thenar web spacers). **G**, Volar wrist–hand–finger stabilizers (resting hand splint). **H**, Dorsal blocking splint. **I**, Tone-reduction orthosis (Snook splint).

II. **Thumb stabilizers**

- **Thumb carpometacarpal stabilizers** (**thumb posts**; Fig. 4.3-12.E) are TOs that stabilize the first CMC and MCP joints in a neutral position to protect the thumb against inadvertent motion. In patients with "duck-bill" deformity (the thumb MCP is hyperflexed and the thumb IP extended), thumb posts maintain the thumb in an opposed, abducted position. Thumb posts may be extended distally to the thumb tip for use as an opposition post (e.g., in paralyzed thumb) or proximally over the midforearm to immobilize the wrist.
- **Thumb web-space stabilizers (thenar web spacers**; Fig. 4.3-12.F) are FOs that consist of a rigid C-shaped splint held firmly in the thumb and index finger web space to increase or maintain the thenar space and prevent contractures (e.g., burns and postrevision of scar).

b. ***Wrist–hand–finger stabilizers (resting hand splints, resting pan splints; static hand splints; functional resting splints)*** are WHFOs that extend from two-thirds of the distal forearm to the tips of the fingers and thumb (sometimes the thumb is left free). They can be volar based (Fig. 4.3-12.G), dorsal based, or circumferential. The wrist is usually positioned in neutral or slightly extended position with the digits in an intrinsic-plus position (i.e., the MCPs are flexed at 70–90°, the IPs in full extension, the thumb CMC in palmar abduction, and the thumb MCP/IP in full extension). Intrinsic-plus position is preferred because MCP and IP collateral ligaments are stretched, thus minimizing future joint capsule contractures. Also, the thumb position facilitates opposition and three-jaw chuck pinch. Intrinsic-plus position is contraindicated in certain conditions, e.g., after an extensor tendon repair that requires that MCPs be positioned in full extension to minimize tension on the suture site during healing.

Wrist–hand–finger stabilizers are used to immobilize and promote tissue healing (e.g., open wounds, cellulitis, arthritis, CTD, flexor/extensor tendinitis, postsurgical conditions of the forearm–wrist–hand such as ORIF, tendon/nerve/artery repair, skin graft, Dupuytren's release), to passively maintain ROM of the wrist and hand (often used at night) in patients with upper motor neuron lesions (e.g., stroke, TBI, and MS), and to maintain stretch on MCP/IP collateral ligaments (e.g., in amyotrophic lateral sclerosis, SCI, poliomyelitis, burns, brachial plexus lesion, and GBS). A variation of the wrist–hand–finger stabilizer is the flexor tendon repair orthoses (e.g., Kleinert splints, Strickland splints, early-controlled motion splints; dorsal blocking splints; see Fig. 4.3-12.H) which are WHFOs placed on the dorsal forearm, wrist, and hand so that the wrist is in 20–45° flexion, the MCPs in 40–70° flexion, and the IPs in full extension to protect and promote healing of flexor tendon reconstructions (e.g., in postsurgical flexor tendon repair between DIP and distal volar forearm).

c. ***Wrist–hand stabilizers***

I. **Volar wrist–hand stabilizers (resting wrist splints and static wrist splints)** are WHOs that extend from two-thirds of the distal forearm to about ¼ inch (0.64 cm) proximal to the distal palmar crease to allow unrestricted MCP flexion and maintain the functional position of the wrist and hand. Resting splints are used to rest the wrist and hand (e.g., acutely inflamed rheumatoid arthritis joints, wrist sprain or contusion, forearm/wrist fractures, flexor/extensor tendinitis, carpal tunnel syndrome, and postsurgical wrist extensor tendon repair, wrist fusion, or skin grafting), prevent flexion contractures of the wrist and IP joint, prevent extension contracture of the MCP, prevent radial and ulnar deviation of the wrist (e.g., in rheumatoid arthritis), reduce spasticity and prevent thumb adduction and wrist flexion contractures, and reduce pain from repetitive stress (e.g., CTDs) or from arthritis. For optimal hand function, the wrist is positioned about 15–30° of extension (usually 20°). In patients with carpal tunnel syndrome, there is controversy on whether to maintain the wrist in neutral or up to 20° extension (although both positions seem to be beneficial, the neutral position is generally preferred as it can theoretically maximize the carpal tunnel lumen and minimize median nerve compression pressure).

II. **Dorsal wrist–hand stabilizers** are WHOs that are used to provide the same functions as volar wrist–hand stabilizers with greater stabilization because of the rigid circumferential hand section. However, they are more difficult to fabricate, fit, and don. They are used by patients with severe spasticity but are not suitable for edematous hands because they cover the hand circumferentially.

d. ***Tone-reduction orthoses*** are used to reduce spastic flexor tone (e.g., upper motor neuron lesions such as stroke, SCI, TBI, MS, and cerebral palsy). They are typically worn 2 hours on and 2 hours off throughout the day. They can either be hand-based WHOs (e.g., hand-cone splints) or forearm-based WHFOs (e.g., Rolyan preformed antispasticity "ball" splints and Snook splints; Fig. 4.3-12.I).

Forearm-based splints are generally more effective because of the extension positioning of the extrinsic finger flexors. An inflatable pressure splint (inflated to a maximum pressure of 40 mmHg) may be worn for 30 minutes several times a day to reduce spasticity.

e. ***Gloves*** are worn circumferentially on the hand and wrist. If needed, the tips or whole fingers of the gloves may be cut off.

I. **Shock absorbing gloves** are used to absorb shock/vibration entering the palm or hand (e.g., CTD and carpal tunnel syndrome) and to prevent CTDs (e.g., flexor tendinitis, manual wheelchair users, and hypersensitive palmar skin/scars). The palmar aspect of the glove and the volar wrist can be padded with soft materials (e.g., silicone gel).

II. **Compression gloves (Isotoner®, Tubigrip®, and Jobst®)** are used to reduce edema (e.g., traumatic hand injuries with edema, burns, reflex sympathetic dystrophy, CTD, SCI, and upper motor neuron lesions such as stroke and TBI) and to reduce hypertrophic scarring (e.g., maturation phase of burns and scars). For edema reduction, a pressure garment with low to moderate compression of 10–15 mmHg capillary pressure is used; however, for scar reduction, high compression of 15–25 mmHg capillary pressure is used. They may be worn throughout the day (e.g., in scar reduction).

3. **Mobilization (corrective) orthoses** are used to increase passive ROM and alter joint alignment by stretching articular or musculotendinous contractures or adhesions (e.g., burns). In general, a submaximal load is applied for long periods either dynamically using traction (i.e., elastics, coils, or springs) or statically by holding the joint on low tension circumferentially [e.g., eggshell finger casts; serial static splints; buddy splints (i.e., taping or strapping the involved finger to the adjacent relatively normal finger to support and increase IP ROM in the involved finger)]. The most commonly used stretching method is dynamic elastic load, specifically rubber bands whose amount of force can be regulated by the rubber tension. Mobilization orthoses are worn for a specific time during the day.

a. ***Finger mobilization orthoses***

I. **Interphalangeal mobilization orthoses**

- **Interphalangeal extension mobilization orthoses** (Fig. 4.3-13.A; dynamic IP extension splints, reverse finger knuckle benders, Capener splints, safety pin splints, spring coil assists, eggshell finger extension casts, serial static finger extension splints, and buddy splints) are FOs used to passively extend the PIP joints, for example in finger IP flexion contracture, boutonnière deformity, and postsurgical release of Dupuytren's contracture.
- **Interphalangeal flexion mobilization orthoses** (Fig. 4.3-13.B; dynamic IP flexion splints, finger knuckle benders, fingernail hook orthoses, eggshell finger flexion casts, IP flexion straps, serial static finger flexion splints, and buddy splints) are FOs used to passively flex the PIP joints, for example in finger IP extension contractures.

II. **Metacarpophalangeal mobilization orthoses**

- **Metacarpophalangeal-extension mobilization orthoses [reverse MCP knuckle benders** (Fig. 4.3-13.C); dynamic MCP extension splints with dorsal outrigger (Fig. 4.3-13.E); MCP extension assists; radial nerve splints] are WHFOs or FOs used to extend the MCP joints, for example in MCP flexion contractures, burns, and post-ORIF of metacarpal fracture. In patients with weak finger extension (e.g., in radial nerve lesion and brachial plexus lesion), they may be used to improve hand function by substituting for paralyzed or weak finger extension.
- **Metacarpophalangeal-flexion mobilization orthoses [MCP knuckle benders** (Fig. 4.3-13.D); dynamic MCP flexion splints with volar outrigger and

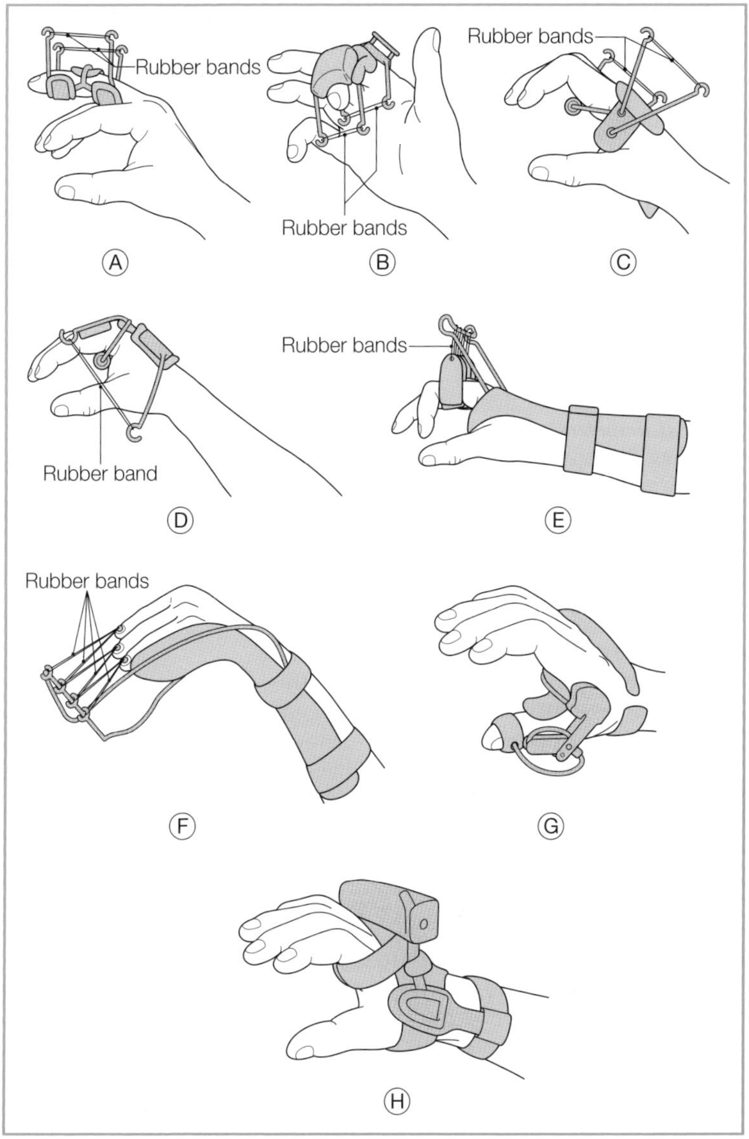

Figure 4.3-13 Mobilization (or corrective) wrist, hand, and finger orthoses. **A**, IP extension mobilization orthosis (reverse finger knuckle bender). **B**, IP flexion mobilization orthosis (finger knuckle bender). **C**, Reverse MCP knuckle bender. **D**, MCP knuckle bender. **E**, Dynamic MCP extension splint with dorsal outrigger. **F**, Dynamic MCP flexion splint with volar outrigger and fingernail hooks. **G**, Dynamic thumb IP extension splints. **H**, Wrist mobilization orthoses.

fingernail hooks (Fig. 4.3-13.F); MCP flexion assists] are WHFOs or FOs used to flex the MCP joints, for example in MCP collateral ligament contractures, extensor tendon shortening, median/ulnar lesion, claw hand, postcapsulotomy, or post-ORIF of metacarpal fracture.

III. **Adjustable wrist–hand orthoses (Swanson postarthroplasty orthoses)** are used to facilitate controlled MCP as well as PIP and DIP motions as needed after arthroplasty and to selectively stabilize joints so there is no undue stretching of unhealed reconstructed tendons and collateral ligaments.

b. ***Thumb mobilization orthoses***

I. **Thumb extension–mobilization orthoses** (Fig. 4.3-13.G; dynamic thumb IP extension splints and serial static thumb extension splints) are TOs used to passively extend the thumb IP joint, for example in thumb IP flexion contracture.

II. **Thumb flexion–mobilization orthoses (dynamic thumb IP flexion splints and serial static thumb flexion splints)** are TOs used to passively flex the thumb IP joint, for example in thumb IP extension contracture.

III. **Thumb abduction–mobilization orthoses (dynamic thumb abduction splints and serial static thumb abduction splints)** are TOs used to passively abduct the thumb, for example in thumb adduction contracture.

c. ***Wrist mobilization orthoses*** (Fig. 4.3-13.H; Ultraflex wrist flexion/extension splints, Dynasplint wrist flexion/extension splints, Phoenix wrist hinge splints, static progressive wrist splints, and turnbuckle wrist splints) are WOs used to passively increase ROM (e.g., in contractures, burns, late phase of fracture, and postrelease of scar). They can also be used to replace or assist weak wrist extensors to enhance function (e.g., radial nerve lesion, SCI, brachial plexus lesion, or poliomyelitis). However, they should not be used in the presence of spastic muscles as they may increase tone.

B. ELBOW, FOREARM, AND WRIST ORTHOSES

1. **Forearm mobilization (corrective) orthoses (dynamic supination/pronation splints)** are elbow–wrist–hand orthoses (EWHOs) consisting of a posterior elbow orthosis and a forearm–wrist or forearm–wrist–hand orthosis. They are used to increase supination or pronation (e.g., in forearm rotational contracture) or increase passive or active-assisted ROM (e.g., upper trunk brachial plexus lesion, or Erb's palsy, and SCI).
2. **Protective elbow, forearm, and wrist orthoses (sugar-tong splints**; Fig. 4.3-14.A) are EWHOs used to immobilize the elbow, forearm, and wrist to promote tissue healing (e.g., CTDs, forearm fractures, postsurgical elbow arthroplasty, or post-transposition of ulnar nerve).

C. ELBOW AND SHOULDER ORTHOSES

1. **Protective elbow and shoulder orthoses** are used to hold the joint in the position opposite the anticipated deformity, limit active motion to reduce pain, guard weak ligaments and muscles from untoward stress, and provide the optimum environment for newly formed skin (which tends to contract as it heals).

a. ***Elbow control orthoses (posterior elbow splints, elbow casts, and elbow air-splint)***, provide mediolateral elbow and forearm rotational stability, limit range of elbow flexion or extension, or both. They are used to promote tissue healing in medial or lateral epicondylitis, cubital tunnel syndrome, olecranon fracture, burns, and postsurgical repair of the elbow.

b. ***Epicondylar straps*** (Fig. 4.3-14.B; tennis or golfer's elbow straps, proximal forearm orthoses, counterforce braces, and forearm bands) are applied circumferentially to the forearm distal to the humeral epicondyles without hindering elbow motion. They are used to reduce pain during activity (e.g., medial or lateral epicondylitis), reduce inflammation, and promote tissue healing at the tendinous origin.

c. ***Shoulder abduction stabilizers (airplane splints***; Fig. 4.3-14.D) are SEWHOs that support the upper arm and shoulder, protect the shoulder from adduction contracture, and relieve tension on the superior aspect of the shoulder. They can

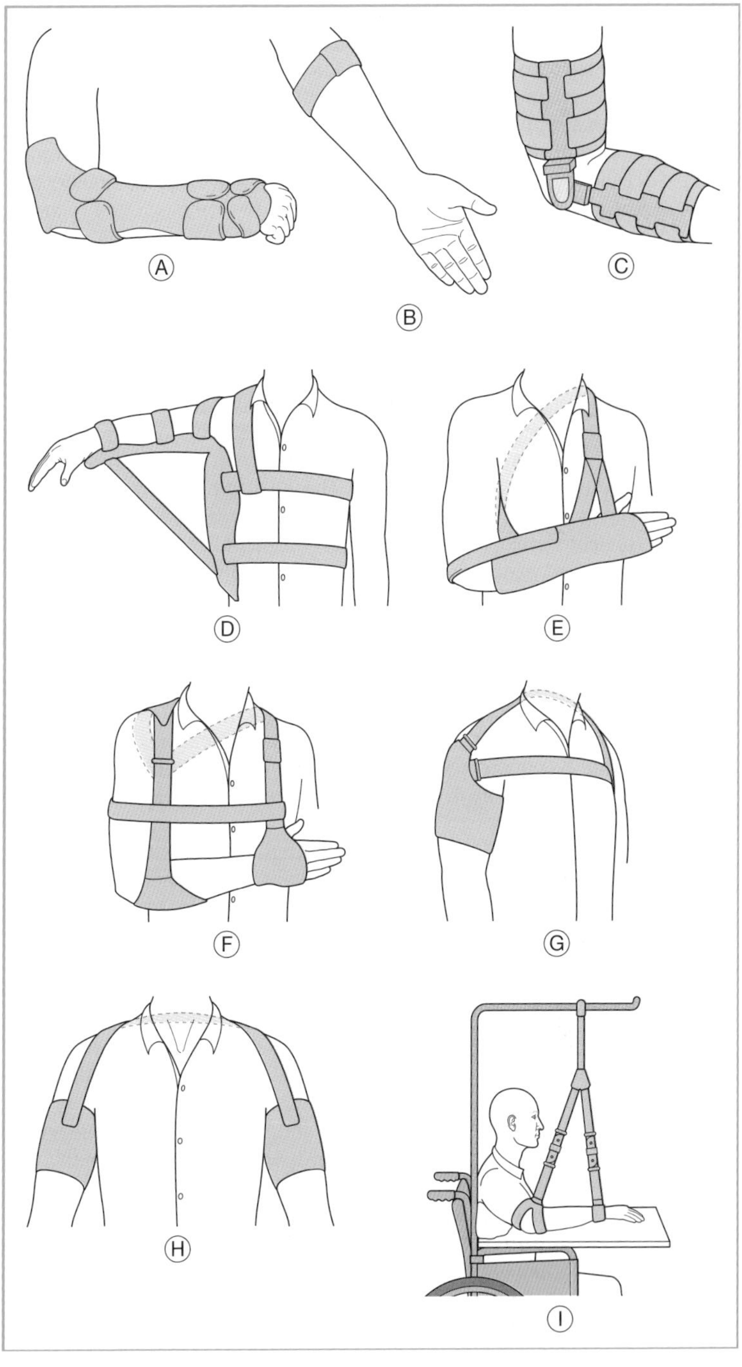

Figure 4.3-14 Protective elbow and shoulder orthoses. **A,** Sugar-tong splint. **B,** Epicondylar strap. **C,** Elbow mobilization orthosis. **D,** Shoulder abduction stabilizer (airplane splint). **E,** Single-strap sling. **F,** Multistrap sling. **G,** Vertical arm sling. **H,** Arm abduction sling. **I,** Arm suspension sling.

be used to stretch the internal rotators and relieve tension on the deltoid and rotator cuff. The shoulder can be maintained in abduction for several weeks after a rotator cuff repair to protect the healing tissues. They are used by patients with axillary burns, contractures, shoulder dislocation, and postsurgery (e.g., shoulder fusion, rotator cuff repair, and axillary scar release).

d. ***Shoulder or arm slings*** are used by patients with shoulder pain or subluxation to protect the shoulder from painful motion (e.g., after injury to shoulder capsule or its supporting muscles). They can be used to promote tissue healing by immobilization (e.g., scapular or humeral fractures, acromioclavicular joint injury, rotator cuff injury, bicipital tendinitis, postsurgical repair of shoulder), prevent overstretching of shoulder muscles or ligaments (e.g., brachial plexus injury), decrease shoulder pain related to glenohumeral distraction and shoulder–hand syndrome (e.g., upper motor neuron lesions and hemiparesis with subluxation), and keep the distal extremity (i.e., hand and forearm) elevated or supported (e.g., edema and cast). They can also be used to protect the flail arm from inadvertent flinging and to place the hand within the patient's immediate visual field. Most arm slings support the forearm with the elbow flexed, and shoulder abducted and internally rotated. The use of arm slings by patients with flexion synergy (e.g., hemiplegia) is controversial. They are discouraged by practitioners of neurodevelopmental techniques (Chapter 4.2, section IV.B.3) as they are believed to encourage flexion synergy, increase flexor tone, and promote contractures.

I. **Single-strap slings** (Fig. 4.3-14.E) are used to support the weight of the arm or a forearm cast, reduce edema, protect the upper limb from inadvertent motion, place the hand in the wearer's visual field, and provide minimal glenohumeral support.

II. **Multistrap slings** (Fig. 4.3-14.F) have the same functions as single-strap slings but also apply vertical forces (e.g., via figure-of-eight suspension) for additional support of the ipsilateral shoulder. They are more difficult to don.

III. **Vertical arm slings** (**Rolyan hemi-arm slings**; Fig. 4.3-14.G) use a humeral cuff with figure-of-eight suspension to provide vertical upward force to support the humerus without restricting the elbow and forearm.

IV. **Arm abduction slings** (**hook hemi-harness slings**; Fig. 4.3-14.H) consist of bilateral humeral cuffs connected by a posterior yoke. The yoke provides a diagonal force to support the shoulders in a slightly abducted position without restricting the elbows and forearms.

V. **Arm suspension slings** (Fig. 4.3-14.I; overhead slings, counterbalance arm slings, deltoid aids, and Swedish slings) are SEWHOs that provide all the functions of the single-strap sling in addition to positioning one or both arms to allow hand use when shoulder and arm muscles have strength of less than fair (e.g., upper motor neuron lesions, proximal myopathy, and GBS); and allowing the arm muscles to be exercised in a gravity-reduced position (e.g., in SCI, muscular dystrophy, and arthrogryposis).

2. Elbow mobilization (or corrective) orthoses (Fig. 4.3-14.C; dynamic elbow splints, Dynasplint elbow splints, Ultraflex elbow splints, Elbow extensionater, static progressive elbow splints, and turnbuckle elbow splints) gently elongate the soft tissues over a long period to attempt to reverse joint malalignment (e.g., contractures, burns, and late phase of fracture). Force is provided by rubber bands, springs, or adjustable mechanisms (e.g., turnbuckles) or by altering the contour of the orthotic frame periodically. They are not used in the presence of spastic muscles as they may increase tone.

a. ***Dorsal elbow-extension mobilization orthoses*** are used to extend the elbow as well as provide mediolateral elbow stability and rotational forearm stability.

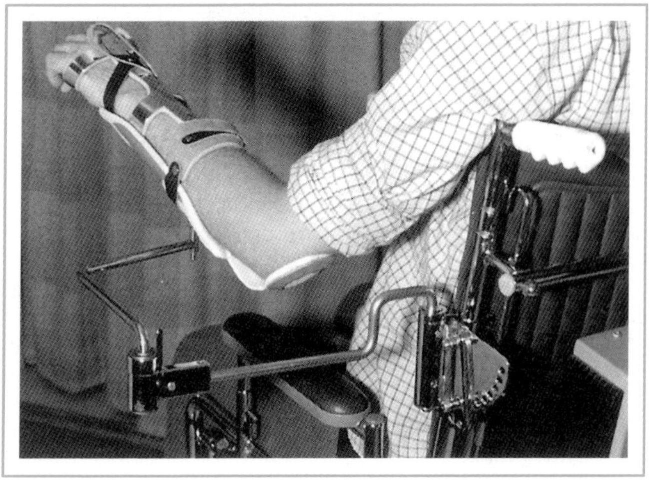

Figure 4.3-15 Balanced forearm orthoses (From Adler C, Pedretti, LW: The balanced forearm orthosis and suspension sling. In Pedretti LW, editor: *Occupational therapy practice skills for physical dysfunction,* ed 4, St Louis, 1996, Mosby-Year Book, p. 345 with permission.)

b. ***Dorsal elbow-flexion mobilization orthoses*** are used to flex the elbow as well as provide mediolateral elbow stability and rotational forearm stability.

3. **Assistive and substitutive elbow and shoulder orthoses** assist upper arm motion thus facilitating wrist–hand functions. They also protect the upper limb from contracture and from secondary trauma as a result of inadvertent motion.

a. ***Elbow and shoulder articulated orthoses*** are used to prevent unwanted motion and to "lock" the upper arm in a position necessary for optimum function. The most commonly used locks are friction locks, ratchet locks (e.g., step-locks), and alternator locks.

b. ***Balanced forearm orthoses or BFOs*** (Fig. 4.3-15; mobile arm supports; ball-bearing feeders; linkage or friction feeders; or "gun-slingers") are SEWHOs that consist of a forearm trough (attached by a hinge joint to a ball-bearing swivel mechanism) and a mount (which can be mounted on the wheelchair, on a table or working surface, or onto a body jacket). BFOs are used to support the forearm against gravity and thereby allow patients with weak shoulder and elbow muscles [i.e., manual muscle testing of at least trace plus (Tr+) to poor minus (P−)] to move the arm horizontally and flex the elbow to bring the hand to the mouth (e.g., patients with SCI, GBS, poliomyelitis, muscular dystrophy, and brachial plexus injury). They also allow patients with spasticity to feed themselves by dampening muscle tone through a friction device.

III. Spinal orthoses and corsets

These use external forces to stabilize, support, and realign the trunk, as well as to protect the spine after acute trauma or spinal surgery. Spinal orthoses and corsets should be properly fitted so the patient can easily don and doff them; rest the desired segment, as well as sit, stand, and perform the prescribed movement comfortably when wearing the orthosis. Also, the orthosis must be functionally, as well as

Table 4.3-4	Percentage of cervical motion restricted by commonly used cervical and cervicothoracic orthoses						
Motion restriction (%)	**Soft**	**Thomas**	**Phila-delphia**	**SOMI**	**Yale**	**4-Poster**	**Halo**
Flexion/extension	26	75*	71	72 NS	87	79	96
Rotation	17	50*	56	66	82	73	99
Side bending	8 NS	75*	34	34 NS	50 NS	54	96

SOMI, sterno-occipital mandibular immobilizer; NS, not statistically significant.
Data adapted from: Johnson RM Hart DL, Simmons EF: Cervical orthoses: a study comparing their effectiveness in restricting cervical motion in normal subjects. J Bone Joint Surg [Am] *59:332–339, 1977.*
**Data adapted from: Hartman JT, Palumbo F, Hill BJ: Cineradiography of the braced normal cervical spine.* Clin Orthoped *109:97–102, 1975.*

cosmetically, acceptable to the patient. When removed, the skin should be unblemished 10 minutes afterwards.

A. **RIGID SPINAL ORTHOSIS** exerts its force via one or more three-point pressure systems through the skin, soft tissue, and ribs to restrict motion, stabilize, and realign the spine. Rigid spinal orthoses can also increase intra-abdominal pressure (IAP), thereby reducing contraction of the erector spinae and consequently reducing the compression of the intervertebral disks. In addition to the general principles applicable to nearly all orthoses (see the beginning of this chapter), rigid spinal orthoses should allow the patient to sit comfortably while wearing the orthosis, and should not restrict breathing, digestion, or chewing. Indications include musculoskeletal pain, instability (trauma, degenerative disease, metastasis), osteoporotic compression fracture of the vertebrae, and postoperative spinal support (e.g., after spinal fusion). Although short-term use of rigid spinal orthoses promotes reduction of muscle spasm, prolonged use should be avoided because they promote atrophy, weakness, decreased flexibility, and psychological dependence. The following classification of rigid spinal orthoses is based on the primary function or control provided by the orthoses.

1. **Cervical and cervicothoracic orthoses** are used to reduce pain because of sprain, strain, or arthritis of the neck; they support the head to allow the patient to see, speak, and eat more easily; and to foster healing of vertebral fracture or surgical arthrodesis. The amount of cervical motion restricted by seven commonly used cervical and cervicothoracic orthoses is shown in Table 4.3-4.

a. ***Cervical flexion–extension (F–E) control orthoses***

I. **Soft cervical collar** (e.g., **Zimmer collar**; Fig. 4.3-16.A) made of polyethylene foam or sponge rubber, limits the least amount of cervical motion. It is fitted high in the back to increase resistance to extension or hyperextension. Through sensory feedback, it reminds the wearer to limit head and neck motions. It also retains body heat, which may help reduce muscle spasm and aid in the healing of soft tissue injuries.

II. **Hard cervical collars** provide more restriction to cervical flexion, extension, rotation, and lateral bending than the soft collars. They have a similar function to the soft collar. Prolonged use of an improperly fitted hard cervical collar may cause an occipital pressure sore.

- **Thomas collar** (Fig. 4.3-16.B) is made of firm plastic with superior and inferior paddings that wrap around the neck and are secured by hook and pile straps (Velcro®).

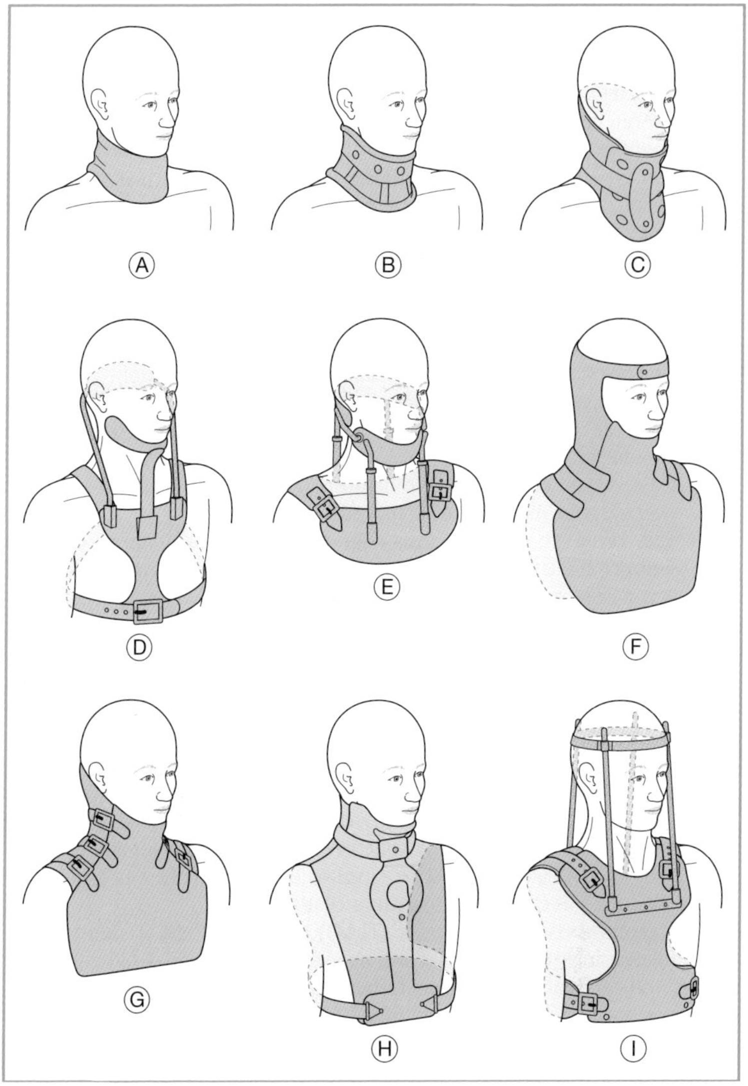

Figure 4.3-16 Cervical orthoses. **A**, Soft cervical collar. **B**, Hard (Thomas) collar. **C**, Hard (Philadelphia) collar. **D**, Sterno-occipital mandibular immobilizer (SOMI). **E**, Post-type cervicothoracic orthosis. **F**, Minerva cervicothoracic orthosis. **G**, Cuirass-type cervicothoracic orthosis. **H**, Yale cervicothoracic orthosis. **I**, Halo-vest cervicothoracic orthosis.

- **Philadelphia collar** (Fig. 4.3-16.C) is made of two pieces of polyethylene foam (Plastazote) secured by hook and pile straps (Velcro®) and is reinforced by rigid anterior and posterior plastic struts. It encompasses the lower jaw and occiput and terminates inferiorly at the proximal thorax. It can be loosened when the patient is eating. Variations of the Philadelphia collar include the Miami-J collar, Aspen collar, StifNeck collar, and NecLoc collar. The NecLoc, followed by the Miami-J collar, was shown to provide the most cervical motion restriction compared with Philadelphia, Aspen, and StifNeck collars (Askins and Eismont, 1997).

b. ***Cervical flexion–extension–rotary (F–E–R) control orthoses (sterno-occipital mandibular immobilizer***; Fig. 4.3-16.D) is a post-type cervicothoracic orthosis in which the uprights supporting the occiput arise anteriorly from a sternal plate. Therefore, it can easily be applied to the supine patient. The mandibular support can be removed so the patient can eat, wash, or shave while supine.

c. ***Cervical flexion–extension–lateral–rotary (F–E–L–R) control orthoses***

I. **Post-type cervicothoracic orthoses** (Fig. 4.3-16.E) have mandibular and occipital plates connected to sternal and thoracic plates by two, three, or four posts. They provide greater motion limitations and can hold the head in extension or flexion by adjusting the length of anterior and posterior posts. They are cooler than cervical collars but are bulkier.

II. **Custom-molded cervicothoracic orthoses** are designed to markedly restrict all neck as well as thoracic motions. They are not frequently used. Instead, a halo-vest orthosis is used for maximum neck motion control.

- **Minerva cervicothoracic orthosis** (Fig. 4.3-16.F) encloses the entire posterior skull, includes a band around the forehead, and extends downward to the inferior costal margin.
- **Cuirass-type cervicothoracic orthosis** (Fig. 4.3-16.G) extends superiorly over the chin, mandible, occiput, and posterior skull.

III. **Yale cervicothoracic orthosis** (Fig. 4.3-16.H) is similar to an extended Philadelphia collar with rigid plastic struts extending down the anterior and posterior thorax with hook and pile strapping (Velcro®) beneath the axillae.

IV. **Halo-vest cervicothoracic orthosis** (Fig. 4.3-16.I) consists of a rigid halo secured to the skull with four external fixation pins. The halo supports four posts that terminate in hardware attached to the front and back of the vest. It provides the greatest control of all cervical motion and is used in patients with high cervical fractures. Its most common complications are pin loosening, pin-site infection, and pressure ulcers. Less common complications are reduced vital capacity, neck pain, brain abscess, and psychological trauma. It is cooler and lighter than the Minerva orthosis. A wrench for quick dismantling of the halo-vest must be taped to the front of the vest in case the patient needs cardiopulmonary resuscitation.

2. **Thoracolumbosacral orthoses (TLSO)** extend from the sacrum to above the inferior angle of the scapulae and are used to support and stabilize the trunk (e.g., truncal paralysis, postspinal fusion, and postscoliotic surgery) and to prevent progression of moderate scoliosis (20–45°) until the patient reaches skeletal maturity. Except for the TLS flexion-control orthoses, TLSOs can increase IAP and consequently reduce compression of the intervertebral disks, thus decreasing low back pain (e.g., in spondylolisthesis, and in intervertebral disk disease). TLSOs are usually worn for 3 months after scoliosis surgery.

a. ***TLS flexion–extension (F–E) control orthosis*** (***Taylor brace***; Fig. 4.3-17.A) consists of two TLS posterior uprights attached inferiorly to a pelvic band. An interscapular band stabilizes the uprights and serves as an attachment for axillary straps. Anteriorly, there is a full-front abdominal support. It decreases trunk flexion and extension and increases IAP. The control of extension is at a higher level (at the thoracolumbar junction) and not at the lumbosacral junction, thus there is less decrease in lordosis.

b. ***TLS flexion–extension–lateral (F–E–L) control*** (***Knight Taylor brace***; Fig. 4.3-17.B) is similar to the Taylor brace except for the addition of lateral uprights and a thoracic band to restrict lateral bending.

c. ***TLS flexion–lateral–rotary (F–L–R) control orthosis*** (***Cowhorn brace***; Fig. 4.3-17.C) consists of pelvic and thoracic bands connected by a pair of lumbosacral posterior uprights and a pair of lateral uprights with abdominal

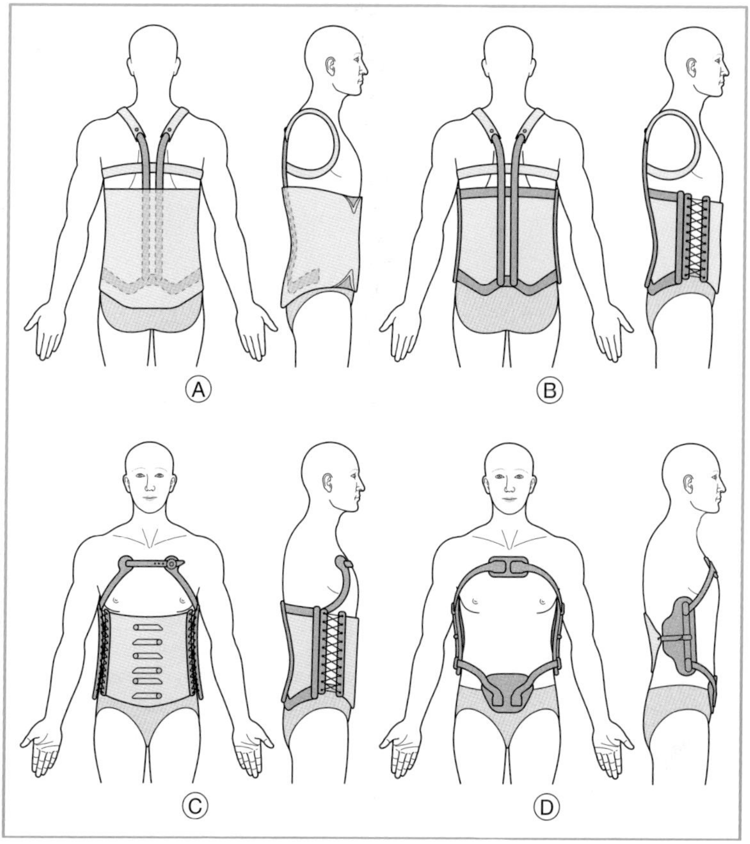

Figure 4.3-17 Thoracolumbosacral (TLS) orthoses. **A**, TLS flexion–extension (F–E) control orthosis (Taylor brace). **B**, TLS flexion–extension–lateral (F–E–L) control orthosis (Knight Taylor brace). **C**, TLS flexion–lateral–rotary (F–L–R) control orthosis (Cowhorn brace). **D**, TLS flexion (F) control orthosis (Jewett or Becker orthoses).

support. The thoracic band extends and curves anteriorly to two subclavicular pads to restrict rotation and flexion. It restricts extension at the lumbar area but not the thoracic area.

d. ***TLS flexion (F) control orthosis*** has anterior metal plates that restrict trunk flexion. It does not increase IAP nor decrease lordosis. It encourages a hyper-extension posture, increases lumbar lordosis, and tends to stabilize the spine to resist lateral and rotary movements.

I. **Jewett or Becker TLSO** (Fig. 4.3-17.D) has a sternal plate, a dorsolumbar plate, lateral uprights, and a suprapubic plate. The suprapubic plate is unacceptable in women because it presses on the bladder. A boomerang band, which applies force on the iliac crest, is used for women instead.

II. **Cruciform anterior spinal hyperextension (CASH) TLSO** (Fig. 4.3-18.A) has cross-shape anterior vertical and horizontal metal or plastic bands. The vertical band joins the sternal and suprapubic plates, while the horizontal band connects the dorsolumbar plate.

e. ***TLS flexion–extension–lateral–rotary (F–E–L–R) control*** (***TLS jacket***; Fig. 4.3-18.B) is made of relatively thick rigid or semi-rigid polyethylene plastic. It is

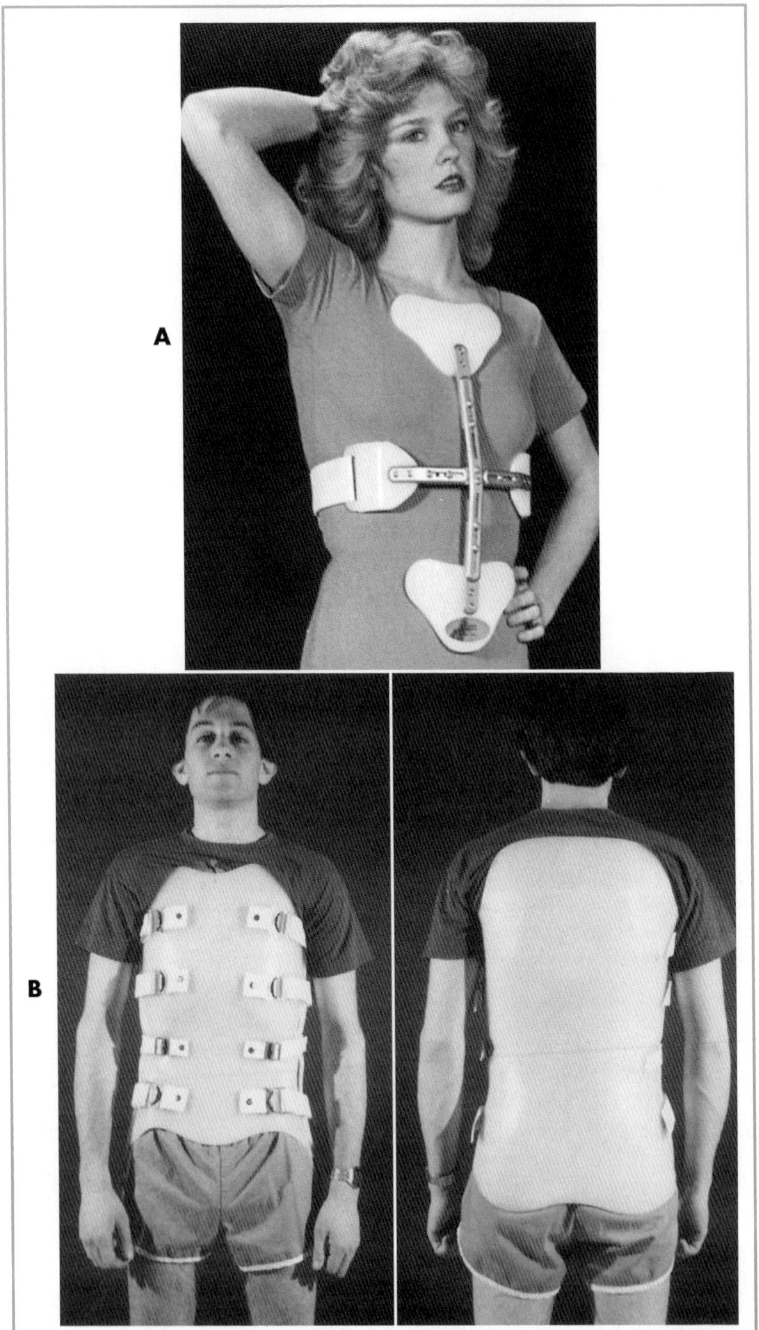

Figure 4.3-18 Thoracolumbosacral orthoses (TLSO). **A**, CASH or cruciform anterior spinal hyperextension TLSO [TLS flexion (F) control orthosis]. **B**, TLS flexion–extension–lateral–rotary (F–E–L–R) control orthosis (TLS jacket). (From Bunch, WH, Keagy RD, Kritter, AE, *et al.*: *American Academy of Orthopedic Surgeons (AAOS) atlas of orthotics: biomechanical principles and application*, ed 2, St Louis, 1985, Mosby-Year Book, pp. 245, 249 with permission.)

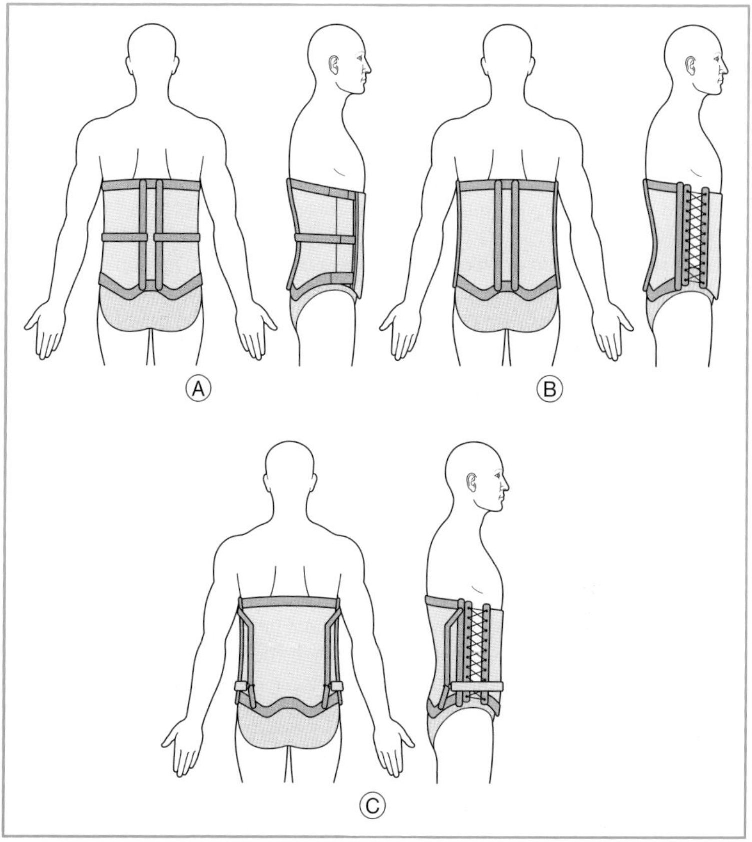

Figure 4.3-19 Lumbosacral (LS) orthoses. **A**, LS flexion–extension (F–E) control orthosis (Chairback orthosis). **B**, LS flexion–extension–lateral (F–E–L) control orthosis (Knight spinal orthosis). **C**, LS extension–lateral (E–L) control orthosis (William's brace).

used for maximum immobilization, for example in unstable fracture involving the posterior vertebral elements.

f. ***Boston TLSO*** is a symmetrical rigid plastic jacket fitted with interior pads used in moderate scoliosis with apex at or below T8.

3. Cervico-thoraco-lumbosacral orthoses (CTLSO) are plastic TLS jackets that extend upward to the mandible and mastoid. The Milwaukee brace, which is a type of CTLSO used for scoliosis, has a rigid plastic pelvic girdle connected to a neck ring over the upper thorax by one anterior and two posterior uprights. Pads strapped to the uprights apply forces to correct the scoliotic curve with apex at or below T6.

4. Lumbosacral orthoses (LSO) extend from the sacrum to the inferior scapular angle.

a. ***LS flexion–extension (F–E) control orthosis*** (***Chairback orthosis***; Fig. 4.3-19.A) consists of two posterior uprights attached inferiorly to a pelvic band and superiorly to a thoracic band. A full-front abdominal support is fastened to the posterior uprights by means of straps. It increases IAP, restricts flexion–extension, and flattens lumbar lordosis.

b. ***LS flexion–extension–lateral (F–E–L) control orthosis*** (***Knight spinal orthosis***; Fig. 4.3-19.B) is similar to the LS F–E control orthosis with the additional restriction of lateral motion by lateral uprights. It has an abdominal support.

c. ***LS extension–lateral (E–L) control orthosis*** (***William's brace***; Fig. 4.3-19.C) consists of pelvic and thoracic bands joined by a pair of lateral uprights, which are pivotably attached to the thoracic bands but not attached to the pelvic band. It has an elastic abdominal support. It increases IAP, decreases lordosis, and decreases extension and lateral bending but does not restrict flexion.

d. ***LSO with hip spica or thigh cuff*** may be used to limit hip motion on one side. It locks the hip joint in extension making it difficult to walk and to climb stairs. It is used by patients with postsurgical screws or fusion of L4 to S1 fractures.

e. ***LS jacket (Boston overlap brace)*** is made of semi-rigid plastic with hook and pile straps (Velcro®). It encases the lower trunk and controls all LS motion.

B. **CORSETS (FLEXIBLE SPINAL ORTHOSES)** are made of fabric with pouches for vertical stays. The vertical staves can be made of rigid (steel) or flexible materials. Corsets are considered flexible (nonrigid) spinal orthoses because the vertical stays are not connected by horizontal bars (i.e., there are no pelvic or thoracic bands). Hence, although corsets create similar forces as in rigid spinal orthoses, they do not restrict motion or realign the spine nearly as much as rigid spinal orthoses do. Corsets increase IAP more than rigid spinal orthoses because the body part is covered snugly without space between corset and skin. Two commonly used corsets are thoracolumbosacral and lumbosacral corsets for patients with low back pain caused by minor spondylolisthesis (grade I without neuropathy). In patients with skin irritations, corsets are contraindicated. As with any spinal orthosis, prolonged used of corsets should be discouraged. The efficacy of corsets remains controversial.

1. **TLS corset** extends anteriorly below the xiphoid process to above the symphysis pubis and posteriorly from the midscapular level to just below the apex of the gluteal bulge for men and lower down to the gluteal fold for women. It can restrict spinal motion at the thoracic and the lumbar spine and can increase IAP, which consequently reduces intradiskal pressure during lifting. Mainly, it is used to remind the wearer to avoid abrupt trunk motion and to lift properly.

2. **LS corset (Richard's corset)** is the most commonly used corset. It has the same design as the TLS corset except that posteriorly it extends to below the inferior angles of the scapulae instead of the midscapular level. It has the same function as the TLS corset but does not restrict thoracic spinal motion.

3. **Sacroiliac (SI) corsets**

a. ***Sacroiliac corset*** extends superiorly from the iliac crest level to the symphysis pubis anteriorly and to the apex of the gluteal bulge posteriorly. Although not effective in restricting motion, it assists in elevating IAP and may be useful for postpartum and post-traumatic stabilization of sacroiliac and symphysis pubis joints. It is also occasionally used temporarily by patients with low back pain with sacroiliac pain.

b. ***Sacroiliac belt*** encircles the pelvis between the iliac crests and the trochanters with perineal straps to prevent upward displacement. The belt passes below the anterior superior iliac spine but should not encroach on the rectus femoris during hip flexion. It is used by patients with postpartum or traumatic separation of the sacroiliac or symphysis pubis or following resection of the symphysis.

c. ***Elastic sacroiliac corset (binder) with plastic insert*** is similar to the SI corset but has a thermoplastic insert contoured to the patient's body and fitted into a posterior pocket with hook and pile straps (Velcro®). It is mainly used to remind the patient to correct back posture. It can also increase IAP.

Further reading

Askins V, Eismont FJ: Efficacy of five cervical orthoses in restricting cervical motion: a comparison study. *Spine* 22(11):1193–1198, 1997.

Bunch WH, Keagy RD, Kritter AS, *et al.*: *American Academy of Orthopedic Surgeons (AAOS) atlas of orthotics: biomechanical principles and application*, ed 2, St Louis, 1985, Mosby-Year Book.

Edelstein JE: Orthotic assessment and management. In O'Sullivan SB, Schmitz TJ, editors: *Physical rehabilitation: assessment and treatment*, ed 4, Philadelphia, 2001, FA Davis, pp. 1025–1060.

Edelstein JE: Orthoses. In Myers RS, editor: *Saunders manual of physical therapy practice*, Philadelphia, 1995, WB Saunders, pp. 1183–1227.

Edelstein JE, Bruckner J: *Orthotics: a comprehensive clinical approach*, Thorofare, NJ, 2002, Slack Inc.

Faculty of Prosthetics and Orthotics, New York University School of Medicine and Post-Graduate Medical School: *Lower-limb orthotics*, New York, 1986, Prosthetic-Orthotic Publications.

Goldberg B, Hsu JD, editors: *American Academy of Orthopedic Surgeons (AAOS) atlas of orthoses and assistive devices*, ed 3, St Louis, 1997, Mosby.

Hennessey WJ, Johnson EW: Lower limb orthoses. In Braddom RL, editor: *Physical medicine and rehabilitation*, ed 2, Philadelphia, 2000, WB Saunders, pp. 326–352.

Lehmann JF: Orthotics. *Phys Med Rehabil Clin North Am* 3(1):1–247, 1992.

Pomerantz F, Durand E: Spinal orthotics. In DeLisa JA, Gans BM, Walsh NE, *et al.*, editors: *Physical medicine and rehabilitation: principles and practice*, ed 4, Philadelphia, 2005, Lippincott, Williams & Wilkins, pp. 1355–1365.

Ragnarsson KT: Lower extremity orthotics, shoes, and gait aids. In DeLisa JA, Gans BM, Walsh NE, *et al.*, editors: *Physical medicine and* rerehabilitation: *principles and practice*, ed 4, Philadelphia, 2005, Lippincott, Williams & Wilkins, pp. 1377–1391.

Redford JB, editor: *Orthotics etcetera*, ed 3, Baltimore, 1986, Williams & Wilkins.

Redford JB: Upper limb orthotic devices. In Braddom RL, editor: *Physical medicine and rehabilitation*, ed 2, Philadelphia, 2000, WB Saunders, pp. 331–352.

Redford JB, Basmajian JV, Trautman P, editors: *Orthotics: Clinical practice and rehabilitation technology*, New York, 1995, Churchill Livingstone.

Sarno JE. Below-knee orthoses: a system for prescription. *Arch Phys Med Rehabil* 54:548–552, 1973.

Uustal H: Upper extremity orthotics. In DeLisa JA, Gans BM, Walsh NE, *et al.*, editors: *Physical medicine and rehabilitation: principles and practice* ed 4, Philadelphia, 2005, Lippincott, Williams & Wilkins, pp. 1367–1376.

CHAPTER 4.4
Prostheses

A prosthesis is an artificial substitute for a missing body part. This chapter deals only with prostheses for missing upper and lower limbs. Lower-limb amputations are 10 times more common than upper-limb amputations. The most common cause of lower-limb amputations in persons older than 50 years is ischemia (e.g., foot gangrene) caused by peripheral vascular diseases (which may result from diabetes mellitus, arteriosclerotic disease, thromboangiitis, venous dysfunction, or a combination of these as well as other vascular problems). Infection (e.g., chronic osteomyelitis) and severe burns may occasionally cause amputations. In younger adults and adolescents, the most common cause is trauma as a result of motor vehicle accidents, work-related injuries, or high-risk recreational activities. Other major causes of lower-limb amputation are malignancy, such as osteosarcoma and chondrosarcoma (peaking in adolescence), and congenital limb (skeletal) deficiency.

Like orthoses, prostheses should be lightweight with reasonable durability, acceptable cosmetically, easy to maintain and clean, easy to don and doff correctly and rapidly, and adjustable to accommodate progression or resolution of concomitant disorders. Most importantly, the patient should be motivated to wear it. Patients perceive their prosthesis as "light" if it suspends well and fits snugly and allows them to sit, stand, and move comfortably. In patients with decreased sensation or impaired circulation, the *residual limb* (formerly called stump) must be checked regularly for redness, trophic changes, abrasions, and dermatitis. Skin redness should disappear 10 minutes after prosthesis removal. Areas that are sensitive to high pressure (e.g., bony prominences) should be accommodated with a concavity within the socket, called a *relief*. In contrast, pressure-tolerant tissues (e.g., patellar tendon) can accept greater loading and should be provided with convexities, called *build-ups* (or *bulges*), within the socket. Selection of the optimal prosthetic component should consider the patient's level of amputation (see Fig. 4.4-1), strength, balance, cardiopulmonary condition, cognitive status, motivation, anticipated vocational and avocational activities, as well as the financial and technical resources available. The energy cost and loss of speed during ambulation using prostheses are shown in Table 4.4-1.

I. Lower-limb prostheses

Lower-limb prostheses substitute for the missing lower-limb segment to restore the amputee's appearance of bodily symmetry and usually perform a major role in ambulation. Except for partial-foot prostheses, all lower-limb prostheses include a foot–ankle assembly. For amputations below the knee (transtibial), the prostheses also include shank, socket, and suspension systems. For amputations above the knee (transfemoral), a knee unit is added. Although gait may be asymmetrical, especially in unilateral amputees, it should not deviate significantly from normal gait. To determine the patients' potential for using lower-limb prostheses, careful assessment of their functional levels of activity and ambulation should be carried out using the Medicare prosthetic K levels (see Table 4.4-2).

Basic prosthetic training includes caring for the residual limb and the prosthesis, instruction in donning the prosthesis correctly, transferring from various chairs,

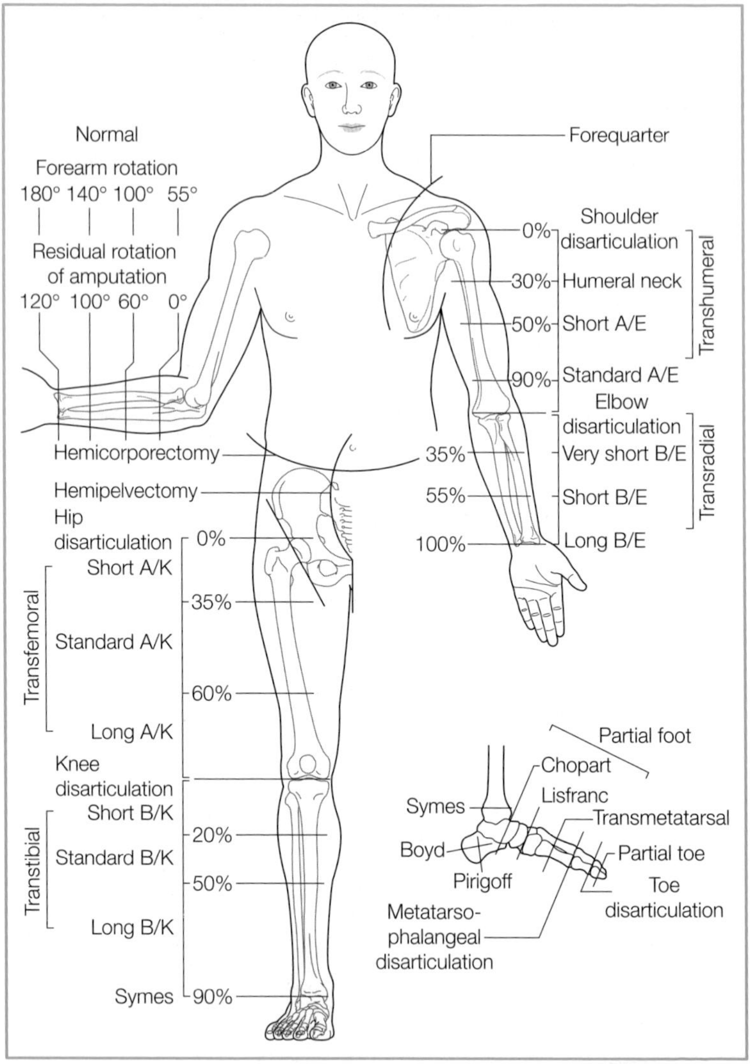

Figure 4.4-1 Levels of upper- and lower-limb amputations. The right upper limb shows the comparison of residual rotation in different levels of amputated forearm vs. normal forearm.

walking, and climbing stairs, ramps, and curbs. An interim (temporary) prosthesis is usually made prior to a definitive (permanent) prosthesis, which is cosmetically finished. The interim prosthesis consists of a socket designed to accept full weight bearing, attached to a pylon and foot. It allows early prosthetic fitting before the residual limb volume is stabilized. It helps in shrinking and shaping the residual limb, allows early gait and functional training with the prosthesis, and allows fine tuning of the prosthetic alignment as the amputee's gait progresses.

A. PARTIAL-FOOT PROSTHESIS is used to restore foot function (particularly walking) and forefoot contour. Small-toe amputation does not significantly affect gait and requires only toe fillers made of cork or plastic foam. Loss of the great toe reduces push-off force during the late stance phase, thus requiring a

Table 4.4-1 Energy cost and speed of ambulation among lower-extremity amputees compared to normal subjects walking at a comfortable speed of 80 m/min or 3 mph (miles per hour)

Walking parameters	TT (BK)	TT + TT (BK + BK)	TF + Crutch (AK + Crutch)	TF (AK)	TT + TF (BK + AK)	TF + TF (AK + AK)
% increase in Ee/unit distance	23	41	92	99	118	186
% decrease in CWS	20	20	51	51	56	60

TT or BK = transtibial or below-knee amputation; TF or AK = transfemoral or above-knee amputation; Ee/unit distance = energy expenditure per unit distance; CWS = comfortable walking speed = 80 m/min or 3 mph.
Adapted from data from multiple sources recalculated and summarized in: Gonzalez EG, Edelstein, JE: Energy expenditure during ambulation. In Gonzalez EG, Myers SJ, Edelstein, JE, et al.: *Downey & Darling's physiological basis of rehabilitation medicine, ed 3, Boston, 2001, Butterworth-Heinemann, p. 433, with permission.*

Table 4.4-2 Medicare prosthetic K levels of functional classification of activity and ambulation used in determining a patient's potential for using lower-limb prostheses

K levels	Description	Activity and prosthetic potential
K-0	Nonambulator (nonprosthetic user)	Has little or no potential for safe transfer or ambulation, with or without assistance
K-1	Household ambulatory (limited or unlimited)	Has the ability or potential to use a prosthesis for transfers or ambulation on level surfaces at fixed cadence
K-2	Limited community ambulatory	Has the ability or potential for ambulation with the ability to traverse low-level environmental barriers (curbs, stairs, or uneven surfaces) at fixed cadence
K-3	Unlimited community ambulatory	Has the ability or potential for ambulation at variable cadence in the community and has the ability to traverse most environmental barriers and may have vocational, therapeutic, or exercise activity that demands prosthetic use beyond simple locomotion
K-4	Exceeds basic ambulation skills	Has the ability or potential for prosthetic ambulation exhibiting high impact, stress, or energy levels (i.e., children, active adult, athletes)

Adapted from: Edwards ML: Lower limb prosthetics. In Olson DA, DeRuyter F, editors: Clinician's guide to assistive technology, St Louis, 2002, Mosby, p. 298, with permission; and Romo HD: Prosthetic knees. In Bussell MH, editor: New developments in prosthetics and orthotics. Phys Med Rehabil Clin North Am 11(3):596, 2000.

resilient toe filler and also a molded insole with an arch support to maintain the alignment of the amputated foot. In transmetatarsal amputation (see Fig. 4.4-1), the hindfoot tends to assume the equinus position, thus requiring a molded socket connected to a rigid sole plate, which extends to a point just posterior to the normal toe break, with a distal padding, a toe break, and a toe filler. If the calcaneus is in varus or valgus position, the molded socket with rigid plate could be extended posteriorly and proximally to encompass and stabilize the heel. For Lisfranc amputation (see Fig. 4.4-1) at the tarsometatarsal junction, the prosthesis used is similar to that for transmetatarsal amputation. In midtarsal amputation

(Chopart's amputation; see Fig. 4.4-1), only the calcaneus and talus remain, thus the prosthesis should extend to the calf in the form of a plastic calf shell strapped around the leg. An alternative is to strap the residual foot to a posterior leaf spring ankle–foot orthosis (AFO) and add a toe filler. Sensitivity of the distal end is common in partial foot amputation, thus shoes should have low heels to prevent the stump from sliding forward. Also, a rocker bottom sole may be used to promote rollover and protect the distal residual limb from pressure. A partial foot prosthesis made of silicone resin was developed by Lawrence Lange to allow for ankle motion, interchangeability of shoes, good cosmesis, comfort and excellent suspension. It is lightweight and flexible and is ankle height with medial and lateral zipper for donning purposes. Its toe resistance can be customized to fit the patient's activities.

B. SYME PROSTHESIS is used for Syme ankle disarticulation (see Fig. 4.4-1), which is a supra-articular or transmalleolar amputation in which all foot bones are removed and the calcaneal fat (heel pad) is attached to the anterior skin flap to cushion the distal end of the lower limb. It consists of a socket strapped onto the calf usually terminating just below the tibial tuberosity or can be higher [e.g., patellar tendon-bearing (PTB) socket] if more proximal weight bearing is needed. If the residual limb is bulbous, the socket needs a removable medial or posterior section to facilitate donning. Otherwise, a nonfenestrated socket may be worn.

1. **Original Syme prosthesis** consists of a leather socket, steel side bars, and a single-axis prosthetic foot. It is rarely used nowadays.
2. **Canadian Syme prosthesis** (see Fig. 4.4-2.A) consists of a plastic laminated socket attached to a modified solid-ankle cushioned-heel (SACH) foot (see section I.C.1.a.1.a) with a removable posterior wall (retained by a strap) to allow donning of the bulbous residual limb.
3. **Removable-window design or Veterans Administration Prosthetics Center (VAPC) Syme prosthesis** (see Fig. 4.4-2.B) is made of a plastic laminated socket with a window cut on the medial aspect to increase prosthetic strength. The window allows donning of the bulbous distal end and can be closed by two straps, thus retaining the residual limb without any additional suspension. Several energy-storing feet are available for low-profile Symes, such as lowprofile FlexFoot.
4. **Flexible posterior build-up Syme prosthesis** (see Fig. 4.4-2.C), designed for a less bulbous residual limb, consists of a nonfenestrated plastic laminated

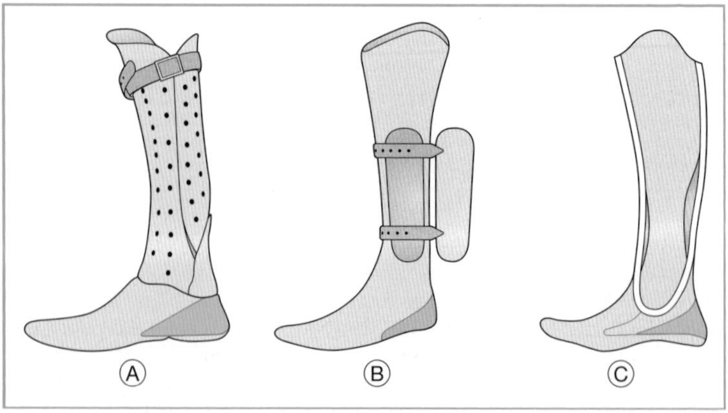

Figure 4.4-2 Types of Symes prostheses. **A**, Canadian Syme prosthesis. **B**, Removable-window design (Veterans Administration Prosthetics Center [VAPC]) Syme prosthesis. **C**, Flexible posterior build-up Syme prosthesis.

socket in which all circumferences are equal to that of the distal residual limb. The void between the socket and the residual limb is filled with relatively soft, flexible build-ups that are either located in the socket or provided in the form of an insert that the amputee dons before slipping into the prosthesis. This design is stronger, but not heavier, than the Canadian or VAPC design because it uses one-piece lamination with unbroken exterior.

C. TRANSTIBIAL (BELOW-KNEE) PROSTHESES are used for amputations above the Syme's site with 5 cm (2 inches) or more of residual tibia. It has four parts: foot–ankle assembly, shank, socket, and suspension.

1. Foot–ankle assembly should resemble the shape of the anatomic foot and provide the basic functions required in walking, i.e., shock absorption during heel strike, ankle plantar flexion in early stance, a stable base of support during midstance, and metatarsophalangeal hyperextension (toe-break action) in late stance to propel the body up and forward. The prosthetic foot yields passively in response to the direction of load applied by the amputee. Some models, however, also move in the transverse and frontal planes. Components called rotators (or shank torque-absorber rotator units) can be placed above the prosthetic foot to absorb shock in the transverse plane and protect the residual limb from chafing, which would occur if the socket is allowed to rotate against the skin. Rotators are not indicated for most transtibial amputees but may be used in those using thigh corsets or who are active athletes encountering discomfort.

a. Nonarticulated prosthetic feet are the most popular types of prosthetic feet. They have streamlined appearance, are relatively lightweight, and have no moving parts that could loosen or become noisy.

I. **Nonenergy-storing prosthetic feet**

- **Solid-ankle cushion-heel (SACH) foot** (see Fig. 4.4-3.A) has a rigid longitudinal keel, the posterosuperior part of which is attached to the shank, has no definite ankle joint, and has a posteroinferior compressible rubber heel wedge, which simulates plantar flexion during early stance. The distal end of the keel permits hyperextension of the foot during late stance. The keel terminates at the site of the metatarsophalangeal joints. It is covered with rubber, which continues distally to form the toe section. During heel strike, the heel wedge compresses up to ¾ to 1 inch (1.9–2.5 cm), plantar flexing the foot, thereby absorbing shock and stabilizing the patient's knee. The heel also compresses on application of medial or lateral loading, such as experienced when walking on uneven terrain. Unlike the normal foot, the SACH version does not dorsiflex at midstance. In late stance, weight advancement causes the foot to hyperextend at the junction between the keel and the toe. The lack of an articulated ankle provides the lever arm to propel the body forward at the end of the stance phase.
- **Stationary attachment flexible endoskeleton foot** (see Fig. 4.4-3.B) has a rigid ankle block attached to the shank, without a definite ankle joint; the anterior part of the block terminates at a 45° angle, abutting a more flexible keel, to permit inversion and eversion and accommodate more readily to irregular surfaces. The distal end of the keel permits hyperextension of the foot during late stance. The heel is cushioned (like a SACH foot) to absorb shock and permit plantar flexion during early stance. It is heavier than a SACH foot.

II. **Dynamic response (or energy-storing) prosthetic feet** have keels that deform slightly during midstance, thus storing potential energy. The stored energy is then released during push-off as the keel recoils to its original shape. Their mechanical efficiency provides significant improvement in the level of function, gait pattern, and overall quality of life of the active amputee. Vigorous amputees are able to run and jump using dynamic response feet (e.g., Flex foot). However, dynamic response feet have not been

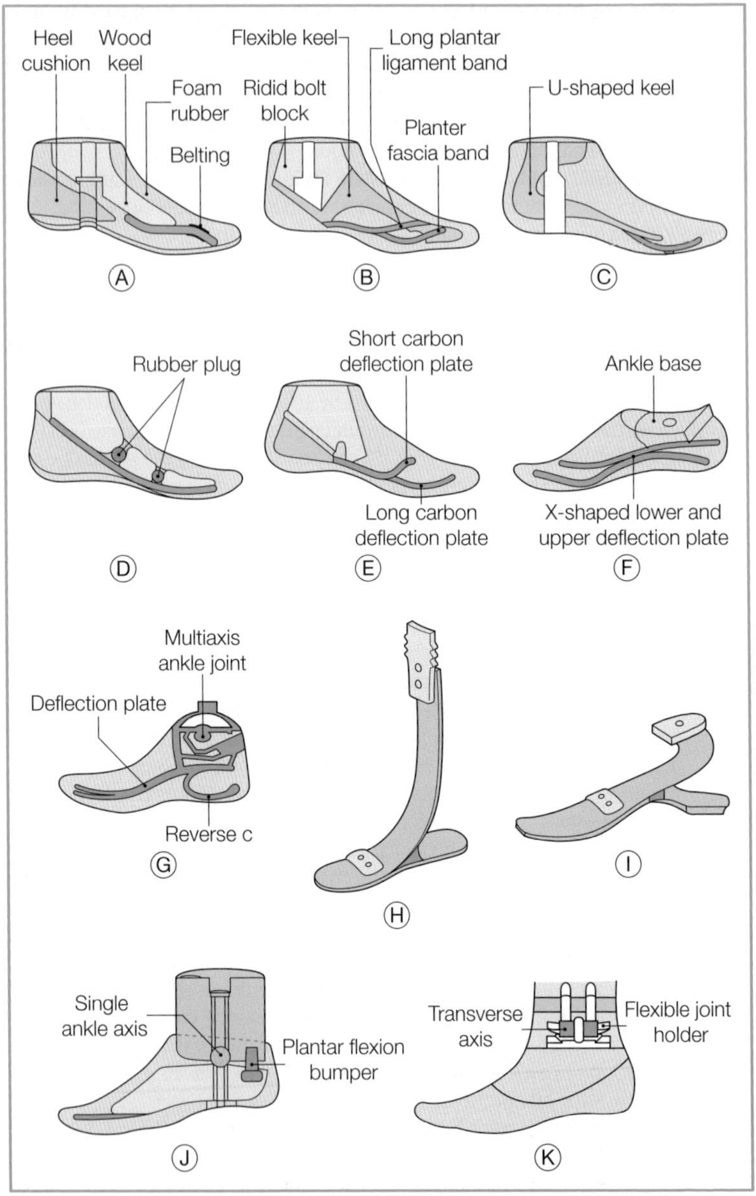

Figure 4.4-3 Foot–ankle assembly for lower-limb prostheses (**A**, **B**, Nonenergy storing nonarticulated prosthetic feet. **C–I**, Energy storing nonarticulated prosthetic feet. **J**, **K**, Articulated prosthetic feet). **A**, Solid ankle cushion heel (SACH) foot. **B**, Stationary attachment flexible endoskeleton (SAFE) foot. **C**, Seattle foot. **D**, STEN (STored ENergy) foot. **E**, Carbon copy II foot. **F**, Quantum modular foot. **G**, Energizer (Dyna-Step) foot. **H**, Flex-foot. **I**, Flex-walk. **J**, Single-axis prosthetic foot. **K**, Multiple-axis prosthetic foot.

shown to reduce metabolic energy consumption when compared to other feet (e.g., SACH), especially at normal walking speed.

- **Seattle foot** (see Fig. 4.4-3.C) has a cantilevered plastic spring keel and Kevlar reinforced toe pad encased in a human-looking polyurethane mold. Body weight after midstance compresses on a U-shaped keel, which acts as a compressed spring. The stored energy is released at push-off. The Seattle foot is wide and heavy and has a relatively high arch, which may interfere with medial–lateral stability. It is useful for the young and middle-aged transtibial and transfemoral amputee.
- **Seattle light foot** provides a dynamic response similar to the Seattle foot at half the weight. The foot has a less pronounced medial arch and a slim profile. This combination provides the patient with some degree of plantar and dorsiflexion and the option of a lightweight endoskeletal system. This foot–ankle system is indicated in the geriatric population.
- **The STEN (STored ENergy) foot** (see Fig. 4.4-3.D) uses a modified SACH mold with a dual, articulated wooden keel and a double-reinforced belting system that permits a smoother transition from midstance to push-off. It weighs and costs more than the SACH foot. The STEN foot is not recommended by the manufacturer for transfemoral amputees because of the soft forefoot, which may cause knee instability.
- **Carbon Copy II foot** (see Fig. 4.4-3.E) consists of a solid-ankle rigid posterior bolt block made of reinforced nylon/Kevlar and combined with two flexible anterior deflection plates, which permit energy storage in accordance with activity level. It is encased in a realistic-looking Elastomer shell. The foot is as light as a geriatric SACH foot. Because the sole of this foot is flat, it improves mediolateral stability. The cost is higher than that of the Seattle foot. It is an excellent foot to be used by active unilateral transtibial and transfemoral amputees. It is 50% lighter than the Seattle foot.
- **Quantum modular foot** (see Fig. 4.4-3.F) consists of a long sole spring, a secondary spring, and an ankle base that are inserted in a hollow cosmetic foot module. It has anterior and posterior deflector plates shaped like an X, a multiple-axis ankle system, and a mechanism inside the cosmetically designed foot. The foot is assembled from stock components, which are chosen according to the patient's foot size, weight, and level of activity. Because it is modular, the foot and knee units are easy to interchange. The system is in the same price and weight range as the Carbon Copy II. It is only available for endoskeletal systems, but with the use of an adaptor, it can be aligned to an exoskeletal system.
- **Energizer (DynaSTEP) foot** (see Fig. 4.4-3.G) has a reversed C-shaped carbon heel that stores the energy of heel strike and transfers it to the pylon, propelling the tibia forward through the end of midstance. It has an extended carbon keel with a toe-plate extension that deflects and stores energy throughout the second half of stance, then releases the energy to provide an active push-off. When compared to the SACH foot, it significantly lowers the amputee's energy demand. It is waterproof and is dependable and durable. It can be used in patients up to 220 lb (100 kg). It can be combined with a multiaxis ankle.
- **Flex-foot** (see Fig. 4.4-3.H) is made from graphite composite to store energy during stance and to release it at toe-off. The Flex-foot keel extends to the bottom of the transtibial socket. The shank is also compressible, thus more energy storing. The foot is custom designed and fabricated for each amputee taking into consideration body weight and level of activity. This foot is light and is indicated for very active unilateral or bilateral transtibial amputees. It is best for runners. Its alignment can be cumbersome and the cost is high.

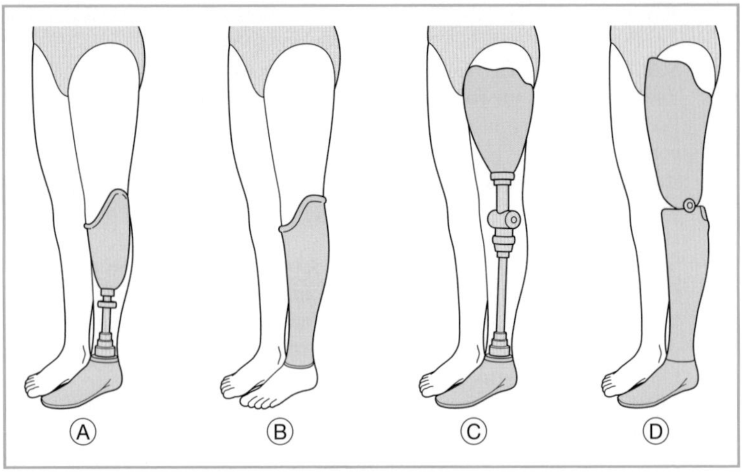

Figure 4.4-4 Endo- vs. exoskeletal lower-limb prostheses. **A**, Endoskeletal transtibial prosthesis (covered with soft rubber foam). **B**, Exoskeletal transtibial prosthesis. **C**, Endoskeletal transfemoral prosthesis (covered with soft rubber foam). **D**, Exoskeletal transfemoral prosthesis.

- **Flex-walk** (see Fig. 4.4-3.I) is a shorter version of the Flex-foot. It is lighter, less expensive, and ideal for less active individuals.

b. ***Articulated prosthetic feet***

I. **Single-axis prosthetic foot** (see Fig. 4.4-3.J) consists of separate foot and distal shank sections joined by a fixed metal axle around which the foot rotates into plantar and dorsiflexion. Ankle excursion is limited by a resilient plantar flexion bumper posteriorly and a moderately firm dorsiflexion stop anteriorly. Toe hyperextension occurs in a manner similar to the SACH foot. It is indicated for transtibial amputees who go up and down stairs and ramps and for transfemoral amputees.

II. **Multiple-axis prosthetic foot** (see Fig. 4.4-3.K) provides slight mediolateral (inversion/eversion) and transverse (rotation) motion in addition to sagittal movement. It is used by active individuals who run and have to ambulate in uneven terrain. The amputee may feel unstable with it because the foot is controlled by the rubber in the prosthesis and not by the patient. It is more complex, heavier, and costlier than the single-axis foot. It needs to be maintained at least every 6 months. Examples are Greisinger Ankle–Foot System, Dual Ankle Spring-Multi Axial Rotation System (DAS-MARS), McKendrick Ankle–Foot System, Masterstep Foot, Multiflex Ankle–Foot or Dynamic Response 2 Foot (Endolite) System, Graph-Lite, Energizer (DynaSTEP) foot/ankle system; and College Park Ankle–Foot System (Trustep foot).

2. **Shank** is the rigid portion of the prosthesis that connects the socket to the prosthetic foot. It restores leg length and shape, and transmits the amputee's body weight from the socket to the foot.

a. ***Endoskeletal shank*** (see Fig. 4.4-4.A) is a rigid metal or plastic pylon usually fitted with an adjustment mechanism to enable making slight changes in prosthetic alignment. The pylon can be covered with foam rubber shaped to resemble the contralateral limb. It is more attractive, lighter and, in the past was less durable than an exoskeletal shank. However, with the use of titanium, its strength is the same as, if not greater than, that of an exoskeletal shank.

b. ***Exoskeletal (crustacean) shank*** (see Fig. 4.4-4.B) is made of rigid material (either plastic foam or hollowed wood) carved to the shape of the contralateral

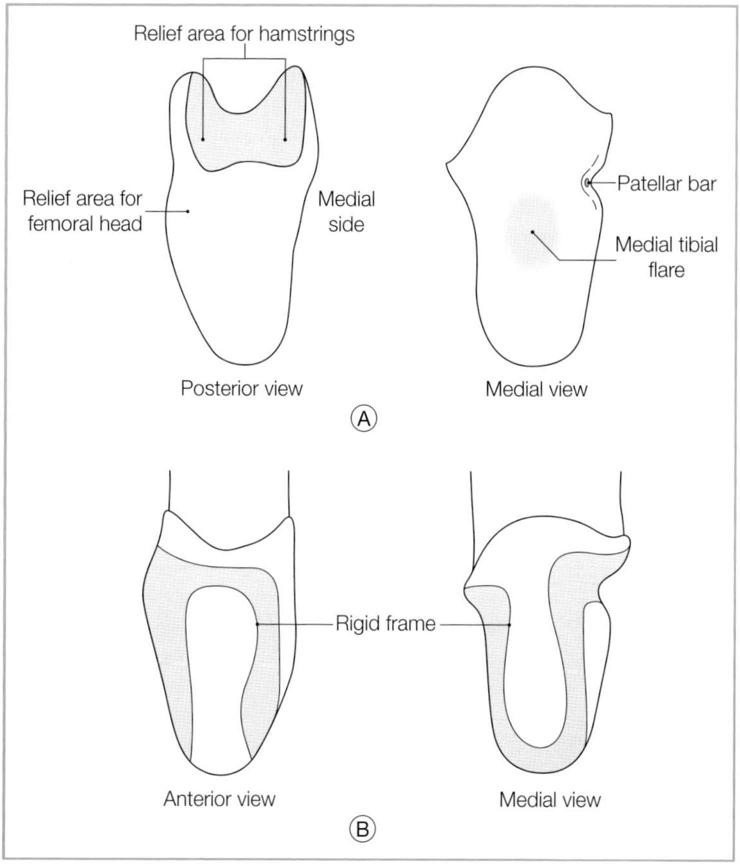

Figure 4.4-5 Transtibial sockets. **A**, Patellar tendon-bearing (PTB) socket. **B**, Icelandic–Swedish–New York University or ISNY socket (molded from a thin, flexible plastic and nested in a rigid padded frame). (From Kapp S, Cummings D: Prosthetic management. In Bowker JH, Michael JW, editors: *American Academy of Orthopedic Surgeons (AAOS) atlas of limb prosthetics: surgical, prosthetic, and rehabilitation principle*, ed 2, St Louis, 1992, Mosby-Year Book, pp. 454, 456 with permission.)

leg and covered with a thin layer of waterproof polyethylene or plastic laminate finish. Recently, acrylic lamination using I-beam construction (i.e., carbon fibers sandwiched between two layers of fiberglass) has become popular because it is lightweight but strong.

3. **Transtibial socket** is a receptacle that receives the transtibial residual limb. It can be molded entirely of rigid plastic with or without a resilient liner. Sockets lined with polyethylene foam liners (Pelite inserts) are used in elderly amputees with poor tissue covering of the residual limb or in amputees with continuing vascular problems, sensitive tissue, or fluctuating residual limb volume. The socket may be unlined (hard socket) for amputees who sweat profusely or whose residual limb is matured and has good tissue covering. An alternative socket design is to mold it from a thin, flexible plastic and nest it in a rigid padded frame [Icelandic–Swedish–New York University (ISNY) design, see Fig. 4.4-5.B]. The ISNY socket conforms more closely to the amputated limb but is not as durable.

a. ***Total contact (PTB socket;** see Fig. 4.4-5.A)* is the most commonly used socket for transtibial amputation. It is a custom-molded plastic socket, which

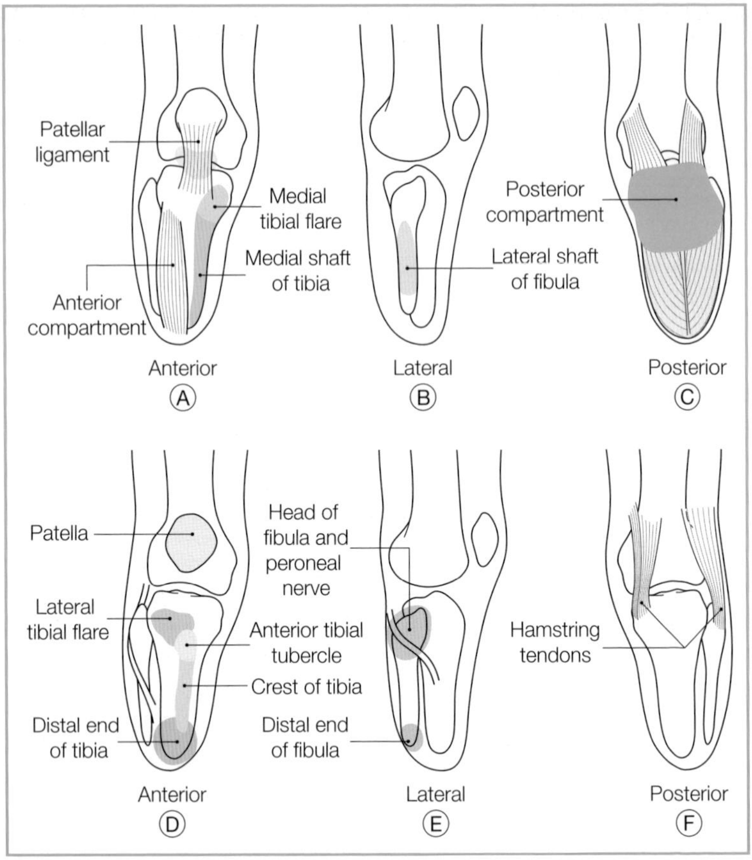

Figure 4.4-6 Pressure-tolerant (**A–C**) and pressure-relief (**D–F**) areas in a patellar tendon-bearing (PTB) socket. (From Kapp S, Cummings D: Prosthetic management. In Bowker JH, Michael JW, editors: *American Academy of Orthopedic Surgeons (AAOS) atlas of limb prosthetics: Surgical, prosthetic, and rehabilitation principle*, ed 2, St Louis, 1992, Mosby-Year Book, p. 468 with permission.)

distributes weight through convex build-ups (bulges) on pressure-tolerant areas (see Fig. 4.4-6.A–C) of the transtibial residual limb (i.e., patellar ligament or tendon, belly of the gastrocnemius, popliteal fossa, area of the pes anserinus, proximomedial tibia, pretibial muscle mass between the tibial crest and the fibula, lateral surface of the fibular shaft, and inferior surface of the medial tibial condyle). Although called a PTB socket, the patellar tendon only bears a moderate load. The socket also provides concavities or reliefs over pressure-sensitive areas (see Fig. 4.4-6.D–F; i.e., patella, tibial crest, anterior tibial tubercle, distal end of tibia, anterodistal tibia, fibular head, lateral distal end of the fibula, common peroneal nerve, and hamstring tendons). The socket is aligned on the shank in slight flexion (about 5°) to enhance loading on the patellar ligament, prevent genu recurvatum, resist the tendency of the residual limb to slide down the socket, and facilitate contraction of the quadriceps muscles. The socket is also aligned with a slight lateral tilt to reduce pressure on the fibular head. The intimate total-contact fit helps prevent edema, provides some additional support, and probably provides greater sensory feedback.

b. ***Total surface-bearing socket*** is less frequently used. It customizes pressure distribution within the socket through careful and extensive checking and adjustment of socket fit using a transparent socket (also called a check socket). Although theoretically better than the PTB socket, its goals are difficult to attain because the skin–socket interface pressure is constantly changing during active use of the prosthesis. Also, the residual limb can change in size and shape because of weight gain or loss, edema, and muscle function.

Recently, a **vacuum-assisted socket system (VASS)** has been incorporated in the total surface-bearing socket (Otto Bock VASS). Aside from a total surface-bearing socket, the Otto Bock VASS includes a urethane interface/liner, sealing sleeves, and a vacuum pump/shock absorber. The VASS is claimed to maintain a balanced volume in an amputee's residual limb, minimize limb movement in the socket, facilitate evaporation of perspiration within the socket, and reduce friction between the limb, liner, and socket. However, more studies are needed to show the effectiveness of the VASS in maintaining limb volume.

4. **Transtibial suspensions** are used to retain the prosthesis on the residual limb during swing phase.

a. ***Supracondylar cuff suspensions***

I. **Supracondylar cuff suspension (without fork strap or waist belt)** (see Fig. 4.4-7.A) is made of an adjustable leather or fabric strap that grips over the proximal patella anteriorly and wraps circumferentially around the thigh immediately above the femoral epicondyles. It is indicated in early prosthetic fittings when effective suspension is essential to protect the skin from shear forces during gait; in new amputees who need adjustable suspension or in whom residual limb shrinkage is anticipated; and in limited ambulators who spend the majority of their time sitting (because the supracondylar cuff is comfortable during sitting). It is contraindicated in patients with severely arthritic hands or limited vision who have difficulty engaging the buckle closure or pressure loop (Velcro) closure of the cuff; in patients who find straps cosmetically unacceptable; in patients with mediolateral knee instability or short residual limbs where problems with mediolateral knee control are anticipated; and in fleshy residual limbs with poor bony definition, hence making it difficult to attain suspension over the patella or femoral condyles.

II. **Supracondylar cuff** with fork strap and waist-belt suspension (see Fig. 4.4-7.B) is essentially a supracondylar cuff with a fork strap attached to the prosthesis distally and to the waist belt proximally. A part of the fork strap is always elastic to allow for the knee to flex during ambulation while maintaining tension for suspension at all times. It is indicated for active amputees with vigorous activities needing additional suspension during athletic activities and for amputees who climb ladders or participate in activities during which the prosthesis is unsupported by the ground for long periods.

b. ***Brim suspension*** retains the prosthesis by rigid extension of the socket brim proximally to cover the femoral epicondyles. It is easy to don and looks good when the wearer sits but is more difficult to fabricate, more expensive, and is not adjustable. It is difficult to suspend if the femoral condyles are not well-defined.

I. **Supracondylar (SC) brim suspension** (see Fig. 4.4-7.C) has medial and lateral walls that extend above the femoral epicondyles to increase the mediolateral knee stability of the prosthesis. The anterior area is cut out to accommodate the patella. The medial wall can either have a removable brim (see Fig. 4.4-7.D) or it can have a removable plastic wedge (see Fig. 4.4-7.E), which is inserted between the medial epicondyle and proximomedial socket wall to retain the prosthesis snugly on the residual limb. Instead of a removable medial brim or wedge, a compressible foam wedge build-up may be incorporated into the soft liner.

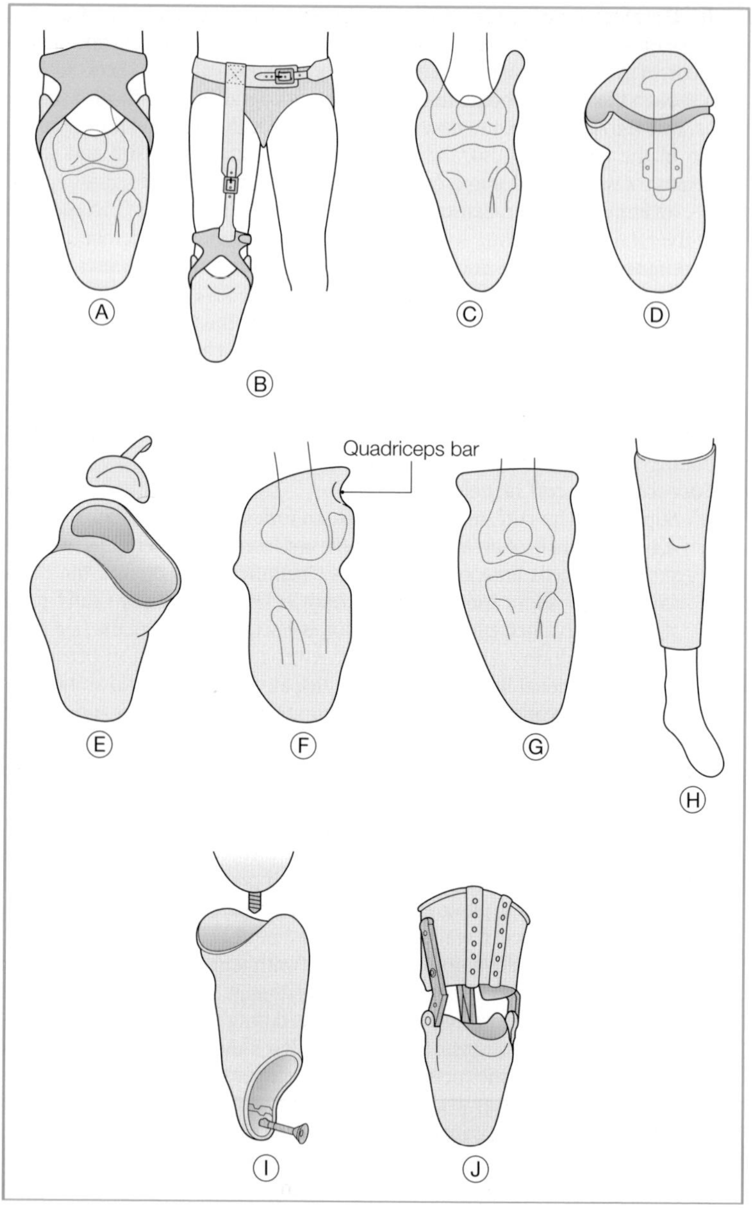

Figure 4.4-7 Knee suspension for transtibial prostheses. **A**, Supracondylar cuff suspension (without fork strap or waist belt). **B**, Supracondylar cuff with fork strap and waist belt suspension. **C**, Supracondylar (SC) brim suspension. **D**, Removable brim. **E**, Removable plastic wedge. **F**, **G**, Supracondylar/suprapatellar (SC/SP) brim suspension. **H**, Sleeve suspension. **I**, Silicone suction suspension (3 S; Residual limb with silicone liner is attached to the socket by a shuttle lock system). **J**, Joint and thigh corset suspension. (From Kapp S, Cummings D: Prosthetic management. In Bowker JH, Michael JW, editors: *American Academy of Orthopedic Surgeons (AAOS) atlas of limb prosthetics: surgical, prosthetic, and rehabilitation principle*, ed 2, St Louis, 1992, Mosby-Year Book, pp. 457, 459–462, with permission; Part I, silicone suction socket, reproduced with courtesy of Fillauer, Inc.)

II. **Supracondylar/suprapatellar (SC/SP) brim suspension** (see Fig. 4.4-7.F,G) is similar to the SC brim suspension with the addition of a high anterior socket margin ("quadriceps bar") that ends above the patella. It is used in transtibial amputations with short residual limb, which have a short lever arm and poor resistance of knee forces. It has more effective suspension and mediolateral knee control than an SC socket and also helps control genu recurvatum. However, the anterior socket bulk interferes with kneeling and looks conspicuous when sitting.

c. ***Sleeve suspension*** (see Fig. 4.4-7.H) uses sleeves of neoprene, latex, or other elastic material either as the primary suspension system or in conjunction with another suspension (e.g., SC suspension). The distal sleeve is rolled over the prosthetic socket, whereas the proximal end of the sleeve is rolled up over the thigh (extending a few inches above the prosthetic sock). This creates a smooth silhouette when the patient stands and sits. Sleeve suspension is accomplished through a combination of longitudinal tension in the sleeve and negative pressure during the swing phase, which results in a suction-type effect. It is indicated as an auxiliary suspension when added security is desired, control of positioning is essential, or when high activity levels create higher suspension demands. It may be used as a primary suspension with standard PTB trim lines for the same population that benefits from a supracondylar cuff. It is contraindicated as a primary suspension with standard PTB trim when mediolateral knee stability is questionable, hyperextension control is required, and when the residual limb is short. It should not be used if the patient has a fleshy thigh, perspires excessively (it may cause skin irritation), and lacks bimanual dexterity or strength to manipulate the sleeve.

d. ***Suction suspension (silicone suction suspension)*** (see Fig. 4.4-7.I) uses a flexible, molded silicone liner rolled directly onto the residual limb and secured to the outer rigid socket by a distal transverse rod or pin. It provides snug suspension without any prosthetic component contacting the thigh skin. Suspension is accomplished through longitudinal tension in the sleeve, tension between the sleeve and the residual limb, and negative pressure during the swing phase, which results in a suction-type effect between the limb and the liner. The liner may be incorporated into a socket with a soft interface material or a hard socket. Prosthetic socks are worn over the liner to accommodate changes in socket fit. Standard PTB trim lines are commonly used, which allow for the combination of a secure suspension with relative freedom of knee movements. It is indicated in amputees with greater suspension demands because of high activity levels, with short residual limbs for which suspension may be difficult, with residual limbs whose skin integrity is susceptible to shear forces and would thus benefit from a secure inherent suspension, and for whom standard PTB trim lines are adequate for knee stability. It is contraindicated in amputees with stability problems who would benefit from an alternative socket design with higher proximal socket walls and who lack the hand dexterity or strength to manipulate the silicone liner and the distal pin.

e. ***Joint and thigh corset suspension*** (see Fig. 4.4-7.J) uses a leather thigh corset connected to the prosthesis through metal joints and side bars. Suspension is achieved through the corset by its grip over the proximal patellar area or with the use of auxiliary suspensions (e.g., fork straps and waist belts). The metal uprights provide maximum mediolateral stability while the leather corset increases the weight-bearing area. It can shunt 40–60% of the body weight from the residual limb to the thigh via the thigh corset and is used when the patellar tendon cannot tolerate weight bearing or when the knee joint is painful or unstable. It is also used to control moderate to severe mediolateral knee instability and to control moderate to severe genu recurvatum by limiting knee extension. However, lacing or strapping the corset complicates donning and continued use can cause atrophy of the thigh muscles.

D. TRANSFEMORAL (ABOVE-KNEE) PROSTHESIS uses the same types of prosthetic feet and shank described under transtibial prosthesis. Prosthetic feet that are stable (e.g., single-axis or SACH-type feet) and shanks that are light (endoskeleton; see Fig. 4.4-3.C) are commonly prescribed for the transfemoral amputee. The socket and suspension components for transfemoral amputees differ from those used in transtibial amputees. In addition, the prosthesis for transfemoral amputees also requires a knee unit. A rotator (or shank torque-absorber rotator unit) may be placed between the knee unit and the socket to absorb shock in the transverse plane and protect the residual limb from chafing in active transfemoral amputees. Based on the prosthetic K levels (see Table 4.4-2), Medicare does not provide a prosthesis for the K-0, nonambulator. For the K-1 and K-2 levels or single-velocity (fixed cadence) ambulators, the knee unit selected must provide a constant friction-type of swing-rate control (see section I.D.1.b.1). Patients at the K-3 and K-4 levels are capable of variable cadence (multiple velocities), thus requiring a fluid-control or fluid-friction knee unit (see section I.D.1.b.2.b).

1. Knee units provide stability during walking (particularly during early stance) and allow the knee to bend when the patient sits and, in most cases, during the swing phase.

a. Knee-unit axes

I. **Single-axis knee unit for transfemoral prosthesis** is in the form of a transverse bolt that allows knee flexion and extension. It is simple to maintain, less costly, and has minimal noise.

II. **Polycentric-axes knee unit** has multiple (usually four-bar) linkage, which constantly shifts the knee axis so that the instantaneous center of rotation remains behind the weight line. Compared to the single-axis knee, it is more stable but is heavier, more costly, and needs more maintenance. It is indicated in amputees with a short transfemoral residual limb, knee disarticulation, or weak hip extensors.

b. Friction mechanisms are devices used in a swing-control knee to dampen the pendular action of the prosthetic knee during the swing phase to reduce the incidence of high heel rise in early swing and decrease terminal impact in late swing.

I. **Constant friction knee unit** applies uniform resistance throughout the swing phase by using a sleeve or split bushing and clamp that slide around the knee bolt. The friction can be adjusted by tightening or loosening the sleeve or bushing. It is the most commonly used friction mechanism because it is simple, low in cost, lightweight, quiet, and easy to adjust and maintain. However, it only allows one cadence and if the amputee walks faster or slower than the preset cadence, the swing becomes asymmetrical.

II. **Variable friction knee unit** applies greater friction at the beginning and at the end of the swing phase and less friction during midswing. It tends to be noisier, more costly, and to require more maintenance.

- **Sliding friction** is applied by contact of two solid structures that resist motion by moving against each other, such as a clamp on the knee bolt. It is rarely used.
- **Fluid friction** consists of an oil-filled hydraulic friction or air-filled pneumatic friction cylinder in which a piston connected to the knee hinge moves up and down. Fluid-friction knee units automatically compensate for changes in walking speed, increasing friction when the wearer walks faster. Recently, microprocessor-controlled knees with both hydraulic stance and swing-phase control have become available (e.g., Otto Bock's C-Leg). The C-Leg uses force sensors in the shin to determine stance phase stability and

a knee-angle sensor for control of the swing phase, angle, velocity, and direction of the moment created at the knee. The sensor information is then transferred to the hydraulic valve, allowing reaction to changing conditions. Although patients perceive C-Legs as favorable, their ability to facilitate walking on uneven ground and stairs remains controversial. C-Legs may reduce energy expenditure, but were not shown to reduce the cognitive effort required for walking (i.e., it did not require less cognitive demand than conventional prostheses).

c. ***Mechanical stabilizers*** increase the stability of the prosthetic knee unit by using a manual lock or a friction brake.

   I. **Manual lock** is a spring-loaded pin that automatically locks when the amputee stands and extends the knee. The knee is kept extended throughout the gait cycle to increase stability. Because of a lack of knee flexion, the prosthesis usually needs to be shortened by 1 cm to allow gait clearance. It is indicated for amputees who need utmost stability because of muscular weakness or poor coordination, for active amputees whose job requires prolonged standing, and for new, unstable amputees temporarily. To sit, the amputee raises the pin manually so that the knee can flex.

   II. **Weight-activated friction brake (stance-stabilized knee, safety knee)** commonly uses a spring-loaded wedge that is forced into a groove upon transfer of body weight to the prosthesis thus resisting knee flexion during early stance when the knee is flexed less than 25°. It is indicated in amputees with poor control of their residual limb. It can also be used by amputees in training who have a residual limb of functional length and who are capable of extending the knee and of ambulating. Several fluid-friction units incorporate stance-phase controls (e.g., the Mauch Hydraulic Swing and Stance unit) and are equipped with locking or braking action. The brake does not interfere with the swing phase or with sitting, but the unit is relatively heavy. Although durable, it must be maintained every 3–6 months.

d. ***Extension aids*** give additional mechanical assistance; they stretch during early swing as the knee flexes and recoil in late swing to aid knee extension and make heel contact more secure. They also help to restrain heel rise.

   I. **Internal extension aid** uses an elastic webbing or an extension lever with compression spring or tension spring attached inconspicuously within the knee unit. It does not protrude when the amputee is seated but can be noisy and difficult to adjust in some knee models.

   II. **External extension aid (fork strap, kick strap)** consists of an elastic strap (can be fork-shaped) placed externally in front of the knee and connected to a waist belt. It is simple, easy to adjust, and low in cost and maintenance.

2. **Transfemoral socket** can be molded in rigid plastic or in the ISNY design (i.e., molded in flexible plastic worn in a rigid frame). The flexible ISNY transfemoral socket is more comfortable, has adaptable shape, provides greater sensory input, and is cooler because body heat dissipates through the thin plastic walls. However, it is more expensive and not as durable as the rigid socket. Virtually all sockets have a total contact configuration with two basic socket shapes: quadrilateral and narrow mediolateral shape.

a. ***Quadrilateral (ischial-gluteal bearing) socket*** (see Fig. 4.4-8) has four distinct sides and corners. It is narrow from anterior to posterior and relatively wide mediolaterally. The posterior socket wall has a proximal brim lying directly under the ischial tuberosity and buttock and is intended for the majority of the weight bearing, thus relieving weight-bearing tasks from the distal pressure-sensitive areas of the residual limb. The anterior wall is higher than the posterior so as to apply posteriorly directed forces to maintain the position of the ischial tuberosity on the posterior brim. There is a prominent bulge over Scarpa's femoral triangle

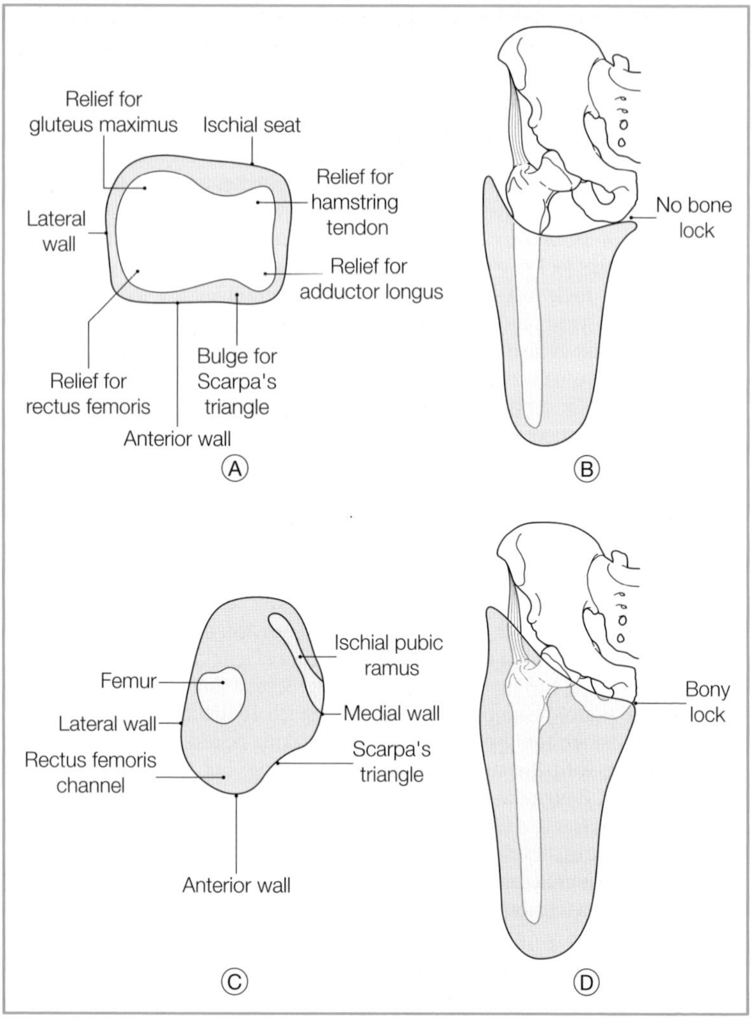

Figure 4.4-8 Transfemoral sockets. **A**, **B**, Quadrilateral transfemoral socket, top and anterior view. **C**, **D**, Ischial containment (or narrow mediolateral) transfemoral socket, top and anterior view. The ischial containment socket has a bony lock. (Adapted from: New York University Prosthetics and Orthotics Staff: *Lower limb prosthetics*, New York, 1993, Prosthetic-Orthotic Publications, p. 140; Sabolich J: Contoured adducted trochanter-controlled alignment method. *Clin Prosthet Orthot* 9:13, 17, 1985; Pritham CH: Biomechanics and shape of the above-knee socket considered in light of the ischial containment concept. *Prosthet Orthot Int* 14:14–15, 1990.)

for wide pressure distribution. Reliefs are located over the sensitive adductor longus and hamstring tendons and greater trochanter. Extra room is provided for expansion of the gluteus maximus when the muscle becomes tense. Although the design is based on sound anatomical and biomechanical principles, it has several problems including skin irritation at the ischium and pubis from the proximal brim, tenderness on the anterior distal femur, discomfort while sitting from either the anterior proximal brim or the rigid posterior socket wall, poor cosmesis with gapping of the lateral socket wall during stance, and frequent lateral lurch when walking.

b. ***Narrow mediolateral (narrow ML) or ischial containment (IC) socket*** (see Fig. 4.4-8) has a mediolateral dimension that is narrower than the anteroposterior measurement. The ischial tuberosity (which lies outside the socket in the quadrilateral design) is contained within the narrow ML (or IC) socket. Weight bearing, therefore, is focused primarily through the medial aspect of the ischium and the ischial ramus instead of the ischial tuberosity. The ischial tuberosity is locked in the socket and the resulting "bony lock" between ischium, trochanter, and lateral distal aspect of the femur gives a more stable mechanism for acceptance of perineal biomechanical forces, thus providing increased comfort in the groin and better control of pelvis and trunk. The narrow ML design is intended to maintain the femur in adduction although this may not always be feasible if the amputee has an uncorrectable deformity because of poor surgical technique. By keeping the femur in relative adduction during the stance phase, the hip abductors are kept in a more stretched and efficient position. The narrow ML socket can decrease neurovascular bundle compression and can be fitted to a short residual limb. It is more expensive and more difficult to fabricate than the quadrilateral socket. First-time prosthetic wearers may accommodate to the narrow ML design more readily than a long-time quadrilateral socket wearer. The narrow ML socket design developed by Ivan Long is called the Normal Shape-Normal Alignment (NSNA) socket while the narrow ML socket design developed by John Sabolich is called the Contoured Adducted Trochanteric-Controlled Alignment Method (CAT-CAM) socket.

3. **Transfemoral suspension mechanism**

a. ***Suction suspension*** (see Fig. 4.4-9.A) is the ideal suspension for patients with a middle to long transfemoral amputation residual limb.

   I. **Total suction suspension** is equipped with a one-way valve at the distal end of the socket that permits air to escape in the stance phase. Thus, pressure within the socket is less than atmospheric pressure so the socket remains on the thigh during the swing phase. It requires a snugly fitted socket worn without any sock because socks interfere with the airtight seal. A donning sock (open-ended stockinette) may be used to help in the donning process by applying it around the residual limb, putting the end of the stockinette through the valve hole. As the residual limb is inserted into the socket, the stockinette is removed by pulling it through the valve hole. An alternative way of donning is to lubricate the thigh and socket with a potato-based cream (e.g., Dry Lite) which dries readily. In most cases, the total suction suspension eliminates the need for wearing any belt around the torso (a silesian belt may be used in a very active individual), thus providing greater control of the prosthesis (particularly in rotation and abduction); increased use of the remaining musculatures; and better cosmesis. It also decreases piston action between limb and socket and is more comfortable. It is indicated in young, active amputees with a well-shaped, fairly strong residual limb. It is unsuitable for the elderly amputee or for those with cardiac conditions or poor cognition or poor balance and general weakness because of the relative difficulty of donning. It is unsuitable if the residual limb fluctuates in volume or has excessive redundant or flabby tissue. The presence of hypertrophic scarring, or deep, fissured scars may allow air to enter the socket, thus diminishing the effectiveness of the total suction suspension.

   II. **Partial suction suspension (silicone suspension)** provides an alternative for patients who cannot tolerate total suction suspension because of difficulty in donning the prosthesis, are unable to tolerate the prosthesis without

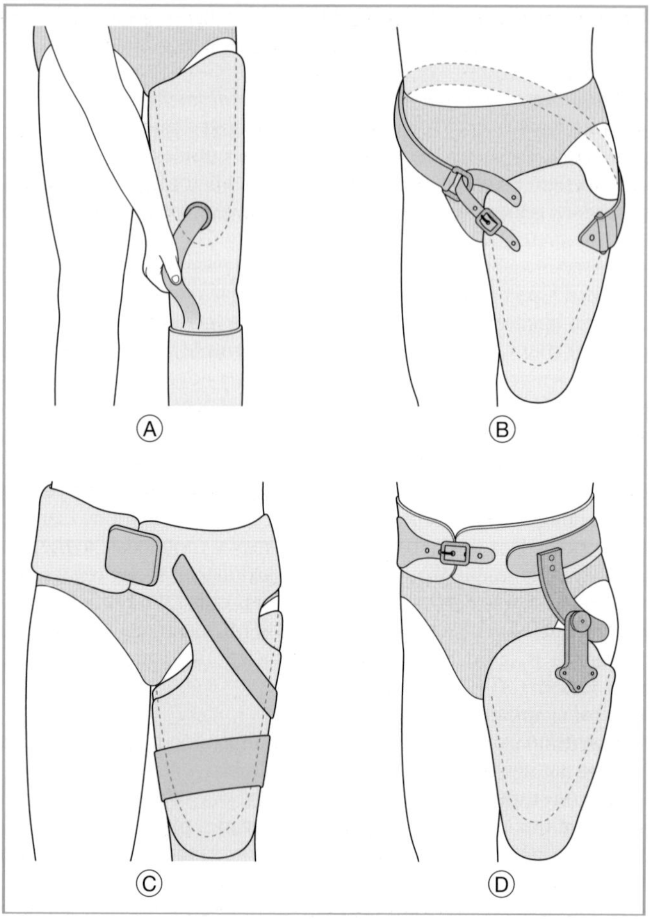

Figure 4.4-9 Transfemoral suspension. **A**, Suction suspension. **B**, Silesian belt. **C**, Total elastic suspension (TES) belt. **D**, Pelvic band and belt suspension with metal hip joint.

a sock, or have residual limbs that fluctuate in volume. It uses a hyperbaric sock with a 1-inch-wide (2.5 cm) silicone ring impregnated around its proximal end to create a seal between sock and socket. The lubricated ring, generally placed 2 inches (5 cm) below the ischium, is pushed into the socket to provide an air seal between socket and skin. A one-way valve in the distal end of the socket is used to expel air, just as in the total suction socket. Different sock piles may be used to accommodate fluctuations in residual-limb volume. Another method is to use a silicone locking liner in a socket with a suction valve, which may have a pin and shuttle lock or a lanyard-type locking system. This allows for volume fluctuation through the addition or removal of prosthetic socks. Longer limbs, however, may not allow sufficient space for the shuttle lock hardware and may result in a knee-center discrepancy. To prevent the prosthesis from dropping off the limb during swing phase (caused by the reduction of the intimate airtight fit because of the use of socks) or to provide rotational control caused by weak muscles or redundant tissue, an auxiliary suspension (usually a silesian belt or occasionally a rigid plastic or metal and leather pelvic band) may be used.

b. ***Nonsuction or belt suspension*** is provided by a socket that has no suction valve (it may have a distal hole that is plugged in case it needs to be converted to a suction type), hence one of the following pelvic belts is needed.

I. **Soft belts**

- **Silesian belt or bandage** (see Fig. 4.4-9.B) is made of leather, cotton webbing, or Dacron materials. It is attached to the socket in the area of the greater trochanter and passes as a belt around the back and opposite iliac crest, where it achieves most of its suspension. It then attaches anteriorly to the socket at either one or two points. It is simple to use, comfortable, and washable. It is used to prevent socket rotation encountered in limbs with significant redundant tissue. It is also used when the total elastic suspension (TES) belt (see below) fails to provide adequate suspension or rotational control. Often, it is used for temporary and intermediate prostheses, where suction is inappropriate because of decreasing limb volume. It is contraindicated in patients with significant hip instability or with weak abduction (in these patients, pelvic band and belt suspension would be a better option). It is also contraindicated in patients with scars, skin grafts, burns, or any other skin condition that would lie beneath the belt (in these patients a TES would be more appropriate).
- **Total elastic suspension (TES) belt** (see Fig. 4.4-9.C) is made of elastic neoprene materials and fits around the proximal 8 inches (20 cm) of the prosthesis and then around the waist and fastens anteriorly with Velcro. Because of its elastic nature, it can allow for vertical prosthetic displacement during the swing phase. It can be used as an auxiliary suspension for the patient who occasionally needs it for higher activities (e.g., sports). It enhances rotational control of the prosthesis and is quite comfortable; however, it retains body heat, has limited durability, and has the tendency to slide or rotate on the socket during strenuous activity. The newer TES (Powerbelt) is made entirely of elastic materials to prevent body heat build-up.

II. **Pelvic band and belt suspension** (see Fig. 4.4-9.D) made of rigid metal or semi-rigid plastic with a leather or fabric strap is connected to a metal hip joint at the lateral superior aspect of the socket. It is indicated for amputees who need rotational and mediolateral pelvic stability; obese amputees or those with significant redundant tissue that is difficult to stabilize; amputees with weak abductors or with short, weak, or poorly shaped amputation limbs. It is heavy and bulky, and tends to interfere with sitting comfort. The hip joint can be noisy, tear clothing, have maintenance problems, and contribute to excessive piston action of the thigh in the socket. The leather belt may absorb perspiration and cause skin problems.

E. DISARTICULATION PROSTHESES

1. **Knee disarticulation prosthesis** is not commonly used in the United States because knee disarticulation accounts for only 1–2% of all lower-limb amputations. A knee disarticulation surgery, as long as it is well-balanced, is preferred over a transtibial amputation surgery with very short residual limb (which is difficult to fit with a prosthesis), because patients with knee disarticulation can be fitted with high-functioning prostheses. The prosthetic feet are similar to those described for the transtibial prosthesis. The socket design is traditionally leather with a laced or buckled anterior opening to facilitate donning if the limb is bulbous. More modern sockets are made of molded polyester laminates with a window to accommodate donning of a bulbous residual limb. If the limb is not bulbous, it can fit readily into a nonfenestrated socket with plastic liner or compressible build-ups, or a removable insert may be used. The shape of the socket is usually quadrilateral to minimize rotation. Ordinarily, the knee disarticulation prosthesis requires no special provision for suspension other than snug fitting of

the socket around the bulbous, irregular contour of the distal residual limb. If the residual limb can tolerate full end bearing through the femoral shaft, the socket does not have to extend to the ischium. To control shank motion during the swing phase, older style prostheses use either side bars with single-axis knee joints and an extension aid or a conventional knee unit distal to the socket. New designs use a compact fluid-friction (hydraulic or pneumatic) unit housed in the hollow shank so that it does not protrude when the patient sits. A polycentric four-bar linkage axis may be used to provide knee stability. The polycentric hinges enable the shank to move behind the thigh section slightly to improve sitting appearance.

2. **Hip disarticulation and hemipelvectomy prostheses** use the "Canadian" design to achieve stance-phase stability while allowing flexion at the hip and knee during the swing phase. It is made of a molded plastic socket, which encloses the ischial tuberosity for weight bearing, extends over the iliac crest to provide suspension during the swing phase, and encases the contralateral pelvis to provide mediolateral trunk stability. The socket is attached to a mechanical hip joint, which is a hinge placed on the anterodistal aspect of the socket so that simple downward weight bearing stabilizes the joints against buckling. A posterior hip bumper is used to resist hyperextension. Any type of knee, shank, and foot may be used. The hip joint and the knee unit may each have an extension aid. An endoskeletal shank and thigh are customarily used to save weight.

II. Upper-limb prostheses

A prosthesis for an upper limb is used either as a cosmetic replacement (if it includes a prosthetic hand), or as a functional assistive device, or both, depending ultimately on the realistic goals of the amputee. For cosmetic purposes, the prosthetic hand should ideally imitate the color, size, and contour of the anatomic hand during activities and at rest. For functional purposes, a hook may be used instead of a hand. For both cosmetic and functional purposes, a mechanized hand with acceptable grasp force may be used. Because prostheses do not provide sensory feedback, many unilateral upper-limb amputees learn to do all their activities of daily living (ADLs) with their good hand and choose to function without any prostheses at all. As with lower-limb prostheses, the upper-limb prostheses should be lightweight, durable, easy to don and doff, comfortable when worn, capable of performing the prescribed function, and capable of providing total socket contact. Upper-limb prostheses should only be prescribed for patients who are motivated and have realistic expectations as to what the devices can do. The skin should be unblemished 10 minutes after prosthesis removal.

Functional upper-limb prostheses may be body controlled with body power (using cables and harness), myoelectrically controlled with electric power, or a combination of the two (hybrid, e.g., body control with electric power). Body-powered devices use proximal muscles to move the prosthesis through cables and harnesses. Myoelectrically operated devices are controlled by electromyographic signals from intact proximal muscles. Because the majority of acquired upper-limb amputations are caused by traumatic work injuries, most of these active amputees are initially fitted with a body-powered prosthesis to accomplish manual work and outdoor activities. After their residual limb has matured, a myoelectrically controlled elbow or hand may be considered for unilateral, proximal arm amputees with white-collar jobs. For the bilateral upper-limb amputee, a myoelectrically controlled elbow with hooks is usually used. However, a body-powered prosthesis should also be available for backup in case of electrical component malfunction in bilateral upper-limb amputees.

Components for above-elbow (see Fig. 4.4-10) and shoulder disarticulation prostheses include a terminal device (hand or hook), a wrist unit, a mechanical elbow

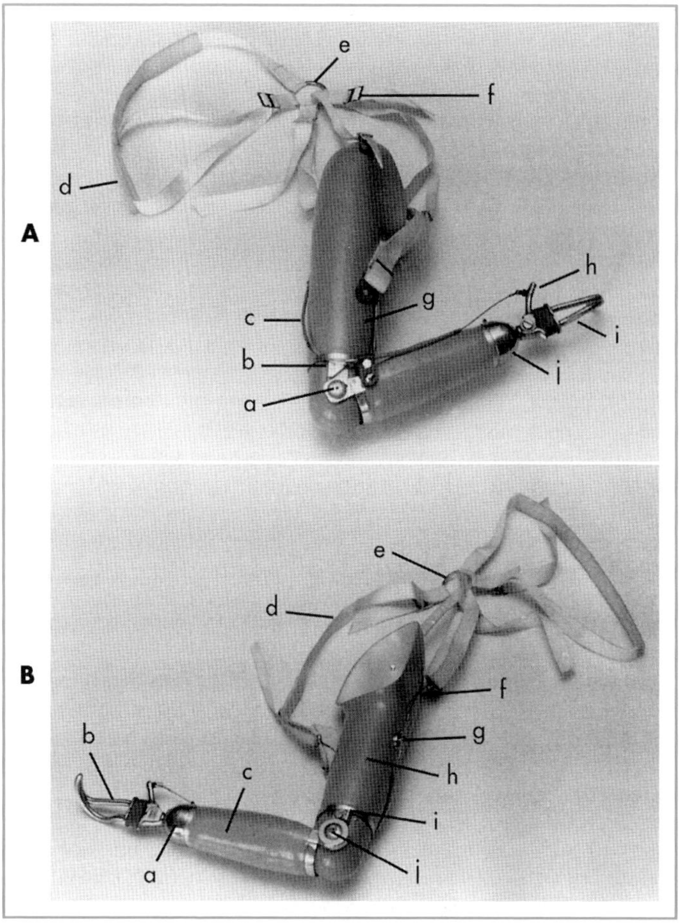

Figure 4.4-10 Transhumeral (above-elbow) prostheses. **A**, Lateral side of transhumeral prosthesis: a, Elbow unit; b, Turntable; c, Control cable; d, Adjustable axilla loop; e, Harness ring; f, Figure-of-eight harness; g, Elbow lock cable; h, Terminal device (TD) thumb; i, Hook TD; j, Wrist flexion unit. **B**, Medial side of transhumeral prosthesis: a, Wrist unit; b, Hook TD; c, Forearm; d, Harness; e, Harness ring; f, Control cable; g, Baseplate and retainer; h, Socket; i, Turntable; j, Spring-loading device. (From Keenan DD, Rock LM: Upper extremity amputations. In Pedretti LW, Early MB, editors: *Occupational therapy practice skills for physical dysfunction,* ed 5, St Louis, 2001, Mosby, p. 933, with permission.)

unit, socket, suspension, upper-arm cuff or pad, and harness and control elements. A below-elbow prosthesis has basically the same components as an above-elbow prosthesis, except that instead of a mechanical elbow unit, it may have an elbow hinge. A wrist disarticulation prosthesis does not have any elbow components at all.

A. PARTIAL HAND PROSTHESIS is prescribed to restore a more normal appearance, protect hypersensitive or fragile areas (e.g., neuroma and grafted skin), and improve grasp (prehension). A cosmetic hand or finger also serves an important functional role by providing opposition to a remaining mobile finger or by lengthening a residual finger that is too short. Partial prostheses used to restore grasp can have static or dynamic configurations. Static devices are nonarticulated and are constructed to perform a specific task under rugged conditions of factory work or manual labor (e.g., handling shovels or rakes). Dynamic devices are articulated and powered by residual motions at the wrist or palm to enhance grasp.

B. TRANSRADIAL (BELOW-ELBOW) PROSTHESIS AND WRIST DISARTICULATION PROSTHESIS

1. **Terminal devices (TDs) or hand substitutes** are used in all upper-limb prostheses for amputation at the wrist level and above (see levels of upper-limb amputation in Fig. 4.4-1).

a. ***Passive TDs*** have no functional mechanism and do not provide grasps. Whether prefabricated or custom made, they should be relatively lightweight.

I. **Passive hand** is intended for cosmetic effect only. It can be covered by a cosmetic glove, which can be custom made or, more often, selected from models manufactured in a wide range of skin tones.

II. **Flexible passive TDs** are mitt-shaped TDs used to absorb shock and store and release energy during ball sports and other activities. They are manufactured by Therapeutic Recreations Systems (Super Sport series).

b. ***Active TDs*** are used to replace the grasp (prehension) function of the hand. The active TD, however, is unable to manipulate objects because of the absence of sensory feedback and the absence of individual control of the individual fingers of the prosthetic hand. In a unilateral amputee, the active TD is used as a helper and is not usually required for intricate movements, which can be done with the good hand. The TDs that open voluntarily are used more commonly than the voluntary-closing TDs.

I. **Hooks** consist of two fingers made of aluminum lined with synthetic rubber (e.g., neoprene) or of steel, in split-hook design that is either canted or lyre-shaped. It provides lateral prehension and is slender enough to be used in restricted areas. It is superior for grasping small objects because it does not obstruct the amputee's visual feedback as much as the bulkier insensate fingers of the prosthetic hand. It is lighter in weight, more durable, has lower cost, and is easier to maintain than a hand TD. Manufacturers of hooks include Dorrance, Army Prosthetic Research Laboratory (APRL), Sierra, Otto-Bock, and Therapeutic Recreation Systems (TRS). Newer, more functional designs include the Grip TD and the Adept TD (both by TRS), the Utah TD (by University of Utah, and the CAPP (Child Amputee Prosthetics Program) TD (by Hosmer). The Lite-Touch Biomechanical Hands with realistic anatomical features on the fingers and thumb are voluntary-closing (VC) hooks available from TRS, Otto-Bach, and Hosmer.

- **Voluntary-opening (VO) hook** is a curved and split hook in which sturdy rubber bands maintain the closed position. The pinch force is determined by the number and type of rubber bands [each rubber band provides about 1 lb of pinch force (450 g)]. The amputee uses cable control powered by proximal muscles to open the hook fingers against the force of the rubber band. The rubber band then acts as a spring to close the hook. In a myoelectrically controlled hook, the electric motor turns in the opposite direction to close the hook.
- **Voluntary-closing (VC) hook** is maintained in an open position and has to be closed voluntarily by cable control or myoelectric control. It is seldom used because it is heavier and less durable than the VO hooks. Most models have a lock to keep them closed (for cosmetic reasons) when not in use. Some models (e.g., Sierra VC hook) have a self-locking feature that automatically locks the hook in the grasp position as soon as the amputee relaxes, enabling the patient to hold on to an object without exerting continued force. This makes it suitable for fine work. However, it has durability and maintenance problems. The Adept VC (by TRS) TD has voluntary closing

function that gives sensory input by allowing the amputee to "feel", by the amount of tension in the cable, how much gripping force is being exerted.

II. **Hands provide palmar prehension** by allowing the amputee to move the thumb, index, and middle finger through body power (using cable) or myoelectric control with electric power. The ring and little fingers remain passive. Compared to hooks, hands are more cosmetic and can be used for grasping a large or round object or just the handle of a tool. However, they are bulkier and heavier than the hooks. The myoelectrically controlled hand initiates palmar tip grasp by contraction of residual forearm flexor musculatures and releases the hand by contraction of residual forearm extensor musculatures. Hence, it is preferred by many patients because it does not require any external harness as in cable-controlled hands. Manufacturers of VO hands are Dorrance, Sierra, Otto Bock, and Becker and Robins Aid.

- **Voluntary-opening hand** operates on the same principle as the VO hooks, i.e., springs in the hand close the fingers and produce a modest grasp force.
- **Voluntary-closing hand** provides control of prehension with automatic locking in various grasp positions.

III. **Nonhand, nonhook (Stanford) design** prostheses that can either be voluntarily opened or voluntarily closed and with improved aesthetics are being developed.

2. **Wrist units** are metal devices used for attaching TDs (hooks or hands) to the anatomic wrist area at the distal end of the socket. They position the TD into the best position for accomplishing a desired activity and also permit interchange of TD from hook to a hand and vice versa. Wrist units can be positioned passively (by using the sound hand or by pushing the TD against any part of the body or any surface) or by electric power [e.g., Otto Bock Electric Wrist Rotator, Sierra Wrist Flexion Unit, Hosmer Flexion–Friction Wrist, and United States Manufacturing Company (USMC) E-Z Flex Wrist].

a. ***Wrist friction (rotation) units*** hold the TD in the desired pronation or supination position by means of friction resistance provided by a rubber washer or a bushing.

b. ***Quick disconnect/locking wrist units*** allow the amputee to quickly interchange TDs. They are useful in amputees who use more than one TD or are routinely performing activities that require the elimination of any unwanted wrist rotation during functional performance. Some models have a locking feature that prevents inadvertent rotation of the TD in the wrist unit when a heavy object is grasped. The lock, however, complicates prosthetic use, because the amputee must lock and unlock whenever repositioning the TD.

c. ***Wrist flexion units*** allow the TD to flex and are used on the dominant side (i.e., the side of the longer residual limb regardless of previous dominance) of the bilateral upper-limb amputees for activities close to the midline of the body (e.g., for buttoning and shaving). The hook on the nondominant side is used to position the unit in 0°, 25°, or 50° of wrist flexion. Wrist flexion units are not useful for unilateral amputees because they generally prefer to use their good hand.

3. **Socket designs** for transradial amputation and wrist disarticulation are determined by the type of suspension desired and the length of the residual limb. All transradial and wrist disarticulation socket designs have "double wall" construction with the inner wall (the socket *per se*) providing a snug, total-contact fit, including the distal end of the residual limb. The outer wall is shaped and sized to match the contours and length of the contralateral forearm. The socket extends proximoposteriorly to the olecranon and proximoanteriorly to the elbow crease. The shorter the residual limb is, the closer is the trimline to the crease. For wrist disarticulation or for long transradial residual limb (see Fig. 4.4-1 for levels of upper-limb amputation), the volar and dorsal walls of the inner socket are compressed distally so as to capture and transmit as much

Table 4.4-3	Recommended elbow hinges for wrist disarticulation and transradial amputations
UE amputations	**Recommended elbow hinges**
Wrist disarticulation	Flexible elbow hinge
Long transradial (55–90%)	Flexible elbow hinge
Short transradial (35–55%)	Single-axis rigid elbow hinge; May use flexible elbow hinge for longer residual limb
Very short transradial (<35%) or if elbow range of motion is limited	Polycentric rigid-elbow hinge or split socket with step-up and locking rigid-elbow hinge

pronation and supination as possible (see Fig. 4.4-1 comparing residual rotation of amputated forearm vs. normal forearm). An alternative socket design is the ISNY flexible socket, which is made of thin translucent polyethylene with a rigid frame consisting of slender medial and lateral laminates. The thin flexible ISNY socket provides increased function, comfort, and sensory feedback.

a. ***Harness-suspended socket design*** uses a harnessing system to suspend the socket from the involved and uninvolved shoulders. The harness is connected to an upper arm half-cuff or a triceps pad, which is then connected to the elbow hinge and socket. The arm half-cuff or triceps pad helps provide socket suspension and stability in addition to serving as an anchor for the control-cable reaction point. The **arm half-cuff** is used in short transradial fittings, while the **triceps pad** is used with long transradial, wrist disarticulation, and with transmetacarpal prostheses.
b. ***Self-suspended socket design*** is less cumbersome and more popular than the harness-suspended socket design. Although harness (usually figure-of-nine harness) is seldom used for suspension, it may still be used for control of a TD.
   I. **Suprastyloid suspension** uses silicone bladder, or window/door suspension with elasticized closure, or soft removable inserts that grip the styloids. It is indicated for wrist disarticulation amputations with prominent styloids.
   II. **Sleeve suspension** uses latex rubber to provide atmospheric pressure suspension, elastic sleeves to provide a skin traction suspension, or neoprene to provide a combination of atmospheric pressure and skin traction suspension.
   III. **Supracondylar brim suspension** retains the prosthesis by enclosing and capturing the humeral epicondyles and the posterior olecranon. It does not allow forearm rotation and sacrifices range of motion for power and stability (i.e., the lesser the range of motion allowed, the greater power it has).
   - **Munster supracondylar socket** is used for short transradial amputation.
   - **Northwestern University socket** is used for midlength transradial amputation.
   - **Modified supracondylar brim with olecranon cutout** is used for long transradial amputations.
   - **Floating brim suspension** is used for long transradial and wrist disarticulation amputations.
   - **Silicone locking liners with locking pin** can also be used in long residual limbs.
c. ***Split socket*** is a special design that consists of a total-contact segment encasing the residual limb and connected by hinges to a separate forearm shell to which the wrist unit and TD are attached. Split socket is used for very short residual limbs so that special elbow hinges (e.g., step-up elbow hinge and locking elbow hinge) can be used.

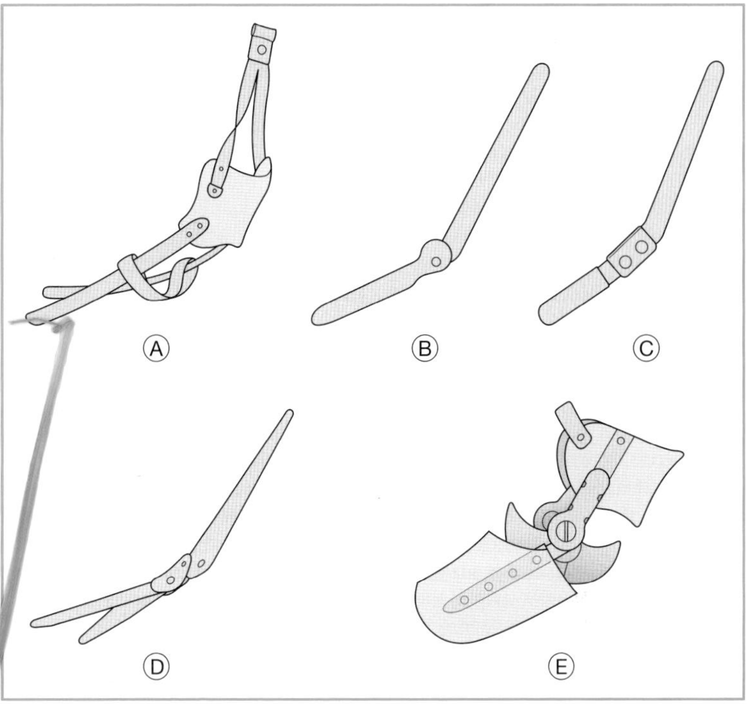

Figure 4.4-11 Elbow hinges for transradial prostheses. **A**. Flexible elbow hinge; **B**. Rigid elbow hinge, single axis; **C**. Rigid elbow hinge; polycentric; **D**. Step-up elbow hinge; **E**. Residual limb-activated locking elbow hinge.

4. **Elbow hinges** connect the socket to a cuff or a pad on the upper arm and are important for suspension and stability. Their selection depends primarily on the site of amputation and the residual function (see Table 4.4-3).

a. ***Flexible elbow hinge*** (see Fig. 4.4-11.A) can be made out of triple-thickness Dacron webbing or flexible metal cable and is used primarily to suspend the forearm socket. It is used where sufficient voluntary pronation and supination (as well as elbow flexion and extension) are available, i.e., in wrist disarticulation and long transradial amputation.

b. ***Rigid elbow hinge*** is used for short transradial amputation where normal elbow flexion is present but little or no voluntary pronation–supination is available and additional stability about the elbow is needed.

   I. **Single-axis rigid elbow hinge** (see Fig. 4.4-11.B) is used to provide stability when socket rotation around the very short transradial residual limb becomes a problem.

   II. **Polycentric rigid elbow hinge** (see Fig. 4.4-11.C) uses a gear that has mating teeth to impart a displacing action to the socket during elbow flexion and provide clearance for bunching of flesh in the crook of the elbow of amputees with fleshy arms.

   III. **Step-up elbow hinge** (see Fig. 4.4-11.D) uses a gear or double-pivot arrangement that permits the residual limb to drive the prosthetic forearm through an increased range of movement. It is connected to a socket with split-socket design and is indicated in amputees with very short transradial residual limbs.

- **Gear-type step-up elbow hinge** has a step-up ratio of 2:1, i.e., the forearm shell of the split socket flexes 2° for every 1° of residual limb flexion. Although the ROM is doubled, the energy cost is doubled also, hence cutting the strength in half.
- **Double-pivot type step-up elbow hinge** has an average step-up ratio of 3:2.

c. ***Residual limb-activated locking elbow hinge*** (see Fig. 4.4-11.E), together with a split socket (see section II.B.3.c) prosthesis and a dual control system, is used for amputees with very short transradial residual limbs and very limited range of motion or lifting force. The cable that operates the TD is used to lift the forearm to the desired position whereupon the elbow is locked by a small amount of residual limb motion. Once the elbow is locked, the cable can then be used to operate the TD.

5. **Harness suspension and control systems** for transradial and wrist disarticulation prostheses are used to suspend the prosthesis from the shoulders so the socket is held firmly onto the residual limb and to transmit force from shoulder and scapular motion via a cable system to operate the TD. The harness is usually unnecessary with passive and myoelectrically controlled prostheses with self-suspended socket.

a. ***Figure-of-eight harness*** (see Fig. 4.4-10.A) is the most commonly used harness in prostheses with harness-suspended socket. It has an axilla loop worn on the sound side, which acts as a reaction point for the transmission of the body force to the TD. The upper strap of the axillary loop runs diagonally across and down the back towards the posterior part of the prosthesis; while the lower strap runs diagonally across and up the back and over to the anterior shoulder of the amputated limb where it connects to the prosthesis via an inverted Y-suspensor strap. This front support strap carries most of the axial loads. The crossing point of the two diagonal straps on the back (which can be connected by an O-shaped metal ring) should be below C7 and slightly to the sound side.

b. ***Cross-chest strap harness with shoulder saddle*** consists of a shoulder saddle on the side of the amputated limb, which is connected to a chest strap looped around the opposite axilla. The shoulder saddle is connected to a loop suspensor, which is then connected to the socket through an arm half-cuff or triceps pad. It is used in amputees who cannot tolerate axillary pressure from an axilla loop or in amputees who do a great deal of heavy lifting. This hardness tends to rotate upon the chest when excessive forces are applied to the control cable.

c. ***Figure-of-nine harness*** consists of an axillary loop on the sound side with a diagonal strap that runs across and down the back and attaches to a control strap on the prosthetic limb. It is lighter and provides greater freedom and comfort by the elimination of usual front support strap, triceps pad, or cuff, etc. It is used in self-suspended transradial socket that requires a harness only for controlling the TD.

6. **TD control system** for transradial prostheses can be either body powered or electrically powered. Body-powered units have moderate costs, are moderately lightweight, are most durable, and provide the highest sensory feedback. However, they require the most body movement and the most harnessing to operate, and they are the least cosmetically pleasing. On the other hand, electrically powered units require the least body movement with moderate or no harnessing to operate and provide more function at proximal levels and moderate cosmesis. However, they are heavy, expensive, delicate, hard to maintain, and have limited sensory feedback.

a. ***Body-powered (cable-activated) TDs*** use forces from the shoulder and scapula transmitted via harnesses and cables to operate the TD. The cable system used is the single-control (Bowden control) cable system, which consists of a single continuous flexible stranded stainless steel cable, which can slide inside a flexible tube or housing. This housing has terminal fittings that connect one end of the cable to a harnessed body-control point and the other end to a point of operation of the TD. When the amputee flexes the ipsilateral shoulder (or abducts the scapulae for functions close to the body midline), the motion tenses the cable attached proximally to the harness and distally to the TD. The length of the control cable is maintained constant by the cable housing, thus the same amount of body motion is required to operate a TD regardless of elbow joint angle.

b. ***Electrically powered TDs*** are controlled by switches or myoelectric signals and are powered with energy supplied from external batteries (e.g., rechargeable nickel cadmium batteries, which can be mounted on or within the prosthesis). The electrically powered TD can be hand-like (Otto Bock System Electric Hands and Steeper Electric Hand) or nonhand-like in appearance (Otto Bock System Electric Greifer, Hosmer NU-VA Synergistic Prehensor, and Steeper Powered Gripper).

I. **Myoelectrically controlled TD** uses surface electrodes placed on the muscles of the residual limb. Myoelectric signals from the muscles are picked up by the surface electrodes, amplified into volts to activate an electric switch (myoswitch), and cause electricity to flow from a battery to an electric motor, thus activating the TD. The TD function (i.e., speed and force) can be controlled either in a constant manner or in proportion to the amplitude of the myoelectric signals (i.e., strength of muscle contraction).

- **Two-site, two-function myoelectric controller** uses two sites for attachment of the electrodes (e.g., the wrist extensors and wrist flexors of the residual limb) to open and close the TD. It is used in Otto Bock Myoelectric Hand, Steeper Electric Hand, Otto Bock System Electric Greifer, Hosmer NU-VA Synergistic Prehensor, and Steeper Powered Gripper.
- **One-site, two-function myoelectric controller ("double channel")** uses a myoelectric signal from one muscle to control both opening and closing of the TD, depending on the amplitude with respect to one of two thresholds (e.g., weak contraction closes the TD and strong contraction opens the TD). It is used in Otto Bock Myoelectric Hand, Steeper Electric Hand, Otto Bock System Electric Greifer, Steeper Powered Gripper, and University of New Brunswick controller.
- **One-site, one-function myoelectric controller** is used if the amputee does not have two good myoelectric sites or in very young limb-deficient children. It is used in Cookie Crusher Hand and Steeper Powered Gripper. The NYU-Hosmer Prehension Actuator uses a single-site, single-function myoswitch to open a cable-actuated VO split hook.

II. **Microswitch-controlled TD** uses either a push-button electromechanical switch, which can be activated by a bony prominence, or a pull-switch, which is incorporated in a harness or cable. It is used in the Otto Bock System Electric Hands and Otto Bock System Electric Greifer.

C. TRANSHUMERAL (ABOVE-ELBOW) PROSTHESIS AND ELBOW DISARTICULATION PROSTHESIS (see Fig. 4.4-10) uses the same TD and wrist units described under transradial (or below-elbow) prostheses. However, the socket, harness, and control systems differ from those used in transradial prostheses. In addition, transhumeral prostheses require an elbow unit. Most upper-limb prostheses are exoskeletal. When active function is not a significant goal, however, an endoskeletal prostheses may be used to improve cosmesis and conserve weight. The endoskeletal prosthesis consists of a TD, a wrist module, and a lightweight forearm and humeral pylon covered with a cosmetic foam interconnected by a manually controlled, ratchet locking elbow unit. The following components are for active and functional transhumeral and elbow disarticulation prostheses.

1. **Sockets** for transhumeral and wrist disarticulation prostheses have a double construction similar to the transradial sockets. The lateral socket wall extends up to the acromion (or higher in the case of unusually short transhumeral residual limbs), while the medial socket wall is flattened below the axilla to help prevent inadvertent socket rotation. Elbow disarticulation prostheses have sockets that are flat and broad distally to conform to the anatomic configuration of the epicondyles of the distal humerus and provide the amputee with active control of humeral rotation. An alternative socket design is the ISNY flexible socket (see section I.C.3).
2. **Elbow units** consist of hinge and cable systems, which can be locked to position and maintain the prosthesis at various elbow flexion angles. Most have an alternator lock, in which one pull of the cable locks the hinge and the next pull unlocks it. The pulling movement used to lock or unlock the unit is usually a combination of shoulder depression, extension, and abduction. The amputee unlocks the elbow unit and selects the desired angle of flexion by exerting tension on the elbow flexion cable. The elbow unit is then locked so that the same cable can be used to activate the TD. Most elbow units also provide passive humeral rotation to enable the TD to be positioned for a desired function. This is accomplished by means of a turntable between the elbow unit and the upper arm shell or socket. As with wrist units, friction between the elbow unit and the turntable allows control of the rotation to maintain the desired plane of elbow operation.

a. ***Elbow flexion-locking system***

I. **External flexion-locking elbow** is used with the elbow disarticulation prosthesis because there is not enough space for the internal locking mechanism.

II. **Internal flexion-locking elbow** is used for transhumeral and shoulder prostheses. An internal spring-assist for elbow flexion may be used by amputees who have difficulty flexing their prosthetic forearms.

b. ***Elbow and TD control system*** (see section II.B.6 for the advantages and disadvantages of body-powered vs. electric-powered control systems).

I. **Body-powered (cable-activated) elbow units** transmit forces from the shoulder and scapula via harnesses and cables to lock and unlock the elbow, flex the elbow, and operate the TD. The cable control used consists of two separate cable systems. The first cable system (single-control cable) is used to lock and unlock the elbow, while the second cable system uses a dual-control (or fair-lead control) cable, which consists of one cable with two functions (i.e., to flex the elbow unit when the elbow is unlocked and to operate the TD when the elbow is locked). The usual sequence of cable control is as follows: the unlocked elbow is flexed to the desired position using the dual-control (fair-lead) cable; then the first single-control cable system is used to lock the elbow (by any two combinations of the following shoulder motions: extension, abduction, and depression; usually shoulder extension and abduction are used). When the elbow is locked, the TD can be activated via the dual-control cable system by either shoulder flexion or scapular abduction or chest expansion. When the desired TD function is accomplished, the elbow can be extended by unlocking it using the single-control cable (the same shoulder movement combination for locking the elbow unit is used to unlock the elbow).

II. **Electrically powered elbow units** are powered from a battery and controlled by myoelectric signals or microswitches.

- **Myoelectrically controlled elbow units** uses amplified myoelectric signals picked up from surface electrodes placed on the residual arm. Examples are the Utah Elbow and the Utah Arm, which use the biceps and the triceps for two-site, two-function, proportional control of the elbow.

- **Microswitch-controlled elbow units** uses push-buttons for activation by a bony prominence or a pull switch, which is incorporated in a harness. They are used in Boston (Liberty Mutual) Elbow and NY-Hosmer Electric Elbow.

III. **Hybrid control system** combines electric and body (cable) control system. The hybrid control/power approach has reasonable proprioceptive qualities and allows simultaneous coordinated control of elbow and prehensor function.

- **Hybrid cable-controlled elbow with myoelectric TD** is used for long transhumeral or elbow disarticulation prostheses. Although it has increased TD pinch strength, the electric TD adds weight to the forearm making it harder to lift.
- **Hybrid electric elbow with cable-controlled TD** uses the Boston (or Liberty Mutual) Elbow in conjunction with a cable-controlled (body-actuated) TD. The cable-controlled TD requires less maintenance but has lower TD pinch strength and is uncosmetic.
- **Hybrid cable-controlled elbow with motorized locks** is used in the Steeper Electric Elbow Lock, but myoelectric or microswitches are used to lock the cable-actuated elbow.

3. **Transhumeral harness and control** suspends the prosthesis from the shoulders and transmits power from the shoulder to flex the prosthetic elbow, to lock and unlock the elbow unit, and to operate the TD. It uses modifications of the basic figure-of-eight harness or a shoulder saddle with chest strap patterns similar to those used for the transradial prostheses.

D. **SHOULDER DISARTICULATION PROSTHESES AND FOREQUARTER PROSTHESES** have prosthetic TD and elbow units similar to the transhumeral prostheses. However, their socket and harness/control systems differ from the transhumeral prostheses. In addition, they have a shoulder unit. Although functional shoulder disarticulation and forequarter prostheses are available, most amputees prefer a cosmetic shoulder cap or an endoskeletal prosthesis, which can be passively positioned by the opposite hand. This is because of the lack of proximal muscles for cable operation on the involved side and the complexity of actions required for the shoulder prostheses to be functional.

1. **Sockets** for shoulder disarticulation and forequarter prostheses extend onto the thorax to suspend and stabilize the prosthesis. They are also suspended by chest straps attached anteriorly and posteriorly to the socket.

a. ***Enclosed socket*** is made of plastic laminate to encircle the shoulder and formed to its contours.

b. ***Frame socket*** uses padded metal strips (or stiff, carbon-reinforced laminates) to form a frame that encompasses the shoulder and the trunk, extending down to the fifth rib. It provides structural mounting points for the prostheses and location and reference points for a variety of controls.

2. **Shoulder unit**

a. ***Motionless shoulder unit*** consists of a monolithic construction in which the humeral section and shoulder socket are laminated together, and no motion between these components is possible.

b. ***Friction-controlled passive-motion shoulder unit*** allows passive positioning of the shoulder joint in flexion–extension and abduction–adduction. Passive abduction of the humeral section is convenient for dressing and for sitting in a chair with arms. An abduction–flexion joint allows abduction and flexion, while the universal shoulder joint can be used to permit motion in all the planes.

3. **Harness suspension and control system** for shoulder prosthesis has a chest strap that is attached to the anterior and posterior aspects of the laminated shoulder section. An elastic suspensor strap helps to stabilize the shoulder section and permits movement of the shoulder girdle. The harness and control assembly usually includes a waist band with a strap connected to the elbow lock

control cable. The waist band stabilizes the distal end of the elbow lock control strap so that shoulder elevation can work the elbow lock.

4. **Control system** for shoulder prostheses commonly uses shoulder girdle flexion (i.e., biscapular abduction) for elbow flexion and TD operation and shoulder elevation for elbow locking and unlocking. Other control mechanisms for operation of the elbow lock include pulling with the good hand or using a "chin-nudge" button.

a. ***Cable-controlled (body-powered) system***

I. **Dual-control (or fair-lead control) cable system** similar to that used in a transhumeral prosthesis is traditionally used for body-powered control of the elbow unit and TD in shoulder prostheses.

II. **Triple-cable system** is a newer alternative in cable control for shoulder prostheses. It uses three cables, each providing a distinct function. One cable, attached to the forearm shell and an axilla loop, provides active elbow flexion when the contralateral shoulder is flexed. A second cable, attached to the chest strap and the TD, provides TD opening with chest expansion. The third cable, attached to the elbow lock and a nudge control, locks and unlocks the elbow when the nudge control is depressed by the chin or contralateral hand.

b. ***Electrically powered control systems*** are usually used because it is difficult to provide body-powered control motion of sufficient strength.

Further reading

Bowker JH, Michael JW, editors: *Atlas of limb prosthetics: surgical, prosthetic, and rehabilitation principles – American Academy of Orthopedic Surgeons*, ed 2, St Louis, 1992, Mosby-Year Book.

Bussell MH, editor: New developments in prosthetics and orthotics. *Phys Med Rehabil Clin North Am* 11(3):477–720, 2000.

Faculty of Prosthetics and Orthotics, New York University School of Medicine and Post-Graduate Medical School: *Upper-limb prosthetics*, New York, 1986, Prosthetic-Orthotic Publications.

Gitter A, Bosker G: Upper and lower extremity prosthetics. In DeLisa JA, Gans BM, Walsh NE, *et al.*, editors: *Physical medicine and rehabilitation: principles and practice*, ed 4, Philadelphia, 2005, Lippincott, Williams & Wilkins, pp. 1325–1354.

Wilson Jr AB: *A primer on limb prosthetics*, Springfield, IL, 1998, Charles C Thomas.

Washington State Department of Labor and Industries: *Technology Assessment*. Available at: http://www.lni.wa.gov/ClaimsInsurance/Providers/TreatmentGuidelines/TechAssess/default.asp. Accessed July 17, 2004.

CHAPTER 4.5
Adaptations for activities of daily living

Functional independence in the performance of activities of daily living (ADL) can enhance the positive self-image and quality of life of the disabled person. Its attainment can be limited by various conditions that cause limitations in range of motion (ROM), strength, endurance, coordination, dexterity, balance, sensation, vision, cognition, and perception. The detailed evaluation of these functional limitations (see Chapter 2.8 for functional scales) as well as their specific ADL adaptations are typically carried out by an occupational therapist (except in certain aspects of ADL, e.g., transfers and functional ambulation, in which the physical therapist is primarily involved) with input from other members of the interdisciplinary rehabilitation team.

The goals for ADL adaptation are generally to improve living space, minimize costs of self-care independence, and decrease the time and energy required to safely perform ADLs. Any ADL adaptation must maximize the patient's function within the constraints of limited time, money, and the patient's potential for improvement. Factors to consider in the long-term selection of adaptive or assistive devices include effectiveness in improving ADL and in attaining functional independence, affordability (aside from the purchase cost, also consider the costs of maintenance and repair), operability (i.e., is it easy to use as well as don and doff? does it respond adequately to demands?), dependability (i.e., does it operate with predictable levels of accuracy under conditions of reasonable use?), disease progression, and, ultimately, the patient's motivation or desire to use it.

This chapter includes the general and specific principles for ADL adaptation as well as specific adaptations for basic ADLs (i.e., self-care tasks) and the more advanced instrumental ADLs (i.e., tasks beyond caring for oneself that involve complex interaction with the physical and social environment, including occupational adaptations). ADL adaptations include disposable medical products, for example, medical, nursing, and urinary supplies, prosthetic devices (see Chapter 4.4), orthotic devices (see Chapter 4.3), durable medical products, such as wheelchairs (see Chapter 4.7), gait aids (see Chapter 4.6), bathing equipment, accessibility products (e.g., lifts, ramps, and hand controls), and self-care adaptive or assistive devices described in this chapter. Although the major focus of the chapter is on adaptations for sensory/motor deficits, it must be noted that all ADL adaptations should also incorporate cognitive–perceptual–visual components. For details on ADL adaptations, the reader is referred to any major textbook in occupational therapy (see Further reading section). For a more comprehensive listing of addresses of vendors of adaptive devices, associations, and other resources for disabled persons, refer to *The complete directory for people with disabilities*, Greyhouse Publishing, Pocket Knife Square, Lakeville, CT 06039, tel. (800) 562-2139 or (860) 435-0868.

I. Principles for ADL adaptation

A. GENERAL PRINCIPLES FOR ADL ADAPTATION

1. Modification of the task, the method of accomplishing the task, and the environment.
2. Instruction and training on joint protection and energy conservation.
3. Safe use of assistive devices (i.e., devices that give support) or adaptive devices (i.e., devices that are made fit or suitable, often by modification).

B. SPECIFIC PRINCIPLES FOR ADL ADAPTATION

1. **Adaptations for limited ROM** include using adaptations to increase reach, eliminate the need to bend over, and compensate for limited grasp; storing frequently used items within reach; and using joint-protection techniques (e.g., in patients with rheumatoid arthritis). From an upright wheelchair sitting position, the vertical range of reach is from 20 to 48 inches (51–122 cm) and the maximum functional horizontal reach is considered 18 inches (46 cm) from the edge of a desk or work surface. In general, patients with good trunk control have greater reaching capacity.
2. **Adaptations for weakness** include using lightweight objects, utensils, and tools; allowing gravity to assist; using adaptive equipment or methods to replace lost functions such as grasp; using powered tools and utensils; using biomechanical principles (e.g., improving leverage in body mechanics and increasing friction to decrease the power needed for pinch or grasp); and using two hands. For hemiplegics, specific principles for ADL adaptations include providing substitution for the stabilizing or holding function of the involved upper limb and adapting bilateral activities so they can be performed unilaterally.
3. **Adaptations for low endurance** include using energy conservation methods, pacing work to prevent fatigue, using principles listed for weakness that reduce workload (e.g., lightweight utensils and powered equipment), matching activity demands to ability, avoiding stressful positions (e.g., bending over, reaching overhead, isometric contractions such as pushing, pulling, and maintained grasp), and environmental stressors (e.g., hot humid environment and overexertion). Energy conservation techniques (see also Chapter 5.12, section IV.B.7) include planning ahead and organizing work; combining tasks to eliminate extra work and eliminating unnecessary tasks; preparing and obtaining all the required equipment before starting a task; using electrical appliances to conserve personal energy; using lightweight utensils and tools; working with gravity assisting, rather than resisting; sitting down when working; and resting before fatigue sets in.
4. **Adaptations for incoordination or poor dexterity** include stabilizing the object being worked on; stabilizing proximal limb segments so that control can be concentrated on the distal limb segments; adding weight to the distal segments; using heavy utensils, cooking equipment, tools, etc.; using adaptive equipment that reduces slipperiness and provides stability; and using adaptations that substitute for lack of fine motor skills.
5. **Adaptations for limited vision** include organizing so everything is kept in its proper place; using Braille labels to distinguish canned goods, clothing colors, etc.; using techniques and devices that magnify words or images and provide high contrast; increasing illumination and using adaptive equipment that provides auditory, tactile, or kinesthetic feedback to compensate for low vision or blindness.
6. **Adaptations for decreased sensation** include protecting the anesthetic part from abrasions, bruises, cuts, burns, and decubiti; substituting vision for poor awareness of limbs and limb movement or to detect texture change; and directing attention to the affected part on a regular basis (e.g., using a long-handled mirror for skin inspection or using a specialized timer that beeps every 15 minutes to remind a person to perform a pressure relief maneuver).

7. **Adaptations for cognitive and perceptual deficits** are discussed in Chapter 5.5, sections I.B and II.

II. Classification of ADLs and their specific adaptations

A. **BASIC ADL (B-ADL)** include mobility, self-maintenance activities (i.e., feeding, grooming, dressing, bathing, personal hygiene, toileting, menstrual care, and skin management), communication, and sexual expression. Driving, which can be considered a component of mobility, is not described here as it involves more advanced skills (see community-living skills under instrumental-ADL in section II.B.2.f).

1. **Positioning** in bed (e.g., when resting or sleeping) or chair (e.g., wheelchair) is important in preventing pressure ulcers, contractures, dislocations, and other deformities. Positioning is also important as preparation for other ADLs (e.g., transfers, dressing, sexual acts, sports, work, etc.), exercises, and other interventions. Specifics on different positioning for orthotics are discussed in Chapter 5.2, section VI.B.1.

a. ***Bed-positioning adaptations*** include hourglass-shaped foam leg spacers (e.g., for maintenance of the lower limb and spine alignment in side-lying positions), supporting wedges for the back or limbs, triangular-shaped hip abduction wedge cushions (with straps), modified pillows (e.g., pillows with recessed center or head cradles and neck rolls), blanket cradles to protect sensitive skin (e.g., healing skin grafts) from weight of the blanket, and modified mattresses and other limb positioners or supporters for the prevention of pressure ulcers (discussed in Chapter 5.2, section VI.B).

b. ***Seating positioning adaptations*** include abductor wedge cushions (with or without straps), padded knee or leg spreaders (made of metal or flexible plastic), and wheelchair seating adaptations (discussed in Chapter 4.7, section I.A.3.b).

2. **Mobility** is the ability to move from one position in space (whether sitting, lying down, standing, etc.) to another position in space regardless of the distance between the two positions. For independent bed mobility and transfers, patients may use webbing loops (applied around legs or thighs so they can be lifted by the upper limbs). A half or quarter bed siderail may also be used for bed mobility or for enabling transfer. However, when using bed siderails, the potential for head or limb entrapment must be carefully assessed.

a. ***Bed mobility*** is the ability to turn over in bed (i.e., rolling side to side), to scoot up, down, or toward either edge of the bed, or to come to a sitting position at the edge of the bed. In addition to motor planning skills, the patient should have adequate head and trunk control as well as upper-limb strength and endurance.

   I. **Overhead trapeze bars** can be used to assist in scooting up or down in bed and in helping the patient come to a sitting position at the edge of the bed. Trapeze bars can be attached onto the bed through an orthopedic frame or can be mounted on the wall for home use.

   II. **Loops** can be attached along the edge of the bed or bed railings to help the patient with inadequate trunk strength to use the upper limbs to pull himself or herself to either side when rolling. Ladder-like loops have rungs spaced for progressive hand or arm placement when the patient is pulling himself or herself up from supine.

   III. **Electric beds** can be used to raise or lower the head of the bed and assist the patient in coming to a sitting position.

b. ***Transfers*** refer to short-distance movements from one surface to another (e.g., to and from bed and wheelchair or commode and to and from wheelchair and tub or car seat). If another person is needed to assist transfers, a transfer or ambulation belt (with or without handles) may be looped around the patient's waist for easy grasping by the assisting person.

I. **Stand-pivot transfer (SPT)** is indicated if weight bearing on the lower limbs is possible or permitted in patients with adequate hip and knee extension and good sitting balance. The patient rises from a seated to a standing position and pivots to the adjacent surface to sit down. This can be done independently or with the supervision or assistance of another person. Prior to SPT, a step stool may be used as an intermediate step between the bed and the floor. If the patient is unable to stand up fully, a variation called bent-pivot transfer may be used in which the patient is kept in a bent-knee position to maintain equal weight bearing as the assisting person provides optimal trunk and lower-limb support during the pivot transfer. Adaptations to assist in sit-to-stand transfers include: cushions to raise up seat height, air or spring cushions that expand posteriorly as the patient leans forward thus assisting patient rise, side rails (home models are also available), and bilateral push-up frames.

II. **Sit-pivot transfer (depression transfer)** is indicated in patients who are unable to bear weight on their lower limbs but have strong upper limbs enabling them to depress their scapulae (and extend elbows) to lift their buttocks off one surface onto another surface without coming to a standing position. The patient should have good sitting balance.

III. **Swivel-trapeze transfer** is indicated in patients who are unable to bear weight on their lower limbs but whose upper limbs are strong enough to lift half of their body weight. The patients hold onto the swivel trapeze bar (attached to the bed via an orthopedic frame or wall-mounted for home use), pull themselves off the bed, then swing their body onto another surface. This may be done independently or with the assistance of another person (to swing the lower part of the body).

IV. **Sliding board transfer (SBT)** is indicated in patients who are unable to bear weight on their lower limbs but whose upper limbs are not strong enough to lift their buttocks off the sitting surface. It uses a sliding board to bridge the gap between transfer sites. The basic sliding board is usually made of a flat, sturdy, smooth wood or rigid plastic, which can either be short (if used for toilet transfers) or long (if used for wheelchair to car transfers). Some modifications of the basic sliding board include slots for easy gripping; notches on one end, which can be secured to the wheelchair armrest for stability; the addition of rolling balls, sliding or rotating disks for ease of transfer; or offset designs that are shaped to fit around the wheel on the wheelchair when the armrest is removed. Once the sliding board is positioned securely between the surfaces, the patient positions his or her buttocks on one end of the board, and, with the aid of the upper limbs (or another person), scoots across the board to the new surface. If strong enough, the patient may do a series of small shoulder depressions instead of "sliding". The patient should have good sitting balance. Powder can be used on the board to diminish friction.

V. **Lift transfer** is indicated if the patient is unable to move at all. It may be carried out with the assistance of one person (e.g., logroll transfer or one-person carry transfer), or more than one person (e.g., two- or three-person carry transfer). It may also be done by using a sling-style lift with a mechanical jack (e.g., Hoyer lift or Trans-Aid lift) or hydraulic lift.

VI. **Floor transfer (e.g., wheelchair-to-floor or floor-to-wheelchair)** is indicated for wheelchair users with sufficient upper-limb strength for transferring to and from the wheelchair and the floor (e.g., for floor mat exercises or in case of a fall). This may be accomplished independently or with the assistance of another person. If necessary, a small bench may be used as an intermediate step between the wheelchair seat and the floor.

c. ***Wheelchair mobility*** is used for attaining functional independence in the community for patients who cannot ambulate or can ambulate only for short distances. Proper positioning in the wheelchair, good sitting tolerance, strength, endurance, and cognitive skills are necessary for efficient and safe wheelchair mobility. Wheelchair and seating prescriptions are described in Chapter 4.7.

d. ***Functional ambulation*** refers to walking with an aid (e.g., walker) to accomplish a task (e.g., putting clothes into the closet). It is described in Chapter 4.6.

3. **Self-maintenance tasks** include feeding, dressing, grooming and personal hygiene, bathing, and toileting. The following sections list the adaptations commonly prescribed for patients with limited ROM, weakness, incoordination, poor dexterity, and/or low endurance. Most patients need lightweight utensils or devices, except patients with incoordination who need weighted or heavy equipment to maintain steadiness. Plastic or unbreakable materials are preferred. Specifications for environmental adaptations related to self-maintenance tasks (i.e., barrier-free architectural designs of bathroom, toilet, sinks, countertops, closets, etc.) are described in section II.B.1.

a. ***Feeding*** requires adequate upper-limb ROM, coordination, and strength to scoop and bring the hand to the mouth from a surface while grasping a utensil or cup. It also requires the ability to manipulate utensils and to cut food, as well as the ability to suck, to close the lips around the utensil, to manipulate the bolus with the tongue, and to chew and swallow the food (for dysphagia care, see Chapter 5.6).

I. **Spoon and fork adaptations** include modified handles to improve grip (e.g., built-up handles with foam; plastic-molded, nylon-coated, or polypropylene handles; flexible or adjustable handles; swivel handles; curved handles; long extension handles; handles with palmar cuffs; handles that fit easily onto utensil holders), spoon–fork combinations or sporks (e.g., regular, offset, or swivel type) for patients with limited wrist supination and radial deviation, weighted and/or coated utensils for patients with incoordination, spatula spoons with flat shallow bowls for soft foods, and holders that grip sandwiches (which can be inserted onto a utensil holder).

II. **Knife adaptations** include modified knives (e.g., rocker knife, which cuts food by rocking down on food, rather than the traditional sliding method, which requires stabilization of the food with a fork in the opposite hand, or roller knife or pizza-cutter knife for one-handed use); knife and fork combinations (e.g., rocker knife with fork edges or fork with cutting edge on the side prong); modified knife handles to improve grip (e.g., nonslip handles, wooden handles, or cuff-handle); and serrated knife to facilitate cutting.

III. **Dish adaptations** include scoop dishes, which are deep bowl-like dishes that prevent food slippage (e.g., round or oval scoop dish, high-sided scoop dish, scooper bowl, scoop plate, plate with inside edge, divided or partitioned scoop dish or scoop plate, scoop dish with lid and bowl, and scoop dish with suction cups or nonskid mat) and food guards, which are C-shaped plastic or stainless steel attachments that can be clipped onto a shallow plate to prevent food slippage.

IV. **Drinking utensil adaptations** include lid adaptations for oral weakness (e.g., lids with snorkel or spout or nipple-shaped lids); drinking utensils with spout, nipple, or a cutout for the nose so a person can drink without neck extension; drinking utensils adapted to assist grasp (e.g., T-shaped handles, bilateral handles, or foam insulation); weighted drinking utensils (for uncoordinated patients); drinking utensil holders, which can be clipped onto the wheelchair; base extensions to prevent tipping of drinking utensils (e.g., when drinking with straws); straws (one-way straws, long straws, reusable straws, or disposable straws); and straw holders.

V. **Self-feeders** include electric self-feeders with elevated set-ups for plate and spoon (which can be activated by slight head movement) for bilateral upper limb weakness, balanced forearm orthoses (also called mobile arm supports, ball-bearing feeder, or linkage feeder; see Chapter 4.3, section II.C.3.b), and suspension arm slings (see Chapter 4.3, section II.C.1.d.5), which support the forearm and arm to assist horizontal arm movement and elbow flexion in patients with weak (at least Tr+ to poor P−) shoulder and elbow muscles.

VI. **General feeding adaptations** include utensil holders, that is splints that can be attached to various utensils, for example universal cuffs with straps, webbings with straps, splints (e.g., long opponens splints or externally powered splints for C5 tetraplegics) with utensil slots, palmar clips or palmar cuffs with utensil pockets, and wrist supports with palmar clips and utensil pockets. General feeding adaptations also include feeding accessories such as plate stabilizers (e.g., nonskid mats, suction bases, or damp dishtowels) and food or crumb catchers (e.g., terry cloth, vinyl, or disposable materials).

b. ***Dressing*** involves putting on and taking off clothing, along with managing fasteners (i.e., buttons, zippers, and snaps) and handling accessories such as belts, socks, and shoes. It is contraindicated in patients with unstable spines; pressure ulcers or a tendency for skin breakdown during rolling, scooting, and transferring; uncontrollable muscle spasms in legs; and 50% or less vital capacity (especially for lower-limb dressing).

The minimum criteria for upper-limb dressing include: (a) fair to good muscle strength in the deltoids, upper and middle trapezii, shoulder rotators, rhomboids, biceps, supinators, and radial wrist extensors; (b) ROM of 0–90° in shoulder flexion and abduction, 0–80° in shoulder internal rotation, 0–30° in shoulder external rotation, and 15–140° in elbow flexion; (c) adequate sitting balance in bed or wheelchair, which may be achieved with the assistance of bedrails, an electric hospital bed, or wheelchair safety belts; and (d) adequate finger prehension, which may be achieved by using tenodesis grasp or wrist-driven flexor-hinge orthosis.

For dressing of the lower limbs, the following are needed in addition to the minimum criteria for upper-limb dressing: (a) adequate balance and strength to pull up underwear, pants, or skirt (i.e., fair to good muscle strength in pectoralis major and minor, serratus anterior, and rhomboid major and minor muscles); (b) adequate ROM to reach the feet to don shoes and socks (i.e., ROM of 0–120° in knee flexion, 0–110° in hip flexion, and 0–80° in hip external rotation); (c) adequate body control for transfer from bed to wheelchair with minimal assistance; (d) ability to roll from side to side, balance in side-lying, or turning from supine to prone position and back; and the ability to lift the buttocks to allow items to be pulled to the waist; and (e) vital capacity of 50% or more. For tips and techniques to make dressing easier in people with disabilities, refer to: *Dressing tips and clothing resources for making life easier,* 933 Chapel Hill Road, Madison, WI 53711, (608) 274-4380.

I. **Dressing material adaptations** include touch fasteners (e.g., Velcro), button hooks (i.e., wire loops, which hook around the button and are then pulled through the button holes; and various handles available including built-up foam handles), large buttons, zipper pulls (hook that attaches to zipper tab, zippers with loops or rings on the tab), combination buttoner–zipper pulls (loops attached to bendable metal cuffs that can be contoured to fit the palm), cuff and collar button extenders, and modified shoelaces (e.g., elastic shoelaces, which are similar to the regular cloth laces except the laces do not need to be untied or retied each time because they stretch as a person places the foot into the shoe; clipped-on shoe fastener units, which tighten or loosen laces by pinching the unit; shoe buttons on which lace can be wrapped to maintain tightness; and lace locks through which laces can be threaded and tightness can be adjusted by sliding a plastic knob to lock the shoelace in position).

II. **Dressing style adaptations** include front-fastening garments (e.g., bra with front closure), cardigan or slip-on garments instead of pull-over garments in patients with inadequate over-head shoulder movement, buttoned items in patients with inadequate over-head shoulder ROM but with fine motor skills to manipulate buttons, large or loose-fitting clothes to facilitate donning and doffing, pants and shorts with elastic waistbands and cuffs, garments with Velcro closures (e.g., bra or trousers), clip-on ties, and slip-on or loafer shoes.

III. **General dressing adaptations** include reachers or grabbers (which are extended sticks, usually made of lightweight aluminum, with a grasping unit at the end, which is operated by squeezing the handle to activate the gripper to open and close; they may be adapted for tetraplegics by using a special orthosis that can activate the reacher through wrist tenodesis), dressing sticks or wands (i.e., long sticks with a hook at the end), trouser pulls (webbing loops that can be hooked onto trouser belts), modified shoehorns (e.g., long-handled or spring-action), and stocking or pantyhose or sock aids (i.e., flexible plastic cores or fabric frames that can hold stockings or pantyhose or socks open, so they can be pulled up the legs via cords attached to the plastic core or fabric frame).

c. ***Grooming and personal hygiene*** consists of grooming (e.g., shaving; hair combing or brushing; caring for nails; application of facial makeup such as face powder, lipstick, and mascara; and application of antiperspirant, cologne, or perfume) and oral hygiene (e.g., brushing of teeth or dentures and flossing) activities. To perform grooming and hygiene skills, a person must have adequate upper-limb ROM and strength, adequate coordination and hand function, and adequate trunk control and sitting balance.

I. **Grooming adaptations** include shaving aids (e.g., electric shavers, universal electric-shaver holders, razor holders with cuffs that can be contoured to the palm, and clamp-on shaving cream dispenser handle), hair grooming aids (e.g., extension comb and hairbrush, hairbrush with Velcro handles, and straps with Velcro fasteners, which can be attached to hairbrushes), nail grooming aids (e.g., nail clippers, files, or brushes which can be stabilized, attached to a board with suction cups; and long-reach angled toenail scissors), facial makeup aids (e.g., spray powder, long handled powder puffs, and weighted wrist-cuffs for steadiness in makeup application), and modified mirrors (e.g., portable mirrors with suction cups, magnification mirrors, and adjustable mirrors with gooseneck).

II. **Oral hygiene adaptations** include toothbrush aids (e.g., electric toothbrush, self-rotating toothbrush with horizontal palm handle, and toothbrush attached to a base with suction cups), toothpaste dispenser aids (e.g., toothpaste pumps with large handles, which dispense a fixed amount of toothpaste; and tube squeezers), floss aids (e.g., large handle base that holds the floss upright), disposable foam tips for oral hygiene, and WaterPiks.

III. **General grooming/personal hygiene adaptations** include universal cuffs or custom-made palmar cuffs, splints with slots for hygiene-care devices, adjustable grooming extenders (e.g., long handles attached to washcloths, combs, or hairbrushes), a cord attached to grooming or hygiene care products (e.g., razor, lipstick, soap, and toothbrush) for easy pickup when dropped, use of spray mechanism (e.g., spray deodorant, spray cologne, hair spray, spray powder, or spray perfume), adapters with large handles for aerosol cans, use of large roll-on deodorants (instead of sprays or creams), short reachers, and balanced forearm orthosis (see Chapter 4.3, section II.C.3.b) or suspension arm slings (see Chapter 4.3, section II.C.1.d.5) for patients with weak (at least Tr+ to poor P−) shoulder and elbow muscles.

d. ***Bathing*** includes body cleaning or washing (e.g., using showers, bathtubs, sponge baths, or body cleaning by the sink), hairwashing or shampooing, and drying after washing. To use the shower or bathtub, the patient needs to perform gross motor mobility skills (i.e., patient needs adequate upper-limb ROM/strength, fine motor coordination, and transfer/sitting balance to get in and out of the bathtub or shower safely, to sit or stand for the activity, and to perform the cleansing activity) in a slippery environment. Environmental adaptations (see section II.B.1.b.3) that assist with bathing and safety include placement of grab bars outside and inside the bathing area, placement of nonskid strips inside the tub, extended handles on faucets, and automatic water temperature controls. For patients with a roll-in shower, a wheelchair commode or shower chair is recommended.

   I. **Bathing mobility adaptations** include a tub transfer bench, which has two legs in the tub and two legs outside the tub for safe means of transfer to and from wheelchair; a cushion inflated with water, which can form a rigid support for transfer; a bath chair, stool, or seat with suction feet; a wheeled shower chair; a bath board, which can be fitted onto the tub for seating; safety rails; wall grab bars; tub grab bars; and nonskid mats.

   II. **Body washing and shampooing adaptations** include long-handled bath sponge or bath brush (the handle may be flexible, straight, or curved); soap aids (e.g., soap-on-a-rope for easy pickup of dropped soap; bath mitt with soap pocket; soap grippers, i.e., finger cuffs with suction cups attached to the soap; pump dispensers); bath mitts (e.g., sponge, mesh, or terrycloth mitts); hair shampoo aids (e.g., pump dispensers, sink trays for shampooing while seated in wheelchair, and shampoo basin for bedside hair washing); finger ring brushes for scrubbing the scalp or hair; a hand-held shower head, which may have a flexible hose or a built-up handle, which may be placed on the side of the tub for easy access; lever-type faucet handles or tap-turning devices; bath supports to hold the person steady in the tub; and inflatable bed baths.

   III. **Drying adaptations** include towels with loops, terrycloth robes, adjustable hair dryers (e.g., with gooseneck), and hands-free hair-dryer holders.

e. ***Toileting*** includes skills necessary to perform bowel and bladder care, that is mobility and transfer skills (e.g., transferring on and off the toilet), sitting balance, upper-limb ROM and strength, hand function (e.g., pinch and grasp), coordination, and lowering or raising of clothing (see dressing skills in section II.A.3.b). It also includes menstrual care. For specific environmental adaptations (e.g., grab bars, toilet-seat height), see section II.B.1.b.3.

   I. **Toileting adaptations** include raised toilet seats (with or without armrests) for patients unable to sit and arise from a low commode; toilet safety frame with arm rests to assist in transfers; high-back toilet supports; commode chairs and potty chairs, which can be used if the patient has difficulty with standard toilets; chair or bed male urinals; female urinals with collector bags; and snap-on toilet-paper holders.

   II. **Bowel-care adaptations** include toilet-paper holders (e.g., wiping tongs, spring clip holders, and extended holders), bidet, digital bowel stimulators, and suppository inserters.

III. **Bladder-care adaptations** include positioning aids for catheterization (e.g., labia spreaders and knee spreaders with mirrors), dynamic splints or catheter inserters, modified catheter clamps, pneumatic or electric leg-bag clamps, modified leg-bag emptiers, modified condom catheter holders (to secure condom catheters), and modified strapping for urinary drainage bags.

IV. **Incontinence adaptations** include disposable underpads or diapers, reusable incontinence garments with easy access (e.g., Velcro), brief or panty liners, waterproof mattress protectors, and absorbent pads or draw sheets.

V. **Menstrual-care adaptations** include the use of sanitary pads that stick to the undergarments instead of tampons.

4. **Communication** is a process by which information is exchanged among individuals. It is discussed in detail in Chapter 5.5. For electronic assistive technologies, the alternative output strategies may include speech synthesis, tactile output, enlarged character display, or telecommunications. Its input strategies may use switches (see classification in section II.A.5.a) or standard or alternative keyboards or a computer mouse.

a. ***Writing adaptations*** include modified pens or pencils (e.g., with built-up foam handles, weighted, enlarged, or special grips; triangular-shaped or round grips; or with permanent attachment to a base for stabilization), pen or pencil holders (e.g., slip-on palmar cuffs; wrist supports or stabilizing bar; and figure-of-eight writing splints), and paper stabilizers (e.g., stabilized clipboard, paperweights, and the use of tape to hold the paper to the writing surface).

b. ***Typing adaptations*** include electric typewriters (may have self-correcting ribbons), word processors or computers, typewriter holders, modified typing sticks (e.g., mouthsticks, long-handle sticks, head-pointer sticks, and splints with a slot or vertical holder for a typing stick), alternative keyboards (e.g., expanded keyboard or a small keyboard), keyguards and a key latch (to facilitate accuracy), speech-to-text software, tremor-dampening mouse, and modified switches (see section II.A.5.a).

c. ***Book-handling and reading adaptations*** include modified sticks with suction cup ends which stick onto the book page (e.g., mouthstick or head wand or stick), book holders, electric page turners, magnifying readers, prism glasses that allow reading while lying flat, and nonslip plastic or rubber stabilizing sheets (e.g., Dycem).

d. ***Telephone-use adaptations*** include speaker phones (may have a quick dial feature), portable cordless phones, headsets, phone holders (e.g., gooseneck holders and clip holders), push-button phones (e.g., use of large button for uncoordinated patients), and mouth sticks for dialing.

e. ***General communication adaptations*** include modified mail handlers (e.g., electric letter openers or letter openers with modified handles), armrests, balanced forearm orthosis (see Chapter 4.3, section II.C.3.b) or suspension arm slings (see Chapter 4.3, section II.C.1.d.5) for patients with weak (at least Tr+ to poor P−) shoulder and elbow muscles, and environmental control units (see section II.A.5.a.3).

5. **Environmental hardware** include switches, faucets, and door hardware (e.g., doorknobs and keys). Environmental modifications for attaining barrier-free architectural designs for the physically handicapped are discussed in section II.B.1.b.

a. ***Switch adaptations for household appliances***

I. **Physical-contact switches** include pneumatic switches (e.g., Sip-and-Puff and air cushion); switches requiring contact, no pressure, or slight movement (e.g., P-switch or sensor, mercury or tilt switches, electromyography, or electro-oculography switches); and pressure switches (e.g., joystick, light touch, tongue, pillow, lead, wobble, plate, tread, rocker, grasp, or mat switches).

II. **Nonphysical-contact switches** include eye movement or gaze switches (e.g., infrared sensors), light-sensitive switches (e.g., light-activated, photoelectric, infrared reflex, and blink switches), voice- or sound-activated switches, electromagnetic switches (e.g., remote radio transmitters), magnetic-finger switches, and switches activated by proximity (e.g., heat sensitive) or a capacitive sensor.

III. **Environmental control units (ECUs)** refer to a centralized panel that allows easy operation of multiple devices such as televisions, radios, lights, telephones, intercoms, and hospital beds.

b. ***Faucet adaptations*** include extended or built-up handles on faucets, and faucets controlled by infrared sensors.

c. ***Door hardware adaptations*** include doorknob adaptations (e.g., lever type, extended, or covered with rubber or friction tape), vehicle door openers (lever type), automatic door openers, lock system adaptations (e.g., push-button and voice- or card-activated locks), and key aids (key holders that are rigid and offer more leverage for turning the key; key lever).

6. **Sexual expression** (e.g., masturbation) is an often neglected part of B-ADL (it may also be considered a more advanced ADL as it may involve tasks beyond caring for oneself with complex interaction with the social environment). Issues related to human sexuality are discussed in Chapter 5.9.

B. **INSTRUMENTAL ACTIVITIES OF DAILY LIVING (I-ADL)** refer to more advanced problem-solving skills, and more complex environmental interactions, including home management, community living skills, health management, safety preparedness, leisure, and work. They also include environmental adaptations for home and community access (i.e., barrier-free architectural design for the physically handicapped) as well as transportation adaptation and driving.

1. **Home management** requires gross motor mobility skills as well as fine and gross motor coordination, strength, and endurance of the upper limbs for the performance of household activities (i.e., meal planning, preparation, service, and clean-up; household maintenance including cleaning and bedmaking; clothing care including laundry and sewing; and childcare). When limitations exist, assistive devices can be used in conjunction with techniques for work simplification and energy conservation. Environmental adaptations to improve home accessibility can also be made.

a. ***Household activities adaptations***

I. **Meal preparation, service, and clean-up adaptations** include cooking appliances, storage, dishwashing, and kitchen utensils. See section II.B.1.b for barrier-free designs for kitchens, for example floor, countertop, and sink.

- **Cooking-appliance adaptations** include electric appliances (i.e., stoves, ovens, and blenders); countertop appliances (e.g., broilers and microwave ovens); push-button controls at the front of appliances; appliances with side doors (rather than top doors), pull-out shelves, burn-proof counters, and insulation of areas that can potentially cause burns; oven-cleaning adaptations (e.g., self-cleaning ovens; covering the oven with aluminum foil, which can easily be peeled and replaced; and using a hand-held cordless vacuum cleaner); push–pull sticks for oven racks; and mirrors angled above the stove to see into the contents of the pots if patient is wheelchair bound.
- **Dishwashing adaptations** include electric dishwashers (i.e., front-loading, front-panel controls with pull-out shelves), rubber mats at sink base, air drying, bottle brushes or scrub brushes with suction bases attached to the sink, soap dispensers, and terrycloth or sponge mitts.

- **Storage adaptations** include two-door, side-by-side model refrigerator and freezer with self-defrosting and automatic ice-dispenser features, pull-out shelves or drawers, turntables (e.g., Lazy Susans), storing items vertically or side-by-side (to avoid the need to lift off top items to retrieve bottom items), and easy-to-open plastic containers for food storage.
- **Kitchen-utensil adaptations** include electric appliances (e.g., choppers, blenders, food processors, mixers, and can openers), one-handed appliances (e.g., can or jar openers, rolling pins, egg-beaters, grapefruit sectioners, and garlic presses), modified openers (e.g., jar-lid openers, can openers, soda tab-grabbers, bottle openers, nonslip stabilizing plastic sheets such as Dycem, plastic-bag openers, box-top opener, and carton openers), modified scissors for opening packages (e.g., electric scissors, quick-clip scissors, and loop-scissors), modified knives (e.g., rocker knives, roller knives or pizza-cutting wheels, right-angle knives, and serrated knives), modified paring or cutting board (e.g., with spikes or corner guards to keep food from sliding away or with suction bases for anchoring), peelers, bagel slicers, graters, adjustable strainers, pan holders or stabilizers, tongs (instead of fork, spatula, or serving spoon), jugs with plastic lids (rather than cartons for milk or juice), carton holders, box toppers, clear beakers with clear markings for measuring liquids, and kitchen timers.
- **General adaptations for meal preparation and service** include modified transporting of items (e.g., wheeled carts, lap apron, basket or apron with large pockets, and wheeled tabletop disks with handles for moving hot pans or dishes), reachers, using convenience and prepared foods, lightweight utensils (except in uncoordinated patients who need heavy utensils for stability), unbreakable utensils, modified handles (e.g., bilateral, built-up, loop, extended, and rubber or plastic covered handles), stability adaptations (e.g., utensils with suction base, and plastic or rubber stabilizing mats or sheets), protective rubber mats or mesh mattings, and well-lit counters that are open underneath.

II. **Household maintenance adaptations** include general housecleaning (see section II.B.1.a.1.a for oven cleaning) and bedmaking. See also section II.B.1.b for barrier-free designs of living rooms, bedrooms, etc.

- **Cleaning adaptations** include vacuum cleaners (e.g., upright vacuum, self-propelled vacuum, cordless vacuum cleaner, and central vacuum-cleaning system); carpet sweeper; modified handles (e.g., extended, flexible, built-up, and cuff for easy grasping) for dustpans, feather dusters, mops, and brooms; dust cloths with a rubber band over a top broom; duster mittens; self-wring mops or sponge mops with squeeze lever on the handle; use of furniture with casters for easy moving; wheeled utility carts for transporting several items at once; lightweight utensils (except for patients with incoordination, who need heavy utensils for stability); nonslip mats; and reachers.
- **Bedmaking adaptations** include modified fitted sheets with touch fasteners or Velcro; lightweight blankets and spreads, satin pillow cases, and quilt covers.

III. **Clothing care adaptations** include laundry (collecting and transportation of clothes; washing, drying, and folding of clothes) and sewing.

- **Laundry adaptations** include automatic washer and raised dryer (top loading for ambulatory patients, or front loading for wheelchair-bound patients); a mirror to see into the tub and a reacher to pull out clothes from front-loader for patients in wheelchairs; push-button controls or large knobs; turning handles for adaptation; premeasured detergents, bleaches, and fabric softeners; heat-resistant pads (so iron does not need to be stored vertically); cord holders; adjustable tables for sorting and folding; wheelchair lapboards; hampers lined with plastic bags with handles; utility carts for transporting several items at once; reachers; and the use of no-iron or permanent-press fabrics.

- **Sewing adaptations** include electric sewing machines (with foot or knee controls), embroidery hoops, and pin cushions or bar of soap to hold needle for threading.

IV. **Childcare adaptations** include feeding, diapering/dressing, bathing, lifting and carrying, and child-safety measures.

- **Feeding adaptations** include breastfeeding (medically preferred and is generally easier than bottle-feeding); modified feeding bottles (e.g., lightweight plastic bottles with screw-on lids, disposable bottle-liners, and premeasured formulas); pillows for supporting the arms and the baby; sturdy highchairs with swing-away trays, one-hand release mechanisms, and safety straps; electric dish warmers; plastic aprons; bibs with pockets and Velcro closures; and rubber-coated spoons to protect the baby's gums and teeth.
- **Diapering/dressing adaptations** include touch fasteners (e.g., Velcro), disposable diapers, loose clothing with full-length openings, changing tables with straps to secure infant, and padded dressing tables.
- **Bathing adaptations** include foam-rubber bath aids, infant bath seats, child's bath support, terrycloth apron, and use of the kitchen sink or portable plastic tubs.
- **Lifting and carrying adaptations** for ambulatory parents include bassinet on wheels or reclining strollers, carriage carts, or cloth infant-carriers; and for wheelchair-bound parents, the child may be placed on the parent's lap supported by soft pillows or strapped to the armrest by touch fasteners to prevent slippage. The side of the crib may be adapted so the child can easily be lifted in and out of the crib.
- **Safety adaptations** include harnesses to keep the child from wandering away, safety devices to protect the child from accidents, reachers (to pick up clothing and toys), nonslip mats, and the use of a playpen or safety gates to confine the child to a safe environment.

b. ***Home accessibility adaptations*** can range from simple modifications (e.g., rearranging the furniture and placing commonly used items within reach) to complex modifications, that is adaptation of a barrier-free architectural design for the physically handicapped. As with any adaptive equipment, factors to be considered for home or building modifications include the support system (are there neighbors or family members who can help or does the patient live alone?); financial and physical resources available to implement the modifications (whether the patient owns or rents the home may also dictate the level of modification possible); condition of the patient (is the condition static or progressive? any age-related changes?); type of adaptation (e.g., does the patient need furniture rearrangement, structural modification, or relocation?); and patient's preference, desire, and ability to be independent. If possible, any suggested modification should be tried (e.g., in a simulated set-up) before actual implementation at home. The following recommendations are based on the American standards for buildings and facilities [i.e., *American National Standard for Building and Facilities – providing accessibility and usability for physically handicapped people,* published by American National Standards Institute, 1430 Broadway, New York, NY 10018, tel. (212) 642-4900] and on the publications of the United States Architectural and Transportation Barriers Compliance Board ["Access Board"; 1331 F Street, NW Suite 1000, Washington, DC 20004-1111 (800) USA-ABLE]. For other resources on accessibility for the disabled, see Appendix G-1.

I. **Access routes** must consist of at least two accessible routes for entrances and exits with emergency evacuation plans.

- **Stairs** for ambulatory patients must have uniform steps of 4–7 inches (10.2–17.8 cm) height with depth of 11 inches (27.9-cm) and nonskid surface; stair nosings or "lips" should be 60° from horizontal with a maximum protrusion of 1.5 inches (3.8 cm), or, if possible, should be removed; there should be continuous handrails (bilateral if feasible) with height of 34–38 inches (86.4–96.5 cm), situated 1.5 inches (3.8 cm) from the wall, with circular cross-section of 1.25–2 inches (3.2–5.1 cm), and with at least one handrail extending 12 inches (30.5 cm) beyond the top and bottom of the ramp runs.
- **Ramps** for wheelchair users must have an incline or slope of 12 inches (30.5 cm) of ramp length for every inch of vertical rise or the least possible slope (the overall rise of any ramp should be <30 inches or 76.2 cm); a width of at least 36–48 inches (91.4–121.9 cm); continuous bilateral handrails with measurements as described for stairs; a landing of 5 × 5 feet (60 × 60 inches or 152.4 × 152.4 cm) if the door swings out, or 5 feet wide (60 inches or 152.4 cm) by 3 feet deep (36 inches or 91.4 cm) if the door swings in; and a nonskid surface, which is protected from the elements if possible. In a long or curved ramp, there must be level rest platforms at 10-foot (120 inches or 304.8 cm) intervals.
- **Mechanical lifts** for wheelchair users may be installed when space for a ramp is not available. A wheelchair lift must have clear floor space of 30 × 40 inches (76.2 × 101.6 cm) with a stable, firm, slip-resistant surface; a forward approach of 36 inches (91.4 cm) or a parallel approach of 60 inches (152.4 cm); gratings of less than 1.5 inches (less than 3.8 cm) in one direction; operable parts within reach ranges; and enclosing walls and interlocked gates. If a vertical lift is used, an upper landing (dimensions as described for ramps) is often needed. If an inclined platform lift is used, it can be post-mounted on tracks along the stairs or on the wall(s) or stairs themselves. **Chair lifts** with built-in seats may be installed for patients who are not wheelchair users but who have difficulty climbing stairs.
- **Elevators** may be installed in the house if the patient can afford them. They must have call-buttons centered 42 inches (106.7 cm) above the floor (maximum height of 60 inches or 152.4 cm) with minimum button size of 3 × 4 inch (1.9 cm); hall signals that are audible and visible (with minimum size of 2.5 inches or 6.35 cm and located 72 inches or 182.9 cm above the floor); automatic doors, which remain open for a sufficient duration (at least 20 seconds) and which reopen when a person or object exerts sufficient force at any point on the door edge; emergency communication systems; sufficient space to enter (at least 32 inches or 81.3 cm for wheelchair users); and sufficient space inside the elevator car for wheelchair maneuvers (minimum diameter for 180° wheelchair turn is 60 inches or 152.4 cm).
- **Doors and doorways** must have a clear width of at least 32 inches or 81.3 cm (for wheelchair users) with level threshold (or if threshold is raised, it must be beveled and have maximal height of 0.5 inch or 1.27 cm); hardware situated 3 feet (36 inches or 91.5 cm) high; and if the door is weighted for easy closing, it should be less than 8 lb (<3.6 kg) with an opening force of about 5 lb (2.3 kg). Doors can be hinged (regular or fold-back), pocket-sliding, sliding, and folding (accordion-type) with automatic or pulley-operated openers and closers. Doorknobs must be easy to grasp (e.g., rubber-covered doorknobs or doorknobs that use lever-operated, push-type or U-shaped mechanisms). For patients unable to use keys, an alternative lock system may be used (e.g., voice- or card-activated, or push-button

system). Kickplates may be positioned 12 inches (30.5 cm) from the bottom of the door or remote controls may be installed. Doors in series should have adequate space between them to permit door swing into space.

- **Hallways** for a single wheelchair user must have a minimum of 3 feet (36 inches or 91.4 cm) with adequate turning space at the beginning and end of each hallway customized for different wheelchairs. For a 180° wheelchair turn, the minimum dimension should be a clear space of 60-inch or 152.4-cm diameter or a T-shaped space within a 60-inch or 152.4-cm square with arms 36 inches (91.4 cm) wide and 60 inches (152.4 cm) long and with sufficient toe and knee clearance.

II. **General living space**

- **Ground and floor surfaces** should be stable, firm, slope-resistant, and non-skid (options for nonskid surfaces include wood, vinyl, and specially treated tile). If there is a change in level of a walking surface greater than 0.25 inch (0.64 cm), a slope or edge treatment is needed. If the floor is carpeted, it must have a level loop or textured loop with level-cut pile or pile texture no greater than 0.5 inch (1.3 cm). If possible, avoid thick carpeting and throw rugs. Gratings must have openings no greater than 0.5 inch (1.27 cm) with long openings placed perpendicular to the dominant direction of travel.
- **Windows** should be easy to operate and open outward when possible. In general, it is easier to operate double-hung and horizontal-sliding windows than casement or awning windows that have cranks.
- **Controls** for lights, drapes, fire alarms, emergency power (fuses and circuit breaker), windows, and heating, ventilating and air conditioning systems should be placed 18–48 inches (45.7–121.9 cm) above the floor. Remote control or an alternative control system (e.g., voice-activated, proximity-activated, or pressure-sensitive switches) are available from hardware stores or could be used from an environmental control unit.

III. **Bathrooms and toilets**

- **Floor space** must have clear and unobstructed wheelchair-turning space of at least 60-inch (152.4-cm) diameter and must be nonskid (bathmats may be used).
- **Toilets** should have a height of 15–19 inches (38.1–48.3 cm) from the floor to the top of the toilet seat and should be mounted adjacent to the side wall or partition with at least an 18-inch (45.7-cm) clearance to and from the centerline of the toilet to the sink and at least a 48-inch (121.9-cm) clear space in front of the bowl and from the side wall. Flush controls and toilet-paper dispenser should be within reach.
- **Countertops and sinks** for wheelchair users must have clear floor space of at least 30 × 48 inches (76.2 × 121.9 cm) in front with maximum of 19 inches (48.3 cm) depth underneath. The countertop should be mounted with a height of 28–34 inches (71.1–86.4 cm) from the floor to the countertop and a knee clearance of at least 29–30 inches (73.7–76.2 cm) from the floor to bottom of the front edge of the countertop. The sink should have a maximum bowl depth of 6.5 inches (16.5 cm) and the same height as for countertops. Built-in sinks should be placed close to the front edge of the countertop. Any exposed pipes and surfaces should be covered to prevent burns.
- **Cabinets** (e.g., medicine cabinet) should be located 36–44 inches (91.4–111.8 cm) from the floor to cabinet bottom.
- **Water controls** should have a maximum activation force of 5 lb (2.3 kg), valves with single-handle control and a lever blade shape that mixes the water to control temperature and adjust flow, and pressure balance and thermostatic controls.

- **Shower areas** can be transfer-type showers [with or without a fixed bench of 17–19 inches (43.2–48.3 cm) height] with a clear floor space of at least 36 × 48 inches (91.4 × 121.9 cm), or it can be a roll-in shower with a clear floor space of at least 36 × 60 inches (91.4 × 152.4 cm). The maximum threshold height should be 0.5 inch (1.27 cm). For roll-in showers, there should be grab bars on the three walls of the shower; whereas for transfer-type showers, there should be grab bars across the control wall and on the back wall to a point 18 inches (45.7 cm) from the water-control wall. Water controls should be at 38–48 inches (96.5–121.9 cm) above the floor mounted on the side wall opposite the seat for transfer-type showers and on the back wall for roll-in showers. The shower spray unit, which can be fixed or hand-held, should have a hose at least 60 inches (152.4 cm) long and an angle lever-type handle.
- **Bathtubs** should have clear floor space of at least 30 × 60 inches (76.2 × 152.4 cm) in front for parallel approach or at least 48 × 60 inches (121.9 × 152.4 cm) for forward approach or at least 30 × 93 inches (76.2 × 236.2 cm) when an in-tub seat is provided at the head end of the tub and a rim height of 17–19 inches (43.2–48.3 cm) from the floor to top of rim. Grab bars should be provided on three walls (back wall, head-end wall, and foot-end wall). Tub benches, bathtub seats, portable seats, built-in seats, and hydraulic seats may be used to facilitate transfer into the bathtub. Water controls should be 33–36 inches (83.8–91.4 cm) above the floor located between rim of tub and grab bar at foot of tub.
- **Grab bars** should be 24–42 inches (61–106.7 cm) long, 1.5 inches (3.8 cm) in diameter, secured to withstand 250 lb (113.6 kg) of pressure, and mounted at 33–36 inches (83.8–91.4 cm) above the floor depending on the patient's transfer style, body mechanics, and equipment used.
- **Accessories** such as dispensers, hand dryers, towel racks, or other fixtures should be 33–48 inches (83.8–121.9 cm) above the floor and should not impede movement. Mirrors should be full length (bottom edge of reflecting surface with maximum of 38 inches or 96.5 cm above the floor) or tilted downwards.

IV. **Kitchens**

- **Floors** should have a clear space of at least 30 × 48 inches (76.2 × 121.9 cm) and should have a smooth, nonskid surface. A U- or L-shaped kitchen design is often most efficient for a wheelchair user.
- **Work surface** should be at least 30 inches (76.2 cm) wide, at least 24 inches (61 cm) deep, and with a height of 28–36 inches (71.1–91.4 cm) from the floor.
- **Countertops, sinks, cabinets, and water controls** have the same specifications as those described for bathrooms. There should be at least 40 inches (101.6 cm) clearance between counters. All storage space should be within the patient's reach. Hardware (e.g., cabinet door handles) and drawers should be easy to operate.

V. **Bedrooms** should have convenient access to the bathroom.

- **Beds** should be stationary and positioned to provide sufficient space for transfers. Bed stability may be improved by placing the bed against a wall or in the corner of the room (except when the patient plans to make the bed). The height of the sleeping surface must facilitate transfer activities (if needed the height can be adjusted by using wooden blocks with routed depressions to hold each leg). The mattress should provide a firm, comfortable surface (to increase firmness, a bed board may be inserted between the mattress and the box spring).
- **Closets** should be large, have wide entry, have open or pull-out shelves, and have low hanging rods hung at a maximum of 54 inches (137.2 cm) from

the floor for wheelchair users or adjustable clothes rod (42–72 inches or 106.7–182.9 cm) for ambulatory patients. The shelf height should be at waist level (up to 45 inches or 114.3 cm) in ambulatory patients or about 28–32 inches (71.1–81.3 cm) for wheelchair users. Wall hooks may be a useful addition to the closet area and should be placed 40–56 inches (101.6–142.2 cm) from the floor.

2. **Community living skills** include shopping, handling of money and finance, safety preparedness (i.e., fire safety awareness, ability to call 911, response to smoke detectors, and identification of dangerous situations), and personal health care (i.e., handling medications, self-monitoring, making medical appointments, and management of home attendant). They also include community mobility, that is barrier-free architectural designs for handicapped accessibility to public buildings, transportation accessibility, and driving. Most of these skills require intact cognition and perception.

a. ***Shopping adaptations*** include modified shopping and transport carts (e.g., carts that attach to the wheelchair, motorized carts, and heavy carts, which can be used for support), lightly packed plastic grocery bags with handles, reachers, use of proper body mechanics, use of shopping lists, and shopping at nonpeak hours.

b. ***Money and finance adaptations*** include modified writing or typing devices to handle paperwork (see section II.A.4.a).

c. ***Personal health-care adaptations***

I. **Medication handling adaptations** include a pillbox with an alarm to remind the patient of the medication schedule, handy compartmentalized storage units containing weekly medications with labels on lids (e.g., Mediplanner and Multi-Med Organizer), pill crusher, pill splitter, push-button pill dispenser, premeasured liquid medicines, premeasured injection shots (e.g., insulin), and one-handed auto-injectors;

II. **Self-monitoring adaptations** include electronic pulse or blood pressure digital monitors (e.g., self-inflating and deflating cuff and finger monitoring), digital thermometers, modified scales (e.g., large digital display, voice readout, and sitting scale), auto-lancet finger-lancing devices, and electronic glucometers (e.g., One-Touch).

d. ***Safety preparedness adaptations*** include prominent display of emergency numbers or emergency exit signs, auto-dial phones, a loud alarm for smoke detectors, Medicalert bracelets, provision of at least two accessible routes for entrance and exit, fire exits, and emergency evacuation plans.

e. ***Community accessibility adaptations*** include environmental modifications (i.e., barrier-free architectural designs) of public buildings that provide access for the physically handicapped into social, religious, educational, cultural, entertainment, medical, employment, and shopping facilities. For information resources on accessibility for the disabled, see Appendix G-1.

I. **External building accessibility**

- **Parking spaces** should be at least 96 inches (243.8 cm) wide, with an access aisle 60 inches wide (152.4 cm) by 20 feet long (240 inches or 609.6 cm) adjacent and parallel to the vehicle pull-up space for loading and unloading. The minimum vertical clearance should be 114 inches (289.6 cm or 9.5 ft). For vans, the parking space should be at least 98 inches (248.9 cm) high and have an access aisle width of 96 inches (243.8 cm). The surface slope should not be steeper than 1 : 48 in all directions (i.e., 1 inch rise for every 48 inches surface length). The location should be reserved and clearly marked as a parking area for the handicapped.
- **Curbs** must be beveled with textured cuts, which should meet the street surface with as little lip as possible.

- **Other access routes** such as ramps, stairs, doors and doorways, and elevators have similar specifications as for home (see section II.B.1.b.1). Any entrance doors that are not accessible should have appropriate directional signs to the nearest accessible entrance. Automatic revolving doors can be built with sufficiently large space to accommodate a wheelchair. Automatic sliding or swinging doors are also useful.

II. **Internal building accessibility** (access routes have essentially the same specification as for home described in section II.B.1.b.1.).

- **Corridors** should be at least 48 inches wide (121.9 cm) and be free of obstructions such as supporting columns and decorative plants. There should also be adequate wheelchair-turning space (see section II.B.1.b.1.f). The floor should have a nonslip hard surface or low-pile carpet (see section II.B.1.b.2.a). Path of travel in all areas (e.g., between desks) should be at least 3 feet (36 inches or 91.4 cm).
- **Rest rooms** that are wheelchair accessible should be provided, at least one each for men and women. There should be at least 48 inches (121.9 cm) between the inside wall and partitions enclosing the toilet. The entrance to the cubicle should be at least 48 inches (121.9 cm), and there should be adequate turning space in the main area of the rest room (6 × 6 feet or 72 × 72 inches or 183 × 183 cm). Specifications for functional access (e.g., grab bars, toilet flush, sink, etc.) are described in section II.B.1.b.3.
- **Water fountains** should not be higher than 36 inches (91.4 cm) from the floor to the level of water flow. They should have buttons or levers for easy activation.
- **Public telephones** should have at least one that is wheelchair accessible (mounted not higher than 48 inches or 121.9 cm) with push-button dialing.
- **Identifying signs and labels** should be easy to view (i.e., of sufficient size and color contrast). Tactile letters and numbers and Braille letters as well as auditory signals in elevators should be provided to identify floor level. Stairs and corridors should have adequate lighting.

f. ***Community mobility adaptations*** refer to commuting (by public transportation or by driving) to visit social, religious, educational, cultural, entertainment, medical, employment, and shopping facilities. Community organizations (e.g., Arthritis Foundation, National Easter Seal Society, Multiple Sclerosis Society, Chamber of Commerce, Veterans Administration, or the school's or campus's disabled student services office) may provide information on transportation services available to the disabled residents.

I. **Public transportation adaptations** include modified buses (e.g., kneeling buses equipped with a hydraulic unit that lowers the entrance to curb level for easier boarding or buses equipped with hydraulic lifts to allow direct entry by a wheelchair user), elevator access to subway trains, and door-to-door cab and van service.

II. **Driving** is a complex task that requires continuous integration of visual, motor, cognitive, and perceptual skills at a high level of functioning. Because driving carries a high potential for harm to the driver and other people, persons with physical handicaps require a predriving clinical screening, a comprehensive driving evaluation (i.e., stationary and behind-the-wheel performance tests and vehicular selection and adaptations). Specifics on evaluation programs vary from state to state and must be obtained through the Department of Motor Vehicles and Licensing for each state. A partial listing of adaptive driving resources and association is provided in the Appendix G-2.

- **Predriving screenings** are generally carried out by physicians to medically clear patients and to identify problems related to driving. The patient's desire to drive should be tempered with an acknowledgment of his or her mental, physical, or emotional limitations. Moreover, the patient's family and support system should be supportive and firm. The history and physical examination should include the following (if the physician has any concern, it must be documented in the evaluation form):

- **History of physical impairment** including its nature, etiology, and progression. The patient should be under the care of a regular physician and should be stable or improving. Patients with spinal fusion may need enough mirrors to provide a 360° field of vision.
- **Medication history** including drug type, side-effects, and reason for use. The patient must show excellent drug compliance and be aware of potential adverse drug effects.
- **Social history.** Patients should not be recreational drug or alcohol abusers.
- **History of temporary loss of consciousness (LOC)** because of epilepsy, diabetes, etc. Diabetic patients should have good control of blood sugar and should be taught how to prevent, recognize, and treat symptoms of hypoglycemia. Epileptic patients should not have had loss of consciousness or seizure episodes (including petit mal) for 6–24 months (this prerequisite varies from state to state). Both epileptic and diabetic patients must be under strict medical supervision and must submit proof of medication compliance (e.g., therapeutic range of medication in the blood or normal level of glycosylated hemoglobin for diabetics).
- **Functional skill examination**, including musculoskeletal skills (i.e., ROM, strength, endurance, coordination, muscle spasms, deformities, reaction time, upper and lower limb mobility skills, hand grip and dexterity, transfer skills, and sitting tolerance) and the ability to use gait aids, prostheses, orthoses, and wheelchairs. The patient must be able to maximize his or her self-reliance in these functional skills. If available, functional assessment may be carried out in a simulated environment using a mock-up vehicle.
- **Vision examination** including acuity, peripheral fields, scanning, color discrimination, glare recovery, depth perception, visual accommodation, and visuospatial perception (including visual organization, visual search and scanning, spatial relations, directionality, and visual processing speed). Evaluation methods for visual–perceptual skills include observation, functional task performance, pencil and paper tasks, computerized assessment programs and paper tasks. Vision and visual–perception skills must meet safety criteria for safe driving (e.g., visual acuity must have a cut-off point of 20/40 to 20/50, depending on the state law) as determined by the State's Department of Motor Vehicles.
- **Communication and hearing examination** including dysarthria, aphasia, and hearing impairment. The patient must meet safety criteria for safe driving as determined by the State's Department of Motor Vehicles.
- **Psychologic examination** including problem-solving skills, decision-making skills, selective and divided attention (distractibility), safety judgment (impulsivity), memory, sequencing, ability to plan ahead, recognition of signs and symbols, number recognition, confusion, agitation, hostility, and suicidal ideation. Patient must be rational, have good judgment, have the ability to recognize signs and symbols, and be emotionally stable (i.e., patient's behavior should not be physically or verbally explosive, aggressive, hostile, paranoid, or suicidal).

• **Vehicular set-up** must be performed prior to predriving or behind-the-wheel assessment to determine optimal driver positioning and ability to manipulate *primary controls* (i.e., steering wheel, accelerator, and brake) and *secondary controls* (i.e., ignition, turn signals, horn, windshield wiper and washer, headlights, headlight dimmer, heater and air-conditioning, power windows, power door locks, electric mirrors, door and lift controls, electric gear selector, electric parking brake, emergency flashers, and electric wheelchair lockdown). In general, recommendations for adaptive equipment should be made only when a driver can demonstrate the ability to use the same general type of device in a behind-the-wheel assessment.

- **Vehicular selections** include a car or a van (full size or minivan). A car is appropriate for patients (e.g., low-level paraplegics) who can enter or exit the vehicle independently and load the mobility equipment. The standard car recommendation is a two-door sedan with power steering, power brakes, automatic transmission, and, if needed, modified car seat or safety harness system. The car should be large enough to allow wheelchair storage behind the front seat or if the patient cannot independently load and unload the wheelchair, it can be modified with a car-top carrier that automatically loads and unloads the wheelchair. The van is appropriate for patients who need to drive from their own wheelchair because of an inability to transfer themselves and their wheelchair independently and safely into the vehicle (e.g., tetraplegic or high-level paraplegic patients using motorized wheelchairs or scooters). The width of the van door and the roof clearance should accommodate the motorized wheelchair or scooter. Entry into the van can be accomplished by a hydraulic lift (e.g., swing-away style or fold-out platform style), which can be mounted onto the rear or side of the van, or by a portable ramp (for safety reasons, the wheelchair or scooter has to be pushed or driven up the ramp by someone other than the user). Wheelchair restraint systems (e.g., manually operated on electric tie-downs) are also available for vans.
- **Primary-controls adaptations** include modified steering wheels for one-handed use or for weak grip (e.g., use of steering aids such as spinner-knobs, V-shaped grips, tri-pins which use three adjusted pins in a triangular arrangement, universal or palmar cuffs, or amputee rings onto which a prosthetic hook can be inserted); modified gas and brake controls, which include pedal extensions (to increase reach), pedal relocation (e.g., left-sided accelerator pedal for right hemiplegia), hand controls for paraplegics (e.g., rotary, push-pull, push-twist, push-right angle pull, push-pull down, or side-to-side motions for manipulating controls), or high-tech adaptations (e.g., operated by vacuum, pneumatic, or computer). All primary controls may be integrated into a single lever (joystick) system for patients with severe disabilities, such as C5 tetraplegics.
- **Secondary-controls adaptations** include quad key holders, elbow switches, head control switches, and touch pads (instead of toggle) switches which may be built up.
- **Other modifications** include a raised roof, mirrors for rear, side, or 360° vision; expanded doorway widths and heights; modified seat belts (and, if needed, chest straps for control of weak trunks); air conditioner (especially for patients with multiple sclerosis); two-way radio; and cellular phones.

• **Stationary (predriving) assessment** includes the evaluation of the following tasks: moving or transferring to the vehicle, inserting and turning a key (or using "keyless" entry operation or remote control), opening and closing the door, entering and exiting the vehicle, loading and unloading mobility devices (cane, walker, wheelchair), adjusting the driver's seat, adjusting the mirrors, and fastening the seat belt (and chest strap if needed). Adaptive devices include special key holders, vehicle door lever-type openers, loops for lower-limb management, a wheelchair strap to extend reach for wheelchair loading, modifications for independent seat belt retrieval, and use of hydraulic lifts or ramps.

- **Behind-the-wheel assessment** can either be simulated or on-the-road. A driving simulator uses a mock-up vehicle to test the patient's defensive driving skills, hazard perception, and emergency procedures as he or she steers and reacts to the simulated driving situation displayed on a movie screen. However, the optimal industry standard of driving competence remains the on-the-road driving test.

3. **Occupational activities** are age specific, for example a preschool child's occupation may be play and learning, whereas a school-age child's occupation is school activity and play, and an adult's occupation is work and leisure activity.

a. ***Leisure*** refers to unoccupied time (free from work and self-care activities) during which a person may indulge in rest and recreational activities. Benefits of participating in recreational activities include physical, emotional, and social well-being through enjoyment, exercise, competition, and socialization. Leisure activities can be used with therapeutic intent (e.g., using principles of reflex maturation and neurophysiology) to help develop skills needed for the patient's occupation or other ADL tasks. It uses a fun-based setting to encourage patients to use their remaining abilities to compensate for their mental limitations and physical disabilities. Adaptations for leisure activities include the use of high- and low-technology aids and devices, as well as modification of the physical environment. There are many organizations that provide programs (e.g., camps and wheelchair-adapted basketball, rugby, tennis, or other sports) especially designed for the disabled (see partial listing in Appendix G-6). This information can also be obtained from the local parks and recreation departments, churches, and other disability-related organizations (see partial listing in Appendix G-4). The following are examples of some common adaptations used for indoor and outdoor recreations.

I. **Indoor recreation adaptations** include bowling (e.g., bowling ball ramp, spring-loaded bowling ball, bowling ball holder mounted to wheelchair), knitting (e.g., embroidery hoop, and knitting needle holder), board games (e.g., enlarged game pieces and weighted pieces for uncoordinated patients), card games (e.g., card holders, automatic card shufflers, and magnetic playing cards and boards), toy modifications (e.g., switch-activated, modified handles, and stabilizing surface), spring-loaded cue stick, and indoor photography (e.g., pneumatic-control camera and camera tripod holder, which can be mounted on the wheelchair).

II. **Outdoor recreation adaptations** include trigger-release archery; raised gardening beds; modified frisbees (e.g., Quad-grip); electric-retrieve fishing reels; upper limb-propelled bicycles (for paraplegics); tricycles with footplates, straps, trunk supports, and extended seats; modified saddles; outrigger skis; modified swings (i.e., swings that can be propelled by pushing and pulling on the handles or using the arms); and outdoor photography (same as for indoor adaptations).

III. **General recreation adaptations** include universal cuffs, splints with slot or vertical holders, Velcro straps and grips, built-up handles (e.g., for tennis rackets and paint brush), mouthsticks (e.g., for painting), clamp frames, recreation belts, and chest straps or body harnesses.

b. ***Work*** refers to activities or tasks performed to provide meaning and support to the self, family, and society. It is learned through the process of socialization, is influenced by one's cultural tradition, and is motivated by one's intrinsic urge to be effective in the environment. Work is used by most people to provide their source of livelihood. It is discussed in Chapter 5.11.

Further reading

Crepeau EB, Cohn ES, Boyt Schell BA, editors: *Willard and Spackman's occupational therapy*, ed 10, Philadelphia, 2003, Lippincott, Williams & Wilkins.
Kent H, Redford JB: Adaptive driving modifications. In Redford JB, Basmajian JV, Trautman P, editors: *Orthotics: clinical practice and rehabilitation technology*, New York, 1995, Churchill Livingstone, pp. 219–234.
Kohlmeyer K: Adaptations in and to the home environment. In Redford JB, Basmajian JV, Trautman P, editors: *Orthotics: clinical practice and rehabilitation technology*, New York, 1995, Churchill Livingstone, pp. 235–255.
Mix CM, Specht DP: Achieving functional independence. In Braddom RL, editor: *Physical medicine and rehabilitation*, ed 2, Philadelphia, 2000, WB Saunders, pp. 517–534.
Pedretti LW, Early MB, editors: *Occupational therapy practice skills for physical dysfunction*, ed 5, St Louis, 2001, Mosby.
Trombly CA, Radomski MV, editors: *Occupational therapy for physical dysfunction*, ed 5, Philadelphia, 2002, Lippincott, Williams & Wilkins.

CHAPTER 4.6
Gait aids and gait patterns

The ability to ambulate (with or without aid) greatly affects a person's level of functional independence. As defined in Chapter 4.5, section II.A.2.d, functional ambulation refers to walking with an aid (e.g., walker) to accomplish some task (e.g., putting clothes into the closet). To become independent in functional ambulation, the patient must have adequate strength, range of motion (ROM), balance, coordination, and cognitive skills (for safety and timing). If the patient has limitations in any of these areas, PM&R intervention is needed. For example, patients may be taught energy- and time-efficient physical compensations (through physical and occupational therapy) and, if needed, they may be prescribed orthoses (see Chapter 4.3), wheelchairs (see Chapter 4.7), gait aids, or any combination of these. This chapter deals with gait aids and gait patterns commonly prescribed by physiatrists.

I. Gait aids

Gait aids (see Fig. 4.6-1) are prescribed to improve balance and stability (by redistributing and widening the weight-bearing or support area), provide sensory feedback, provide small propulsive forces to assist acceleration during locomotion, and reduce lower limb pain (by decreasing the load on musculoskeletal structures). Because they are considered to be an extension of the upper limb, good upper-limb strength and coordination are needed. The important muscle groups include shoulder depressors (latissimus dorsi, lower trapezius, pectoralis minor), shoulder flexors, elbow and wrist extensors, and finger flexors. Trunk muscles are also necessary to improve balance and endurance. Strengthening and coordination exercises of these muscle groups should be started while the patient is nonambulatory or preoperatively if surgery is elective.

A gait aid and gait pattern should be prescribed according to the patient's general functional ability, ability to maintain the body erect, and the amount of balance and weight-bearing assistance needed. In general, walkers provide the most stability, crutches provide moderate stability, and canes provide the least stability. Walkers are prescribed for patients with more significantly decreased balance, strength, or coordination. The body weight transmitted away from the affected lower limbs is: axillary crutches, up to 80%; nonaxillary crutches, 40–50%; and canes, 20–25% (i.e., in unilateral canes used opposite the affected side). When compared to normal unassisted gait, the energy expenditure per unit distance is about 18–36% greater for partial weight-bearing gaits using either crutches (axillary or forearm) or a cane and 41–61% greater for nonweight-bearing gaits using either axillary or forearm crutches. All patients should be trained in the proper use of the gait aid. In general, crutch ambulation needs more skill than the other gait aids.

A. WALKERS (see Fig. 4.6-1.M–R) are made of lightweight, durable, tubular aluminum or other tubular metal, with plastic handgrips, and four rubber-tipped legs. They are relatively easy to use, provide greater support and safer gait than canes and crutches, and are often used in the early phase of gait training (e.g., in

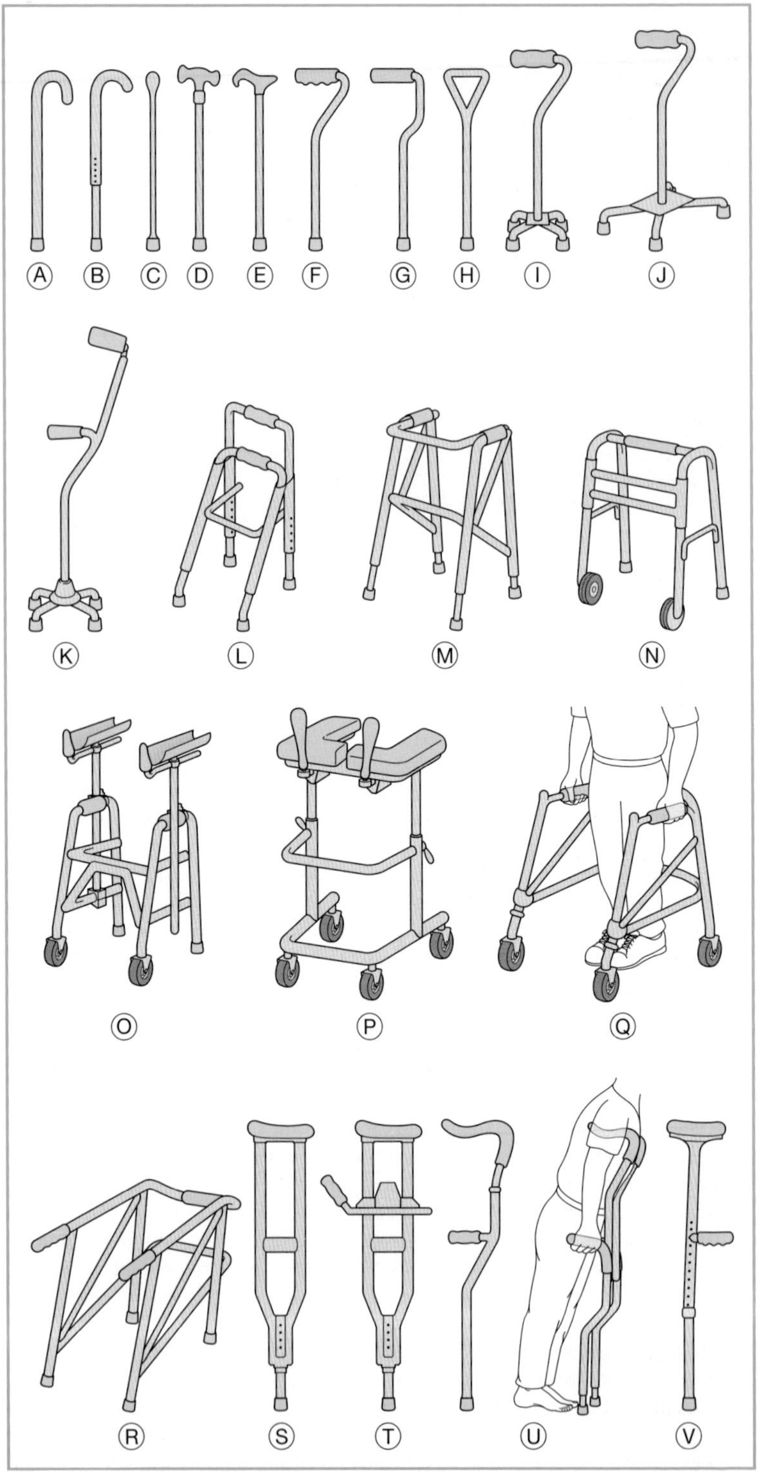

(Continued)

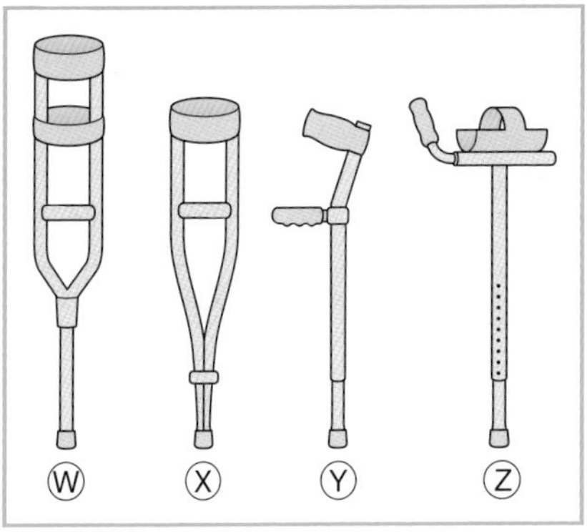

Figure 4.6-1 Gait aids. **A,** C-handle (J-handle or crook-top) wooden straight cane. **B,** C-handle adjustable aluminum straight cane. **C,** Ball-top straight cane. **D,** Functional grip cane. **E,** Slant-handled straight cane. **F,** Curved-top straight cane. **G,** Adjustable offset cane (e.g., Ortho-cane). **H,** Shovel-handle (stirrup-like) straight cane. **I,** Narrow-based quadruped ("quad") cane. **J,** Wide-based quadruped ("quad") cane. **K,** Forearm quad cane. **L,** Walk-cane or Hemi-walker or side-stepper cane. **M,** Non-folding standard walker (folding type not shown). **N,** Rolling or gliding walker. **O,** Bilateral platform walker. **P,** Rolling triceps walker. **Q,** Reverse rollator or posture-control walker. **R,** Stair-climbing walker. **S,** Adjustable axillary crutch (aluminum or wooden). **T,** Axillary crutch with platform. **U,** Ortho-crutch. **V,** Telescoping underarm (axillary) aluminum crutch. **W,** Triceps crutches (e.g., Canadian elbow extensor crutches). **X,** Forearm crutch with closed cuff (e.g., Kenny stick). **Y,** Adjustable forearm crutch (Lofstrand crutch). **Z,** Platform crutch or forearm support crutch.

hemiplegic or ataxic patients) to help the patient gain more balance and confidence prior to progressing to crutches or canes. In patients with lower-limb incoordination but good upper-limb strength, weights (e.g., sandbags) may be added to the cross-pieces of the walker for greater stability. The main disadvantages of walkers are that they cause a slow and awkward gait, and, in prolonged use, patients may assume bad posture and walking habits. Also, in most cases, the use of a walker is limited to indoor activities. Unless patients are strong enough to use a stair-climbing walker, they are unable to climb stairs using walkers. Walkers are made in several sizes, both for pediatric and adult groups. A walker is fitted by placing it about 10–12 inches (25.4–30.5 cm) in front of and partially surrounding the patient. With the patient standing straight, shoulders relaxed, and elbows flexed to between 15° and 20° degrees, the height of the walker should be adjusted so that the handle lies at the ulnar styloid.

1. **Standard walkers** (see Fig. 4.6-1.M) have telescopic or adjustable legs, and the height can be adjusted to most individual patients. Some models fold for easy transportation (e.g., via car trunk). For very tall patients, a tall design may be necessary. The patient needs good standing balance and upper-limb strength to lift the walker to advance it forward. The patient should also have sufficient hand strength and range of motion to grip the walker.
2. **Rolling or gliding walkers** (see Fig. 4.6-1.N) have wheels on the front legs to help facilitate movement of the walker for patients who lack coordination or strength in the upper limbs and trunk (hence, with difficulty in lifting and advancing crutches or standard walkers). By slightly raising the back legs off the floor, patients may be able to push this walker; however, the wheels may provide some instability, and patients may require supervision.

3. **Platform walkers** have a platform type of forearm support, which can be attached to either a standard walker or a rolling walker (see Fig. 4.6-1.O). It is used in patients with flexion contracture of the elbow or pain or deformities of the wrist and hand; however, they are generally quite heavy.
4. **Rolling triceps walker** (see Fig. 4.6-1.P) is a four-wheeled walker with padded platforms. It is used by persons with limited upper-limb strength and range of motion. The patient's forearms, which rest on the pads, accept the patient's weight as the lower limbs take steps. The wheels allow the walker to be pushed forward without lifting.
5. **Reciprocal walker** has swivel joints allowing reciprocal action as each side of the walker moves alternately. It allows a longer stride and a less awkward gait. It is commonly used by patients with bilateral hip replacements.
6. **Reverse walker**(see Fig. 4.6-1.Q) is used to facilitate extension posture by a person who tends to maintain a flexed posture while standing. It is commonly used in spastic cerebral palsy children with crouched gait.
7. **Stair-climbing walker** (see Fig. 4.6-1.R) has a U-shaped front extension with extra supports to provide stability in stair climbing. It is useful primarily in well-motivated patients with good balance and superior strength in their upper limbs, such as young paraplegics.

B. CRUTCHES (see Fig. 4.6-1.S–Z) have two points of contact with the body and thus provide better stability than canes. Crutches have rubber tips for absorbing shock and preventing slippage. The clinician must make sure that the crutch tips are not worn out. If needed, special crutch tips (e.g., for rainy and icy conditions) may be prescribed. Padded hand grips are used to reduce pressure on the hands and to help prevent slippage of grip. Crutches should only be prescribed to patients with enough strength to extend the elbows and raise the body 1–2 inches (2.5–5.1 cm) off the floor.

1. **Axillary crutches** (see Fig. 4.6-1.S–V) provide better trunk support than non-axillary crutches. They are prescribed for short-term use by patients with good balance and coordination. Patients using axillary crutches can free their hands for opening doors by leaning on the shoulder piece. However, they should be instructed to refrain from leaning their axilla against the axillary pads for prolonged periods as this may cause compressive radial neuropathy leading to "crutch palsy". Other compressive neuropathies (e.g., median and ulnar) may occasionally occur in the upper arm or in the hand and wrist.

   Crutch length (from the top of the axillary pad to the crutch tip) can quickly be estimated by taking the patient's height and subtracting 16 inches (40 cm) or, alternatively, by making the crutch length equal to 77% of the patient's height. To measure crutch length in the supine position, measure from the anterior axillary fold to a surface point 4–6 inches (10–15 cm) lateral to the anatomic heel or, alternatively, take the distance from the anterior axillary fold to the heel (without shoes) and add 2 inches (5.1 cm). When standing upright (with the shoulders relaxed), crutch length can be measured by taking the distance from the anterior axillary fold to a point 6 inches (15 cm) anterior and 2–4 inches (5–10 cm) lateral to the foot. It is important to keep the axillary pad about 1.5–2 inches (4–5 cm; i.e., two finger-breadths) below the axilla.

   The crutches' hand bars are adjusted in each case to give about 15–30° of elbow flexion with the wrist in maximal extension, and the fingers forming a fist. This is measured after the total crutch length is determined with the crutch 3 inches (7.6 cm) lateral to the foot. A quick alternative way of determining hand bar placement is to position the hand bar so that its distance from the bottom of the axillary piece equals the distance from the patient's olecranon to outstretched thumb.

a. ***Standard axillary crutches*** (see Fig. 4.6-1.S) have double uprights with a shoulder piece and handgrip or bar. They can be made of wood or tubular aluminum and their length can be adjusted. They can also be adapted for patients with poor handgrip by attaching a forearm platform (see Fig. 4.6-1.T).

b. ***Single-upright crutches*** can either be straight [e.g., telescoping underarm (axillary) aluminum crutch; see Fig. 4.6-1.V] or have a curved upper half (e.g., Ortho-crutch; see Fig. 4.6-1.U). They usually have a contoured underarm piece and an adjustable hand piece. Some patients find the Ortho-crutch to be more comfortable than standard axillary crutches.

2. **Nonaxillary crutches (forearm or arm canes**; see Fig. 4.6-1.W–Z) are prescribed for long-term use in patients with good trunk balance and confidence in ambulation (e.g., paraplegics who may require bracing with ambulation).

a. ***Forearm (Lofstrand) crutches*** (see Fig. 4.6-1.Y) are the most popular nonaxillary type. They are made of tubular aluminum with a padded hand bar and forearm cuff. The forearm cuff (which is open at the front or side) helps to stabilize the forearm and wrist during weight bearing to make ambulation easier and safer. They are most often used bilaterally and provide less support than axillary crutches for ambulation. They are more useful than bilateral canes because they allow the patient to free a hand (without dropping the crutches) to perform certain tasks such as grasping a stair rail, opening a door handle, or adjusting clothes. Forearm crutches are measured to provide 15–30° of elbow flexion in a standing position with the tip of the crutch positioned at a point 6 inches (15 cm) anterior and 2–4 inches (5–10 cm) lateral to the foot. The cuff of the forearm crutch should lie on the proximal third of the forearm (i.e., about 1–1.6 inches, or 2.5–4 cm, below the olecranon process).

b. ***Platform crutches*** (see Fig. 4.6-1.Z) have a platform on the top level of the crutch on which to rest the forearm and a vertical handgrip at the distal end of the platform. They are often used by arthritic patients with flexion contracture of the elbow and also by those with a weak grip because of pain and deformities of the hand and wrist. Velcro straps around the forearm may assist in holding the crutch in those with poor grip. Their advantage is that the body weight is borne mostly on the forearm instead of the hand. The handgrip can also be contoured to adapt to the deformities. It is measured by having the patient stand upright with the shoulders relaxed and the elbows flexed to 90°. The distance from the ground to the forearm rest is the proper length.

c. ***Forearm crutches with closed cuff*** (***Kenny Stick***; see Fig. 4.6-1.X) are similar to the Lofstrand crutches except that instead of an open cuff, they have a closed leather band, which ensures that the patient (more so than with the Lofstrand forearm orthosis) will not drop the crutches. They were designed for polio patients who had satisfactory proximal upper-limb musculature but who may have been weak distally and unable to effectively hold and control the crutches. They are prescribed for children who need total contact around their forearm.

d. ***Triceps crutches*** (***or Canadian Elbow Extensor Crutches***; see Fig. 4.6-1.W) have a single shaft attached to bilateral uprights, which extend above the elbow. They resemble the style of standard axillary crutches, but they end proximally at the mid-arm level. They have two cuffs: an upper cuff contacting the proximal third of the arm, about 2 inches (5 cm) below the anterior fold of the axilla; and a lower cuff lying 0.4–1.6 inches (1–4 cm) below the olecranon process (to avoid bony contact and yet provide adequate stability to the arm). Both cuffs support the arm with the elbow extended (thus preventing elbow buckling) during gait. They are useful for patients with triceps weakness (e.g., poliomyelitis patients).

C. **CANES** (see Fig. 4.6-1) have only a single point of contact with the body and provide less support than other gait aids. Hence, they are not appropriate in patients needing more than partial weight relief or support. The cane is held in the hand on the side of the unaffected lower limb to widen the base of support and reduce the load on the affected hip as well as to simulate a more physiological gait (i.e., in normal walking the opposite leg and arm move together). Without a cane, the load on the hip is increased by four times the body weight during stance phase of the gait because of the gravitational forces and the gluteus medius and minimus force exerted across the weight-bearing hip. With the use of a cane, the upper limb exerts force on the cane thus minimizing pelvic drop on the side opposite the weight-bearing lower limb and shifting the center of gravity to the unaffected side. This results in decreased work of the gluteus medius–minimus complex and reduced load generated across the affected hip joint. The length of the cane is measured with the patient in an upright position (and the elbow is flexed to about 20–30°) so that the highest point of the cane is at the level of the greater trochanter. A short cane will tend to hold the elbow in complete extension (hence reducing support during the stance phase and increasing stress on the lumbosacral region); and a long cane will force the elbow into too much flexion causing the user to lean forward (hence increasing fatigue by putting excessive demands on the triceps and shoulder muscles).

1. **Regular (straight-tip) canes** can be made of wood or aluminum. The aluminum canes have adjustable notches (Fig. 4.6-1.B) while the wooden cane needs to be cut to the patient's height. There are several varieties of cane handles. The C-handle cane (crook-top cane or J-cane; see Fig. 4.6-1.A,B) is the most commonly used. A functional grip cane (shaped to fit the approximate contour of a gripping hand; see Fig. 4.6-1.D) may offer a more comfortable grip than that of the C-cane for some patients. Other straight-cane handles include ball-shaped (Fig. 4.6-1.C), slant-handled (Fig. 4.6-1.E), and shovel-handle (or stirrup-like; see Fig. 4.6-1.H). Canes with a curved staff at the top are claimed to provide better balance for the patient (Fig. 4.6-1.F,G). The Ortho-cane (Fig. 4.6-1.G), which has a plastic palm grip and a curved staff at the top, was designed to provide better grip in addition to better balance for the patient.
2. **Quad canes** (Fig. 4.6-1.I,J) have four prongs at the base and are prescribed for patients (e.g., hemiplegics) who need more stability than that provided by other canes. The gait of patients using a quad cane is relatively slow. However, this slowing is negligible in most patients (e.g., hemiplegics) whose gait is slow to start with. The quad cane's base of support can either be narrow (Fig. 4.6-1.I) or wide (Fig. 4.6-1.J). In using the quad cane, the lateral two prongs should be directed away from the body. A variation of the quad cane is the forearm quad cane (Fig. 4.6-1.K), which is essentially a Lofstrand crutch with four-prong base.
3. **Walk-canes (hemi-walkers or side-steppers**; Fig. 4.6-1.L) combine the features of a walker and a quad cane. They are made of tubular aluminum and are foldable (hence more compact than the quad cane). Their bases of support are wider than that of quad canes and provide significantly better lateral support. They are used by hemiplegics who no longer need parallel bars but are not ready to use the quad cane.

II. Basic gait patterns using gait aids for level ground

These should emphasize normal heel-to-toe progression of the affected limb. The choice of gait pattern depends on the patient's strength, balance, coordination, and on the walking surface. Each patient should be trained with more than one type of gait pattern.

A. WALKER GAIT PATTERNS are more stable than those of crutch or cane. The patient should pick up and place down the walker on all four legs simultaneously (without tipping the walker on two legs) to achieve maximum stability.

1. **Full-weight-bearing walker gait** sequence is walker is lifted and moved forward, one foot is moved forward, then the other foot is advanced past the first foot.
2. **Partial-weight-bearing walker gait** sequence is walker is lifted and moved forward, the affected lower limb is moved forward, weight is shifted onto the walker (through the upper limbs) and partially onto the affected lower limb, then the unaffected lower limb steps past the affected limb.
3. **Nonweight-bearing walker gait** sequence is walker is lifted and moved forward (the affected lower limb, which does not bear any weight, may be advanced together with the walker or following the walker), weight is shifted through the upper limbs to the walker, and the unaffected lower limb steps forward.

B. CRUTCH GAIT PATTERNS

1. **Point gaits**

a. ***Four-point gait*** sequence is right crutch, left foot, left crutch, right foot. This is a very stable gait because three points are always in contact with the floor. It is used by patients with ataxia and by those with marked lower-limb weakness. However, the gait is relatively slow, and it is more difficult to learn than the other gait patterns.

b. ***Three-point gaits*** have only three points of support in contact with the floor and generally require good balance. They are commonly used by patients with lower-limb fractures or amputations.

I. **Nonweight-bearing crutch gait** sequence is both crutches are advanced (the affected lower limb, which does not bear any weight, may be advanced together with the crutches or following the crutches), weight is shifted onto the crutches, and the unaffected lower limb steps forward.

II. **Partial weight-bearing crutch gait** sequence is both crutches are advanced (the affected lower limb may be advanced together with the crutches or following the crutches), weight is shifted onto the crutches and partially to the affected lower limb, then the unaffected lower limb steps past the crutches.

c. ***Two-point gait or two-point alternate gait*** sequence is simultaneous advancement of right crutch and left foot, followed by simultaneous advancement of the left crutch and right foot. This is faster than the four-point gait and is fairly stable. It is used for reduction of weight bearing on the lower limbs.

d. ***Tripod (drag-to) gaits*** are initially used by paraplegic patients. When they improve their balance, they progress to a swing gait. Tripod gaits are stable but slow and laborious.

I. **Tripod alternate gait** sequence is right crutch, left crutch, then both lower limbs are dragged to the crutch level.

II. **Tripod simultaneous gait** sequence is both crutches are advanced simultaneously, then both lower limbs are dragged to the crutch level.

2. **Swing gaits**

a. ***Swing-to gait sequence*** is both crutches are advanced simultaneously, then the arms push down, and both lower limbs lift and swing *to* the level of the crutches. It is easy to learn and is used by most paraplegic patients.

b. ***Swing-through gait*** sequence is both crutches are advanced simultaneously, then the arms push down, and both lower limbs lift and swing *beyond* the level of the crutches. It is the fastest gait (even faster than able-bodied walking) but is very energy-demanding and difficult to do. The patient needs good trunk balance (with functional abdominal muscles) and good strength in the upper limbs.

C. CANE GAIT PATTERNS uses only point gaits. When only one cane is used, it should be held contralateral to the affected lower limb. The patient should always have the relatively "good" or unaffected lower limb assume the first full weight-bearing step.

1. **One-cane gait** sequence is the cane and affected lower limb are advanced simultaneously, weight is shifted onto the cane (through the upper limb) and partially onto the affected lower limb, then the unaffected lower limb is advanced.
2. **Two-cane gaits** are similar to the point gaits used in crutch walking (see section II.B.1).

III. Gait patterns using gait aids for elevation activities

These gait patterns involve stair climbing with a stair-climbing walker, crutches, or cane. Any gait aids may be used for negotiating ramps or curbs, although cane and crutches are more maneuverable than the walker. In general, the sequence for going upstairs or up a curb is to lead up with the unaffected ("good") lower limb followed by both the gait aid and the affected lower limb. When going down stairs or curbs, the sequence is reversed, that is both the affected ("bad") lower limb and gait aid are simultaneously lowered first, followed by the good or unaffected lower limb. The mnemonic is the "good" goes up to heaven and the "bad" goes down to hell.

IV. Gait training program

The gait training program should be individualized based on patient's diagnosis, contraindications, and goals. Some of the following activities may be contraindicated for some patients (e.g., leg-crossing activities that involve hip adduction should not be used by patients with total hip replacements).

A. PREAMBULATION PROGRAMS are used to improve strength, coordination, and ROM; facilitate proprioceptive feedback; develop postural stability; develop controlled mobility in movement transitions; and develop dynamic balance control and skills. Standing aids may be used for passive standing to control orthostatic hypotension and altered sense of body balance, to facilitate antigravity muscle action, to inhibit spasticity, to improve psychologic state, to decrease lower-limb contractures, to prevent or retard osteoporosis, and to provide positioning for functional activities. Several designs of standing aids (stationary or mobile) exist including tilt tables, standing frames, and parapodiums.

1. **Basic mat activities** in different postures use the following progression: side-lying and rolling; prone-on-elbows and prone-on-hands; hook-lying and bridging; quadruped; short and long sitting; kneeling and half-kneeling; modified plantigrade (modified standing position with trunk slightly flexed so that weight is supported on both hands resting on the table or a plinth and on both feet standing on the floor; the hips are slightly flexed, knees extended, and ankles dorsiflexed); and standing (if patient has postural or orthostatic hypotension, a tilt table may be needed; see section IV.A).
2. **Concurrent activities** include strengthening and coordination exercises, transfer training, and wheelchair management and mobility.

B. PARALLEL BARS ACTIVITIES PROGRESSION

1. **Basic parallel bars activities.** Moving from sitting to standing and reverse, standing balance and weight-shifting activities, hip-hiking, standing push-ups,

stepping forward and backward, forward progression, use of appropriate gait pattern, and turning.

2. **Intermediate parallel bars activities** (if activities are not feasible within the parallel bars because bar width is not adjustable, these activities may be performed outside and next to the parallel bars for added security). Moving from sitting to standing, and reverse, with an assistive device; standing balance and weight-shifting activities with assistive device; and use of assistive device (with selected gait pattern) for forward progression and turning.
3. **Advanced parallel bars activities** include walking sideward (side-stepping), walking backward, proprioceptive neuromuscular facilitation braiding (combination of crossed and side-step progression), and resisted forward progression (i.e., therapist provides manual resistance on the patient's pelvis or shoulder as patient walks forward) activities.

C. INDOOR PROGRESSION includes instruction and training use of assistive device for ambulation on level surfaces; elevation activities, including climbing stairs (if crutches or canes are used for stair climbing, handrails, if present, should be used), and if available indoors, negotiating ramps and curbs; opening doors and passing through doorways (including elevators) and over thresholds; and falling techniques (generally included for active ambulators requiring long-term use of assistive device).

D. OUTDOOR PROGRESSION includes instruction and training in opening doors and passing through thresholds that lead outdoors; use of assistive device for ambulation on outdoor surfaces and uneven terrain; elevation activities, including climbing stairs, and negotiating ramps and curbs; crossing a street within the time allocated by a traffic light; and getting in and out of private and public transportation.

Further reading

Goldberg B, LeBlanc M, Edelstein J: Cane, crutches, and walkers. In Goldberg B, Hsu JD, editors: *American Academy of Orthopedic Surgeons (AAOS) atlas of orthoses and assistive devices*, ed 3, St Louis, 1997, Mosby, pp. 557–573.

Hennessey WJ, Johnson EW: Lower limb orthoses. In Braddom RL, editor: *Physical medicine and rehabilitation*, ed 2, Philadelphia, 2000, WB Saunders, pp. 326–352.

Nash DL, Thompson JM: Ambulatory aids. In Sinaki M, editor: *Basic clinical rehabilitation medicine*, St Louis, 1994, Mosby-Year Book, pp. 462–470.

Ragnarsson, KT: Lower extremity orthotics, shoes, and gait aids. In DeLisa JA, Gans BM, Walsh NE, *et al.*, editors: *Physical medicine and rehabilitation: principles and practice*, ed 4, Philadelphia, 2005, Lippincott, Williams & Wilkins, pp. 1377–1391.

Schmitz TJ: Preambulation and gait training. In O'Sullivan SB, Schmitz TJ, editors: *Physical rehabilitation: assessment and treatment*, ed 4, Philadelphia, 2001, FA Davis, pp. 411–444.

Varghese G: Crutches, canes, and walkers. In Redford JB, editor: *Orthotics etcetera*, ed 3, Baltimore, 1986, Williams & Wilkins, pp. 453–463.

CHAPTER 4.7
Manual and powered mobility systems

Wheeled mobility systems can be manually propelled (manual wheelchairs and attendant-propelled wheelchairs) or externally powered (e.g., powered wheelchairs, scooters). From a 1992 survey, there were more than 1 million users of wheeled mobility systems in the United States, 75% of whom used manual wheelchairs. Standards for the performance and safety of wheeled mobility systems have been established by the Rehabilitation Engineering Society of North America (RESNA), 1700 North Moore Street, Suite 1540, Arlington, VA 22209-1903, tel. (703) 524-6686, website: www.resna.org, and can be accessed from publications by the National Rehabilitation Information Center (NARIC), 4200 Forbes Blvd, Suite 202, Lanham, MD 20706, tel. (800) 346-2742 or (301) 459-5900, website: http://www.naric.com.

I. Manual wheelchairs

Manual wheelchairs are designed to be manually propelled by a patient with sufficient strength in both upper limbs (e.g., paraplegic or lower-limb amputee patients) or in at least one upper or lower limb (e.g., hemiplegic patients who can be taught to use foot-drive or one-hand-drive wheelchairs). They are indicated for patients whose ambulation is either *inadvisable* (e.g., when lower limbs are contraindicated from weight bearing or from assuming dependent positions such as during fracture healing; when prolonged walking is contraindicated because of poor endurance from various cardiopulmonary neuromusculoskeletal conditions; when walking is unsafe because of lower limb or postural instability) or *not functionally possible* (e.g., conditions involving loss of lower-limb function such as spinal cord injury, bilateral amputation, multiple sclerosis, stroke, traumatic brain injury, cerebral palsy, poliomyelitis, muscular dystrophy, arthritis, etc.).

Absolute contraindications to manual wheelchairs include ischial pressure ulcers grade three or four, blindness, and poor judgment. Other **relative contraindications** include surgical or postoperative conditions of the pelvis or proximal femur, vertebral fractures, disk and nerve root compression, truncal weakness, and postural defects. If the wheelchair is contraindicated because of ischial pressure ulcers, a gurney (adapted for self-propulsion in the prone position) might be considered.

Complications of manual wheelchair use include: back pain and deformities (can be prevented by proper positioning or seating), pressure ulcers (can be prevented by frequent weight shifting or reclining wheelchairs), lower-limb contractures (can be prevented by frequent stretching of tight structures around pelvis, hips, and knees), and dependent lower-limb edema (can be prevented by elevating the legs and using compression garments).

Wheelchair and seating prescriptions should be made with a team approach that includes the patient, the patient's family or support system, the physician, physical and occupational therapists, orthotist, rehabilitation engineer, rehabilitation technology supplier, social worker, case manager, nurse, and other allied health-care professionals. The factors to consider in the prescription of manual wheelchairs and seating systems include:

- Patient's diagnosis and residual abilities (including endurance, vision, cognition, intelligence level, judgment, perception, and motivation), that is need for attendant-propelled wheelchair, manually propelled wheelchair, or powered mobility systems;
- Patient's expected duration of disability to determine if the wheelchair should be purchased or rented (consider renting if the patient is expected to regain ambulation ability within a short period, e.g., 9–12 months, or if the patient only needs the wheelchair periodically such as for prolonged trips);
- Patient's bodily dimensions, i.e., need for a standard, heavy, lightweight, or ultralight wheelchair;
- Patient's active or sedentary life-style as well as vocation and avocation;
- Proposed use of the wheelchair, that is as a primary means of mobility at home, school, work, and community, or as a backup system such as when bilateral leg prostheses are in for repair or when leg prostheses cannot be worn because of residual-limb ulcer, or for use only when showering, toileting, or when the walking terrain is hazardous (e.g., icy sidewalk);
- Need for wheelchair portability, that is folding vs. nonfolding, or lightweight vs. standard-weight wheelchair;
- Environmental accessibility in home, office, school, and recreational or other community facilities; consider the entrance, door width, turning radius in bathroom and hallways, floor surface, workspace design, etc. (see Chapter 4.5, sections II.B.1.b and II.B.2.e for environmental adaptations for wheelchair accessibility);
- Financial resources, that is bottom-of-the-line vs. top-of-the-line wheel-chair; and
- Other factors such as availability of wheelchair parts, wheelchair repair, and wheelchair trial opportunity.

If the manual wheelchair is prescribed for temporary use, patients must be encouraged to learn to walk when indicated (with appropriate braces, prostheses, crutches, and hard work) so as not to make them dependent on the wheelchair. Unlike prescription of wheelchairs for children, growth in length is no longer an important factor; however, adult wheelchairs may need adjustability for changes in girth or progression of disease [e.g., amyotrophic lateral sclerosis (ALS), or multiple sclerosis]. Two other major considerations in manual wheelchair prescription are proper wheelchair fitting (see Fig. 4.7-1 for critical wheelchair measurements) and proper wheelchair seating and positioning.

Goals of proper wheelchair seating and positioning include prevention of deformities and pressure ulcers, tone normalization, promotion of function (e.g., promote efficient use of upper limbs for propelling a manual wheelchair or for activating switches of a power wheelchair), increasing sitting comfort and tolerance, optimizing respiratory function, and provision of proper body alignment not only for propelling the manual wheelchair or for moving within the wheelchair, but also for keeping the patient alert and comfortable. For details on wheelchair seating and positioning prescription, refer to textbooks by Letts or Mayall and Desharnais (see Further reading section).

Manual wheelchair checkout and training. Prior to writing the wheelchair prescription, it is advisable to have the patient try a comparable wheelchair (both indoors and outdoors) to evaluate his or her ability to learn to use the wheelchair and to help the patient decide whether that particular type of wheelchair is appropriate. After the prescribed wheelchair is delivered, the clinician must test drive the wheelchair to check the wheelchair's performance as well as the function and

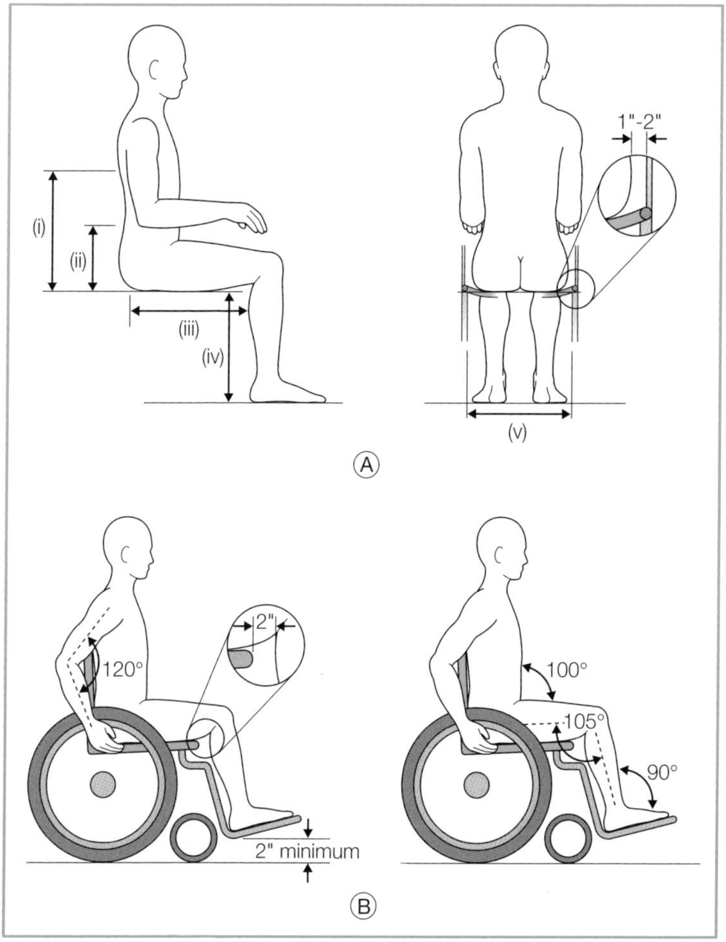

Figure 4.7-1 A. Critical measurements for wheelchair prescription. **(i)**, Back height (from seat) = distance from bottom of buttocks to level of scapulae. **(ii)**, Arm height = distance from bottom of buttocks to olecranon with elbow fixed to 90°. **(iii)**, Seat depth = distance between popliteal and back of buttocks (add 1–2 inches or 2.5–5 cm so that the popliteal fold is clear from the anterior edge of seat; alternative method for providing clearance of popliteal fold is to adjust the back cushion or footrest). **(iv)**, Seat height (from floor) = length of leg from bottom of heel to popliteal fold (add 2 inches or 5 cm to provide clearance of footrest when approaching slopes and ramps; alternative method for providing clearance of footrest is to adjust seat cushion or footrest). **(v)**, Seat width (between uprights) = widest distance across hips (add 1–2 inches or 2.5–5 cm to take into account the patient's clothing or braces). **B**. The bottom figures show proper elbow, hip, knee, and ankle angles as well as proper footrest and popliteal clearance. (Adapted from Wilson A: *Wheelchairs: a prescription guide*, New York, 1992, Demos Medical Publishing, with permission.)

safety of its parts. If everything meets the approval of the prescribing physician, the patient tests the wheelchair and necessary modifications can be made. The patient and caregivers are then trained in the safe use of the newly prescribed wheelchair both indoors and outdoors (including traffic situations if appropriate), transfer techniques, wheelchair transport (e.g., wheelchair assembly and disassembly), wheelchair maintenance (e.g., regular lubrication and cleaning of moving parts, bearing replacements, brake or lock adjustments, caring for batteries of power mobility systems, putting power mobility systems out of gear when not in use), and troubleshooting of common wheelchair problems.

Important biomechanical and ergonomic principles of wheelchair design and propulsion include:

- **Rolling resistance** refers to the inherent resistance to rolling, which is affected by the weight distribution between the front and the rear wheels. Rolling resistance is reduced by: 1) moving the seat (the center of gravity) rearward or by moving the wheel axle forward; 2) type of tire (solid tires have lower rolling resistance than pneumatic tires; narrower tires have less rolling resistance than wider tires); 3) wheel alignment (symmetric toeing error with a misalignment of as little as 2° can increase rolling resistance quite dramatically; see section I.A.2.a for description of "toe-in" vs. "toe-out") and 4) type of floor or ground surface (a flat, hard surface provides the lowest rolling resistance, while carpeting, rough terrain, and even small inclines or slopes greatly increase rolling resistance and the energy cost of wheelchair propulsion).
- **Propulsion efficiency** is improved by positioning the user more rearward (so the center of gravity is closer to the axle and the elbows are flexed at about 120° during propulsion; see Fig. 4.7-1). This minimizes energy consumption and uses gravity to aid the recovery phase of propulsion, thus making the return to the starting position of the stroke more horizontal and more efficient. In contrast, wheelchairs that position the user more anteriorly make propulsion strokes predominantly downward; the user then requires excessive internal rotation, extension, and elevation of the shoulders during the recovery phase to grab the rim for the next stroke of the wheel.
- **Downhill-turning tendency (side-slope effect)** refers to the tendency of the wheelchair to turn downhill when the wheelchair moves longitudinally along an inclined surface such as on a slightly tilted sidewalk (this is ever prevalent because most outdoor surfaces have a 1° to 2° slope to aid in drainage). A 2° slope results in a nearly twofold increase in effort required for forward propulsion. This increased propulsion effort can be reduced by moving the seat and center of gravity rearward relative to the rear-wheel axle and also by widening the camber (see description below).
- **Yaw-axis control (maneuverability)** refers to the ease of altering the direction of the wheelchair and involves overcoming the polar moment of inertia of the wheelchair (i.e., the greater the moment of inertia, the more difficult it is to change wheelchair direction). To increase yaw-axis control, the moment of inertia can be reduced by moving the seat rearward, thereby decreasing the distance from the main axis to the center of gravity (i.e., by providing a shorter lever arm).
- **Pitch-axis control (wheelie control or dynamic stability)** refers to rotation at the axle in an anterior and posterior direction, thereby affecting the ease of tipping the wheelchair backward during propulsion or while "popping wheelies". Wheelies, which are performed by the wheelchair user (e.g., when negotiating curbs), refer to the lifting of the front casters off the ground while balancing and/or turning on the rear wheels. During wheelies, the wheelchair user leans the trunk forward to counterbalance the backward tipping force. The ease of performing wheelies can be increased by moving the seat rearward, however, this also increases the backward tipping tendency of the wheelchair, which can be detrimental to users with poor trunk balance and control.

- **Static stability** refers to the tipping angle or stability in the forward-to-rear and side-to-side directions while the chair is stationary (both with and without the wheels locked). The side-to-side static stability can be determined by the camber (see below), while the forward-to-rear static stability can be determined by the relation of the seat or center of gravity to the rear-wheel axle. The longer the distance between the rear-wheel axle and the center of gravity (i.e., by placing the seat in a relatively forward position), the greater the forward-to-rear static stability. In contrast, placing the seat in a relatively rearward position decreases forward-to-rear static stability. For active users with good trunk balance and control, a rearward seat position is recommended (despite the decrease in static stability, which is easily compensated by leaning forward) because it improves pitch-axis control and decreases angular displacement.
- **Camber** refers to a position in which the bottom parts of the propelling wheels are further apart than the top parts of the wheels (see Fig. 4.7-3.H). The camber of a standard wheelchair is 7° (range 3–9°), but in sports wheelchairs, the camber is usually widened (i.e., the tilt angle is increased) by adding different camber washers. A wider camber leads to increased side-to-side as well as forward stability of the wheelchair, increased ease of wheelchair rolling at higher speeds (camber has little or no effect on rolling resistance at regular speed), decreased wheelchair turning radius (i.e., increased wheelchair maneuverability), reduced downhill-turning tendency, and also increased protection of the user's hands from doorways or other players in sports. The disadvantages of a wide camber include greater wear and tear on the tires and wheel bearings; the need for a wider track, which may cause difficulty in tight spaces; increased tendency of the wheelchair to toe-out during a wheelie in proportion to the wheelie angle (even if the wheels are perfectly aligned when all four wheels are on the ground); and decreased rear stability. The decrease in rear stability is associated with a 3.9-fold increased risk of injuries because of instability unless compensatory measures are taken, such as moving the rear-wheel axle rearward, positioning loads closer to the front, or using antitipping devices.
- **Weight/portability.** The weight of the wheelchair can be heavy (>50 lb or 23 kg), standard (40–50 lb or 18–23 kg), lightweight (20–40 lb or 9–18 kg), or ultralight (15–20 lb or 7–9 kg, e.g., "sports" wheelchairs; see section I.B.4). Wheelchair weight is important when considering wheelchair transportability, but it does not have a significant effect on the overall energy cost of wheeling when propelling on a flat surface. When propelling uphill, however, wheelchairs with lighter weight are more energy efficient. Other factors such as weight distribution in the wheelchair and efficiency of propulsion have a greater impact on wheelchair function than simply considering the overall weight of the wheelchair. Although lighter wheelchair models are generally technologically superior and more energy efficient, they tend to be more expensive and are not indicated for every wheelchair user. The standard wheelchair is indicated for temporary use, short-distance dependent mobility, or for some part-time users who have some walking ability. The heavy wheelchairs are indicated for persons over 250 lb (>114 kg) or needing more than 20 inches (>51 cm) wheelchair width.

A. PARTS AND SUBTYPES OF MANUAL WHEELCHAIRS (see Fig. 4.7-2)

1. Frame

a. ***Folding (X-shaped) frame wheelchairs*** are the most common frames for manual wheelchairs because they are easy to fold and transport. They also provide a smoother ride than rigid-frame wheelchairs because their greater flexibility makes it more likely that all four wheels will remain in contact with uneven

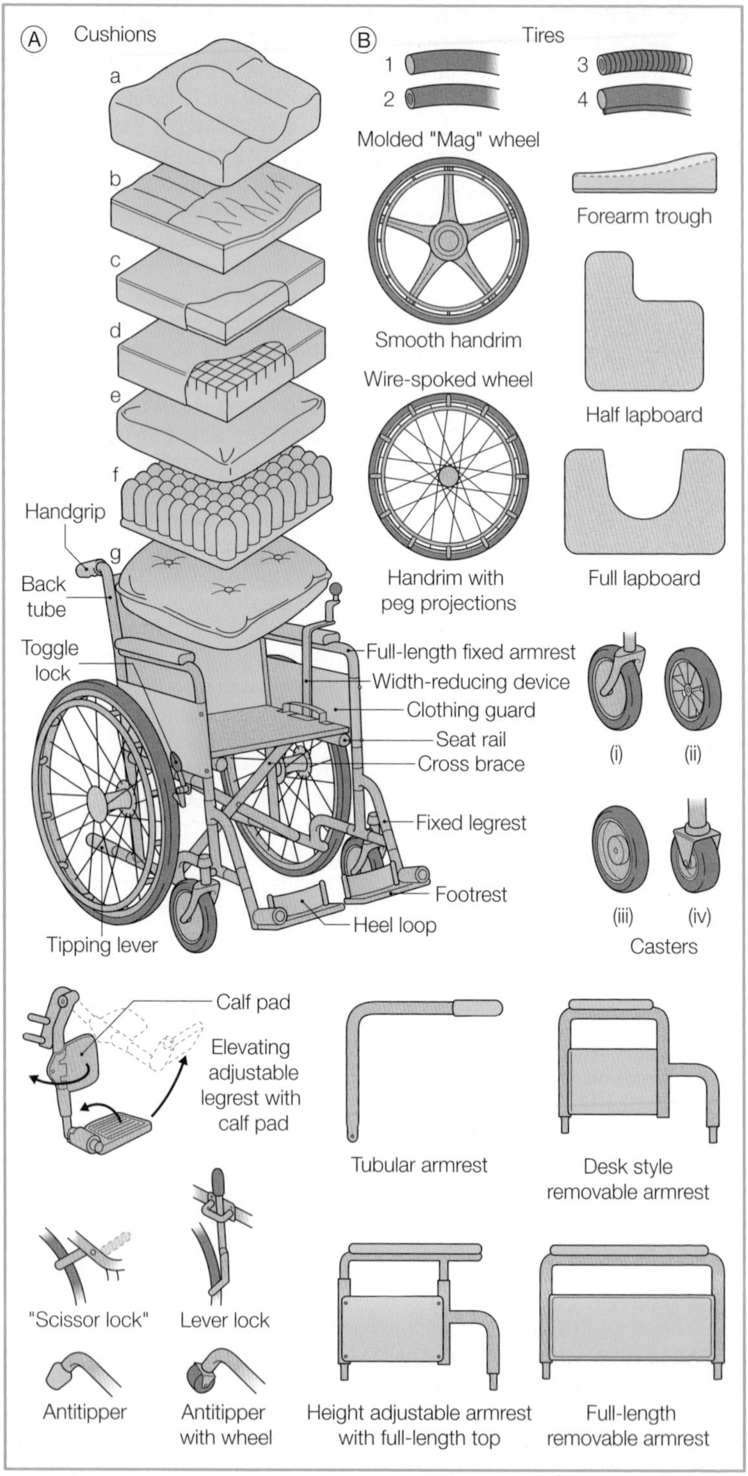
A
Cushions
a
b
c
d
e
f
g
Handgrip
Back tube
Toggle lock
Tipping lever
Full-length fixed armrest
Width-reducing device
Clothing guard
Seat rail
Cross brace
Fixed legrest
Footrest
Heel loop
B
Tires
1
2
3
4
Molded "Mag" wheel
Smooth handrim
Wire-spoked wheel
Handrim with peg projections
Forearm trough
Half lapboard
Full lapboard
(i)
(ii)
(iii)
(iv)
Casters
Calf pad
Elevating adjustable legrest with calf pad
Tubular armrest
Desk style removable armrest
"Scissor lock"
Lever lock
Antitipper
Antitipper with wheel
Height adjustable armrest with full-length top
Full-length removable armrest

Figure 4.7-2 Parts of a manual wheelchair. **A**. Types of pressure-relief seat cushions: **a**, Contoured foam (Veterans Administration Spinal Injury Orthosis [VASIO]); **b**, Contoured foam base with gel-filled pad (Jay cushion); **c**, Viscoelastic foam with casing; **d**, Polyurethane foam; **e**, Gel enclosed in a nonbreathing plastic casing; **f**, Air-filled villous ROHO cushion; **g**, Water-filled seat cushion. **B**. Types of tires: **1**, Solid hard rubber tire; **2**, Pneumatic inner tube; **3**, Semi-pneumatic tire with coil-reinforced zero pressure tire (ZPT) inner tube; **4**, Semi-pneumatic tire with solid foam ZPT inner tube. **A** Types of casters: **i**, Standard 8-inch (20 cm) diameter with solid rubber tire; **ii**, 8-inch diameter with semi-pneumatic tire; **iii**, 8-inch diameter with pneumatic tire; **iv**, 5-inch (13 cm) diameter with solid rubber tire.

terrain. However, they have more moving parts and are thus heavier and less energy efficient (because propelling energy is lost or wasted to the torque in the cross-frame) than rigid-frame wheelchairs. The folding wheelchair can be made narrower temporarily by a few inches by turning the crank of the narrowing (or width-reducing) device (see Fig. 4.7-2) which through a gear mechanism provides the necessary force to slightly fold the wheelchair frame.

b. ***Rigid-frame wheelchairs*** are nonfolding and are thus more difficult and cumbersome to transport, despite models with quick-release wheels and a fold-down back. Rigid-frame wheelchairs are commonly used in institutions and are used in "sports" wheelchairs (see section I.B.4). Due to their energy efficiency compared to X-frame wheelchairs, the wheels of rigid wheelchairs are easier to align precisely resulting in less rolling resistance and in greater propelling efficiency. The applied forces (for propulsion and turning) are also not damped because of the wheelchair's rigidity.

2. Propulsion

a. ***Propelling wheels***. The diameter of the propelling wheels of rear-wheel-drive wheelchairs is usually 24 inches (61 cm). To decrease the wheelchair height, smaller diameter propelling wheels [e.g., 20- or 22-inch (51- or 56-cm) rear wheels] can be used. The alignment of the propelling wheel also affects the wheelchair's function. The propelling wheel can either be "toed-in" (i.e., the front parts of the wheels are closer to each other than the back parts) or "toed-out" (opposite of "toe-in"). A symmetric toeing error increases rolling resistance, while a nonsymmetrical toeing error may cause the wheelchair to deviate persistently to one side. In wheelchairs with axle-adjustment plates, the toeing error can be corrected by adding washers under the front or back bolts, but in wheelchairs with axles housed in a tube of fixed alignment, the tube can be rotated.

I. **Wheel placement**

- **Rear-wheel-drive wheelchair** (see Fig. 4.7-3), which has propelling wheels placed at the rear behind the casters, is the most common type of manual wheelchair.
- **Front-wheel-drive wheelchair** (unjustifiably known as the "traveler" or "indoor" wheelchair; see Fig. 4.7-3), which is typically used indoors, especially in small rooms, but may also be used outdoors if there are no curbs. It has the advantage of being 1–3 inches (2.5–7.6 cm) shorter in length (thus requiring less space for turning) and being better balanced posteriorly, decreasing the risk of tipping backwards, especially in lower-limb amputees, than the rear-wheel-drive wheelchair. The large propelling wheels of the front-wheel-drive wheelchair, which usually have a diameter of 26 inches (66 cm), help overcome the irregularities of streets and roads, leading to a smoother wheelchair ride with less vibration; however, when compared to rear-wheel-drive wheelchairs, they tend to veer from side to side and, in general, are much more tiring to propel and more difficult to maneuver for the

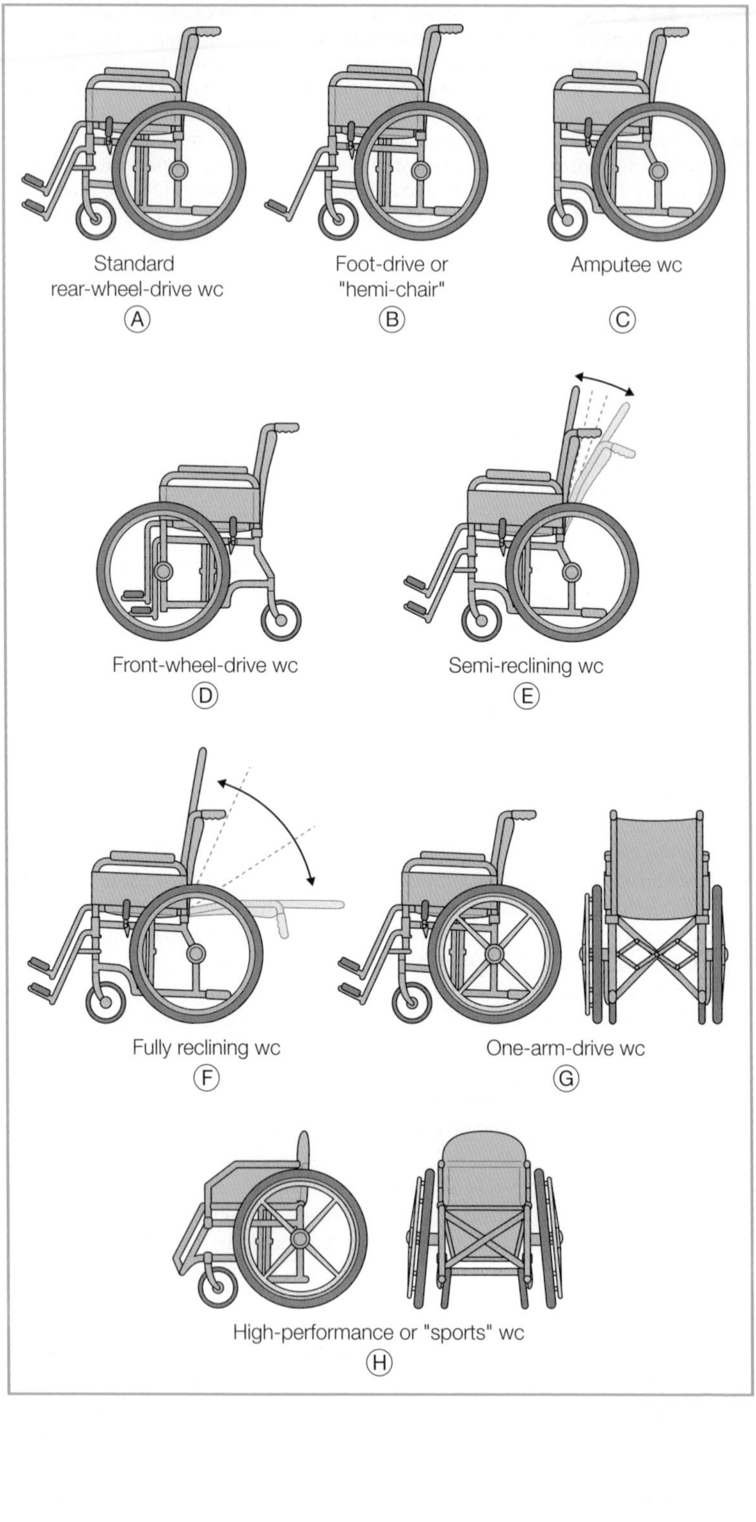
Standard
rear-wheel-drive wc
A
Foot-drive or
"hemi-chair"
B
Amputee wc
C
Front-wheel-drive wc
D
Semi-reclining wc
E
Fully reclining wc
F
One-arm-drive wc
G
High-performance or "sports" wc
H

Figure 4.7-3 Types of manual wheelchair (wc). Foot-drive or hemi-chair (**B**) has about 2-inch (5 cm) lower seat than standard wheelchair (**A**) and has only one front rigging. Amputee wheelchair (**C**) has rear wheels moved about 1.25–2 inches (3–5 cm) toward the rear to compensate for the posterior shift of the center of gravity of seated bilateral amputees. The front-wheel-drive wheelchair (**D**) is typically used indoors. The semi-reclining wheelchair (**E**) has back upholstery 5 inches (13 cm) higher than that of a standard wheelchair, and the wheel is set back 1.25 inches (3 cm) toward the rear. The fully reclining wheelchair (**F**) has back upholstery 7 inches (17 cm) higher than that of a standard wheelchair, and the wheel is set back 5 inches (12 cm) toward the rear. The (**G**) one-hand-drive wheelchair (wheelchair in illustration is left-hand drive) has driving wheels interconnected so that either or both can be controlled from one side through a dual set of handrims. The high-performance or "sports" wheelchair (**H**) is very light and has wider camber (i.e., lower part of wheel is tilted outwards).

occupant as well as for the person pushing when used over curbs and particularly over stairs.

II. **Wheel construction** (see Fig. 4.7-2)

- **Molded (plastic-molded) wheels**, also called "**mag**" **wheels**, because they were originally made primarily out of magnesium, are the most commonly used wheels in nonsports wheelchairs. They are heavier but more durable and need less maintenance than spoked wheels.
- **Wire-spoked wheels** are lighter (preferred in most sports wheelchairs), less durable (because the spokes tend to bend with heavy use), need greater maintenance (e.g., to tighten loosened spokes), and are less safe for elderly patients whose fingers may get caught in the spoked wheels.

b. ***Rear-wheel axles***. The rear-wheel axles can be fixed or adjustable. In patients who are expected to progress in their rehabilitation, an adjustable rear-wheel axle is preferred because the optimal site of axle placement may change as the patient improves. Axle placement can be adjusted either in the vertical direction [i.e., up or down to vary wheelchair height, improve positioning, and allow the user to reach the floor with the "good" foot (e.g., in wheelchairs used by hemiplegics)] or in the horizontal direction (i.e., anterior or posterior placement). The horizontal adjustment of the axle relative to the seat or the center of gravity determines the wheelchair's stability and efficiency. The most important factor to consider in axle placement is safety. Other factors include the height, weight, build, and functional abilities of the wheelchair user. An inappropriate axle position relative to the center of gravity can lead to accidental wheelchair tipping and falls. Tipping, in fact, accounts for the majority of wheelchair accidents and falls happen to 3.3% of wheelchair users each year.

I. **Posteriorly placed axle**. The seat or center of gravity is relatively anterior which increases wheelchair rear stability (advantageous for the elderly or patients with poor trunk stability, for amputees, and for reclining or posterior tilting wheelchairs). However, there is a tradeoff of increased wheelchair rolling resistance, greater turning radius (i.e., decreased wheelchair maneuverability), increased downhill turning tendency, and decreased ease of doing wheelies (because of the difficulty of tilting the wheelchair backwards).

II. **Anteriorly placed axle**. The seat or center of gravity is relatively posterior, which increases wheelchair's anterior stability and leads to decreased rolling resistance, decreased turning radius (with greater maneuverability), and decreased downhill turning tendency. However, it increases the tendency of the wheelchair to tip backwards when accelerating quickly or going up ramps. Anteriorly placed axles are advantageous for active paraplegic patients with good trunk balance and control who do wheelies to negotiate curbs. However, they are undesirable for patients with bilateral lower-limb amputations, because the lack of forward-placed lower-limb weight puts the sitting center of mass farther backward and makes it even easier for the wheelchair to tip backward.

c. ***Handrims*** (see Fig. 4.7-2), which are used for self-propulsion of the wheelchair, are smaller in diameter than the propelling wheel and are attached slightly lateral to the propelling wheel to permit wheelchair control without soiling the hands. Handrims can be modified for patients with poor handgrip by increasing the handrim's thickness (disadvantage of adding weight and width to the wheelchair); adding rubberized coatings to the handrim (disadvantage of the coating wearing off with time, discoloring the hands, or becoming rough, thus causing hand injuries); or attaching knobby projections (pegs or lugs; see Fig. 4.7-2) to the handrim with varied spacing and angle (e.g., vertical or oblique) for easy gripping and handrim control by patients with tetraplegia or hand deformities. In most cases, the best way to improve handrim grip is simply by having the patient wear a pair of sports gloves.
   I. **Large handrim diameters** make it easier to propel the wheelchair and are used in most wheelchairs because they provide greater power and maneuverability. However, more arm strokes are required to cover a given distance.
   II. **Small handrim diameters** are used in sports wheelchairs to maximize the distance covered with each stroke although more force is required to propel them.

d. ***Casters*** (see Fig. 4.7-2) are the small steering wheels found on the front of the rear-wheel-drive wheelchairs or on the back of front-wheel-drive wheelchairs. Front casters on rear-wheel-drive wheelchairs are easily damaged, have downhill-turning tendencies, and tend to flutter (shimmy) at higher speeds. Caster shimmy is not only annoying but can also increase rolling resistance and may cause an unintentional change in wheelchair direction. Caster shimmy at normal rolling speeds can be reduced by decreasing the size and weight of the caster, increasing the caster trail (i.e., the distance on the ground between the two casters), or increasing the proportion of the weight on the casters.
   I. **Large and wide casters.** For most purposes, 8-inch (20-cm) diameter casters of relatively wide configuration are optimal because these are easier to use on rougher outdoor terrain. Larger diameter casters also make it easier to climb curbs but have more of a tendency to flutter or shimmy. However, large and wide casters provide increased rolling resistance on smooth, level surfaces.
   II. **Small and narrow casters.** Casters of 5-inch or 13-cm diameters (often used in sports wheelchairs) and narrow widths are easier to maneuver and are suited for smooth, level surfaces. However they perform poorly on rough outdoor terrain, as they can get stuck on uneven terrain or soft ground, thus causing the chair to tip forward.

e. ***Tires*** (see Fig. 4.7-2) refer to wheel parts fitted onto the rims of the propelling wheels and casters. Narrow tires have less rolling resistance and are suitable for use on hard, flat, indoor surfaces but require much more force to propel through uneven surfaces and are thus not suited for outdoor use. Wide tires are easier to propel on uneven outdoor surfaces but have greater rolling resistance.
   I. **Solid (hard rubber) tires** (see Fig. 4.7-2) with smooth treads are very durable and have a low rolling resistance, especially on flat, smooth, and hard indoor surfaces but are relatively heavy and yield a harsh ride when used on uneven, outdoor terrain. They are recommended if the wheelchair is to be

used mostly indoors (e.g., in the hospital or nursing home) because the cushioning provided by pneumatic tires is not required for indoor use.

II. **Pneumatic tires** (see Fig. 4.7-2), which use an outer tire casing with an air-filled inner tube, are relatively lighter and provide the cushioning needed for outdoor use on uneven terrain not only to give a smooth comfortable ride but also to reduce the wear and tear on the wheelchair when used under normal outside conditions. If treaded pneumatic tires ("clincher" tires) are used, they also improve traction. The "all-terrain" tire has a wider tire with a different tread. The disadvantages of pneumatic tires include high rolling resistance on flat, smooth surfaces and also the tendency to develop a "flat" tire. To minimize this "flat" tire problem, thorn-resistant inner tubes may be used.

III. **Semi-pneumatic tires** (see Fig. 4.7-2) use flat-free inserts (zero-pressure tubes or ZPTs), which eliminate the flat-tire problem. The ZPTs can either be a coil type of soft rubber, latex gel, or a solid inner tube of foam (see Fig. 4.7-2), which replaces the inner tubes. They provide slightly rougher rides than pneumatic tires and also add weight to the wheelchair.

3. **Seating systems**. Fig. 4.7-1 shows the critical measurements needed for wheelchair fitting. The usual measurements for a standard adult wheelchair are seat height above the ground (19.5–20.5 inches or 49.5–52.0 cm), seat width (16–18 inches or 41–46 cm), and seat depth (16–18 inches or 41–46 cm). If orthotics are worn, a clearance of 1–2 inches (2.5–5.0 cm) is required on each side. Seat depth is important because if it is too short, the thighs are poorly supported and the area over which forces are distributed is reduced thus causing more pressure; however, if it is too deep, pressure ulcers may develop in the popliteal space, or the patient may tend to slide forward thus increasing sacral pressure and promoting kyphotic postures. The seat-plane angle (i.e., angle of the seat plane relative to the horizontal plane), which is usually 1–4° higher in front, may be increased to reduce spasticity, exaggerated lumbar lordosis, and the tendency of the patient to slide forward on the seat. However, it puts more pressure on the ischial tuberosities and makes transfers more difficult.

a. Seat types

I. **Sling (hammock) seats** consist of a tautly stretched flexible upholstery suspended between the wheelchair seat rails (see Fig. 4.7-2). They are the most commonly used wheelchair seats and can be considered a "planar seating" because they provide a flat seating surface in contact with the body. They are lightweight and easy to fold but provide little support, cannot adequately stabilize the pelvis, and thus can cause an increased incidence of posterior pelvic tilt (because of the tendency of the hips to slide forward), pelvic obliquity, internal rotation, and adduction at the hips (a position generally to be avoided by patients with total hip replacement as it may lead to hip dislocation). The upholstery commonly used is vinyl, which is inexpensive, durable, easy to clean, and comes in a number of colors; however, vinyl tends to cause heat buildup and promote perspiration. Vinyl will also stretch after long use and cause an undesirable "hammocking" effect on the seat. Alternatives to vinyl are Dacron and nylon, which are lighter in weight and more breathable, but are less easy to clean.

II. **Solid seats** are usually indicated for posture control. The solid seat design can be: 1) planar or linear (i.e., use of flat support surfaces such as flat foam seats); 2) contoured seats with human contours, e.g., buttocks, shaped by carving or sculpting foams, building with pads and blocks, or using preformed shapes based on research about human contours; 3) modular (i.e., use of prefabricated planar or contoured designs with adjustable and removable components for positioning and stabilization); 4) custom-molded seats created from the casted shape or mold taken from the individuals body contours; indicated for patients with complex seating and positioning needs; may utilize CAD–CAM, i.e., computer-assisted design and computer-assisted manufacturing.

- **Removable solid seats** can consist of a firm foam insert with a convex lower surface, a flat upper surface, and a cushion on top, or, alternatively, a cushioned plywood base. They are often placed on top of the sling seat to provide better support and decrease sling sagging.
- **Nonremovable solid seats** may be used, but they are not easily modified and they also add weight to the wheelchair. They can have a folding design for easy transportability.
- **Drop seat base (drop-hook seats)** are used to lower a solid seat surface below the level of the seat rails (usually up to a maximum of 5 cm or 2 inches) so as to provide a level base of support and prevent build-up of the seat height when cushions are added. Suspension hooks may be used to lower the seat base.

b. ***Pressure-relief seat cushions*** (see Fig. 4.7-2) are designed to counteract or to minimize stresses that act perpendicular to the skin (i.e., loading pressure) as well as stresses that act parallel to the skin (i.e., shear forces or stresses), both of which may lead to pressure ulcers. The common causes of pressure ulcers in wheelchair users include the patient's inability to shift weight; minimal adipose tissue and/or loss of muscle mass over the buttocks; pelvic obliquity (seen in "wind-swept" deformities in which one hip is abducted and one hip adducted causing the legs to appear unequal in length) caused by the "hammock effect" of sling seats, which leads to shearing forces; slumped sitting postures (i.e., sacral sitting) or posterior pelvic tilt, which can cause increased sacral pressure; and poor health or nutritional status. Aside from patient factors (e.g., bowel or bladder continence or presence of spasticity or flaccidity), other important factors to consider in cushion selection include moisture resistance (especially in incontinent patients or in places with hot, humid weather), ease of cushion maintenance and cleaning, weight of the cushion (if it is necessary to transport the cushion), and the cushion's durability and cost.

The design of pressure-relief cushions can either be total contact (to equalize or redistribute weight bearing over a maximal surface area), or specific pressure relief (achieved by carving out the cushion under bony prominences), or a combination of both. Static as well as dynamic pressure-relief cushions are available (see Chapter 5.2, section VI.B.3.a for descriptions, advantages, and disadvantages). The standard wheelchair cushion is a foam cushion; however, for wheelchair users with high risk of developing pressure ulcers, the two most commonly used static pressure-relief cushions are air- or fluid-filled cushions. At present, studies have shown that no single type of cushion is superior at relieving all types of pressure ulcers for all patients. Each cushion has its own advantages and disadvantages, which should be considered before prescribing any particular type of cushion. The decision about the cushion to be used should be made early because it affects other dimensions of the wheelchair (e.g., backrest, armrest, and seat height). The following are some of the common static pressure-relief wheelchair seat cushions, which can be customized to provide optimal pressure distribution while helping to control posture:

I. **Foam seat cushions** (see Fig. 4.7-2) are used in standard wheel-chairs because they are lightweight, inexpensive, and have breathable coverings. However, they are not washable, they wear out faster than other types of cushion, and they are not good dissipators of heat (because foams are heat insulators). Foam cushions are usually made of 3-inch (7.5-cm) medium-density polyurethane foams. They can also be made of viscoelastic foams (see Fig. 4.7-2.C) which are less resilient than polyurethane foams (see Fig. 4.7-2.D). The shape of foam cushions can be modified by placing a ramp on the anterior part of the cushion or by using a wedge-shaped foam cushion anteriorly (to promote hip flexion as well as transfer weight from the sacral, coccygeal, and ischial regions to the thighs for a better pelvic position, control, and stability, which may be beneficial in patients with spasticity); by using a preischial bar (to counteract forward sliding and transfer pressure from the sacral, coccygeal, and ischial regions to the thighs); by using cutout designs in the areas underlying bony prominences to relieve pressure; or by coating the cushion and contouring it to the shape of the buttocks to decrease skin-to-cushion interface pressures. An example of contoured foam is the Veterans Administration Spinal Injury Orthosis (VASIO) (see Fig. 4.7-2.A), in which foams of two different densities are combined and contoured to meet the needs of the paraplegic patient. The use of a foam coating increases the foam cushion's durability and ease of cleaning but also increases heat buildup and is more expensive. Wedge-shaped foam cushions attached to a solid plywood base are also commercially available (e.g., KSS Seat Base).

II. **Gel-filled seat cushions** consist of a firm emulsion (gel) enclosed in a "non-breathing" plastic casing (see Fig. 4.7-2.E). They are used to decrease peak pressures over bony prominences, accommodate movement and position shifts of the user, and provide postural stability. The most popular commercial brand is the Jay cushion (see Fig. 4.7-2.B), which consists of a contoured foam base (that can incorporate medial and lateral thigh as well as hip support) and a fluid-filled pad which pockets into the depression created for the ischial tuberosities and is covered with a washable cover. The gel of the newer Jay-2 cushion has a "memory" that provides optimal conformation. Jay cushions can also be fitted with modular components. They are durable, easy to maintain and clean, and have high heat capacity. Fluids are moderate conductors of heat and so they help dissipate skin heat buildup (decreasing the risk of skin breakdown through overheating). However, they are expensive; tend to be heavy (their weight varies from 8 to 35 lb, or 3.6 to 15.9 kg), which may hinder portability; and some patients may find difficulty with transfer techniques because of the contouring that they provide.

III. **Air-filled villous (ROHO) seat cushions** (see Fig. 4.7-2.F), consist of multiple balloon-like air cells, which the patient sits "in" to assure maximum skin contact and conformity. The high-profile ROHO cushion (with 10-cm- or 4-inch-high air cells) is the cushion of choice in preventing and healing pressure ulcers in long-term or high-risk sitting. The low-profile ROHO cushion (with 5-cm- or 2-inch-high air cells) is used for active patients with less potential for development of pressure ulcers. ROHO cushions can also be custom contoured for asymmetric patients (e.g., unilateral amputees). ROHO cushions are lightweight, easy to clean, and easy to transport. They are expensive, however, and do not provide good seating stability. They are, therefore, not recommended for patients who tend to slide forward in their wheelchair or who have a poor sitting position because of increased extensor tone. The ROHO seating stability can be improved by decreasing air-cell inflation. Patients – especially those with decreased lateral stability because of trunk weakness – may have difficulty transferring sideways to another surface because of the ROHO's soft and freely moving surface. The ROHO air pressure needs to be maintained regularly for skin protection and seating stability. In terms of their ability to control heat and moisture collection, air cushions are rated between fluid and foam cushions. Care must be taken to prevent punctures by avoiding pins or other sharp objects resting on them.

IV. **Water-filled seat cushions** (see Fig. 4.7-2.G) consist of a plastic or rubber membrane filled with chemically treated water or other liquid. The overall effect varies with the amount of water used. They adjust to body movements, are easy to clean, and can decrease temperature on the support surface. They may, however, leak if punctured and are relatively more heavy and difficult to transport.

V. **Combination air- and fluid-filled seat cushions (e.g., Bard Flotation cushion)** consist of a water-filled cushion (to assure even pressure distribution) and an air-filled frame (which prevents sacral sitting and sliding forward in the wheelchair by maintaining the femurs parallel to the seat). They are effective in preventing sacral sliding when 100° of hip flexion cannot be achieved because of mild extension contractures or when patients have increased extensor tone or extensor spasm in the lower limbs or of the whole body. However, they are relatively heavy and difficult to transport.

c. ***Seat support and positioning aids*** include antithrust designs, pelvic wells, pelvic stabilizers, pelvic bars, pelvic belts, lateral pelvic supports, anterior pelvic supports, medial thigh supports, lateral thigh supports, thigh troughs, abductor wedges, medial knee blocks (abductor pommels), and lateral knee blocks (adductor cushion). A key goal in wheelchair seating is to stabilize the pelvis because, during upright seating, 80% of the trunk weight is borne directly by the pelvis. Patients with pelvic obliquities or other deformities may need special custom-molded seats. Often the seat can be designed to place the patient in a position in which gravity helps stabilize the trunk and the head into the contours of the seat. Although firmer cushions generally provide a better base of support, they may be inappropriate in some patients who are insensate.

4. **Head and neck support and positioning systems** include foam headrests (flat, curved, three-piece, occipital supports, circumferential collars, horseshoe collars, customized), hook-on headrests (i.e., backrest extensions), telescopic headrests, pillow headrests, crown head supports (with headbands), and commercially available head and neck support systems (e.g., QA2 Headrest, KSS Neck Support, and Otto Bock Head and Neck Supports). A reclining wheelchair (see section I.B.5) or tilt-in-space wheelchair (see section I.B.6) may be used to hold the head back.

5. **Trunk support system**

a. ***Primary trunk supports (backrests)*** can be slings attached to the wheelchair back frame posts (i.e., back tubes; see Fig. 4.7-2). They are made of similar upholsteries as those used in sling seats (described in section I.A.3.a.1). They can also be solid (i.e., removable and placed over sling seats or folding), adjustable (i.e., in height and tension), or customized. The frame posts for the backrests are usually fitted with push handles to allow another person to propel and maneuver the wheelchair. Some wheelchair users, however, prefer not to have push handles because they connote a certain amount of dependence. The backrest height determines the wheelchair user's desired level of control and mobility, that is higher backrests give more support (to the spine and also to the head) but less freedom of mobility. Lower backrests, however, provide greater freedom of movement to the upper body and trunk but give almost no spinal or head support at all and can lead to a slumped "sacral seating" posture with a tendency toward development of thoracic kyphosis.

An ideal backrest height should provide sufficient support to the user, maintain good posture, and prevent fatigue over an extended time, while affording as much movement as possible without forcing the user into poor posture. In all cases the backrest should provide good support for the lumbosacral spine. In a standard wheelchair, the backrest height is usually 16–16.5 inches (41–42 cm) with about 8° of backward tilt from the vertical. This backrest height reaches up to the mid-back at about 1–2 inches (2.5–5 cm) below the inferior angles of the scapulae to minimize scapular irritation from rubbing during propulsion. The backrest width is similar to the seat width. In general, tetraplegic patients require higher backrest heights, but paraplegic patients (with normal trunk control, strong arms, and no spinal deformity) usually do well with a standard or lower backrest height. Wheelchair users with varying needs throughout the day can be given wheelchairs with adjustable backrest heights.

b. ***Secondary trunk positioning and support aids*** include foam side cushions, hook-on headrests, padded chest restraints (with or without shoulder straps), chest belts, Posey "Y" wheelchair safety belts, Otto-Bock sternal supports, Otto-Bock spherical side thoracic supports, lateral supports with padded armrests, padded lateral supports, back cushions, lumbar backrest cushions, soft T-foam back cushions, firm contoured back supports (e.g., Jay Active Back, KSS Back, QA2 Seatback with thoracic support, Jay Back, Jay Care Back, and Avanti Personal Back), modular back supports (e.g., Jay Modular Back), and sacral supports. A reclining wheelchair (see section I.B.5) or tilt-in-space wheelchair (see section I.B.6) may be used to support the back. Wheelchair restraints for maintaining posture and stability should only be used as a last resort as they make it almost impossible to do weight-shifting maneuvers for pressure relief.

6. Upper-limb support and positioning systems

a. ***Primary arm supports (armrests)*** are used to provide not only support for the patient's arms in a resting attitude (for maintaining balance and stability) but also to provide lateral support as well as serve as points of push-off for weight shifting (to assist in transfers or for relief of buttock pressure). The wheelchair armrest height should be such that the wheelchair user does not lean to either side when using the wheelchair armrest, and it should not interfere with arm movement, hand function, manual propulsion of the wheelchair. These conditions are easily met by using adjustable height armrests (although they weigh more than any other armrests). The armrest height of the standard adult wheelchair is 9 inches (23 cm). Prior to specifying the wheelchair's armrest height, the thickness of the seat cushion must be taken into account. Some models of sports wheelchairs have lightweight tubular armrests (see Fig. 4.7-2) or no armrests at all. The following are different types and styles of armrests, which can be combined to produce at least 12 different styles (except, obviously, for the "fixed style with adjustable height" combination).

I. **Fixed vs. nonfixed armrests**

- **Fixed armrests** (see Fig. 4.7-2) are continuous parts of the wheelchair frame and are not detachable. They are inexpensive and cannot be lost; however, they make wheelchair fitting more difficult, limit the proximity of the wheelchair to the table or desk surface, and prohibit side transfers (thus they are impractical if the patient is unable to stand for a brief period). They are usually found in wheelchairs used in airports or train stations or for hospital transport and are rarely found in prescription wheelchairs (except in some sports wheelchair models).
- **Nonfixed armrests**

– **Removable armrests** (see Fig. 4.7-2) are commonly used because they can be detached to allow for side transfers (in patients who are unable to stand up for transfers) and to increase the proximity of the wheelchair to the table or desk surface. However, they increase the wheelchair weight as well as wheelchair width the simplest type of removable armrest adds nearly 2 inches or 5 cm to the overall width of the standard wheelchair. Removable armrests (see Fig. 4.7-2) are usually height adjustable and can have either full-length or desk-style designs. To reduce the wheelchair width, an offset design or a wrap-around design may be used.

- **Flip-up (or swing-away) armrests** have the same features as removable armrests except that instead of detaching the armrest, it is swung away or flipped up when performing side-approach transfers.
- **Wrap-around or space-saver armrests** reduce the width of the wheelchair by attaching the armrest behind the backrest frame rather than next to the seat. They can generally be swung away or detached for transfers. They also allow the rear wheels to be placed closer to the wheelchair frame thus narrowing the outside width of the wheelchair without narrowing the seat width. The single functional disadvantage of the wrap-around design is that the desk-style armrest cannot be reversed or turned end-for-end.

II. **Full-length vs. desk-style armrests**. Both are available in fixed, nonfixed, or adjustable height models.

- **Full-length armrests** (see Fig. 4.7-2) extend from the backrest to the front of the wheelchair. They are indicated when the patient needs the full height of the front of the armrest to provide the leverage required to stand up from the wheelchair or when lordosis, obesity, or some other physical factors make it necessary to use the front part of the armrest for support while the patient is sitting in the wheelchair. However, they interfere with the ability to maneuver the wheelchair close to table or desk surfaces.
- **Desk-style armrests** (see Fig. 4.7-2) extend forward only partially (i.e., it is foreshortened by the forward one-third) to allow the user to get close enough to a desk or table top for good working conditions. The removable desk-style armrests, which are the most popular, are usually reversible, i.e., they can be used to provide the desk-style feature, or turned end-for-end to the reversed position (i.e., with the foreshortened part at the back) to allow sit-to-stand transfers or provide better access of the arms to the wheels for propulsion. However, when desk-style armrests are used in the reversed position, there is no lateral support of the trunk through the armrests.

III. **Fixed-height vs. adjustable height armrests**

- **Fixed-height armrests** (see Fig. 4.7-2) are found in wheelchairs with fixed armrests and nonfixed armrests (full-length or desk-style models). Their main disadvantage is their inability to accommodate individuals of different sizes.
- **Adjustable height armrests** (see Fig. 4.7-2) generally have adjustments ranging from 5 to 12 inches (12.7–30.5 cm) above the seat to accommodate the arm-positioning needs of individuals of different sizes. They are usually found in nonfixed armrests (full-length or desk-style models).

b. ***Secondary arm support and positioning aids*** include arm troughs (see Fig. 4.7-2), which hold the forearms in place [arm troughs can be padded, flat, elevated (to control edema), and molded)], swinging armrests (e.g., Otto-Bock Armrests and balanced forearm orthosis), shoulder support (anterior, posterior, superior), and elbow supports (elbow blocks).

c. ***Laptrays or lapboards*** are table-like surfaces (half- or full-size; see Fig. 4.7-2), which are either attached to the armrests or used as a substitute for regular armrests. They are usually detachable or may have swing-away capabilities. They can be used for eating, reading, writing, and other activities as well as for holding objects (e.g., a communication board or a daily schedule) and for supporting the upper limbs and preventing shoulder subluxation (e.g., in hemiplegic patients). When properly adjusted for height, they promote good posture (particularly when the patient would otherwise have to lean forward to reach a working surface). Laptrays can be made of wood, plywood, opaque plastic, or clear plastic that allows visualization of the lower limbs, the front rigging of the wheelchair, and the floor, thus helping to reduce the possibility of injuring the feet or toes.

For certain activities, a laptray with an extra shelf may be useful. Laptray use in front-wheel-drive wheelchairs makes wheelchair propulsion slightly more difficult.

7. **Lower-limb support and positioning systems.** Optimal lower-limb support and positioning (see Fig. 4.7-1 for proper angulation of the hips, knees, and ankle joints) play important roles in improving the distribution of pressure over the sacrum and ischial tuberosities. In an upright seated position, the forces produced at the weight-bearing surfaces of the buttocks are equal to the body weight minus the supporting forces provided by the footrests or floor. The lower legs (calves) usually do not require direct support if there is proper support of the thighs (seating surface) and feet (foot rest). In most wheelchairs, the knees are positioned at a maximum of 60–70° flexion. However, some wheelchair models allow the knees to be hyperflexed (at >90° flexion) to provide tighter turns, get closer access to objects (counter, bathtub, or bed), protect the feet, ease transport of the wheelchair, and inhibit spasticity. Some of the disadvantages of a hyperflexed knee position include difficulty in accommodating users with long legs, a need for smaller caster diameters to avoid the footrests hitting the swiveling casters when changing direction, and decreased effectiveness of the footrests as forward antitipping devices.

a. ***Primary lower-limb support (front rigging).*** *Front rigging* is a collective term for the legrest and footrest. Aside from supporting the lower limbs, the front rigging acts as a forward antitipper (i.e., it increases rearward stability). It may consist of fixed bars, nondetachable and nonelevating (see Fig. 4.7-2), that are continuous with the wheelchair frame. Fixed front riggings have no "elevating legrest" but have footrests that may consist of footplates with heel hoops or may simply consist of a single horizontal bar with heel loops as seen in sports wheelchairs. Although fixed front riggings generally make the wheelchair lighter and allow more freedom of movement of the lower limb for propulsion or other function, they may interfere with transfers and wheelchair portability. Most wheelchairs have nonfixed front riggings, which consist of the following:

I. **Legrests.** Legrests (see Fig. 4.7-2) refer to "elevating legrests" and the calf pads, which support the legs when the legrests are elevated. Legrests usually consist of elevating support brackets with swing-away or detachable mechanisms so they can be moved aside or detached when needed (e.g., for transfers; wheelchair transport; and getting closer to a counter, bathtub, or bed). Some medical or surgical conditions that require leg elevation include dependent lower-limb edema, postsurgery of lower limb (e.g., to allow knee arthrodesis to fuse), knee contracture (i.e., elevating the legrest may help extend the knee), and leg in a cast. By elevating the legrests, there is decreased forward static stability because the center of gravity is shifted forward, increased rolling resistance, and more difficulty maneuvering in tight places. The legrests may be elevated up to the level of the seating surface (i.e., a low pivot-point style) or they may project higher than the seat (i.e., goose-neck style). The goose-neck style is less desirable as it can interfere with transfers and provides a point of pressure contact with the leg.

II. **Footrests.** Footrests (see Fig. 4.7-2) consist of footplates that can be swung up 90° so that they are vertical to the floor to permit easy access to the chair by patients who can stand. They keep the feet off the floor with the ankle in the neutral position and they hold the posterior aspect of the distal thighs of paralyzed patients at a height above the front edge of the seat to maintain lower-limb circulation. The lowest point on the footrests (see Fig. 4.7-1) should be at least 2 inches (5 cm) above the floor to avoid being caught on obstacles and on incline transitions. Footrests should not be positioned so high above the floor as to force more weight backward onto the ischial tuberosities and increase the risk of ischial pressure ulcers; nor should they be positioned so low (or removed) as to increase the pressure at the distal thighs, increasing the chance for posterior pelvic tilt, and providing less support for forward leaning. The distance between the footplates and the front edge of the seat can be adjusted to alter the distribution of the loads over the thighs and buttocks.

b. ***Secondary lower-limb support and positioning aids*** include anterior knee supports, anterior leg supports, knee protectors for elevating legrests, legrest panels, board supports on legrests (legrest board, leg and footrest board), padded wooden legrests, amputee cushions, knee abductors, elevating blocks on footplates, footplate extensions, heel straps, foot positioners, wooden foot supports with posterior extensions, foot straps (figure-eight foot straps, ankle straps), ankle-positioning aids (ankle-positioning blocks, footplates with adjustable angle setting), and heel loops (heel loops, instead of calf supports of the legrest units, are often used in sports wheelchairs as they reduce wheelchair weight).

8. **Safety components**

a. ***Parking locks (wheel locks)*** are devices that put pressure on the propelling wheels or tires (or occasionally the casters as well, for greater stability) to lock them into position (while parked) and prevent unintended rolling of the wheelchair, either on an incline or during transfers. Parking locks should not be used nor be erroneously referred to as "brakes" because they are not intended to slow down a moving wheelchair (this not only subjects the tires to unnecessary wear and tear but may cause sudden stopping and overturning of the wheelchair). If the moving wheelchair needs to be slowed down, the "brake" should be applied by the hand(s) on the handrim(s). Parking locks are usually attached to the sideframe of the wheelchair and are available in either a push-to-lock or a pull-to-lock mechanism. Either mechanism has no distinct advantage as whatever is pushed to lock needs to be pulled to unlock and vice versa. In some wheelchair models, the lock may be placed in the rear of the chair where it can be activated only by an attendant or caregiver and not by the patient with cognitive deficits. Parking locks can be mounted in a high position with long handles for easy access (e.g., hemiplegic patients), or they can be mounted in a low position with short handles (preferred by active wheelchair users because they do not interfere with their long pushing strokes or get in the way during transfers).

   I. **Toggle locks** (see Fig. 4.7-2), which are used in most wheelchairs, have a preset locking "power", which is turned on or off by moving the activating toggle. The activating toggle can consist of a vertical handle bar, or it can consist of a flat horizontal bar [i.e., a scissors-type lock (see Fig. 4.7-2) used in sports wheelchairs as they present less hazard to the thumbs and hands during vigorous pushing].

   II. **Lever locks** (see Fig. 4.7-2) can be set at different notches to provide varying degrees of holding power. They are advantageous for parking on steep inclines, but their use requires greater upper limb control and strength than toggle locks.

b. ***Grade aids (or "hill holders")*** are spring-loaded devices that are activated only on uphill inclines to prevent the wheelchair from rolling backward but do not interfere with forward motion. They are useful for patients with poor strength or endurance when propelling uphill (because they prevent the wheelchair from rolling backwards between forward thrusts). Grade aids should not be used by active, strong wheelchair users because they can become accidentally activated while the user is performing a wheelie, thus causing a backward tipping fall.

c. ***Antitip bars (antitippers; see Fig. 4.7-2)*** are extensions for the lower rail installed in the rear of the wheelchair to prevent at-risk patients (e.g., above-knee amputees with a more posterior center of gravity) from falling backward in the wheelchair. They can be fixed, removable, or can be turned to the "up" position to help the wheelchair user in negotiating curbs or incline transitions where the device might interfere or "ground" the wheelchair. Antitippers may have wheels at their ends, which will come in contact with the floor upon tipping, thus avoiding a sudden deceleration. Antitippers are generally not used by active wheelchair users who practice wheelies to climb up curbs. The front rigging of the wheelchair can be considered an antitipping device as this increases rear stability. To prevent the wheelchair from tipping forward, antitipping devices may be attached to the front rigging.

d. ***Seat belts, safety vests, and harnesses*** are described above under seat support and positioning systems as well as secondary support and positioning systems for the trunk and extremities.

B. CLASSIFICATION BY WHEELCHAIR-USER NEEDS

1. The standard (conventional or basic) adult wheelchair (see Fig. 4.7-3) is typically made of steel tubings with a sling seat and back; has two large wheels in the rear, each fitted with a concentric handrim, which is turned by the wheelchair user; has two small swiveling wheels (casters) in front; has a front rigging (with legrest and footrest); has a back height of 16–16.5 inches (41–42 cm), a seat depth and seat width of 16–18 inches (41–46 cm), a seat height of 19.5–20.5 inches (49.5–52 cm) from the floor, a weight of about 40–50 lb (18–23 kg), and usually an X-frame that allows for folding of the wheelchair. The standard wheelchair is generally indicated for temporary use, short-distance dependent mobility, or for some part-time users who have some walking ability. For obese patients wanting manual wheelchairs, a wider than standard seat and heavy duty frame must be prescribed. Seat width is critical: seats wider than 24 inches will not go through standard doors. Hence, a powered chair may be the only choice in the very obese.

2. Hemiplegic or one-arm amputee wheelchairs

a. ***One-arm-drive (or mono-drive) wheelchairs*** (see Fig. 4.7-3) are designed to be operated with one arm, either right or left. Both handrims are typically mounted on one side. The first handrim is the usual handrim close to the wheel with which it is connected directly. The second handrim is mounted outside the first but is connected by an axle to the wheel on the other side. Turning both handrims moves the wheelchair straight ahead, while turning one or the other handrim steers the wheelchair. An alternative to this design is the use of a single hand-lever propulsion mechanism. The disadvantage of one-arm-drive chairs is their increased width and weight. They are rarely used successfully by hemiplegic or one-arm amputee patients, as propelling them requires a fairly high degree of strength and coordination. However, some two-handed patients may find them useful when it is important to have one hand free (e.g., for work) while the other propels the chair.

b. ***Foot-drive (or low-seat) wheelchairs or "hemi-chairs"*** (see Fig. 4.7-3) are practical alternatives to one-arm-drive wheelchairs (which are difficult to propel). The hemiplegic patient uses one handrim and one "good" foot (both feet may be used if feasible) to help propel and steer the wheelchair. For the foot or feet to reach the ground, the seat is lowered by 2 inches or 5 cm [thus the seat height from the floor is about 17.5–18.5 inches (44.5–47 cm)], and one or both of the front riggings is removed. Lowering of the seat height can be accomplished by using 22-inch (56-cm) diameter wheels (which lower seat height by 1 inch, or 2.5 cm) or by using drop-hook seats (see above section I.A.3.a.2.c).

3. Lower-limb amputee wheelchairs (see Fig. 4.7-3) are indicated for patients who have lost both lower limbs or significant parts of them or for those whose lower limbs are significantly atrophied. The center of gravity of a bilateral lower-limb amputee in the seated position, even with lower-limb prostheses which are usually lighter than the amputated extremities, is at least an inch further to the rear than for nonamputees. To maintain stability and compensate for the loss of weight in the absent or atrophied lower limbs, the rear axle and the propelling wheels of the lower-limb amputee wheelchairs should be moved further posteriorly (usually by 1.25–2 inches or 3–5 cm). By moving the rear wheel posteriorly, the wheelchair turning radius is increased slightly, but this is compensated when the front rigging is removed for those not wearing lower-limb prostheses. Other alternatives to moving the rear-wheel axle posteriorly are to put 10–15 lb (4.5–6.8 kg) of sandbags on the front rigging of a standard wheelchair to re-establish the lost counterweight or to attach two special axles (amputee attachments) behind the original ones.

4. **High-performance wheelchairs** (see Fig. 4.7-3) are lightweight (20–40 lb or 9–18 kg) or ultralightweight (15–20 lb or 7–9 kg) wheelchairs. The ultralightweight wheelchairs are generally known as sports wheelchairs, and although they are typically used by athletic paraplegics patients, they can also be used by nonathletic patients. Sports wheelchairs have rigid frames of high strength and durability, fixed front riggings (usually consisting of a horizontal bar with heel loops rather than footplates), lower and firmer backrests (may be detachable), lower armrests (may use detachable tubular armrest or have no armrest at all), lower and firmer seats positioned more rearward in relation to the rear-wheel axle, spoked wheels that are cambered, small-diameter handrims, and small and narrow casters. They are much more energy efficient during propulsion (i.e., they require about 17% less energy to propel than standard wheelchairs) and are not as easy to transport and store as the X-frame wheelchairs. There are different sports wheelchairs for specific sporting events (e.g., racing or basketball).
5. **Reclining wheelchairs** cause an increase in the sagittal angle of the backrest in relation to the seat surface via the use of either manual controls (operated by an attendant caretaker) or motorized controls (may be activated by the patient). As the backrest is lowered during a recline maneuver, the legrests generally elevate at the same rate as the descent of the backrest. Reclining wheelchairs are used to improve trunk control and spinal alignment, reduce ischial pressure in proportion to the extent of the recline (especially useful for patients who cannot adequately shift their own weight), reduce orthostatic hypotension, increase mobilization of pulmonary secretions, alleviate back pain (because of the decreased effect of gravity on the spine), facilitate catheterizing a patient in the wheelchair, reduce the need for additional transfers during the day for rest periods, and allow some patients with insufficient hip flexion who might not otherwise fit into a wheelchair to "sit" in a wheelchair.

   The disadvantages of reclining wheelchairs include increased wheelchair weight, width, and bulk; increased difficulty of wheelchair transportation; reclining may trigger spasticity because of the change in the relative positions of the user's body parts; and reclining may cause increased shear stress over the back and sacrum during position changes (this is particularly true when simple hinge-reclining wheelchairs are used because the mechanical axis of the backrest with variable recline is usually below and behind the anatomic axis of the user's hip joint). If the shear force is not minimized, the process of reclining and resuming the upright posture tends to slide the patient forward onto the seat and into a poor sitting position especially when there is significant spasticity. To minimize this shear force particularly for persons at risk for pressure ulcers, any or all of the following measures may be taken: slide the seat of the wheelchair anteriorly while reclining; slide the back of the chair downward while reclining; align the axis of movement of the reclining back with the anatomic axis of hip flexion and extension; use a special low-shear or zero-shear reclining wheelchair (which consists of a double-back arrangement that allows the user to adhere to the forward-most back of the chair, while shear force is concentrated between the "front" and "rear" backs of the chair); or use a tilt-in-space wheelchair (see below).

a. ***Semi-reclining wheelchair*** (see Fig. 4.7-3) reclines about 30° from vertical and locks in several positions. It has a back upholstery, which is 5 inches (13 cm) higher than a standard adult wheelchair; a detachable 10-inch (25-cm) telescopic headrest; and rear wheels set back 1.25 inches (3 cm) to maintain good balance and stability of the wheelchair. Its armrests and legrests must provide support for the limbs in all positions. The semi-reclining wheelchair relieves part of the pressure from the ischia but not from the sacrum where shearing forces can still lead to sacral pressure ulcers.

b. ***Fully reclining wheelchairs*** (see Fig. 4.7-3) may be locked in any position between the vertical and horizontal and, therefore, permit conversion from a wheelchair to a stretcher. These have a back upholstery, which is 7 inches (17 cm) higher than a standard adult wheelchair; detachable 10-inch (25-cm) telescopic headrests; and rear wheels set back 5 inches (12 cm) to maintain wheelchair stability and balance. These provide better relief of pressure from the ischia and sacrum than semi-reclining wheelchairs.

6. **Tilt-in-space wheelchairs** provide alternatives to the reclining wheelchairs. They use a system (usually hydraulic, sometimes manual or motorized) by which the entire seat and back are tilted posteriorly as a single unit in the sagittal plane, thus the angle between seat, backrest, and leg- or footrest remains the same in all positions, and the relative position of the user's body parts remains unchanged. Like reclining wheelchairs, they improve trunk control and spinal alignment, as well as reduce spinal and ischial pressure (in proportion to the extent of the tilt), reduce orthostatic hypotension, and allow for increased mobilization of pulmonary secretions. The advantages of tilt-in-space wheelchairs over reclining wheelchairs include lack of shear stress during tilting movements, less likelihood of triggering spasticity in patients with increased tone or spasticity problems, and better repositioning when the upright position is resumed. However, they tend to be unstable with large persons, require a higher seating position, do not allow the patient's body to straighten toward the supine position, and are difficult to transport.
7. **Stand-up wheelchairs** allow the patient to stand within the frame of the wheelchair. They are used for medical reasons (e.g., to provide weight-bearing benefits on bone or provide pressure relief) as well as other reasons such as improved psychological outlook and increased work access). They are usually available in both motorized and manual versions. Their main disadvantages are increased weight, width, cost, and complexity.
8. **Manual wheelchairs with add-on power-pack units.** Although technically considered a motorized wheelchair (see section III.A), these are classified under manual wheelchairs because they are mainly indicated for manual wheelchair users who are progressively losing strength or who occasionally need power assistance for long-distance travel or rough terrain. The add-on power-pack units (which consist of a pair of drive motor and battery, or set of batteries, and a proportional joy stick-type control) are attached to a manual wheelchair (which can either have a folding or a rigid frame) to convert it into a motorized wheelchair. Because the power-pack units can easily be removed, the transportability of the manual wheelchair is retained. Although they are less expensive (especially if the patient already owns a manual wheelchair), they are also less durable, provide less power (because of the smaller batteries), and are less adaptable than other motorized wheelchairs.

II. Attendant-propelled wheelchairs

Attendant-propelled wheelchairs are designed to be pushed by another person because of the patient's short- or long-term inability to propel a manual wheelchair or operate a powered-mobility system in a functional or safe manner. Attendant-propelled wheelchairs may be used on a short-term basis for long-distance transportation in the community or when the patient's power-mobility system is being repaired or cannot be used because of space constraints (e.g., in airline aisles). An example of a long-term indication for attendant-propelled wheelchairs includes demented patients who are unable to walk because of various medical conditions (e.g., lower limb contractures and deformities). The attendant-propelled wheelchairs can be full-sized wheelchairs with four small wheels (e.g., posture-care chairs or "gerichairs"), or front-wheel-drive manual wheelchairs (used for their maneuverability in limited indoor spaces such as in nursing homes; see above section I.A.2.a.1.b), or they may be smaller and created for use in limited spaces, e.g., folding stroller-type wheelchairs. Many rear-wheel-drive manual wheelchairs (see section I.A.2.a.1.a), such as standard-sized manual wheelchairs, can also serve as attendant-propelled wheelchairs. Factors to consider in ordering an attendant-propelled wheelchair include not only the fit and comfort of the patient but also accommodating the person pushing the wheelchair.

III. Powered mobility systems

A. MANUAL WHEELCHAIRS WITH ADD-ON POWER-PACK UNITS are described in section I.B.8 under manual wheelchairs.

B. POWERED OR MOTORIZED WHEELCHAIRS (INTEGRAL-POWER MOBILITY SYSTEMS) refer to wheelchairs with integrated power-drive systems (direct-drive vs. belt-drive; see below), battery power sources, and user-operated controls, in addition to other similar features essentially found in manual wheelchairs, such as seating systems, positioning and support systems, and safety components.

Indications. They are indicated for patients with physical limitations not compatible with manual wheelchair propulsion, i.e., those who cannot propel a wheelchair using either the hands or feet because of limb absence, paralysis, deformity, or other neuromusculoskeletal problems and those with poor endurance (because of cardiopulmonary or neuromusculoskeletal conditions) who must conserve their energy for other functions (e.g., vocational work). Some common conditions that might warrant powered wheelchairs include high-level spinal cord injury (e.g., C4 and above); advanced muscle weakness because of amyotrophic lateral sclerosis, multiple sclerosis, or muscular dystrophy; and poor coordination in all limbs (e.g., cerebral palsy). Powered wheelchairs are usually indicated for outdoor use (rarely for indoor use) in patients of all ages who have to travel long distances (usually without help) and who tire easily. Patients with powered wheelchairs generally need standard wheelchairs for indoor use and as backups when their powered wheelchairs are being repaired or cannot be transported. The indoor use of manual wheelchairs also provides beneficial exercise for many patients.

User requirements. To safely use a powered wheelchair, patients must have at least one reproducible movement (using the upper limb or other part of the body) to access the control system; a basic understanding of cause and effect and directionality; sufficient vision, perceptual ability, and judgment to permit movement through the environment; and proper motivation. Even children as young as 2–3 years can be taught to safely operate a powered wheelchair. Potential candidates (even those with severe physical disabilities or cognitive limitations) must be given a trial with a similar powered wheelchair, not necessarily to assess whether the patient can drive the system but to determine the patient's ability to learn to use it.

Potential benefits of powered wheelchairs include an increased independence level at school and work, increased efficiency of mobility, sparing of the upper limb joints (especially shoulder joints) from repetitive stress injury induced by manual wheelchair propulsion or from premature deterioration (e.g., musculoskeletal complications such as arthritis of the upper limb joints), and improved self-esteem generated by greater independence.

The **potential disadvantages** of powered wheelchairs include the following: relatively high cost, heavy weight, transportation difficulty, relatively high maintenance, technological dependence, and limited environmental accessibility. Patients also do not get as much needed exercise as manual wheelchair users.

Contraindications to powered mobility systems include inability to securely execute the motions of the control lever or switch, involuntary motions or inattention which might result in activating the controls unintentionally, blindness, lack of judgment, and irresponsibility – all of which count much more than in a manually propelled chair.

Prescription guidelines for a powered wheelchair are based on the same general wheelchair prescription principles described above (see introduction to this chapter) but with greater emphasis on the safety (of the user and of others) and performance of the powered wheelchair. Although it uses the same seating and positioning principles as those described for manual wheelchairs, the positioning of the upper limbs or other body parts is critical for placement of the wheelchair control system. The main factors to consider in powered wheelchair prescription include:

- Primary use, i.e., usually for outdoor use; consider the type of terrain and the need for "all-terrain wheelchairs";
- Stability, i.e., lower seat and wider wheelchair base have more stability;
- Overall weight and portability, i.e., ease of assembly and disassembly, if appropriate; the weight, size, and transportability of each disassembled part;
- Availability of adapted vehicles for wheelchair transportation, e.g., vans with ramps or hydraulic lifts;
- Environmental barriers, i.e., need for extensive environmental modifications; dimensions required for turning (in small spaces, short-based wheelchairs are easier to maneuver);
- Battery life, i.e., the range (or distance capability) of the powered wheelchair based on a single battery charge;
- Power adjustability, e.g., speed, acceleration, and deceleration (high acceleration or deceleration may cause problems in persons with poor trunk control);
- Type and placement of the wheelchair control system, e.g., joystick on the right-side armrest or Sip-and-Puff controls on the left-side mouth angle;
- Safety features, e.g., brakes, parking locks, safety harnesses, and antitippers;
- Availability of other equipment and features, e.g., communication aids, powered recliners, and platforms for respiratory aids;
- Durability, i.e., consider wheelchair maintenance requirements as well as availability of parts and technical support;
- Other factors, e.g., cost (financial resources), noise factors, and ride quality.

The following are essential components of powered wheelchairs that are not found in manual wheelchairs:

1. Power-drive systems

a. Direct-drive powered wheelchairs (or power-base wheelchairs; see Fig. 4.7-4.A,B) consist of a rigid mainframe (that contains the batteries and drive

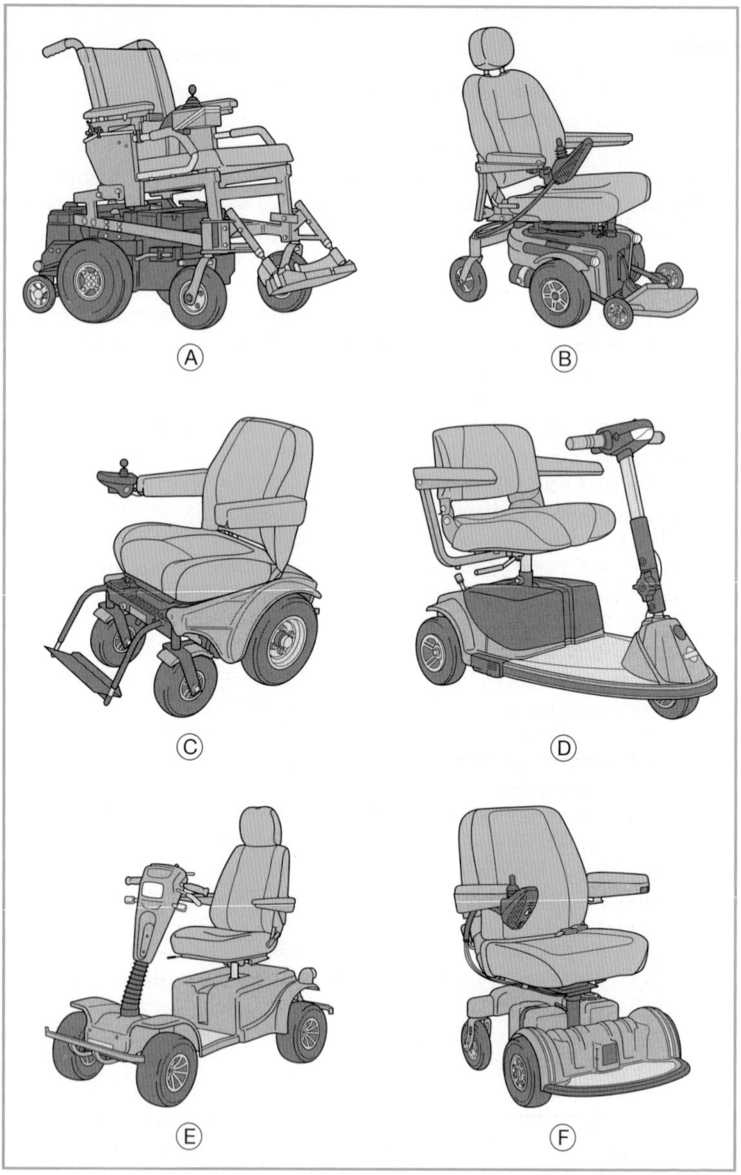

Figure 4.7-4 Types of powered wheelchair (wc): **A**, Direct-drive powered wheelchair or power-base wheelchair, rear-wheel drive; **B**, Direct-drive powered wheelchair or power-base wheelchair, front-wheel drive (this is more maneuverable than rear-wheel drive); **C**, Belt-driven powered wheelchair; **D**, Three-wheeled scooter; **E**, Four-wheeled scooter; **F**, Hoveround (note the round power base and single steerable rear wheel). Sources: A. Quickie P200 Electric Wheelchair by Sunrise/Quickie Electric Wheelchairs (*http://www.spinlife.com*); B. Jet 3 Ultra Electric Wheelchair by Pride Electric Wheelchairs (*http://www.spinlife.com*); C. Prairie Cruiser Power Chair by Wheelchairs of Kansas (*http://glad.net*); D. 2004 Revo 3-wheel Scooter by Pride Scooters (*http://www.spinlife.com*); E. Wrangler PMV Electric Scooter by Pride Scooters (*http://www.spinlife.com*); F. Hoveround MPV4 by Hoveround (http://www.Hoveround.com).

mechanisms); a seat, which is positioned directly above the power base on a pedestal attached to the rigid mainframe; and four small balloon tires (diameter of 8–10 inches or 20–25 cm and width of 3 inches or 7.6 cm; some newer models have slightly larger wheels, either in the rear or front). They are durable and better suited for rough terrain (because of their low center of gravity and wider tires). However, they are less maneuverable indoors or on carpets, and the large caster wheels have a tendency to wrinkle and roll carpeting, especially small rugs.

b. ***Belt-driven powered wheelchairs*** (see Fig. 4.7-4.C) have comparable rigid mainframe and seating system as direct-drive wheelchairs but usually have two large rear wheels and two small front casters (the wheels of belt-driven powered wheelchairs look almost like those of manual wheelchairs). They are more versatile (i.e., their frames are better suited to modification and the addition of different components), more stable, and are generally capable of reaching greater speeds than direct-drive wheelchairs; however, they tend to be less durable.

2. **Control systems** can be activated by any reproducible movement of the body such as those involving the upper extremity (i.e., hand, wrist, arm, fingertip, or upper limb residual limb) or non-upper-limb body parts (e.g., head, chin, mouth, lips, tongue, and lower limbs). The activating devices commonly used include joysticks (i.e., a small pressure-sensitive stem attached to a control box; joystick-stem modifications include T-bar handles, knobs, long extension handles, mouthstick, etc.), chin- or head-pressure controls, and pneumatic controls (e.g., Sip-and-Puff, which uses soft or intense inspiration, the sip, or expiration, the puff). Other special controls include the leaf switch, touch plate, toggle switch, voice-activated switch, myoelectric control switch, proximity sensing system, and scanning system (i.e., a control option that presents grouped or single choices one at a time until the user selects it by activating a switch). In general, the controls have a high and low range as well as options to increase power (e.g., when negotiating carpeted floor, grassy ground, or rough terrain). If possible, the control system of the powered wheelchair should be compatible with the patient's environmental control unit (see Chapter 4.5, section II.A.5.a.3).

a. ***Primary controls*** are used for changing wheelchair direction and speed, as well as for braking.

I. **Proportional controls** respond to pressure in a similar fashion to a car accelerator, i.e., an increase in the amount (or direction) of pressure applied to the control mechanism (most commonly a joystick) proportionately increases such wheelchair parameters as speed, acceleration, or direction change (i.e., forward, reverse, right, left, and all variations in between). They give the greatest degree of wheelchair control and provide the smoothest ride; however, the user must have fair to good motor control, as determined by manual muscle testing.

II. **Nonproportional (momentary or latching) controls** use microswitch controls, which operate by the all-or-none principle (the switch is either "on" or "off" like a light switch). The user applies any degree of pressure and as soon as the switch is activated, the system operates at the preset speed and/or direction (i.e., forward, reverse, right, and left). Multiple switch controls (e.g., a series of Sip-and-Puff switches) may be used. They are less responsive than proportional controls and generally require fewer skilled movements to achieve control, although learning to use such controls is not simple.

b. ***Secondary controls*** usually consist of nonproportional (on/off) controls (e.g., scanning systems) for operating reclining or tilt-in-space wheelchair functions, call signals, communication aids, environmental control units, or personal computers.

3. **Battery systems** can either be made of gel or lead. The recommended battery is usually a deep-cycle lead acid battery, either wet or sealed cell type. Most

batteries are based on 12- or 24-volt electrical systems: 24-volt power is used for outdoor wheelchairs, which need charging on a daily basis. The battery life determines the range (or distance capability) of the wheelchair, which is approximately 20 miles during the course of a day for most batteries. The range in turn depends on the user's driving habits (e.g., fast vs. slow; use of frequent quick starts), type of terrain covered (rough vs. flat), and adequacy of tire inflation. The batteries should be conveniently placed for easy access (e.g., for removal when transporting wheelchair) and should have indicators showing when the charge is low.

4. **Brake and parking lock systems.** Most powered wheelchairs have an electromechanical brake (that slows down the moving wheelchair. The braking speed may be adjusted for patients with unsteady balance) and a parking lock (that holds the wheelchair still when it comes to a stop). Both must be easily activated either manually or through an automatic switch.
5. **Special powered features** include elevating and lowering seats; reclining and/or tilt-in-space seats; standing mechanisms (to raise the wheelchair user to a standing position); mechanism to negotiate uneven surfaces and stairs; and mechanism to use wheelchair as a lift or in transferring.

C. **ELECTRIC CARTS (SCOOTERS)** differ from powered wheelchairs by their use of a front tiller or steering column (which has forward, reverse, turning, and stop controls) and their seat design, which is usually a bracket-type seat (with or without armrests) mounted on a central pedestal, which can be easily adjusted in height or swiveled for easy transfers and for working at a desk. Unlike other types of wheelchairs, they have less "custom-fitting" flexibility and generally do not have as good a seating position. Also they have a tendency to be top-heavy and can easily topple, especially when operating at high speed. Compared to powered wheelchairs, they are generally easier to mount and dismount, have better cosmetic appearance, have good suspension and power for travel over rough terrain, and have longer service range. Some units are large, heavy (weighing between 225 and 250 lb or 102 and 114 kg or more), and difficult to transport. Others, however, are modular and can be disassembled and loaded in the trunk of a car or back of a station wagon. However, certain parts could be as heavy as 50 lb or 23 kg and usually require a hydraulic lift to load and unload. They are indicated for patients who can ambulate, transfer, and perform most activities of daily living but who need the scooter for traveling long distances outside the home (in urban environments) because of lack of endurance or inability to use a manual wheelchair. They are also for patients who must avoid overuse of their limbs.

Scooter users (e.g., patients with rheumatoid arthritis, severe cardiac or degenerative disease, or early stages of multiple sclerosis or motor neuron or neuromuscular junction disease) are generally less disabled than the users of the other power-mobility systems. In general, the user must have good sitting balance, good eye–hand coordination, adequate spatial and figure-ground perception, and good judgment. Although reduced endurance and strength, especially of the lower extremities, are the main indications, the user must have good control of the upper trunk and at least one upper limb to manually steer the unit. Scooters are usually used in conjunction with walkers, canes, or manual wheelchairs. Like golf carts, they may not be absolutely necessary, but they can help save the user's energy and provide an element of pleasure and fun.

1. **Three-wheeled scooters** (see Fig. 4.7-4.D) have three 6-inch (15-cm) diameter wheels (two wheels in the rear and a third wheel in the front). A rear-wheel-drive type (more powerful but bulkier, heavier, and less maneuverable in tight spaces) is generally recommended for outdoor use, while a front-wheel-drive type (lighter, smaller, and more maneuverable in tight spaces but less powerful)

is recommended for indoor use. In both types, the controls and steering of the scooters are the same (i.e., the tiller is located above the front wheel). Three-wheeled scooters are generally indicated for users who are less disabled than users of the four-wheeled wheelchairs.

2. **Four-wheeled scooters** (see Fig. 4.7-4.E) are available in both rear-wheel- and front-wheel-drive models. They have the same tiller mechanism, advantages and disadvantages as do similar three-wheeled models. They are more stable than the three-wheeled models but are less compact and less portable. They are indicated for patients who are more disabled than the users of the three-wheeled scooters.

D. HOVEROUNDS (see Fig. 4.7-4.F), have configurations similar to that of a power-base chair, but with features and options more frequently found on scooters. Their unique features include their round power base (which allows for an extremely tight turning radius) and their one steerable rear wheel.

E. ADAPTED VANS AND CARS can be considered sources of powered mobility systems for disabled patients and their wheelchair or scooter. The driver's seat of the van may be removed so that it can be substituted with the patient's wheelchair or scooter for driving. A selection of vehicles is described in Chapter 4.5, section II.B.2.f.

Further reading

ABLE-DATA: Powered wheelchair. Fact Sheet No. 24, July 1994. Available at: http://www.abledata.com. Accessed July 18, 2004.

Adler C, Tipton-Burton M: Wheelchair assessment and transfers. In Pedretti LW, Early MB, editors: *Occupational therapy practice skills for physical dysfunction*, ed 5, St Louis, 2001, Mosby, pp. 507–525.

Bergen AF: The prescriptive wheelchair: An orthotic device. In O'Sullivan SB, Schmitz TJ, editors: *Physical rehabilitation: assessment and treatment*, ed 4, Philadelphia, 2001, FA Davis, pp. 1061–1092.

Boninger ML, Cooper RA, Schmeler M, *et al.*: Wheelchairs. In DeLisa JA, Gans BM, Walsh NE, *et al.*, editors: *Physical medicine and rehabilitation: principles and practice*, ed 4, Philadelphia, 2005, Lippincott, Williams & Wilkins, pp. 1289–1305.

Brittell CW: Wheelchair prescription. In Kottke FJ, Lehmann JF, editors: *Krusen's handbook of physical medicine and rehabilitation*, ed 4, Philadelphia, 1990, WB Saunders, pp. 548–563.

Buschbacher R, Adkins J, Lay B, *et al.*: Prescription of wheelchair and seating system. In Braddom RL, editor: *Physical medicine and rehabilitation*, ed 2, Philadelphia, 2000, WB Saunders, pp. 370–391.

Deitz J, Dudgeon B: Wheelchair selection process. In Trombly CA, editor: *Occupational therapy for physical dysfunction*, ed 4, Baltimore, 1995, Williams & Wilkins, pp. 599–609.

Enders A, Hall M, editors: *Assistive technology source book*, Washington, DC, 1991, RESNA.

Gettel AH, Redford JB: Wheelchairs and wheeled mobility. In Redford JB, Basmajian JV, Trautman P, editors: *Orthotics: clinical practice and rehabilitation technology*, New York, 1995, Churchill Livingstone, pp. 171–217.

Kirby RL: Manual wheelchairs. In O'Young B, Young MA, Stiens SA, editors: *PM&R secrets*, ed 2, Philadelphia, 2002, Hanley & Belfus, pp. 589–593.

Letts RM, editor: *Principles of seating the disabled*, Boca Raton, 1991, CRC Press.

Mayall JK, Desharnais G: *Positioning in a wheelchair: a guide for professional caregivers of the disabled adult*, ed 2, Thorofare, NJ, 1995, Slack.

Miller NE: Wheelchair prescriptions and types of wheelchairs. In Sinaki M, editor: *Basic clinical rehabilitation medicine*, St Louis, 1994, Mosby-Year Book, pp. 449–461.

Redford JB: Seating and wheeled mobility in the disabled elderly population. *Arch Phys Med Rehabil* 74:877–885, 1993.

Trudel G, Kirby RL, Ackroyd-Stolarz A, *et al.*: Effects of rear-wheel camber on wheelchair stability. *Arch Phys Med Rehabil* 78(1):78–81, 1997.

Warren CG: Powered mobility and its implications. In Todd SP, Gianini MJ, editors: Choosing a wheelchair system. *J Rehabil Res Dev* 25 (suppl 2):74–85, 1990.

Wilson A: *Wheelchairs: a prescription guide*, New York, 1992, Demos.

CHAPTER 4.8
Pharmacologic agents

In prescribing drugs, the physician should know the metabolism, route of excretion, indications, contraindications, precautions, and major adverse effects associated with each drug used. Adverse drug reactions (ADRs) may be allergic, idiosyncratic, or dose-related extensions of known effects. The ADRs occur frequently and the rate of occurrence increases in proportion to the number of drugs taken. Drug dosages should be individualized according to the patient's age and weight as well as kidney and liver function. Drugs are always contraindicated in patients with known hypersensitivity to the drug or component of the drug or its vehicle (e.g., propylene glycol found in most injectable forms).

In the clinical setting, half-life is usually the most relevant pharmacokinetic parameter. It generally takes about four to five half-lives to reach a steady-state plasma level and about the same time for the drug to be eliminated after drug discontinuation. Hence, a loading dose is usually needed for drugs with a long half-life (unless such a dose produces intolerable side-effects). Also, if possible, any drug with a long half-life should be avoided in the elderly because it takes longer for the drug to be eliminated in case of toxicity. Drug effects generally continue to increase in intensity until a steady-state plasma level is achieved (the relationship between drug effect and plasma level varies in different individuals). In some drugs (e.g., tricyclic antidepressants or nonsteroidal anti-inflammatory agents), the drug effect may continue to increase for days to weeks after achieving steady-state plasma levels (thus, clinicians should wait for at least 1–2 weeks longer before further drug titration or drug discontinuation). To increase compliance and ensure adequate therapeutic trials, patients must be educated about the titration process, delay in clinical benefit, and anticipated side-effects.

I. Analgesics

Analgesics are used to temporarily relieve pain and help improve patient's function. Because pain is subjective, analgesic therapy should be individualized. When possible, nonopioid preparations should be used. In patients with chronic pain refractory to analgesics, nonpharmacologic modalities (e.g., nerve blocks, sympathectomy, and relaxation therapy) should be considered (see Chapter 5.10, section VI).

A. NONOPIOID (OR NON-NARCOTIC) ANALGESICS (see Tables 4.8-1 and 4.8-2)

1. **Acetaminophen** (see Table 4.8-1) has antipyretic and analgesic properties similar to aspirin (see section I.A.3.a) but does not inhibit platelet function. Its anti-inflammatory effect is probably insignificant. Although its mechanism of action (MOA) is unknown, its primary action appears to be in the central nervous system (CNS). Acetaminophen is approximately equianalgesic with aspirin, but unlike aspirin and other nonsteroidal anti-inflammatory drugs (NSAIDs), it does not cause gastric toxicity (although chronic use can cause dyspepsia) or renal toxicity (except in prolonged use). Also, it does not exacerbate encephalopathy or congestive heart failure. In patients with bleeding diathesis or with renal insufficiency who need nonopioid analgesics, acetaminophen is safer than other NSAIDs (long-term use of acetaminophen should be avoided by patients with renal pathology). Acetaminophen should be used cautiously by patients with

Table 4.8-1 Recommended dosage of acetaminophen, tramadol, and salicylate NSAIDs

Generic	Selected brand names	Available preparations (mg)	Dosage (mg), route, frequency	MDD (mg)
1. **Acetaminophen**	*Tylenol, Tylenol ES, Panadol, Tempra, Anacin-3*	tab 160,325,500,650; chew tab 80; cap 325, 500; supp 120,325, 650; elix (per 5 mL) 120,160,320; liq 160/5 mL; 500/15 mL; drop 80 mg/0.8 mL	650–1000 po/pr q4–6h	4000
2. **Tramadol**	*Ultram*	tab 50	50–100 po q4–6h	400
	Ultracet	tab 37.5/325 acetaminophen	2 tabs q4–6h	8 tabs
3. **Acetylated salicylate**				
Aspirin*	*ASA; Bayer Ascriptin Ecotrin Empirin*	tab 81,325, 500,600,650, 800,975; cap 325,500	325–650 po q4–6h	6000§
4. **Non-acetylated salicylate**†				
Choline Mg trisalicylate	*Trilisate*	tab 500,750,1000; liq 500 mg/5 mL	750–1500 po bid/tid; 3000 po qd	3000§
Diflunisal	*Dolobid*	tab 250,500	1000 po initially, then 250–500 po q8–12h	1500
Salsalate‡	*Disalcid; Salflex*	tab 500,750; cap 500	500–750 po bid/tid	3000§

** Plasma half-life for ASA is 9–16 hours.*
† Plasma half-life: choline Mg trisalicylate is 9–17 hours, diflunisal is 8–12 hours, and salsalate is 3–16 hours.
‡ Analgesia indication is not listed by manufacturer.
§ Determined by measurement of serum salicylate level. For optimal anti-inflammatory effects, blood levels between 20 and 30 mg/dL and a total daily dose of 3–6 g are usually required.
MDD = maximum daily dose; ES = extra-strength.

liver pathology (fatal hepatic necrosis has been reported in acute acetaminophen overdosage, i.e., 10–15 g). Acetaminophen is available in oral and suppository forms. When combined with NSAIDs (see section I.A.3) or opioids (see sections I.B), it provides greater pain relief than acetaminophen or the other agents alone. Patients should be advised to refrain from alcohol intake while taking acetaminophen.

2. **Tramadol (Ultram; Ultracet)** (see Table 4.8-1) is a centrally acting oral synthetic nonopioid analgesic agent. It probably acts by binding weakly to opioid receptors (i.e., μ-receptors) and by inhibiting reuptake of norepinephrine and serotonin. Although its affinity for μ-receptors is 10 times less than that of codeine and 6000 times less than that of morphine, it is still considered a strong analgesic, and can be used in moderate to moderately severe pain. Adverse drug reactions include dizziness, somnolence, nausea, constipation, sweating, and pruritus. Seizure and orthostatic hypotension have also been reported. Compared to morphine, it causes less respiratory depression, does not cause histamine release, and has milder physical tolerance with less severe withdrawal symptoms. It has no effect on heart rate, left ventricular function, or cardiac index. It can be given without regard to food intake. It is contraindicated in persons with acute alcohol intoxication. It must be used with caution in patients

Table 4.8-2 Selected nonsalicylate NSAIDs classified by half-life duration				
Generic	**Selected brand names**	**Available preparations (mg)**	**Dosage (mg), route, frequency**	**MDD (mg)**
I. Short half-life*				
Diclofenac	*Cataflam IR* *Voltaren EC*	IR tab 50 EC tab 25,50,75	IR/EC:50 po bid/tid EC: 75 po bid; 25 po qid + hs	150
	Voltaren XR *Arthrotec*[¶]	XR tab 100 tab 50,75	XR: 100 po qd tab: 50 po bit/tid; 75 po bid	
Fenoprofen[§]	*Nalfon*	cap 200,300; tab 600	200–600 po tid/qid	2400
Flurbiprofen	*Ansaid*	tab 50,100	50–100 po tid	300
Ibuprofen[§]	*Motrin, Medipren, Advil, Nuprin, Rufen*	tab 200,300,400, 600,800; liq 100 mg/5 mL	200–800 po tid/qid	3200
Indomethacin	*Indocin, Indocid, Indocin SR*	cap 25,50; supp 50; susp 25 mg/5 mL SR cap 75	25–50 po tid, pc; 50, pr, bid; SR: 75 po qd/bid	150
Ketoprofen[§]	a) *Orudis* b) *Oruvail*	a) cap 25,50,75 b) cap 100,150,200	a) 25–75 po q4–8h; b) 200 po qd	300
Ketorolac[§]	*Toradol*	tab 10 Inj 15,30,60	10 po q4–6h; 30–60 IM initially, then 15–30 IM/IV q6h	tab 40 inj 120
Meclofenamate[§]	*Meclomen*	cap 50,100	50 po tid/qid	400
Mefenamic acid*	*Ponstel*	cap 250	500 po initially, then 250 po q6h	1000
Tolmetin	*Tolectin*	tab 200,600; cap 400	200–600 po tid	1800
II. Intermediate[†]				
Etodolac§	a) *Lodine;* b) *Lodine XL*	a) cap 200,300,400 b) tab 400, 600	a) 200–400 po bid/qid b) 400–1000 po qd	1200
Sulindac	*Clinoril*	tab 150, 200	150–200 po bid, pc	400
III. Long half-life[‡]				
Naproxen[§]	*Naprosyn; Aleve; EC-Naprosyn*	tab 200,250,375, 500; susp 125 mg/5 mL	500 po initially, then 250–500 po bid	1025
Naproxen Na[§]	a) *Anaprox* b) *Naprelan CR*	a) tab 275,550 b) tab 375,500	275–550 po bid; 750–1000 po qd	a) 1375 b) 1500
Nabumetone	*Relafen*	tab 500,750	500–750 po bid; 1000 po qd/bid	2000
Oxaprozin	*Daypro*	cap 600	1200 po qd	1200
Piroxicam	*Feldene*	cap 10,20	20 po qd	20
Meloxicam	*Mobic*	tab 7.5,15	7.5–15 po qd	15
Celecoxib	*Celebrex*	cap 100,200	OA: 200 po qd; RA: 100–200 po bid Dysmen: 400–600 po qd initially, then 200 po bid	600

** Short half-life = <6 hours; [†] intermediate half-life = 6–10 hours; [‡] long half-life = >10 hours;*
[§] NSAIDs with primary indications as analgesics; The slow- or extended-release forms or enteric-coated forms (e.g., EC-Naprosyn) have delayed time-to-peak concentration and are not recommended for primary analgesic use.
[¶] Arthrotec is combined with 200 mg of misoprostol.
MDD = maximum daily dose; DR = delayed release; IR = immediate release; SR = sustained release; CR = controlled release; ER or XL = extended release; EC = enteric coated; DS = double strength; OA = osteoarthritis; RA = rheumatoid arthritis; Dysmen = primary dysmenorrhea; Ac pain = acute pain.

taking hypnotics, central acting analgesics, opioids, or psychotropic drugs (e.g., tricyclic antidepressants). Because its MOA is similar to that of opioids, its use may produce some of the same tolerance, dependence, and abuse issues associated with opioid use (see section I.B).

To decrease the likelihood of ADRs, tramadol (Ultram) should be initiated at 50 mg, po, qd/bid, then increased every 3–7 days by 50–100 mg/day in divided doses as tolerated. Its maximum daily dose is 100 mg, po, qid. An adequate trial requires 4 weeks. In elderly high-risk patients, it should be given at 25 mg/day and increased by 25 mg every 3 days, with maximum daily dose of 300 mg/day in divided doses. In patients with advanced liver disease, it should be reduced to 50 mg, po, bid up to a maximum dose of 100 mg/day. In patients with renal insufficiency (i.e., creatinine clearance of 30 mL/min or less), it should be reduced to 50–100 mg, po, bid up to a maximum dose of 100–200 mg/day. Ultracet, which has 37.5 mg of tramadol combined with 325 mg of acetaminophen is not recommended in patients with liver disease, but may be given at a dose of 2 tablets, po, bid for patients with creatinine clearance of 30 mL/min or less.

3. **Nonsteroidal anti-inflammatory drugs**, which are the most widely used drugs in the world, exhibit anti-inflammatory, antipyretic, and analgesic activities. They are primarily used for treating inflammatory conditions of the musculoskeletal system (particularly rheumatoid arthritis and other autoimmune arthritides, as well as osteoarthritis, which may be associated with an inflammatory component). Selected drugs have also been formally approved for the treatment of shoulder bursitis/tendinitis (e.g., naprosyn, indomethacin, and sulindac), dysmenorrhea (e.g., ibuprofen, diclofenac, and mefenamic acid), postoperative pain [e.g., intramuscular (IM) ketorolac], and other conditions. A number of NSAIDs have primary indications as analgesics (see Table 4.8-2) and have been used on pain associated with noninflammatory conditions (e.g., neuropathic pain), with chronic or frequently recurrent headache, and with cancer pain (particularly bone pain related to cancer). The NSAIDs are also used to supplement a primary analgesic agent (e.g., morphine) to decrease the required dosage of opioid, and thereby minimize the opioid side-effects.

   Mechanism of action. The major MOA of NSAIDs is the inhibition of the synthesis of prostaglandin (PG), specifically PGE_2 via the blocking of cyclooxygenase (COX), which is the enzyme that converts arachidonic acid into PG (see Fig. 4.8-1). Prostaglandins do not themselves activate nociceptors but they lower the threshold to noxious stimulation, i.e., they sensitize the nociceptors to the actions of other noxious endogenous substances (e.g., bradykinin, histamine, substance P, and serotonin). In soft tissues, PGE_2 causes pain and inflammation. In the gastrointestinal (GI) tract, PGE_2 is cytoprotective, that is, it increases the secretion of mucus and bicarbonates and decreases secretion of gastric acids and digestive enzymes; whereas in the kidney, PGE_2 enhances renal salt and water excretion by acting as a vasodilator of small arterial blood vessels. Other possible MOAs of NSAIDs are inhibition of lipo-oxygenase activity and leukotriene production, membrane stabilization, and a supraspinal (central) analgesic effect, which is separate and distinct from the action in the inflamed peripheral tissues. In the arachidonic cascade (see Fig. 4.8-1), the COX enzymes can be subdivided into COX-1, which is responsible for PGE_2 production in the GI tract and the kidney, and COX-2, which is responsible for inflammatory PG synthesis during tissue injury. However, there is controversy in determining COX-1 or COX-2 selectivity because of the lack of standardization of the methods for evaluating relative COX-2/COX-1 inhibitory activity. It is generally believed that glucocorticoids selectively block COX-2 and have less ulcerogenic side-effects. Acetylsalicylic acid (ASA), however, causes irreversible inhibition of both COX-1

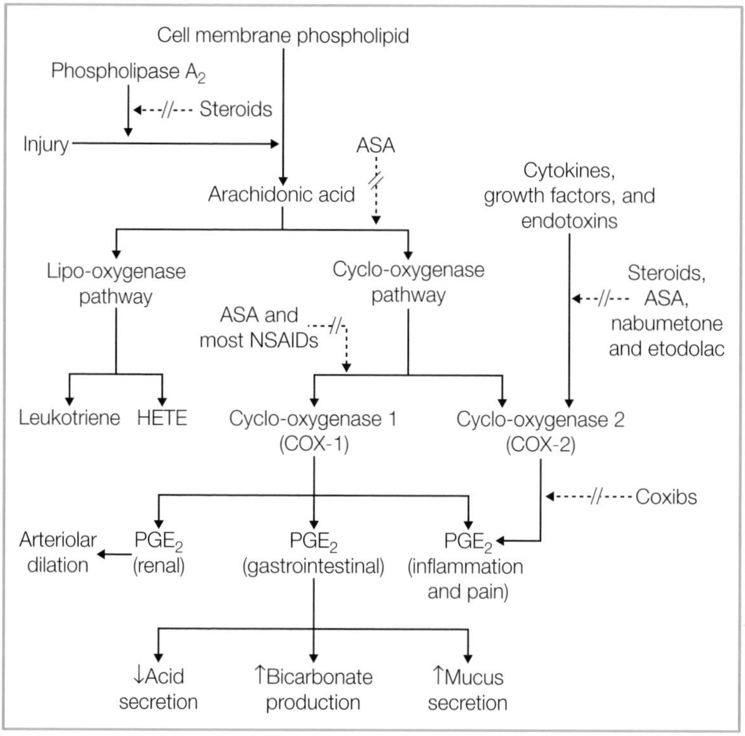

Figure 4.8-1 Effects of steroids and NSAIDs on the arachidonic cascade. There are two major routes of metabolism of arachidonic acid: the lipo-oxygenase pathway which leads to the production of leukotrienes and HETE; and the cyclo-oxygenase pathway which leads to the production of prostaglandins, specifically PGE_2. The PGE_2 responsible for inflammation as well as for renal and GI protection is activated by the COX-1 pathway which in turn is blocked by ASA and most NSAIDs. The PGE_2 responsible for inflammation and pain (but not for GI protection or kidney arteriolar dilation) is activated by the COX-2 pathway. COX-2 is induced by cytokines, growth factors, and endotoxin, an effect blocked by glucocorticoids, ASA, and some NSAIDs (nabumetone, etodolac). COX-2 receptors, which are selectively blocked by coxibs, can theoretically cause less GI ulceration. ASA, on the other hand, completely blocks the cyclo-oxygenase pathway and has relatively higher incidence of GI ulceration. Note that aside from acting on the cyclo-oxygenase pathway, steroids also inhibit arachidonic acid formation by blocking phospholipase A_2. Note also that recent data indicated that coxibs can suppress the formation of prostaglandin I_2 (which is COX-2-dependent) and might predispose patients to myocardial infarction or thrombotic stroke. Broken lines (-//-) indicate inhibitory effects.

and COX-2 and is ulcerogenic. Most of the other NSAIDs serve as reversible, competitive inhibitors of COX activity, and either nonselectively inhibit the COX-1 and COX-2 enzymes or have selectivity for the COX-1 isoform; hence, they are all ulcerogenic. The possible exceptions are the new classs of NSAIDs called coxibs, which selectively inhibit COX-2 (see section I.A.3.b.7) and, hence, have theoretically less (but not absent) ulcerogenic side-effects. However, coxibs can also suppress the formation of another type of prostaglandin (PGI_2) and might be expected to elevate blood pressure, accelerate atherogenesis, and predispose patients receiving coxibs to an exaggerated thrombotic response to the rupture of an atherosclerotic plaque, especially in patients with intrinsic risk of cardiovascular disease (see FitzGerald, 2004).

Adverse drug reactions. Most NSAIDs have similar ADRs. These include GI intolerance in 10% of NSAID users (e.g., nausea or dyspepsia); GI ulceration (i.e., gastric and also duodenal) in 2% of NSAID users; inhibition of PG-mediated renal function, that is inhibition of antidiuretic hormone, increased renal reabsorption of chloride, and enhanced reabsorption of K^+ [thus fluid retention in patients with congestive heart failure, hepatic cirrhosis with ascites, chronic renal disease (analgesic toxic nephropathy with medullary ischemia), hypertension or hypovolemia, and hyperkalemia]; renal injury (interstitial nephritis, papillary necrosis, or, rarely, acute renal failure); bleeding (because of the inhibition of platelet aggregation or gastric erosion and ulceration); inhibition of uterine smooth muscle motility (prolongation of gestation); hypersensitivity reaction; and a vague sense of dizziness and confusion especially in elderly patients. Although not contraindicated, NSAIDs must be used with caution in the elderly and in patients with impaired renal or hepatic function. In addition, the United States Food and Drug Administration (FDA) have added potential risks of cardiovascular events (including myocardial infarction [MI], stroke, and death; especially in long-term use of high doses of NSAIDs) and skin reactions to all NSAIDs.

Hepatic toxicity. The risk factors for hepatic toxicity include advanced age, decreased renal function, multiple drug use, higher drug dosages, and increased duration of therapy. Agents with high hepatotoxic risk include diclofenac and sulindac; while those with lower risk include ibuprofen and ketoprofen. Hence, with institution of a new agent, it is advisable to monitor liver function during the first 4–6 weeks in patients with increased risk of hepatotoxicity.

Renal toxicity. Risk factors for NSAID nephrotoxicity include age over 60 years with atherosclerotic cardiovascular disease and concurrent diuretic therapy, renal insufficiency (serum creatinine above 2.0 mg/dL), and states of renal hypoperfusion (e.g., sodium depletion, diuretic use, hypotension, nephrotic syndrome, and congestive heart failure). High-risk patients should be hydrated and treated with the lowest effective dose of the least potent renal COX inhibitor (e.g., sulindac or a nonacetylated agent), and the creatinine and electrolyte levels must be monitored at baseline and after 5–7 days of treatment.

GI toxicity. Therapy with NSAIDs is associated with upper GI symptoms in 25% of patients, causing ulcers or erosions in 40% of patients, increasing the risk of ulcer bleeding or perforation three- to four-fold, and increasing the rate of hospitalization or death from a GI complication five-fold. It also causes lower GI complications (i.e., 10–15% of NSAID users experience diarrhea). In spite of the high frequency of ulceration, the risk of developing GI complications while taking an NSAID remains relatively low (1–5% per year). GI irritation, erosion, and mucosal ulceration are thought to be the result of the NSAID inhibition of PGs (see Fig. 4.8-1). Prostaglandins are known to provide GI cytoprotection by suppressing gastric acid secretion and maintaining the mucosal barrier. An increased risk of developing a GI ulcer from NSAID use has been strongly associated with a history of either ulcer disease or previous GI complications from NSAIDs, elderly patients (over 70 years old), and concomitant administration of corticosteroids or anticoagulants. Other factors include the use of high NSAID doses, history of cardiac disease, and history of rheumatoid arthritis. Smoking and/or alcohol consumption, in the absence of other risk factors, have been suggested as risk factors of NSAID-induced ulceration but these remain controversial.

In patients with high risk for GI toxicity who need NSAID therapy, the following are recommended: (a) use of the lowest effective dosages of NSAIDs or use of selective COX-2 inhibitor NSAIDs (see section I.A.3.b.7), (b) avoidance of NSAIDs with high levels of enterohepatic recirculation (e.g., indomethacin, sulindac, and meclofenamate), (c) use of a nonacetylated salicylate when possible, and (d) concomitant use of a proton-pump inhibitor (PrPI, see next paragraph) or misoprostol (Cytotec). Misoprostol, a PG analog, is a mucosal protective agent approved by the FDA for use in prevention of both NSAID-induced gastric and duodenal ulcers. It can be started at 100 μg, po, qid, after meals, then gradually increased to 200 μg, po, qid (gradual titration is used to prevent diarrhea). It has been shown to reduce the risk of serious NSAID-induced ulcers to less than 1.5% (after 3 months of NSAID therapy) without reversing the desired anti-inflammatory and analgesic effects. However, its long-term use can be costly, thus it should only be considered in patients with high risk for GI toxicity (as listed in the previous paragraph) or in patients who are unable to tolerate a GI complication (e.g., presence of severe comorbid conditions). Misoprostol is contraindicated in pregnant women because it may induce spontaneous abortion. It may only be used in a woman of childbearing potential who has had a negative serum pregnancy test within 2 weeks prior to beginning therapy; is capable of complying with effective contraceptive measures; has received both oral and written warnings of the hazards of misoprostol, the risk of possible contraceptive failure, and the danger in other women of childbearing potential should the drug be taken by mistake; and will begin misoprostol only on the 2nd or 3rd day of her next normal menstrual period.

In patients with NSAID-induced ulcers, the treatment of choice is NSAID discontinuation (which in most cases will lead to ulcer healing) and treatment with one of the acid inhibitory agents, i.e., histamine-2 receptor blockers [H_2 blockers, e.g., nizatidine (Axid), 300 mg, po, at bedtime (hs)] or PrPIs [e.g., omeprazole (Prilosec), 20 mg, po, qd]. During this period, other analgesic (e.g., acetaminophen or opioids) or anti-inflammatory (e.g., corticosteroid) agents may be used. If NSAID discontinuation is not possible, a short-term therapy (usually 4–8 weeks) using PrPI is recommended for healing gastric or duodenal ulcers. In patients with gastric ulcer, higher doses and/or prolonged therapy with PrPI (e.g., up to 8–12 weeks) may be needed. If GI symptoms persist for more than 2 weeks or if patients have evidence of complications (e.g., iron-deficiency anemia, GI bleeding, unexplained weight loss, and dysphagia), endoscopic evaluation is indicated. In the presence of *Helicobacter pylori* infection in patients with active ulcer or with past history of peptic ulcer disease, Prevpac (lansoprazole, clarithromycin, and amoxicillin), po, bid for 14 days or Helidac (bismuth subsalicylate, tetracycline, and metronidazole), po, qid with PrPI or H_2-blocker for 14 days may be used for *H. pylori* eradication. The use of antacids, which may help relieve NSAID-induced dyspepsia, has not been shown to be effective in preventing or treating NSAID-induced ulcers.

Nausea and abdominal pain raise concerns about the potential for ulceration, but are actually poor predictors. To decrease GI distress, NSAIDs should be taken with food or milk, and, in some cases, antacids may be used. The use of pro-drugs (which need to be metabolized in the liver to become active) and enteric-coated drugs as well as the concomitant use of acid-reducing agents can decrease the local GI injury effects of NSAIDs, because the gastric or intestinal mucosa is not exposed to high concentrations of its active metabolite during oral ingestion. However, local injuries such as superficial gastritis and submucosal hemorrhage are not predictive of symptoms, are rarely clinically significant, and may resolve with continued NSAID use. As the drug is activated and becomes available systemically, it can eventually cause GI ulceration especially in long-term use. Clinical evidence seems to indicate that parenteral or rectal administration of NSAIDs can produce the same GI complications as oral administrations. Patients with NSAID-induced nausea, can be given hydroxyzine (Atarax,

Vistaril), 25–50 mg, po, q4–6 hours. Hydroxyzine is an antihistamine agent, which not only acts as an antiemetic but also as a coanalgesic (see section VI.A).

Contraindications and precautions. The NSAIDs are contraindicated in patients with allergies to aspirin or NSAIDs, active bleeding, high coagulation time, peptic ulcers, or in women who are pregnant (may cause miscarriages in pregnant women and also palate deformities in the fetus). For lactating women, some NSAIDs, such as ASA, should be used with caution, while others, such as ibuprofen and naproxen, can be safely used because their drug level in the milk is negligible. (For more information about which drugs are safe for pregnant or lactating women, see Briggs GG, Freeman RK, Yaffe SJ, editors: *Drugs in pregnancy and lactation*, ed 6, Philadelphia, 2002, Lippincott, Williams & Wilkins.)

In patients with known "triad" symptoms (aspirin hypersensitivity, rhinitis/nasal polyps, asthma), NSAIDs can cause bronchospasm, laryngeal edema, and urticaria. The NSAIDs are protein-bound after absorption and may displace other drugs or be displaced themselves, thereby potentiating the effects of protein-bound drugs such as oral hypoglycemics (sulfonylureas), warfarin, digoxin, anticonvulsants (phenytoin), methotrexate, and sulfonamides (e.g., sulfamethoxazole). Thus, the combination of most NSAIDs with warfarin and some NSAIDs with sulfonylureas should be used with extreme caution or avoided if possible. Other drug–drug interactions include increased GI toxicity when NSAIDs are used with ethanol, increased lithium concentration with concomitant NSAID use, and decreased NSAID excretion with the use of probenecid. Moreover, the use of PG-inhibiting NSAIDs can decrease the antihypertensive and diuretic effects of diuretic drugs (e.g., thiazides and furosemide). They can also decrease the antihypertensive effects of β-blockers and angiotensin-converting enzyme inhibitors. In general, when using NSAIDs in patients taking antihypertensive drugs (i.e., ACE inhibitors or angiotensin II receptor antagonists), there should be adequate hydration and periodic monitoring of renal function to avoid the risk of renal failure, especially in patients who are elderly or dehydrated. On April 6, 2005, the FDA recommended that the labeling for all NSAIDs (COX-2 selective and non-selective NSAIDs, including both prescription and nonprescription NSAIDs) should be revised to include more specific information about the potential CV and GI risks, as well as warning of potential skin reactions. In addition, the FDA recommended that, pending the availability of additional data, the labeling for all prescription NSAIDs should include a contraindication for use in patients immediately postoperative from coronary artery bypass graft (CABG) surgery.

Drug administration guidelines. Optimal NSAID selection should be based on the therapeutic goals and the actual need for peripheral anti-inflammatory effect vs. central analgesia. The NSAIDs such as mefenamic acid, ketorolac, and etodolac have insufficient peripheral anti-inflammatory activity (hence are not indicated in the treatment of rheumatoid arthritis) but have significant central analgesic properties (hence are useful for pain relief). Generally, NSAIDs with a longer half-life (see classification in Table 4.8-2) allow better patient compliance, but do not afford as quick an analgesic effect after the dose is taken. Although the half-life itself does not increase the inherent toxicity of the NSAIDs, use of NSAIDs with long half-lives is more likely to result in excess accumulation and serious ADRs.

The dose–response relationship for the NSAIDs is characterized by a ceiling dose for analgesia, i.e., doses higher than the ceiling do not provide additional analgesia but presumably increase the risk of dose-related toxicity. The ceiling dose as well as the minimal effective dose and toxic dose of different NSAIDs have large individual variations. This, in combination with the fact that the recommended therapeutic doses of NSAIDs are based on dose-ranging studies in relatively healthy populations, suggests the need for individual titration of

NSAIDs in the clinical setting. The same NSAID should be considered if the patient had a favorable response to its previous use for similar indications because of interindividual variability in NSAID response. Although the use of NSAIDs can be titrated against symptoms, around-the-clock dosings are usually more effective than "as needed" (prn, or *pro re nata*) dosings.

For patients with mild to moderate pain and for those with a relatively increased risk of NSAID toxicity (e.g., the elderly, or those on multiple drugs or with renal insufficiency), a relatively low starting dose of NSAID should be given (i.e., one-half to one-third of the recommended dose). For patients with acute severe pain, an initial loading dose of 1.5 to 2 times the conventional starting dose may be given (e.g., when giving ketorolac for postoperative pain). In most other patients, conventional starting doses can be used. The NSAID dose is gradually titrated with at least 1 week (or up to a few weeks) of observation period between dose adjustments. Dose titration should stop when analgesia is adequate, the ceiling dose is reached (i.e., there is no increased analgesia after the dose is titrated), side-effects occur, or the dose approaches a conventionally accepted maximum (usually 1.5 to 2 times the average recommended starting dose). To minimize dose-related side-effects, the dose may be lowered to the previous level prior to the ceiling dose level. If the patient is unable to achieve balance between analgesia and side-effects at a dose below the maximal safe dose, the drug should be discontinued and another NSAID (even from the same chemical class) should be tried because there is a marked variation in the response of individuals to different but closely related NSAIDs.

There is no indication for the use of two NSAIDs simultaneously (e.g., aspirin and another NSAID or two nonaspirin NSAIDs), as there is no additive effect. Moreover, the addition of a second NSAID increases cost and the incidence of side-effects. Because most NSAIDs are equipotent, the only justification for choosing a more costly drug is the convenience of dosing, or if the drug is better tolerated and has better efficacy for that given patient. (Note that while all NSAIDs have anti-inflammatory effects, not all are effective as primary analgesics; see Table 4.8-2 to determine which NSAIDs have primary analgesic indications.) In long-term NSAID therapy, the following tests should be monitored regularly: hemoglobin and hematocrit, hepatic function, and renal function (blood urea nitrogen/creatinine). Occult fecal blood may also be monitored. The frequency of monitoring ranges from every 6–12 months for most patients, to more frequent monitoring (e.g., monthly or bimonthly) for patients who are predisposed to side-effects and who are receiving relatively high doses of NSAIDs.

a. ***Salicylate NSAIDs*** (see Table 4.8-1) have analgesic, antipyretic, and anti-inflammatory effects. In addition to the ADRs common to other NSAIDs, salicylates can also cause tinnitus, hearing loss, vertigo, metabolic acidosis, and hyperglycemia. In patients receiving concomitant corticosteroids, salicylate serum levels may be decreased because corticosteroids may increase the clearance of serum salicylates. When the corticosteroid is tapered or withdrawn, salicylate toxicity may occur.

I. **Acetylsalicylic acid (ASA) or aspirin** is the most commonly used salicylate NSAID. Aspirin is indicated as an analgesic and anti-inflammatory agent (for rheumatoid arthritis, osteoarthritis, and related rheumatic disorders) as well as an antiplatelet agent (see section VII.B.2). It produces more GI toxicity and less anti-inflammatory effect than the other NSAIDs (except for a few, e.g., piroxicam, which has relatively more GI toxicity than ASA). Although ASA does not generally cause liver damage in healthy adults, it may exacerbate pre-existing liver disease. It has been implicated in Reye's syndrome and is, therefore, not recommended in children. It may also exacerbate pre-existing kidney disease and cause salicylate toxicity, especially among the elderly. For optimal anti-inflammatory effect, a total daily dose of 3–6 g of ASA with blood levels between 20 and 30 mg/dL is usually needed. The maximum tolerated dose must be reached slowly, often with 1 week between alterations in dosage. However, for relief of mild to moderate pain in nonarthritic patients, its optimal dose may be less than the 650 mg given every 3 to 4 hours. At dosages above 1 g, the analgesic effect does not increase although toxicity rises dramatically. To avoid toxicity, the interval between doses should be increased as the dose is increased. Aspirin has the additional effect of inhibiting platelet aggregation and in low doses can be used for stroke prophylaxis. Buffered ASA tablets (containing either absorbable bicarbonate or nonabsorbable antacids) are not necessarily associated with reduced GI bleeding. Enteric-coated ASA tablets often cause less dyspepsia and less occult GI blood loss, but their absorption rates are more variable than either buffered or nonbuffered tablets. Time-release ASA tablets have delayed absorption and possibly more sustained plasma levels.

II. **The nonacetylated salicylates** produce minimal PG inhibition and minimal platelet effects. They also have less potential for GI ulceration than other NSAIDs.

- **Salsalate (Disalcid)** is indicated for use in rheumatoid arthritis, osteoarthritis, and related rheumatic disorders. It has been used to relieve mild to moderate pain, although analgesia is not listed by the manufacturer as a primary indication.
- **Diflunisal (Dolobid)** is indicated for use in rheumatoid arthritis and osteoarthritis and as an analgesic for mild to moderate pain. It is longer acting and has more auditory side-effects than other salicylates.
- **Choline magnesium trisalicylate (Trilisate)** is indicated for use in rheumatoid arthritis and osteoarthritis, and as an analgesic for mild to moderate pain (e.g., acute painful shoulder).

b. ***Nonsalicylate NSAIDs*** can generally be subdivided into six chemical classes. They are available in many oral preparations and are available in injectable and suppository forms (see Table 4.8-2).

I. **Indole and indene acetic acid NSAIDs**

- **Indomethacin (Indocin)** is primarily indicated for acute gout, rheumatoid arthritis, osteoarthritis, ankylosing spondylitis, and acute painful shoulder (bursitis/tendinitis) but is not approved as a primary analgesic. It can be given orally, as a suppository, and intravenously. The oral form is also available as a sustained-release capsule (this form is not recommended for acute gout). The intravenous (IV) form is only indicated for closure of patent ductus arteriosus. Indomethacin has high GI toxicity and has a higher incidence of headache than other NSAIDs.
- **Sulindac (Clinoril)** has the same indications as indomethacin. It is also not approved as an analgesic. It has half the potency of indomethacin but is longer acting and may have less renal toxicity than indomethacin. It is a pro-drug with less GI toxicity in short-term use; however, in long-term use (more than 5–14 days), it may increase the risk of GI toxicity.
- **Etodolac (Lodine; Lodine XL)** is indicated for use in rheumatoid arthritis and osteoarthritis. The short-acting form, Lodine, which is also approved for analgesic use, has been shown to produce analgesia approximately 30 minutes after oral administration with relief lasting 4–6 hours (this is comparable to aspirin and acetaminophen with codeine). Etodolac has a lower risk of producing GI complications (less than 0.1%) probably because of selective inhibition of COX-2. Etodolac seems to be well-tolerated, especially by elderly patients.

II. **Arylpropionic acid NSAIDs**

- **Fenoprofen (Nalfon)** is used in rheumatoid arthritis and osteoarthritis, as well as being an analgesic. It has greater renal toxicity than other NSAIDs and is therefore contraindicated in patients with impaired renal function.
- **Flurbiprofen (Ansaid)** is used in rheumatoid arthritis and osteoarthritis but is not approved for analgesic use.
- **Ibuprofen (Motrin, Advil, and others)** has the advantage of causing less epigastric pain, less GI occult blood loss, and less hepatotoxicity. Ibuprofen (and also diclofenac) has the lowest risk for GI ulceration and bleeding. Aside from its indication for rheumatoid arthritis and osteoarthritis, it is also used as an analgesic for mild to moderate pain and is effective in dysmenorrhea.
- **Ketoprofen (Orudis, Oruvail)** is indicated for use in rheumatoid arthritis and osteoarthritis. The short-acting form, Orudis, is also approved for analgesic use and for dysmenorrhea. The controlled-release preparation, Oruvail, which can be given once a day, is not recommended for acute pain. Oruvail is pH-dependent and is released in the intestine, thus minimizing gastric irritation. Ketoprofen is reported to have less hepatotoxicity.
- **Naproxen (Naprosyn, Anaprox, Aleve, Naprelan)** has a long half-life and is more potent than the other propionic acid NSAIDs. It is indicated for rheumatoid arthritis, osteoarthritis, ankylosing spondylitis, juvenile arthritis, acute gout, and for mild to moderate pain (e.g., for dysmenorrhea, bursitis, and tendinitis). The controlled-release form, Naprelan, can be given once daily. All formulations (including Naprelan) are recommended for analgesic use in acute pain except the enteric-coated form (EC-Naprosyn) because of its delayed absorption.
- **Oxaprozin (Daypro)** has a 40–50-hour half-life and can be given once a day. It is approved for use in rheumatoid arthritis and osteoarthritis but not as an analgesic.

III. **Heteroaryl acetic acid NSAIDs**

- **Diclofenac (Voltaren, Cataflam; Arthrotec)** is more potent than the indole and proprionic acid NSAIDs. It is available in a delayed-release (enteric-coated) form (Voltaren), in an immediate-release form (Cataflam), and in combination with misoprostol (Arthrotec). Both are primarily indicated for rheumatoid arthritis, osteoarthritis, and ankylosing spondylitis, whereas only Cataflam has the additional indication as an analgesic and for dysmenorrhea. In addition to the other ADRs of NSAIDs, diclofenac can cause hepatic toxicity, hence liver enzymes should be monitored in the first 8 weeks of treatment. Diclofenac has a relatively low risk of causing bleeding GI ulcers.
- **Tolmetin (Tolectin)**, which is primarily indicated for rheumatoid arthritis and osteoarthritis in adults, is also indicated for children (over 2 years old) with juvenile rheumatoid arthritis. It is not approved as an analgesic.
- **Ketorolac (Toradol)** is a potent analgesic but is only moderately effective as an anti-inflammatory drug. It is available in both oral and IM forms (in the United States, ketorolac is the only available injectable nonsalicylate NSAID). It is indicated for short-term use in the relief of acute pain (up to 5–days for the IM form or up to a week for prn use of the oral form because of increased incidence of GI complications when used longer than 5–7 days). Intramuscular ketorolac is effective in relieving moderate to severe pain. Thirty milligrams of ketorolac is equipotent to 12 mg of morphine sulfate or 100 mg of meperidine.

IV. **Fenamate (anthranilic acid) NSAIDs** include **meclofenamate (Meclomen)** and **mefenamic acid (Ponstel)**. Both are comparable to aspirin and are primarily indicated as analgesics for moderate pain and for dysmenorrhea (mefenamic acid being more effective). They should not be used for more than 1 week because prolonged use may increase GI toxicity.

V. **Enolic acid (oxicams) or benzothiazine derivative NSAIDs** include **piroxicam (Feldene)** and **meloxicam (Mobic)**. Piroxicam has the longest half-life (50 hours) and can be given once a day. It is approved for use in rheumatoid arthritis and osteoarthritis but not as an analgesic. It has high GI toxicity (greater than ASA). Meloxicam, which was shown *in vitro* to selectively inhibit COX-2, has less GI toxicity compared to nonselective COX inhibitors. *In vivo* testing of meloxicam, however, showed that its selectivity to inhibit COX-2 compared to COX-1 was only about 10-fold. It has been approved for use in osteoarthritis (but not as an analgesic), and can be given once a day. Another oxicam is phenylbutazone, but this is no longer used because it can cause death due to aplastic anemia and agranulocytosis.

VI. **Alkanone NSAIDs** include **nabumetone (Relafen)** which, like sulindac (see section I.A.3.b.1), is a pro-drug. Nabumetone has a long half-life (24 hours) and can be given once a day. It has a lower risk of producing GI complications (less than 0.1%) probably because of selective inhibition of COX-2. It is approved for use in rheumatoid arthritis and osteoarthritis but not as an analgesic.

VII. **Diaryl-substituted COX-2 inhibitors (coxibs)** have similar efficacy to matching high-dose NSAIDs, but can theoretically offer improved GI safety and tolerability. In the United States, three coxibs – rofecoxib (Vioxx), celecoxib (Celebrex), and valdecoxib (Bextra) – were previously available. However, both rofecoxib and valdecoxib were recently withdrawn from the market. Hence, celecoxib is the only coxib available as of May 2005. According to the FDA, all three coxibs are associated with an increased risk of serious adverse CV events compared with placebo (the available data do not permit a rank ordering of these three drugs with regard to CV risk). However, it has not been clearly demonstrated that the coxibs confer a greater risk of serious adverse CV events than non-selective NSAIDs. Among the three coxibs, only rofecoxib (which was subsequently withdrawn from the market by the manufacturer) has been shown to reduce GI complications compared with naproxen. Although all three coxibs have been shown to reduce the incidence of GI ulcers visualized at endoscopy compared with certain non-selective NSAIDs, the clinical relevance of this finding as a predictor of serious GI bleeding has not been confirmed. When used simultaneously with low-dose aspirin, the advantage of coxibs in preventing or reducing GI complications was offset. Thus, in patients susceptible to GI complications, gastric protection therapy (see section I.A.3 under GI toxicity) is required when taking coxibs and aspirin prophylaxis. In general, coxibs should not be used in patients with renal or hepatic insufficiency or in patients with established coronary or cerebrovascular disease. A small percentage of patients taking coxibs can develop weight gain, peripheral edema, and hypertension.

The decision to prescribe a coxib (celecoxib) should be based on the assessment of the individual patient's overall risk, i.e., their GI risk must outweigh their cardiac risk. The use of coxib is a rational choice for patients at a low cardiovascular risk who have had serious GI complications (especially while taking traditional or nonselective NSAIDs), or who are not responding to traditional (nonselective) NSAIDs. It should be avoided in patients who have cardiovascular disease or who are at risk for it. When coxibs are prescribed, the lowest effective dose should be used for the shortest duration possible because cardiovascular risk of treatment may increase with dose and duration of exposure. If there is insufficient relief from symptoms, an increased dose may be tried for 2 weeks. If there is no increase in therapeutic benefit after 2 weeks, other therapeutic options should be considered. In all cases, the patient's response and risk to therapy should be re-evaluated periodically.

- **Diaryl-substituted furanone**, i.e., **rofecoxib (Vioxx)**, has a half-life of 17 hours. It has been voluntarily withdrawn from the market by its manufacturer (Merck) on September 30, 2004 due to safety concerns of an increased risk of serious adverse CV (including MI and thrombotic stroke) in patients on rofecoxib.
- **Diaryl-substituted pyrazole**, i.e., **celecoxib (Celebrex)**, has a half-life of 11 hours and is indicated for acute pain, osteoarthritis, rheumatoid arthritis, and primary dysmenorrhea. It is contraindicated in patients with aspirin-sensitive asthma, or allergic reactions to aspirin or other arthritis medicines or sulfonamides. On April 6, 2005, the FDA recommended that the package insert of celecoxib should include a boxed warning about the potential of increased risk of serious adverse CV events.
- **Diaryl-substituted isoxazole**, i.e., **valdecoxib (Bextra)**, is a second-generation coxib with a half-life of 8–11 hours. It was withdrawn from the market by the manufacturer (Pfizer) on April 7, 2005 upon the recommendation of the FDA due to safety concerns regarding serious, and potentially life-threatening, skin reactions (e.g., Stevens–Johnson syndrome, toxic epidermal necrolysis, and erythema multiforme) and the fact that there are no data that demonstrate that valdecoxib offers any therapeutic advantage over other NSAIDs.
- **Other second-generation coxibs**, including **etoricoxib (Arcoxia)**, **parecoxib (Dynastat, Rayzon, Xapit)**, and **lumiracoxib (Prexige)** are undergoing clinical trial and are not yet available in the United States.

4. Non-narcotic analgesic combinations. Caffeine is added to some of the opioid with nonopioid analgesic or muscle relaxant combinations to increase their analgesic potency and to enhance mood.

a. Acetaminophen with caffeine is used for migraine headaches. A common combination is 325 mg acetaminophen, 50 mg butalbital, and 40 mg caffeine (Fiorecet, Esgic), 1 to 2 tablets (tabs), po, every 4 hours (q4h).

b. Acetylsalicylic acid with caffeine can also be used for migraine headaches. Examples are Fiorinal (ASA/butalbical/caffeine 325/50/40 mg), 1 to 2 tabs, po, q4h; Norgesic (ASA/orphenadrine/caffeine 385/25/30 mg), 1 to 2 tabs, po, tid/qid; and Norgesic Forte (ASA/orphenadrine/caffeine 770/50/60 mg), 0.5 to 1 tab, po, tid/qid.

c. Acetylsalicylic acid with muscle relaxants is used to relieve pain in patients with muscle spasms. Examples are Robaxisal (ASA/methocarbamol 325/400 mg), 2 tabs, po, qid and Soma Compound (ASA/carisoprodol 325/200 mg), 1 to 2 tabs, po, qid.

B. OPIOID (OR NARCOTIC) ANALGESICS refer to drugs that are pharmacologically similar to opium or morphine. They provide analgesia without antipyretic or anti-inflammatory action. They are indicated for short-term use in patients with acute severe or moderate-to-severe pain (e.g., postsurgical or post-traumatic pain or acute phase of myocardial infarct) and for long-term use in cancer patients with chronic pain. Their use in noncancer chronic pain remains controversial (see Chapter 5.10, section VI.E.1.b). If possible, they are used in combination with nonopioid analgesics (e.g., NSAIDs) to reduce the need for the opioid and minimize the opioid side-effects. For details on guidelines for the use of opioids in pain management refer to Chapter 5.10, section VI.E.1.b. Aside from their primary use as analgesics, opioids can also be used clinically to provide sedation, suppress coughs (e.g., in intubated patients), and control diarrhea.

Mechanism of action. All opioid drugs bind to opioid receptors and produce analgesia and other effects by mimicking the actions of endogenous opioid compounds at opioid receptors. These opioid receptors are highly concentrated on the second and third layers of the substantia gelatinosa and are in the cerebral cortex, hypothalamus, medial thalamus, amygdala, extrapyramidal regions, and sympathetic preganglionic neurons. In humans, the opioid receptors have been classified according to their pharmacologic effect and their location into (a) *μ-receptors*, primarily distributed in the brain and spinal cord and associated with supraspinal analgesia (they are further subclassified into *μ1-receptors*, which mediate somatic and visceral analgesia, and the *μ2-receptors*, which are associated with respiratory depression, bradycardia, decreased GI motility, euphoria, and dependence); (b) *δ-receptors*, which modulate μ activity and mediate somatic (but not visceral) analgesia as well as some respiratory depression; (c) *κ-receptors*, which function at the spinal and supraspinal levels, where they have some direct (and primarily visceral) analgesic function in addition to sedation; (d) *σ-receptors*, which are associated with dysphoria, psychotomimetic effects, and other excitatory phenomena (e.g., tachycardia, tachypnea, mydriasis, and hypertonia); and (e) *ε-receptors*, which are not well-defined but appear to be stimulated by β-endorphin and are possibly involved in the control of heat-related antinociception.

Opioid classification. Based on their effect on the opioid receptors, exogenous opioids can be classified into pure agonist opioids, agonist–antagonist opioids, and pure antagonist opioids. Pure agonist opioids bind and activate μ-receptors. Examples are the opium-related alkaloids (i.e., morphine and codeine) and their semi-synthetic (e.g., hydrocodone, hydromorphone, oxycodone, oxymorphone, and dihydrocodeine) as well as synthetic derivatives (e.g., methadone, meperidine, lovorphanol, fentanyl, sufentanil, alfentanil, and propoxyphene). The pure agonist opioids are preferred over the agonist–antagonist opioids in the management of pain, because the pure agonists do not have a "ceiling" effect, and their analgesic effect can accrue until side-effects limit their dosage. In contrast, the agonist–antagonist opioids have a "ceiling" effect for analgesia (i.e., increasing the dose above a certain level will not produce increased analgesia); this then limits efficacy for pain management, especially for severe pain.

The agonist–antagonist opioids can be subclassified into partial agonists (e.g., buprenorphine) and mixed agonist–antagonists (e.g., butorphanol, nalbuphine, pentazocine, and dezocine). The partial agonist buprenorphine has limited analgesic efficacy because it partially stimulates the μ-receptor to a level below its maximum level. The mixed agonist–antagonist opioids act simultaneously on different subtypes, with the potential for agonist action on one or more subtypes (e.g., agonists at κ-receptors) and antagonist action on one or more subtypes (e.g., antagonists at δ-receptors and weak antagonists at μ-receptors). The selective action of agonist–antagonist opioids at the opioid receptors is responsible for producing less respiratory depression and lowering the risk of abuse (because they do not produce euphoria). Their selective actions can also be responsible for their weak-to-moderate analgesic effect and, except possibly for dezocine, for their increased psychotomimetic side-effects (e.g., hallucination and dysphoria). Although agonist–antagonist opioids have lower abuse potential in addict populations, they can still produce withdrawal symptoms or pain recurrence in opioid-dependent patients (because of their antagonistic effects). The lower abuse potential of agonist–antagonist opioids is of little clinical significance because most patients who have no prior history of substance abuse have very low risk of this outcome regardless of the opioid chosen. Hence, the only apparent advantage to agonist–antagonist opioids in pain management is their possible use in patients with substantial pulmonary compromise and the availability of unique routes of administration for patients who cannot tolerate oral or other routes (e.g., intranasal butorphanol for acute headache).

The pure antagonist opioids, which competitively displace the opiate agonists from the μ, κ, δ, and σ-receptors, are not analgesics but are clinically used to reverse the life-threatening adverse effects (e.g., respiratory depression and hypotension) caused by overdosage from other opioid drugs. Opioid antagonists should not be used to reverse nonlife-threatening effects such as confusion or sedation because opioid reversal can result in acute withdrawal, which may be complicated by excruciating pain and seizures. Examples of pure opioid antagonists are naloxone (Narcan), naltrexone (ReVia, Trexan), and nalmefene (Revex). Naloxone is used to reverse life-threatening side-effects (e.g., respiratory depression; see next paragraph); whereas naltrexone and nalmefene, which can be given orally, are used as an adjunct to the maintenance of the opioid-free state in detoxified formerly opioid-dependent patients.

Adverse drug reactions. Opioids do not produce major organ toxicity from acute or chronic administration (except isolated cases of pulmonary edema in severely ill patients). Adverse drug reactions include CNS effects (e.g., sedation, dysphoria, confusion, sleep disturbances, and seizures), respiratory depression (rarely occurs except in opioid-naive patients and those with significant pulmonary disease), cardiovascular effects (e.g., hypotension, orthostatic hypotension, dysrhythmias, and bradycardia), gastrointestinal effects (e.g., constipation, nausea and vomiting, and toxic megacolon in patients with inflammatory bowel disease), genitourinary effects (e.g., increase in the tone of the bladder, ureter, and sphincter; and urinary retention), and others (e.g., miosis, dry mouth, pruritus, skeletal muscle rigidity, sexual dysfunction, inappropriate secretion of antidiuretic hormone, and physical dependence). True hypersensitivity reactions to opioids (e.g., urticaria, rash, and anaphylaxis) are rare. If patients experience such reactions, it is often possible to administer an opioid from another subclass safely, i.e., from the phenanthrene derivatives (e.g., morphine, codeine, hydromorphone, and oxycodone) to phenylpiperidine derivatives (e.g., meperidine and fentanyl) or to diphenylheptane derivatives (e.g., methadone). Drugs that potentiate the adverse effects of opioids include phenothiazines, antidepressants, benzodiazepines, alcohol, and other psychotropic drugs.

The opioid side-effects can be managed as follows:

- For mild constipation, increase dietary fiber and use a mild osmotic laxative (e.g., milk of magnesia); for severe constipation, use daily oral hyperosmotic agents (e.g., lactulose) or stimulant laxatives plus stool softeners (e.g., senokot plus docusate) or stimulant suppositories (e.g., bisacodyl). See Chapter 5.8, section VI.B.3.a.5.a.2 for details;
- For persistent opioid-induced sedation, try to reduce the opioid in each dose and increase the dosage frequency to decrease the peak concentration in the blood and brain while maintaining the same total dose. In some patients, switching to another opioid may reduce the sedation. If the above strategy is ineffective, add a psychostimulant drug, for example, caffeine; methylphenidate (Ritalin), 5–10 mg, po, bid/tid; dextroamphetamine (Dexedrine), 2.5–7.5 mg, po, bid; or pemoline (Cylert), 18.5–37.5 mg, po, qd; or modafinil (Provigil), 200 mg, po, qd;
- For nausea associated with early satiety, give metoclopramide (Reglan), 10 mg, IV/IM, q2–3h or 5–20 mg, po, tid/qid; for nausea associated with vertigo or if markedly exacerbated by movement, give antivertiginous drug, e.g., scopolamine (Transderm Scop), one patch (0.5 mg) behind ear, q72h, meclizine (Antivert), 25 mg, po, q6h, or dimenhydrinate (Dramamine), 50 mg po/IM/IV, q4h; in other cases of nausea, try an antihistamine agent, e.g., hydroxyzine (Vistaril), 25–100 mg, IM, q4–6h or a dopamine antagonist drug, e.g., prochlorperazine (Compazine), 10 mg, po/IM, tid/qid, or 25 mg, PR, q12h, chlorpromazine (Thorazine), 10 mg, po/IM, bid/tid/qid, haloperidol

(Haldol), 1–2 mg, IM/po, bid/tid. If the patient complains of nausea after opioid administration has begun, it is often helpful to give an antiemetic on a fixed schedule for several days, after which as-needed dosing is usually adequate. Depending on the antiemetic chosen, patients should be monitored for the possibility of increasing sedation.

- For respiratory depression, give naloxone (Narcan), 0.01 mg/kg or 0.4–2.0 mg or more, IV/IM/SC or via endotracheal route. Naloxone should be given incrementally in doses that improve the respiratory function but do not reverse analgesia. A dilute solution of naloxone (0.4 mg in 10 mL of saline) may be given as 0.5 mL (0.02 mg) boluses every minute. Alternatively, an infusion of two ampules (total of 0.8 mg) in 250 mL of 5% dextrose in water may be continually titrated toward this goal.
- For pruritus, an antihistamine, e.g., diphenhydramine (Benadryl), 25–50 mg, IV/IM/po, q6h or hydroxyzine (Atarax, Vistaril), 25 mg, po, tid/qid may be used.

Physical dependence. With chronic opioid use, tolerance and physical dependence may occur even after as little as a few days of therapy. When the drug is abruptly stopped, physically dependent patients can develop withdrawal or abstinence syndromes (e.g., anxiety, nervousness, agitation, narcotic craving, tachycardia, hypertension, GI distress, temperature instability, diffuse musculoskeletal pain, piloerection, pupil dilation, diaphoresis, lacrimation, and rhinorrhea). Likewise, if an opioid antagonist (e.g., naloxone) has been given, the patient may go into withdrawal even after only 3 days of opioid therapy. Withdrawal or abstinence syndromes are rarely life-threatening, and once withdrawal is complete, dependence ceases. To minimize abstinence syndromes, opioids should be tapered slowly over 3–5 days, for example, taper by 50%, then decrease further by 25% q2d; once the dose is tapered to equianalgesic oral morphine dose of 0.6 mg/kg/day for patients above 50 kg, or 30 mg/day for patients below 50 kg, then the opioid can be stopped. If a faster dose reduction is required, sympathetic overactivity during withdrawal can be blocked by coadministration of an α_1-adrenergic blocker, e.g., clonidine (Catapres), 0.1 mg, po bid, or 0.1 to 0.2 mg/day transdermally.

Contraindications and precautions. Aside from being contraindicated in patients with known hypersensitivity to the drug or component of the drug or its vehicle, opioids are also not used if the pattern and degree of pain are important diagnostic signs in the acute stage of the disease [e.g., in patients with traumatic brain injury (TBI) or abdominal pain]. They should be used with caution in the elderly, neonates, and in patients with impaired renal or hepatic function, respiratory disease (e.g., chronic obstructive pulmonary disease, asthma, kyphoscoliosis, severe obesity, and chronic cor pulmonale), head injury (increased opioid sensitivity because of alterations in blood–brain integrity), hydrocephalus, hypothyroidism, Addison's disease, hypopituitarism, anemia, severe malnutrition, or debilitation. They must also be used with caution (because of the potential for addiction) in patients with a prior history of drug abuse or severe personality disorder.

Drug administration guidelines. The use of opioids or other analgesics should always be done in conjunction with adjunctive pharmacologic and nonpharmacologic therapies (see Chapter 5.10, section VI). The dose, drug, and route of administration of opioids are chosen according to the severity of the pain, location, cause, risk of potential side-effects, and the patient's psychophysiologic condition. Oral administration is as effective as parenteral in appropriate dosages and should be used whenever oral medications are tolerated. In patients with dysphagia, emesis, and decreased GI absorption, opioids may be given rectally (used as if dose is equianalgesic to oral dose) or parenterally. Subcutaneous (SQ) or IV administration is the parenteral route of choice for opioids (e.g., after major surgery). This may be accomplished by bolus or by patient-controlled analgesia using special infusion pumps (which can deliver opioid intravenously, epidurally, intrathecally, or subcutaneously); although effective, epidural and intrathecal administration should be monitored as they may result in delayed, significant respiratory depression. Patient-controlled analgesia has been shown to improve pain relief, decrease anxiety, and allow less total drug to be given in postoperative patients and in cancer patients. The old standard, IM administration should be avoided as it is painful and drug absorption is unreliable. Opioids for long-term pain management (e.g., in cancer patients) can also be given transdermally (available for fentanyl).

The type of opioid used should preferably be a pure agonist opioid. The initial dose should be the lowest recommended dose (see Tables 4.8-3 and 4.8-4 for recommended starting dose for treating severe pain in patients who are opioid-naive or with limited prior opioid exposure). The initial dose can be increased gradually until a favorable balance between analgesia and side-effects is attained. After 24 hours, if the pain is not 90% controlled, the opioid dose can be increased by 50%. The absolute opioid dose is immaterial and is considered right for the patient if it provides adequate relief for 4 hours without unacceptable adverse effects. Drug treatment for side-effects (see above, under Adverse Drug Reactions) such as nausea, sedation, and constipation may enhance patient comfort and allow opioid dose escalation into an effective range. If possible, opioids should be supplemented with a coanalgesic to help decrease the need for opioids and minimize the opioid side-effects (especially in patients with a significant risk of hypoxia and who are at increased risk of respiratory depression or sedation, e.g., patients with morbid obesity, sleep apnea, intrapulmonary shunts, or who are ventilator-dependent). The coanalgesic can either be a nonopioid analgesic (e.g., NSAIDs) or an antihistamine agent (e.g., hydroxyzine, which also has antiemetic properties; see section I.B). It has been reported that regularly scheduled NSAIDs for only 72 hours can significantly reduce opioid requirement in the acute postoperative or post-traumatic phase.

In patients with constant pain, continuous (around-the-clock) analgesia is indicated with a supplementary or prn dose (also called the "rescue" dose) for breakthrough pain (i.e., pain that occurs between the regularly scheduled analgesic regimen, which may be associated with activity or treatments). The rescue opioid could be another weak or strong opioid, usually one with rapid onset and short half-life (e.g., parenteral hydromorphone; or if using slow-release oral morphine, an immediate-release oral morphine or injectable morphine sulfate could be used as the rescue opioid). The rescue dose is given q2h or more frequently at a dose equal to 5–15% of the total daily opioid requirement. If the patient requires frequent "rescue" doses, then the regular dosage should be increased or the interval between doses should be decreased. In patients receiving continuous opioid infusions, the rescue dose is usually 50–200% of the continuous hourly rate. If there is inadequate relief and no significant toxicity noted, then the rescue dose may be increased by a 50% increment. If six or more rescue doses are needed in 24 hours, then the infusion rate should be increased by using the rescue doses taken in the previous 24 hours, i.e., 10 × 5 mg rescues × 24 hours divided by 24 = rate of increase in infusion by mg/h, or the infusion may be increased by 50%.

If the maximum recommended dose of one narcotic is attained without adequate analgesia, or if the side-effects are intolerable, then another opioid preparation should be used. It is inadvisable to prescribe simultaneously two weak opioids or two strong opioids. If changing from a short half-life opioid to another short half-life opioid, start at 50% of the equianalgesic dose and titrate

Table 4.8-3 Pure agonist opioids commonly used for management of pain

Pure agonist opioids	Selected brand names	Available preparations (mg)	Dosage (mg), route, frequency
I. Short half-life*			
Morphine sulfate	*MSO_4 injection; MS-IR; Roxanol*	inj 1,5,8,10,15/mL MS-IR tab or cap 15,30; MS-IR sol 10, 20/5 mL; 10,20/mL; Roxanol liq 20,100/5 mL; 10/2.5 mL; 30/1.5 mL; 20/mL Roxanol supp 5,10,20,30	0.1–0.2/kg up to 15 IV/SQ/IM q3–4h; 10–30 po q3–4h prn breakthrough pain
Morphine sulfate (sustained release)	*MS-Contin; Oramorph; Kadian; Avinza*	MS-Contin tab 15,30,60,100,200; Oramorph tab 30,60,100; Kadian cap 20,50,100 Avinza cap, 30,60,90,120	1 tab po q8–12h Avinza: 1 cap po qd
Hydromorphone	*Dilaudid; Palladone ER*	Dilaudid inj 1,2,4,10/mL Dilaudid tab 1,2,3,4 Dilaudid supp 3 Palladone ER cap 12,16,24,32	1–1.5 IM/SQ/IV q34h; 2–8 po q3–4h; 3 PR q4h Palladone ER 12–32 po qd
Meperidine[†]	*Demerol*	inj 25.50,100/mL; tab 50,100; liq 50/5 mL	1–1.8/kg up to 150 or 50–150 SQ/IM/po q3–4h
Codeine[‡]	*Codeine*	inj 30/mL; 60/mL tab 15,30,60	0.5–1/kg up to 60 po/IM q3–4h
Oxycodone	*Roxicodone* *OxyIR* *OxyFast* *Oxycontin*	tab 5; liq 5/5 mL OxyIR cap 5 OxyFast liq 20/mL Oxycontin tab 10,20,40	0.2/kg up to 20 po q3–4h; 5 po q6h prn breakthrough pain; 0.25 mL q6h prn breakthrough pain; Oxycontin 10–40 po q12h
Oxymorphone	*Numorphan*	inj 1,1.5/mL supp 5	0.02/kg or 1–1.5 IM/SQ/IV q3–4h; 5 PR q4h

(Continued)

Table 4.8-3 *(Continued)*

Pure agonist opioids	Selected brand names	Available preparations (mg)	Dosage (mg), route, frequency
Propoxyphene	*Darvon*	tab 65	65 po q4h
Fentanyl	*Duragesic TD patch*[§];	TD patch: 25,50,75,100 μg/h	1 patch q48–72h (maximum of 300 μg/h per day)
	Actiq[¶]	Oral TM unit: 200,400,600,800,1200,1600 μg	200 μg initial dose, titrated up q15 min after finishing last unit (maximum of 4 units per day)
II. Long half-life			
Levorphanol	*Levo-Dromoran*	inj 2/mL tab 2	0.02–0.04/kg up to 2–4 po/SQ q6–8h
Methadone	*Dolophine*	inj 5, 10/5 mL tab 5, 10	0.1–0.2/kg IM/SQ q6–8; 10–20 po q6–8h

** Hydrocodone and dihydrocodeine, both of which have short half-life, are available only in combination with NSAIDs (ASA or acetaminophen). See sections I.B.2.a and I.B.2.b for recommended dosage.*

[†] Meperidine may be useful for brief courses (e.g., few days) to treat acute pain and to manage rigors (shivering) induced by medication but should be avoided for pain management because of its need for repeated dosing which can lead to CNS toxicity (tremor, confusion, dysphoria, or seizure).

[‡] Codeine doses above 65 mg are often not appropriate because of diminishing incremental analgesia with increasing doses but continually increasing nausea, constipation, and other side-effects; IV codeine can cause hypotension.

[§] *Transdermal fentanyl* (Duragesic TD patch) *is used in more chronic (not acute) pain. Doses above 25 μg/h should not be used in opioid-naive patients.*

[¶] Oral Transmucosal fentanyl (Actiq) is used for breakthrough cancer pain in opioid-tolerant patients. It must be placed between cheek and lower gum (to be sucked but not chewed or swallowed) so the unit slowly dissolves in about 15 minutes.

Table 4.8-4 Recommended starting dose (oral and parenteral) of opioids in (A) adults >50 kg body weight and (C) children (excluding babies <6 months old) or adults <50 kg body weight

Opioid agonists	Equianalgesic oral dose	Equianalgesic parenteral dose	Starting dose§ (oral)	Starting dose§ (parenteral)
I. "Strong"*				
Morphine	30 mg q3–4h (ATC dosing); 60 mg q3–4h (single dosing)	10 mg q3–4h	A: 30 mg q3–4h C: 0.3 mg/kg q3–4h	A: 10 mg q3–4h C: 0.1 mg/kg q3–4h
Hydromorphone	7.5 mg q3–4h	1.5 mg q3–4h	A: 6 mg q3–4h C: 0.06 mg/kg q3–4h	A: 1.5 mg q3–4h C: 0.015 mg/kg q3–4h
Levorphanol	4 mg q6–8h	2 mg q6–8h	A: 4 mg q6–8h C: 0.04 mg/kg q6–8h	A: 2 mg q6–8h C: 0.02 mg/kg q6–8h
Methadone	20 mg q6–8h	10 mg q6–8h	A: 20 mg q6–8h C: 0.2 mg/kg q6–8h	A: 10 mg q6–8h C: 0.1 mg/kg q6–8h
Fentanyl†	N/A	100 μg q30 min–1h	N/A	A: 25–75 μg q30 min C: 0.5–1.5 μg/kg q30 min
II. "Weak"*				
Codeine‡	130–200 mg q3–4h	75–130 mg q3–4h	A: 60 mg q3–4h C: 1 mg/kg q3–4h	A: 60 mg q2h (IM/SQ) C: NR
Hydrocodone	30 mg q3–4h	N/A	A: 10 mg q3–4h C: 0.2 mg/kg q3–4h	N/A
Oxycodone	30 mg q3–4h	N/A	A: 10 mg q3–4h C: 0.2 mg/kg q3–4h	N/A

(*Continued*)

Table 4.8-4 *(Continued)*

Opioid agonists	Equianalgesic oral dose	Equianalgesic parenteral dose	Starting dose[§] (oral)	Starting dose[§] (parenteral)
Oxymorphone	N/A	1 mg q3–4h	N/A	A: 1 mg q3–4h C: NR
Meperidine	300 mg q2–3h	100 mg q3h	NR	A: 100 mg q3h C: 0.75 mg/kg q2–3h

* *Classification of opioids into "weak" opioids (for use in mild to moderate pain) and "strong" opioids (for use in moderate to severe pain) is made principally on the grounds of common patterns of use and not on any pharmacological differences (i.e., there is no pharmacological difference between a high dose of codeine and an equianalgesic low dose of morphine).*

† *Available as transdermal patches (*Duragesic*) in four sizes (25, 50, 75, or 100 μg/h) given q72h for chronic pain use.*

‡ *Codeine dose above 65 mg is often not appropriate because of diminishing incremental analgesia with increasing doses but continually increasing nausea, constipation, and other side-effects; published equianalgesic dose varies.*

§ *Recommended starting doses do not apply to patients with renal or hepatic insufficiency or other conditions affecting drug metabolism or kinetics.*

(A) *dose for adults >50 kg body weight;* **(C)** *dose for children (excluding babies <6 months old) or adults <50 kg body weight; ATC = around the clock; N/A = not available; NR = not recommended.*

Adapted from: Acute Pain Management Guideline Panel: Acute pain management in infants, children, and adolescents: Operative and medical procedures. Quick reference guide for clinicians. *AHCPR Pub. No. 92-0020, Rockville, MD, 1992, Agency for Health Care Policy and Research, US Department of Health and Human Services, with permission.*

to the desired response (except in circumstances such as severe pain and absence of CNS side-effects, which may necessitate starting at 100% of the equianalgesic dose). If changing from a short half-life to a long half-life opioid, start at only 25% of the equianalgesic dose and titrate to the desired response. The equianalgesic dose, which is shown in Table 4.8-4, does not indicate the efficacy of the drug, but is useful to know when one is switching opioid drugs or routes of administration. Published tables vary in the suggested doses that are equianalgesic to morphine. The criterion that must be applied for each patient is the clinical response, which needs to be titrated for each patient. If the patient feels that he or she does not need the prescribed amount of medication, the dose should be reduced. Also, if the cause of the pain is eliminated or lessened (e.g., after cordotomy), the opioid dose should be lowered because patients who previously appeared to be tolerant to adverse opioid effects can suddenly develop adverse drug reactions.

The following is a classification of clinically useful opioid analgesics, i.e., pure agonist opioids and combination opioid with nonopioid analgesic drugs. Heroin (Diamorphine), which is also a pure agonist opioid, is illegal in the United States and is not discussed. As mentioned before (under opioid classification), the agonist–antagonist opioids are of little benefit in pain management in the PM&R setting and are therefore not discussed below (except for pentazocine, which is available orally in combination with nonopioid analgesics).

1. Pure agonist opioids

a. Opium alkaloids (phenanthrene derivatives)

I. **Morphine** is the standard against which all other opioids are often compared. It is classified as a "strong" opioid analgesic (see Table 4.8-4) and is indicated for use in patients with moderate to severe pain. Its potency is the basis for the construction of the equianalgesic table (see Table 4.8-4), which helps facilitate appropriate dose adjustment when another opioid of different potency is used. Morphine is available in oral (MS-IR, Roxanol), suppository (Roxanol), and injectable (morphine sulfate) forms. When given parenterally, the SQ or IV route of administration is preferred because the rate of absorption from the IM route is variable and unreliable. The oral form is also available in slow-release form (MS-Contin, Oramorph SR; Kadian; Avinza). Although the slow-release preparations do not increase the bioavailability of the morphine, they play a significant role in the relief of chronic and malignancy-related pain. Because of the advent of the slow-release morphine, there is now less reason for choosing an opioid other than morphine on the grounds of longer duration of effect.

II. **Codeine or methylmorphine** is usually administered in combination forms with nonopioid analgesics or muscle relaxants, e.g., Tylenol with codeine, Fiorecet with codeine, Empirin with codeine, and Soma compound with codeine (see section I.B.2.b.1.c). Codeine is classified as a "weak" opioid and is indicated for use in mild to moderate pain (Table 4.8-4). Codeine doses above 65 mg are often not appropriate because of diminishing incremental analgesia, continually increasing nausea, constipation, and other side-effects with increasing doses.

b. Semi-synthetic pure agonist opioids include hydromorphone (Dilaudid, Palladone), oxymorphone (Numorphan), oxycodone (Roxicodone, Oxycontin), hydrocodone, and dihydrocodeine. Both hydrocodone (e.g., Vicodin, Lortab, Lorcet, Anexsia, Zydone, Norco, Vicoprofen) and dihydrocodeine (Synalgos-DC) are available only in oral forms in combination with nonopioid analgesics (see section I). Oxycodone is also available as a controlled-release single formulation (Oxycontin) and in combination with nonopioid analgesics (e.g., Percocet, Percodan, Tylox, Combunox). All semi-synthetic pure agonist opioids are classified as "weak" opioids and are indicated for use in mild to moderate pain, except hydromorphone, which is a "strong" opioid indicated for use in moderate to severe pain (Table 4.8-4). Hydromorphone has a shorter duration and more sedation but produces less euphoria than morphine. It is available in oral, parenteral, as well as suppository forms. Hydromorphone can be used in cases of morphine toxicity in patients with renal disease. The other semi-synthetic pure agonist opioid available in suppository form is oxymorphone, which is also available in injectable but not in oral forms.

c. ***Synthetic pure agonist opioids*** include levorphanol (Levor-Dromoran), methadone (Dolophine), propoxyphene (Darvon), and the phenylpiperidine opioids, which consist of meperidine (Demerol), fentanyl (Sublimaze, Duragesic; Actiq), and the two fentanyl derivatives, sufentanil (Sufenta) and alfentanil (Alfenta). Sufentanil and alfentanil, which are both intravenous drugs with rapid onset and short duration, are primarily used in general anesthesia. They play no role in physiatric pain management. Among the synthetic pure agonist opioids, levorphanol, methadone, and fentanyl are classified as "strong" opioid analgesic drugs (Table 4.8-4) and are indicated for use in patients with moderate to severe pain; whereas meperidine and propoxyphene are classified as "weak" opioid analgesics (Table 4.8-4) and are used in patients with mild to moderate pain.

Levorphanol and methadone are two of the pure agonist opioids with the longest half-life (12–16 hours and 15–40 hours respectively). Because of their long half-lives, they must be used with caution as they can accumulate and cause delayed respiratory and CNS depression. However, because biologic half-lives do not always correspond to analgesic half-lives, methadone and levorphanol can have much shorter analgesic duration despite the long elimination half-life. They are both available in oral and injectable forms. Oral methadone is the drug of choice for the suppression of narcotic withdrawal symptoms and is a good choice for patients with chronic intractable pain.

Fentanyl is available in an IV form (Sublimaze), a transdermal form (Duragesic), and an oral transmucosal form (Actiq). The IV form is primarily used in general anesthesia. Transdermal (TD) delivery bypasses GI absorption and has been shown to be an effective, noninvasive route, which can reach the same peak concentrations in the blood as with IV administration. Each Duragesic patch contains a 48- to 72-hour supply of fentanyl, which is passively absorbed through the skin over this period. Fentanyl, which has high lipid solubility is deposited in the subcutaneous tissue and subsequently absorbed into the systemic circulation. Over a period of 12–18 hours after patch placement, the fentanyl levels in plasma rise slowly (this can continue even after patch removal because of subcutaneous deposition). The prolonged time between patch application and the achievement of adequate serum levels producing analgesia makes it inappropriate for use in acute pain. TD fentanyl should be considered when patients already on opioid therapy have relatively constant pain and infrequent episodes of breakthrough pain such that rapid increases or decreases in pain intensity are not anticipated. As with other long-acting analgesics, all patients with breakthrough pain should be provided with oral, oral transmucosal, or parenteral opioids that act rapidly with short duration. The maximum daily dose of TD fentanyl is 300 μg/h. If patients require larger doses, they should be switched to an equianalgesic dose of an oral or subcutaneously administered opioid. The most commonly reported ADRs of TD fentanyl administration are nausea, mental clouding, drowsiness, and skin irritation.

Fentanyl is not available in an oral form because of low oral bioavailability caused by its high hepatic clearance. However, it is available in an oral transmucosal (OTM) form (Actiq). OTM fentanyl is indicated only for the management of breakthrough cancer pain in patients who are opioid tolerant (i.e., taking at least 60 mg morphine/day, 50 μg/h TD fentanyl, or an equianalgesic dose of another opioid for a week or longer). Because life-threatening hypoventilation could occur at any dose in patients not taking chronic opiates, OTM fentanyl is contraindicated in acute or postoperative pain.

Propoxyphene is clinically equivalent to codeine when given regularly but is structurally related to methadone (which is a diphenylheptane derivative). Propoxyphene is available orally as a single formulation or in combination with nonopioid analgesics or muscle relaxants (Darvocet-N, Wygesic, Darvon compound). Its analgesic efficacy is minimal (with an analgesic potency equivalent to 600 mg of aspirin), and it may be useful as an analgesic for mild pain that is not responsive to aspirin alone. Like meperidine and codeine, it is not indicated in the management of more severe pain because of relatively increased toxicity at higher doses.

Meperidine (Demerol) has a short duration of action and may be useful for brief courses (e.g., a few days) to treat acute pain and to manage rigors (shivering) induced by medication; however, it should not be used if continued opioid use is anticipated. Its active metabolite (normeperidine) can accumulate in patients given repeated dosing for pain control or in patients with renal failure or those taking monoamine oxidase inhibitors (MAOI). This can lead to CNS toxicity, which causes tremor, confusion, dysphoria, or seizure. Moreover, meperidine is difficult to titrate to a steady state because of large fluctuations in plasma concentrations. Meperidine is available in both oral and injectable forms.

2. **Opioid with nonopioid analgesic combinations** are available in oral preparations and are recommended if optimal analgesia is not attained by nonopioid analgesics alone. The combination enhances the analgesic efficacy by combining two analgesics with different MOA and by reducing ADRs (i.e., adequate analgesia can often be achieved while keeping the dose of each constituent below the threshold that causes adverse effects). They should not be given in quantities that exceed the maximal safe amount of the nonopioid coanalgesics (e.g., 4 g of acetaminophen per day). Caffeine is added in some of the opioid with nonopioid analgesic combinations to increase the drugs's analgesic potency and to enhance mood. All of the following are pure agonist opioids except pentazocine, which is a mixed agonist–antagonist opioid.

a. ***Opioids with acetaminophen combination***

I. **Codeine**

- **Tylenol with codeine** [acetaminophen 300 mg + codeine 15 mg (#2), 30 mg (#3), 60 mg (#4)]: 1–2 tabs, po, q4 h; pediatric elixir (acetaminophen 120 mg and codeine 12 mg per 5 mL): 5 mL/dose if 3–6 years old; 10 mL/dose if 7–12 years old.
- **Fioricet with codeine** (acetaminophen/butalbital/caffeine/codeine 325/50/40/30 mg): 1–2 tabs, po, q4h.

II. **Hydrocodone**

- **Anexsia** (hydrocodone/acetaminophen 5/500 mg): 1–2 tabs, po, q4–6h; (7.5/650 mg): 1 tab, po, q4–6h.
- **Lortab** (hydrocodone/acetaminophen 2.5/500; 5/500 mg): 1–2 tabs, po, q4–6h; (7.5/500; 10/500 mg): 1 tab, po, q4–6h; elixir (2.5/167 mg per 5 mL): 15 mL, po, q4–6h.
- **Lorcet HD** (hydrocodone/acetaminophen 5/500 mg): 1–2 tabs, po, q4–6h; **Lorcet Plus** (7.5/650 mg) and **Lorcet 10/650** (10/650 mg): 1 tab, po, q4–6h.
- **Vicodin** (hydrocodone/acetaminophen 5/500 mg): 1–2 tabs, po, q4–6h; **Vicodin ES** (7.5/750 mg) and **Vicoden HP** (10/660 mg): 1 tab, po, q4–6 h.
- **Zydone** (hydrocodone/acetaminophen 5/400 mg): 1–2 tabs, po, q4–6h; (7.5/400; 10/400 mg): 1 tabs, po, q4–6h.
- **Norco** (hydrocodone/acetaminophen 5/325 mg): 1–2 tabs, po, q4–6h; (7.5/325, 10/325 mg): 1 tab, po, q4–6h.

III. **Oxycodone**
- **Percocet** (oxycodone/acetaminophen 2.5/325. 5/325 mg): 1–2 tabs, po, q4–6h; (7.5/325, 10/325, 7.5/500, 10/650 mg): 1 tab, po, q4–6h.
- **Tylox** (oxycodone/acetaminophen 5/500 mg): 1 tab, po, q6h.

IV. **Propoxyphene** is available as propoxyphene hydrochloride (Darvon, Wygesic) and propoxyphene napsylate (Darvocet-N). The napsylate form is more stable in liquid and tablet formulations. Because of the difference in molecular weight, however, a dose of 100 mg of propoxyphene napsylate is needed to supply an amount of propoxyphene equivalent to that present in 65 mg of propoxyphene hydrochloride (HCl).
- **Darvocet N-50** (propoxyphene napsylate/acetaminophen 50/325 mg), 2 tabs, po, q4h; **Darvocet N-100** (100/650 mg), 1 tab, po, q4h.
- **Wygesic** (propoxyphene HCl/acetaminophen 65/650 mg), 1 tab, po, q4h.

V. **Talacen** (pentazocine/acetaminophen 25/650 mg): 1 tab, po, q4h.

b. Opioid with aspirin (ASA) combination

I. **Codeine**
- **Empirin with codeine** [ASA 325 mg and codeine 30 mg (#3), 60 mg (#4)]: 1–2 tabs, po, q4h.
- **Fiorinal with codeine** (ASA/butalbital/caffeine/codeine 325/50/ 40/30 mg): 1–2 tabs, po, q4h.
- **Soma compound with codeine** (ASA/carisoprodol/codeine 325/200/ 16 mg): 1–2 tabs, po, q4–6h.

II. **Percodan** (oxycodone/ASA 5/325 mg): 1 tab, po, q4–6h.

III. **Darvon compound** (propoxyphene HCl/ASA/caffeine 65/389/32.4 mg): 1 tab, po, q4h.

IV. **Synalgos-DC** (dihydrocodeine/ASA/caffeine 16/356.4/ 30 mg): 2 caps, po, q4h.

V. **Talwin compound** (pentazocine/ASA 12.5/325 mg): 2 tabs, po, q6–8h.

c. Opioid with ibuprofen combination

I. **Vicoprofen** (hydrocodone/ibuprofen 7.5/200 mg): 1 tab, po, q4–6h.

II. **Combunox** (oxycodone/ibuprofen 5/400 mg): 1 tab, po, q6h.

C. ADJUVANT ANALGESICS (i.e., drugs primarily approved for the treatment of conditions other than pain but are analgesic in selected circumstances) are described in Chapter 5.10, section VI.E.2.

II. Skeletal muscle relaxants

These are "antispasmodic" drugs, which are indicated for short-term relief of acute musculoskeletal pains, some of which are characterized by "muscle spasms", which may result in pain and anxiety, thus interfering with the physical rehabilitation process. Their use in the treatment of chronic pain remains controversial (see Chapter 5.10, section VI.E.2.g). The "muscle spasms" that occur in the setting of nerve or muscle (or myofascial) injury represent focal areas of increased muscle activity associated with tenderness and splinting of the painful part. This should be distinguished from the terms *spasticity* and *spasms*.

Spasticity (see Chapter 5.4) is a component of the upper motor neuron syndrome characterized by a velocity-dependent increase in muscle tone with exaggerated tendon jerks; whereas spasms are spontaneous uncontrolled movements (such as painful flexor or extensor spasms, which in turn may precipitate or aggravate spasticity) or other hyperactive spinal reflexes (e.g., such as cramps, dystonia, and rigidity). Except for diazepam, the antispasticity drugs (i.e., baclofen, dantrolene, clonidine, tizanidine) discussed in Chapter 5.4, section III.D.1, are not FDA-approved for treating "muscle spasms" for which the "skeletal muscle relaxants" are indicated. Likewise, drugs classified as "skeletal muscle relaxants" are not indicated for the treatment of spasticity. The only drug that qualifies both as "antispastic" and truly as a "skeletal muscle relaxant" is diazepam. To add to the above confusion, all the drugs commonly referred to as "skeletal muscle relaxants" (except perhaps for diazepam) have not been proved to actually relax the skeletal muscles of human beings in the clinical setting. Nevertheless, many clinicians continue to use antispastic drugs (such as tizanidine and baclofen) and "skeletal muscle relaxants" in patients with musculoskeletal pain probably because of their ability to cause relaxation through depression of the central nerve pathway and possibly through their effect on higher centers.

Mechanism of action. The precise MOA of "skeletal muscle relaxants" remains unknown, although it is likely related to a central depressant effect with little or no direct effect on skeletal muscles. In animal models, these drugs have been shown to inhibit polysynaptic spinal myogenic reflexes, but the relationship between these actions and any possible analgesic effect is unknown. It is unclear if these drugs have analgesic effects that are selective for musculoskeletal pain problems or if relaxation of the "muscle spasm" is a necessary condition for their analgesic effectiveness.

Adverse drug reactions. At the doses used clinically, the "skeletal muscle relaxants" are generally well tolerated. The most common side-effects include drowsiness, dizziness, ataxia, tremor, headache, and changes in temperament. They are usually transient and resolve as the patient develops tolerance to them. Other ADRs include rash, hypotension, dyspnea, chest pain, and syncope. Additional ADRs are discussed under each specific drug.

Contraindications and precautions. They should be used with caution by patients for whom mental alertness is required (e.g., machinery operators or drivers) because of the side-effect of drowsiness. Patients should also refrain from concurrent intake of alcohol or other CNS depressants. Aside from general contraindications in patients with known hypersensitivity to the drug or component of the drug or its vehicle, additional contraindications and precautions for each drug are discussed below.

Drug administration guidelines. "Skeletal muscle relaxants" should be started at a low dose and gradually increased (up to the recommended maximum daily dose) if the response is inadequate and side-effects minimal. If treatment is ineffective or if side-effects are intolerable with one drug, it is reasonable to switch to another drug. Use should ideally be limited to 10–14 days (or up to 3 weeks) because of their potential for abuse (reported in some patients with noncancer chronic pain). Also, long-term effects have not been fully evaluated.

"Skeletal muscle relaxants" are marketed alone and in combination with other compounds (usually with aspirin or codeine).

A. SINGLE FORMULATIONS

1. **Cyclobenzaprine (Flexeril)** probably exerts its effects centrally, primarily in the brainstem and not in the spinal cord. It is chemically related to the tricyclic antidepressants (see section V.A.1) and possesses many of their adverse effects, including CNS depression, anticholinergic effects, and GI effects (e.g., nausea, vomiting, altered taste, constipation or diarrhea, anorexia, and abdominal pain). It has been reported to be effective in patients with fibromyalgia (see Chapter 4.11; Chapter 5.10, Table 5.10-1). Its use is contraindicated in many forms of heart disease (e.g., acute myocardial infarction) or in patients with hyperthyroidism, symptomatic prostatic hypertrophy, or narrow angle glaucoma. It should not be used concurrently or within 2 weeks of MAOI use. The starting dose is 5 or 10 mg, po, tid, which can be increased up to a maximum of 60 mg/day. Flexeril is available only in oral form (5- or 10-mg tablets).
2. **Carisoprodol (Soma)** probably acts by blocking interneuronal activity in the descending reticular formation and spinal cord (thus causing CNS depression). It has a rapid onset which lasts for 4–6 hours. Idiosyncratic drug reactions include extreme weakness, transient tetraplegia, temporary vision problems, mydriasis, dysarthria, agitation, euphoria, confusion, and disorientation. It must be used

with caution in patients with hepatic and renal impairments. It is contraindicated in acute intermittent porphyria. Soma is available only for oral use (350-mg tablets) at a dose of 350 mg, po, tid/qid. It is also available in combination with ASA and/or opioids (see below).

3. **Chlorzoxazone (Parafon Forte)** probably acts at the spinal cord and subcortical levels, by inhibiting multisynaptic reflex arcs that may be associated with painful muscle spasms. This drug is usually well-tolerated with rare ADRs. The starting dose is 250–500 mg, po, tid/qid, which can be increased up to 750 mg, po, tid/qid. Parafon Forte is available only in oral forms (250- and 500-mg caplets).
4. **Methocarbamol (Robaxin)** probably exerts its effects by generalized CNS depression. It is available in both oral (500- and 750-mg tablets) and parenteral forms (100 mg/mL in 10-mL single-dose vial). The initial oral dose is 1500 mg qid, which can be maintained at 1000 mg qid. It is usually given at 6 g/day for the first 48–72 hours, then reduced to 4 g/day. The maximum daily oral dose for severe conditions can be as high as 8 g. The oral form is also marketed in combination with opioids and/or ASA (see below). The injectable form contains polyethylene glycol in the vehicle, which is contraindicated in patients with renal pathology (because polyethylene glycol can increase pre-existing acidosis and cause urea retention). Intravenous injections have also been reported to cause seizures. The parenteral form can be given as 1 g, IM/IV, q6h as needed (maximum rate of IV injection is 3 mL/min; maximum dose is 3 g/day).
5. **Orphenadrine (Norflex)** probably acts in the reticular formation of the brainstem. It is also classified as an antihistaminic agent and has mild anticholinergic effects (dose-related). Its use is contraindicated in patients with glaucoma, pyloric or duodenal obstruction, stenosing peptic ulcers, prostatic hypertrophy or obstruction of the bladder neck, cardiospasm (megaesophagus), or myasthenia gravis. Norflex is available in both oral (100-mg tablet) and parenteral (60 mg/2 mL ampule) forms. The oral dose is 100 mg, po, bid; while the parenteral dose is 60 mg IM/IV, q12h. Oral orphenadrine is also available in combination with ASA and/or opioids (see below).
6. **Metaxalone (Skelaxin)** probably exerts its effects by generalized CNS depression. Additional ADRs include GI upsets (nausea, vomiting), leukopenia, hemolytic anemia, and jaundice. It is contraindicated in patients with significant renal and hepatic impairment, or with known tendency to drug-induced hemolytic or other anemia. It is available only for oral use (400- and 800-mg tablet) at a dose of 400–800 mg, po, tid/qid.
7. **Diazepam (Valium),** discussed in section V.C.1.b.1. and in Chapter 5.4, section III.D.1.c, can be used to relieve muscle spasm at a dose of 2–10 mg, po, tid/qid.
8. **Tizanidine (Zanaflex),** discussed in Chapter 5.4, section III.D.1.e, can be used to provide muscle relaxation at a dose of 2–4 mg, po, qd/bid/tid.
9. **Baclofen,** discussed in Chapter 5.4, section III.D.1.a, can be used to provide muscle relaxation at a dose of 5 mg, po, bid/tid, then gradually titrated up to 30–90 mg/day.
10. **Chlorphenesin carbamate (Maolate, Mycil, Rinlaxer),** a central-acting skeletal muscle relaxant that is structurally and pharmacologically similar to methocarbamol, is not commercially available in the United States. The usual adult daily dose is 1600 mg in divided doses (up to a maximum of 8 weeks). It should not be used in patients with liver dysfunction.

B. COMBINATIONS WITH ASA, OPIOID, OR BOTH. The analgesic effect of ASA and/or opioid can be potentiated by combining them with "skeletal muscle relaxants".

1. **Carisoprodol**. Soma compound (carisoprodol/ASA 200/325 mg), 1–2 tabs, po, qid; **Soma compound with codeine** (carisoprodol/ASA/codeine 200/325/16 mg): 1–2 tabs, po, q6h.

2. **Orphenadrine. Norgesic** (orphenadrine/ASA/caffeine 25/385/30 mg): 1–2 tabs, po, tid/qid; **Norgesic Forte** (orphenadrine/ASA/caffeine 50/770/60 mg): 0.5–1 tab, po, tid/qid.
3. **Methocarbamol: Robaxisal** (methocarbamol/ASA 400/325 mg), 2 tabs, po, qid.

III. Corticosteroids

Corticosteroids are one of the two steroids (the other being androgen) synthesized by the adrenal cortex. There are two kinds of corticosteroids: glucocorticoids and mineralocorticoids. In humans, the main glucocorticoid is hydrocortisone (cortisol), and the main mineralocorticoid is aldosterone. The corticosteroids referred to in this chapter are mainly glucocorticoids. Glucocorticoids have potent anti-inflammatory, hormonal, and metabolic effects. They are capable of suppressing many disease manifestations, both articular and systemic. In the PM&R setting, they are primarily used in treating neuromuscular diseases (e.g., acute disk herniation with radiculopathy), rheumatic and collagen disorders, acute spinal cord injuries, acute exacerbation of chronic obstructive pulmonary disease (COPD), and cerebral edema (e.g., after brain surgery, head injury, or stroke). Their possible role as an analgesic is discussed in Chapter 5.10, section VI.E.2.J.

Mechanism of action. Corticosteroids suppress inflammation by blocking phospholipase A_2 thus inhibiting the formation of arachidonic acid, which is the precursor of prostaglandins (see Fig. 4.8-1). They also inhibit humoral and cell-mediated immune processes as well as stabilizing lysosomal membranes.

Adverse drug reactions. Corticosteroids provide multisystem benefits and likewise cause multisystem ADRs. The ADRs and complications are time- and dose-related, hence long-term or high-dose corticosteroid therapy should be avoided unless it produces a definite advantage. The possible ADRs of corticosteroids include:

- Fluid and electrolyte disturbances, e.g., fluid retention (with weight gain), congestive heart failure, hypertension, and hypokalemic alkalosis;
- Musculoskeletal effects, e.g., muscle weakness and atrophy, tendon rupture, steroid myopathy, osteoporosis, vertebral compression fracture, aseptic necrosis of femoral and humeral heads, and pathologic fracture of long bones;
- Gastrointestinal effects, e.g., peptic or gastric ulcers with possible bleeding (for GI protection, see section I.A.3 under GI toxicity), ulcerative esophagitis, pancreatitis, abdominal distension, and nausea;
- Dermatologic effects, e.g., impaired wound healing, thin fragile skin, petechiae, ecchymoses, acne, hirsutism, striae, purpura, and suppression of reactions to skin tests;
- Endocrine effects, e.g., cushingoid state, manifestations of latent diabetes mellitus, glucose intolerance, increase need for hypoglycemics, growth arrest, secondary amenorrhea, impotence, and suppression of the hypothalamic–pituitary–adrenal axis;
- Ophthalmic effects, e.g., cataract, glaucoma, and exophthalmos;
- Neurologic and psychological effects, e.g., convulsions, increased intracranial pressure, vertigo, headache, behavior disturbance, and steroid psychoses;
- Immune system effects, e.g., increased susceptibility to infection, and activation of old infection (e.g., tuberculosis or amebiasis);
- Other effects, e.g., thromboembolism, changes in leukocyte and lymphocyte count, protein catabolism, myocardial rupture following recent myocardial infarction, malaise, and increased appetite.

Contraindications and precautions. Aside from its contraindication in patients with known hypersensitivity to the drug or component of the drug or its vehicle, corticosteroids are also contraindicated in patients with systemic infection (especially fungal). They must be used with caution in patients with diabetes mellitus, hypertension, pregnancy, psychotic tendencies, renal impairments, osteoporosis, active or latent peptic ulcer, ulcerative colitis, or ocular herpes simplex. The steroid effects are enhanced in patients with cirrhosis and in those with hypothyroidism.

Drug administration guidelines. In general, nonsteroidal agents are tried before corticosteroids are begun. However, in some cases (e.g., acute disk herniation with radiculopathy, acute spinal cord injuries, tumors, vasculitis, acute exacerbation of COPD) corticosteroids are tried first. When possible, less hazardous agents should be used concurrently to allow the lowest possible dose of corticosteroid. The concurrent use of NSAIDs, however, is not recommended because of the high risk of GI toxicity. In long-term corticosteroid therapy, periodic determinations of blood sugar, electrolytes, complete blood counts (CBCs), stool guaiacs, blood pressure, and body weight should be obtained. Drug dosage varies widely according to the specific disease, its severity, as well as the corticosteroid preparation and the patient's response. The route of systemic corticosteroid therapy can be oral or parenteral (IM/IV). Dosages of oral and parenteral preparations are generally comparable. High-dose parenteral therapy is often used for severe illnesses. IM administration may provide a sustained or depot action, which can be used to supplement or replace initial oral therapy. Some corticosteroid preparations [e.g., triamcinolone (Aristocort Forte) or dexamethasone (Decadron-LA)] may be effective from 4–7 days up to 3–4 weeks when given as a single IM dose four to seven times the daily oral dose in selected noncompliant patients. Corticosteroids can also be administered locally by topical applications, by iontophoresis (see Chapter 4.1, section V.A.1.a) or by injecting it into the lesion (e.g., keloids), soft tissues, or joints (see Chapter 4.9). Local corticosteroid administration may be absorbed systemically and cause systemic ADRs. Also, repeated intra-articular or soft tissue injections of corticosteroid may lead to disruption and weakening of cartilage and supporting soft tissue structures as well as possibly causing a crystal-induced transient synovitis.

Daily regimen guidelines. Corticosteroids can be given daily in divided doses or in a single morning dose. In most illnesses, the therapeutic effect of a single morning dose is the same as daily divided doses. For short treatments (<1 month), the dosage schedule does not matter. However, when chronic daily therapy is required, the single morning dose is preferred. This is because of the diurnal rhythm of the hypothalamic–pituitary–adrenal axis (HPAA), i.e., there is maximal activity of the adrenal cortex between 2 a.m. and 8 a.m. and minimal activity between 4 p.m. and midnight. Hence, exogenous corticosteroids suppress the HPAA the least when given at the time of maximal activity (i.e., in the morning). Also, it probably does not increase susceptibility to infection (as does daily divided doses). However, neither single nor divided daily doses have been shown to prevent iatrogenic Cushing's syndrome in long-term therapy. Only short- or intermediate-acting corticosteroids are suitable for single morning-dose therapy because long-acting corticosteroids (i.e., dexamethasone and betamethasone) constantly suppress adrenal activity and do not allow a sufficient period of low steroid level in the blood to prevent side-effects.

Alternate-day therapy (ADT) guidelines. In the ADT schedule, corticosteroid is given at twice the amount of the daily dose on alternate mornings. This is indicated in patients requiring long-term corticosteroid therapy because it minimizes certain adverse effects such as HPAA suppression, iatrogenic Cushing's syndrome, corticoid withdrawal symptoms, and growth suppression in children. There is also evidence that ADT does not increase the susceptibility to infection. As with single morning-dose therapy, long-acting corticosteroids (i.e., dexamethasone and betamethasone) are not suitable for ADT. If an acute flare-up occurs during ADT, it may be necessary to return to a full suppressive daily divided dose for control.

Once control is re-established, ADT may be reinstituted. To change from a daily single dose to ADT, the dosage can be increased gradually on one day, while the dosage is reduced by the same amount on the alternate day. In the case of divided daily doses, the frequency of the dose is reduced until the whole dose is given in the morning.

Stress dose guidelines. A brief dosage of steroid boost called "stress dosing" or "steroid coverage" is traditionally given in patients on long-term corticosteroid therapy (i.e., >5 mg/day of prednisone or its equivalent) during situations that cause acute physiologic stress, e.g., surgery, trauma, infection, or severe illness. This is given to prevent potential secondary adrenaline insufficiency, which can be life-threatening. In general, the stress dose should be proportionate to the severity of the stress and should be tapered over 1–3 days. For surgical patients with no complications, the recommended perioperative hydrocortisone "stress dose" is: 25 mg/day for 1 day for minor surgery (e.g., inguinal herniorrhaphy); 50–75 mg/day for 1–2 days for moderate surgery (e.g., total joint replacement); and 100–150 mg/day for major surgery (e.g., cardiopulmonary bypass) (see Salem *et al.*, 1994).

Discontinuation guidelines. When chronic corticosteroid therapy is discontinued, the following problems may arise: suppression of the adrenal gland or HPAA yielding corticosteroid withdrawal symptoms and acute exacerbation of the underlying disease. Suppression of HPAA should be considered in any patient who has received more than 10 mg of prednisone or its equivalent for longer than 1 week. With doses closer to the physiologic level, HPAA suppression may not occur for a month. Complete recovery from HPAA suppression may take from months up to a year. These patients usually need no replacement therapy but may require corticosteroid supplementation ("stress dose") during periods of stress, such as surgery, trauma, acute infection.

Corticosteroid withdrawal symptoms include anorexia, nausea, vomiting, lethargy, headache, fever, arthralgia, myalgia, and weight loss, which may occur after chronic treatment is discontinued. It is treated symptomatically and/or with small doses (10 mg) of cortisol for several weeks.

Acute exacerbation (flare-ups) of the underlying disease can be prevented by very gradual dose reduction. The rate of corticosteroid taper is determined by the disease activity. Monitoring of the HPAA is usually not necessary. If symptoms consistent with adrenal insufficiency develop, the rate of tapering can be decreased or glucocorticoid replacement can be empirically reinitiated.

Classification. Oral or parenteral corticosteroid preparations can be classified according to their biological half-lives (see Table 4.8-5). Table 4.8-5 also shows the equivalent anti-inflammatory dose, as well as the relative glucocorticoid and mineralocorticoid potency of each agent. The short-acting fludrocortisone (Florinef) is not included among the glucocorticoids because it is used only for its mineralocorticoid effects (although it also has glucocorticoid effects). For short-duration oral administration, prednisone is commonly used; however, the inactive prednisone (and also cortisone) needs to be activated in the liver. In patients with liver impairment, therefore, the active parenteral forms (prednisolone or cortisol) should be used instead. Methylprednisolone (Solumedrol) is used for exacerbations of multiple sclerosis and in the first 24 hours after acute spinal cord injury. The long-acting dexamethasone (Decadron), which has slight or absent mineralocorticoid effect (i.e., no sodium retention effect), is used in patients with cerebral edema.

IV. Anticonvulsants

Anticonvulsants are used in the PM&R setting for seizure prophylaxis and/or treatment (e.g., in patients with head trauma, brain tumor, or stroke) and for treatment of chronic neuropathic pain (see Chapter 5.10, section VI.E.2.b).

Table 4.8-5 Selected oral and parenteral (IV/IM) glucocorticoid preparations classified according to half-lives. For intra-articular preparations, see Table 4.9-1 in Chapter 4.9

Generic	Selected brand names	Available preparations (mg)	Initial daily dose (mg) and route[§]	Equiv-dose[¶]	Gluco-pot.**	Mine-Pot.[††]
A. Short*						
Cortisol or Hydrocortisone	a) *Hydrocortone* b) *Solu-cortef*	a) tab 10,20; b) inj 100,250/2 mL; 500/4 mL,1000/8 mL	a) 20–240 po; b) 100–500 IV/IM q2–6h prn	20	1	1
Cortisone	*Cortone*	tab 25 inj 50/mL	25–300 po/IM	25	0.8	0.8
B. Intermediate[†]						
Prednisone	a) *Prednisone* b) *Liquid Pred*	a) tab 1,2.5,5,10,20,50; b) liq 5/5 mL	a) and b) 5–60 po	5	4.0	0.8
Prednisolone	a) *Pediapred* b) *Prelone* c) *Hydeltrasol*	a) liq 5/5 mL; b) liq 15/5 mL; c) inj 20/5 mL	a) and b) 5–60 po; c) 4–60 IV/IM	5	4.0	0.8
Methyl-prednisolone	a) *Medrol;* b) *Solumedrol*[‡‡] c) *Depomedrol*	a) tab 2,4,8,16,24,32; b) inj 40/mL, 125/2 mL, 500/4 mL, 1 g, 2 g/8 mL; c) 20, 40, 80/mL	a) 4–48 po; b) 10–40 IM/IV[‡‡] c) 4–48 IM/day or 40–120 IM q1–4 wk	4	5	0
Triamcinolone	*Aristocort*	tab 1, 2, 4, 8 inj 40/mL (*Forte*)	4–48 po/IM	4	5	0
C. Long[‡]						
Dexamethasone	*Decadron;* *DecadronLA*[§§]	tab 0.25,0.5,0.75,1.5,4,6; liq 0.5/5 mL inj 4/mL; 24/mL (IV only); 8/mL (*LA*).	0.75–9 po 0.5–9 IM/IV *LA* 8–16 IM q1–3 wks as needed	0.75	20–30	0
Betamethasone	*Celestone*	inj 6/mL	0.5–9.0 IM	0.6	20–30	0

* *Short half-life = 8–12 hours;* [†] *intermediate half-life = 12–36 hours;* [‡] *long half-life = 36–72 hours.*
[§] *Dose varies widely according to the specific disease and its severity as well as the patient's response.*
[¶] *Equivalent anti-inflammatory dose (in mg);* ** *relative glucocorticoid potency;* [††] *relative mineralocorticoid potency.*
[‡‡] Solumedrol *may be given in high dose therapy at 30 mg/kg, IV over at least 30 min, repeated q4–6h for 48h (e.g., within the first 48 hours of spinal cord injury).*
[§§] *LA = long-acting.*

Mechanism of action. The specific MOA of anticonvulsants is unknown. Some proposed mechanisms for their antiseizure and analgesic effects include: blockade of sodium channels and/or calcium channel to stabilize neuronal membrane and reduce neuronal hyperexcitability (through suppression of spontaneous paroxysmal neuronal discharges and their spread from the site of origin); inhibition of the release of excitatory amino acid (e.g., glutamate and aspartate); and/or enhancement of the effects of γ-aminobutyric acid (GABA), which is the predominant inhibitory neurotransmitter in the CNS.

Adverse drug reactions. Common ADRs (mostly dose-related) include CNS effects (e.g., somnolence, fatigue, dizziness, confusion, ataxia, slurred speech, tremors, and vision difficulties, such as nystagmus and diplopia) as well as GI effects (e.g., nausea and vomiting). Other rare but serious ADRs include blood dyscrasias, bone marrow depression, and hepatic toxicity. Because anticonvulsants rely on hepatic metabolism for elimination, they may accumulate and lead to toxicity in patients with hepatic impairment. Additional ADRs are listed below under each specific drug.

Contraindications and precautions. As with any drug, anticonvulsants should not be used in patients with known hypersensitivity to the drug or component of the drug or its vehicle. Specific contraindications and precautions are listed below under each drug. They should be used with caution in patients simultaneously taking another anticonvulsant or other drugs (as listed below under the specific drug).

Drug administration guidelines. In general anticonvulsant drugs should be initiated at low doses, except possibly for phenytoin which is usually well tolerated during a cautious oral or intravenous loading regimen. Low-dose titration also minimizes side-effects. Once therapeutic range is reached, the dose should be maintained. To discontinue anticonvulsants, they should be gradually withdrawn over a minimum of 1–2 weeks to minimize the risk of withdrawal seizures and status epilepticus. Patients who are maintained on the first-generation anticonvulsants [i.e., the hydantoins (phenytoin and fosphenytoin), carbamazepine, carboxylic acids (valproic acid and divalproex sodium), clonazepam] should undergo periodic monitoring of laboratory parameters (CBC and differential count; liver and renal function tests) as well as regular medical evaluations. The second-generation anticonvulsants (i.e., gabapentin, tiagabine, lamotrigine, topiramate, oxcarbazepine, zonisamide, and leveracetam) with the exception of felbamate are generally not associated with life-threatening side-effects. Tiagabine (Gabatril), however, has been reported to cause new-onset seizures and status epilepticus in patients with no history of epilepsy. Unless anticonvulsants are used for acute seizure therapy (see section V.C.1.b.1), their dosage should be gradually raised to build tolerance to side-effects.

The following discussion concentrates on anticonvulsants which have also been used by physiatrists as adjunctive analgesics in chronic neuropathic pain (see also Chapter 5.10, section VI.E.2.c). Sedatives with anticonvulsant effects, e.g., phenobarbital (Luminal) and diazepam (Valium), are discussed under sections V.C and V.D. Recommended dosages of selected oral anticonvulsants used in PM&R are shown in Table 4.8-6.

A. HYDANTOINS, INCLUDING PHENYTOIN AND ITS PRECURSOR, FOSPHENYTOIN

1. **Phenytoin (Dilantin)** is indicated in generalized tonic–clonic seizures, partial seizures, and for seizure prophylaxis as well as in the treatment of acute seizures. It may be used to treat trigeminal neuralgia in patients in whom carbamazepine is ineffective or poorly tolerated. Its MOA is believed to be related to sodium-channel blockade. Aside from common anticonvulsant ADRs (see section IV under ADRs), its prolonged use can cause gingival hyperplasia, hypertrichosis, maculopapular rash, systemic lupus erythromatosus, Stevens–Johnson syndrome, lymphadenopathy, progressive encephalopathy, osteomalacia, hepatic failure, and, rarely, permanent cerebellar degeneration. Blood dyscrasias

Table 4.8-6 Recommended dosage of selected oral anticonvulsants used in PM&R

Generic	Selected brand names	Available preparations (mg)	Dosage (mg), route, frequency	MDD* (mg)
I. First-generation[†]				
A. Phenytoin*	*Dilantin Infatabs;* *Dilantin kapseals ER*	tab 50 liq 30,125/5 mL ER cap 30,100	100, po, tid, increase q 2 wks to maintain serum level of 10–20 μg/mL	10–20 μg/mL serum
B. Carbamazepine	*Tegretol* *Tegretol ER* *Carbatrol ER*	tab 100,200 liq 100/5 mL ER cap 100,200,400 ER cap 200,300	100–200 po bid, increase by 100–200 mg q 3–7 days until 400–800 mg/day (for pain) or 800–1200 mg/day (for seizure) given tid/qid	1200–1600
C. Carboxylic acid				
1. Valproic acid*	*Depakene*	cap 250 liq 250/5 mL	10–15 mg/kg/day, increase by 5–10 mg/kg/wk up to 60 mg/kg/day given bid/tid	50–100 μg/mL serum
2. Divalproex sodium	*Depakote*	tab 125,250,500 ER tab 250,500 sprinkle cap 125	10–15 mg/kg/day, increase by 5–10 mg/kg/wk up to 60 mg/kg/day given bid/tid Migraine: 500, po, qd x 1 wk, increase to 500, po, bid	50–100 μg/mL serum 1000
D. Clonazepam	*Klonopin*	tab 0.5,1,2 wafers 0.125,0.25,0.5,1,2	0.5 mg, po, tid, increase by 0.5–1 mg q 3 days	20
II. Second-generation				
A. GABA analog				
1. Gabapentin	*Neurontin*	cap 100,300,400; tab 600,800; liq 250/5 mL	300, po, qhs, on day 1; 300, po, bid, on day 2; and 300, po, tid, on day 3, may increase to 600–800, po, tid	3600
2. Tiagabine	*Gabitril*	tab 2,4,12,16,20	2 po bid or 4 po qd, increase q 1 wk by 4–8 mg up to 32–56 mg/day (in 2–4 divided doses)	56

(*Continued*)

Table 4.8-6 *(Continued)*

Generic	Selected brand names	Available preparations (mg)	Dosage (mg), route, frequency	MDD* (mg)
B. Lamotrigine	*Lamictal*	tab 25,100,150,200 chew tab 2,5,25	25 po bid × 2 wks, increase to 50 po bid × wks, then increase by 100 mg/day q 1 wk to 150–250 po bid	600
C. Topiramate†	*Topamax*	tab 25,100,200 sprinkle cap 15,25	25 po qd/bid, increase q 1 wk by 25–50 mg/week up to 200, po, bid	400
D. Oxcarbazepine†	*Trileptal*	tab 150,300,600 liq 300/5 mL	300, po, bid, increase q few days by 150–300	2400
E. Levetiracetam†	*Keppra*	tab 250,500,750; liq 100/mL	500 po bid, increase q 2 wks by 1000 mg/day every 2 weeks	3000
F. Zonisamide†	*Zonegran*	tab 100	100 mg/day, increase q 2 wks by 100 mg/day	400

**MDD = maximum daily dose. The MDDs of phenytoin and valproic acid are determined by their effectiveness, side-effects, and serum drug level.*

† First-generation anticonvulsants require periodic laboratory monitoring [e.g., complete blood count (CBC) with differential count, liver and/or renal function tests] due to their side-effects. Levetiracetam needs periodic CBC with differential count due to reports of blood dyscrasias. Oxcarbazepine needs periodic blood sodium level due to reports of hyponatremia. Topiramate and zonisamide need periodic renal monitoring due to reports of nephrolithiasis.

(agranulocytosis, aplastic anemis) have also been reported, thus warranting periodic monitoring of CBC with differential count.

Some common drugs that affect phenytoin levels are drugs that may *increase* serum phenytoin level (acute alcohol intake, chlordiazepoxide, diazepam, estrogens, fluoxetine, H_2-blockers, isoniazid, methylphenidate, phenothiazines, salicylates, sulfonamides, tolbutamide, trimethoprim, trazodone), drugs that may *decrease* serum phenytoin level (carbamazepine, chronic ethanol abuse, folic acid, reserpine, rifampin, sucralfate), and drugs that may increase or decrease the serum phenytoin level (phenobarbital, valproic acid). Phenytoin may impair the efficacy of the following drugs: corticosteroids, digitoxin, doxycycline, estrogens, furosemide, levodopa, oral contraceptives, quinidine, rifampin, theophylline, thyroid hormones, vitamin D, and warfarin.

The initial dose of phenytoin is 300 mg/day (usually in bid/tid dose; if to be taken once a day, the extended release preparation is preferred; suspension requires more frequent dosing every 6 hours). It is then adjusted to maintain a serum concentration of 10–20 μg/mL. When dosage exceeds 300 mg/day, it should be increased at intervals of 2 weeks or more. Phenytoin levels have been reported to rise from subtherapeutic to toxic with as little as a 50-mg/day increment. Hence, blood level of free dilantin should be monitored. Phenytoin is available in both oral forms (50-mg tablets; 30- and 100-mg extended capsules; 30- and 125-mg/5 mL oral suspension) and parenteral forms (50 mg/mL in 2- and 5-mL vials). Intravenous phenytoin (given slowly not to exceed 50 mg/min) may be used for controlling status epilepticus (however, IV fosphenytoin is preferred because of the better tolerability; see section IV.A.2).

2. **Fosphenytoin (Cerebyx)** is a pro-drug that is rapidly converted to phenytoin after IV or IM injection. It is indicated for short-term parenteral use when oral phenytoin is unavailable or less advantageous; for control of status epilepticus; and for preventing and controlling seizures during neurosurgery. It can be given parenterally (IM or IV) in neuropathic pain (e.g., trigeminal neuralgia) if an oral dose of phenytoin is not possible. Compared to IV phenytoin, it has low risk of tissue irritation and is better tolerated. It is 100% bioavailable and attains therapeutic serum levels of phenytoin with 10 minutes of IV infusion. Because of its effect on ventricular automaticity, it is contraindicated in patients with sinus bradycardia, sinoatrial block, second- and third-degree atrioventricular block, and Stokes–Adams syndrome. Some of its more common ADRs include pruritus, nystagmus, dizziness, somnolence, ataxia, nausea, tinnitus, and hypotension. Up to 64% of patients experience groin discomfort on IV administration, which usually subsides within 60 minutes. Doses of fosphenytoin are expressed as their phenytoin sodium equivalents or PE. A 150-mg PE dose of fosphenytoin is equivalent to 100 mg of phenytoin. For patients with status epilepticus, 22.5–30 mg PE/kg of IV fosphenytoin is given at a rate of 100–150 mg PE/min. For seizure prophylaxis and for neuropathic pain, an IV or IM loading dose of 15–30 mg PE/kg is followed by a daily maintenance dosage of 6–12 mg PE/kg.

B. **CARBAMAZEPINE (TEGRETOL; CARBATROL)** is indicated for generalized tonic–clonic seizures and partial seizures with complex symptomatology (psychomotor or temporal lobe), as well as for trigeminal neuralgia. Like phenytoin, its MOA is believed to be related to sodium-channel blockade. Serious ADRs include leukopenia and thrombocytopenia (in approximately 2% of patients) and, rarely, agranulocytosis and aplastic anemia. Other rare adverse effects of carbamazepine include hepatotoxicity, inappropriate secretion of antidiuretic hormone, cardiovascular effects (e.g., congestive heart failure, arrhythmias, and orthostatic hypotension), hypersensitivity reactions (Stevens–Johnson syndrome), pancreatitis, and eye changes (cortical lens opacity, conjunctivitis). Carbamazepine should not be used in patients with previous bone marrow suppression or in patients taking concurrent MAOI drugs. Because carbamazepine is structurally related to the tricyclic antidepressants of the imipramine class, caution similar to the other tricyclics should be exercised (see section V.A.1). Drugs that may increase serum carbamazepine levels include calcium-channel blockers, cimetidine, erythromycin, fluoxetine, isoniazid, and propoxyphene.

Baseline CBC, differential count, liver and renal function tests, as well as eye examination (slit-lamp, fundoscopy, and tonometry) need to be monitored before drug therapy. CBC and differential counts should be repeated 2–3 weeks after initiation of therapy, and monthly for 3 months, followed by biannual counts if there is no evidence of bone marrow suppression. A leukocyte count below 4000 cells/mm^3 is a contraindication to treatment. After therapy is begun, the drug should be discontinued if the white blood cell count falls below 3000 cells/mm^3, the absolute neutrophil count declines below 1500 cells/mm^3, or if there is significant thrombocytopenia or if other blood elements become abnormal. Liver and renal function tests as well as eye examination should be monitored periodically.

The initial dose of carbamazepine is 100–200 mg, po, bid, which can be increased by 100–200 mg every 3–7 days until the usual dose (given tid or qid) of 400–800 mg/day for pain control or 800–1200 mg/day for seizure control. The maximum daily dose in most adults is 1200 mg or up to 1600 mg in rare instances. Common ADRs can be obviated by starting at 100 mg bid and slowly titrating up in 100-mg doses. Plasma levels can be used for monitoring compliance and for adjusting dosage (therapeutic range is 4–12 mg/mL for antiseizure and analgesic response). Carbamazepine is available only in oral forms as Tegretol (100- and 200-mg tablets; 100-, 200-, and 400-mg extended release capsules; and 100 mg/5 mL oral suspension) and as Carbatrol (200- and 300-mg extended release capsules).

C. CARBOXYLIC ACIDS (VALPROIC ACID AND DIVALPROEX SODIUM) are indicated in the treatment of absence seizures as well as partial complex seizures. Their MOA is believed to be related to enhancement of GABA effects on the CNS. Aside from common anticonvulsant ADRs (e.g., somnolence, fatigue, dizziness, nausea, dyspepsia, diarrhea), their idiosyncratic reactions include hepatotoxicity (with reports of fatality), teratogenicity, pancreatitis (life-threatening), encephalopathy, hematologic abnormalities (e.g., thrombocytopenia, aplastic anemia, agranulocytosis), dermatitis or rash, Stevens–Johnson syndrome, alopecia, and a rare hyperammonemia syndrome (in patients with urea cycle disorders or UCDs). Liver function tests (LFTs) and CBCs with differential count should be monitored before starting therapy and at frequent intervals thereafter, especially during the first 6 months. In addition, patients should be monitored for serum ammonia, which can be elevated without abnormalities in the LFTs. In patients with abdominal pain, nausea, vomiting, and/or anorexia, pancreatitis should be ruled out. In women of childbearing potential, its benefit should be weighed against the fetal teratogenic risk. It is contraindicated in patients with significant liver dysfunction and known UCDs. In the treatment of neuropathic pain, they have better tolerability compared to carbamazepine or phenytoin.

1. **Valproic acid (Depakene; Depacon)** may also be used in the management of phantom limb pain syndromes, lancinating neuropathic pain (trigeminal neuralgia), and postherpetic neuralgias. Its initial dose is 15 mg/kg/day in two or more divided doses, which can be increased by 5–10 mg/kg/day until either seizure control or pain relief is achieved or the patient experiences side-effects, up to a maximum of 60 mg/kg/day. Pain relief may be felt at doses lower than

those required to achieve the therapeutic anticonvulsant serum concentrations of 50–150 μg/mL. Valproic acid is available in oral forms as Depakene (250-mg capsules and 250-mg/5 mL syrup) and in IV form as Depacon (100 mg/mL in 5-mL vials). The IV form is used if the oral form is temporarily not feasible.

2. **Divalproex sodium (Depakote)** is composed of sodium valproate and valproic acid. In the GI tract it dissociates into the valproate ion and has similar pharmacologic action and drug interaction with valproic acid. It has been approved by the FDA for prophylaxis of migraine headaches. It has been used in the management of polyneuropathy, herpetic neuralgia, facial pain, and central pain. When combined with baclofen, it can be used to treat spasticity-related chronic pain. Its initial dose is 15 mg/kg/day in two or more divided doses, which can be increased by 5–10 mg/kg/day until either seizure control or pain relief is achieved or the patient experiences side-effects, up to a maximum of 60 mg/kg/day. Pain relief may be felt at doses lower than those required to achieve the therapeutic anticonvulsant serum concentrations of 50–150 μg/mL. For migraine headache, the starting dose is 500 mg, po, qd for one week, which may be increased up to 1000 mg/day. It is only available orally as 125-, 250-, and 500-mg delayed-release tablets; as 250- and 500-mg extended-release tablets; and as 125-mg sprinkle capsules.

D. **CLONAZEPAM (KLONOPIN)** is a benzodiazepine (see section V.C.1), which is primarily indicated for absence, myoclonic, and akinetic seizures. It has been reported to help reduce pain in patients with trigeminal neuralgia, paroxysmal postlaminectomy pain, and post-traumatic neuralgia. It has anxiolytic and sedative effects, which may be beneficial in chronic pain patients with anxiety or insomnia. Its MOA is believed to be mediated through enhancement of GABA. Rare idiosyncratic reactions include dermatitis, hepatotoxicity, and hematologic effects (blood dyscrasias). Hence, periodic blood count and LFTs are advisable, especially in long-term use. Clonazepam is contraindicated in patients with allergy to benzodiazepines. As with other benzodiazepine drugs, it should not be abruptly discontinued (especially at high doses), as doing so may lead to a withdrawal syndrome. Its starting dose is 0.5 mg, po, tid, which can be increased by 0.5–1 mg every 3 days until seizure or pain is controlled or side-effects limit use. Maximum daily dose is 20 mg. It is available only in oral forms (0.5-, 1-, and 2-mg tablets or 0.125-, 0.25-, 0.5-, 1-, 2-mg wafers, i.e., orally disintegrating tablets).

E. **GABA ANALOG (GABAPENTIN and TIAGABIN)** are indicated as adjunctive therapy in partial seizures (with or without secondary generalization). It is believed that gabapentin acts by binding to calcium channels and modulating calcium influx as well as influencing GABAergic neurotransmission; whereas tiagabine acts as a selective GABA reuptake inhibitor. A new GABA analog, **pregabalin**, which is related to gabapentin, is currently under review by the FDA for the management of generalized anxiety disorder, neuropathic pain associated with diabetic peripheral neuropathy, and herpes zoster (postherpetic neuralgia), and as adjunctive therapy in the treatment of partial seizures. However, reports of incidence of tumor in mice have delayed trials of pregabalin on neuropathic pain in humans.

1. **Gabapentin (Neurontin)** has recently been approved by the FDA for the management of postherpetic neuralgia. Although not FDA-approved, it has been used in the management of other types of neuropathic pain (e.g., diabetic neuropathy, trigeminal neuralgia, complex regional pain syndrome, nerve trauma, brachial and lumbosacral plexus pain syndromes, phantom limb pain, Guillian–Barré syndrome, and acute and chronic pain from spinal cord injury), radiation myelopathy, as well as for prophylaxis of vascular headaches. It is recommended as the first-choice drug for neuropathic pain, especially when there

is a potential for tricyclic antidepressant-related side-effects or toxic drug–disease or drug–drug interactions. It has positive effects on mood and quality of life and can improve sleep. It has no documented long-term toxicity, active metabolites, hepatic enzyme induction, or major drug interactions. Its ADRs are minimal, dose dependent, and similar to other anticonvulsants (i.e., somnolence, fatigue, dizziness, ataxia, tremor, nausea, nystagmus, and diplopia). When taken concurrently with antacids, its bioavailability is reduced by 20%, thus 2 hours should be allowed to elapse after using antacids and before taking gabapentin. The effective dose range is 300–600 mg, po, tid, which can be titrated as needed up to 2400 mg (or even as high as 3600 mg) per day. To avoid or minimize ADRs, it can be given at 300 mg, po, qhs, on day one; 300 mg, po, bid, on day two; and 300 mg, po, tid, on day three. It is only available orally as capsules (100-, 300-, or 400-mg), tablets (600- or 800-mg) and oral solution (250 mg/5 mL).

2. **Tiagabine (Gabitril)** has been used as adjunctive therapy in patients with neuropathic pain alone or with comorbid anxiety disorders. However, post-marketing reports have shown its use to be associated with new onset seizures and status epilepticus in patients without epilepsy. It is believed that dose may be an important predisposing factor in the development of seizures, although seizures have been reported in patients taking daily doses of tiagabine as low as 4 mg/day. In most cases, patients were using concomitant medications (antidepressants, antipsychotics, stimulants, narcotics) that are thought to lower the seizure threshold. Some seizures were reported to occur near the time of a dose increase, even after periods of prior stable dosing. Hence, off-label use of tiagabine (e.g., for patients with neuropathic pain) is discouraged by its drug manufacturer (Cephalon). Its starting dose is 4 mg/day (in one or two divided doses), which can be increased by 4–8 mg at weekly interval up to a maximum of 32–56 mg/ day (in two to four divided doses). Tiagabine is only available orally as 2-, 4-, 12-, and 16-mg tablets.

F. LAMOTRIGINE (LAMICTAL) is indicated as an adjunctive therapy for partial seizures. It is considered a second-line drug in the treatment of neuropathic pain because of human immunodeficiency virus (HIV) sensory neuropathy, painful diabetic neuropathy (PDN), central poststroke pain, and pain from incomplete spinal cord lesions. It can also be used (probably as a third-line drug) in the treatment for refractory trigeminal neuralgia, postherpetic neuralgia, peripheral neuropathy, migraine with aura, multiple sclerosis pain, and central pain. However, it has not been shown to be effective for the treatment of radiculopathy, atypical head pain, and failed back syndrome. Its MOA is believed to be related to blockade of sodium channels (thus stabilizing the neuronal membrane) and inhibition of the release of excitatory amino acids (e.g., glutamate and aspartate). It has mild sedating and psychomotor effects but does not impair cognition. However, serious potentially life-threatening rashes (Stevens– Johnson syndrome; hypersensitivity syndrome) have been reported, especially when used with valproic acid. Hence, it should not be combined with valproic acid and it should be discontinued at the first sign of rash. Its starting dose is 25 mg, po, bid, for 2 weeks, which can be increased to 50 mg, po, bid for an additional 2 weeks, and then increased by 100 mg/day weekly to a maintenance level of 150–250 mg, po, bid. Its maximum dose is 600 mg/day. It is only available orally as 25-, 100-, 150- and 200-mg tablets and as 2-, 5-, 25-mg chewable dispersible tablets.

G. TOPIRAMATE (TOPAMAX) is indicated as adjunctive therapy in partial onset seizure or primary generalized tonic–clonic seizures. It has recently been approved by the FDA for prophylaxis of migraine headaches. It has been reported to be effective in treating refractory intercostal neuralgia. Its MOA is believed to be related to blockade of sodium channels and enhancement of GABAergic transmission. Its ADRs are similar to those of other anticonvulsants (i.e., somnolence, dizziness, fatigue, confusion, ataxia, slurred speech, tremors, and vision difficulties) but unlike other anticonvulsants, its somnolence and dizziness effects do not appear to be dose-related. It can also cause memory difficulties and paresthesias. It is associated with an increased risk of nephrolithiasis, which may be the result of carbonic anhydrase inhibition. Hence, it should not be used concomitantly with other carbonic anhydrase inhibitors such as dichlorphenamide (Daranide) or acetazolamide (Diamox). Its starting dose is 50 mg/day given in the evening, which can be increased by 25–50 mg/week until a dosage of 200 mg, po, bid is reached (its maximum daily dose is 400 mg/day). It is only available orally as 25-, 100- and 200-mg tablets and as 15- and 25-mg sprinkle capsules.

H. OXCARBAZEPINE (TRILEPTAL) is indicated in the treatment of partial seizures. It has also been used to treat trigeminal neuralgia, painful diabetic neuropathy, and neuropathic pain refractory to other anticonvulsants (e.g., carbamazepine and gabapentin). Its MOA is believed to be related to sodium-channel blockade. Compared to carbamazepine, it has comparable analgesic effect with fewer ADRs. Some of its more common ADRs include somnolence, fatigue, vertigo, dizziness, ataxia, diplopia, nausea, vomiting, and abdominal pain. It can also cause hyponatremia, which may require fluid restriction to reduce the risk of precipitating seizures secondary to low serum sodium. Updated warnings include serious dermatological reactions, such as Stevens–Johnson syndrome, and toxic epidermal necrolysis. Its starting dose is 300 mg, po, bid, which can be increased every few days by 150–300 mg up to a maximum of 2400 mg/day. It is only available orally as 150-, 300- and 600-mg tablets and as 300 mg/5 mL oral suspension.

I. LEVETIRACETAM (KEPPRA) is indicated as adjunctive treatment in partial onset seizures. When used alone and in combination with other treatments (e.g., with tricyclic antidepressants, other anticonvulsant drugs, and/or long-acting narcotics), it can be effective in treating neuropathic pain, migraine headaches, and multiple sclerosis pain. Its MOA is believed to be related to the inhibition of negative modulators of GABA. Some of its more common ADRs include somnolence, fatigue, and dizziness. Idiosyncratic reactions include anemia, leukopenia, neutropenia, pancytopenia, and thrombocytopenia. Thus CBC with differential count should be monitored periodically. Its starting dose is 500 mg, po, bid, which can be increased by 1000 mg/day every 2 weeks up to a maximum dosage of 3000 mg/day. It is only available orally as 250-, 500- and 750-mg tablets and as a 100 mg/mL oral solution.

J. ZONISAMIDE (ZONEGRAN) is indicated as treatment in partial onset seizures. It has been used in managing neuropathic pain, when first-line medications are ineffective or not tolerated. Its MOA is believed to be blockade of the sodium and calcium channels. Some of its more common ADRs include somnolence, fatigue, dizziness, confusion, difficulty with memory and concentration, ataxia, tremor, agitation/irritation, paresthesia, depression, insomnia, speech abnormalities, vision difficulties (diplopia, nystagmus), GI effects (e.g., anorexia, nausea, diarrhea), headache, and abdominal pain. Idiosyncratic reactions include nephrolithiasis, status epilepticus, and sudden unexplained deaths. Its starting dose is 100 mg/day, which may be increased every 2 weeks by 100 mg/day, up to 400 mg/day. It is only available orally as 100-mg tablets.

K. FELBAMATE (FELBATROL) is generally *not* recommended (except for seizures uncontrolled by other drugs) because of its increased potential for aplastic anemia and hepatic failure, both of which can cause death.

L. VIGABATRIN (SABRIL) is believed to increase GABAergic activities by irreversible inhibition of GABA-transaminase. It is used world-wide, except in the United States because of visual field deficits as a result of retinal damage and reports of white-matter damage in animals.

V. Psychotropic drugs

A. ANTIDEPRESSANTS are used in PM&R primarily as an adjunct to psychotherapy in patients with secondary depression (e.g., associated with stroke, multiple sclerosis, spinal cord injury, head injury, and Parkinson's disease) and as a multipurpose adjuvant analgesic (see Chapter 5.10, section VI.E.2.a) in patients suffering from chronic pain including neuropathic pain [e.g., postherpetic neuralgia, central pain syndromes, phantom pain, complex regional pain syndrome (CRPS) type I (formerly called reflex sympathetic dystrophy), and painful polyneuropathies or mononeuropathies including diabetic neuropathy], musculoskeletal pain (e.g., fibromyalgia, myofascial pain syndromes, chronic osteoarthritis, chronic low back pain, and mixed arthritic disorders), headaches (e.g., migraine, cluster, or tension headaches), chronic facial pain, cancer pain, post-traumatic encephalopathies, and psychogenic pain. The only chronic pain syndrome that possibly does not respond well to antidepressants is pure lancinating neuropathic pain (e.g., trigeminal neuralgia), which has been shown to respond better to anticonvulsant therapy.

Mechanism of action. Antidepressants increase the availability of neurotransmitters (e.g., serotonin and norepinephrine), which are reported to be decreased in patients with depression and chronic pain. Most of them block the reuptake of the neurotransmitters at the neuronal membrane, except probably for MAOIs, which enhance neurotransmitters (i.e., dopamine, serotonin, and norepinephrine) through a different pathway involving the inhibition of the MAO enzyme. The enhancement of neurotransmitter availability elevates the mood and improves depression. Mood elevation in patients with concomitant pain may also contribute to the analgesia; however, analgesia can occur independent of mood elevation because the primary analgesic dose occurs at a dose lower than that required to treat depression.

Other suggested mechanisms of analgesia include raising the pain threshold, allowing improved sleep, and altering the perception of pain. The sedating effects of some antidepressants (e.g., tricyclic antidepressants) probably help in improving the disturbed sleep cycle of patients with depression and/or chronic pain (e.g., in patients with fibromyalgia). Antidepressants also potentiate the analgesic effectiveness of concomitant opioids and NSAIDs. Other proposed and less commonly accepted mechanisms of analgesic action of antidepressants include an anticonvulsant mechanism, an anti-inflammatory mechanism, and an antispasmodic mechanism.

Classification. Antidepressants can be classified according to the pathway in which they increase neurotransmitters (i.e., non-MAOIs vs. MAOIs). The non-MAOIs can be subclassified into tricyclic antidepressants (TCAs), selective serotonin reuptake inhibitors (SSRIs), and other antidepressants. The non-MAOI antidepressants (especially the TCAs) interact with other types of receptors (e.g., acetylcholine and histamine receptors). Their inhibition of acetylcholine receptors probably contributes to the analgesic as well as anticholinergic effects of TCAs. Some antidepressants are more selective toward the blockade of serotonin reuptake (e.g., SSRIs) whereas others are selective toward norepinephrine blockade (e.g., TCAs with secondary amines). Other antidepressants also block dopamine in addition to serotonin and norepinephrine (e.g., amoxapine, buproprion, and the MAOIs). In general, the TCAs with secondary amines and SSRIs are less sedating than the TCAs with tertiary amines. The SSRIs have lesser anticholinergic effects and also less potent analgesic effects (both probably because of their significantly diminished inhibitory effects on acetylcholine receptors) than the TCAs. The "other" antidepressants are unrelated and pharmacologically distinct from the remaining classes of antidepressants but also enhance serotonin, norepinephrine, and dopamine availability.

Adverse drug reactions. The side-effect profiles for different antidepressants are summarized in Table 4.8-7. In general, ADRs of antidepressants include anticholinergic effects (e.g., dry mucous membranes is the most common; other more serious but less common anticholinergic effects include urinary retention, precipitation of acute-angle-closure glaucoma, obstipation, and delirium), cardiovascular effects (e.g., arrhythmia, hypotension, orthostatic hypotension, and reflex tachycardia), CNS effects (e.g., excessive sedation, insomnia, agitation, anxiety, confusion, tremor, seizure, and occasional development of extrapyramidal symptoms), and other effects (e.g., GI distress, weight gain or loss, respiratory depression, hematologic disturbances, transient elevation in serum transaminase levels, jaundice, hepatitis, endocrine effects, sexual dysfunction, and hypersensitivity reactions). Elderly patients taking antidepressants have increased risk of falls and hip fractures, probably due to ADRs of antidepressants, such as sedation, orthostatic hypotension, confusion, and cardiac irregularities. Many drugs (e.g., norepinephrine, alcohol, and barbiturates) may potentiate toxicity of the antidepressants. The occurrence of serious ADRs during antidepressant therapy is relatively rare, particularly at the low doses typically used to treat pain. Moreover, many patients develop tolerance to the ADRs within several weeks after treatment is initiated.

Contraindications. Concurrent use of any antidepressant with a MAOI antidepressant is contraindicated because their interaction can lead to hyperpyretic crises, severe convulsions, and even death. Patients taking MAOI must discontinue use for at least 2 weeks prior to starting another class of antidepressant. All antidepressants (except possibly SSRIs) should be avoided by patients with recent myocardial infarction, heart failure, left bundle branch block, or other significant cardiac conduction abnormalities. Antidepressants are also contraindicated in patients with symptomatic prostatic hypertrophy, or narrow-angle glaucoma.

Drug administration guidelines. Start at a low dose and gradually titrate upward until a therapeutic response is reached with the least amount of side-effects. Only one drug should be added or titrated at a time. For use as an analgesic, the dosing guideline of amitriptyline is discussed in Chapter 5.10, section VI.E.2. The variability in patient response to different antidepressants is well known and sequential trial of different antidepressants (even within the same class) is justified. Because of the arrhythmic effects of TCAs, any patients with known cardiac disease or those with no known cardiac disease but who are older than 40 years should have a baseline electrocardiogram (ECG) prior to starting TCAs. Older patients should undergo serial ECG if doses are increased to relatively high levels (e.g., at least 150 mg of amitriptyline per day). Some ECG effects of TCAs include: increased heart rate, prolongation of the PR interval, intraventricular conduction disturbances, increase in QTc interval, and flattening of T waves.

To further reduce the risk of adverse effects associated with unexpectedly high levels (even with low dose in some elderly patients), the plasma drug concentration and its primary metabolite should be monitored if available (e.g., nortriptyline, desipramine, amitriptyline and its metabolite, and imipramine and its metabolite). Cardiovascular status should also be monitored closely for hypotensive or orthostatic hypotensive effects. Bedside evaluation of the depth of the anterior chamber (to determine narrow-angle glaucoma) should be considered before starting TCAs. Prescription of TCAs should be limited to a total of 1 g, without any refills, in the early stages of therapy especially when the patient appears to be suicidal. It is also advisable to check laboratory tests (e.g., CBC,

Table 4.8-7 Relative frequency of adverse drug reactions (ADRs) of antidepressant drugs commonly used for management of depression and chronic pain

Drug	Anticholinergic*	Drowsiness	Insomnia/ agitation	Seizures	Orthostatic hypotension	Cardiac arrhythmia	GI distress†	Weight gain‡
Tertiary amine TCAs								
Amitriptyline	+++	+++	0/+	++	+++	+++	0/+	++
Clomipramine	+++	++	0/+	+++	++	+++	+	+
Doxepin	++	+++	0	++	+++	++	0/+	++
Imipramine	++	++	0/+	++	++	+++	0/+	++
Trimipramine	+++	+++	0/+	++	++	+++	0/+	++
Secondary amine TCAs								
Amoxapine	+	+	0/+	++	++	++	+	+
Desipramine	+	0/+	0/+	+	+	++	0/+	+
Nortriptyline	+	+	0/+	+	+	++	0/+	+
Protriptyline	++	0/+	0/+	++	+	+++	0/+	+
Maprotiline	++	++	0/+	+++	++	++	0/+	+
SSRIs								
Fluoxetine	+	+	++	0	0	0/+	++	0
Paroxetine	+	++	++	0	0	0	++	0
Sertraline	+	+	++	0	0	0	+++	0
Fluvoxamine	0	++	++	0	0	0	+++	0
Citalopram	+	+	0	0	0	0	++	0
Escitalopram	0	+	+	0	0	0	++	0

(Continued)

Table 4.8-7 *(Continued)*

Drug	Anticholinergic*	Drowsiness	Insomnia/ agitation	Seizures	Orthostatic hypotension	Cardiac arrhythmia	GI distress†	Weight gain‡
Atypical								
Bupropion	0/+	0	++	++++	0/+	0/+	0/+	0
Nefazodone	0/+	+++	+	0	+	0/+	+	0/+
Trazodone	0/+	+++	0	0/+	++	+	0/+	+
Venlafaxine§	0/+	++	+	0	0/+	0/+	+	+
Mirtazapine	+	+++	0	0	0/+	+	0/+	+
Duloxetine	++	+	+	0	0	0	+	0
MAOI¶								
Phenelzine	0/+	+	++	0/+	+++	0	++	+
Tranylcypromine	0/+	+	++	0	++	0	++	+

Note: 0 = negligible; 0/+ = minimal; + = mild; ++ = moderate; +++ = moderately severe; ++++ = severe. This table should not be used to predict ADR incidence. TCA = tricyclic antidepressant; SSRI = selective serotonin reuptake inhibitor; MAOI = monoamine oxidase inhibitor.

* *Urinary retention, constipation, blurred vision, glaucoma aggravation, dry mouth.*

† *Nausea, diarrhea, vomiting.*

‡ *Weight gain of >6 kg.*

§ *Venlafaxine is a SSRI at low doses. At high doses, it is a potent inhibitor of serotonin and norepinephrine reuptake.*

¶ *All MAOIs can have potentially fatal interaction with vasoconstrictors, decongestants, meperidine, methyldopa, levodopa, other antidepressants, other narcotics (possibly), and dietary substances (e.g., tyramine).*

differential count, and liver and renal function tests) before starting treatment and periodically thereafter.

1. **Tricyclic antidepressants** (see Table 4.8-8 for dosage), aside from their use in patients with depression, are the most common nonanalgesic medications used in the treatment of chronic pain. In general, doses lower than depression doses are used to help chronic pain patients (e.g., those with neuropathic pain, diabetic neuropathy, postherpetic neuralgia, and cancer-related pain). The most widely studied TCA in the management of chronic pain is amitriptyline.

a. ***TCA with tertiary amines*** generally block norepinephrine as well as serotonin reuptake. Compared to other antidepressants they have relatively high incidence of sedation, anticholinergic effects (thus use with caution in neurogenic bladder and bowel), orthostatic hypotension, and cardiac arrhythmias. They can also cause weight gain and seizure.

   I. **Amitriptyline (Elavil, Endep)** is available in both oral and parenteral (IM) forms. It is indicated for depression and in the treatment of most chronic pain syndromes (e.g., fibromyalgia, chronic low back pain, arthritis, postherpetic neuralgia, central pain, phantom pain, painful diabetic neuropathy, migraine and other types of headache, and psychogenic pain) except lancinating neuropathic pain (where its effectiveness is variable, and where anticonvulsants are more effective). The initial dose for treatment of depression is 75–100 mg titrated up to 150–200 mg/day or more. For pain management, the starting dose is usually 10 mg in the elderly or 25 mg in younger patients, then titrated up to 25–100 mg/day. It usually takes an average of about 2–4 weeks before the analgesic effect is felt (the delay is probably longer for its antidepression effect). Dosing guidelines for amitriptyline in chronic pain management are given in Chapter 5.10, section VI.E.2.a. It is available in combination with chlordiazepoxide (Limbitrol; see section V.C.1.b.2).

   II. **Doxepin (Adapin, Sinequan)** is given orally for either antidepressant or analgesic effects. It is effective in patients with headache, low back pain, and in pain with coexisting depression. It can also be used as an anxiolytic (see section V.C.2.e) especially in anxiety accompanied by symptoms of depression.

   III. **Imipramine (Tofranil)** is indicated for depression and nocturnal enuresis. It has also been reported to be beneficial in patients with chronic osteoarthritis, rheumatoid arthritis, low back pain, headache, and painful diabetic neuropathy. It is available in both oral and injectable forms.

   IV. **Clomipramine (Anafranil)** has been reported favorably in both neuropathic and non-neuropathic pain syndromes. Aside from its use in patients with depression and pain, it is indicated in patients with obsessive–compulsive disorders. It is available in an oral form.

   V. **Trimipramine (Surmontil)**, which is available in an oral form, is primarily used for depression.

b. ***The TCAs with secondary amines include desipramine (Norpramine), nortriptyline (Pamelor, Aventyl), protriptyline (Vivactil), Maprotiline (Ludiomil), and amoxapine (Asendin).*** They are selective in inhibiting norepinephrine reuptake (except amoxapine, which additionally blocks dopamine receptors) and have relatively fewer anticholinergic effects than TCAs with tertiary amines. They can be used in patients with significant risk for anticholinergic effects (e.g., symptomatic prostatism and narrow-angle glaucoma) or in patients who are unable to tolerate the side-effects of tertiary amines (e.g., drowsiness and orthostatic hypotension). Among the TCAs, desipramine (which has the least sedative effect) and nortriptyline have better side-effect profiles and are commonly used, particularly for chronic pain patients with depression. Desipramine has been reported to be effective in postherpetic neuralgia, while nortriptyline, in combination with fluphenazine (Prolixin), has been reported to

Table 4.8-8 Recommended starting dosage of selected antidepressants used in PM&R. Most of them have also been used in treating chronic pain patients

Generic	Selected brand names	Available preparations (mg)	Initial dosage (mg), route, frequency	MDD (mg)
A. Tertiary amine tricyclics*†				
1. Amitriptyline	*Elavil; Endep*	tab 10,25,50,75, 100,150 inj 10/mL	10–75 po qhs or 25 po tid; 20–30 IM qid	300
2. Clomipramine	*Anafranil*	tab 25,50,75	25 po qd	300
3. Doxepin	*Sinequan; Adapin*	tab 10,25,50,75, 100,150 liq 10/mL	10–25 po tid; or 75 po qhs	300
4. Imipramine	*Tofranil*	tab 10,25,50	75 po qhs	300
5. Trimipramine	*Surmontil*	tab 25,50,100	25 po tid	300
B. Secondary amine tricyclics*†				
1. Amoxapine	*Asendin*	tab 25,50,100,150	25–50 po bid/tid	400
2. Desipramine	*Norpramin*	tab 10,25,50,75,100,150	10–50 po qhs	300
3. Nortriptyline	*Pamelor; Aventyl*	cap 10,25,50, 75 liq 10/5 mL	25 po tid/qid	150
4. Protriptyline	*Vivactil*	tab 5,10	5 po tid	60
5. Maprotiline	*Ludiomil*	tab 10,25,50,75	25 po bid/tid	225
C. SSRI*				
1. Fluoxetine	*Prozac*	tab 10,20 liq 20/5 mL	20 po qd	80
	Prozac weekly	pulvule 10,20,40 cap 90	1 cap q 1 wk	
2. Paroxetine	*Paxil*	tab 20,30 liq 10/5 mL	20 po qd	60
	Paxil CR	CR tab 12.5	25 po qd	
3. Sertraline	*Zoloft*	tab 25,50,100 liq 20/mL	50 po qd	200
4. Fluvoxamine	*Luvox*	tab 50,100	50 po qd	300
5. Citalopram	*Celexa*	tab 10,20,40 liq 10/5 mL	20 po qd	60
6. Escitalopram	*Lexapro*	tab 5,10,20 liq 5/5 mL	10 po qd	30
D. Atypical*				
1. Bupropion	*Wellbutrin; Zyban*	tab 75,100	100 po bid	450
	Wellbutrin SR	SR tab 100,150	150 po bid	
	Zyban SR	Zyban SR tab 150	150 po bid	
	Wellbutrin XL	XL tab 150,300	150 increase to 300 po qd	
2. Nefazodone	*Serzone*	tab 100,150,200,250	100 po bid	600
3. Trazodone	*Desyrel*	tab 50,100,150,300	50 po tid	600
4. Venlafaxine‡	*Effexor*	tab 25,37.5,50,75,100	25 po tid or 37.5 po bid;	375
	Effexor XR	XR cap 37.5,75,150	37.5 increase to 75 po qd	
5. Mirtazapine	*Remeron*	tab 15,30,45	15 po qhs	45
6. Duloxetine‡	*Cymbalta*	Cap 20,30,60	20 po bid	60
E. MAOI§				
1. Phenelzine	*Nardil*	tab 15	15 po tid	90
2. Tranylcypromine	*Parnate*	tab 10	10 po tid	60
3. Isocarboxacid	*Marplan*	tab 10	10 po qd/bid	60

**All non-MAOI antidepressants have potentially fatal drug interaction with MAOI.*
† TCAs have potentially fatal drug interaction with antiarrhythmics.
‡ Vanlafaxine (at high dose) and duloxetine are selective serotonin and norepinephrine reuptake inhibitors (SSNRIs). At low dose, venlafaxine is a SSRI.
§ All MAOI have potentially fatal interaction with vasoconstrictors, decongestants, meperidine, methyldopa, levodopa, other antidepressants, other narcotics (possibly), and dietary substances (e.g., tyramine).
SSRI = selective serotonin reuptake inhibitors; MAOI = monoamine oxidase inhibitor.

be effective in treating painful diabetic neuropathy. Nortriptyline is also effective in treating secondary depression (e.g., stroke and parkinsonism). Protriptyline, which is primarily used for depression, also has activating properties that make it particularly suitable for withdrawn patients. Amoxapine is indicated for depression accompanied by anxiety and agitation. Maprotiline, which is indicated for the treatment of depressive neurosis, and manic-depressive illness and major depression, can also be used for relieving anxiety associated with depression. The analgesic efficacy of maprotiline was suggested in controlled studies that evaluated patients with idiopathic pain and postherpetic neuralgia. Maprotiline is contraindicated in known or suspected seizure disorder, or in the acute phase of myocardial infarction. All are available in oral forms.

2. **Selective serotonin reuptake inhibitors (SSRIs) include fluoxetine (Prozac), paroxetine (Paxil), sertraline (Zoloft), fluvoxamine (Luvox), citalopram (Celexa), and escitalopram (Lexapro)**. They consist of straight-chain phenylpropylamines, which are unrelated and pharmacologically distinct from other antidepressants. They interact minimally with α-adrenergic, histaminic, and acetylcholinergic receptors and, thus, have relatively fewer anticholinergic and sedative effects. They also have absent or rare cardiac arrhythmic effects and infrequent orthostatic hypotension effects. The following side-effects, however, are relatively common: CNS stimulation (e.g., insomnia and agitation), GI distress (e.g., nausea and diarrhea), headache, weight loss, and sexual dysfunction. To avoid insomnia, they should be taken early in the day. There have been reports of SSRIs increasing spasticity. SSRIs are primarily indicated for depression (fluoxetine and fluvoxamine are also indicated for obsessive–compulsive disorders) and are used by patients with significant risk for anticholinergic effects (e.g., symptomatic prostatism). Paroxetine has been reported to have analgesic benefits in patients with painful polyneuropathy, while studies on fluoxetine and sertraline did not show any analgesic effects. However, because of their relatively low incidence of sedative effects, SSRIs may be useful in chronic pain management of depressed patients already taking opioid analgesics. If SSRIs are used, they should be given in the morning as they may cause insomnia. The SSRIs are available in oral forms. See Table 4.8-8 for dosage.

3. **Monoamine oxidase inhibitors (MAOIs), including phenelzine (Nardil), tranylcypromine (Parnate), and isocarboxacid (Marplan)** are not used as first-line drugs because of their association with potentially fatal hypertensive crises, when used in conjunction with other medications (e.g., vasoconstrictors, decongestants, meperidine, methyldopa, levodopa, other antidepressants) and dietary substances (e.g., tyramine). They should not be used in unreliable patients who cannot follow a diet, those who consume alcohol, and those with severe cardiovascular, hepatic or renal disease, or pheochromocytoma. They are used for treatment of atypical depression unresponsive to other antidepressants. They have also been reported to be of some benefit in patients with headache, atypical facial pain, or pain complicated by depression (especially atypical depressions) in whom other treatments have failed or other antidepressants are contraindicated. For dosage recommendation, see Table 4.8-8.

4. **Atypical antidepressants** (see Table 4.8-8 for dosage) do not have a chemical structure similar to the SSRIs, TCAs, or MAOIs. They are available only in oral forms. Except for trazodone, these drugs are relatively new with few clinical studies on their analgesic effects in chronic pain patients.

a. ***Bupropion (Wellbutrin; Zyban)*** is an aminoketone, which is a relatively weak inhibitor of neuronal reuptake of norepinephrine, serotonin, and dopamine, and does not inhibit MAO. Its MOA is presumed to be mediated by noradrenergic and/or dopaminergic mechanisms. It is mainly indicated for major depression and has been approved for use in smoking cessation. It appears to have no effect on sedation, weight change, or sexual dysfunction. However, compared to other antidepressants, it is associated with higher incidence of seizures, especially at high dose and in patients with bulimia or anorexia nervosa. It has been reported to be effective in patients with neuropathic pain resistant to other therapies.

b. ***Nefazodone (Serzone)*** is a phenylpiperazine, which inhibits neuronal reuptake of serotonin and norepinephrine. It is indicated for major depression. Compared to SSRIs, sexual dysfunction and sleep disturbances are infrequent in patients taking nefazodone. However, it is associated with adverse hepatic events including liver failure requiring transplantation as well as life-threatening hepatic failure. Thus, it should not be used in patients with active liver disease or with elevated baseline serum transaminases. It should also *not* be used in patients who are taking terfenadine, astemizole, carbamazepine, cisapride, triazolam, pimozide, or MAOIs.

c. ***Trazodone (Desyrel)*** is a triazolopyridine, which provides weak inhibition of serotonin reuptake. It is indicated for depression with or without anxiety. It can also be used as a sedative (see section V.D.2.d). It may be associated with priapism. It has been shown to be effective in patients with poststroke depression, head injury, and cancer pain. However, a well-controlled trial in patients with dysesthetic pains because of traumatic myelopathy failed to demonstrate favorable effects.

d. ***Venlafaxine (Effexor)***, which is a phenylethylamine, is a serotonin reuptake inhibitor at low doses. However, at high doses, it is a selective serotonin and norepinephrine reuptake inhibitor (SSNRI). It is mainly indicated for depression, but has also been used for treating neuropathic pain and for pain and suffering associated with fibromyalgia. It has been associated with sustained hypertension and sexual dysfunction.

e. ***Mirtazapine (Remeron)*** is a tetracyclic belonging to the piperazino-azepine group, which stimulates central release of norepinephrine and serotonin. It is mainly indicated for major depression. It has relatively high sedating effect. It can also cause sexual dysfunction.

f. ***Duloxetine (Cymbalta)*** is a thiophenepropylamine, which like venlafaxine is considered a SSNRI. It is mainly indicated for major depression. It has been used in diabetic neuropathy pain. It is associated with an increased risk of mydriasis; hence, it should be avoided in patients with uncontrolled narrow-angle glaucoma. It can also cause sexual dysfunction.

B. NEUROLEPTIC DRUGS are used in psychiatry to treat psychotic disorders and as tranquilizers. In the PM&R setting, they are used in the management of refractory chronic pain (see Chapter 5.10, section VI.E.2.e); for controlling nausea, vomiting, and intractable hiccups; for sedating or calming patients with organic brain syndrome and in patients with sundown syndrome (i.e., confusion in the evening); and for controlling severe refractory aggression in patients with traumatic brain injury.

Mechanism of action. Their MOA is unknown. They probably act by postsynaptic blockade of dopaminergic receptors, which may lead to the development of extrapyramidal (parkinsonism) reactions. They also act by blocking cholinergic receptors, histamine receptors (producing sedation), and α-adrenergic receptors (producing hypotension). Some neuroleptics (e.g., prochlorperazine and Haldol) provide antiemesis by inhibiting the chemoreceptor trigger zone in the CNS.

Adverse drug reactions. Although addiction does not occur and overdosage rarely results in death, the following ADRs are common: sedation, orthostatic hypotension, dizziness, and anticholinergic effects (e.g., dry mucous membranes and precipitation of acute-angle-closure glaucoma, obstipation, and urinary retention). In some cases, they can also cause neuroleptic malignant syndrome (i.e., hyperthermia, rigidity, autonomic instability, and encephalopathy, which is potentially lethal; dantrolene and bromocriptine may be required to treat severe cases) and extrapyramidal reactions including acute dystonic reactions, akathisia, parkinsonism, and possibly irreversible tardive movement disorders (e.g., dyskinesia, dystonia, tics, and myoclonus). Rare idiosyncratic reactions such as blood dyscrasias, dermatoses (e.g., photosensitivity, urticaria, and maculopapular rashes), hepatic damage (e.g., cholestatic jaundice), and galactorrhea have also been reported. Management for the extrapyramidal reactions includes benztropine (Cogentin) or diphenhydramine (Benadryl) for acute dystonic reaction, benzodiazepines such as clonazepam (Klonopin) for akathisia, and antidopaminergic drugs [e.g., bromocriptine (Parlodel)] for tardive dyskinesia. At the first signs of any tardive syndrome (which usually develops after months or years of treatment but can occur at any time during treatment), the drugs should be tapered and discontinued. It is advisable to check laboratory tests (e.g., CBC, differential count, and liver and renal function tests) before starting treatment and periodically thereafter.

Contraindications. They should not be used in patients who are comatose or have Parkinson's disease. They can be used with caution in patients with cardiovascular instability or a history of seizures or abnormal electroencephalogram activity (because of its effect on lowering the seizure threshold). In addition, phenothiazines should be used with caution in patients with impaired hepatic or renal function.

The following are neuroleptics with possible use in the PM&R setting:

1. **Phenothiazines**

a. ***Chlorpromazine (Thorazine)*** is used for the relief of intractable hiccups at a dose of 10–25 mg, po, q4–6h or if symptoms persist for 2–3 days, give 25–50 mg IM q3–4h or 25–100 mg rectal suppository q6–8h. It can also be used for controlling nausea and vomiting at 10 mg, po/IM, bid/tid/qid, prn. There is no evidence that this drug has any analgesic effect.

b. ***Prochlorperazine (Compazine)*** is mainly used as an antiemetic. It also has mild analgesic properties. It is rarely used for the treatment of anxiety, agitation, and delirium because of its high incidence of extrapyramidal reactions. For the treatment of nausea and vomiting, the dose is 5–10 mg, po/IM, tid/qid, or 25-mg rectal suppository q12h. It is usually given prn.

c. ***Methotrimeprazine (Levoprome)*** has been shown to have unequivocal analgesic properties and may be used in patients with refractory chronic pain and cancer pain (see Chapter 5.10, section VI.E.1.e). It also has antiemetic and anxiolytic effects.

d. ***Fluphenazine (Prolixin)*** has mild analgesic properties and, when combined with a TCA (e.g., amitriptyline), has been reported to be beneficial in patients with deafferentation pain (see Chapter 5.10, section VI.E.2.e).

2. **Butyrophenone**, e.g., **haloperidol (Haldol)**, is used for managing patients with agitated delirium or with sundown syndrome at a starting dose of 0.25 mg, po/IM, which can be titrated up as needed at 20–30-minute intervals until the desired level of calmness is reached. It also has antiemetic use (1–2 mg, po/IM, bid/tid) and has been suggested to have coanalgesic properties (given at 0.5–1.0 mg, po, bid/tid). At these low doses, it rarely causes excessive sedation, hypotension, or cardiovascular compromise, and it can be given safely to the elderly. Once the condition has stabilized, haloperidol can be tapered over 2–5 days before being discontinued. Although low-to-moderate doses of Haldol may be used in acute aggression, its usefulness in the management of chronic aggression in patients with head injury has recently been surpassed by newer, shorter-acting, and more efficacious agents [e.g., buspirone (Buspar) described in section V.C.2.a; see also section V.F for antiaggression drugs].

3. **Other heterocyclic antipsychotic drugs** include **olanzapine (Zyprexa), risperidone (Risperdal), quetiapine (Seroquel), ziprasidone (Geodon)**, and **clozapine (Clozaril)**. In general, olanzapine, risperidone, and quetiapine have less toxicity than phenothiazines and butyrophenones. In the PM&R setting, they may be helpful in the management of neurologic patients (e.g., traumatic brain injury, Parkinson's disease, stroke), and as adjunctive medications in a variety of chronic or episodic pain syndromes. Olanzapine should not be used in elderly patients with dementia-related psychosis because of increased risk of cerebrovascular adverse events (e.g., stroke, transient ischemic attack), including deaths. Ziprasidone (which has greater capacity to prolong QT/QTc interval can cause torsade de pointes-type arrhythmia, a potentially fatal polymorphic ventricular tachycardia, and sudden death) and clozapine (which has significant risk for agranucytosis, and is associated with seizure, myocarditis, and orthostatic hypotension) are generally not used in the PM&R setting.

a. ***Olanzapine (Zyprexa).*** The initial oral dose for Zyprexa is 2.5 or 5.0 mg, po, qd, which can be increased (preferably by 5.0-mg increments) after intervals of several days (i.e., >24 hours) up to 10–15 mg, po, qd (maximum dose is 20 mg, po, qd). For control of agitation, Zyprexa IntraMuscular may be injected initially at 2.5–5.0 mg, IM. If agitation persists, subsequent IM doses up to 10 mg may be given (not to exceed a total of 30 mg, or three doses of 10 mg IM injections given 2–4 hours apart). After injection, patients should remain recumbent if drowsy or dizzy until examination has ruled out postural hypotension and/or bradycardia. It is available in oral forms as Zyprexa tablets (2.5-, 5.0-, 7.5-, 10-, 15-, and 20-mg) and as Zyprexa Zydis orally disintegrating tablets (5.0-, 10-, 15-, and 20-mg). It is also available in IM injectable form as Zyprexa IntraMuscular (10 mg/vial).

b. ***Risperidone (Risperdal).*** The initial dose is 0.5 mg, po, bid, which can be increased at intervals of at least 1 week in increments of no more than 0.5 mg, po, bid, up to 3 mg, po, bid (maximum dose is 8 mg, po, qd). It is available in oral forms as Risperdal tablets (0.25-, 0.5-, 1.0-, 1-, 2-, 3-, and 4-mg), as Risperdal oral solution (1 mg/mL), and as Risperdal M-Tab (0.5-, 1-, and 2-mg orally disintegrating tablets).

c. ***Quetiapine (Seroquel).*** The initial dose is 25 mg, po, bid, which can be increased in increments of 25–50 mg, po, bid/tid on the 2nd and 3rd day, as tolerated, to a target dose of 300–400 mg/day by the 4th day, given bid or tid. It is only available in oral forms as 25-, 100-, 200-, 300-mg tablets.

C. **ANXIOLYTICS** (Table 4.8-9) are primarily indicated for the management of anxiety disorders (which may be part of the symptom complex seen in major depression, panic disorders, metabolic disturbances, and drug toxicity or withdrawal) as well as reactionary agitation seen as part of the total "pain" problem in patients suffering from trauma (e.g., head trauma) and acute illness. They can also be used to calm down (and sedate) patients during imaging procedures (e.g., prior to computed tomography or magnetic resonance imaging) as well as other diagnostic (e.g., endoscopy) and therapeutic (e.g., cardioversion) procedures. The antegrade amnesia effect of anxiolytics (i.e., benzodiazepines) may be beneficial in patients undergoing procedures because it diminishes the patient's recall of the procedure. Most anxiolytics (especially those belonging to the benzodiazepine class) also have sedative-hypnotic effects (which can be beneficial if the patient also has insomnia), as well as the potential for physical dependence and abuse. Whenever possible, nonpharmacologic treatments (e.g., behavioral methods, relaxation training, biofeedback, and cognitive restructuring) should be tried first, adding anxiolytics as an adjunct if these methods are unsuccessful. Anxiolytics generally do not produce sustained improvement in patients with chronic, nonspecific anxiety. It is best to treat the underlying cause of the anxiety.

Table 4.8-9 Recommended dosage of selected anxiolytics used in PM&R

Generic	Selected brand names	Available preparations (mg)	Initial dosage (mg), route, frequency	MDD§ (mg)
I. Benzodiazepines (short half-life)*				
Alprazolam	*Xanax*	tab 0.25,0.5,1,2	0.25–0.5 po bid/tid	4
	Xanax XR	XR tab 0.5,1,2,3	0.5–3.0 po qd	6
Lorazepam	*Ativan*	a) tab 0.5,1,2 b) and (c) inj 0.5/mL; 2/mL, 4/mL	a) 1–3 po bid/tid b) 0.05/kg IM c) 0.044/kg IV	a) 10 b) 4 c) 2
Oxazepam	*Serax*	tab 15 cap 10,15,30	10–15 po tid/qid	120
II. Benzodiazepines (long half-life)†				
Chlordiaz-epoxide	*Librium;* *Libritabs* *Limbritol¶* *LimbritolDS¶*	cap 5, 10, 25 inj 100/5 mL tab 5/12.5 DS tab 10/25	5–10 po bid/tid/qid; 15–100 IM/IV then 25–50 tid/qid prn; 1 tab tid/qid	300 6 DS tabs
Clorazepate	*Tranxene;* *Tranxene SD*	tab 3.75, 7.5, 15 SD-tab: 11.25, 22.5	tab 3.75–15 po tid SD: 11.25–22.5 po qd	90
Diazepam	a) *Valium* b) *Valrelease*	a) tab 2,5,10; inj 5/mL b) cap 15	a) 2–10 bid/qid; 2–10 IM/IV q3–4hs prn; b) 15–30 po qd	80
III. Non-benzodiazepines				
Buspirone	*BuSpar*	tab 5,10	5 po tid	60
Chlormezanone	*Trancopal*	cap 100, 200	100–200 po tid/qid	800
Doxepin‡	*Adapin;* *Sinequan*	tab 10,25,50,75,100, 150; liq 10/mL	10–25 po tid; or 75 po qhs	300
Hydroxyzine	a) *Atarax;* b) *Vistaril*	a) tab 10,25,100; liq 10/5 mL b) cap 10,25,100; liq 25/5 mL; inj 25, 50/mL; 100/2 mL	25–100 po/IM qid	400
Meprobamate	*Miltown*	tab 200,400,600	400 po tid/qid	2400

**Short half-life = <20 hours.*
† Long half-life = >40 hours.
‡ Dosages given for doxepin are initial dose which may be titrated up or down.
§MDD = Maximum daily dose for anxiolytic use (may be higher in closely monitored patients or for other uses).
¶ Limbritol has 5 mg chlordiazepoxide and 12.5 mg amitriptyline; Limbritol DS has 10 mg chlordiazepoxide and 25 mg amitriptyline.

1. **Benzodiazepines** can be used primarily as anxiolytics or as sedative-hypnotics (discussed in section V.D.1). Their role in pain management (acute musculoskeletal pain and chronic pain) is discussed in Chapter 5.10, section VI.E.2.f.1. In general, they play a very limited role in pain management unless anxiety is the overriding clinical symptom. They are generally not indicated for patients with TBI except for those whose anxiety is associated with muscle tension and insomnia. The role of some benzodiazepines as anticonvulsants (e.g., diazepam and clonazepam) is discussed in section IV.

   Mechanism of action. Benzodiazepines act as CNS depressants, probably by directly potentiating the inhibitory effects of the GABA neurotransmitters throughout the CNS. Studies seem to indicate that they deplete serotonin and can theoretically increase pain perception. They generally do not cause autonomic blockade nor do they produce extrapyramidal side-effects (except transient ataxia at high doses).

Adverse drug reactions. Elderly and critically ill patients are especially at risk for ADRs, because a reduction in renal or hepatic function increases the potential for drug toxicity. Benzodiazepine ADRs include CNS effects (e.g., excessive sedation, morning drowsiness or hangover, incoordination or ataxia, confusion, dizziness, fatigue, anterograde amnesia, and impairment of cognitive and motor behavior), paradoxical excitation (e.g., irritability, agitation, anxiety, auditory and visual hallucinations, delirium, or hostility), respiratory depression (especially in large doses given to elderly patients and those with chronic pulmonary disorders), cardiovascular effects (e.g., hypotension, bradycardia, and even cardiac arrest, especially with IV administration), and other adverse effects (e.g., blurred vision, myalgias, nausea and hiccups, constipation, changes in urination patterns, urticaria, rash, photosensitivity, thrombophlebitis, jaundice, and blood dyscrasias). The effect (and toxicity) of benzodiazepines may be potentiated by concurrent intake of alcohol, other CNS depressants (e.g., opioids, phenothiazines, barbiturates, MAOIs, and other antidepressants), and possibly cimetidine. Although ADRs may occur with initial doses, they diminish as tolerance develops with continued therapy. If ADRs are intolerable, the dose may be decreased or an alternative agent may be used instead. All benzodiazepines have the potential for habituation and may be difficult to withdraw in chronic use.

Physical dependence. Prolonged use of benzodiazepines (usually at least 4 weeks) can lead to tolerance and physical dependence. When the drug is abruptly stopped in physically dependent patients, withdrawal or abstinence syndromes (see section I.B under Opioid physical tolerance) may begin within 1–10 days and may last for several weeks. Likewise, patients given benzodiazepine antagonists [e.g., flumazenil (Romazicon)] may also go into withdrawal syndromes. The probability and intensity of the withdrawal effects are greatest with short-acting drugs and least with long-acting preparations. Withdrawal syndromes can be prevented in chronic benzodiazepine users by decreasing the dose by 5–10% every 5 days. Those taking long-acting benzodiazepines can be tapered more quickly.

Contraindications and precautions. Benzodiazepines are contraindicated in patients with acute narrow-angle glaucoma (because of possible mydriatic effects) or during the first trimester (because of increased risk of congenital fetal malformations). They are also not recommended in patients with primary depressive disorders, psychosis, or patients in confusional states (as they make the existing delirium worse). Patients whose mental alertness is required for safety (e.g., machinery operators and drivers) should be warned about the possibility of psychomotor impairment even after a single dose of benzodiazepine. Patients should also refrain from concurrently taking alcohol or other CNS depressants.

Drug administration guidelines. Benzodiazepines should only be used for short-term treatment. Aside from greater abuse potential and increased incidence of ADRs, the long-term use of most benzodiazepines (i.e., more than 4 months) has not been assessed by clinical studies. Patients treated with benzodiazepines should be followed regularly to reassess their drug need and to gradually taper off the drug as soon as possible. Dosing must take into account the patient's degree of daytime sedation from the medication or from the insomnia itself. In general, benzodiazepines with long half-lives and/or active metabolites should be avoided by the elderly (or patients with hepatic or renal impairment) because of greater ADR potential because of drug accumulation by repeated dosing (made worse by the fact that drug half-lives may be increased two- to fourfold in these patients). Periodic laboratory tests (e.g., CBC and LFT) are advisable during prolonged treatment because of occasional reports of blood dyscrasias and jaundice. Serum blood urea nitrogen/creatinine or urinalysis may be done also to determine kidney function (responsible for drug elimination).

a. ***Short-acting delayed-onset anxiolytic benzodiazepines*** (with half-lives of less than 20 hours) have a delayed onset of action when compared with the long-acting anxiolytic benzodiazepines listed below (and hence may not be as useful in acute agitation). However, lorazepam and oxazepam have no active metabolites and are generally safer in patients with liver impairment and in the elderly (i.e., if given at its lowest possible dose; see section V.D.1.a for advantages of short-acting benzodiazepines).
   I. **Lorazepam (Ativan)** is also indicated for anxiety associated with depressive symptoms. It has inactive metabolites and is generally well-tolerated by the elderly. The initial dosage in the elderly should not exceed 2 mg to avoid oversedation. It is available in both oral and injectable forms. The injectable form contains propylene glycol and should be administered intravenously at a maximum rate of 2 mg/min.
   II. **Oxazepam (Serax)** is also indicated for anxiety associated with depressive symptoms and anxiety associated with alcohol withdrawal. It has inactive metabolites and has been found to be particularly useful in the management of anxiety, tension, agitation, and irritability in elderly patients (at a dosage of 10 mg, po, tid). Hypotension may occur in rare cases, and Serax must be used with caution by elderly patients prone to hypotension. Serax is only available in oral form.
   III. **Alprazolam (Xanax)** is also indicated for anxiety associated with depression and for panic disorders (with or without agoraphobia). Unlike lorazepam and oxazepam, it produces active metabolites and, in patients with liver disease, its half-life can be prolonged (up to 65 hours). It has possible analgesic effects in cancer patients with neuropathic pain (see Chapter 5.10, section VI.E.2.f) and in patients with fibromyalgia (see Chapter 5.10, Table 5.10-1). It is only available in oral form.

b. ***Long-acting rapid-onset anxiolytic benzodiazepines*** (with half-lives of 48–96 hours) have rapid onset of action and can be used for the acutely agitated patient. These drugs produce active metabolites and must be used with caution (i.e., lowest dose and longest interval possible) in patients with liver impairment and in the elderly (see section V.D.1.b for disadvantage of long-acting drugs).
   I. **Diazepam (Valium)** is also used as a sedative-hypnotic (see section V.D.1), anticonvulsant (i.e., in acute treatment of status epilepticus), "skeletal muscle relaxant" (see section II.A.7), and antispasticity agent (see Chapter 4, section III.B.2.c), as well as in minimizing the effects of acute alcohol withdrawal. Diazepam has the disadvantage of producing several active metabolites with long elimination half-lives and should be used with caution in the elderly. It is available in oral forms (short-acting and slow-release) and injectable forms. The injectable form contains propylene glycol and should be administered intravenously at a maximum rate of 5 mg/min. Parenteral diazepam is usually used as an adjunct in status epilepticus (at a dose of 1–2 mg/min IV, given slowly to a total dose of 5–10 mg), as a premedication prior to procedures, and in controlling severe anxiety.
   II. **Chlordiazepoxide (Librium, Libritabs; Limbitrol)** is also useful in managing delirium tremens and early signs of alcohol withdrawal. Unlike other benzodiazepines, it is not listed as being contraindicated in patients with acute, narrow-angle glaucoma. It is available in both oral and injectable forms. The oral form is marketed either as a single agent (Librium, Libritabs) or in combination with amitriptyline (Limbitrol or Limbitrol DS; see section V.A.1.a.1).

III. **Clorazepate** (**Tranxene**) is also indicated for symptomatic relief of acute alcohol withdrawal and as an adjunct in the management of partial seizures. It is available only in an oral form.

2. **Nonbenzodiazepine anxiolytics**

a. ***Buspirone (BuSpar)*** is an azapirone, which has high affinity for serotonin receptors and moderate affinity for D_2-dopamine receptors. It has no significant affinity for benzodiazepine receptors and does not affect the GABA neurotransmitter. It is an anxiolytic agent with few side-effects (and lesser cognitive effects than benzodiazepines); however, its clinical benefit may not be evident until after weeks of drug administration. Buspirone is less sedating than other anxiolytics and does not produce significant functional impairment. It has limited interaction with ethanol. There is no evidence that it causes either physical or psychological dependence. Although it binds to dopamine receptors, it has not been shown to cause extrapyramidal symptoms. Its ADRs include dizziness, nausea, headache, nervousness, lightheadedness, diarrhea, excitement, paresthesias, and sweating. Its only contraindication is in patients with known hypersensitivity to the drug or components of the drug.

Buspirone is more effective when anxiety is associated with anger and hostility or with depression. In TBI patients, it is preferred over benzodiazepines or haloperidol in managing anxiety disorders (with no accompanying muscle tension or insomnia). It is also effective in managing TBI patients with aggression (see section V.F). Buspirone is not cross-tolerant with benzodiazepines, hence it does not prevent benzodiazepine withdrawal. Switching from benzodiazepine to buspirone can be done safely by adding buspirone at 5 mg tid and then gradually tapering the benzodiazepine. Buspirone is only available in oral forms. It is given at 5 mg, po, tid, increasing by 5 mg every 2 days to a maximum of 50–60 mg/day.

b. ***Hydroxyzine (Atarax, Vistaril)*** is an antihistamine (see section VI), which is also indicated for anxiety associated with psychoneurosis and other organic disease.

c. ***Chlormezanone (Trancopal)*** is indicated for the treatment of mild anxiety (its MOA is unknown). Its common ADRs include drowsiness, drug rash, dizziness, flushing, nausea, depression, edema, inability to void, weakness, excitement, tremor, confusion, and headache. Rare cases of erythema multiforme, Stevens–Johnson syndrome, toxic epidermal necrolysis, and cholestatic jaundice have been reported. Its only contraindication is patients with known hypersensitivity to the drug or components of the drug. It is only available in an oral form.

d. ***Meprobamate (Miltown)*** is an anxiolytic whose MOA is unknown (it acts at multiple sites in the CNS of animals). The ADRs include CNS depression (e.g., drowsiness, ataxia, dizziness, and slurred speech), GI disorders (e.g., nausea and diarrhea), cardiovascular effects (palpitations and hypotension), and other allergic or idiosyncratic reactions (e.g., Stevens–Johnson syndrome and blood dyscrasias). It can cause physical dependence and can cause potentiation of CNS depression with alcohol or other CNS depressants. It is contraindicated in patients with acute intermittent porphyria or patients with hypersensitivity to the drug or related compound (e.g., carisoprodol). It is only available in an oral form.

e. ***Doxepin (Adapin, Sinequan)*** is an antidepressant also indicated for anxiety (with or without depression) in patients with organic disease or those with alcoholism. It is discussed in section V.A.1.a.2.

f. ***Propranolol (Inderal)*** may be used to control somatic symptoms of anxiety (e.g., tachycardia and performance anxiety). It is described under antiaggression drugs (see section V.F).

g. ***Phenothiazines*** such as prochlorperazine (Compazine) and trifluoperazine (Stelazine) have anxiolytic properties but are not recommended because of potentially serious ADRs (e.g., extrapyramidal reactions; see section V.B).

Table 4.8-10	Recommended dosage of selected sedative-hypnotics used in PM&R			
Generic	Selected brand names	Available preparations (mg)	Dosage (mg), route, frequency	MDD‡ (mg)
I. Benzodiazepines (short half-life)*				
Estazolam	*Prosom*	tab 1,2	0.5–2 po qhs	2
Temazepam	*Restoril*	cap 7.5,15,30	7.5–15 po qhs	30
Triazolam	*Halcion*	tab 0.125,0.25	0.125–0.25 po qhs	0.5
II. Benzodiazepines (long half-life)†				
Fluorazepam	*Dalmane*	cap 15,30	15–30 po qhs	30
Quazepam	*Doral*	tab 7.5,15	7.5–15 po qhs	15
III. Nonbenzodiazepines				
Chloral hydrate	*Chloral hydrate; Noctec; Aquachloral supp*	cap 500,1000 liq 500,1000/10 mL supp 325,650	500–1000 po qhs	1000
Ethchlorvynol	*Placidyl*	cap 200,500,750	200–750 po qhs	1000
Zolpidem	*Ambien*	tab 5,10	5–10 po qhs	10
Zaleplon	*Sonata*	cap 10	5–20 po qhs	20
Eszopiclone	*Lunesta*	tab 1,2,3	1–3 po qhs	3

** Short half-life = <20 hours.*
† Long half-life = >40 hours.
‡ MDD = maximum daily dose for sedative-hypnotic use (may be higher in closely monitored patients).

D. SEDATIVE-HYPNOTICS (Table 4.8-10) are primarily indicated for the treatment of insomnia characterized by complaints of difficulty in falling asleep, frequent awakenings, and morning awakenings. They are beneficial in hospitalized patients who frequently complain of insomnia because of hospital noise, frequent monitoring and medication administration by the staff, and unfamiliar surroundings. In a rehabilitation ward, sedative-hypnotics given at bedtime can be helpful in keeping the insomniac patient from feeling drowsy during daytime rehabilitation sessions. All insomniac patients must be evaluated for a variety of underlying medical or psychiatric disorders (e.g., depression) for which there is a more specific treatment. As with anxiolytics, nonpharmacologic treatments (e.g., behavioral methods, relaxation training, and biofeedback) should be tried, whenever possible, before drug therapy is initiated. If sedative-hypnotics are used, they must be used for a short period (less than 1–2 weeks) and if possible, a nonbenzodiazepine should be used to avoid the potential for abuse common among benzodiazepine users. They must be used with caution in the elderly, or in patients with CNS insults or who are already drowsy or lethargic from surgery. They should not be prescribed in quantities exceeding a 1-month supply. They should be ingested prior to going to sleep (generally within 30 minutes).

1. **Benzodiazepines** are discussed in section V.C.1. The MOA, ADR, contraindications, and precautions of the following sedative-hypnotic benzodiazepines are essentially similar to those of anxiolytic benzodiazepines. They are all available in oral forms.

a. ***Short-acting sedative-hypnotic benzodiazepines*** have elimination half-lives of less than 20 hours. They include temazepam (Restoril), triazolam (Halcion), and estazolam (Prosom). They are primarily used for the short-term treatment of insomnia (generally 7–10 days). The advantage of short half-lives is that the drug and its metabolites are cleared before the next dose is ingested, hence daytime sedation and performance impairment are minimal or absent (in short-term use). Both temazepam and triazolam have inactive metabolites but estazolam has an active metabolite. In the rehabilitation ward, temazepam (Restoril) is one of the commonly used benzodiazepine sedative-hypnotics. Elderly patients on temazepam should be started at a low dose (7.5 mg) to avoid oversedation.

b. ***Long-acting sedative-hypnotic benzodiazepines*** have elimination half-lives of more than 40 hours. They include fluorazepam (Dalmane) and quazepam (Doral), both of which have active metabolites. They can be used briefly in patients with recurring insomnia or poor sleeping habits, and in acute or chronic medical conditions requiring restful sleep. The disadvantage of long half-lives is that the drug and its metabolites may accumulate during repeated dosage intervals of less than 24 hours and may be associated with impairments of cognitive or motor performance during waking hours. Also the possibility of interaction with other psychoactive drugs or alcohol will be enhanced. In the elderly in whom the half-life may be increased two- to four-fold, benzodiazepines with long half-lives are generally not indicated.

2. Nonbenzodiazepine sedative-hypnotics

a. ***Zolpidem (Ambien)*** is indicated for the short-term treatment of insomnia (generally 7–10 days). Although its structure is nonbenzodiazepine, it interacts with the GABA–benzodiazepine receptor complex. However, unlike benzodiazepines (which nonselectively bind to and activate all types of GABA receptors), zolpidem selectively binds with the ω-1 GABA–benzodiazepine receptor, thus probably accounting for its lack of myorelaxant and anticonvulsant effects. It has a short elimination half-life (2.6 hours) and its metabolite is inactive. Its clearance time is 7–8 hours. The more common ADRs include daytime drowsiness, dizziness, incoordination, headache, nausea, vomiting, diarrhea, amnesia, confusion, vertigo, visual disturbance, palpitations, and dry mouth. As with benzodiazepines, zolpidem can cause physical dependence and should not be withdrawn abruptly after prolonged use. Its only contraindication is in patients with known hypersensitivity to the drug or its component. It has not been shown to accumulate in elderly patients following nightly oral doses of 10 mg for 1 week. This gives an adequate safety margin for the recommended bedtime dose of 5 mg in the elderly. Zolpidem is only available in an oral form. It is one of the most commonly used sedative-hypnotics in the rehabilitation ward (possibly because of its general lack of residual next-day effect during rehabilitation sessions).

b. ***Zaleplon (Sonata)*** is indicated for the short-term treatment of insomnia (generally 7–10 days), specifically to decrease time to sleep onset. Like zolpidem, its structure is nonbenzodiazepine but it probably acts by selectively binding with a specific GABA-receptor (i.e., ω-1 GABA–benzodiazepine receptor), which probably accounts for its lack of myorelaxant and anticonvulsant effects. It has a short elimination half-life (1 hour) and its metabolite is inactive. It has a rapid clearance of 2–4 hours. The more common ADRs include daytime drowsiness, dizziness, lightheadedness, and incoordination. As with benzodiazepines, zaleplon can cause physical dependence and should not be withdrawn abruptly after prolonged use. Its only contraindication is patients with known hypersensitivity to the drug or its component. Zaleplon is only available in an oral form. Like Zolpidem it generally lacks residual next-day effect.

c. ***Chloral hydrate (Noctec)*** is a rapidly effective hypnotic that may be useful because it has little effect on normal sleep cycles. Its specific MOA remains unknown, although it appears to induce a general depression of CNS functions. In routine doses, it has relatively fewer adverse respiratory and cardiovascular effects than benzodiazepines. It also seldom produces excitement or hangover. However, in high doses and in long-term administration, it may cause CNS effects (excessive or prolonged sedation, headache, dizziness, ataxia, hallucinations, malaise, and paradoxical excitation), cardiovascular effects (e.g., supraventricular and ventricular arrhythmias following the ingestion of toxic quantities), GI effects, (e.g., nausea, vomiting, hemorrhage, necrosis, and perforation of the stomach), skin reactions (e.g., rash), and other effects (e.g., leukopenia, eosinophilia, ketonuria, apnea, and laryngospasm). Tolerance and physical dependence may also be seen with chronic ingestion. There have been reports of fatal interaction with ethanol and a short-term increase in the effect of warfarin. It is contraindicated in patients with significant hepatic or renal impairments.

d. ***Ethchlorvynol (Placidyl)*** is indicated for the short-term treatment of insomnia of up to 1 week. Its MOA is unknown. The ADRs include hematologic effects (e.g., thrombocytopenia, with one case of fatality), GI effects (e.g., nausea and vomiting), neurologic effects (e.g., dizziness and facial numbness), miscellaneous effects (e.g., blurred vision, hypotension, and mild "hangover"), and other idiosyncratic responses. It can also cause physical dependence and should not be withdrawn abruptly. It is contraindicated in patients with porphyria. Ethchlorvynol is only available in an oral form.

e. ***Trazodone (Desyrel)***, 50–300 mg (up to a maximum of 600 mg/day), po, qhs has been found to be beneficial in TBI patients whose insomnia is attributed to "racing thoughts" as they lie down and try to sleep. Trazodone, which is primarily indicated for the management of depression is discussed in section V.A.4.d. The manufacturer does not include sedative-hypnotic as its major effect, although sedation is listed as one of its major side-effects.

f. ***Diphenhydramine (Benadryl)*** can be given at 25–50 mg, po, qhs for periodic sedation although sedation is only listed as its side-effect (not a primary indication). See section VI.B for details about diphenhydramine.

g. ***Barbiturates*** have low therapeutic indices and are not recommended as sedative-hypnotics or anxiolytics. They induce sleep that is deficient in rapid-eye-movement periods, resulting in inadequate rest. They also have a high potential for adverse effects (e.g., respiratory depression, hypersensitivity reactions, cardiovascular depression, paradoxical excitement, and increased sensitivity to pain). Their usefulness as sedative-hypnotics (and also as anxiolytics) has been surpassed by other safer drugs described above (nonbenzodiazepines and benzodiazepines). Barbiturates such as phenobarbital (Luminal) or mephobarbital (Mebaral) are generally used as anticonvulsants (see section IV), while other barbiturates such as secobarbital (Seconal), pentobarbital (Nembutal), thiopental (Pentothal), and methohexital (Brevital) are generally used for preoperative or procedural sedation.

h. ***Eszopiclone (Lunesta***; formerly **Estorra**) is indicated for the treatment of insomnia to help decrease sleep latency and improve sleep maintenance. Unlike other sedative-hypnotics, which are generally limited to 7–10 days of use, eszopiclone can be prescribed for long-term use. Its structure is nonbenzodiazepine and it probably acts by interacting with GABA-receptor complexes at binding domains located close to or allosterically coupled to benzodiazepine receptors. Its elimination half-life is 6 hours. It has no known contraindication. It has no reported serious withdrawal syndrome. Its more common ADRs include headache, unpleasant taste, dry mouth, dyspepsia, nausea, vomiting, somnolence, anxiety, depression, nervousness, dizziness, dysmennorhea, gynecomastia, rash, and respiratory infection. It is only available in an oral form.

E. PSYCHOSTIMULANTS are used to improve attention and concentration (which in turn can probably help improve memory and learning) and to counteract the sedative effects of other drugs (e.g., opioids; see section I.B; see also Chapter 5.10, section VI.E.2.k). They may be beneficial in patients with cognitive communication impairments (e.g., TBI; see Chapter 5.5, section I.B for details on cognitive communication impairment). They should be used only as an adjunct to nonpharmacological measures (i.e., psychological, educational, and social). They should not be given at high doses (may impair performance) and should not be stopped abruptly (may cause withdrawal symptoms).

1. **Amphetamines** are noncatecholamine, sympathomimetic amines with CNS stimulant activity. Peripheral sympathomimetic effects include hypertension and weak bronchodilator and respiratory stimulant actions.

   Mechanism of action. The exact MOA for producing the mental and behavioral effects is unknown. They probably act via direct release of dopamine and norepinephrine, blockade of catecholamine reuptake, and reduction in catecholamine turnover.

   Adverse drug reactions include CNS effects (e.g., overstimulation, restlessness, dizziness, insomnia, euphoria, dyskinesia, dysphoria, tremor, headache, psychotic episodes, and exacerbation of tics), GI effects (e.g., dry mouth, diarrhea, constipation, and anorexia), and other effects (e.g., urticaria and impotence). Amphetamines cause tolerance and physical dependence and have been extensively abused.

   Contraindications and precautions. Amphetamine use is contraindicated in patients with advanced arteriosclerosis, symptomatic cardiovascular disease, moderate to severe hypertension, hyperthyroidism, glaucoma, agitation, history of drug abuse, concurrent intake of MAOIs, and known hypersensitivity or idiosyncrasy to sympathomimetic amines.

   Drug administration guidelines. Patients should initially be monitored for tachycardia, hypertension, anorexia, dysphoria, and insomnia. Prolonged use should be avoided because of their abuse potential.

   a. ***Dextroamphetamine (Dexedrine)*** is indicated for narcolepsy and in attention deficit disorder with hyperactivity. There is some evidence of its short-term effects on cognitive and behavior sequelae of patients with TBI. If given in moderate dosage, it can probably improve long-term memory, attention, distractibility, disorganization, and impulsivity seen after TBI. Although not listed as an indication by its manufacturer, it has also been used (and abused) as a weight-loss pill in obese patients. It is available in an oral form (5- and 10-mg tablets and 5 mg/5 mL elixir). Its dosage is 2.5–5 mg, po, bid (administered morning and at midday) and gradually increased up to 30–60 mg/day.

   b. ***Methamphetamine (Desoxyn)*** is indicated for attention deficit disorder with hyperactivity and for short-term use in exogenous obesity. It is available in an oral form (5- and 10-mg tablets) and is given at 5 mg, po, qd/bid (administered morning and at midday) and gradually increased weekly up to 20–25 mg/day.

2. **Methylphenidate (Ritalin; Metadate ER)** is a mild CNS stimulant whose exact MOA is unknown (probably similar to that of amphetamines except for the increased catecholamine turnover). It is indicated for narcolepsy and in attention deficit disorder with hyperactivity and may be helpful in improving attention and concentration in TBI patients (especially if with hypoarousal). Its ADRs include CNS effects (e.g., nervousness, insomnia, dizziness, headache, drowsiness, dyskinesia, psychotic episodes, and exacerbation of tics), GI effects (e.g., nausea, anorexia, and abdominal pain), cardiovascular effects (e.g., tachycardia, palpitations, increased or decreased blood pressures, and cardiac arrhythmias), hypersensitivity and idiosyncratic reactions (e.g., rash, urticaria, leukopenia, and cerebral arteritis or occlusion). It should not be abruptly stopped as it may cause a severe withdrawal syndrome. It can be potentially abused in emotionally unstable patients. It is contraindicated in patients with marked anxiety, tension, agitation, glaucoma, severe depression, motor tics, Tourette's syndrome, or concurrent intake of MAOIs. Methylphenidate is available only in an oral form and can be short-acting (e.g., Ritalin, 5-, 10-, or 20-mg

tablets; Ritalin SR, 20-mg or Metadate ER, 10- or 20-mg sustained- or extended-release tablets) or long-acting (e.g., Ritalin LA, 20-, 30-, or 40-mg capsules). The short-acting forms can be given at 5–10 mg, po, bid/tid, before meals (may be increased up to 40–60 mg/day). The long-acting form can be given once a day, then adjusted by 10 mg weekly up to a maximum of 60 mg/day. Patients should initially be monitored for tachycardia, hypertension, insomnia, and anorexia. Periodic CBC and differential count are advisable.

3. **Pemoline (Cylert)** is a CNS stimulant with minimal sympathomimetic effects. It is unrelated to dextroamphetamine and methylphenidate. Its exact MOA is unknown (probably acts on dopaminergic receptors and decreases catecholamine turnover). It is indicated in patients with attention deficit disorder with hyperactivity. It may be helpful in improving attention and concentration in TBI patients. ADRs include hepatic effects (hepatitis, jaundice, rare cases of hepatic-related fatalities), CNS effects (insomnia, convulsive seizures, exacerbation of tics, hallucinations, dyskinesia, nystagmus, mild depression, dizziness, increased irritability, headache, drowsiness), GI effects (anorexia, nausea, stomach ache), other effects (e.g., aplastic anemia, increased acid phosphatase, and growth suppression in children). It is contraindicated in patients with hepatic impairment. It has the potential of being misused in emotionally unstable patients. It is available only in an oral form (18.75-, 37.5-, and 75-mg tablets). It can be given at 37.5 mg qd (in the morning), which can be increased by 18.75 mg at 1-week intervals up to a maximum of 112.5 mg/day. Its clinical benefit may not be evident until the third or fourth week of drug administration. Patients should be monitored for liver function tests (LFTs) before starting the drug, and LFTs and CBC should be monitored periodically.
4. **Other drugs** that may possibly improve attention as well as memory and learning include tricyclic antidepressants (e.g., **protriptyline** or **desipramine** may be used for mildly impaired patients with attention difficulties; see under tricyclic antidepressants in section V.A.1), **physostigmine** (2 mg, po, tid, increased over 1 week up to 3.5–4.0 mg, po, tid; its MOA is probably via decreased destruction of acetylcholine; it may improve retrieval of long-term memory), **amantadine** (**Symmetrel**, 50 mg, po, bid, increased weekly to a maximum of 400 mg/day; it may be helpful in TBI patients with low energy or with depression and may improve cognitive function in selected TBI patients during early recovery stages based on its effects on agitation; however, seizures have been reported in TBI patients taking amantadine; see section XIII.B for discussion of amantadine), **donepezil** [**Aricept**, 5 mg or 10 mg, po, at bedtime; a reversible acetylcholinesterase (AchE) inhibitor used in the treatment of mild to moderate dementia of the Alzheimer's type], **rivastigmine** (**Exelon**, 3–6 mg, po, bid; another reversible AchE inhibitor used in the treatment of mild to moderate dementia of the Alzheimer's type), **ergoloid mesylate** (**Hydergine**, 1 mg, po, tid; indicated for patients over 60 years old with symptomatic decline in mental capacity), nootropics or "cognitive activators" [e.g., **piracetam** (**Nootropil**), 400 mg, po, tid or **pramiracetam** (**Neupramir, Pramistar**), 600 mg, po, qd/bid; probably increases turnover of acetylcholine in the hippocampal cholinergic nerve terminals; may be effective in treating memory and other cognitive problems in patients with long-term stable losses in memory and cognition]; **gangliosides** (probably induce neural regeneration; experimental), and **thyrotropin-releasing hormones**. Tacrine (Cognex), an older AchE inhibitor, is no longer used due to hepatotoxicity.

F. ANTIAGGRESSION DRUGS may be used as an adjunct to nonpharmacologic measures (e.g., behavioral therapy) in patients with chronic aggression (e.g., TBI patients). For acute management of agitation, neuroleptive drugs (e.g., IM olanzapine, see section V.B.3) or long-acting rapid-onset anxiolytic benzodiazepines (e.g., Valium, see section V.C.1.b) may be used. Drugs used in chronic aggression span a broad range, including anticonvulsants, antidepressants, antihypertensives, antipsychotics, anxiolytics (benzodiazepines, buspirone), psychostimulants, and amantadine. The drug is chosen based on the type and frequency of target behaviors. Ideally, it should minimize the patient's aggression without impairing arousal and cognition. If possible, it should also treat a coexisting condition. During treatment, the target behavior and adverse effects of the drug should be carefully monitored by family and the treating team.

A drug commonly used in the PM&R setting for controlling chronic aggression in TBI patients is **buspirone (Buspar)** because of its favorable side-effect profile (see section V.C.2.a); however, it takes weeks of daily administration before its clinical benefits become evident. The most widely studied antiaggression drug is **propranolol (Inderal)**, a β-blocker that is used for controlling chronic aggressive behavior. Its dose is 60 mg/day, which can be increased by 60 mg every 3 days to a maximum of 420 mg/day. The clinical benefit of propranolol may not be evident until after 6–8 weeks of drug administration. It is contraindicated in patients with asthma, pulse less than 60/min, hypotension, conduction defects, diabetes, or patients on concurrent intake of MAOIs. Another β-blocker used for controlling chronic aggression is **pindolol (Visken)**, which can be given at 5 mg, po, bid up to a maximum of 60 mg/day. Pindolol has the same contraindications as propranolol. It causes less hypotension and bradycardia than propranolol but may cause excitement and agitation.

Other drugs used in chronic aggression include: **anticonvulsants** (e.g., **carbamazepine, valproic acid**; or low-dose **clonazepam** combined with clonidine; see section IV for details on anticonvulsants); **antidepressants** (e.g., **trazodone, amitriptyline**; see section V.A); **neuroleptics** [e.g., low-to-moderate doses of **haloperidol (Haldol)** which can be used to calm down acutely aggressive or agitated patients; see section V.B.2]; **benzodiazepines** (e.g., **lorazepam;** see section V.C.1.a.1); **psychostimulants** (e.g., **methylphenydate; dextroamphetamine**; see section V.E); **verapamil** (**Calan; Isoptin**; see section IX.B), a calcium-channel blocker which can be given at 40 mg, po, tid/qid up to 240–320 mg/day; **clonidine (Catapres)**; see section IX.A.1); and **amantadine** (see sections V.E.4 and XIII.B). Toxic drugs such as lithium are best avoided because of the high potential for serious adverse effects.

VI. Antihistamines

Antihistamines are generally indicated for allergy, pruritus, and for periodic sedation. Some also have antiemetic, antianxiety, and nonspecific analgesic effects. As a result of their low potency, they are often used in conjunction with other therapies. Their usefulness is often limited by adverse effects.

Mechanism of action. Antihistamines act by blocking histamine release through competitive inhibition at histamine H_1-receptors. Many antihistamines also possess anticholinergic effects.

Adverse drug reactions. The ADRs include CNS effects (e.g., excessive sedation, dizziness, ataxia, headaches, and muscle weakness), paradoxical excitation (e.g., restlessness, insomnia, tremors, delirium, and possibly seizures), respiratory depression (secondary to generalized CNS depression after administering large drug doses), cardiovascular effects (e.g., hypotension, hypertension, tachycardia, and other arrhythmias; overall incidence is low), and other adverse effects (e.g., nausea, vomiting, changes in bowel habits, hypersensitivity, flushing, dryness of the mouth, dysuria, urinary retention, impotence, vertigo, blurred vision, and tinnitus). Tolerance to these adverse effects frequently occurs after repeated use.

Contraindications and precautions. Antihistamines with pronounced anticholinergic activity, should be used with caution in patients with narrow-angle glaucoma, cardiovascular instability, difficulty with urination (e.g., symptomatic prostatism), or myasthenia gravis. Its only contraindication is in patients with hypersensitivity to the drug or the components of the drug or its vehicle.

A. HYDROXYZINE (ATARAX, VISTARIL) has antihistaminic with anticholinergic, anxiolytic, sedative, antispasmodic, and antiemetic effects. It also has some analgesic effects (see Chapter 5.10, section VI.E.2.f.2) either alone or in combination with morphine. The combination of an NSAID or opioid with hydroxyzine (25–50 mg q4–6 h) given orally on a regular basis is useful in controlling moderate pain and the nausea often associated with NSAID (see section I.A) or opioid use (see section I.B). Hydroxyzine is available in oral forms (Atarax, Vistaril) and parenteral forms (Vistaril IM solution, 25- and 50-mg/mL vials and 100-mg/2 mL vials). To provide sedation and anxiolytic effects, a dose of 50–100 mg, po/IM, qid may be given.

B. DIPHENHYDRAMINE (BENADRYL) has antihistaminic with anticholinergic, sedative, antiparkinsonism, and antimotion-sickness effects. Additional ADRs include thickening of bronchial secretions with wheezing and nasal stuffiness (thus it should be used with caution in asthmatic patients). Diphenhydramine is available in both oral forms (25 and 50-mg capsules) and injectable forms (50-mg/mL ampule or syringe). The oral dose is 25–50 mg, po, tid/qid, and the parenteral dose is 10–50 mg (or up to 100 mg), IM/IV, q4h (up to a maximum of 400 mg/day).

VII. Hematological agents

The hematological agents commonly used in PM&R are antithrombotic agents (anticoagulant and antiplatelet drugs), which interrupt the progression of the thrombotic process with the ultimate goal of preventing pulmonary embolism (PE). Anticoagulant drugs used for deep-vein thrombosis (DVT) prophylaxis include SQ low-molecular-weight heparin (LMWH; fixed dose), SQ low-dose unfractionated heparin (LDUH; using fixed dose), SQ fondaparinux (using fixed dose), and oral warfarin. For treatment of DVT and PE, anticoagulant drugs used include LMWH (given SQ in total body weight-adjusted dose), adjusted-dose unfractionated heparin (ADUH; given SQ for DVT treatment or IV for DVT or PE treatment), and oral warfarin. Specific recommendations of DVT and PE prophylaxis and treatment based on the recommendations of the Seventh American College of Chest Physicians (ACCP) Conference on Antithrombotic and Thrombolytic Therapy (Buller *et al.*, 2004), are discussed in Chapter 5.3. Thrombolytic agents [e.g., streptokinase, urokinase, tissue plasminogen activator (Alteplase), human antithrombin III concentrate (ATnativ, Thrombate III)], which actively resolve the thrombus, are not discussed in this book because their use is beyond the expertise of most physiatrists.

A. ANTICOAGULANT THERAPY is indicated in patients with atrial fibrillation, deep venous thrombosis (DVT; see Chapter 5.3, sections IV.B.1 and V.A), pulmonary embolism (see Chapter 5.3, sections VI.A.3), vertebral basilar insufficiency, stroke caused by cardiogenic embolus, prosthetic heart valves (especially mechanical valves or complicated bioprosthetic valves; anticoagulant therapy is controversial in uncomplicated bioprosthetic valves), and unstable angina and acute myocardial infarction (especially anterolateral wall). It is also indicated in patients who have cardiac surgery under cardiac bypass; in those who have vascular surgery; during and after coronary angioplasty; in patients with coronary stents; and in selected patients with disseminated intravascular coagulation.

It is absolutely contraindicated in patients with subarachnoid or cerebral hemorrhage, serious active bleeding (postoperative, spontaneous, or associated with trauma; except selected cases of disseminated intravascular coagulation); severe thrombocytopenia, recent brain, eye, or spinal cord surgery; or malignant hypertension. It is relatively contraindicated in other conditions with increased danger of bleeding, that is cardiovascular conditions (severe hypertension, subacute bacterial endocarditis), surgical conditions (during and immediately following spinal tap, spinal anesthesia, or surgery other than those listed under absolute contraindications due to potential risk of spontaneous neuraxial bleeding), hematologic conditions (thrombocytopenia, hemophilia, and some vascular purpuras), gastrointestinal conditions (bleeding as a result of ulcerative lesions of the stomach or small intestines), or other conditions (menstruation, liver disease with impaired homeostasis, and severe renal failure). It must be used with extreme caution in patients prone to falling (e.g., elderly or debilitated patients) or those with poor compliance. During anticoagulation, invasive procedures and intramuscular injections should be minimized and NSAIDs should be avoided. Moreover, the following must be monitored regularly: coagulation time [prothrombin time (PT)/activated partial thromboplastin time (aPTT)], CBC (hematocrit/hemoglobin, platelet), urinalysis (hematuria), and stool guaiac.

1. **Warfarin** (**Coumadin, Panwarfin**; see Chapter 5.3, sections IV.B.1.a and V.A.2) is the most widely used oral vitamin K antagonist for long-term anticoagulation. It prevents the activation of prothrombin in the coagulation cascade by acting in the liver to deplete and inhibit the production of four vitamin K-dependent clotting factors (II, VII, IX, X) and at least two vitamin K-dependent anticoagulant factors (proteins C and S). Warfarin's anticoagulation effect is not immediate because time is needed to clear the normal coagulation factors already present in the plasma and to replace them with newly synthesized dysfunctional vitamin K-dependent proteins. Depending on the dose given, the delay in anticoagulation may range from 2 to 7 days.

   Warfarin is bound to plasma proteins and can be easily displaced by other medications (see Table 4.8-10 for classes of drugs that can interact with warfarin). Many endogenous conditions can potentiate warfarin, including a vitamin K-deficient diet, diarrhea, steatorrhea, hypermetabolic states (fever, hyperthyroidism), liver disease, cancer, collagen disease, and congestive heart failure. Endogenous conditions that can inhibit warfarin are edema, hyperlipidemia, hypothyroidism, and hereditary warfarin resistance. Because patients may be exposed to the above factors, their response to warfarin may be unpredictable. Hence warfarin administration must be monitored regularly using the prothrombin time test, which reflects the warfarin dose given 24–48 hours earlier.

   The standard reporting of PT is in international normalized ratio (INR). The recommended INR is 2.0–3.0 for all indications except for patients with mechanical prosthetic heart valves in which case an INR of 2.5–3.5 is recommended. If the INR is above therapeutic range, refer to the ACCP guidelines described in Table 5.3-3 in Chapter 5.3. Duration of warfarin treatment varies from 3 to 6 months (e.g., patients with slow-resolving risk factors, such as prolonged immobilization) to a lifetime (e.g., patients with chronic atrial fibrillation). Warfarin (Coumadin) is available in 1-, 2-, 2.5-, 5-, 7.5-, and 10-mg tablets and is given once a day (usually at bedtime). Adverse drug reactions include bleeding and, rarely, cutaneous microvascular thrombosis (with subsequent skin necrosis). Warfarin crosses the placenta and should not be used during pregnancy, particularly during the first trimester. When anticoagulation is needed in pregnancy, LMWH or unfractionated heparin is preferred.

   Although commonly practiced, starting warfarin therapy with a loading dose is unnecessary. If a rapid anticoagulant effect is needed, an initial dose of

Table 4.8-11 Classes of drugs that can potentially interact with warfarin

Effect on warfarin	Drug class
Potentiation (i.e., causes increased INR)	Adrenergic stimulants (central); Alcohol abuse reduction preparations; Analgesics; Anesthetics (inhalation); Anticoagulants; Antimalarial agents; Antiparasitic drugs; Antiplatelets; Beta-adrenergic blockers; Bromelains; Cholelitholytic agents; Diabetic agents (oral); Gastrointestinal (ulcerative colitis) agents; Gout treatment agents; Hemorrheologic agents; Hepatotoxic drugs; Hyperglycemic agents; Hypertensive emergency agents; Monoamine oxidase inhibitors; Narcotics (prolonged use); Nonsteroidal anti-inflammatory drugs; Psychostimulants; Pyrazolones; Salicylates; Steroids (anabolic); Thrombolytics; Thyroid drugs; Uricosuric agents; Vaccines
Inhibition (i.e., causes decreased INR)	Adrenal cortical steroid inhibitors; Antacids; Antianxiety agents; Antihistamine; Antipsychotic drugs; Barbiturates; Enteral nutritional supplements; Immunosuppressives; Oral contraceptives (estrogen-containing)
Potentiation or Inhibition	Antiarrhythmics; Antibiotics; Anticonvulsants; Antidepressants; Antineoplastics; Antithyroid drugs; Diuretics; Fungal medications (systemic); Gastric acidity and peptic ulcer agents; Hypnotics; Hypolipidemics; Steroids (adrenocortical); Tuberculosis agents; Vitamins

Data adapted from the Physicians' desk reference, *ed 58, Montvale, NJ, 2004, Thomson PDR, pp. 1049–1050.*

IV unfractionated heparin (see section VII.A.2) should be used and overlapped with warfarin for at least 5 days (during which time both anticoagulants are given in combination). The heparin can be discontinued when the INR has been in the therapeutic range for 2 consecutive days. If anticoagulation is not urgent (e.g., chronic stable atrial fibrillation), it is safer to start with an estimated maintenance dose of 5 mg/day of warfarin, which usually results in the patient reaching an INR of 2.0 in about 5 days and achieving a steady-state anticoagulant effect in about 14 days.

Prothrombin time (INR) is monitored daily until therapeutic range has been achieved and maintained for at least 2 consecutive days, then two to three times weekly for 1–2 weeks. Thereafter, if the INR remains stable, the interval of testing can be reduced to weekly or biweekly and eventually to once every 4–6 weeks. If dose adjustments are required, then the cycle of more frequent monitoring is repeated until a stable dose response is again achieved. Unexpected fluctuations in dose response could be attributed to changes in diet (e.g., high vitamin K diet) or undisclosed drug use (see Table 4.8-11 for drug and food interaction), inaccuracy of prothrombin time testing, poor patient compliance, surreptitious self-medication, or intermittent alcohol consumption.

2. **Unfractionated heparin** (**UH**; previously referred to as **heparin**; see Chapter 5.3, sections IV.B.1.b and V.A.2) enhances the activity of antithrombin III which in turn inactivates factor IIa (thrombin) and, to a lesser degree, factors Xa and IXa. It also inhibits the activation of factors V and VIII by thrombin. It is prescribed in international units (IU) and can be given either by IV or SQ routes. Fixed, low-dose unfractionated heparin (LDUH) at 10000–15000 IU/day or 5000 IU q8–12 h can be given SQ for the prevention of DVT. Adjusted-dose unfractionated heparin (ADUH) can be given by SQ or IV route at a high dose (25000–35000 IU/day) to treat DVT or PE or to prevent recurrent thrombosis.

The anticoagulation effect of SQ ADUH is delayed for about 1 hour and peak levels occur at about 3 hours. If the ADUH is given by SQ route, a high initial dose should be used (35 000 IU/24 hours in two divided doses) to overcome the poor bioavailability of moderate doses, or if immediate anticoagulation is needed, the SQ injection should be preceded by an IV bolus of 5000 IU. The anticoagulation effect of ADUH is monitored q6h after injection using the aPTT, which is sensitive to the inhibitory effects of heparin on thrombin, factor Xa and factor IXa. Fixed, SQ LDUH does not require aPTT monitoring. Routine CBC is needed in all patients receiving heparin to detect bleeding and thrombocytopenia.

Adjusted-dose unfractionated heparin (ADUH) by IV bolus can be used when a rapid (immediate) anticoagulant effect is needed and for the treatment of PE and DVT. ADUH is usually indicated for short-term anticoagulation. Long-term ADUH (given SQ) may occasionally be used (e.g., when anticoagulant therapy is needed in pregnancy and in the rare patient who develops recurrent venous thromboembolism while being treated with appropriate doses of warfarin). Length of ADUH anticoagulation is 5–10 days with warfarin administered jointly with heparin for 5 days. When the INR is therapeutic, ADUH may be discontinued. Administration of ADUH must be monitored and its dosage adjusted as needed (see Chapter 5.3, Table 5.3-5 for ADUH dose adjustment using body weight). If body weight is not available, an alternative method is to load 5000 IU of IV ADUH then infuse 25 000 IU in 250 mL 5% dextrose in water or normal saline (i.e., 100 IU/mL) at 800–1000 IU/h (8–10 mL/h) and adjust at the rate 100 IU/h as needed until the therapeutic dose (aPTT of 1.5–2.3 × the control value) is reached.

Adverse drug reactions of heparin include bleeding, hematoma at subcutaneous injection sites, thrombocytopenia (incidence is 1–5%; usually benign and reversible; more common with bovine than porcine heparin; heparin should be stopped if platelet count is <100 000/mL), paradoxical thrombotic events, skin lesions (urticarial lesions, erythematosus papules and plaques, and skin necrosis), osteoporosis, hypersensitivity reactions, and increases in transaminases (59% incidence). If bleeding occurs (e.g., GI or CNS), protamine sulfate, 10–50 mg IV over 10 minutes (0.5–1 mg protamine sulfate neutralizes about 100 IU heparin) is used to reverse the anticoagulation.

3. **Enoxaparin (Lovenox) and dalteparin [Fragmin]** (see Chapter 5.3, sections IV.B.1.c and V.A.3) are low-molecular-weight heparins (LMWHs) that weigh about one-third of the unfractionated heparin. They were developed in an attempt to reduce the risk of major bleeding that accompanies treatment with unfractionated heparins. Because of their low molecular weight, they do not inhibit thrombin (IIa); however, they retain their ability to inhibit factor Xa and are, therefore, factor Xa specific. With more predictable anticoagulant responses, LMWHs have longer plasma half-life than standard unfractionated heparin. LMWHs can be given once or twice daily and, generally, without aPTT monitoring (although routine CBC may be checked to determine thrombocytopenia). In certain clinical situations (e.g., severe renal failure or pregnancy), where LMWH dose might need to be adjusted, plasma anti-Xa assay may be monitored (with a target range of 0.6 to 1.0 IU/mL) 4 hours after administration of LMWH.

   LMWHs can be used for DVT prophylaxis in moderate- to highest-risk patients (see Table 5.3-1 and 5.3-2 in Chapter 5.3). They have currently replaced ADUHs as the preferred anticoagulant for treatment of suspected or confirmed DVT or PE. Their side-effects (including bleeding, thrombocytopenia, and osteopenia) are similar to those of unfractionated heparin, but the incidence is generally lower. Like unfractionated heparin, LMWHs do not cross the placental barrier and thus can be used in pregnancy. Commercially available LMWHs in the United States are enoxaparin (Lovenox) and dalteparin (Fragmin). For DVT prophylaxis, a fixed dose of enoxoparin (30 mg, SQ, qd, where 1 mg of enoxaparin = 100 IU of antifactor Xa) or dalteparin (2500 IU, SQ, qd) may be given (see Table 5.3-1 and 5.3-2 in Chapter 5.3). For treatment of suspected and confirmed acute DVT or pulmonary embolism, total body weight (TBW)-adjusted doses of LMWHs are used instead of fixed dose (see Table 5.3-4 in Chapter 5.3). Other LMWH (e.g., nadroparin and tinzaparin) are not available in the United States.

4. **Fondaparinux (Arixtra)** is a synthetic pentasaccharide whose structure is similar to the heparin sequence that binds to antithrombin and enhances its indirect inhibition of factor Xa. By selectively inactivating factor Xa, fondaparinux inhibits thrombin generation without any direct effect on thrombin activity. Fondaparinux can be given once-daily SQ with rapid onset of action and predictable duration of effect. It can be used for the prevention of venous thromboembolism in the highest risk patients (see Tables 5.3-1 and 5.3-2 in Chapter 5.3). It is contraindicated in patients with severe renal impairment because it is eliminated primarily by the kidneys. However, in patients with moderate renal dysfunction, dose adjustment or laboratory monitoring is not required. Fondaparinux is commercially available as Arixtra, administered at a dose of 2.5 mg SQ once daily, with the initial dose given 6–8 hours after surgery (after establishing hemostasis).
5. **Danaparoid (Orgaran)** is a heparinoid consisting of heparan sulfate, dermatan sulfate, and chondroitin sulfate but no heparin or heparin fragment. It acts by inhibiting factor Xa and decreasing thrombin. Compared to LMWH, it has less platelet activity and less cross reactivity to antibodies correlated with heparin-induced thrombocytopenia or HIT (it therefore can be used to treat persons at high risk for thrombosis who have history of HIT). Its dose is 400 to 6400 IU/day. The ACCP recommends it for acute ischemic stroke (see Table 5.3-2 in Chapter 5.3) at an initial IV bolus dose of up to 1000 IU, then 750 IU SQ q12 h (or using body weight: <90 kg = 750 IU q8 h; >90 kg = 1250 IU q12 h) for 14 days. Its dose should be reduced in patients with severe renal impairment. However, in the elderly, the usual dose can be given because clearance is not changed.
6. **Other new drugs** include direct thrombin inhibitors [hirudin; recombinant hirudin or lepirudin (Refludan); argatroban; bivalirudin (Angiomax)], direct factor Xa inhibitors, activated protein C (APC), tissue factor pathway inhibitor (TFPI), and nematode anticoagulant peptide c2 (NAPc2). They need further clinical testing to define their role in the prevention and treatment of venous thromboembolism. Lepirudin and argatroban have been used in patients with heparin-induced thrombocytopenia.

B. ANTIPLATELET THERAPY, in the PM&R setting, is strongly recommended after stroke/transient ischemic attack. But it is not recommended for primary stroke prevention. For primary prevention, one should consider all major vascular events (including myocardial infarction and stroke), and hence whether antiplatelet therapy (e.g., low-dose aspirin) should be advised concerns more than its effect on stroke.

1. **Dextran-40 solution (10%)** is a low molecular weight (40 kDa) polysaccharide originally used as a plasma volume expander, but it was found to have antithrombotic effects related to its ability to decrease platelet adhesion and fibrin polymerization. It also forms a coating on the endothelial walls, thereby inhibiting nidus formation. It is ineffective in preventing DVTs in stroke patients. In other high-risk patients (e.g., after total hip or knee replacement), its antithrombotic effects are controversial. Adverse drug reactions include increased risk of congestive heart failure, volume overload, anaphylaxis (hence, test dose must be done), renal insufficiency, phlebitis from IV insertion, and

about 14% incidence of postoperative bleeding (e.g., GI bleeding and wound hematomas). It is given intravenously at 20 mL/kg up to 500 mL.

2. **Aspirin** (see section I.A.3.a) is the most commonly used antiplatelet drug. It is a relatively weak drug that interferes with platelet activity by inhibiting only one of many platelet activators, i.e., thromboxane A_2. Aspirin is indicated in patients with stable angina, unstable angina, acute myocardial infarction, transient cerebral ischemia, thrombotic stroke, and peripheral arterial disease. It is also indicated in patients with atrial fibrillation in whom warfarin is contraindicated. A dose of 75–100 mg/day of ASA is generally used chronically for all indications, although an initial dose of 160–325 mg may be used in acute settings. For patients with cerebrovascular disease, a dose of 75 mg/day is effective (whether higher doses are more effective remains controversial). A dose of 100 mg/day may be combined with warfarin in patients with mechanical prosthetic heart valves who develop systemic embolism while on warfarin. For stroke prophylaxis after transient ischemic attack or stroke, the consensus among US experts (e.g., American Heart Association Stroke Council, American College of Chest Physician, FDA) favors a low-to-intermediate ASA dose (50–35 mg daily). For DVT prophylaxis, ASA is generally not recommended because it is not as effective as other DVT prophylaxis methods.
3. **Dipyridamole (Persantine)** is a platelet inhibitor, which, at 225 mg/day, is indicated as an adjunct (not as sole therapy) to warfarin anticoagulation in the prevention of thromboembolism in patients with prosthetic heart valves who develop systemic embolism while on warfarin and who cannot tolerate aspirin. Dipyridamole has not been shown to be effective (and is thus not recommended) in DVT prophylaxis. The ADRs include dizziness, abdominal distress, headache, and rash. It is available in oral forms (25-, 50-, and 75-mg tablets) and is given at 75–100 mg, po, tid/qid. It has also been combined with ASA (**Aggrenox**, 25 mg ASA/200 mg extended-release dipyridamole, 1 cap., po, bid) to reduce the risk of stroke in patients who have had transient ischemia of the brain or complete ischemic stroke because of thrombosis. Aggrenox was shown to prevent twice as many strokes as ASA.
4. **Ticlopidine (Ticlid)** inhibits platelet aggregation by inhibiting adenosine diphosphate (ADP)-induced platelet–fibrinogen binding and subsequent platelet–platelet interaction. This inhibitory effect is delayed for 24–48 hours, thus it may not be used when a rapid antiplatelet effect is required. Ticlopidine is indicated instead of aspirin in ischemic stroke patients with aspirin allergy or aspirin intolerance and in patients who develop recurrent thromboembolism despite aspirin. The ADRs include GI complaints, rash, abnormal LFTs, reversible neutropenia, and other blood dyscrasias (e.g., agranulocytosis, thrombotic thrombocytopenic purpura, aplastic anemia, leukemia). Hence CBC and LFTs must be checked biweekly, especially during the first 2–3 months of therapy. It is available in 250-mg tablets and is given at 250 mg, po, bid with food.
5. **Clopidogrel (Plavix)** is an antiplatelet drug with similar MOA as ticlopidine. Compared to ticlopidine, clopidogrel has a better safety profile and its antiaggregating properties are several times higher. It has similar overall tolerability to ASA but has a more favorable effect on clinical outcome than ASA. It is FDA-approved for reducing the risk of of heart attack, stroke, or cardiovascular death in patients with a history of recent heart attack, recent stroke, or established peripheral arterial disease. The ADRs include pruritus, purpura, diarrhea, rash, and, infrequently, intracranial hemorrhage or severe neutropenia. Thrombotic thrombocytopenic purpura has also been reported but is rare. Clopidogrel should be used with caution in patients who may be at risk of increased bleeding from trauma, surgery, or other pathological conditions (particularly GI and intraocular). It is contraindicated in active pathological bleeding such as peptic

ulcer or intracranial hemorrhage. It is available in 75-mg oral tablets and is given at 75 mg, po, qd. It may be combined with ASA to achieve greater antiplatelet effect.

VIII. Bone-metabolism regulators

Regulators of bone metabolism are used in conjunction with other nonpharmacologic treatments of osteoporosis, including exercise.

A. ANTI-BONE-RESORPTION AGENTS act by decreasing the rate of bone resorption through inhibition of bone osteoclasts. They are generally useful for the type I ("high-turnover" or involutional) type of osteoporosis (e.g., postmenopausal osteoporosis).

1. Estrogen replacement is the most effective preventive strategy in the management of postmenopausal osteoporosis in women, whether the menopause is natural or surgically induced (e.g., oophorectomy before age 50). It has been shown to inhibit bone resorption, slow the loss of bone mass, and partially reduce (i.e., by 50%) the risk of fractures in postmenopausal women. Also, for the most part, bone that has already been lost after menopause cannot be replaced (despite retardation of bone loss).

Mechanisms of action. Estrogen decreases bone response to parathyroid hormone; promotes synthesis of calcitonin; and enhances the availability of vitamin D. It probably also acts directly on specific estrogen receptors in osteoblasts.

Adverse drug reactions. The ADRs of estrogen replacement include menstrual bleeding, weight gain, nausea, headache, and breast tenderness – all of which can be alleviated by a reduction in estrogen dose. Estrogen replacement can also increase the risk of endometrial cancer and possibly breast cancer (these risks can be reduced or eliminated by cyclic therapy with added progestin; however, the coronary artery disease risk of adding progesterone is unknown). There is no evidence of hypertension or increased risk of thromboembolism in postmenopausal estrogen replacement.

Contraindications and precautions. Contraindications to estrogen replacement include a history of breast or endometrial cancer, recurrent thromboembolic disease, acute liver or gallbladder disease, or unexplained vaginal bleeding. Relative contraindications include fibrocystic disease of the breast, uterine myomata or fibroids, endometriosis, or a family history of breast cancer. In the PM&R setting, it should be discontinued during prolonged immobilization or <4–6 weeks before surgery of the type associated with increased risk of thromboembolism (e.g., total hip or knee replacement).

Drug administration guidelines. Estrogen replacement is indicated for all women with premature menopause and no contraindications. Patients who have had a hysterectomy may take estrogen daily without the addition of progesterone.

In postmenopausal women without hysterectomy, a cyclic regimen including estrogen and a progesterone should be used, giving estrogen on days 1 to 25 of each month with the addition of progesterone [e.g., medroxyprogesterone (Provera), 10 mg, po, qd] started between days 12 and 15 through to day 25 of each monthly cycle. Estrogen preparations and their doses include conjugated estrogens (Premarin), 0.625 mg, po, qd; estropipate (Ogen), 0.625 mg, po, qd; ethinyl estradiol, 20 mg, po, qd; or estradiol (Estrace), 1 mg, po, qd. In women who have side-effects at these doses, conjugated estrogen (Premarin), 0.3 mg, po, qd, may be tried. Patients on estrogen replacement should be given calcium supplements (1500 mg/day; see section VIII.A.5). An alternative to oral estrogen replacement is transdermal estradiol (Estraderm patch, 0.05–0.10-mg patch twice a week), which bypasses the GI system and circumvents the possible GI ADRs but still adequately delivers to the skeletal system. If noncycled estrogen without progesterone is used in women with an intact uterus, an endometrial biopsy should be taken regularly (at least every 2 years).

Estrogen replacement should begin as soon as possible after the menopause to delay the rapid phase of bone loss; however, therapy may be beneficial as late as age 70 (beyond this age, there is little evidence to support its usage). The optimal duration of therapy is not established, but there is consensus that it should continue for at least 10 years (or up to age 70). Women with premature menopause should be treated at least until the time of normal menopause (about age 50). Regular evaluation should include breast examinations, annual mammography, and prompt evaluation of unexpected vaginal bleeding with endometrial biopsy.

2. **Raloxifene (Evista)** is a selective estrogen receptor modulator (SERM), which decreases resorption of bone and reduces biochemical markers of bone turnover to the premenopausal range. It is indicated for the treatment and prevention of postmenopausal osteoporosis. It also has the added benefit of lowering total cholesterol by about 7% and low-density cholesterol by about 11%. It is contraindicated in lactating women, women who are or may become pregnant, or women with active or past history of venous thromboembolic events. It can be used with caution in patients with hepatic insufficiency, congestive heart failure, or active malignancy. Unlike estrogen replacement, it does not cause breast tenderness or vaginal bleeding and it has no increased risk of breast or uterine cancer. The ADRs include hot flushes, leg cramps, and increased risk of venous thromboembolism. In the PM&R setting, it should be discontinued <72 hours prior to and during prolonged immobilization and should be resumed only after the patient is fully ambulatory. The recommended dose is 60 mg, po, qd. It is available only in oral form (60-mg tablet).
3. **Calcitonin (Calcimar, Miacalcin)** can be used in women over 70 years of age (because estrogen is ineffective in women over 70), postmenopausal women in whom estrogen is contraindicated, women or men with established osteoporosis (especially "high-turnover" osteoporosis), women with medical or chemical oophorectomy, persons with low bone mass, amenorrheic athletes, painful vertebral crush fractures, and lytic disease of the weight-bearing bones. Calcitonin also has analgesic properties (e.g., in cancer patients with bone pain or in elderly patients in whom the CNS side-effects from analgesics are contraindicated; see Chapter 5.10, section VI.E.2.l). The role of calcitonin in osteoporosis prevention is under investigation. Calcitonin has not been shown to reduce the risk of fracture.

Mechanisms of action. Calcitonin is a polypeptide hormone with receptors in osteoclasts that decrease bone resorption, inhibit osteoclasts, and may be helpful in rapid bone losers. Aside from its direct action on bone, it also has direct renal effects and actions on the GI tract.

Adverse drug reactions. Side-effects include nausea, flushing, and, rarely, allergic reactions (e.g., urticaria and local reactions at injection sites). These may diminish or disappear after continued administration or may be alleviated by an antiemetic or antihistaminic agent.

Contraindication. Its only contraindication is in patients with known hypersensitivity to the drug or to the components of the drug or its vehicle.

Drug administration guidelines. There are three forms of injectable calcitonin: salmon calcitonin (Calcimar, Miacalcin), human calcitonin (Cibacalcin), and eel calcitonin. Both salmon and human calcitonins are FDA-approved for postmenopausal osteoporosis. It has high activity, low antigenicity, and costs less than the other preparations. Salmon calcitonin (Calcimar or Miacalcin,

200 IU/mL in 2-mL vials) is given at 50–100 IU, IM or SQ, qd or qod for at least 1–3 months. Prior to administration, skin testing for allergy should be done. When an adequate response is achieved (usually after several months), the dosage is decreased to 50 IU, SQ, three times a week for at least 3–6 months (it is not clear if treatment beyond a total of 12–18 months is beneficial). Aside from injectable forms, salmon calcitonin is also available as a nasal spray (i.e., Miacalcin nasal spray, 200 units intranasally daily in alternate nostrils; patient should be monitored for nasal ulcers or rhinitis). If resistance to salmon calcitonin develops, human calcitonin (Cibacalcin), 0.5 mg, SQ or IM, qd or qod, is often effective. Patients on calcitonin need adequate vitamin D (e.g., 400 IU/day; see section VIII.A.6) and calcium intake (1500 mg/day; see section VIII.A.5) to prevent progressive loss of bone mass in postmenopausal osteoporosis. Periodic urinalysis for sediments or casts is also recommended.

4. **Bisphosphonates** can be used instead of calcitonin in women over 70 years of age, postmenopausal women for whom estrogen is contraindicated, and women and men with established osteoporosis. It can also be used in Paget's disease of bone (osteitis deformans) and in heterotopic ossification. Bisphosphonates inhibit bone turnover by interfering with the function of osteoclasts and the dissolution of hydroxyapatite. In high doses, however, they can impair bone mineralization and promote osteomalacia as well as preventing the formation of heterotopic ossification (see section VIII.C). They may cause upper GI disorders, such as dysphagia, esophagitis, and esophageal or gastric ulcer.

a. ***Oral bisphosphonates*** should only be taken by patients with an adequate intake of vitamin D (e.g., 400 IU/day; see section VIII.A.6) and calcium (e.g., 1500 mg/day; see section VIII.A.5). Both alendronate and risedronate must be taken with plain water in an upright position (i.e., patients should not lie down for 30 minutes after intake) and on an empty stomach (i.e., 30 minutes before any other beverage or medication) to maximize their absorption.

I. **Etidronate (Didronel)** is primarily indicated for the management of heterotopic ossification and Paget's disease of bone. It is not FDA-approved for the treatment of osteoporosis (although it has experimentally been shown to be beneficial for postmenopausal osteoporosis by increasing vertebral bone density and decreasing the rate of vertebral fracture). In patients with, or predisposed to, heterotopic ossification, it is given in high doses for prevention of bone mineralization (see section VIII.C). In Paget's disease, it is given at a dosage of 5–10 mg/kg/day for a period not to exceed 6 months or 11–20 mg/kg/day, not to exceed 3 months. It may be repeated after a didronel period of >90 days if Paget's disease is still active and symptomatic. The ADRs, contraindications, precautions, preparations, and administration guidelines for etidronate are given in section VIII.C.

II. **Alendronate (Fosamax)** is 200 times more potent than etidronate. Because of its high potency, it provides effective inhibition of bone resorption at doses that do not impair mineralization. It is indicated for treatment of postmenopausal osteoporosis or of men with osteoporosis (10 mg, po, qd or 70 mg, po, weekly); for prevention of postmenopausal osteoporosis (5 mg, po, qd or 35 mg, po, weekly); for treatment of glucocorticoid-induced osteoporosis (5 mg, po, qd); and for treatment of Paget's disease of bone (40 mg/day for 6 months; may be repeated following a 6-month post-treatment evaluation showing elevated serum alkaline phosphatase). The ADRs include GI upset, musculoskeletal pain, and headache. It is contraindicated in patients with hypocalcemia, inability to stand or sit upright for 30 minutes, esophageal abnormalities which delay esophageal emptying (e.g., stricture or achalasia), patients at increased risk of aspiration (this contraindication is for the oral solution), or severe renal dysfunction (creatinine clearance of <35 mL/min). However, for less severe renal insufficiency, it may be given without dose adjustment. It is available in tablet form (5- ,10-, 35-, 40-, and 70-mg) or oral solution (70-mg).

III. **Risedronate (Actonel)**, which is more potent than alendronate, also provides effective inhibition of bone resorption at doses that do not impair mineralization. It is indicated in the treatment and prevention of postmenopausal osteoporosis (5 mg, po, qd or 35 mg, po, weekly), as well as treatment of glucocorticoid-induced osteoporosis (5 mg, po, qd) and Paget's disease of bone (30 mg, po, qd for 2 months, which may be repeated if serum alkaline phosphatase is not normalized). The ADRs include back or joint pain, abdominal pain, and GI upset. It is contraindicated in patients with hypocalcemia or inability to stand or sit upright for 30 minutes, or severe renal dysfunction (creatinine clearance of <30 mL/min). It is available in 5-, 30-, and 35-mg tablets.

b. ***Intravenous bisphosphonates, i.e., pamidronate (Aredia)*** are indicated for treatment of patients with osteolytic bone metastases of breast cancer (90 mg in 2-h IV infusion given every 3–4 weeks in conjunction with standard antineoplastic therapy), with osteolytic bone lesions of multiple myeloma (90 mg in 4-h IV infusion on a monthly basis), moderate-to-severe hypercalcemia of malignancy (60–90 mg in a single-dose IV infusion over 2–24 hours; a minimum of 7 days should elapse before retreatment), and moderate-to-severe Paget's disease (30 mg daily administered as 4-h IV infusion on 3 consecutive days for a total of 90 mg). In patients with bone pain because of metastatic breast cancer, it can also act as an adjuvant analgesic (see Chapter 5.10, section VI.E.2.l). The ADRs include local soft tissue symptoms (e.g., redness, swelling, induration), fluid overload, generalized pain, hypertension, headaches, bone pain, abdominal pain, GI upset, urinary tract infection, and laboratory abnormality (e.g., anemia, hypokalemia, hypomagnesemia, hypophosphatemia). It should be used with caution in patients with renal insufficiency (i.e., dose should not exceed 90 mg to prevent renal toxicity). It should not be used in pregnant patients.

5. **Calcium** is the major inorganic component of bone. It structures the human skeleton along with collagenous fibers, and it regulates many cellular activities. It also decreases the effect of parathyroid hormone on bone resorption. Foods high in calcium include milk, buttermilk, yogurt, cheese, ice cream, sardines (with bones), shrimp, salmon, broccoli (cooked), tofu (bean curd), and turnip greens (cooked). The intestinal absorption of dietary calcium is reduced as the person ages and in women with estrogen deficiency. The recommended calcium intake for premenopausal women and men is 1000 mg/day and for postmenopausal women is 1500 mg/day. To achieve this level of intake, most women need calcium supplements, 500–1000 mg/day. Calcium supplementation can slow the loss of bone mass in postmenopausal women with low calcium intake. Side-effects of calcium supplementation include dyspepsia, constipation, and hypercalciuria. It can also cause digitalis toxicity. It is contraindicated in patients with kidney stones or those who are prone to form kidney stones. Among calcium preparations, calcium carbonate (e.g., Os-Cal, 250 or 500 mg elemental calcium per tablet, Tums Extra-strength, 400 mg elemental calcium/5 mL, or various generics) is probably the best and least expensive. Calcium citrate (Citracal) may also be used.

6. **Vitamin D** allows increased calcium absorption from the GI tract. While some studies found it useful in maintaining bone mass, others suggest that it can actually accelerate bone loss. Hence it should only be supplemented if the patient has vitamin D deficiency (shown by testing serum 25-hydroxy vitamin D). Dietary vitamin D deficiency can initially be treated with vitamin D, 50 000 IU po weekly for several weeks to produce replete body stores, followed

by long-term therapy with 400–800 IU/day. If vitamin D deficiency is caused by malabsorption, the dose ranges from 50 000 IU po weekly to daily. For both dietary deficiency and malabsorption deficiency, the dose should be adjusted to maintain serum 25-hydroxy vitamin D levels within the normal range. Calcium supplements (e.g., 1500 mg/day; see section VIII.A.5) are usually required during vitamin D supplementation. Vitamin D preparations include calcium supplements containing vitamin D (e.g., Os-Cal + D, 125 IU/250- or 500-mg tablet), many multivitamins (400 IU/tablet), and vitamin D drops (200 IU/drop or 8000 IU/mL). The combination calcium/vitamin D tablets (e.g., Os-Cal + D) should be used with caution because the ratio may lead to vitamin D toxicity.

Elderly people may tolerate two to three times the recommended daily allowance of vitamin D if cutaneous generation of vitamin D, mediated through sun exposure, is reduced. Some clinicians advocate 5–10 minutes of sunshine three times per week rather than supplementation. If the patient does not respond to high doses of vitamin D, calcifediol (Calderol, 20 or 50 mg/capsule), 20–100 mg, po, qd, may be better absorbed (the dose is then reduced depending on serum 5-hydroxy vitamin D levels). Patients on vitamin D supplementation should be monitored every 3–6 months for serum 25-hydroxy vitamin D, serum calcium, and 24-hour urine calcium.

B. BONE-FORMATION AGENTS stimulate bone growth and are generally useful in type II (or "low-turnover" or senile) osteoporosis.

1. **Vitamin D** stimulates bone growth and prevents bone resorption. It is described in section VIII.A.6.
2. **Fluoride** stimulates osteoblastic cells to form new bone and increases trabecular bone density (but not cortical bone density). Its effect on the incidence of fracture is controversial and might be dose dependent (i.e., larger doses result in bones with impaired mineralization, which are more likely to fracture). Although used in Europe, fluoride use in osteoporosis has not been formally approved in the United States. It may be indicated for the treatment of established vertebral osteoporosis with symptomatic fractures that will not respond to other therapies. The ADRs include GI problems (gastric irritation, nausea, recurrent vomiting, and peptic ulcer); rheumatologic problems (e.g., plantar fasciitis, synovitis, arthralgias, and questionable increased risk of hip fractures), and anemia. It may be given as sodium fluoride (e.g., Luride, 2.2 mg/tablet or 1.1 mg/mL) at 25 mg, po, qd with food, increasing slowly to 25 mg tid as tolerated over a few weeks. It should be given with calcium (1500 mg/day) and vitamin D (400 IU/day).
3. **Anabolic steroids (androgens)** can increase bone mass perhaps by increasing bone formation; however, their prolonged use in osteoporotic patients is generally not recommended because of their androgenic (virilizing) effects as well as adverse effects on carbohydrate, lipid metabolism, and liver function. Studies have shown that 10–20% of men with osteoporosis have partial or complete hypogonadism of various causes. In osteoporotic men with low plasma testosterone, androgen (e.g., testosterone enanthate) may be used under the supervision of an endocrinologist.

C. ANTI-BONE-MINERALIZATION AGENTS are used in preventing heterotopic ossification. Heterotopic ossification is characterized by metaplastic osteogenesis and can be associated with traumatic conditions (e.g., spinal cord injury, TBI, burns, severe thigh bruises, as well as surgical trauma such as total hip replacement) or nontraumatic conditions (e.g., infection of the CNS and peripheral neuropathy; association with various benign and malignant neoplasms). The bisphosphonate etidronate (see section VIII.A.4), when given in high dose, prevents or retards heterotopic ossification by inhibiting bone mineralization through chemical absorption of calcium hydroxyapatite crystals and their amorphous precursors, thus blocking the aggregation, growth, and mineralization of these crystals. Etidronate is indicated in the prevention and treatment of heterotopic ossification (e.g., after total hip replacement and spinal cord injury). Studies show that in patients with total hip replacement, etidronate does not promote loosening of hip prostheses or impede trochanteric reattachment; and in spinal cord injury, it does not inhibit fracture healing or stabilization of the spine. The ADRs of etidronate include GI problems (e.g., diarrhea and nausea) and rarely blood dyscrasias. The GI problems can usually be alleviated by dividing the daily total dose. Etidronate is contraindicated in patients with clinically overt osteomalacia. It should be used with caution in patients with renal impairment.

Etidronate disodium (**Didronel**; see section VIII.A.4) is available orally in 200- and 400-mg tablets. It is given as a single oral dose (may be divided if patient has GI upset) on an empty stomach to maximize absorption. Food should be avoided within 2 hours of dosing (especially high-calcium food such as milk; or vitamins with mineral supplement or antacids which are high in metals such as calcium, iron, magnesium, or aluminum). Patients also need to have adequate intake of vitamin D (see section VIII.A.6) and calcium (see section VIII.A.5). For the prevention and treatment of heterotopic ossification in total hip replacement patients, the dose is 20 mg/kg/day for 1 month before and 3 months after surgery (4 months in total). For the prevention and treatment of heterotopic ossification in spinal cord injury patients, the dose is 20 mg/kg/day for 2 weeks followed by 10 mg/kg/day for 10 weeks (12 weeks total). Treatment should begin prior to any evidence of heterotopic ossification because etidronate does not affect mature heterotopic ossification. Ideally it should be started in the hypervascular precursor phase (demonstrated when the flow and pool phases of a three-phase bone scan are positive).

IX. Cardiovascular drugs

Cardiovascular drugs prescribed by physiatrists for noncardiac indications include the following.

A. ADRENERGIC DRUGS

1. **Centrally acting adrenergic agonists**, which include **clonidine (Catapres; Duraclon)**, **methyldopa (Aldomet)**, **guanabenz (Wytensin)**, and **guanfacine (Tenex)**, are primarily used as antihypertensive agents. Among these drugs, only clonidine is described as it is a multipurpose drug commonly used in the PM&R setting. Clonidine is an α_2-adrenergic agonist as well as an α_1-adrenergic blocker. It is used in the management of pain (see Chapter 5.10, section VI.E.2.i), spasticity (see Chapter 5.4, section III.D.1.d), aggression (see section V.F), and sympathetic overactivity during opioid withdrawal (see section I.B) or autonomic dysreflexia (see Chapter 5.7, section V.F). Its ADRs include cardiovascular effects (e.g., hypotension, syncope, dizziness, palpitation, bradycardia, and rarely arrhythmias), CNS effects (e.g., sedation, mental depression, agitation, nervousness, vivid dreams, and nightmares), GI effects (dry mouth, constipation, nausea, vomiting, and anorexia), and other effects (e.g., weight gain, malaise, rash, decreased sexual activity, and weakness).

   The risk of serious adverse cardiovascular effects appears to be low in younger patients without a significant associated medical disorder. In the elderly, there is higher risk of serious adverse cardiovascular effects, especially those predisposed to hypotensive effects, those receiving other drugs with additive effects on blood pressure, and those with concurrent diseases such as renal or cardiac failure. Its only contraindication is in patients with known hypersensitivity to the drug or component of the drug or its vehicle (e.g., contact sensitivity to the transdermal patch).

Clonidine is available in oral form (Catapres) and transdermal form (Catapres TTS) at 0.1-, 0.2-, and 0.3-mg strengths. It is also available in an injectable form (Duraclon) at 100- and 500 μg/mL. Th IV form is given intrathecally (epidurally) for treating chronic intractable pain such as in cancer patients (see Chapter 5.10, section VI.E.2.i.1). The choice between the oral and transdermal forms is based on patient preference. The oral form is taken twice daily, and the transdermal patch is changed every week. The starting dose is 0.1–0.2 mg/day, which can be gradually increased (every few days for oral route and every 1–2 weeks for transdermal route) to a usual dose of 0.2–0.6 mg/day and a maximum dose of 2.4 mg/day depending on the patient's response (especially blood pressure). For the oral route, the higher dose should be taken at bedtime to minimize the transient effects of dry mouth and drowsiness. Prior to discontinuation, tapering is required to prevent rebound hypertension.

2. **Peripherally acting adrenergic blockers**, e.g., **guanethidine (Ismelin)** and **reserpine (Serpasil)**, are primarily used as hypertensive agents; however, their parenteral forms (available only for experimental use) can also be used as ganglionic blocking agents for IV regional sympathetic blocks in patients with CRPS type I (formerly called reflex sympathetic dystrophy; see Chapter 4.10, section IV.B.4).
3. **Selective α_1-adrenergic blockers, e.g., prazosin (Minipress), terazosin (Hytrin),** and **doxazosin (Cardura)**, are primarily used as antihypertensive agents but can also be used to improve bladder-emptying function (see Chapter 5.7, section IV.D.4.a). Prazosin has also been used as an adjunct analgesic in patients with neuropathic pain (see Chapter 5.10, section VI.E.2.i).
4. **Nonselective α_1- and α_2-adrenergic blockers**, for example **phenoxybenzamine (Dibenzyline)**, are primarily used to control hypertension in patients with pheochromocytoma but have been reported to be effective in selected cases of CRPS type I (see Chapter 5.10, section VI.E.2.i.3).
5. **Nonselective β_1- and β_2-adrenergic blockers**, which are primarily used as antihypertensive agents, can also be used in the management of pain (see Chapter 5.10; section VI.E.2.i), aggression (see section V.F), and anxiety (see section V.C.2.f). They include **propranolol (Inderal)** and **pindolol (Visken)**, both of which are described in section V.F.

B. CALCIUM-CHANNEL BLOCKERS, which are primarily used as antihypertensive, anti-ischemic (or antianginal), and antiarrhythmic agents, include **verapamil (Calan, Isoptin), diltiazem (Cardizem), isradipine (DynaCirc), amlodipine (Norvasc)**, and **nicardipine (Cardene). Nifedipine (Procardia, Adalat)** is also a calcium-channel blocker but is primarily used as an anti-ischemic agent for the emergency management of hypertensive crises (e.g., in autonomic dysreflexia; see Chapter 5.7, section V.F) and for management of CRPS type I, CRPS type II (causalgia), and Raynaud's phenomenon (see Chapter 5.10, section VI.E.2.i.5). Among the other calcium-channel blockers, verapamil is used in the PM&R setting as an antiaggression agent (see section V.F) and as an adjunct analgesic in patients with neuropathic pain (see Chapter 5.10, section VI.E.2.i.5). The ADRs of verapamil include cardiovascular effects (e.g., hypotension, syncope, dizziness, palpitation, bradycardia, atrioventricular block, angina pectoris, myocardial infarct, and congestive heart failure), CNS effects (e.g., headache, sedation, insomnia, paresthesia, confusion, equilibrium disorders, stroke, and psychotic symptoms), GI effects (dry mouth, constipation, diarrhea, nausea, and gingival hyperplasia), and other effects (e.g., rash, impotence, blurred vision, and fatigue). Verapamil is contraindicated in patients with severe left ventricular dysfunction; hypotension (systolic blood pressure below

90 mmHg) or cardiogenic shock; arrhythmias such as sick sinus syndrome, second- or third-degree atrioventricular block (except in patients with a functioning artificial ventricular pacemaker); atrial flutter or fibrillation; or accessory bypass tract (e.g., Wolff–Parkinson–White and Lown–Ganong–Levine syndromes). Verapamil is available in oral (immediate and sustained release) and parenteral forms. It is usually started at 40 mg, po, tid/qid, and titrated up to 240–320 mg/day.

C. **ANTIARRHYTHMIC DRUGS** can also be used as local anesthetics in the management of chronic pain (see Chapter 5.10, section VI.E.2.c). They include intravenous local anesthetics [e.g., **lidocaine (Xylocaine)**, **procaine (Procan)**] and oral local anesthetics [e.g., **mexiletine (Mexitil)**, **tocainamide (Tonacard)**, and **flecainide (Tumbocor)**]. Lidocaine is also used as a patch (**Lidoderm 5% Patch**; see Chapter 5.10, section VI.E.2.c), as a topical anesthetic cream (e.g., **EMLA**, **Ela-Max; LMX**, see Chapter 5.10, section VI.E.2.c), and an iontophoresis agent (see Chapter 4.1, section V.A.1.a)

X. Gastrointestinal drugs

Drugs used for bowel problems (i.e., antidiarrheal and laxative drugs) are described in Chapter 5.8, sections VI.A.2 and VI.B.3 respectively.

Other GI medications are discussed in different sections of this chapter, for example, antiemetic drugs used to treat nausea in patients taking opioids (see section I.B. under Adverse drug reactions), and antiulcer drugs used for GI protection when taking NSAIDs (see section I.A.3 under GI toxicity).

XI. Neurourologic drugs

Neurourologic drugs commonly used in treating voiding dysfunction are described in Chapter 5.7, section IV.D. They include anticholinergic, cholinergic, α-adrenergic agonist, and α-adrenergic blocking agents.

XII. Pulmonary drugs

Pulmonary drugs are primarily used in patients with chronic obstructive pulmonary disorder (see Chapter 5.12).

XIII. Parkinson's disease (PD) drugs

Parkinsonism (an extrapyramidal disorder characterized by rigidity, tremor at rest, bradykinesia, and loss of postural reflexes) can be classified into: primary (i.e., idiopathic Parkinson's disease); secondary or acquired [which can be caused by drugs (e.g., neuroleptic drugs, metoclopramide, prochlorperazine, reserpine), toxins (e.g., carbon monoxide, manganese, 1-methyl-4-phenyl-tetrahydropyridine or MPTP), infections (e.g., encephalitis lethargica, Creutzfeldt–Jacob disease, acquired immunodeficiency disease), hypoparathyroidism, cerebrovascular disease (e.g., basal ganglia lacunes), repeated head trauma]; and parkinsonism-plus [i.e., parkinsonism in association with other multisystem degenerative diseases, such as Alzheimer's disease, normal pressure hydrocephalus, Wilson's disease, rigid variant of Huntington's disease, multiple systems atrophy (e.g., Shy–Drager syndrome)]. This section deals only with drugs used in managing idiopathic Parkinson's disease (PD). In the PM&R setting, the use of PD drug therapy is only one component of its interdisciplinary treatment approach, which includes physical therapy, occupational therapy, speech therapy, swallowing therapy, and others.

PD drugs can be broadly classified into drugs aimed at increasing the availability of dopamine in the CNS (e.g., dopaminergic agents, dopamine-reuptake inhibitors, dopamine-breakdown inhibitors) and drugs aimed at improving the symptoms of PD by other means (e.g., anticholinergics, antihistamines, benzodiazepines). Increasing dopamine level is essential in the management of PD because the neurotransmitter dopamine (which facilitates execution of movement and helps suppress unwanted movement) is deficient in the corpus striatum of PD patients due to neurodegeneration of dopamine-producing cells in the substantia nigra.

A. DOPAMINERGIC AGENTS

1. **Levodopa (L-dopa)** is still considered the most effective symptomatic treatment of PD despite the availability of newer agents (e.g., dopamine agonists) as first-line therapy for PD. A dramatic initial response to L-dopa is helpful in confirming the diagnosis of PD and differentiating it from other parkinsonian syndromes which have partial response to L-dopa. Most experts recommend that L-dopa only be used when other drug alternatives (e.g., dopamine agonists) fail to provide sufficient relief. The use of L-dopa in early PD in patients younger than 65 years remains controversial. However, there is general consensus about its early use in PD patients over 65 years old because: a) the motor complications of L-dopa are less likely to occur in the elderly; and b) elderly patients have higher risk of having cognitive side-effects of confusion and hallucinations from other PD drugs (e.g., dopamine agonists).

   Mechanism of action. L-dopa is the immediate metabolic precursor of dopamine. It is used instead of dopamine itself because of L-dopa's ability to cross the blood–brain barrier (BBB). Given alone, most of L-dopa (>95%) is converted to dopamine in the periphery (i.e., extracerebral tissues) by dopa decarboxylase, with minimal active dopamine crossing the BBB. Thus, L-dopa is combined with a peripheral dopa decarboxylase inhibitor, **carbidopa** [as carbidopa-levodopa combination (**Sinemet**)], to potentiate the CNS effect of L-dopa and to minimize the side-effects caused by peripheral dopamine (especially nausea and vomiting).

   Adverse drug reactions. The most common ADRs of L-dopa include dyskinesia, nausea, hallucinations, confusion, dizziness, depression, urinary tract infection, and headaches. Other ADRs include dream abnormalities, dystonia, vomiting, upper respiratory infection, dyspnea, "on–off" phenomena, back pain, dry mouth, anorexia, diarrhea, insomnia, orthostatic hypotension, shoulder pain, chest pain, muscle cramps, paresthesia, urinary frequency, dyspepsia, and constipation. Cardiac arrhythmias and neuroleptic malignant syndrome have also been reported. Dyskinesia, i.e., involuntary movements associated with loose muscle tone, typically begin to develop in milder forms after 3–5 years of L-dopa treatment, and are more severe after 5–10 years of treatment. In patients with the "on–off" phenomenon, there are unpredictable swings from mobility to immobility due to abrupt changes in muscle tone, switching from rigidity ("off") to a normal or dyskinetic state ("on") and then back to rigidity ("off") within minutes. Changing the amount or timing of the L-dopa dose may help prevent ADRs.

   Contraindications and precautions. L-dopa is contraindicated in patients taking nonselective MAO inhibitors and in patients with narrow-angle glaucoma or history of melanoma. It should be used cautiously in patients with severe cardiovascular or pulmonary disease, bronchial asthma, renal, hepatic or endocrine disease, peptic ulcers. Periodic evaluations of hepatic, hematopoietic, cardiovascular, and renal function are recommended during extended therapy. Patients should be advised of possible garment discoloration due to dark discoloration of bodily fluids.

Drug administration guidelines. Carbidopa/levodopa (Sinemet) can be orally administered as immediate-release (IR) or controlled-release (CR) formulation. Sinemet IR has a faster onset (usually 20 to 40 min) but a shorter duration of action (2–4 hours in more advanced stages of PD), whereas Sinemet CR has a delayed onset but a longer duration of action. Both formulations are equally effective in treating the symptoms of PD, although some patients prefer the CR formulation. Sinemet CR, which has a more steady plasma L-dopa concentration, was hypothesized to decrease incidence of motor fluctuations or dyskinesia. However, clinical studies (see Koller *et al.*, 1999) failed to demonstrate this. Both formulations tend to be more effective when used in combination, e.g., use of Sinemet IR as the first dose of the day (due to its faster onset of action) and use of Sinemet CR at bedtime (due to its longer duration of action).

Sinemet IR is formulated in doses of 10/100, 25/100, and 25/250 mg tablets of carbidopa/levidopa. The starting dose is 25/100 mg, one tablet, po, tid, increasing by one tablet every day or every other day, as necessary, up to 2 tablets, po, qid. If the 10/100 mg tablet is used, the starting dose may be one tablet, po, tid/qid, increasing by one tablet every day or every other day, as necessary, up to 2 tablets, po, qid.

Sinemet CR is formulated in 1:4 carbidopa/levidopa ratio as 25/100 (nonscored) and 50/200 (scored) tablets. When replacing Sinemet IR, it is necessary to increase the dosage of Sinemet CR by 10 to 30% per day (i.e., Sinemet CR daily dose = Sinemet IR daily dose × 110% to 130%) due to its reduced GI absorption and lower bioavailability (by approximately 80%) when compared to Sinemet IR. It can be titrated up to 400 to 1600 mg of L-dopa per day (2400 mg or more have been used but are not usually recommended), given in divided doses at intervals ranging from 4–8 hours during the waking day. The effect of its first morning dose may be delayed up to 1 hour compared to Sinemet IR. Sinemet CR should not be chewed or crushed.

2. Dopamine agonists

a. ***Oral dopamine agonists*** are generally recommended (instead of carbidopa/levodopa) in younger PD patients (less than 65 years old) to delay the onset of dyskinesia. They are not quite as effective as L-dopa in the symptomatic treatment of PD, but they provide excellent relief of symptoms and delay the onset of motor complications when used as monotherapy early in the disease.

Mechanism of action. Dopamine agonists mimic the action of dopamine by stimulating all five types of dopamine receptors (D1 to D5) in the corpus striatum to varying degrees.

Adverse drug reactions. Common ADRs of oral dopamine agonists include nausea, vomiting, dizziness, orthostatic hypotension, edema, psychosis (with visual hallucinations), cognitive effects, and drowsiness. Sudden sleep onset ("sleep attack") has also been reported in patients taking nonergot dopamine agonists (i.e., pramipexole and ropinirole). Edema and psychosis, which are more common than with the use of levodopa, may be more significant than mild dyskinesia, especially in older patients. The ADRs of dopamine agonists tend to occur most commonly during the first few weeks after initiation of treatment. Their incidence is higher when taken with L-dopa than when taken as monotherapy. In addition, the ergot-derived dopamine agonists (i.e., bromocriptine and pergolide) have associated risks of retroperitoneal and pulmonary fibrosis, heart valve fibrosis, and erythromelalgia (redness and burning pain in the distal extremities, usually the feet). These effects however, appear to reverse when the drug is withdrawn.

Contraindications and precautions. Caution is advised in prescribing dopamine agonists to elderly patients or patients who have already experienced hallucinations, confusion, or cognitive impairment.

Drug administration guidelines. Dopamine agonists may be taken alone (as monotherapy) or in combination with L-dopa. Generally, dopamine agonists are prescribed as monotherapy in the initial treatment of PD, then L-dopa is added after a variable time period (ranging from months to years) when the patient's symptoms cannot be controlled sufficiently. In patients already taking L-dopa, dopamine agonists should be initiated when patients are still taking a low to medium dosage of L-dopa (i.e., <600 mg/day) to avoid ADRs. In patients who do not respond to L-dopa, it is unlikely that they will respond to dopamine agonist monotherapy. When started, dopamine agonists must be given at a low dosage level and gradually titrated to therapeutic levels. In general, the combined use of dopamine agonists with L-dopa appears to result in a lower incidence of motor complications than L-dopa alone, because they allow a lower dosage of L-dopa to be used.

I. **Nonergot oral dopamine agonists** are newer medications, and are safer and more effective than the ergot dopamine agonists. Because the newer dopamine agonists, particularly ropinirole, are better tolerated and do not have the same risks of long-term complications as L-dopa therapy, ropinirole is often the first choice of treatment for PD.

- **Ropinirole (Requip)** is available as 0.25-, 0.5-, 1-, 2-, 3-, 4-, and 5-mg tablets. The initial dose is 0.25 mg, po, tid, on the first week, which is increased weekly up to 1.5 mg/day on the second week, 2.25 mg/day on the third week, then 3.0 mg/day on the fourth week. After the fourth week, if necessary, daily dosage may be increased by 1.5 mg/day on a weekly basis up to a dose of 9 mg/day, and then by up to 3 mg/day weekly to a total dose of 24 mg/day.
- **Pramipexole (Mirapex)** is available as 0.125-, 5-, 1-, and 1.5-mg tablets. The initial dose is 0.125 mg, po, tid, which is increased weekly by 0.125 or 0.25 mg/day, aiming for a therapeutic dose of 1.5 to 4.5 mg/day.

II. **Ergot-derived oral dopamine agonists**

- **Bromocriptine (Parlodel)** is available as 2.5-mg tablet and as 5-mg capsule. The initial dose is 1.25 mg, po, bid, with meals, increasing at 2–4-week intervals by 2.5 mg/day up to a maximum of 10–40 mg daily.
- **Pergolide (Permax)** is available as 0.05-, 0.25-, and 1-mg tablets. The initial dose is 0.05 mg for the first 2–3 days increasing by 0.10 or 0.15 mg/day every third day over the next 12 days. The dose can then be increased by 0.25 mg/day every third day, aiming for a therapeutic dosage of 0.75 mg to 3 mg/day, given in three divided doses.
- **Cabergoline** is not yet available in the United States.

b. ***Injectable dopamine agonist,*** **i.e., apomorphine (Apokyn)**, is nonergot. It is indicated for the acute, intermittent ("rescue") treatment of hypomobility, "off" episodes ("end-of-dose wearing off" and unpredictable "on–off" episodes) associated with advanced PD. It is available only in subcutaneous injection form at 10 mg/mL. Its onset of action is approximately 10 min, and lasts approximately 90 min (shorter than L-dopa's). It can be used up to 10 times per day. Its dosage must be titrated on the basis of effectiveness and tolerance, starting at 0.2 mL (the dose is always expressed in mL to avoid confusion) and up to a maximum recommended dose of 0.6 mL. Most common ADRs are nausea and vomiting. Hence, an antiemetic agent (trimethobenzamide, 300 mg, po, tid is preferred) is recommended for 3 days prior to beginning apomorphine and continued for at least during the first 2 months of therapy. Other ADRs include syncope, QT prolongation and potential for proarrhythymic effects, symptomatic hypotension, falls, hallucinations, falling asleep during activities of daily living (ADL), coronary events, and injection-site reactions. Apomorphine is contraindicated in patients concomitantly taking drugs of the $5HT_3$ antagonist class (including ondansetron, granisetron, dolasetron, palonosetron, and alosetron) because of reports of profound hypotension and loss of consciousness.

B. DOPAMINE REUPTAKE INHIBITORS include **amantadine (Symmetrel)**, which is also an antiviral agent. Aside from dopamine reuptake inhibition, other proposed mechanism of action of amantadine include release of dopamine from central neurons, blockade of N-methyl-D-aspartate (NMDA) receptors, and anticholinergic effects. Amantadine, which has a longer half-life than L-dopa, appears to act synergistically with L-dopa. Although it has a mild symptomatic effect on the motor symptoms of PD, it has a more significant effect on the reduction of dyskinesia associated with L-dopa therapy. In up to one-third of patients, however, amantadine may be ineffective for dyskinesia. ADRs of amantadine include confusion and memory problems, hallucinations, insomnia, agitation, difficulty concentrating, nausea, dry mouth, ankle swelling, skin mottling (livedo reticularis), and orthostatic hypotension. The usual dose is 100 mg, po, bid to qid. It is available in 100-mg capsules.

C. DOPAMINE BREAKDOWN INHIBITORS

1. Monoamine oxidase B (MAO-B) inhibitors prevents the conversion of the neurotoxin MPTP (1-methyl-4-phenyl-tetrahydropyridine) to MPP + (1-methyl-4-phenylpyridinium ion). MPP+, which causes oxidative damage and also generates free radicals directly, is associated with the development of experimental parkinsonism in animal models.

a. Selegiline (Eldepryl; Deprenyl) is indicated as an adjunct in the management of PD patients being treated with carbidopa/levodopa who exhibit deterioration in the quality of their response to this therapy. The use of selegiline as monotherapy is controversial. Aside from its antioxidant properties, it may also slow the progression of PD, particularly early in the course of the disease. ADRs of selegiline include headache, sweating, and insomnia, as well as dopaminergic reactions such as orthostatic hypotension, nausea, vomiting, and hallucinations. It should not be given to patients who are taking other MAO inhibitors and/or meperidine (Demerol). It should be used cautiously in patients taking serotonergic agents [e.g., sumatriptan (Imitrex)] or nonadrenergic agents [e.g., amitriptyline (Elavil)] and in patients with peptic ulcer disease and cardiovascular disease. There were reports that it may increase mortality in PD patients, but a recent meta-analysis failed to support this finding. Its dose is 5 mg, po, bid given at breakfast and lunch because later dosing can cause insomnia. At more than 10 mg/day, it can cause a hypertensive crisis when foods rich in tyramine are ingested. After 2–3 days of selegiline treatment, an attempt may be made to reduce the dose of carbidopa/levodopa (typically a reduction of 10 to 30% can be achieved). It is available in 5-mg capsule.

b. Rasagiline (Agilect) is still in clinical trials and not available in the United States.

2. Catechol O-methyltransferase (COMT) inhibitors prevent breakdown of dopamine and its precursor, L-dopa, thus enhancing the amount of L-dopa that reaches the CNS. This mechanism parallels that of carbidopa, but because a different enzyme is involved, COMT inhibitors can be taken concurrently with the carbidopa/levodopa combination (Sinemet). Two COMT inhibitors are approved in the United States, entacapone (Comtan) and tolcapone (Tasmar). Both are indicated as an adjunct to carbidopa/levodopa to decrease the duration of "wearing-off" time (i.e., the period of time at the end of dose of carbidopa/levidopa when PD symptoms are present) in PD patients with significant "off" time. Tolcapone is more effective than entacapone, reducing "off" time in clinical trials by 2–3 hours, vs. 1–2 hours for entacapone. Both usually allow reduction of carbidopa/levodopa dose, in the range of 20% to 30%. In addition to dyskinesia and ADRs related to dopaminergic reactions (such as orthostatic hypotension, nausea, vomiting, and hallucinations), they can commonly cause diarrhea. They may also turn urine bright yellow.

a. ***Entacapone (Comtan),*** a less potent COMT inhibitor than tolcapone, does not cross the BBB well, and has a very short half-life. Monitoring of liver function is recommended but not required. It is available in 200-mg tablet and is dosed at 200 mg with each carbidopa/levodopa dose up to a maximum of 8 times daily (1600 mg/day). Aside from dopaminergic reactions and diarrhea (which may be so severe in up to 5% of patients as to eliminate this drug as a treatment option), it can also cause severe rhabdomyolysis. A combination of carbidopa, levodopa, and entacapone in a single tablet (**Stalevo**) is also available as Stalevo 50 (with 12.5/50/200 mg of carbidopa/levodopa/entacapone), Stalevo 100 (with 25/100/200 mg of carbidopa/levodopa/entacapone), and Stalevo 150 (with 37.5/150/200 mg of carbidopa/levodopa/entacapone). In general, Stalevo is used as a substitute for patients already stabilized on equivalent doses of carbidopa/levodopa and entacapone. It may also be used as a way of adding entacapone in some patients who have been stabilized on a given dose of carbidopa/levodopa.

b. ***Tolcapone (Tasmar),*** a very potent COMT inhibitor with high lipid solubility, crosses the BBB well. Aside from dopaminergic reactions and diarrhea (which may be so severe in up to 15% of patients as to eliminate this drug as a treatment option), it was also reported to cause hepatocellular injury, acute fulminant hepatic necrosis, severe rhabdomyolysis, and deaths. Hence, it should only be used in PD patients whose symptoms cannot be adequately controlled without it. When prescribed, informed consent is required, including patient education about the restricted indications and the symptoms of hepatic dysfunction. Frequent liver function monitoring is required (every 2 weeks for the first year, then every 4 weeks for the next 6 months, and every 8 weeks thereafter). It is available in 100- and 200-mg tablets. The initial dose is 100 mg, po, tid, always as an adjunct to carbidopa/levodopa therapy. It may be increased up to 200 mg, po, tid. However, if a patient fails to show the expected incremental benefit on the 200-mg dose after a total of 3 weeks of treatment, it should be discontinued due to potential risk of liver failure.

D. OTHER DRUGS THAT IMPROVE THE SYMPTOMS OF PD BY OTHER MEANS

1. **Anticholinergics** are generally used for treating mild tremors of early PD. They have little effect on rigidity and bradykinesia. Their use is often limited by their ADRs (such as dry mouth, urinary retention, constipation, memory and thinking impairment, confusion, hallucination, delirium, sedation, and narrow-angle glaucoma), especially in older people. In patients who have been taking anticholinergics regularly, it is extremely difficult to withdraw these drugs. They include:

a. ***Trihexyphenidyl (Artane)*** is available in 2- and 5-mg tablets and as 2 mg/5 mL elixir. The starting dose is 1 mg, po, on the first day, increased by 2-mg increments at intervals of 3–5 days, until a total of 6–10 mg/day (given bid or tid at mealtimes).

b. ***Benztropine (Cogentin)*** is available in 0.5-, 1-, and 2-mg tablets. The starting dose is 0.5–1 mg, po, hs, increased gradually to 4–6 mg/day (given bid or tid).

c. ***Procyclidine (Kemadrin)*** is available in 5-mg tablet. The starting dose is 2.5 mg, po, tid, after meals, and is increased gradually to 5 mg, po, tid or qid.

d. ***Ethopropazine (Parsitan)*** is available in 50- and 100-mg tablets. The starting dose is 50 mg, po, qd/bid up to 600 mg/day (given bid or tid).

2. **Botulinum toxin** type A (Botox; see Chapter 5.4, section III.D.2.a.3) may be useful for alleviating the blepharospasm and limb dystonias that are frequently associated with PD even when other manifestations are successfully controlled by medications.

3. Other drugs that affect motor tone and control, including diphenhydramine (see section V.D.2.f), **benzodiazepines** (see section V.C.1), **anticonvulsants** (see section IV), and **antispasticity agents** [e.g., baclofen (Lioresal) see Chapter 5.4, section III.D.1.a], should be used with caution in patients with PD. For example, baclofen is effective in managing hemifacial spasm and possibly blepharospasm associated with PD, but it may lower the seizure threshold and produce muscle weakness.

Further reading

Acute Pain Management Guideline Panel: *Clinical practice guideline: acute pain management*, AHCPR Pub. No. 92-0032, Rockville, MD, Feb, 1992, Agency for Health Care Policy and Research.

Ansell J, Hirsch J, Poller L, *et al.*: The pharmacology and management of the vitamin K antagonists. The Seventh ACCP Conference on Antithrombotic and Thrombolytic Therapy. *Chest Suppl* 126(3):204S–232S, 2004.

Aronoff GM, editor: *Evaluation and treatment of chronic pain*, Baltimore, 1992, Williams & Wilkins.

Bjorkman DJ: Nonsteroidal anti-inflammatory drug-induced gastrointestinal injury. *Am J Med* 101 (suppl 1A):25S–32S, 1996.

Brooks PM, Day RO: Nonsteroidal antiinflammatory drugs differences and similarities. *N Engl J Med* 324:1716–1725, 1991.

Buller HR, Agnelli G, Hull RD, *et al.*: Antithrombotic therapy for venous thromboembolic disease. The Seventh ACCP Conference on Antithrombotic and Thrombolytic Therapy. *Chest Suppl* 126(3):401S–428S, 2004.

Cardenas DD, McLean Jr A: Psychopharmacologic management of traumatic brain injury. *Phys Med and Rehab Clin North Am* 3(2):273–290, 1992.

Chuang C, Waters C: Initial therapy of Parkinson's disease. In Samuels MA, Feske SK, editors: *Office Practice of Neurology*, ed 2, Philadelphia, 2003, Churchill Livingstone, pp. 743–748.

Consensus Development Conference: Osteoporosis Prevention, Diagnosis, and Therapy, *NIH Consensus Statement* 17(1):1–36, March 27–29, 2000.

Dalen J, editor: *Venous thromboembolism*, New York, 2003, Marcel Dekker.

Dean BZ, Williams FH, King JC, Goddard MJ: Pain rehabilitation. 4. Therapeutic options in pain management. *Arch Phys Med Rehabil* Suppl 75:21–30, 1994.

FitzGerald GA: Coxibs and cardiovascular disease. *N Engl J Med* 351:1709–1711, 2004.

Frishman WH, Lerner RG, Klein MD, *et al.*: Antiplatelet and antithrombotic drugs. In Frishman WH, Sonnenblick EH, Sica DA, editors: *Cardiovascuar pharmocotherapeutics*, ed 2, New York, 2003, McGraw Hill, pp. 259–299.

Geerts WH, Graham FP, Heit JA, *et al.*: Prevention of venous thromboembolism. The Seventh ACCP Conference on Antithrombotic and Thrombolytic Therapy. *Chest Suppl* 126(3):338S–400S, 2004.

Hamill RJ, Rowlingson JC, editors: *Handbook of critical care pain management*, New York, 1994, McGraw-Hill.

Hardman JG, Limbird LE, editors: *Goodman and Gilman's the pharmacological basis of therapeutics*, ed 10, New York, 2001, McGraw-Hill.

Hirsch J, Raschke: Heparin and low-molecular weight heparin: The Seventh ACCP Conference on Antithrombotic and Thrombolytic Therapy. *Chest Suppl* 126(3):188S–203S, 2004.

Kasper DL, Braunwald E, Fauci AS, *et al.*, editors: *Harrison's principles of internal medicine*, ed 16, New York, 2005, McGraw-Hill.

Koller WC, Hutton JC, Tolosa E, *et al.*: Immediate-release and controlled-release carbidopa/levodopa in Parkinson's disease: A 5-year randomized multicenter study. *Neurology* 53:1012–1019, 1999.

Miller MA, Burnett DM, McElliott JM: Congenital and acquired brain injury. 3. Rehabilitation interventions: cognitive, behavioral, and community reentry. *Arch Phys Med Rehabil* 84(3) suppl 1:S12–S17, 2003.

Mysiw WJ, Jandel, ME: The agitated brain injured patient. Part 2: Pathophysiology and treatment. *Arch Phys Med Rehabil* 78:213–220, 1997.

Physicians' desk reference, ed 59, Montvale, NJ, 2005, Thomson PDR.

Portenoy RK, Kanner RM, editors: *Pain management: theory and practice*, Philadelphia, 1996, FA Davis.
Salem M, Tainsh RE, JR., Bromberg J, *et al.*: Perioperative glucocorticoid coverage: a reassessment 42 years after emergence of a problem. *Ann Surg* 219:416–425, 1994.
The Publications Committee for the Trial of ORG 10172 in Acute Stroke Treatment (TOAST) Investigators: low molecular weight heparinoid, ORG 10172 (Danaparoid), and outcome after acute ischemic stroke. A randomized controlled trial. *JAMA* 279(16):1265–1272, 1998.
Tollison CD, Satterthwaite JR, Tollison JW, editors: *Practical pain management*, ed 3, Philadelphia, 2002, Lippincott, Williams & Wilkins.
Topol EJ: Arthritis medicines and cardiovascular events – "House of coxibs." *JAMA* 293(3):366–368, 2005.
United States Food and Drug Administration: COX-2 selective and non-selective non-steroidal anti-inflammatory drugs (NSAIDs). Available at http://www.fda.gov/cder/drug/infopage/cox2. Accessed May 15, 2005.
Wall PD, Melzack R, editors: *Textbook of pain*, ed 4, Edinburgh, 1999, Churchill Livingstone.
Worldwide Education and Awareness for Movement Disorders (WE MOVE): *Parkinson's disease*. Available at http://www.wemove.org/par. Accessed March 30, 2005.

CHAPTER 4.9
Joint and soft tissue injections

This chapter deals with joint and soft tissue injections for diagnostic purposes (e.g., arthrocentesis and joint arthrography) as well as for therapeutic purposes (e.g., injection of corticosteroid or combination of corticosteroid with local anesthetic agents into the joint, bursa, and tendon for the relief of inflammation and pain and for the restoration of joint functions). Most injection therapies do not have well-controlled trials but are based on anecdotal and empirical evidence. When performed judiciously by a skilled practitioner, joint and soft tissue injections are relatively safe procedures. They are considered adjuncts to the overall management of musculoskeletal disorders and are generally performed after other conservative methods (e.g., physical modalities, oral analgesics, or anti-inflammatory agents) have failed.

I. Supplies

A. **"INTRA-ARTICULAR" CORTICOSTEROIDS** are suspensions of insoluble particles whose anti-inflammatory effect is profound only where the material is deposited. It can be injected into acutely inflamed joints or soft tissues (e.g., synovitis, bursitis, tenosynovitis, epicondylitis, and adhesive capsulitis) of patients with rheumatoid arthritis, spondyloarthropathies, gout, pseudogout, systemic lupus erythematosus, and other forms of arthritis. Their usefulness in patients with osteoarthritis remains controversial. Many clinicians believe that they are beneficial in osteoarthritis patients in whom an effusion can be identified or from whom synovial fluid can be aspirated.

Mechanism of action (MOA). The exact MOA by which corticosteroids inhibit local joint or soft tissue inflammation is not fully known. Pharmacologically, corticosteroids are known to inhibit the process of chemotaxis, decrease capillary permeability, decrease vasodilation, prevent release of arachidonic acid and its metabolites, decrease fibroblast and collagen deposition, stabilize lysosomal membranes, and inhibit macrophage function. For details about the MOA of corticosteroids, see Chapter 4.8, section III.

Adverse drug reactions (ADRs). The injection of corticosteroid into joints or soft tissues seldom causes permanent deleterious effects when performed using accepted guidelines. The ADRs (and prevalence) include postinjection flare [2–5%; attributed to the microcrystalline structure of the steroids or joint trauma of injection; joint appears inflamed or even infected within 2–4 hours after injection and subsides spontaneously in 24–72 hours; give supportive care, ice, and nonsteroidal anti-inflammatory drugs (NSAIDs)]; steroid arthropathy of weight-bearing joints (0.8% occurring after multiple steroid injections; can lead to aseptic osteonecrosis); tendon rupture (less than 1%); facial flushing (less than 1%); benign but uncosmetic skin changes (less than 1%; e.g., depigmentation, scarring, and skin depression as a result of atrophy of the underlying subcutaneous tissues; may remit over 5 years); and infection (less than 0.1%; avoided by sterile technique). Rare complications include transient paresis of the injected limb, hypersensitivity, asymptomatic periarticular calcification in finger joints, and sickle cell crisis. If injections are frequently repeated (especially using long-lasting corticosteroids) or if the patient is receiving concomitant oral corticosteroid therapy, there is the possibility of systemic corticosteroid effects and suppression of the pituitary–adrenal axis (see Chapter 4.8, section III for the systemic effects of corticosteroids).

Contraindications and precautions for corticosteroid injections include infection (systemic and local), bleeding diathesis, uncontrolled brittle diabetes, extreme obesity, severe joint destruction (e.g., osteoporosis) or soft tissue destruction, traumatic arthritis secondary to fracture through the joint, unstable joints, joint prosthesis, inaccessible joints, soft tissue or bony tumors at or near the underlying joint, failure to respond to previous injections, and hypersensitivity to the corticosteroid or its vehicle. Patients taking an anticoagulant may be injected carefully after checking the prothrombin time and informing the patient of its risks and benefits.

Drug administration guidelines. The "intra-articular" corticosteroid preparations are shown in Table 4.9-1. They have low hormonal side-effects and do not dissipate rapidly from the joint. None of these preparations appears to have any superiority over another; however, triamcinolone hexacetonide (Aristospan) is the least water-soluble preparation with the longest duration of action within the peripheral joint space (it also causes less postinjection flare). The choice of a particular corticosteroid preparation depends on its duration of action, solubility, potency, onset of action, and intended purpose. The more insoluble the preparation, the longer is its duration of action, but the longer is the delay in its onset of action. To overcome the lack of immediate response, some clinicians combine short-acting with delayed-acting steroid preparations, and others suggest the addition of a short-acting anesthetic agent (e.g., lidocaine) to form insoluble materials. The combination of corticosteroid and anesthetic agents, however, has been associated with crystal-like formations in the joint, which can cause postinjection flares. Crystal-like formations are attributed to the preservatives (e.g., methylparaben, propylparaben, and phenol) in the anesthetic agents reacting with the steroid; hence, preservative-free anesthetic agents must be used.

For long-term suppression of an inflammatory process such as rheumatoid arthritis, the low-solubility and intermediate- to long-acting triamcinolone hexacetonide (Aristospan) or triamcinolone acetonide (Kenalog) would be preferable. If the patient's condition requires a long-acting agent with faster relief of symptoms, the betamethasome phosphate and acetate preparation (Celestone Soluspan) would be preferable. The short onset from the phosphate preparation and the long duration from the acetate preparation make this a desirable choice. For more rapid onset of therapy, the shorter acting methylprednisolone acetate (Depo-Medrol) would be the drug of choice. Aristospan, Kenalog, and Celestone seem to remain within the joint cavity longer than Depo-Medrol, and their systemic effect is limited because of their low serum levels and release over a prolonged period of time.

The number of injections per joint or soft tissue should be limited so as to avoid joint damage (steroid arthropathy) and soft tissue damage. Large (e.g., weight-bearing) joints should not be injected more than three times per joint per year up to a maximum of 10 cumulative injections. Small joints should be injected less often, i.e., not more than twice per joint per year up to a maximum of four cumulative injections. Although multiple joint injections interfere with normal cartilage protein synthesis, it has been shown that patients with long-standing rheumatoid arthritis who do not receive intra-articular corticosteroids have joint disuse and decreased function much sooner than those who receive the injections. For pain reduction in osteoarthritis as well as an adjunct in the mobilization of the adhesive capsulitis, injections at the rate of one every 4–6 weeks for a maximum of three injections is the most commonly accepted regimen.

Table 4.9-1 Corticosteroid preparations for joint and soft tissue injection and their dosages for different joints

"Intra-articular" corticosteroids (*brand name*)	Solubility	Preparation (mg/mL)	Hip (mg)	Knee/shoulder (mg)	Wrist/elbow/ankle (mg)	Small joints (mg)
I. Short-acting*						
Hydrocortisone acetate (*Hydrocortone*)	High	25	30–40	25–40	12.5–37.5	10–25
II. Intermediate-acting†						
Prednisolone sodium phosphate (*Hydeltrasol*)	Intermediate	20	15–20	10–20	5–10	5
Methylprednisolone acetate (*Depo-Medrol*)	Intermediate	20, 40, 80	40–100	20–80	10–40	4–10
Triamcinolone diacetate (*Aristocort*)	Low to intermediate	25, 40	30–40	20–40	10–25	5–15
III. Intermediate/long-acting‡						
Triamcinolone hexacetonide (*Aristospan*)	Low	20	15–20	10–20	5–10	1–5
Triamcinolone acetonide (*Kenalog*)	Low	10, 40	20–40	20–40	5–10	5
IV. Long-acting§						
Dexamethasone acetate (*Decadron-LA*)	Low	8	4–6	2–4	1–2	0.5–1.5
Betamethasone phosphate and acetate (*Celestone soluspan*)	Low	6	6–12	6–9	3–6	3

* *Short half-life = 8–12 hours.*
† *Intermediate half-life = 12–36 hours.*
‡ *Intermediate/long half-life = 12–72 hours.*
§ *Long half-life = 36–72 hours.*

B. LOCAL ANESTHETICS without epinephrine are usually combined with "intra-articular" corticosteroids for injection into the joint and soft tissues. This combination provides a larger volume of injectable material with which to bathe the joint more adequately, in addition to providing immediate (although temporary) pain relief. Some clinicians prefer to use corticosteroids alone without anesthetic agents because the anesthetic effect can obscure the exact site of the needle tip (on which these clinicians rely to determine the point of maximal tenderness for injection of the corticosteroid).

The local anesthetics commonly used in combination with corticosteroids include short-acting agents [e.g., 0.5, 1.0, or 2% lidocaine (Xylocaine) or procaine (Novacain)] and longer-acting agents [e.g., 0.25 or 0.5% bupivacaine (Marcaine, Sensorcaine)]. Lidocaine and bupivacaine may be combined to obtain an early onset of action with prolonged anesthesia. The anesthetic dosages vary widely with the size of the joint. Usually, the smaller joints, such as the acromioclavicular, sternoclavicular, and elbow joints, would take 1–2 mL of 1% lidocaine combined with the corticosteroid. The glenohumeral, knee, and hip joints would take 2–4 mL of anesthetic agent. Bupivacaine is often preferable for nonweight-bearing joints, such as the shoulder, elbow, acromioclavicular, and sternoclavicular joints, as long as these joints can be somewhat immobilized for several hours. Lidocaine injection is preferred for weight-bearing joints, such as the knee, because its duration is much shorter and, thus, the joint is subject to less postinjection trauma by noncompliant patients. Longer-acting anesthetics should not be used on noncompliant patients as they may "feel cured" and proceed to use the anesthetized joint indiscriminately. The ADRs, contraindications, and precautions of local anesthetics are discussed in Chapter 5.10, section VI.E.2.

C. STERILE NEEDLES range from gauge 16 to 24 (for hip, knee, and shoulder joints), gauge 20 to 22 (for wrist, ankle, elbow, and facet joints), and gauge 25 to 27 (for small and superficial joints). For aspiration of inflamed joint or soft tissues with thick fluids, a large-bore needle may be necessary. For patient comfort, a gauge 25, 1–1.5 inch-long needle should be used; however, when a needle >1.5 inch-long is used or when the joint is to be aspirated, a gauge 22 needle is used.

D. STERILE SYRINGES range from 3 to 50 mL. Choice of syringe depends on the joint and amount of effusion to be tapped.

E. OTHER SUPPLIES include aseptic skin preparation materials (sterile gloves, Betadine solution, alcohol solution, sterile gauze pads, and Band-Aids) and tubes for synovial fluid analysis (e.g., chemistry tube for glucose, hematology tube with ethylenediaminetetraacetic acid or EDTA for cell and differential count, sterile tube for cultures and smears, heparinized tube for crystal analysis, and cytology bottle if neoplasm is suspected). Make sure that the heparinized tubes do not use powdered anticoagulants as these may interfere with crystal identification.

II. General injection techniques

A. INFORMED CONSENT. Prior to the procedure, the patient must sign an informed consent form, which should include the possible benefits, common side-effects, and risks of the procedure, as well as alternative treatments if the procedure is not pursued.

B. MEDICATION PREPARATION. Single-dose vials are preferred as they eliminate the possibility of contamination from previous withdrawal of steroid or anesthetic from the vial. When an anesthetic and steroid are given together, the mixing should be done in the injection syringe. If multiple-dose vials are used, draw the steroid in first, followed by the anesthetic so the anesthetic will not be introduced inadvertently into the vial of steroid. The mixture must be used immediately and any unused portion must be discarded.

C. SKIN PREPARATION. Use universal precautions by wearing gloves to prevent contact with blood-borne pathogens. Select the site of injection based on available bony landmarks. Bony landmarks are used because they are more stable than soft tissue landmarks. Using an indelible felt pen, carefully outline the site with a circle (as a target) at least 3 cm in diameter. A less preferable alternative (if a felt pen is unavailable) is to use skin markings made by fingernail pressure. Clean the area with three swipes of povidone-iodine (Betadine) and one swipe of 70% isopropyl alcohol, taking care not to erase the markings. The antiseptics should be allowed to dry for about 2 minutes to maximally reduce cutaneous bacteria and to prevent the injection of the antiseptic into the body (povidone–iodine can be toxic to the cells when injected). The presence of hair should not alter the method of skin decontamination. Hair shaving should be avoided as it increases wound infection rate (if absolutely necessary, hair may be clipped or depilatory cream may be used). After skin decontamination, the prepared area should not be touched. With this technique, no drapes or sterile room is required.

D. POSITIONING. Before, during, and after the injection procedure, both patient and practitioner should be properly positioned. The patient should be positioned so that the injection site is accessible and he or she is as comfortable as possible. The recumbent procedure is preferred for comfort and safety. If the patient is seated, make sure the patient can be supported in case of fainting. The practitioner should also be comfortable and, if needed, the table should be raised to minimize bending or reaching.

E. GENERAL INJECTION TECHNIQUES. The syringe is gripped close to its tip like a pencil (between the thumb and index finger) with the hypothenar part of the hand resting on the patient (and only the fingers moving) for maximum control. If a longer needle is used (e.g., 3.5 inch), the bore of the needle may be gripped with sterile gloves. Inject an anesthetic [e.g., 1% lidocaine (Xylocaine)] into the epidermis (creating a small wheal) using a 0.75- to 1.0-inch, 25- to 30-gauge needle with 1 mL syringe. If the patient is particularly apprehensive about the injection procedure, topical anesthetics such as vapocoolant spray (e.g., ethyl chloride or fluorimethane) or EMLA cream (see Chapter 5.10, section VI.E.2.e.2; EMLA cream must be applied at least 1 hour before injection) may be applied on the skin. If the joint is distended with fluid or if the joint is superficial (e.g., acromioclavicular, sternoclavicular, and interphalangeal joints), use a topical anesthetic rather than raising a skin wheal for skin anesthesia. After raising a skin wheal, use another needle (e.g., 1.5-inch, 18–22 gauge) attached to an anesthetic-filled syringe and insert it through the wheal. Stop and aspirate every 0.5 cm and, if no clear or bloody aspirate is drawn up, inject another small bolus of anesthetic. For proper aspiration, the needle must be rotated 180° (because of the beveled tip of the needle) and then reaspirated.

When the joint capsule is entered (or when the needle is placed at the tender site of soft tissues), the hub of the needle should be clasped securely with a clean (or sterile) hemostat (an alternative is to use an intravenous catheter extension). The anesthetic-filled syringe is then removed, and it is replaced with an aspirating syringe (for arthrocentesis) or a syringe with the injectate (for soft tissue injections). For arthrocentesis, the joint may be "milked" by using steady pressure with the opposite hand on the joint itself and kneading the skin toward the site of aspiration. After all of the available fluid is aspirated, a separate syringe containing the injectate is attached to the needle. The hub of the needle should not be grasped for syringe exchange with the fingers so as to prevent needle shaft contamination.

When depositing the injectable material, use slow, steady pressure on the plunger. If resistance is met during the time of the injection, the needle should be withdrawn up to the subcutaneous tissue (without exiting the skin) and then redirected in 5° increments (otherwise it will just bend the needle). The syringe is then reaspirated (make sure blood or air is not drawn up) prior to reinjection. If corticosteroid is injected, a slight amount of lidocaine is used to flush the needle before withdrawal to avoid leaving a needle tract of cortisteroid through the adipose tissue and skin, which may cause depigmentation or subcutaneous necrosis. After the injection, the needle is quickly withdrawn and mild pressure is applied with a sterile gauze pad followed by a Band-Aid to prevent bleeding. Before getting up, the patient is assessed carefully for vasovagal response, and appropriate measures are taken to prevent any secondary harm, e.g., falling as a result of transient hypotension. Patients should also be advised to rest the joint (especially weight-bearing joints) for at least 1 day to prevent joint destruction because of premature resumption of vigorous exercise.

III. Specific injection procedures

A. JOINT INJECTION TECHNIQUES for arthrocentesis and for therapeutic intra-articular injections are the same. In arthrocentesis the joint is aspirated and the synovial fluid is sent for analysis as part of the initial evaluation and to rule out superimposed infection vs. crystal-induced arthritis in an already diseased joint (especially in patients with monoarthritis). If joint infection is strongly suspected (e.g., purulent synovial fluid), corticosteroid should not be injected until the final culture report is back. However, if the possibility of joint infection is slight, steroid injection may be given after aspirating the joint for culture (injecting an infected joint may delay the diagnosis but not necessarily cause increased joint damage). The aim of therapeutic joint injection is to relieve pain by drainage of an effusion, installation of medication, and drainage of aseptic joints or hemarthroses (after first correcting coagulation disorders).

1. Upper limb

a. Glenohumeral joint. The patient is seated with hands in the lap and the shoulder muscles relaxed.

I. **Anterior approach.** Palpate the glenohumeral joint by placing one's fingers between the coracoid process and the humeral head. Internally rotate the shoulder to feel the inward turning of the humeral head and the joint space, which can be felt as a groove just lateral to the coracoid. Insert a 20- or 22-gauge needle lateral to the coracoid and avoid the thoracoacromial artery (which runs on the medial aspect of the coracoid). Direct the needle dorsally and medially into the joint space, then slightly superiorly to avoid the neurovascular bundle.

II. **Posterior approach.** Place the patient's ipsilateral hand on the opposite scapula (as if hooking a bra) to maximally internally rotate the shoulder. Place a finger posteriorly along the acromion and insert a 20- or 22-gauge needle about 1 cm inferior to the posterolateral tip of the acromion and direct it anteriorly and medially (aimed toward the coracoid process, which can be anteriorly marked with the index finger). This approach is usually used for adhesive capsulitis and synovitis or chronic osteoarthritis.

b. Acromioclavicular (AC) joint. With the patient sitting or supine and the shoulder propped on a pillow, locate the tip of the distal clavicle and insert a 25-gauge needle either from a superior angle or an anterosuperior angle into the AC joint space (located about 0.5 cm medial to the tip of the acromion). The AC joint may be injected for diagnostic purposes (using local anesthetics) to delineate the source of pain in the shoulder. A vapocoolant spray or EMLA cream may be used for superficial skin anesthesia.

c. ***Sternoclavicular (SC) joint***. The patient is supine or seated. The SC joint is palpated just lateral to the sternal notch where the clavicle attaches to the sternum. It cannot be readily entered by a needle, hence a 25- or 27-gauge needle is superficially inserted adjacent to it (taking care not to hit the brachiocephalic veins, which are immediately posterior to the SC joint). A vapocoolant spray or EMLA cream may be used for superficial skin anesthesia (the EMLA cream must be applied at least 1 hour before injection).

d. ***Elbow joint***. Do not use the medial approach (because of the potential for ulnar nerve injury) or the anterior approach (because of the hazard to the biceps tendon, brachioradialis tendon, median nerve, radial nerve, and branches of the radial artery). The position of the elbow is between 50 and 90° of flexion with the palm facing the patient.
   I. **Posterolateral approach**. Palpate the triangular bony landmark consisting of the olecranon process, the head of the radius, and the lateral epicondyle. Insert a 22- or 25-gauge needle perpendicular to the elbow joint just anterior to the center of this triangle and posterior to the head of the radius.
   II. **Posterior approach**. Palpate the posterior olecranon and the lateral olecranon groove located just posterior to the lateral epicondyle. Insert a 22- or 25-gauge needle above the superior aspect of and lateral to the olecranon.

e. ***Wrist joint***. The hand and wrist are relaxed in a slightly flexed position (e.g., over a rolled towel). The approach used should be based on the area of maximal point tenderness or site of inflammation and specific anatomic structures underlying the region to be infiltrated. After joint injection, medication diffusion can be facilitated by range-of-motion exercises.
   I. **Radial or dorsal approach**. Palpate the joint space at the distal edge of the radius just medial to the extensor pollicis longus tendon and insert a 22- or 25-gauge needle perpendicularly into the joint space from the dorsal aspect (midpoint of radius and ulna). The dorsal or radial approach is preferred to avoid any major arteries, veins, and nerves.
   II. **Dorsal snuffbox approach**. Palpate the joint space between the edge of the distal radius and the carpal bones. Then insert a 22- or 25-gauge needle into the joint space dorsally and just medial to the anatomic snuffbox.
   III. **Ulnar approach**. Palpate the joint space just distal to the lateral ulnar margin and insert a 22- or 25-gauge needle directed in a volar and radial direction.

f. ***Intercarpal joints***. Connect an imaginary line between the ulnar and radial styli to define the proximal row of carpal bones. Insert a 25-gauge needle into the intercarpal joint space at the point of maximal tenderness. Fluoroscopic guidance may be needed for precise location of a specific carpal joint, which has its own synovial cavity.

g. ***Carpometacarpal (CMC) joint of the thumb***. Hold the thumb in slight flexion and insert a 25-gauge needle into the point of maximal tenderness from the dorsal aspect of the radial side of the CMC joint. Avoid the radial artery and the extensor pollicis brevis tendon.

h. ***Metacarpophalangeal (MCP) joint of the thumb and fingers***. Have the patient make a fist so the knuckles protrude. Palpate the MCP joint, which is distal to the apex of the knuckles. Insert a 25-gauge needle into the joint space distally at about a 60° angle (not directly laterally or directly superiorly) to avoid the digital nerve, artery, and vein and the extensor tendon apparatus on the superior aspect of each digit.

i. ***Interphalangeal (IP) joints (proximal and distal)***. Use a vapocoolant spray or EMLA cream for superficial skin anesthesia. Palpate the dorsal borders of the IP joint (just distal to the skin crease) and insert a 25- or 27-gauge needle from the dorsal aspect and directed slightly distally into the area just beyond the apex of the IP joint. Inject less than 2 mL of medication into the adjacent subcutaneous tissue where it can eventually be transported into the inflamed capsule and synovium. Postinjection splinting of the affected joint may be needed for resolution of the inflammation.

2. **Facet joint injection**. The patient is prone (with pillow under the hip). Insert a 22-gauge, 3.5-inch needle into the appropriate facet joint under fluoroscopic or computed tomography scan guidance. Inject 1–2 mL of local anesthetic followed by 20–25 mg of triamcinolone diacetate (Aristocort) or, in the presence of a synovial cyst at the facet joint, the facet joint may be aspirated.

3. **Lower limb**

a. ***Hip joint***. Fluoroscopic guidance is necessary to confirm needle placement because the hip joint is deep and difficult to infiltrate or aspirate. To verify needle placement in the hip joint bursa, a small injection of radiopaque dye may be necessary. An 18- to 20-gauge, 3–4-inch long (7.6–10.2 cm) needle is used, and depending on joint integrity, 2–4 mL of medication may be injected. A major potential complication of hip injection of corticosteroid is avascular necrosis.

   I. **Anterior approach**. The anterior approach is preferred. Position the patient in a supine position with the lower limb externally rotated. Palpate the area 2 cm distal to the anterior superior iliac spine and 3 cm lateral to the palpated femoral artery at a level corresponding to the superior margins of the greater trochanter. Insert the needle at an angle 60° posteromedially through the tough capsular ligaments into the bone, then slightly withdraw it.

   II. **Lateral approach**. The patient lies on the uninvolved side with the leg externally rotated. Insert the needle just anterior to the greater trochanter of the femur and walk it medially along the neck of the femur until the joint is reached.

b. ***Sacroiliac joint***. The sacroiliac joint should be injected under fluoroscopic guidance.

c. ***Knee***. Aside from corticosteroids, the knee may be injected with hyaluronate (Hyalgan, 2 mL or 20 mg each knee, once a week at a weekly interval for a total of 3–5 injections) or hylan G-F 20 (Synvisc, 2 mL or 16 mg each knee, once a week at weekly interval for a total of 3 injections) for the treatment of osteoarthritic knee pain. The patient is positioned supine with the knee comfortably extended to relax the quadriceps muscle (a small pillow may be used under the knee). Grasp the patella and rock it gently side to side to determine adequate relaxation. A 19-gauge needle (or a larger bore needle if the effusion is thick) is inserted at the point of maximal effusion or through one of the following approaches:

   I. **Medial approach**. The medial approach is generally easier for aspiration. Slightly displace the patella laterally to increase the medial gap between the patella and femur. The traditional route of entry is through the medial side of the patella in a direction parallel to the plane of the posterior surface of the patella midway between the superior and inferior margins of the patella. However, this traditional point of entry leaves very little room between the femur and patella, hence the needle commonly hits the joint surfaces, causing the patient to contract the quadriceps muscle in pain, further narrowing the joint space. An alternative route is to insert the needle medial to the patella just superior to the superior margin of the patella on the medial aspect of the knee (this site should be low enough to allow direction of the needle below the quadriceps tendon). The medication is then easily introduced into the suprapatellar pouch, which is contiguous with the synovial cavity and which lies below the quadriceps tendon (thus there is no undue pain or contraction of the quadriceps muscle).

II. **Lateral approach**. It uses similar traditional and alternative routes of entry as that of the medial approach except that the patella is displaced medially to increase the lateral gap between the patella and femur, and the needle is inserted lateral to the patella.

III. **Anterior approach** is used only if the patient cannot extend the knee, if the patient is obese, or if there are osteophytes around the patella. The knee is flexed to 90° and the needle is inserted just inferior to the inferior patellar pole either from the lateral or medial side of the patellar tendon. The needle is then advanced parallel to the tibial plateau until the joint space is entered. The risk of puncturing the articular cartilage is much higher, as is the risk to the infrapatellar fat pad for necrosis. Moreover, it is hard to obtain synovial fluid from this position because the fluid migrates posteriorly during knee flexion.

d. ***Ankle mortise***. The foot is positioned at about a 45° angle of plantar flexion.

I. **Anteromedial approach**. Insert a 22-gauge needle about 1 inch proximal and lateral to the distal end of the medial malleolus with the flexor hallucis longus tendon just lateral to this point. Direct the needle 45° posteriorly, slightly upward, and laterally.

II. **Anterolateral approach**. Insert a 22-gauge needle about 0.5 inch proximal and medial to the distal end of the lateral malleolus. Direct the needle 45° posteriorly, slightly upward, and medially.

e. ***Subtalar joint***. The patient is prone with feet extending over the end of the examination table so that the ankle is in the neutral position. Insert a 22-gauge needle halfway between a line drawn from the most prominent aspect of the lateral malleolus posteriorly to the Achilles tendon and parallel to the plantar aspect of the neutrally positioned foot. Direct the needle toward a point inferior and medial to the medial malleolus.

f. ***Intertarsal joint***. A 22-gauge needle is used and as with intercarpal bones, fluoroscopic needle guidance is needed.

g. ***Metatarsophalangeal joints***. Insert a 22-gauge needle from the dorsal aspect with the toes plantar flexed and the needle directed distal to the largest palpable part of the joint. The needle should not be inserted laterally or superiorly, but between these two planes to avoid essential structures.

h. ***Interphalangeal joints***. The technique is similar to those used for IP joint injection of the hands (see section III.A.1.i).

B. BURSAL INJECTION TECHNIQUES. Bursae are synovial-like tissues that form fluid-filled sacs and are usually located adjacent to joints. Their function is to reduce irritation at friction-prone areas between muscles, tendon, skin, and bone. They can get inflamed during repetitive activities as a result of poor body mechanics or from direct trauma. As with joint injections, bursal injections serve both diagnostic and therapeutic roles. A local anesthetic may initially be injected alone for diagnostic purposes (i.e., to determine the source of pain). If the bursa is aspirated, the fluid should be screened for increased leukocytes, Gram-negative or positive bacteria, or crystals. When a septic bursa has been ruled out, corticosteroid and anesthetic agents may be injected therapeutically into the inflamed bursa. The lowest effective dose is used and the volume injected is adjusted to the size of the bursa (see Table 4.9-2). Corticosteroid is usually given about 14–21 days after bursal injury and should be avoided during the first 7 days as this may theoretically inhibit the healing process. After bursal injection, additional treatment should include ice, NSAIDs, soft tissue mobilization, stretching and strengthening exercises, as well as proper body mechanics. In severe or recurrent bursitis, surgical incision and drainage may be needed.

Table 4.9-2 Guidelines for bursal injections

Bursae*	Anesthetic volume† (mL)	Corticosteroid volume† (mL)	Needle‡ length (inch)
Subacromial	4.0–6.0	0.5–1.0	1.5
Trochanteric	4.5–9.0	0.5–1.0	1.5–3.5
Iliopectineal	4.0–4.5	0.5–1.0	3.5
Ischial	2.5–4.0	0.5–1.0	3.5
Anserine	2.5–4.5	0.25–0.5	1.5
Prepatellar	Variable§	0.5–1.0	1.5

** Fluoroscopic guidance may be necessary to increase accuracy of bursa injection. A bursogram may be a useful tool, increasing the diagnostic and therapeutic value of injections.*

† The volume refers to the capacity of the bursa, and the clinician should select a corticosteroid or anesthetic concentration appropriate for the bursal volume.

‡ A gauge 20 to 22 needle is usually used but the clinician may prefer an 18-gauge needle initially for aspiration if gelatinous fluid is anticipated and then change to a finer gauge for instillation of pharmacologic agents.

§ The prepatellar bursa is often multiloculated, and its capacity may vary.

From: Olsen NK, Press JM, Young JL: Soft tissue injections. In Lennard TA, editor: Pain procedures in clinical practice, Philadelphia, 2000, Hanley & Belfus, p. 145, with permission.

1. **Upper limb**

a. ***Subacromial (subdeltoid) bursitis*** usually coexists with or is secondary to rotator cuff tendinitis or shoulder impingement syndrome. The subacromial bursa rests on the supraspinatus tendon and is covered by the acromion, the coracoacromial ligament, and the deltoid muscle. Although an anterior, posterior, or lateral approach may be used, the posterolateral approach is usually easier to perform. Palpate the tip of the acromion and insert a 25-gauge, 1.5-inch needle approximately 1.5 cm beneath it and superior to the humeral head. Initially inject a total volume of 4–6 mL of local anesthetic (e.g., a mixture of 1% lidocaine with 0.5% bupivacaine). If there is a 50% reduction of pain with improved strength (supporting the diagnosis of shoulder impingement, supraspinatus tendinitis, or subdeltoid bursitis), this can be followed by injecting corticosteroid (e.g., 1 mL betamethasone). If the initial blind injection is unsuccessful or if the diagnosis is unclear, subacromial bursography may be performed. If the bursogram is normal, the diagnosis of subacromial impingement is doubtful.

b. ***Olecranon bursitis (draftsman's elbow)*** is commonly seen in rheumatologic disorders (e.g., gout). Insert an 18-gauge needle (because the fluid is usually gelatinous) perpendicular to the central swelling of the enlarged bursa overlying the olecranon process of the ulna. A low-dose corticosteroid injection may be given after aspiration.

2. **Lower limb**

a. ***Greater trochanteric bursitis*** is common in the elderly and usually manifests as lateral thigh pain (which may radiate down to the leg or up to the buttock) during ambulation. The pain may be elicited by applying deep pressures to the posterior and superior aspects of the greater trochanter in an externally rotated and abducted lower limb. For injection therapy, the patient is placed in a side-lying position (the site to be injected is on top) with the hips and knees flexed to about 45°. A 3.5-inch, 22-gauge needle is inserted perpendicularly into the skin at the point of maximal tenderness overlying the greater trochanter. Once the needle has touched bone, it is slightly withdrawn and a mixture of corticosteroid and anesthetic is injected. If pain persists despite injection therapy and comprehensive rehabilitation (including stretching of the long constrictors of the hip, such as tensor fascia lata, hamstring, and rectus femoris muscles), the clinician should consider other sources of pain (e.g., from the lumbar spine, hip joint, and distal joints).

b. ***Ischial bursitis (tailor's or weaver's bottom)*** is associated with prolonged sitting on a hard surface or may be seen in adolescent runners in conjunction with ischial apophysitis (pain is aggravated during uphill running or with contraction of hamstring muscles). The ischial bursa is located between the inferior part of the ischial tuberosity and the gluteus maximus. If the patient does not respond to rest, ice, NSAIDs, change in sitting duration and surface, or modification in running styles and intensity, then injection therapy may be warranted. The patient is placed in the side-lying position with the knee fully flexed to relax the hamstrings. Palpate the point of maximal tenderness overlying the ischial tuberosity and horizontally insert a 3-inch, 22-gauge needle directed toward it. Fluoroscopic guidance may be needed to carry out a bursogram and to verify needle placement.

c. ***Iliopsoas (or iliopectineal) bursitis***, which is relatively uncommon, manifests as pain referred to the anterior thigh (following the distribution of the femoral nerve). The patient usually externally rotates and flexes the hip to relieve pressure on the inflamed bursa and avoids extension of the lower limb during ambulation. A 20- to 22-gauge, 3.5-inch needle is inserted to the point of maximum tenderness (elicited by passive extension of the patient's hip) usually under fluoroscopic guidance for diagnostic and therapeutic purposes.

d. ***Prepatellar bursitis (housemaid's knee)*** is often the result of frequent kneeling. Despite the presence of effusion, the patient rarely complains of pain unless direct pressure is applied to the bursa. A 20- to 22-gauge, 1.5-inch needle is inserted to the area of maximal fullness at the middle to superior pole of the patella (either medially or laterally). Repeat injections may be required because the prepatellar bursa is often multiloculated. The patient should be advised to avoid kneeling and to use knee pads when pressure must be applied to the patella.

e. ***Tibial collateral ligament (TCL) bursitis*** should be considered in any patient with medial joint line tenderness (usually with no evidence of new ligamentous or capsular instability). The TCL is located between the deep and superficial aspects of the tibial collateral ligament. It does not adhere to the medial meniscus, and it appears to reduce friction between the superficial layer of the TCL and the medial meniscus. A 20- to 22-gauge, 1.5-inch needle is inserted perpendicularly to the medial joint line at the point of maximal tenderness where medication (e.g., 2-mL mixture of lidocaine and triamcinolone) is injected.

f. ***Anserine bursitis.*** The anserine bursa is located approximately 5 cm distal to the tibial joint line on the medial aspect of the tibia and somewhat posterior. It separates the three conjoined tendons of the pes anserinus (i.e., semitendinosus, sartorius, and gracilis muscles) from the medial collateral ligament and the tibia. Anserine bursitis is commonly seen in women with heavy thighs and osteoarthritis of the knees or in athletes (especially soccer players) because of direct knee trauma. Patients usually complain of pain below the anteromedial surface of the knee during stair ascension. This pain can be reproduced by moving the patient's knee in flexion and extension while the leg is internally rotated. In addition to a comprehensive rehabilitation program (including ice, NSAIDs, and exercise), injection therapy may be given. The knee is fully extended, and a 1- to 1.5-inch, 22-gauge needle is inserted perpendicular to the skin over the point of maximal tenderness on the medial tibial flare where the pes anserinus tendon and bursa lie. The tip of the needle is slightly withdrawn once its tip touches bone surface and a 1- to 3-mL combination of anesthetic and corticosteroid is injected. Athletes at risk for repetitive trauma may also benefit from padded protection about the knee.

g. ***Retrocalcaneal (subtendinous) bursitis.*** The retrocalcaneal bursa is located between the posterior surface of the calcaneus and the tendon of the triceps surae. It may be inflamed during overstraining (e.g., early assumption of increased mileage in a runner or an ill-fitting shoe resulting in pressure from a restricting heel counter). Pain can be elicited by placing the thumb and index finger on the anterior edges of the Achilles tendon and applying pressure. The first step in treatment is footwear modification combined with ice and NSAIDs. This is followed by daily stretching of the triceps surae. If these measures fail, then a 20- to 22-gauge, 1- to 1.5-inch needle may be inserted with an anterior angle of 15–20° to the point of greatest bursal distension, which is often on the lateral aspect of the heel. Care must be taken to avoid instilling corticosteroid into the Achilles tendon because of risk of tendon rupture.

h. ***Achilles (or subcutaneous) bursitis*** is common in women who wear high-heeled shoes that apply direct pressure on the bursa that lies subcutaneous to the posterior surface of the Achilles tendon. A midline swelling is usually noted where the upper edge of the heel counter comes in contact with the heel cord. Treatments include changing the patient's shoes and the use of ice and NSAIDs. If these fail, the point of maximal tenderness or distension may be injected with a corticosteroid and anesthetic mixture via a 20- to 22-gauge, 1- to 1.5-inch needle. Care must be taken to avoid instilling corticosteroid into the Achilles tendon because of the risk of tendon rupture.

i. ***Calcaneal bursitis*** is common in elderly patients with a calcified heel spur that irritates the bursa during prolonged walking or running. Treatment includes the use of an appropriate walking or running shoe (with good heel cushion) and the use of a heel cup. Athletes are encouraged to change their running shoes every 200–300 miles (or 320–480 km; this amount of mileage usually causes mid-sole breakdown). If these measures fail, a 20- to 22-gauge, 1- to 1.5-inch needle may be inserted to the point of maximal tenderness for diagnostic and therapeutic purposes.

C. TENDON AND TENDON SHEATH INJECTIONS. A tendinitis or tenosynovitis may be caused by either an acute injury or chronic overuse. Injection therapy may be used to facilitate, or as part of, the overall rehabilitation program (which includes work or environmental modification, proper body mechanics, use of splints, stretching and flexibility exercises, NSAIDs, etc.). Corticosteroid injection for tendinitis or tenosynovitis should be limited to a maximum of three in a given area. It may be injected into the tendon sheath but not directly into the substance of the tendon to avoid tendon rupture. When injecting into the tendon sheath, there is generally no significant resistance felt over the plunger of the syringe. To alleviate the pain of injection, a vapocoolant spray (e.g., ethyl chloride or fluorimethane) or EMLA cream may be used for superficial skin anesthesia.

1. Upper limb

a. ***Supraspinatus tendinitis (impingement syndrome, rotator cuff tendinitis).*** Palpate the supraspinatus tendon, which is usually located approximately 2.5 cm medial to the most lateral aspect of the spine of the scapula. Insert a 22-gauge needle to the point of maximal tenderness and inject the mixture of corticosteroid and anesthetic in the proximity of the tendon. After the injection, advise the patient to avoid heavy lifting and excessive overhead work for at least 2 days.

b. ***Biceps tendinitis***. The corticosteroid and anesthetic mixture is injected into the immediate proximity of the tendon (not into the tendon substance) through the anterior approach using a 22-gauge needle. After the injection, the patient is advised not to do heavy lifting or vigorous exercises for 48–72 hours. In general, steroid injection into the bicipital groove is discouraged because of the possibility of promoting eventual tendon rupture.
   I. **Long head of the biceps tendons**. Insert the needle at the point of maximum tenderness located at the bicipital groove located in the head of the humerus.
   II. **Short head of the biceps tendon**. Insert the needle at the point of maximum tenderness, which is usually right on top of the coracoid process.

c. ***Lateral epicondylitis (tennis elbow)*** is usually associated with pain when making a fist, doing backhand shots in tennis, lifting objects, using a screwdriver, and when the patient extends the wrist against resistance. Injection therapy may be tried only after conservative treatments (e.g., NSAIDs, tennis-elbow band, exercises, proper body mechanics, and environmental or work modifications) have failed. The elbow is flexed to about 90° and a 22-gauge needle is inserted just below and medial to the lateral epicondyle into the common extensor tendon origin. Deposit about 0.5 mL mixture of local anesthetic into the point of maximal tenderness, and if the symptoms improve, follow this with a corticosteroid preparation (e.g., 10-20 mg of triamcinolone). After injection, the elbow is fully extended and pronated and the wrist is simultaneously flexed to stretch the common extensor tendon. A wrist splint may be beneficial to help immobilize the wrist extensor tendons for a few days.

d. ***De Quervain's syndrome*** refers to the stenosing tenosynovitis of the first dorsal wrist compartment, which typically transmits the tendons of both the abductor pollicis longus (APL) and extensor pollicis brevis (EPB). Place the forearm in a neutral position with the wrist in 15–20° of ulnar deviation. Insert a 25-gauge needle to the point of maximal tenderness at the level of the distal end of the radius tangential to the skin along the length of the APL and EPB. Inject a small amount of local anesthetic, and look for a small fusiform swelling along the length of the tendons to indicate that the needle is in the tenosynovium. Carefully disconnect the syringe and replace it with a tuberculin syringe containing corticosteroids (e.g., DepoMedrol) and inject about 0.125 mL of the steroid. Other clinicians believe that any attempt to enter a tendon sheath causes more damage than benefit and thus recommend that the corticosteroid be injected intradermally above the site of tenderness and allowed to diffuse into the inflamed tendon sheath.

e. ***Trigger thumb or trigger digit*** is a stenosing flexor tenosynovitis for which corticosteroid (mixed with anesthetic) injection is a primary treatment. Insert a 25-gauge needle tangentially and just proximal to the fusiform swelling at about the level of the metacarpal head and inject a small amount of local anesthetic and steroid mixture into the tendon sheath (there should be no resistance felt over the syringe plunger). A more conservative method is to inject intradermally above the site of tenderness and to let the medication diffuse into the inflamed tendon sheath.

2. **Lower limb**. Although quadriceps (infrapatellar) tendinitis and Achilles tendinitis may be treated by injecting corticosteroid and anesthetic, many clinicians avoid injection therapy in these weight-bearing structures because of fear of tendon rupture.

a. ***Hip abductor tendinitis***. The technique for patient positioning and injection is similar to that described for trochanteric bursitis (see section III.B.2.a). A 20- or 22-gauge needle is inserted at the point of maximal tenderness and the mixture of corticosteroid and anesthetic is injected into the proximity of the hip abductor tendon.

b. ***Iliotibial band tendinitis***. The patient lies on their side. Using a 20- or 22-gauge needle, inject a mixture of corticosteroid and anesthetic around the insertion of the iliotibial band at the proximal, lateral tibia, or, depending on the site of symptoms, where it passes over the prominence of the lateral femoral condyle.

c. ***Plantar fasciitis***. Palpate for the exact site of inflammation or point of maximal tenderness (usually at the attachment of the plantar fascia to the calcaneus) and approach it perpendicularly from the plantar aspect of the foot (usually slightly off center, closer to the medial border of the foot). Insert a 22-gauge needle until it touches the underlying bone, then withdraw it slightly by 1–2 mm and deposit the mixture of local anesthetic and steroid (e.g., 0.5 mL of DepoMedrol and 1 mL of lidocaine). Steroid injection should be considered only after other measures (e.g., stretching exercises, NSAIDs, and shoe modification) have failed because it can theoretically cause atrophy of the specialized fat pads of the heel leading to a significant disability (especially in athletes).

D. OTHER SOFT TISSUE INJECTIONS (FOR TRIGGER POINT INJECTIONS SEE CHAPTER 4.11)

1. **Carpal tunnel syndrome (CTS)** is an entrapment syndrome of the median nerve at the wrist which manifests as pain and paresthesia at the median nerve distribution. The pain usually occurs at night-time or after frequent use of the hands or fingers. Carpal tunnel syndrome is often caused by overuse of the hand (e.g., forceful gripping or repetitive hand/wrist motions). Corticosteroid injection is considered only after conservative measures (e.g., wearing of wrist splints, in neutral position, during sleeping hours for 4–8 weeks, work and activity modification, and NSAIDs) have failed. One method of carpal tunnel injection is to inject 0.5 mL (20 mg) of triamcinolone hexacetonide (Aristopan) without anesthetics (to avoid accidental injection into the median nerve after the area becomes anesthetized). A 25-gauge needle is pointed distally toward the carpal tunnel and inserted at a 35° angle on the ulnar side of the palmaris longus tendon, a few millimeters beyond the distal wrist crease. Another approach is to draw a line connecting the pisiform and trapezoid bones to approximate the position of the transverse carpal ligament. The needle is then inserted through the transverse carpal ligament approximately 6 mm below the surface of the skin. If the patient complains of paresthesias, the needle should be redirected laterally and more superficially.
2. **Morton's neuroma**, which is neither a neuroma nor a neoplasm, is a degenerative process of the nerve characterized by tenderness with distal paresthesia (because of hypertrophic fibrosis of the digital nerve) usually located between the distal metatarsal bones of the second and third or third and fourth digits of the foot. The corticosteroid preparation is injected through the foot dorsum into the point of maximal tenderness via a 22-gauge needle. Morton's neuroma has a tendency to recur.

Further reading

Cyriax J, Russell G: *Textbook of orthopedic medicine, vol. 2. Treatment by manipulation, massage, and injection*, ed 9, Baltimore, 1977, Williams & Wilkins.

Gray RG, Gottlieb NL: Intra-articular corticosteroids: an updated assessment. *Clin Orthop* 177:235–236, 1983.

Hasselbacker P: Synovial fluid analysis. In Utsinger PD, Zvaifler JK, Erlich GE, editors: *Rheumatoid arthritis*, Philadelphia, 1985, JB Lippincott.

Hollander JL: Intrasynovial corticosteroid therapy in arthritis. *Maryland State Med J* 19:62–66, 1970.

Lennard TA, editor: *Pain procedures in clinical practice*, Philadelphia, 2000, Hanley & Belfus.

Nicholas JJ, Lennard TA: Joint and soft tissue injection techniques. In Braddom RL, editor: *Physical medicine and rehabilitation*, ed 2, Philadelphia, 2000, WB Saunders, pp. 498–514.
Pfenninger JL: Injections of joints and soft tissue: Part I: General guidelines. *Am Fam Physician* 44:1196–1202, 1991.
Pfenninger JL: Injections of joints and soft tissue: Part II: Guidelines for specific joints. *Am Fam Physician* 44:1690–1701, 1991.
Rifat SF, Moeller JL: Basics of joint injection: general techniques and tips for safe, effective use. *Postgrad Med* 109(1):157–166, 2001.
Sandrock NJG, Warfield CA: Epidural steroids and facet injections. In Warfield CA, Bajwa ZH, editors: *Principles and practice of pain management*, New York, 2003, McGraw-Hill, pp. 401–412.
Stern R: Arthrocentesis and intraarticular injection. In Paget S, Gibofsky A, Beary III JF, editors: *Manual of rheumatology and outpatient orthopedic disorders*, ed 4, Philadelphia, 2000, Lippincott, Williams & Wilkins, pp. 32–37.
Waldman SD: *Atlas of pain management injection techniques*, Philadelphia, 2000, WB Saunders.
Walsh NE, Rogers JN: Injection procedures. In DeLisa JA, Gans BM, Walsh NE, *et al.*, editors: *Physical medicine and rehabilitation: principles and practice*, ed 4, Philadelphia, 2005, Lippincott, Williams & Wilkins, pp. 311–367.
Zuckerman JD, Meislin RJ, Rothberg M: Injections for joint and soft tissue disorders: when and how to use them. *Geriatrics* 45:45–55, 1990.

CHAPTER 4.10
Nerve blocks

In physical medicine and rehabilitation, nerve blocks should only be used as an adjunct in the comprehensive treatment of the patient. They refer to the administration of a local anesthetic agent or neurolytic agent to interrupt the nerve's somatic function (motor, sensory, or both) and/or sympathetic functions. Motor nerve blocks are used to relax specific muscles such as for the treatment of spasticity (see Chapter 5.4, section III.D.2) or trigger points (see Chapter 4.11). Sensory nerve blocks are commonly used for providing anesthesia to facilitate surgical procedures and for pain management. Sympathetic blocks are generally used to dilate blood vessels (e.g., in patients with ischemic rest pain) and for the treatment of sympathetically maintained pain (SMP). This chapter presents an overview of nerve blocks primarily used in pain management for diagnostic, pre-emptive, prognostic, and therapeutic purposes. Although commonly placed by anesthesiologists, nerve blocks are becoming popular among physiatrists who specialize in pain management and who have received additional training in performing these procedures. Clinicians performing nerve blocks should be knowledgeable about the recognition, treatment, and prevention of potential side effects and complications of nerve blocks (Table 4.10-1). The risk of significant complications is generally low but can be potentially fata, Hence, clinicians performing nerve blocks should have resuscitation equipment at hand and should be able to perform cardiac/respiratory resuscitation according to the Advanced Cardiac Life Support (ACLS) protocols. For specific injection techniques and for specific diagnosis and treatment of side-effects and complications of nerve blocks, the reader is referred to standard anesthesiology textbooks or other standard textbooks on pain management. For general injection procedures, see Chapter 4.9, section II.

I. Diagnostic nerve blocks

Diagnostic nerve blocks are used to ascertain specific nociceptive pathways, to help determine the possible mechanism of chronic pain syndromes, to aid in the differential diagnosis of the site and cause of pain, and to determine the patient's reaction to pain relief. They use varying volumes (depending on the nerve and anesthetic concentration, it may vary from 0.5 mL for nerve block of the medial branch of the posterior ramus up to 10 mL for sciatic nerve block) of local anesthetics (e.g., lidocaine, bupivacaine, procaine, and tetracaine), which are injected through disposable 21- to 27-gauge, 3.5-inch needles or, for deeper structures (e.g., lumbar sympathetic and celiac plexus blocks), via 5- or 6-inch needles. The different local anesthetic agents used should have different durations which should be correlated with the duration of subjective pain relief (placebo blocks may be included). Neurolytic agents (e.g., chemical agents such as phenol and absolute alcohol) are rarely used for diagnostic nerve blocks because of their destructive effects. For spine procedures, accurate needle placement is recommended by using fluoroscopy or computed tomography (CT) scan with or without prior injection of contrast medium. For peripheral nerve blocks, electrical stimulators are generally used for localizing

Table 4.10-1	Common side-effects and complications of nerve blocks and their general prevention and treatment
Side-effects and complications	**General prevention (P) and treatment (Tx)**
Systemic toxic reaction (e.g., tonic–clonic seizures; cardiovascular and/or respiratory depression)	**P:** Aspirate before injecting to avoid intravascular injection; premedicate with diazepam or midazolam to increase seizure threshold **Tx:** General cardiovascular* and/or ventilatory† supportive measures; IV diazepam (5–10 mg) for seizures
Other systemic reactions	
• Epinephrine reaction	**P:** Avoid epinephrine in patients who are hypertensive, hyperthyroid, or arrhythmic; do not use epinephrine for blocks of fingers, toes, or penis **Tx:** Fast acting barbiturate or vasodilator if needed
• Vasovagal reaction	**Tx:** Put patient in Trendelenberg position and remove painful stimuli; general cardiovascular* and/or ventilatory† supportive measures, if needed
• Allergic reaction	**P:** Do intradermal skin test by injecting diluted (1 : 1000) followed by undiluted local anesthetic **Tx:** Administer epinephrine or antihistamine; general cardiovascular* and/or ventilatory† supportive measures
Accidental spinal block	**P:** Avoid subarachnoid or epidural blockade when doing intercostals nerve blocks, sympathetic blocks, or nerve root injections **Tx:** General supportive measures to maintain cardiovascular and ventilatory functions
Concurrent medical episode	
• Infection	**P:** Aseptic and sterile technique **Tx:** Antibiotics abscess drainage
• Pneumothorax	**Tx:** Supplemental O_2, O_2 saturation and vital sign monitoring, and when needed, needle aspiration of air and/or chest tube thoracostomy and vacuum drainage
• Nerve injury	**P:** Infiltrate around the nerve and not directly into the nerve; use short beveled needles **Tx:** Immediate cessation for the injection and repositioning of the needle
Other complications	
• Hypotension	**P:** Avoid sympathetic blockade; make sure patient is not hypovolemic **Tx:** General cardiovascular supportive measures*
• Arterial puncture	**Tx:** Prolonged direct pressure to prevent hematoma
• Methomoglobinemia	**P:** Avoid large doses of prilocaine **Tx:** IV methylene blue

** General cardiovascular supportive measures include administration of intravenous (IV) fluid; proper positioning (e.g., leg elevation), and vasopresors (e.g., ephedrine, 12.5–25 mg, IV).*

† General ventilatory supportive measures include supplemental O_2 monitoring of O_2 saturation and vital signs, airway maintenance (including endotracheal intubation and artificial ventilation, if needed).

Data tabulated from Walsh NE, Rogers JN: Injection procedures. In DeLisa JA, Gans BM, Walsh NE, et al., *editors:* Physical medicine and rehabilitation: principles and practice, *ed 4, Philadelphia, 2005, Lippincott, Williams & Wilkins, pp. 311–367.*

peripheral nerves. For more accurate results, patients should be given little or no analgesic medication during diagnostic blocks. Although placebo responses to nerve blocks may suggest pain of psychogenic origin, nerve blocks should never be used to make definitive diagnoses of psychogenic pain. Diagnostic nerve blocks should produce consistent results for two or three nerve block sessions before any decisions are made about their effectiveness.

A. DIAGNOSTIC SYMPATHETIC AND SOMATIC NERVE BLOCKS are used to differentiate between sympathetic and somatic pain for the diagnosis of complex regional pain syndrome (CRPS; formerly called reflex sympathetic dystrophy) with SMP features and the localization of somatic nerve pain.

1. **Diagnostic anatomic nerve blocks** utilize the presumed anatomic differences in the sympathetic and somatic nerve pathways to determine the source of pain. One method is to start proximally (i.e., with sympathetic blockade) and proceed distally (i.e., with somatic blockade). A placebo block is placed first by injecting 5–10 mL of normal saline into the sympathetic pathway. If pain is relieved, a placebo effect is assumed. If not, then 10–15 mL of local anesthetic (e.g., lidocaine and/or bupivacaine) is injected. If pain is relieved, the sympathetic pathway is probably the source of the pain, but if pain is persistent, then a somatic block to the painful area is performed. Another method of anatomic nerve blockade is to start distally with a somatic block then proceed proximally toward a sympathetic blockade.

a. ***For head, neck, and upper limb pain,*** use the stellate (cervicothoracic) ganglion for sympathetic blockade. For somatic blockade, the nerves used are the trigeminal nerve for the head, the cervical roots for the neck, and the brachial plexus for the upper limb.

b. ***For upper chest and thoracic pain,*** use the stellate ganglion for sympathetic blockade and the intercostal nerves for somatic blockade.

c. ***For upper abdominal pain,*** use the intercostal nerves for somatic blockade followed by sympathetic blockade using the celiac plexus.

d. ***For lower back and lower limb pain,*** use the lumbar sympathetic nerves for sympathetic blockade. For somatic blockade, the lumbar paravertebral nerves are used for the lower back pain, and either the lumbar paravertebral nerves or the trans-sacral S1 nerves are used for the lower limb.

2. **Diagnostic pharmacologic (or neurophysiologic) nerve blocks** utilize the differential sensitivities of sympathetic and somatic nerve fibers of different sizes to the blocking effect of local anesthetics. Injection of 0.25% procaine or 0.5% lidocaine selectively blocks the type B, myelinated preganglionic autonomic fibers, while 0.5% procaine or 1% lidocaine blocks the type C, unmyelinated postganglionic fibers and the type A-δ myelinated fibers responsible for touch, pressure, pain, and temperature. A higher dose of procaine (1%) or lidocaine (2%) blocks the type A (α, β, and γ) myelinated fibers responsible for motor function. The following differential blocks are used to distinguish the character of a pain state and to help differentiate somatic sensory from sympathetic, central, or probable pain of psychogenic origin. It must be noted that these procedures are in part theoretical.

a. ***Differential spinal blocks*** consist of sequential injections of 5–10 mL of normal saline followed by 0.25%, 0.5%, and 1% of procaine (or 0.5%, 1%, and 2% of lidocaine) to determine the source of pain. The same volume of local anesthetic (5–10 mL) is used for each injection. The injection may be given via the subarachnoid space (**subarachnoid block**) or the epidural space (**epidural block**). Subarachnoid blocks are generally made at the mid-thoracic level or caudally because of the cervical origin of the phrenic nerve. Epidural blocks have more limited areas of effect than subarachnoid blocks and these can be performed virtually at any point in the spinal cord. However, epidural blocks are seldom used for diagnostic purposes because bilateral effects usually occur and it is more difficult to control their area of action. Relief by normal saline suggests a placebo effect or probably pain of psychogenic origin. If there is no relief, then 0.25%, 0.5%, and 1% procaine (or 0.5%, 1%, and 2% lidocaine) solutions are sequentially injected until the patient reports pain relief. Pain relief from 0.25% procaine (or 0.5% lidocaine) suggests sympathetic pain (e.g., CRPS with SMP features) whereas pain relief from 0.5% procaine (or 1% lidocaine) suggests somatosensory pain. The 1% procaine (or 2% lidocaine) is used to provide motor block. If there is no pain relief after all four injections are completed, an intravenous test for centrally mediated pain (see section I.C) may be carried out.

b. ***Modified differential spinal blocks*** take advantage of the fact that a complete block wears off in the following sequence: motor, sensory, then sympathetic. A local anesthetic agent (2 mL of 5% procaine, 10–20 mL of 2% lidocaine, or 3% chloroprocaine) is injected into the subarachnoid space to induce a complete motor block. If there is no pain relief, then an intravenous test for centrally mediated pain may be performed. If there is pain relief, the origin of the pain is identified by assessing which sensation returns during the time when the pain is returning (as the anesthetic effect wears off). For example, if the pain recurs at the time when pinprick and temperature sensations return, the source of pain is most likely somatosensory (type A-δ or type C fibers). However, if the pain recurs long after the return of pinprick and temperature sensations, then the pain is most likely sympathetic. The modified method is more practical than the original spinal blockade method because it is less time consuming and the patient does not need to stay immobile for long.

B. DIAGNOSTIC PERIPHERAL NERVE BLOCKS

1. **Diagnostic selective nerve root blocks** involve the injection of 0.5–1 mL of local anesthetic into the lateral margin of a neuroforamen. They are used to determine classic monoradicular pain for which neuroradiologic studies either fail to provide a structural explanation or show an abnormality related only to an adjacent nerve root. In the first case, blocking of the suspected nerve root should abolish the pain, while in the second case, blocking of the adjacent nerve root (with neuroradiologic abnormality) should not abolish the pain. They can also be used to distinguish pain whose clinical picture is suggestive of both nerve root and distal nerve origin. If the pain has a distal origin, blockade of a single root should not completely abolish pain because of dermatomal overlap.
2. **Diagnostic motor nerve blocks** involve the selective injection of a local anesthetic agent (e.g., lidocaine or bupivacaine) or, on some occasions, a neurolytic agent (e.g., phenol or alcohol) around a peripheral motor or mixed nerve (identified by electrodiagnostic techniques) to effectively paralyze those muscles innervated by the nerve. They are used to simulate or approximate the clinical outcome of a proposed tenotomy or neurectomy in patients with spasticity so that potential muscle imbalance or voluntary motor control can be assessed. When the blockade is done at the point proximal to or near the terminal innervation within the muscle, it is called a motor point block or intramuscular neurolysis. The nerves commonly assessed are the median, ulnar, and musculocutaneous nerves for the upper limbs and the obturator, femoral, posterior tibial, and common peroneal nerves for the lower limbs.

C. INTRAVENOUS (IV) TESTS FOR CENTRALLY MEDIATED PAIN are performed if the sequential, differential spinal blockade (original or modified method) fails to provide pain relief. These tests remain controversial.

1. **Intravenous thiopental test (barbiturate test)** is based on the assumption that a patient's response to typical pain should be the same during barbiturate sleep as when awake. It is done by slow IV infusion of thiopental until the

patient falls into a light sleep. The infusion is then stopped and as the patient awakens slowly, a stimulus other than that which elicits the typical pain (e.g., pressure over the sternum or anterior tibia) is given periodically. If the patient feels the pain, then a stimulus that is known to elicit the typical pain is given. If the patient does not respond to the typical stimulus, then the pain is probably psychogenic.

2. **Intravenous lidocaine test** uses 1.2–2 mg/kg of IV lidocaine, injected until the patient complains of mild toxicity (tingling or dizziness). Relief of pain (2 minutes after toxicity occurs) suggests pain of central origin.
3. **Intravenous phentolamine test** is used in the diagnosis and prognosis of CRPS. CRPS patients with transient relief from IV phentolamine will likely respond to regional IV guanethidine sympathetic blocks.

D. **DIAGNOSTIC FACET INJECTIONS** are indicated in patients whose posterior spinal elements are suspected as the primary source of pain or in conjunction with discogenic disease. A local anesthetic (e.g., lidocaine or bupivacaine) and a steroid (e.g., methylprednisolone) are injected into the intra-articular facets (most commonly the lumbar facets or zygapophyseal joints) under fluoroscopic or CT guidance. If the facet is the source of back pain, there is immediate relief of pain, which may last for about 24 hours. Following the intra-articular injection, anesthetic injections of the medial branch of the posterior ramus (i.e., medial branch blocks) are done to predict the response to denervation procedures. To anesthetize a single joint, medial branch blocks are done at two levels because of dual innervation of the zygapophyseal joints.

II. Prognostic nerve blocks

Prognostic nerve blocks are used to predict the effects of neurolytic blocks or neurosurgery and allow the patient to experience the sensory changes (e.g., numbness) and other side-effects that follow destructive procedures (neuroablative surgical procedures or neurolytic blocks) and help the patient decide whether or not to undergo the procedure. As with diagnostic blocks, little or no analgesic medication should be given to the patient during prognostic blocks; and precise needle placement is determined by fluoroscopy or CT scan with or without prior injection of contrast medium. Prognostic blocks can be used to determine any changes in behavior and effect in the absence of pain and analgesic medication; the amount of physical activity tolerated and the degree of physical limitation unrelated to pain; evidence of narcotic dependence and its severity; and the development of new pain in other locations previously unnoticed but now unmasked. Prognostic nerve blocks are limited in predicting long-term effects. In general, prognostic nerve blocks performed for 2 to 3 days (i.e., using continuous techniques such as indwelling catheters) provide more useful information than a single block.

III. Pre-emptive (or prophylactic) nerve blocks

Pre-emptive nerve blocks involve blockade of the proposed site of the operation to prevent or reduce the incidence and intensity of pain and the delay of normal functional activity that follows postoperatively. Clinical evidence has shown regional nerve blocks for several days prior to limb amputation can decrease the incidence of phantom limb pain, CRPS, and other chronic pain syndromes; thus, resulting in earlier functional rehabilitation, prevention or reduction of complications, and shorter hospitalization.

IV. Therapeutic nerve blocks (or specific regional blocks)

Therapeutic nerve blocks are performed only after the nature and location of the pain has been established by diagnostic blocks. They involve the administration of local anesthetic agents or neurolytic agents into the somatic nerves, sympathetic ganglia, or localized pain-sensitive trigger points (see Chapter 4.11 for trigger point injections). In general, they are used in combination with other therapeutic modalities to control severe acute postoperative pain (e.g., postoperative thoracotomy pain) or post-traumatic pain (e.g., fracture of the ribs) or postinfectious pain (e.g., herpes zoster neuralgia); to provide pain relief and allow normalization of posture to occur through muscle relaxation by breaking the vicious cycle involved in chronic pain syndromes; and to allow the patient to perform other therapeutic measures (e.g., weight-bearing exercises) during the period of symptomatic pain relief.

Therapeutic blocks using local anesthetics (see Chapter 5.10, section VI.E.2.d) are indicated for providing anesthesia for procedures, treatment of inflammatory compression neuropathies in combination with corticosteroids (see Chapter 4.8, section III), and in the following pain situations: presence of a sympathetic component in a pain state with a positive response to diagnostic sympathetic block (a series of sympathetic blocks are usually needed); presence of somatic pain which is unilateral, well-localized, and confined to a small number of dermatomes; and in patients in whom such blocks are associated with minimal risk and morbidity. Although the mechanism of pain relief from a series of therapeutic nerve blocks using local anesthetic is unknown, a variety of factors may contribute, such as transient increases in tissue blood flow; interruption of abnormal neuronal impulse transmission; isolation or disruption of nociceptive foci, particularly in scar tissue or fascial layers; and an occasionally prolonged placebo response or spontaneous resolution of pain.

Therapeutic blocks use neurolytic agents, including chemical agents (e.g., phenol, ethyl alcohol), cold agents (e.g., cryoprobe), and heat agents [e.g., radiofrequency (RF) coagulation]. They are commonly used in patients with cancer pain because of their limited duration of action (the effects of neurolytic nerve blocks range from 8 days to a year and are rarely, if ever, permanent) and potential side-effects (e.g., loss of motor, bowel and/or bladder control, small vessel thrombosis and ischemic tissue damage, and chemical neuritis, which may develop into a deafferentation pain syndrome). Therapeutic blocks (in particular, RF coagulation) have also been used in relieving spasticity (see Chapter 5.4, section III.D.2.a.2) and in relieving pain in selected patients with noncancer chronic pain as a result of peripheral vascular disease (particularly elderly patients with lower limb claudication), trigeminal neuralgia, CRPS, chronic pancreatitis, severe angina pectoris, or other chronic disorders in patients who cannot tolerate a neurosurgical operation. Both RF coagulation and chemical neurolysis can cause neuritis. However, RF coagulation is more accurate and selective and, in recent years, has replaced chemical neurolysis for pain management. The therapeutic effect of RF coagulation tends to diminish with time. Anecdotally, pain relief following RF coagulation for zygapophyseal joint pain continues for at least 12–14 months in the lumbar spine and 9–12 months in the cervical and thoracic spine, with most patients having pain recurrence after 2–3 years (Dreyfuss and Rogers, 2000).

Compared with systemic analgesics, nerve blocks can improve local blood flow and prevent the central effects of sedation, drowsiness, and respiratory depression. Absolute contraindications for therapeutic nerve blocks include anticoagulation, regional infection, and lack of technical expertise. Relative contraindications include pain with documented psychogenic or psychiatric origin, language barrier or inability to grasp the concept of a pain-rating scale or questionnaire, uncooperative patients, unstable narcotic addiction, poor stress or pain tolerance, poorly localized pain, episodic pain, lack of proper equipment, and anatomical distortion of injection site.

A. SOMATIC NERVE BLOCKS

1. **Peripheral local blocks** include infiltration of wound margins or incision irrigation with long-acting local anesthetics (e.g., bupivacaine) to decrease incisional or wound pain; local blocks (e.g., upper limb block, lower limb block, trunk block, head block, and penile nerve block) for anesthesia or analgesia for surgical procedures, nerve entrapment syndrome, or other severe painful conditions; trigger point injections (see Chapter 4.11); nerve blocks for controlling spasticity (e.g., peripheral nerve blocks and motor point blocks; both described in Chapter 5.4, section III.D.2.b), and injection of local anesthetic and corticosteroids into joints and soft tissues (see Chapter 4.9). In using local infiltration of wound margins, a more proximal blockade of the same nerve is usually recommended because the wound's acidic milieu limits the amount of anesthetic passing through the neuronal membrane.
2. **Cranial nerve blocks** are useful in managing severe intractable pain of the head and neck region, which is mostly seen in trigeminal neuralgia or in cancer patients (because of local spread of the tumor, neural infiltration of the tumor, or tumor-related nerve injury). Therapeutic cranial nerve blocks commonly performed include blockade of the trigeminal nerve and its branches (e.g., mandibular and maxillary branches), gasserian ganglion blocks (if more than one division of trigeminal nerve is involved), facial nerve blocks, glossopharyngeal nerve blocks, and vagus nerve blocks. All cranial nerve blocks must be performed under fluoroscopic or CT guidance and only after prior diagnostic and prognostic blocks with local anesthetics. Side-effects include inadvertent injection of or diffusion of the drug to neighboring structures such as motor fibers of the jaw, eye, or the upper cervical sympathetic ganglion or internal jugular vein. Hematoma, permanent neurologic sequelae, and alcoholic neuritis have also been reported.
3. **Spinal nerve blocks**

a. ***Occipital nerve blocks*** provide analgesia in the distribution of the posterior division of the C2 spinal nerve for patients who have suffered musculoskeletal trauma or have occipital headaches. There are no side-effects other than those that occur with accidental intra-arterial injection. Although rare, there are case reports of deaths and seizures reported with intra-arterial anesthetic injections into the occipetal artery during a greater occipital nerve block .

b. ***Paravertebral blocks*** are used to temporarily provide sensory analgesia of selected spinal nerves for the relief of severe pain (e.g., because of musculoskeletal pathology such as fracture) by the placement of local anesthetic distal to the intervertebral foramen. A successful block is denoted by anesthesia and pain relief in the desired distribution; however, overlapping innervation usually necessitates blocks of one or two neighboring segments. Use of neurolytic agents on the spinal nerves is not recommended for pain of nonmalignant disease because most spinal nerves are mixed nerves and neurolytic blocks affect both motor and sensory modalities to the same extent. Moreover, alcohol and, to a lesser degree, phenol can cause a chemical neuropathy, which in itself may create a pain syndrome. Complications are associated with needle penetration of neighboring structures, for example, accidental injection into the vertebral artery with resultant seizures and/or transient paralysis of vital centers and often unconsciousness. Accidental injection into the subarachnoid space with consequent total spinal anesthesia, concomitant block of the cervical sympathetic chain with development of Horner's syndrome, involvement of the superior aspect of recurrent laryngeal nerves and perhaps even the trunk of vagus, and pneumothorax have all been reported. All of these can be avoided by using proper techniques (with fluoroscopic or CT-scan guidance) and small amounts of solutions.

c. ***Intercostal blocks*** are used for the relief of severe acute post-traumatic (e.g., rib or sternal fractures), postoperative (e.g., poststernotomy, postmastectomy, or post-thoracotomy), or postinfectious (e.g., acute herpes zoster) pain in the thoracic or abdominal wall. The nerves are blocked as they course along the underside of the ribs. The most important complications of intercostal blocks are pneumothorax and systemic toxic reactions (e.g., sudden hypotension and cardiorespiratory compromise). Disadvantages include the limited duration of action of a single dose of local anesthetic (6–8 hours) and the subsequent need for repeated injections, which are painful for the patient and labor intensive for the physician. An alternative to intercostal block is intrapleural administration of local anesthetic via a catheter placed over the T7 or T8 rib to simulate the effect of multiple intercostal blocks and reduce the labor intensiveness of repeated injections.

d. ***Subarachnoid neurolytic blocks*** involve segmental injections of small amounts of phenol or alcohol into the subarachnoid space at L2–L5 to produce a chemical posterior rhizotomy (primarily for cancer pain, e.g., pelvic cancer pain). Exact positioning and careful choice of the injection level and volume allow selective sensory anesthesia with sparing of motor fibers. Major complications include permanent weakness and urinary or rectal sphincter dysfunction, chemical meningitis, arachnoiditis, headaches, and neuropathies. Several injections may be necessary, and the duration of action varies from an average of 3 months with alcohol injections to only 3–4 weeks with phenol injections.

e. ***Epidural blocks,*** when compared with subarachnoid blocks, allow for blockade of spinal nerve roots over a more limited area and needle insertion at virtually any point in the spine (including cervical segments) because of the lower risk of penetrating the spinal cord. Unlike subarachnoid drugs, epidural fluids do not flow freely or predictably with changes in patient position. Therapeutic indications of epidural local anesthetics blocks include the management of acute pain in trauma, surgery, and obstetrics.

In chronic pain patients, epidural blocks may be performed using an opioid (with or without local anesthetic) for relief of chronic cancer pain or using a corticosteroid (e.g., 80 mg of methylprednisolone, which should not be repeated if there is relief of pain but may be repeated up to a maximum of three injections at 3-week intervals if there is no pain relief). Epidural corticosteroid injections reduce acute local edema and nerve root compression and may be beneficial in acute back pain as a result of diskogenic disease; however, efficacy in patients with spinal stenosis, scoliosis, spondylolysis, or spondylolisthesis or in those who have had laminectomies remains controversial with highly variable success rates. The variable success rates are attributed to variations in technique, ancillary care, patient selection, and follow-up period. In patients with nonspecific low back pain, several controlled studies showed that epidural steroid injection showed no significant immediate or long-term improvement.

The techniques most commonly used in lumbosacral epidural blocks are the midline and paramedian epidural approaches, which can be used effectively for pain management at the level of pathology in patients with disk herniations, degenerative disk disease, central stenosis, or compression fractures. An alternative technique is the transforaminal or selective nerve root block used in patients with disk herniations with or without radiculopathies, foraminal stenosis, or discogenic disease. In postoperative patients, the transforaminal approach is preferred over the midline or paramedian approaches because scar tissues are typically found in the midline. Another technique is the caudal or transsacral epidural block used in discogenic disease, disk herniations, or central stenosis involving the lower lumbar disk, i.e., at L5-S1 and also at L4-5. Unlike the translumbar approaches, the risk of thecal sac injection is avoided in the caudal epidural approach. Complications of epidural blocks include dural puncture, intravascular injection (with systemic toxicity such as cardiorespiratory compromise, nausea, and vomiting), hypotension (from sympathetic blockade), motor block, pruritus, bladder dysfunction (e.g., urinary retention), epidural abscess, and meningitis.

f. ***Intravenous regional (Bier) somatic block*** is a technique for producing anesthesia of a limb using an ischemic isolation with a tourniquet and refilling the vascular system with local anesthetics for surgical anesthesia. With local anesthetics, the duration of action is only minutes longer than the tourniquet time. The therapeutic indication of Bier somatic block is anesthesia of the distal limb for orthopedic or soft tissue surgery. It is contraindicated in patients with infection in the limb, those who do not have an intact venous system, and those who cannot tolerate a tourniquet. The complications of Bier blocks involve local anesthetic toxicity if the tourniquet fails or leaks or if the tourniquet is deflated before 30 minutes have elapsed since the primary injection. Tourniquet leak may manifest as tinnitus, circumoral numbness, and dizziness. Careful individual observation with various doses of anesthetics should be done to determine anesthetic toxicity.

4. **Plexus blocks** include brachial plexus blocks, which provide sensory, motor, and sympathetic blockade of the ipsilateral upper limb, depending on the volume and concentration of local anesthetic drug used; cervical plexus blocks (superficial and deep), which provide sensory and motor block of the distal C1–C4 nerves prior to surgery in the neck and supraclavicular area; and lumbar plexus blocks, which provide sensory and motor block of the anterior thigh and quadriceps muscle (L1–L4). The complications for brachial and cervical plexus blocks include pneumothorax, Horner's syndrome, and phrenic nerve block. For lumbar plexus blocks, complications include accidental injection into the subarachnoid space (causing total spinal anesthesia) and improper needle placement (leading to retroperitoneal hemorrhage and injury to the kidney, ureter, or renal pelvis). Systemic toxicity (e.g., hypotension and cardiorespiratory compromise) can also occur with plexus blocks.

B. SYMPATHETIC NERVE BLOCKS

1. **Stellate ganglion (cervicothoracic) sympathetic blocks** are aimed at the sympathetic outflow from the upper four to six thoracic sympathetic ganglia and the lower cervical sympathetic ganglion located in a fascial plane at approximately the C7 level in the neck lateral to the vertebral spine. It is important that at least the upper four thoracic ganglia be blocked to obtain complete sympathetic block of the upper limb because not all sympathetic fibers to the upper limb pass through the stellate ganglion. The procedure is usually carried out with local anesthetics; for prolonged action, an indwelling catheter can be used. The use of neurolytic agents, although rarely performed, may be carried out using fluoroscopy and contrast solutions. The block is successful if it affects: (a) the ipsilateral upper quadrant of the body (above T8), including the face and head with miosis, mild ptosis, flushed dry skin, and blocked nasal passage; (b) the upper limb with absence of sweating, measurable skin temperature rise, visible vasodilation (with measurable plethysmographic evidence of increased blood flow), and loss of skin conductance response (or galvanic skin response); and (c) the ipsilateral hemithorax, including visceral pleura and sympathetic supply to the heart.

Therapeutic indications of stellate ganglion sympathetic blocks include chronic conditions such as CRPS involving the upper limb and the face, central pain, phantom pain, post-traumatic pain syndromes, postamputation pain, shoulder–hand syndrome, chronic obstructive vascular disease, ischemic rest pain, chronic herpetic neuralgia, idiopathic neuralgia, painful invasive lung tumors, collagen vascular diseases (e.g., scleroderma, systemic lupus erythematosus, and Raynaud's disease), atypical facial neuralgias, myofascial syndromes, and whiplash injuries. The advantages of stellate ganglion sympathetic blocks compared with other upper limb blocks include the absence of sensory and motor block and the resultant improved blood flow. The potential complications include spinal or epidural block, toxic reaction to the local anesthetic drug because of vertebral artery injection, seizures, bradycardia (with right-sided blocks), pneumothorax, recurrent laryngeal nerve block, which causes temporary hoarseness; brachial plexus block; hematoma formation; and orthostatic hypotension. The presence of temporary miosis may interfere with the neurologic evaluation of a patient with an elevated intracranial pressure.

2. **Lumbar sympathetic blocks** are aimed at the lumbar sympathetic chain of the ipsilateral lower limb, which lies on the anterolateral surface of the bodies of the L2, L3, and L4 vertebrae adjacent to the aorta and vena cava. A single needle insertion is sufficient for temporary blocks, while multiple insertions are safer if neurolytic agents are used. When prolonged sympathectomy is indicated, continuous epidural infusion of a local anesthetic may be used. The block is successful if there is absence of sweating, measurable skin temperature rise, loss of skin conductance response (or galvanic skin response), and visible vasodilation (with measurable plethysmographic evidence of increased blood flow) in the lower limb.

   Therapeutic indications of lumbar sympathetic block include lower limb CRPS with SMP features, post-traumatic pain syndromes, compromised peripheral vascular disease, intermittent claudication, circulatory insufficiency (ischemic rest pain), herpes zoster, renal colic, intractable pelvic and urogenital pain, phantom limb pain, amputation or stump pain, and carcinomatous invasion of nerves and plexi. For lower limb CRPS with SMP features, one of the commonly used protocols is daily blocks for 1 week, followed by every other day, twice a week, and then weekly blocks in combination with early mobilization and aggressive physical and occupational therapy. Complications include spinal or epidural anesthesia (with postural headaches); injection into a root sleeve; lumbar plexus block; intravascular injection precipitating a systemic toxicity (e.g., sudden hypotension and cardiorespiratory compromise); L2, L3, or L4 neuralgic pain; neuropathy of the genitofemoral nerve; retroperitoneal hemorrhage (with injury to the spleen, intestines, and liver); and injury to the kidney, ureter, or renal pelvis.

3. **Celiac plexus sympathetic block** is aimed at the sympathetic ganglia located approximately at the L1 level, anterior to the aorta, anterolateral to the celiac artery, and posterior to the pancreas. Blockade of the celiac plexus provides intra-abdominal visceral analgesia. Therapeutic indications include the management of visceral pain associated with abdominal malignancy (e.g., chronic pancreatitis) and postoperative pain selectively after abdominal surgery. Complications include spinal or epidural anesthesia, subarachnoid injection (with paraplegia), intravascular injection, neuralgic pain in the upper lumbar roots, diaphragmatic irritation (with pleuritic and shoulder pain), urinary difficulties or renal trauma, pneumothorax, hematoma, hemorrhage, splanchnic vasodilation (hypotension), and systemic toxicity (e.g., cardiorespiratory compromise and unchecked parasympathetic tone with increased bowel motility and diarrhea).

4. **Intravenous regional (Bier) sympathetic block** is similar to the Bier somatic block using local anesthetics described in section IV.A.3.f. When sympathectomy is the goal, a sympathetically active drug (e.g., bretylium or guanethidine) is added to the local anesthetic. Even without the use of local anesthetics, however, peripheral sympathectomy can last for 1–2 weeks. Bier sympathetic

block is indicated in patients with SMP syndromes (e.g., CRPS with SMP features). Complications are similar to that of Bier somatic block except that the addition of a sympathetic blocking drug can further cause orthostatic hypotension and headache.

Further reading

Aronoff GM, editor: *Evaluation and treatment of chronic pain*, Baltimore, 1992, Williams & Wilkins.

Cousins MJ, Bridenbaugh PO, editors: *Neural blockade in clinical anesthesia and management of pain*, ed 3, Philadelphia, 1998, Lippincott-Raven.

Dreyfuss P, Rogers CJ: Radiofrequency neurotomy of the zygapophyseal and sacroiliac joints. In Lennard TA, editor: *Pain procedures in clinical practice*, ed 2, Philadelphia, 2000, Hanley & Belfus, p. 417.

Hamill RJ, Rowlingson JC, editors: *Handbook of critical care pain management*, New York, 1994, McGraw-Hill.

Lennard TA, editor: *Pain procedures in clinical practice*, Philadelphia, 2000, Hanley & Belfus.

Loeser JD, Butler SH, Chapman CR, *et al.*, editors: *Bonica's management of pain*, ed 3, Philadelphia, 2001, Lippincott, Williams & Wilkins.

Nicholas JJ, Lennard TA: Joint and soft tissue injection techniques. In Braddom RL, editor: *Physical medicine and rehabilitation*, ed 2, Philadelphia, 2000, WB Saunders, pp. 498–514.

Portenoy RK, Kanner RM, editors: *Pain management: theory and practice*, Philadelphia, 1996, FA Davis.

Raj PP, editor: *Practical management of pain*, ed 3, St Louis, 2000, Mosby.

Sinatra RS, Hord AH, Ginsberg B, *et al.*, editors: *Acute pain: mechanism and management*, St Louis, 1992, Mosby-Year Book.

Tollison CD, Satterthwaite JR, Tollison JW, editors: *Practical pain management*, ed 3, Philadelphia, 2002, Lippincott, Williams & Wilkins.

Waldman SD: *Interventional pain management*, ed 2, Philadelphia, 2001, WB Saunders.

Wall PD, Melzack R, editors: *Textbook of pain*, ed 4, Philadelphia, 1999, WB Saunders.

Walsh NE, Rogers JN: Injection procedures. In DeLisa JA, Gans BM, Walsh NE, *et al.*, editors: *Physical medicine and rehabilitation: principles and practice*, ed 4, Philadelphia, 2005, Lippincott, Williams & Wilkins, pp. 311–367.

Warfield CA, Bajwa ZH, editors: *Principles and practice of pain management*, ed 2, New York, 2003, McGraw-Hill.

CHAPTER 4.11
Trigger point therapy

Trigger points are small, localized tender areas found within skeletal muscles, fascia, tendons, ligaments, periosteum, and pericapsular areas. When "active", they radiate pain into a specific distant area or a zone of **referred pain**. The zone of referred pain, which is constant in its distribution for any given muscle (although it does not always follow a segmental neurological pattern) can be activated by pressure, by piercing with a needle, during activity, or even spontaneously during rest. If there is no zone of referred pain, then the localized tender area is called a **tender spot**. Trigger points and tender spots can be caused or perpetuated by local factors (e.g., sport- or work-related injuries, sprains, strains, overuse or repetitive injuries, compressed nerves, disk disease, arthritis, or muscle tension related to nonphysiologic posture or stress) or systemic factors [e.g., hypothyroidism, metabolic electrolyte disorders (such as hypokalemia and hypocalcemia), vitamin deficiencies (such as vitamin B complex or C deficiencies), chronic infections, and, possibly, estrogen deficiency].

The trigger points in the muscles may involve the fascia and are thus called myofascial trigger points. The symptoms and dysfunctions caused by one or more myofascial trigger points are referred to as myofascial pain syndrome (MPS). In MPS, trigger points are found within palpable **taut bands**. Taut bands run parallel to the orientation of the muscle fibers and represent a constantly contracted group of muscle fibers. When taut bands are snapped by a palpating finger or when they are pierced by a needle, a local twitch response (i.e., transient contraction of the taut band) can be elicited. Electromyographic studies show that although the taut band is electrically silent, the trigger points within the taut band show distinctive spontaneous electrical activity (i.e., motor end-plate-like potentials with high frequency and spikes). In chronic cases (6–8 weeks after injury), the taut band usually hardens because of fibrosis. Trigger points within a taut band can be detected by using a dolorimeter or algometer (see Chapter 5.10, section IV.C.1.a), which shows pain thresholds that are 2 kg/cm^2 lower than those of the normal side. The muscles that are commonly involved in MPS include suboccipital muscles, neck muscles (near the transverse processes of the C4–C6), trapezius muscles, levator scapulae muscles, supraspinatus and infraspinatus muscles, rhomboid muscles, extensor communis muscles near the lateral epicondyle, sacrospinous and quadratus lumborum muscles, gluteal muscles, tensor fascia lata, vastus medialis muscles, gastrocnemius muscles, and soleus muscles.

In contrast to MPS, the tender areas found in patients with fibromyalgia are generalized, diffuse, involving bilateral and symmetrical muscles, typically located in nonmuscular tissues (e.g., suboccipital muscle insertion, C5–C6 intertransverse space, second rib costochondral junction, lateral humeral epicondyle, greater trochanter, and medial knee fat) as well as muscular tissues (e.g., trapezius, supraspinatus, and gluteus muscles), with no zone of referred pain or taut bands. Patients with fibromyalgia can be treated by adjuvant analgesics (see Chapter 5.10, section VI.E.2) such as amitriptyline (see Chapter 4.8, section V.A.1.a.1) and cyclobenzaprine (see Chapter 4.8, section II.A.1), NSAIDS (see Chapter 4.8, section I.A.3), and also trigger point therapy (if there are concomitant myofascial trigger points).

Trigger point therapy encompasses injection therapy as well as noninjection therapy (e.g., spraying with vapocoolants followed by therapeutic exercises; relaxation exercises; electrical stimulation; and other physical modalities). Although there are many variations of trigger point therapy (e.g., Travell and Simon technique and Kraus technique), this chapter deals primarily with the eclectic approach taught by Dr Andrew Fischer. As with other treatment modalities, trigger point therapy should only be used as one of the components of the overall management of the patient (which includes elimination of etiological and contributing factors such as bad posture, poor body mechanics, highly stressful life-style, hypothyroidism, and vitamin deficiencies). Although studies have confirmed the existence of trigger points, data about the effectiveness of trigger point therapy remain mostly empirical. Clinical studies with proper controls on the effectiveness of trigger point therapy are still lacking.

I. Trigger point and tender spot injections

Both trigger point and tender spot injections involve needling (i.e., repetitive insertion and withdrawal of the needle), which is theorized to mechanically break up fibrotic pockets that have entrapped the nerve endings along with sensitizing substances, thus allowing blood to enter and wash away the sensitizing substances, leading to interruption of the "vicious cycle" of pain. The primary sites of injections are areas with the most intense pain and most tenderness and which are functionally important. Some of the functionally important muscles are as follows: for walking – quadratus lumborum, gluteus medius, and gastrocnemius, for shoulder movements – supraspinatus, and for normal postures – quadratus lumborum, levator scapulae, and upper trapezius. Depending on the number of trigger points, the size of the taut bands, and on patient tolerance, at least one or two (up to 10) injections per session may be given. The injection sessions are usually two to three sessions per week (with injections in different areas during the acute pain stage and once per week or once every 2 weeks during the recovery stage. To be effective, injection therapy should be combined with noninjection therapy (particularly exercises and proper body mechanics) as well as the elimination of the perpetuating factors. The contraindications for injection therapy include bleeding disorders (e.g., coagulopathies and thrombocytopenia), anticoagulant therapy, local infection, immunosuppression, certain psychiatric conditions (e.g., anxiety, paranoia, and schizophrenia), and inability to avoid heavy activity on the injected body part for 2–3 days following the procedure. Depression is not a contraindication for injection therapy (in fact, pain relief from the injection may relieve depression). For general injection procedures see Chapter 4.9, section II.

A. BLOCKING INJECTION TECHNIQUES. Prior to needling, paraspinous block and preinjection block can be administered to induce pre-emptive analgesia and help increase the effectiveness of trigger point or tender spot needling.

1. **Paraspinous block (PSB)** consists of anesthetic infiltration administered at the level of the **spinal segmental sensitization (SSS)** to instantaneously relieve segmental pain and to reverse the SSS to normal sensitivity. SSS represents a state of hyperactivity that spreads from the sensory component of the spinal segment to the anterior horn cells that control the myotome and also to the sympathetic centers located in the involved spinal level. SSS is believed to be induced by

the **pentad** (vicious circle) **of diskopathy–radiculpathy**, which consists of (a) narrowed disk space and neural foramen on imaging studies; this is manifested clinically by (b) narrowed space between spinous processes and (c) a sprained supra/interspinous ligament. There is (d) palpable paraspinal muscle spasm, which causes (e) nerve root compression, which leads to radicular dysfunction, which then induces SSS. In the above pentad, the supra/interspinous ligament sprain component serves as an irritative focus causing SSS. Thus, in patients with SSS, it was observed that blocking nociceptive impulses from the supra/interspinous ligament relieves paraspinal muscle spasm, which in turn relieves the radicular symptoms and reverses the SSS to normal sensitivity.

In PSB, a 25-gauge needle, 38 mm or longer, is used to slowly infiltrate 1% lidocaine proximally and distally along the spinous processes (at the affected level) into the loose connective tissue without penetrating the muscles. This is then followed by needling and infiltration of the sprained supra/interspinous ligament. In the cervical region, about 1.5 mL/segment is used over one or two levels per session (not to exceed 3 mL per session). In the thoracic level, about 2 mL/segment is used over two or three segments per session. In the lumbosacral region, about 3–5 mL/segment is used over two or three segments per session. If there is persistent severe pain of another unattended level, then the additional level can be injected after waiting about 45–60 minutes (during the waiting period, the patient can receive physical therapy).

2. **Preinjection block (PIB)** consists of anesthetic infiltration of branches of sensory nerves supplying the tender spot or trigger point along the taut band being prepared for needling and infiltration (NandI). It is done so that NandI can be carried out without causing much pain, thus helping prevent central sensitization caused by needling or injecting a sensitized area such as a trigger point or tender spot. PIB can also shrink the taut band to about 15–20% of its original thickness (because of the relief of neurogenic contraction of the muscle fibers), so that NandI can concentrate upon the remaining "fibrotic core", which is the only target of the mechanical breakup by NandI.

   In PIB, a 25-gauge needle, 38–10.5 cm long, is used to slowly infiltrate 3–8 mL of 1% lidocaine into the region next to the trigger point or tender spot. The needle penetration on PIB should be limited to nontender, normal tissue surrounding the taut band to prevent pain and further sensitization. This goal, however, cannot always be achieved because the bands may be too wide and the anesthesia is ineffective if PIB is performed too far from the sensitized tissue. The spreading of the anesthetic in PIB should be on the side where the nerve supply enters the taut band, trigger point, or tender spot. Thus, if PIB along one side of the taut band has not been successful, then the other side should also be tried. To prevent nerve damage and muscle paralysis, the main nerve should never be blocked in PIB. Instead, only the branches supplying the taut band being prepared for NandI should be blocked in PIB.

B. NEEDLING TECHNIQUES. Needling should only be performed after PIB. A 22- to 25-gauge needle is usually large enough for needling. A length of 1.5 inches (38 mm) is usually long enough to reach deeper than the trigger points or tender spots except for the thicker muscles of the lumbar paraspinal and gluteal muscles, which may need about 2- to 3.5-inch (9 cm) needles. For long-term effect, needling should extend throughout the taut band (not just be confined to the trigger point or tender spot) and should include its attachment to the bone at both sides (i.e., origin and insertion) of the muscle. The following describes general needling techniques. For needling of specific muscles, refer to the textbooks by Travell and Simons or by Kraus (see Further reading section).

1. **Dry needling** is similar to the fluid-injection technique described in section I.A.2 except for the absence of fluid infiltration. The needle is inserted directly

into the trigger point locations, as opposed to the distant points or meridians used in acupuncture. It is generally not recommended because it is painful and is not well-tolerated by patients.

2. **Needling combined with fluid infiltration** (NandI) potentiates the mechanical effects of needling alone and is preferred to dry needling because it is more effective and more comfortable. The most commonly used fluid is a local anesthetic (e.g., 1% lidocaine or 0.5% procaine; about 3–8 mL per session), which blocks the pain and the irritation resulting from tissue damaged by the needling. The total amount of 1% lidocaine used (for PSB, PIB, and NandI) should not exceed 5 mL in the neck or 15–20 mL per session over the entire body. Although their anesthetic effect usually lasts only for about 45–60 minutes, the use of local anesthetics has been reported to reduce the intensity and duration of postinjection soreness as well as postinjection spasm in the surrounding muscles. If the patient is allergic to local anesthetics, however, isotonic saline solution may be used (because ultimately it is the needling, not the infiltrated fluid, that is believed to break up the taut band and trigger points). The use of corticosteroids (alone or in combination with local anesthetics) is generally not recommended (unless for injection into inflamed passive soft tissues like bursa and tendon sheaths; see Chapter 4.9) because trigger points are usually caused by muscular sensitization irritation rather than inflammation. Moreover, corticosteroids are associated with greater potential for side-effects including local myopathy.

After explaining the procedure to the patient, the point of maximal tenderness is located by asking the patient to point with one finger, by clinician's palpation, or by using a dolorimeter (see dolorimeter description in Chapter 5.10, section IV.C.1.a). The patient is positioned to allow proper access to the trigger point and the muscle around it is palpated to find the entire taut band (which may span from the origin to the insertion of the muscle). The taut band and trigger point are marked using an indelible felt pen or using fingernail impressions. The skin is then prepared using the technique described in Chapter 4.9, section II. After the skin is decontaminated, the entire taut band area is sprayed with a vapocoolant (e.g., ethyl chloride or fluorimethane). When the skin is slightly frosted, the needle is quickly inserted aiming directly at the point of maximal tenderness. An alternative to vapocoolant anesthesia is to pinch the skin in the area to be injected (to distract the sensory pathways) followed immediately by needle insertion.

Once the needle reaches the taut band, a fibrotic type of resistance (gritty, sandpaper-like) is usually felt. The syringe is aspirated and if it is clear of blood, a small amount (0.1–0.3 mL) of fluid is deposited while the taut band or fibrotic area is mechanically needled. Any time that blood is drawn during syringe aspiration, the injection therapy for that site should be terminated. The needling is continued several times or until normal muscle is reached, i.e., when the pain and fibrotic resistance ceases. Upon reaching normal muscles, deposit 0.1–0.3 mL of fluid into the normal muscle and redirect the needle. The redirection of the needle should be done under the skin surface, that is, by gently pulling the needle up to the subcutaneous level (without removing or pulling the needle out of the skin) and redirecting it by either a few millimeters or by 1- to 3-cm increments along the plane of the taut band. As the needle pierces each new area in the taut band, infiltrate 0.1–0.3 mL of fluid (making sure no blood is aspirated prior to each fluid deposition). This process is repeated until the entire taut band (including the myotendon junction) is needled and infiltrated; usually up to 10 local infiltrations can be performed in one session depending on the patient's tolerance.

To cover the entire taut bands of large muscles, the needle may need to be pulled out of the skin and reinserted at another site. Otherwise, the remaining parts of the taut band can be injected after a period of about 1 week (to allow for tissue healing). Muscles that are constantly active (e.g., masseters and gluteus medius) should only be given minimum needling per session and may, therefore, need several sessions for complete treatment. The total amounts of fluid used per muscle are as follows: 1–3 mL for head, neck, hand, or foot muscles; 2–5 mL for shoulder muscles; 3–4 mL for trunk muscles; 6–10 mL for lumbar paraspinals or gluteal muscles; and 3–7 mL for leg muscles. If 1% lidocaine is used, the maximum amount per session is 20 mL. When the needle is pulled out, the injected site should be compressed for about 2 minutes to prevent bleeding and then covered with a Band-Aid. After injection, the patient is instructed to perform active full range of motion (ROM) exercises to the injected muscle at least three times in positions with gravity eliminated or reduced (e.g., in a side-lying position for hip flexion and extension).

C. **POSTINJECTION CARE** is crucial to the success of trigger point injection therapy. For the next 3 consecutive days, the patient should avoid heavy use of the injected muscle (e.g., long walks, long driving, or sports activities). If the muscle soreness is excessive, cyclo-oxygenase-2 inhibitors (e.g., celecoxib, valdecoxib), ibuprofen, or acetaminophen may be prescribed for 3–5 days. The patient should also receive 3 consecutive days of physical therapy consisting of the following:

1. **Local heat,** for example, moist hot packs for 20 minutes.
2. **Electrical stimulation** for 15 minutes using sinusoidal surging current to induce muscle squeezing actions (i.e., slow, strong contractions) of the injected muscles with alternating periods of contraction and rest. If there is muscle spasm, a tetanizing current may be applied followed by a sinusoid surging current to induce periodic contractions for 10 minutes each.
3. **Exercises** that follow a pattern of relaxation, warm-up, limbering/stretching (to be repeated only three to five times each movement), and cooling off. The exercises include the following:

a. ***Relaxation exercises,*** such as controlled breathing with eye-movement technique (see Chapter 4.2, section VI.A.1.b), Jacobson's progressive relaxation exercises (see Chapter 4.2, section VI.A.2), or active inhibition techniques (see Chapter 4.2, section I.C), such as hold–relax, agonist contraction with reciprocal inhibition of the antagonist, and hold–relax–contract. When doing active inhibition techniques, breathing can be timed so that stretching is performed during exhalation when the muscles are relaxed.

b. ***Spray and active limbering exercises*** (see section II.A.1.a) or spray and stretch exercise (see section II.A.1.b); and

c. ***Customized home exercise program,*** which consists of limbering exercises and passive stretching to be performed every hour for the first 2–3 days after injection, then gradually reduced in frequency until they are performed at least three times a day. If the patient received an injection to the lower body, he or she is instructed to get up and walk or at least contract and relax the muscles in the sitting position every 2 hours for about 5 minutes to prevent stiffness and to maintain circulation.

II. Noninjection trigger point therapy

Noninjection trigger point therapy should be included in the comprehensive management of trigger points or tender spots. It may be used solely if injection therapy is contraindicated (see section I) or is refused by the patient. It is useful in complex cases involving many muscles in one or more regions of the body because it permits the release of several closely related muscles at one time.

A. THERAPEUTIC EXERCISES

1. **Exercises in combination with vapocoolant spray.** The vapocoolant spray (ethyl chloride or fluorimethane) is used to inactivate the trigger point and facilitate stretching. Its mechanism of action is unclear but it probably works indirectly via skin afferent nerves (rather than by direct cooling of the muscles) to inhibit pain and spinal stretch reflexes thus reflexively relaxing the muscle and allowing it to be adequately stretched. If ethyl chloride is used, fire hazards must be eliminated, and the patient should not inhale the heavy vapors. In contrast, the same caution is not necessary for fluorimethane, which is nonflammable, nonexplosive, chemically stable, nontoxic, and does not irritate the skin.

a. ***Spray and limber protocol (Kraus).*** Ethyl chloride (preferred by Kraus) is sprayed (with very slight frosting) over the area concentrating on the point of maximum tenderness. The patient is then asked to do limbering exercises by actively and slowly moving the joint of the sprayed muscle through its full ROM three to five times with minimal effort in a position with gravity eliminated or reduced. This can be combined with deep breathing exercises to induce muscle relaxation. After the exercise, check if the pain is still present or if it has shifted to another location. Repeat the spraying process followed by limbering exercises to full active ROM until pain is relieved completely or no further increase in ROM or relief of pain can be obtained. In this protocol, all movements are done actively with no passive stretching.

b. ***Spray and stretch protocol*** (Travell and Simons; see Figures 4.11-1 to 4.11-7). Fluorimethane (preferred by Travell and Simons) is sprayed until the skin is cool but without frosting; wait until the skin warms before repeating the application. Use a unidirectional sweeping pattern (one or two sweeps) in the direction of the muscle fibers at a slow rate of 10 cm or 4 inches per second from an angle of 30° and a distance of 45 cm (18 inches) over the entire muscle including the zone of referred pain. While spraying, the muscle is passively stretched (for about 30 seconds slowly) using gentle, smooth, steady tension applied by the patient or the clinician's free hand. Then warm the skin using a hot moist pack for a few minutes followed by having the patient perform slow, active, full ROM exercise through both the fully shortened and fully lengthened positions for the muscle group under treatment. This process is repeated five times. The stretching may be timed to the exhalation phase of controlled breathing exercise.

2. **Customized home exercise program.** Combine relaxation exercises (see section I.B.3.a) with limbering and stretch exercises.

B. PHYSICAL MODALITIES (see Chapter 4.1) include electrical stimulation to primarily reduce muscle spasms (e.g., high-voltage monophasic pulsed current; see Chapter 4.1, section V), ice application (see Chapter 4.1, section II), ultrasound (see Chapter 4.1, section I.B.1), biofeedback (see Chapter 4.1, section VI), and massage (e.g., deep, kneading or friction massage; see Chapter 4.1, section IX).

C. ADJUNCT TREATMENT WITH MEDICATIONS. Non-narcotic analgesics (e.g., NSAIDs, acetaminophen, tramadol; see Chapter 4.8, section I.A.3) and mild narcotic analgesics (e.g., hydrocodone, oxycodone; see Chapter 4.8, section I.B) are the first choice, especially after trigger point injection. Adjuvant analgesics (see Chapter 5.10, section VI.E.2) such as amitriptyline (see Chapter 4.8, section V.A.1.a.1) and cyclobenzaprine (see Chapter 4.8, section II.A.1) may be helpful, especially if the patient has concomitant fibromyalgia. Corticosteroids are ineffective and therefore not used in MPS.

D. ELIMINATION OF ETIOLOGICAL AND CONTRIBUTING FACTORS, such as poor posture, poor body mechanics, leg-length discrepancy, vocational and avocational overuse, highly stressful living, poor sleep, and poor physical fitness, should be addressed.

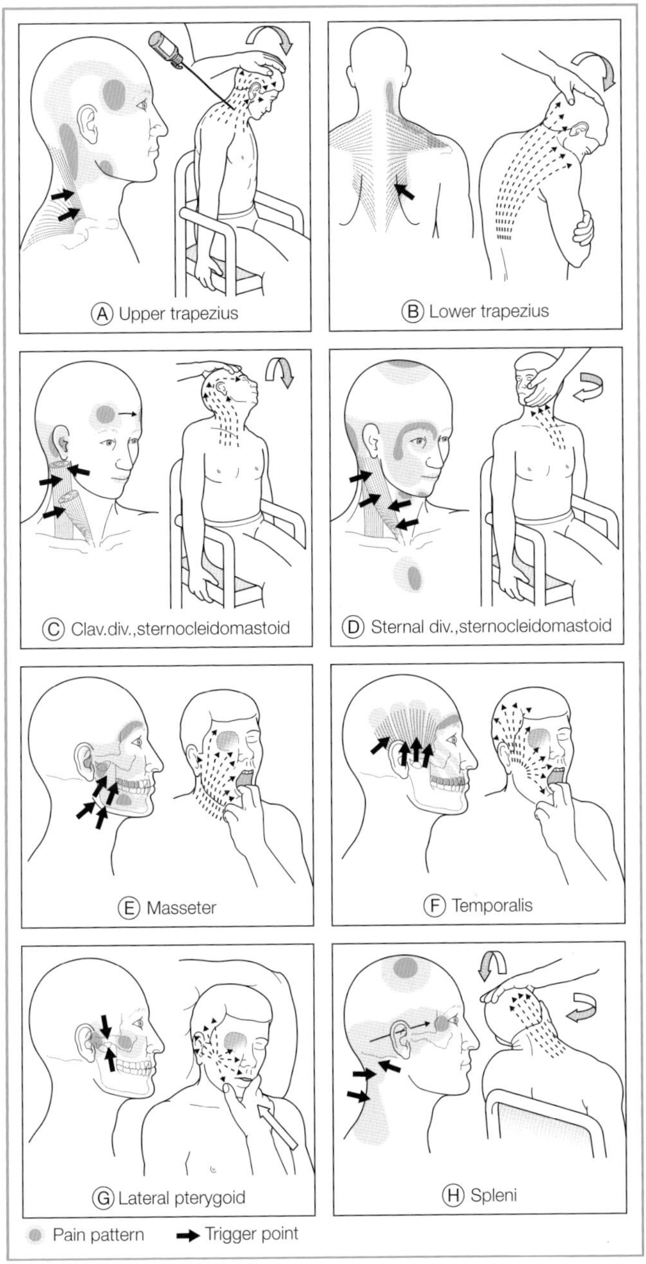

Figure 4.11-1 Location of trigger points (*solid black arrows*) and pain patterns (*gray stipples*), stretch positions and spray patterns (*dashed arrows*) for muscles that cause head and neck pain. Curved white arrows show the direction of pressure applied to stretch each muscle, and dashed arrows trace the path of parallel sweeps of vapocoolant spray to release tension and permit stretch of each muscle. In **H**, broken arrow in pain pattern deep to ear indicates pain deep in head radiating to back of eye. (Redrawn from: Simons DG: Myofascial pain syndromes. In Basmajian JV, Kirby RL, editors: *Medical rehabilitation*, Baltimore, 1984, Williams & Wilkins, p. 314.)

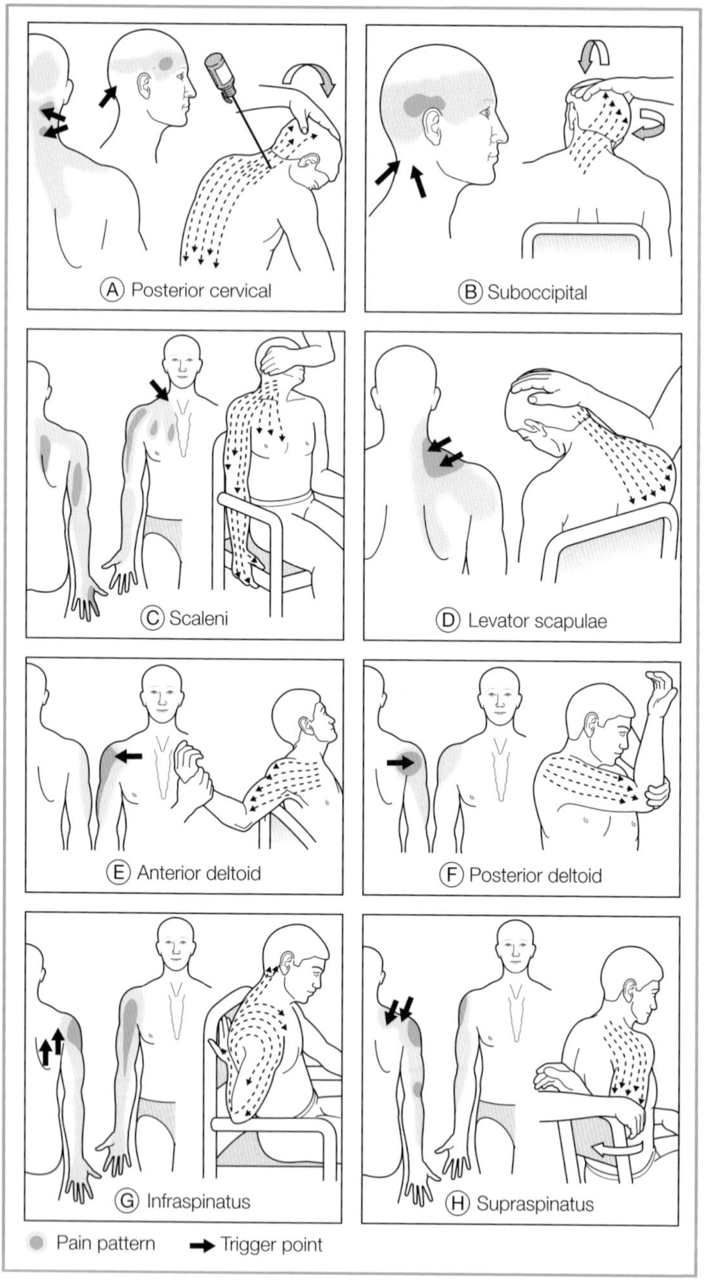

Figure 4.11-2 Location of trigger points (*solid black arrows*) and pain patterns (*gray stipples*), stretch positions and spray patterns (*dashed arrows*) for two muscles producing head and neck pain (**A** and **B**) and six muscles causing shoulder and upper limb pain (**C** to **H**). Curved white arrows identify the direction of pressure applied to stretch the muscle. The dashed arrows trace impact of the stream of vapocoolant spray applied to release the muscular tension during stretch. (Redrawn from: Simons DG: Myofascial pain syndromes. In Basmajian JV, Kirby RL, editors: *Medical rehabilitation*, Baltimore, 1984, Williams & Wilkins, p. 315.)

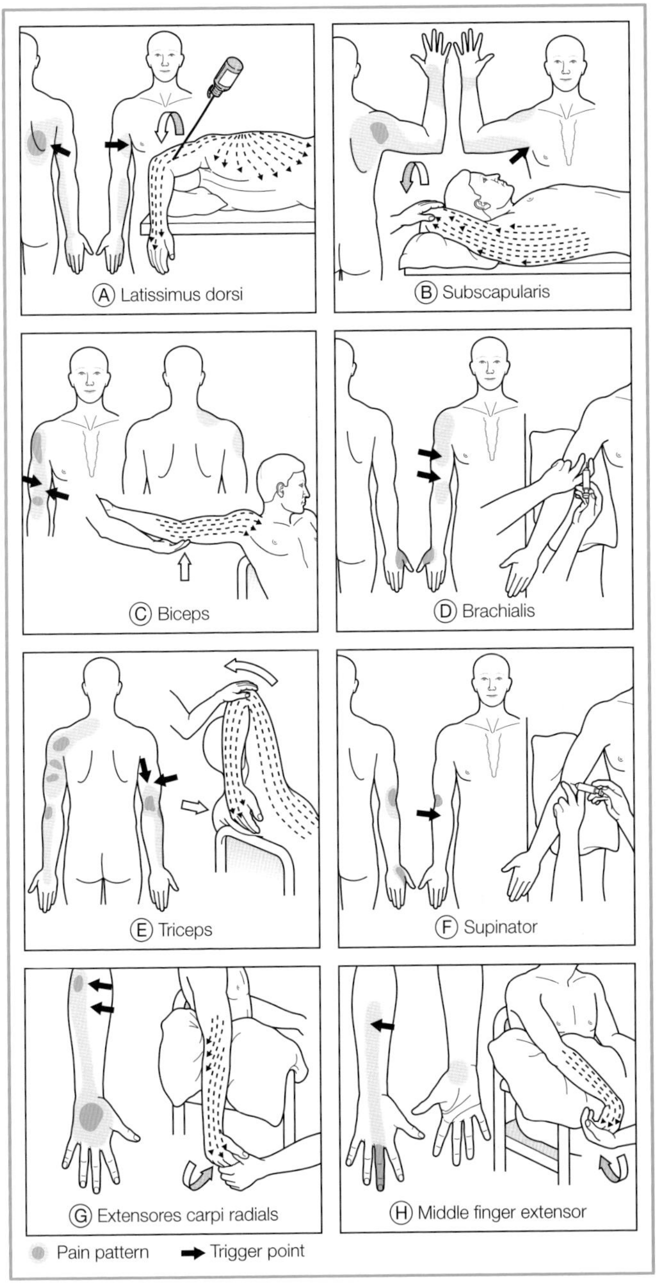

Figure 4.11-3 Location of trigger points (*solid black arrows*) and pain patterns (*gray stipples*), stretch positions and spray patterns (*dashed arrows*) for eight muscles responsible for shoulder and upper limb pain. Curved white arrows identify the direction of pressure applied to stretch the muscle. Dashed arrows trace impact of stream of vapocoolant spray applied to release muscular tension during stretch. (Redrawn from: Simons DG: Myofascial pain syndromes. In Basmajian JV, Kirby RL, editors: *Medical rehabilitation*, Baltimore, 1984, Williams & Wilkins, p. 316.)

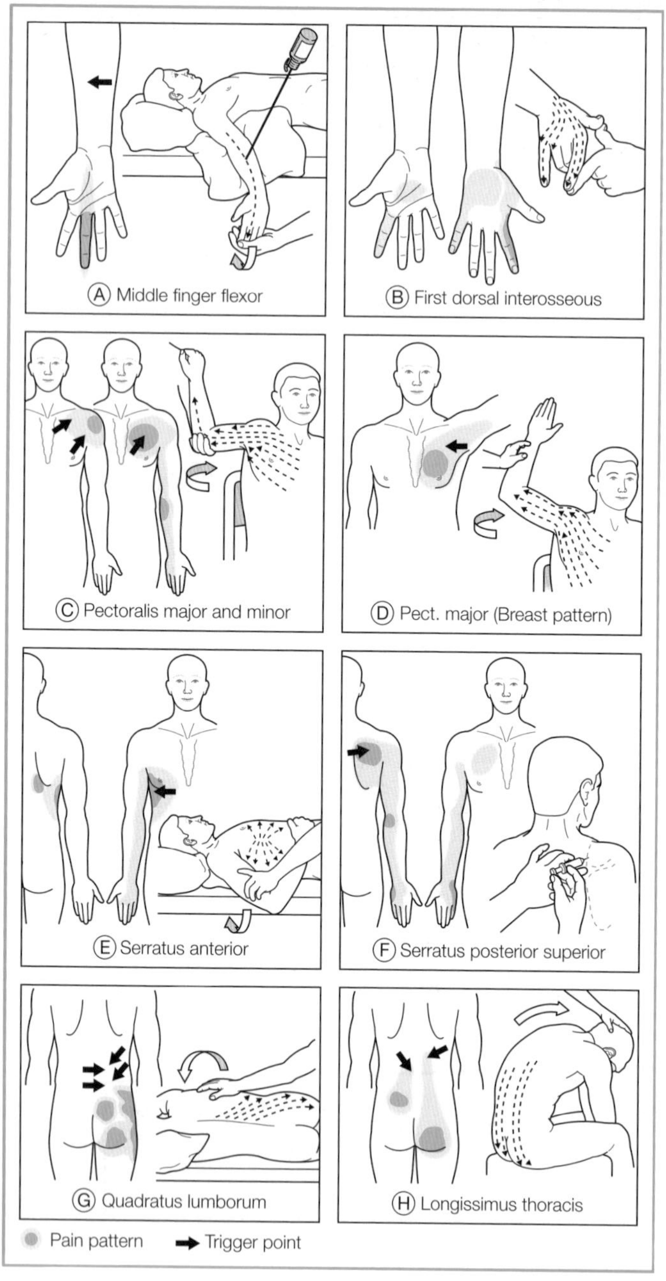

Figure 4.11-4 Location of trigger points (*solid black arrows*) and pain patterns (*gray stipples*), stretch positions and spray patterns (*dashed arrows*) for two muscles producing shoulder and upper limb pain (**A** and **B**) and six muscles causing trunk and back pain (**C** to **H**). Curved white arrows identify the direction of pressure applied to stretch the muscle. Dashed arrows trace impact of stream of vapocoolant spray applied to release muscular tension during stretch. (Redrawn from: Simons DG: Myofascial pain syndromes. In Basmajian JV, Kirby RL, editors: *Medical rehabilitation*, Baltimore, 1984, Williams & Wilkins, p. 317.)

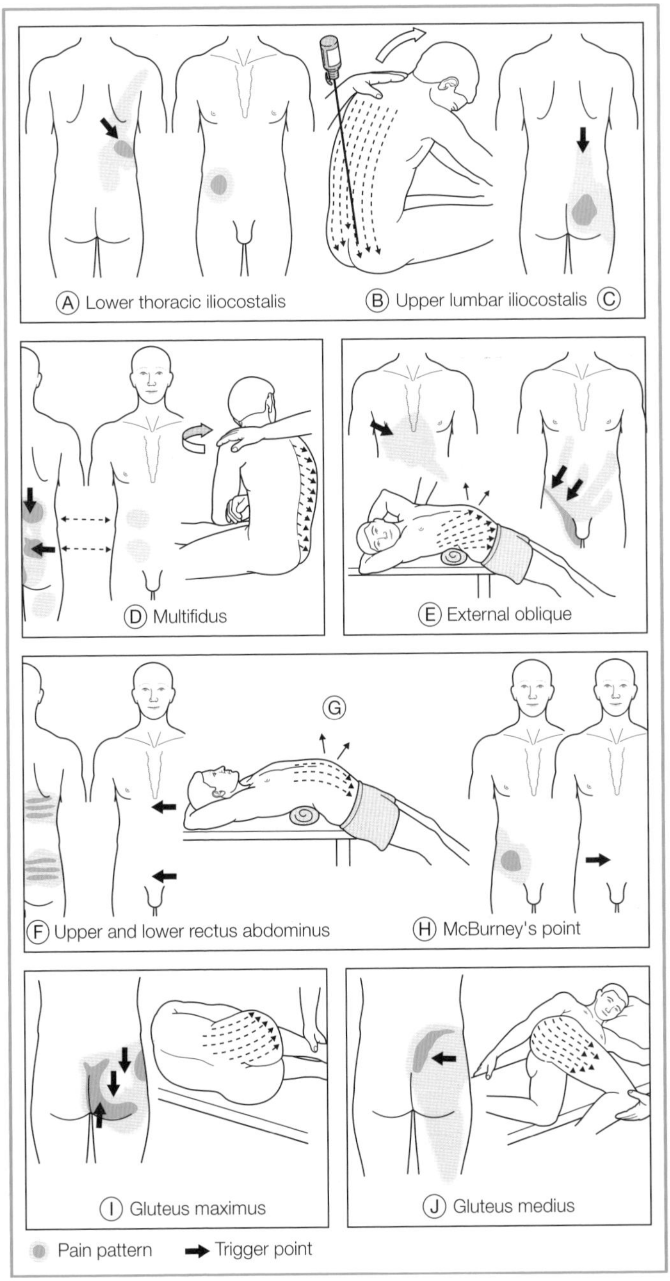

Figure 4.11-5 Location of trigger points (*solid black arrows*) and pain patterns (*gray stipples*), stretch positions and spray patterns (*dashed arrows*) for five muscles producing trunk and back pain (**A** to **H**) and two muscles responsible for lower limb pain (**I** and **J**). Curved white arrows identify the directions of pressure applied to stretch the muscle. Dashed arrows trace impact of stream of vapocoolant spray applied to release muscular tension during stretch. (Redrawn from: Simons DG: Myofascial pain syndromes. In Basmajian JV, Kirby RL, editors: *Medical rehabilitation*, Baltimore, 1984, Williams & Wilkins, p. 318.)

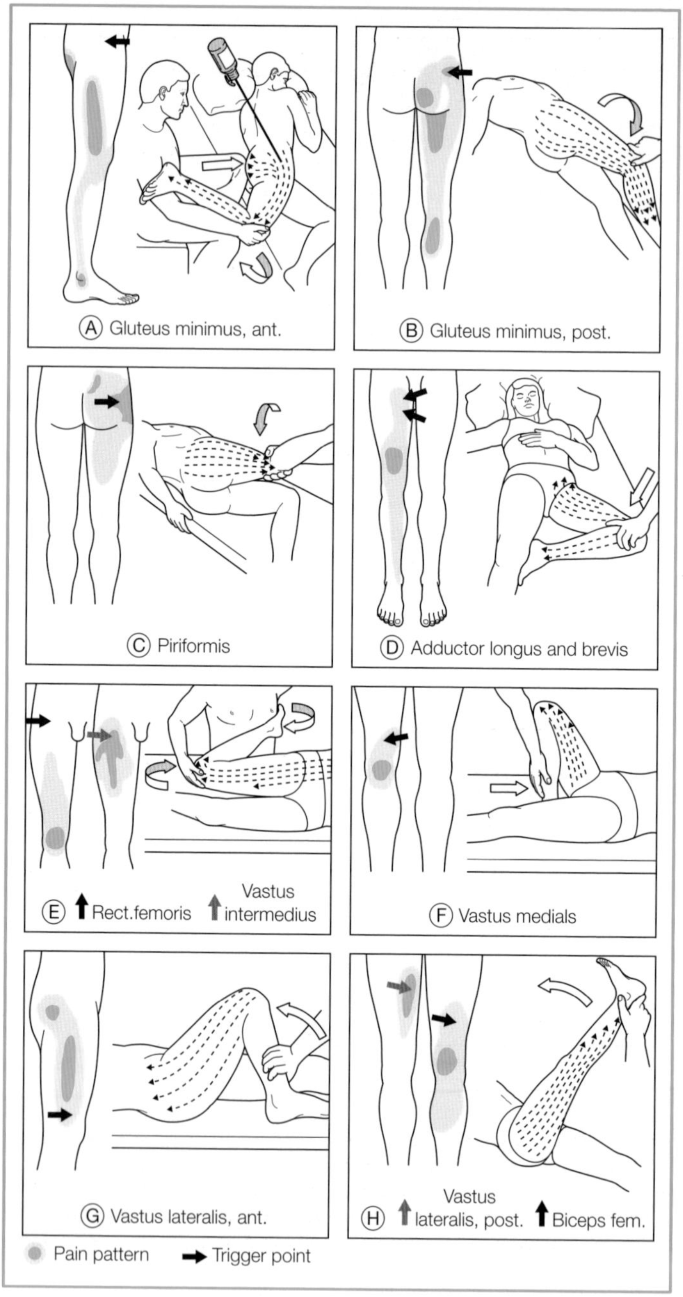

Figure 4.11-6 Location of trigger points (*solid black arrows*) and pain patterns (*gray stipples*), stretch positions and spray patterns (*dashed arrows*) for ten muscles causing lower limb pain. Curved white arrows identify the directions of pressure applied to stretch the muscle. Dashed arrows trace impact of stream of vapocoolant spray applied to release muscular tension during stretch. (Redrawn from: Simons DG: Myofascial pain syndromes. In Basmajian JV, Kirby RL, editors: *Medical rehabilitation*, Baltimore, 1984, Williams & Wilkins, p. 319.)

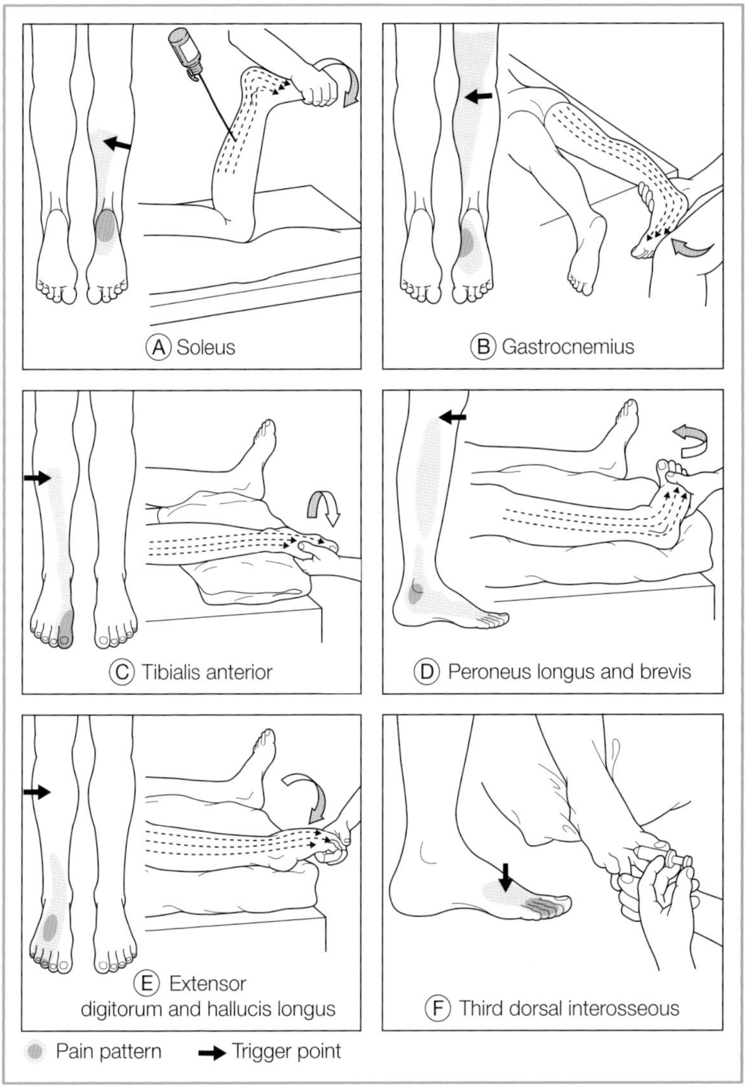

Figure 4.11-7 Location of trigger points (*solid black arrows*) and pain patterns (*gray stipples*), stretch positions and spray patterns (*dashed arrows*) for eight muscles producing lower limb pain. Curved white arrows identify the directions of pressure applied to stretch the muscle. Dashed arrows trace impact of stream of vapocoolant spray applied to release muscular tension during stretch. (Redrawn from: Simons DG: Myofascial pain syndromes. In Basmajian JV, Kirby RL, editors: *Medical rehabilitation*, Baltimore, 1984, Williams & Wilkins, p. 320.)

Further reading

Fischer AA: New injection techniques for treatment of musculoskeletal pain. In Rachlin ES, Rachlin IS, editors: *Myofascial pain and fibromyalgia: trigger point management*, ed 2, St Louis, 2002, Mosby, pp. 403–419.

Fischer AA: Trigger point injection. In Lennard TA, editor: *Pain procedures in clinical practice*, ed 2, Philadelphia, 2000, Hanley & Belfus, pp. 153–161.

Fischer AA: Local injections in pain management: trigger point needling with infiltration and somatic blocks. *Phys Med Rehab Clin North Am* 6(4):851–870, 1995.
Fischer AA, Cassius DA, Imamura M: Myofascial pain and fibromyalgia. In O'Young BJ, Young MA, Stiens SA, editors: *Physical medicine and rehabilitation secrets*, ed 2, Philadelphia, 2002, Hanley & Belfus, pp. 369–378.
Fischer AA, Imamura M: New concepts in the diagnosis and management of musculoskeletal pain. In Lennard TA, editor: *Pain procedures in clinical practice*, ed 2, Philadelphia, 2000, Hanley & Belfus, pp. 213–229.
Kraus H: *Diagnosis and treatment of muscle pain*, Lombard, IL, 1988, Quintessence Publishing.
Rachlin ES, Rachlin IS: *Myofascial pain and fibromyalgia: trigger point management*, ed 2, St Louis, 2002, Mosby.
Simons DG: Muscular pain syndromes. In Fricton JR, Awad, EA, editors: *Advances in pain research and therapy*, New York, 1990, Raven, pp. 1–41.
Simons DG: Myofascial pain syndromes due to trigger points. In Goodgold J, editor: *Rehabilitation medicine*, St Louis, 1988, Mosby-Year Book, pp. 686–723.
Simons DG, Simons LS: Chronic myofascial pain syndrome. In Tollison CD, Satterthwaite JR, Tollison JW, editors: *Practical pain management*, ed 3, Philadelphia, 2002, Lippincott, Williams & Wilkins, pp. 556–577.
Simons DG, Travell JG, Simons LS: *Travell & Simon's Myofascial pain and dysfunction: The trigger point manual. Upper half of body*, vol. 1, ed 2, Philadelphia, 1999, Lippincott, Williams & Wilkins.
Travell JG, Simons DG: *Myofascial pain and dysfunction: the trigger point manual. The lower extremities*, vol. 2, Philadelphia, 1993, Lippincott, Williams & Wilkins.

PART V

BASIC PHYSICAL MEDICINE AND REHABILITATION PROBLEMS

CHAPTER 5.1
Deconditioning

Immobilization is the physical restriction of movement involving a body segment or the entire body. Common causes of immobilization in PM&R include neuromusculoskeletal disorders and injuries (e.g., paralysis as a result of stroke or spinal cord injuries); orthopedic casts, body jackets, and splints, usually after trauma or fracture; critical illness requiring bed rest (e.g., after acute myocardial infarction, cardiac dysrhythmia, or septic shock); and prolonged stays in a recumbent position (e.g., chronic low back pain) or sitting position (e.g., wheelchair sitting). Immobilization as a result of prolonged bed rest results in a clinical entity called **deconditioning**, which is separate from the original process that led to the immobilization. In deconditioning, there is a reduced functional capacity of multiple body systems, especially the musculoskeletal system. The reduced functional capacity of the musculoskeletal system leads to further inactivity and perpetuates the vicious cycle. The severity of deconditioning is dependent on the degree and duration of immobilization. It affects any age and gender, particularly the chronically sick, aged, and disabled population. The adverse clinical manifestations of prolonged immobilization are described below together with the recommended rehabilitation measures to counteract or prevent its deleterious effects. Obviously, prevention is much more cost-effective and is preferable to treatment.

I. Musculoskeletal changes

A. CONTRACTURE is the lack of full active or passive range of motion (ROM) because of a joint, soft tissue, or muscle limitation. Conditions producing limited joint ROM include pain (e.g., trauma, inflammation, infection, joint degeneration, ischemia, and hemorrhage), muscle imbalance (e.g., paralysis and spasticity), capsular or periarticular tissue fibrosis, primary muscle damage (e.g., polymyositis and muscular dystrophy), or mechanical factors (e.g., improper bed positioning, and casting or splinting in a foreshortened position). The muscle fibers and connective tissues which are maintained in a shortened position (e.g., for 5–7 days) adapt to the shortened length by contraction of collagen fibers and a decrease in muscle fiber sarcomeres. In 3 weeks or more, the loose connective tissue in muscles and around joints gradually changes into dense connective tissue, causing contracture on the relaxed side of the joint. Contractures occur most commonly at the lower limb with involvement of muscles that cross two joints in the hips, knees, and ankles. In the upper limbs, the shoulders, elbows, wrists, and fingers are most susceptible.

Contractures are prevented by proper positioning (using pillows, trochanter rolls, hand rolls, or resting splints), active or passive ROM exercises (see Chapter 4.2, section I.A), and early mobilization and ambulation (see Chapter 4.6, section IV). In the supine position, the anterior neck and upper chest should be extended; the trunk and lower limbs should be neutral with the hips extended and slightly abducted; the knees should be extended; and the ankle should be in a neutral position with the toes pointing towards the ceiling (and no pressure at the heels). The shoulders should be in 30° of flexion and 45–90° of abduction, the elbows extended, the wrists in 20–30° extension, and the hands in the functional position (i.e., the thumb should be abducted and the first web space should be preserved by using a hand roll or resting splint; and the metacarpophalangeal and interphalangeal joints should be flexed 30° or the metacarpophalangeal joints flexed and interphalangeal joints extended in patients with dorsal hand burns). A prone or side-lying position may also be used. Nurses or family members should be instructed on how to provide ROM for preventing contractures.

Bed treatment of contractures includes passive ROM (see Chapter 4.2, section I.A) with terminal stretch at least twice daily; prolonged stretch using low passive tension and heat; sustained stretch using continuous passive mobilization; progressive, sustained stretching for 2 hours or more (e.g., dynamic splinting or serial casting); treatment of spasticity (see Chapter 5.4, section III); and surgical release (e.g., tendon lengthening, osteotomies, and joint replacements). In spastic patients, a more aggressive ROM exercise three to four times per day may be necessary, along with medical management of spasticity with medications (see Chapter 5.4, section III.D.1), and nerve or motor point blocks (see Chapter 5.4, section III.D.2.b).

B. MUSCLE WEAKNESS AND ATROPHY are usually seen in the antigravity muscles of the lower limbs (e.g., gastrocnemius-soleus) and the back muscles. Large muscles lose strength twice as quickly as smaller ones. Type I (slow-twitch) muscle fibers tend to atrophy more predominantly than type II (fast-twitch) muscles. In flaccid paralysis caused by lower motor neuron disease, muscle bulk is reduced by 90–95%. In spastic paralysis caused by upper motor neuron disease, muscle bulk is reduced by only 30–35% because of the increased tone caused by spasticity. With total inactivity there is a 10–20% decrease in isometric muscle strength per week, or about 1–3% per day. After as little as one day, muscle fiber atrophy can occur. In 3–5 weeks, complete immobilization can lead to a 50% decrease in muscle strength. Strength that is lost in 1 week may take 4 weeks to regain even with a maximal strengthening program. To prevent disuse weakness and atrophy, a muscle must exert 20–30% of its maximal capacity for several seconds each day. Muscle exertion at 50% of maximum capacity performed for 1 s/day is even more effective. Neuromuscular electrical stimulation can prevent or retard muscle weakness and atrophy if the muscle is not denervated (see Chapter 4.1, section V). Another technique for maintaining or increasing muscle strength and for preventing or retarding atrophy is proprioceptive neuromuscular facilitation (see Chapter 4.2, section IV.B.1).

C. DISUSE (IMMOBILIZATION) OSTEOPOROSIS is the loss of bone density because of increased resorption caused by lack of stimulus (e.g., weight bearing, gravity, and muscle activity) on bone mass. The adverse effects of prolonged immobilization on the endocrine system cause increased urinary excretion of calcium and hydroxyproline and increased excretion of calcium in the stool which contributes to disuse osteoporosis. Disuse osteoporosis is more marked in the subperiosteal region, in contrast to senile osteoporosis, which develops from the marrow outward. Disuse osteoporosis initially involves the cancellous bone at the metaphysis and epiphysis, and later extends to the entire diaphysis. Bone density is reduced by 40–45% after 12 weeks of bed rest. By the 30th week, more than 50% of bone density is lost. In patients with disuse osteoporosis, minor trauma or falls may lead to compression fractures of vertebral bodies, or fractures of the hip or other weight-bearing long bones. In patients with neurogenic paralysis (e.g., from spinal cord injury), disuse osteoporosis is accelerated.

Osteoporosis can only be prevented by weight-bearing standing (see Chapter 4.6, section IV.A). Nonweight-bearing exercise in bed is in itself not effective in preventing or treating osteoporosis. A standing frame or tilt table may be used in patients who are unable to stand unsupported. As soon as the patient is stable, tilt-table conditioning should begin at a 30° tilt for 1 minute. Gradually the tilt can be increased by 10° every 3–5 days or earlier as tolerated, until the patient is able to tolerate a 70° tilt for 30 minutes. Then the patient progresses to standing in parallel bars, and finally, to ambulation (see Chapter 4.6, section IV). A general exercise program (see Chapter 4.2), including strengthening, endurance, and coordination exercises, and resumption of activities of daily living should be started as early as possible.

D. CARTILAGE DEGENERATION occurs in immobilization because of cessation of joint imbibation (i.e., the regular loading and unloading of pressure, which draws fluid into and out of the cartilage). Thus the hyaline cartilage in synovial joints (which is avascular) is only able to obtain its nutrients by diffusion, which is inadequate. Cartilage degeneration caused by immobilization affects both the opposing joint surfaces that are in contact with each other (leading to necrosis and erosions) and those that are not (leading to fissures and loss of smoothness). The cartilage stiffens because of proteoglycan imbalance. There is compensatory cartilage proliferation and formation of osteophytes as the joint tries to repair itself. There is also synovial atrophy and biofatty infiltration of the joint cavity. In the presence of extra-articular connective tissue contracture, it can eventually cause ankylosis. In the early stages, this cartilage degeneration is reversible to some extent, hence early mobilization is imperative.

II. Cardiovascular changes

A. ORTHOSTATIC (POSTURAL) HYPOTENSION is the result of the impaired ability of the circulatory system to adjust to the upright position. As the person stands, blood pools in the lower limbs causing an immediate drop in venous return, which reduces stroke volume and cardiac output. Normally, there is immediate vasoconstriction and increase in heart rate (HR) and systolic blood pressure. However, prolonged bed rest causes the person to lose this adaptation which is manifested in the following clinical signs and symptoms: tingling, burning in the lower limbs, dizziness, lightheadedness, fainting, vertigo, increased pulse rate (20 or more beats per minute), decreased systolic blood pressure (20 or more mmHg), and decreased pulse pressure.

Treatment includes early mobilization (ROM exercises, strengthening exercises, ambulation, and calisthenics); abdominal strengthening and isotonic–isometric exercises of the legs (to reverse venous stasis and pooling); providing the wheelchair with elevating leg rests and a reclining back; use of the tilt table (gradual tilt up to 75° for 20 minutes); use of Ace bandage wraps, full-length elastic stockings, and abdominal binders; use of sympathomimetic pressor agents [ephedrine, 10–25 mg slow intravenous (IV) infusion which may be repeated every 5–10 minutes; or phenylephrine (Neo-Synephrine); 100–200 mg, IV, for severe hypotension or infusion of 20 mg in 250 mL 5% dextrose in water (80 mg/mL) at 40–180 mg/min (35–160 mL/h)]; use of mineralocorticoid [fludrocortisone (Florinef), 0.1 mg, po, qd] to help maintain blood pressure; and maintaining an adequate salt and fluid intake to prevent further blood-volume contraction and worsening of hypotension.

B. CHANGES AS A RESULT OF CARDIAC DECONDITIONING take at least as long or twice as long to recover as they took to deteriorate. Hence early mobilization is important.

1. **At rest,** cardiac changes caused by deconditioning include increased resting HR by one beat per minute every 2 days for the first 3–4 weeks of immobilization; decreased resting stroke volume up to 15% after 2 weeks of bed rest, which is related to a decrease in blood volume by 7% after 20 days of bed rest; decreased

cardiac size by 11%; and decreased left ventricular end-diastolic volume. The cardiac output (CO) remains unchanged or is slightly decreased. Resting systolic and mean blood pressure remain unchanged. Both the oxygen uptake (VO_2) at rest and the arteriovenous oxygen difference remain unchanged.

2. **With exercise,** the cardiac changes caused by deconditioning include increased HR response to submaximal exercise (up to 30–40 beats per minute greater than expected after 3 weeks of bed rest), although maximal HR remains unchanged or slightly increased; decreased stroke volume at submaximal and maximal exercise (30%); decreased CO (slightly at submaximal exercise and up to 26% at maximal exercise); decreased maximum oxygen uptake (VO_2max) by 27%, which indicates reduced aerobic fitness and reduced endurance; increased arteriovenous oxygen difference at submaximal exercise but not at maximal exercise.

C. **CHANGES IN FLUID BALANCE** in the recumbent position include increased CO by 24%; increased cardiac work by 30%; shift of 700 mL of blood volume to the thorax; delayed shift of extravascular fluid into the circulation; and compensatory diuresis, which leads to decreased plasma volume with subsequent loss of plasma mineral and protein. By day 4 of bed rest, plasma volume loss is about 13% of the pre-bed-rest level. It continues to decline because of a reduced hydrostatic blood pressure and decreased secretion of antidiuretic hormone until it plateaus at 70% of normal plasma volume and 60% of normal blood volume. Treatment using isotonic exercise (see Chapter 4.2, section II.B.2) is almost twice as effective as isometric exercises in preventing plasma volume reduction.

D. **VENOUS THROMBOEMBOLISM** (see Chapter 5.3) may develop as a result of venous stasis, increased blood viscosity, and hypercoagulability (caused by the decline in plasma volume while red blood cell mass remains unchanged). Preventive measures (see Chapter 5.3, section IV) include active exercise (e.g., calf or ankle pumps and walking) which have been shown to clear contrast medium injected into the veins four times faster than those on bed rest; use of elastic compression stockings (knee- or thigh-high); use of intermittent pneumatic compression devices; and, depending on the level of risk (see Chapter 5.3, Table 5.3-1), the use of low molecular-weight heparin (e.g., enoxaparin [Lovenox], 30 mg, SQ, qd; dalteparin [Fragmin], 2500 IU, SQ, qd) or low-dose unfractionated heparin (5000 IU, SQ, q8–12 h) or Fondaparinux (2.5 mg, SQ, qd), or oral warfarin (target INR = 2–3).

III. Respiratory changes

Respiratory changes as a result of bed rest are caused by mechanical restriction of breathing (caused in part by reduced chest excursion because of progressive reduction of ROM in the costovertebral and costochondral joints) which subsequently results in rapid, shallow breathing. Pulmonary function parameters, such as tidal volume, minute volume, vital capacity, and maximum voluntary ventilation, are all reduced. The overall reduction in muscular strength and endurance of deconditioned patients results in reduced movement of the diaphragmatic, intercostal, and abdominal muscles.

In the supine patient, mucus secretions accumulate in the dependent (i.e., posterior) respiratory segments, whereas the nondependent (i.e., anterior) respiratory segments become dry, rendering the mucociliary mechanism ineffective in clearing secretions. Both the ciliary malfunction and weakness of the abdominal muscles are responsible for the impaired cough. As dependent areas become poorly ventilated and overperfused, there are regional changes in the ventilation–perfusion ratio, and significant arteriovenous shunting with lowered arterial oxygenation. If metabolic demand is increased, hypoxia can occur. Ultimately, the bed-ridden patient may develop atelectasis and hypostatic pneumonia. Preventive measures (see Chapter 5.12, section IV.B) include: early mobilization; frequent change in position; chest physical therapy (deep breathing exercises, incentive spirometry, assisted coughing, and/or chest percussion and vibration may be indicated, depending on the patient's needs); and adequate pulmonary hygiene.

IV. Skin changes

A. PRESSURE ULCERS are fully discussed in Chapter 5.2.

B. DEPENDENT EDEMA can predispose to cellulitis. Preventive measures include adequate mobilization and elevation, use of elastic stockings or gloves, pressure gradient compression, and massage.

C. SUBCUTANEOUS BURSITIS occurs when there is excessive pressure on the bursae (usually prepatellar or elbow bursae). It can be prevented by removal of aggravating pressure on the bursae. Treatment measures include use of non-steroidal anti-inflammatory drugs (see Chapter 4.8, section I.A.3), percutaneous drainage, corticosteroid injections (see Chapter 4.9, section III.B), and surgery in refractory cases.

V. Gastrointestinal changes

Gastrointestinal changes include decreased appetite, decreased gastric secretion, atrophy of the intestinal mucosa and glands, slower rate of absorption, distaste for protein-rich food (which can lead to nutritional hypoproteinemia), and constipation because of decreased gastric and intestinal motility (caused by increased adrenergic stimulation, which inhibits peristalsis and causes sphincter contraction). The loss of plasma volume and dehydration aggravates the constipation. Desire to defecate is also reduced because of embarrassment at using the bedpan. Treatment of constipation (see Chapter 5.8, section VI.B) or fecal impaction (see Chapter 5.8, section VIII.A) includes laxatives, enemas, manual extraction, or in extreme cases, surgical interventions. Preventive measures include adequate fluid intake and fiber-rich diet (raw fruits and vegetables); use of stool softeners and bulk-forming agents; avoidance of narcotics because they produce slowed peristalsis; and limited use of hyperosmotic (e.g., glycerin) or peristalsis-stimulating (e.g., bisacodyl) suppositories combined with a regularly timed bowel program.

VI. Genitourinary changes

Genitourinary changes include increased diuresis and mineral excretion, stone formation, and urinary tract infection. Stones (struvate and carbonate apatite are the most common) are found in 15–30% of immobilized patients as a result of urinary stagnation (incomplete bladder emptying), hypercalciuria (in patients with spinal cord injury and fractures), altered ratio of citric acid to calcium, and increased excretion of phosphorus. Bladder stones promote bacterial growth because of irritation and trauma to the bladder mucosa, leading to increased incidence of urinary tract infection. Long-term immobilization may lead to a decreased glomerular filtration rate and decreased ability to concentrate urine. There also appears to be decreased spermatogenesis and androgenesis.

Preventive measures include adequate fluid intake, use of the upright position for voiding, and strict avoidance of bladder contamination during instrumentation. In patients with high postvoid residual, an external (condom) catheter (see

Chapter 5.7, section IV.B.1) or intermittent catheterization (see Chapter 5.7, section IV.C) may be used. Any urinary tract infection should be treated with appropriate antibiotics based on urine culture and sensitivity (see Chapter 5.7, section V.A). Other therapeutic approaches include acidification of the urine through the use of vitamin C (to prevent growth of *Proteus* organisms), use of urinary antiseptics, and, in those patients at highest risk for stone formation, a urease inhibitor. Treatment of stones after they have formed (see Chapter 5.7, section V.B) includes surgical removal or the use of lithotripsy.

VII. Metabolic and nutritional changes

Changes in metabolism and nutrition include decreased lean body mass, increased body fat, disorders of nitrogen balance, and mineral and electrolyte losses (nitrogen loss, calcium loss, phosphorus loss, sulfur loss, and potassium loss). Hypercalcemia as a result of immobilization is associated with osteoporosis, especially in young adult males with traumatic injuries who were physically active prior to immobilization. As their bones are reabsorbed, serum calcium levels rise. This is associated with hypercalcemic metabolic alkalosis and may lead to renal failure and ectopic calcification. Hypercalcemia manifests clinically as headache, nausea, lethargy, constipation, and weakness. It is treated by achieving adequate calcium excretion through hydration with 0.9% or 0.45% saline and diuresis with furosemide (Lasix, 1 mg/kg up to 20–40 mg IV or 20–80 mg, po, qd/bid). If hypercalcemia is refractory, etidronate di-sodium (Didronel, 7.5 mg/kg in 250 mL normal saline given IV over 2 hours daily for 3 days) or pamidronate (Aredia, 60–90 mg IV single dose over 2–24 hours) may be used.

VIII. Endocrine changes

Altered responsiveness of hormones and enzymes causes endocrine changes. These changes include glucose intolerance; altered circadian rhythm; altered temperature and sweating responses; and altered regulation of parathyroid hormone, thyroid hormone, adrenal hormones, pituitary hormones, growth hormone, androgens, and plasma renin activity. The glucose intolerance (noted after 8 weeks of immobility) is the result of a reduction in insulin-binding sites which causes decreased sensitivity of the peripheral muscle to circulating insulin. Glucose intolerance induced by bed rest can be improved by isotonic but not isometric exercises of the large muscle groups in the legs. After 2 weeks of bed rest, it takes about 2 weeks of resumed activity before glucose response returns to normal.

IX. Neurological, emotional, and intellectual changes

These include the effects of sensory deprivation (decreased attention span, confusion and disorientation to time and space, decreased hand-to-eye coordination); decreased intellectual capacity; emotional and behavioral disturbances (anxiety, depression, autonomic lability, restlessness, decreased pain tolerance, irritability, hostility, insomnia, and lack of motivation); increased auditory threshold and decreased visual acuity; impaired balance and coordination (probably as a result of neural factors rather than muscle weakness); and compression neuropathies.

Preventive measures include encouraging the patient to interact with staff, other patients, and family members, and recreational therapy for psychosocial integration, resocialization, and adjustment to independent functioning. Nerve compression can be prevented by proper positioning to relieve pressure from the nerve.

Further reading

Akeson WH, Amiel D, Abel MF, *et al.*: Effects of immobilization on joints. *Clin Orthop* 219:28–37, 1987.

Baker JH, Matsumoto DE: Adaptation of skeletal muscle to immobilization in a shortened position. *Muscle Nerve* 2:231–244, 1988.

Buschbacher RM, Porter CD: Deconditioning, conditioning, and the benefits of exercise. In Braddom RL, editor: *Physical medicine and rehabilitation*, ed 2, Philadelphia, 2000, WB Saunders, pp. 702–726.

Chan AS, Vallbona C: Immobilization. In Garrison SJ, editor: *Handbook of physical medicine and rehabilitation basics*, ed 2, Philadelphia, 2003, Lippincott, Williams & Wilkins, pp. 152–160.

Dolkas CB, Greenleaf JE: Insulin and glucose responses during bed rest with isotonic and isometric exercise. *J Appl Physiol* 43:1033–1038, 1977.

Downs FS: Bed rest and sensory disturbances. *Am J Nurs* 74:434–438, 1974.

Haines RF: Effect of bed rest and exercise on body balance. *J Appl Physiol* 36:323–327, 1974.

Halar EM, Bell KR: Immobility and inactivity: physiological and functional changes, prevention, and treatment. In DeLisa JA, Gans BM, Walsh NE, *et al.*, editors: *Physical medicine and rehabilitation: principles and practice*, ed 4, Philadelphia, 2005, Lippincott, Williams & Wilkins, pp. 1447–1467.

Leadbetter WF, Engster HE: Problems of renal lithiasis in convalescent patients. *J Urol* 53:269, 1957.

Minare P: Immobilization osteoporosis: a review. *Clin Rheumatol* 8:95–103, 1989.

Mueller EZ: Influence of training and of inactivity on muscle strength. *Arch Phys Med Rehabil* 51:449–462, 1970.

Saltin B, Blomquist G, Mitchell JH, *et al.*: Response to exercise after bed rest and after training. A longitudinal study of adaptive changes in oxygen transport and body composition. *Circulation* 38(Suppl VII):1–78, 1968.

Spencer WA, Valbona C, Carter RE: Physiologic concepts of immobilization. *Arch Phys Med Rehabil* 46:89–100, 1965.

Taylor HL: The effects of rest in bed and of exercise on cardiovascular function. *Circulation* 38:1016–1017, 1968.

Van Beaumont W, Greenleaf JE, Juhos L: Disproportional changes in hematocrit, plasma volume, and proteins during exercise and bed rest. *J Appl Physiol* 33:55–61, 1972.

CHAPTER 5.2
Pressure ulcers

Pressure ulcers (also called decubitus ulcers, pressure sores, or bedsores) are localized areas of tissue damage (with ischemia and/or necrosis) caused by prolonged, unrelieved, externally applied pressure, which almost always occur over bony prominences. In the PM&R setting, they are most frequently seen in the elderly disabled who are bed- or chair-bound in nursing homes or at home; in patients with decreased mobility because of paralysis (e.g., spinal cord injury, multiple sclerosis, stroke, or traumatic brain injury), fractures (e.g., hip fracture), or surgery; and in patients on steroids or chemotherapy. For details on specific recommendations for the prevention and treatment of pressure ulcers, refer to the Further reading section for guidelines published by the Agency for Health Care Policy and Research (Bergstrom 1992 and 1994) and by the Consortium for Spinal Cord Medicine (2001). The prevention of pressure ulcers must be emphasized throughout the care of the disabled because, not only are pressure ulcers preventable, but prevention is more cost-effective than treatment.

I. Pathophysiology

Pressure ulcers are caused by unrelieved local external pressure (often over bony prominences). Pressures applied for 30 minutes or less cause hyperemia (skin redness), which disappears 1 hour after pressure is removed. If pressure is applied for 2–6 hours, ischemia occurs, and the redness takes 36 hours to disappear after the pressure is relieved. If pressure is applied continuously for 6–12 hours, a blue demarcation is detected, which does not disappear. Two weeks after necrosis, skin breakdown results in ulceration.

II. Epidemiology

In the United States, pressure ulcers occur in 1 million people per year at a cost of $6 billion in hospitalized patients alone for 1991. Every year, 60 000 people die from the complications of pressure ulcers. In hospitalized patients, the incidence ranges from 2.7 to 29.5% with a prevalence of 3.5–69%. In chronic or long-term facilities, the incidence is 10.8% with a prevalence of 2.6–24%. In critical-care units, the incidence is 33% with a prevalence of 41%. In elderly patients admitted for femoral fracture, the incidence is 66%. In patients with spinal cord injury, the incidence is 25–66% with a prevalence of 60% in tetraplegic patients.

III. Risk and etiologic factors

A. **BIOMECHANICAL FACTORS** include pressure, shear, friction, moisture, and temperature. Prolongation of normal activities, such as sitting and lying, can result in extremely high tissue stresses because small volumes of flesh are compressed between the bony skeleton and an external surface. In the development of pressure ulcers, the duration of pressure is more critical than the intensity of pressure, hence if pressure duration is long enough (even with relatively small loads or small applications of pressure), tissue necrosis results. Other common causes of increased pressure, shear, or friction include use of deteriorated or inappropriate wheelchair cushions, activities involving sitting on uncushioned surfaces (e.g., floor), and continuing to sit after bruising the skin (e.g., from transfer). A slumped sitting posture or the shearing forces created by the posterior pelvic tilt as the patient tends to slide out of the wheelchair, also contribute to the formation of sacral ulcers. Increased skin temperature with resulting perspiration can increase the metabolic demands of cells in a local region, thus predisposing to skin breakdown. Moist skin (e.g., from bowel or bladder incontinence and excessive perspiration) may adhere to clothing and bed linen, causing shearing maceration through direct trauma or exposure to pressure. Fecal and urinary incontinence can also cause chemical irritation of the epidermis, which can lead to infection.

B. BIOCHEMICAL FACTORS include poor nutrition, which can result in weight loss with loss of fat padding over bony prominences; negative nitrogen balance and poor vitamin intake, which can compromise normal tissue integrity; hypoproteinemia, which can lead to edema causing decreased skin elasticity thus making it more susceptible to inflammation; and anemia with low serum iron and low serum iron binding hence leading to decreased oxygen and nutrients to the tissues. Other biochemical factors include poor collagen metabolism (with increased susceptibility to skin breakdown), heterotopic ossification (possibly because of increased bony areas against which the tissue can be compressed), and poor circulation (decreased tissue oxygen and nutrient supply).

C. MEDICAL FACTORS include any trauma, illness, or disease that decreases mobility, especially if there is associated malnutrition (hypoalbuminemia, vitamin deficiency), anemia, ischemia, infection, severe spasticity, contracture, muscle atrophy, edema, decreased level of consciousness, decreased or absent sensation (e.g., diabetic neuropathy and spinal cord injury), and psychological stress and depression. Elderly patients are particularly susceptible to pressure ulcers because their skin loses its elasticity and vascularity, and it becomes more dry and fragile.

IV. Classification

Pressure ulcers are graded or staged according to the degree or extent of tissue damage (see Table 5.2-1). The Shea classification is traditionally used. In this chapter, all references to staging are based on the National Pressure Ulcer Advisory Panel classification.

V. Diagnosis

A. INSPECTION of skin over bony prominences (see Fig. 5.2-1). The most common sites of pressure ulcers are the ischium (28%), sacrum (17–27%), greater trochanters (12–19%), and the heels (9–18%). Other common sites include the malleoli, plantar forefeet, anterior knees (tibial crests, patellae), posterior knees, anterior superior iliac spines, perineum, elbows, shoulders, scapulae, thoracic region (costal margins, spinous processes), rim of ears, side of the head, and occiput. Ischial ulcers are most common in paraplegics, and sacral ulcers are most common in tetraplegics. In elderly and diabetic patients, heel ulcers are common. In ambulatory patients, pressure ulcers can occur at the plantar forefoot (the most common site being the metatarsal heads in patients with diabetic neuropathy) and in bodily parts in contact with orthotic or prosthetic devices.

Table 5.2-1 Comparison of three classification systems for clinically grading or staging pressure ulcers. For accurate classification, eschar or slough must be removed so that the wound base is visible

Shea[1] classification	Yarkony–Kirk[2] classification	National Pressure Ulcer Advisory Panel[3,4] classification
1. Erythema or induration overlying a bony prominence without ulceration (i.e., an incipient ulcer)	1. Red area (possible sites of future breakdown) 1a: present >30 min but <24 hours 1b: present >24 hours	Stage I*: Non-blanchable erythema of intact skin not resolved in 30 min; the heralding lesion of skin ulceration
2. Shallow full thickness skin ulcer involving dermis extending to junction of subcutaneous fat	2. Epidermis and/or dermis ulcerated but subcutaneous fat is not seen	Stage II: Partial thickness skin loss involving epidermis and/or dermis; presents as an abrasion, blister, or shallow crater
3. Ulcer extending into subcutaneous tissue, obliterating fat but limited by the deep fascia and does not extend into muscle	3. Subcutaneous fat observed but muscle is not seen	Stage III: Full thickness skin loss with damage or necrosis of subcutaneous tissue which may extend down to, but not through, underlying fascia; presents as a deep crater with or without undermining of adjacent tissue
4. Ulcer extending into or through muscle tissue exposing the underlying bony prominence at its base; "closed pressure sore," i.e., large cavity accessible through a small skin sinus (could be grade 3 or 4)	4. Muscle/fascia observed but bone is not seen	Stage IV: Full thickness skin loss with extensive destruction, tissue necrosis or damage to muscle, bone or supporting structures (e.g., tendon, joint capsule, etc.)
	5. Bone is seen but joint space is not involved	
	6. Joint space involved; pressure ulcer healed	

**An observable pressure-related alteration of intact skin whose indicators as compared to an adjacent or opposite area on the body may include changes in one or more of the following: skin temperature (warmth or coolness), tissue consistency (firm or boggy feeling), and/or sensation (pain, itching). The ulcer appears as a defined area of persistent redness in lightly pigmented skin, whereas in darker skin tones, the ulcer may appear with persistent red, blue, or purple hues.*

Adapted from:

[1] *Shea JD: Pressures classification and management.* Clin Orthop *112:89–100, 1975.*

[2] *Yarkony G, Kirk PM, Carlson C,* et al.: *Classification of pressure ulcers.* Arch Dermatol *126:1218–1219, 1990.*

[3] *National Pressure Ulcer Advisory Panel: Pressure ulcers – prevalence, cost, and risk assessment: Consensus Development Conference Statement.* Decubitus *2(2):24–28, May 1989.*

[4] *Cuddigan J, Frantz RA: Pressure ulcer research: pressure ulcer treatment. A monogram form the National Pressure Ulcer Advisory Panel.* Adv Wound Care *11:294–300, 1998.*

B. PHYSICAL EXAMINATION. Measure the ulcer in centimeters, and determine its depth by inserting a cotton swab to the deepest part of the wound and measuring it in centimeters. Check for signs of infection (redness, induration, exudates, edema, malodor). Probe the ulcer using a sterile cotton swab to rule out

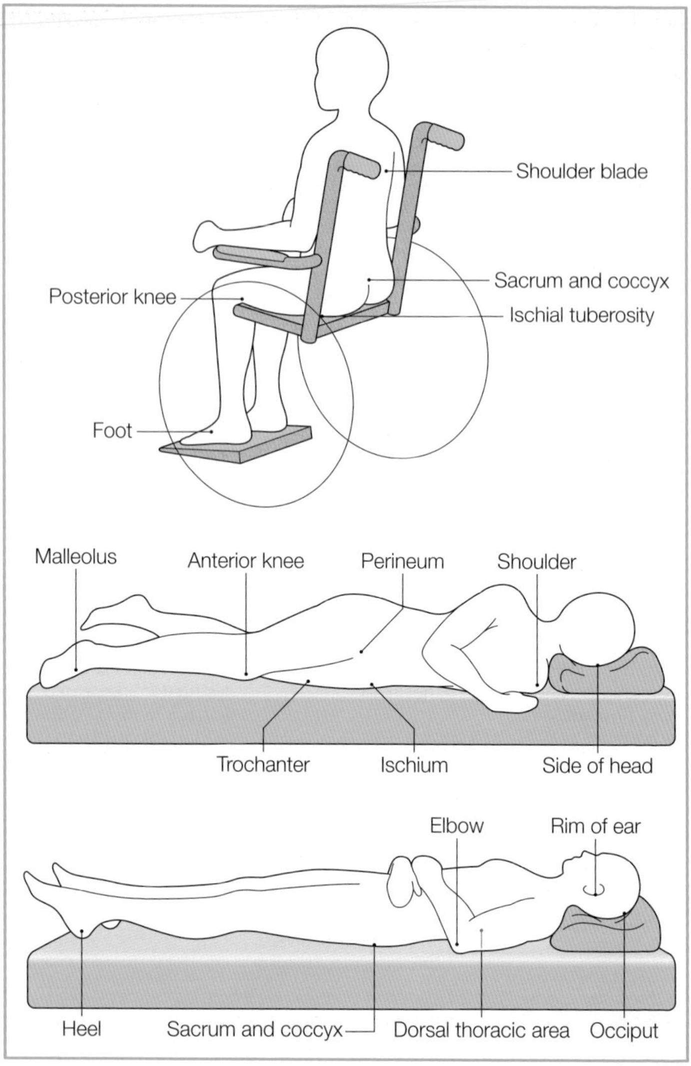

Figure 5.2-1 Bony prominences of the body vulnerable to pressure ulcer development (From Consortium for Spinal Cord Medicine: Pressure ulcer prevention and treatment following spinal cord injury: A clinical practice guideline for health care professionals. *J Spinal Cord Med*, 24 [suppl 1]:S59, 2001, with permission from the American Paraplegia Society.)

communication of ulcers with joint spaces or bony cavities. A Polaroid photograph is useful for documenting pressure ulcers and following their progress. Check for predisposing factors such as urinary or fecal incontinence, severe spasticity, contractures, or malnutrition.

C. LABORATORY WORK-UP includes complete blood count (CBC), prothrombin time (PT), activated partial thromboplastin time (aPTT), total proteins, albumin/globulin ratio, and blood urea nitrogen (BUN). Erythrocyte sedimentation rate (ESR) may be measured to follow the progression of osteomyelitis. Levels of iron, folate, vitamins B_6 and B_{12}, and zinc may also be checked to determine the need for supplementation.

D. BACTERIOLOGY reveals that the most common bacteria present in pressure ulcers are a mix of Gram-positive and Gram-negative flora, namely *Staphylococcus aureus*, *Proteus mirabilis*, *Pseudomonas aeruginosa*, and *Escherichia coli*. Anaerobic cultures often show *Bacteroides* and *Clostridia*.

1. **Qualitative wound culture and sensitivity tests** (C/S) may be performed to guide antibiotic choice.

a. ***Swab culture*** only indicates what organisms are present in the wound fluid. These organisms are usually microbes that have colonized the wound (without causing tissue infection) from the gastrointestinal tract or the surrounding skin. They do not always concur with deep tissue culture.

b. ***Irrigation–aspiration*** is carried out immediately after thorough cleansing of the wound. It has 98% concordance for aerobes and 92% concordance for anaerobes compared to tissue biopsy.

2. **Quantitative wound culture (tissue biopsy)** involves the removal of 1 g of wound tissue followed by the counting of the micro-organisms in it. If the number of bacteria exceeds 10^5/g of tissue, infection exists.

E. DIAGNOSTIC TESTS include bone radiographs to rule out osteomyelitis and heterotopic calcification. Bone biopsy with trochar needle is the definitive diagnostic procedure for ruling out osteomyelitis. Bone scans and computed tomography or magnetic resonance imaging are not routinely indicated but may be used as an adjunct to rule out osteomyelitis or abscess. Bone scans are nonspecific and have high false-positive results. The sensitivity of a bone scan in diagnosing osteomyelitis is increased when a triple-phase bone scan is performed or in conjunction with a gallium or indium scan. Contrast sinography may evaluate the presence and extent of wound tunneling or sinus tracts.

F. PRESSURE ULCER RISK ASSESSMENT SCALES can be used to identify at-risk individuals so that risk factors can be reduced through intervention. These individuals should be assessed on admission to the acute- or long-term-care facility and reassessed at periodic intervals. Despite their limitations, their use ensures systematic evaluation of individual risk factors.

1. **Braden scale** assesses the patient's physical activity, mobility, sensory perception, degree to which the skin is exposed to moisture, nutrition status, and friction and shear. In hospitalized adult patients, a score of 16 or below is considered at risk for developing pressure ulcers. This scale has been tested extensively in diverse sites such as medical-surgical units, intensive-care units, and nursing homes. It has good validity and interrater reliability.

2. **Norton scale** assesses the patient's physical condition, mental condition, activity, mobility, and continence. A score of 12 or below signifies patients at risk of developing pressure ulcers. This scale has been extensively studied on elderly persons in the hospital setting. However, its validity and reliability have not been fully established.

VI. Prevention of pressure ulcers

Prevention of these ulcers involves an integrated team management approach with the emphasis on good medical and nursing care, proper training and education of patients, family, and caregivers, encouragement of patient compliance, and the proper prescription of support surfaces. It is more cost-effective than the treatment of pressure ulcers.

A. SKIN INSPECTION AND SKIN CARE as part of the patient's daily routine are the basis of pressure ulcer prevention. The patient's skin must be examined regularly each morning and evening and each time the patient is turned or receives a specific treatment. Specific attention must be directed to bony prominences, which are vulnerable to pressure ulcer development (see Fig. 5.2-1). Potential signs of impending ulcer formation include color variation (redness, skin discoloration), blisters, rashes, swelling, temperature variation, pimples and ingrown hairs, bruises, surface breaks, and dry, flaky skin. If any of these signs are present, all pressure from that area must be removed immediately. The patient and family must be taught the importance of these routine skin checks and care.

The patient's skin should be washed and dried twice daily. Any areas where perspiration, urine, or feces collect should be washed several times daily with mild soap, then rinsed with warm water, and patted dry. Apply a skin moisturizer and massage it well into the skin immediately after washing or bathing the patient. The patient's skin, after a washing or a bath, is well-hydrated so moisturizers applied at this time provide the optimal moisturizing and protective effect. Moisturizing cream and protective ointments are preferred over lotions because they contain a lower proportion of water and offer better barrier protection. Avoid leaving any moist areas as they may cause skin irritation and maceration.

B. PRESSURE REDUCTION MEASURES

1. **Positioning, turning, and transferring**. Patients at risk for developing pressure ulcers should be turned and repositioned at least every 2 hours around the clock: 2 hours on the side, 2 hours on the back, and 2 hours on the other side regardless of the type of support surface. When lying on the side, the patient should avoid direct pressure on the trochanter by using a 30° lateral-inclined position instead. Elevate the head of the bed as little as possible (maximum of 30°) and for as short a time as possible. If able to tolerate it, the patient should sleep in the prone position because the anterior part of the body has larger low-pressure areas and smaller high-pressure areas. Positioning devices such as pillows or foam wedges may be used to keep bony prominences (e.g., knees or ankles) from direct contact with one another. The heels should be raised off the bed by placing a pillow under the calf. Donut-type devices should *not* be used because they create larger areas of ischemia at the center of the donut. Chair-bound patients must be repositioned every hour. If possible, patients must be taught to raise themselves off the seat for 15 seconds every 30 minutes (e.g., push-up exercises or leaning side to side). Sitting uninterrupted for more than 2 hours should *not* be allowed. During transfers, the patient should not be dragged across the bed. Instead the patient should be lifted using a draw sheet under the patient, or the patient can assist by pulling on the bed trapeze.
2. **Skin protectors** may help prevent skin friction and shear but are usually *not* very helpful in reducing pressure. They include padded dressings, sheepskin mats or pads, silicone gel pads, elbow pads, heel pads, and bunny boots.
3. **Pressure-reducing support surfaces** keep pressures lower than that of the standard hospital bed or standard wheelchair seat, but *not* consistently below capillary closing pressure of 32 mmHg. They consist of a supporting medium ("the core material") and an enclosing membrane, which separates the patient's skin from the supporting medium. The ideal supporting medium should have high compliance, minimum shearing force, high porosity, and should be light, easy to clean, and durable. Although high compliance is essential for uniform pressure distribution, it makes it difficult for the patient to maintain proper bed positioning that ensures spinal support, prevents contractures, and permits transfer activities. Hence, a firm supporting medium is preferred to a highly compliant medium. Ideally, the enclosing membrane should have low stiffness, a low coefficient of friction, high porosity, and high absorbency so that it can

Table 5.2-2	Consortium for Spinal Cord Medicine guidelines on the selection of pressure-reducing support surfaces for individuals who are at risk of or who have pressure ulcers
Pressure-reducing bed support surfaces	**Recommendations**
1. Static support surface	• For individuals who can be positioned – without weight bearing on an ulcer, and – without bottoming out on the support surface
2. Dynamic support surface	• For individuals who cannot be positioned without pressure on an ulcer, or • When a static support surface bottoms out, or • If there is no evidence of ulcer healing, or • If new ulcers develop
3. Low-air-loss and air-fluidized beds	• For treatment of pressure ulcers if one or more of the following conditions exist: – pressure ulcers on multiple turning surfaces – compromised skin temperature and moisture control in the presence of large stages III or IV pressure ulcers

Data tabulated from: Consortium for Spinal Cord Medicine: Pressure ulcer prevention and treatment following spinal cord injury: a clinical practice guideline for health care professionals, J Spinal Cord Med, *24 (suppl 1):S85, 2001.*

prevent skin friction and shear, and decrease the temperature and moisture at the skin surface. Obviously, no one product fulfills all of these requirements all of the time. In choosing the appropriate product to meet individual patient needs, recognize the advantages, disadvantages, and limitations of the different surfaces. For guidelines on the selection of pressure-reducing support surfaces for patients at risk of developing pressure ulcers, refer to Table 5.2-2.

a. ***Static overlays*** attempt to provide pressure reduction by their material and design. They do not eliminate, however, the need for pressure relief by preventive repositioning (see section VI.B.1 above) and do not decrease pressures of the ischium below capillary pressure. Currently no clear evidence supports one static overlay over another.

I. **Functional types of static overlays**

- **Mattress overlays** are placed directly over a regular mattress. A mattress overlay should be 3–4 inches (7.6–10.2 cm) thick with 25% indentation load deflection (ILD) of 30 lb (13.6 kg), a density of 1.3 lb/ft^3 or more, and modulus of 2.5 or more. A 25% ILD is the force needed to compress a 4-inch piece of foam until it is 3 inches tall. Density measures how much material is in the foam, while the modulus of the foam is the ratio of the 65% ILD to 25% ILD.
- **Static seat cushions** are usually placed over a wheelchair seat. They are used to relieve pressure in vulnerable anatomical areas by providing an additional protective layer between the support surface and the body. They distribute the body's weight away from bony prominences and stabilize the body for balance and functional pelvic positioning. They should be durable and moisture resistant for incontinent persons. Although firmer cushions provide a better base of support, they may be inappropriate in insensate patients.

II. **Types of static overlays by materials or contents** (see Chapter 4.7, section I.A.3.b for pressure-relief seat cushions used in wheelchairs).

- **Polyurethane foam overlays** are blocks or layers of foam whose compliance, firmness, and density can be varied from supersoft to extra firm. Combinations with soft foam on the top and firm below can provide both high compliance and good support. Foams can be shaped like egg cartons or they can be split in parts (split-foam) so that separate sections support the trunk, the thighs, and the legs. With split-foams, all pressure points from heel to sacrum can be positioned in a space between the mattress sections so that they are free from pressure and air circulates freely by them in any lying position. Foams used as wheelchair cushions can also be contoured to reduce pressure and improve posture and balance. Unlike the gel- or water-filled overlays, compression of a foam overlay on one area has little effect on other areas, and the pressure distribution depends on the design and firmness of the foam. Foams are lightweight; can be cut into any size, shape, or thickness; are easy to transfer; and can provide stability and good balance; however, they wear out quickly (average of 6 months), cannot be washed or cleaned, can retain moisture, and can increase the temperature of the support surface.

- **Gel-filled (flotation-gel) overlays** are plastic or rubber membranes filled with a plastic-like material that simulates body fat tissue. They adjust to body movements and can act as a shock absorber. They can maintain skin temperature, but cooling of the cushion is necessary every 3 hours to maintain this effect. They can also resist puncture more than water- or air-filled overlays; however, they are heavy, difficult to transfer, and expensive.
- **Air-filled overlays** are inflatable membranes. They are lightweight, easy to clean, can be customized in multiple heights, and can be compartmentalized (with multiple valves). Air-filled overlays with multiple cells (e.g., ROHO overlays, which consist of a series of vertical balloons filled with air) can increase the humidity and temperature of the support surface, but less so than a foam cushion. They are subject to puncture, not easily repaired, require monitoring of the air pressure, and may cause balance or transfer problems.
- **Water-filled (flotation-water) overlays** are plastic or rubber membranes filled with chemically treated water or other liquid. They adjust to body movements and are easy to clean and can decrease temperature on the support surface; however, they are heavy, may leak if punctured, and are difficult to transfer.

b. ***Dynamic overlays or mattresses*** are designed to reduce the duration of pressure by alternating pressure pads, which provide alternating periods of high and low pressure. They are used if the patient cannot assume a variety of positions without bearing weight on the ulcer, or if the patient fully compresses the static support surface, or if the ulcer does not show evidence of healing. They are dependent on an external power source (e.g., battery or wall socket), however, and their use as wheelchair cushions is limited because they can interfere with the patient's functional independence and mobility. They are also noisy and are subject to puncture and breakdown.

I. **Dynamic overlays**

- **Low air-loss overlays** are attached to motorized pumps that maintain a constant inflation. The pump also provides slight air movement against the skin to prevent moisture buildup. These overlays have a fabric covering that reduces shear and friction and is air permeable, bacteria impermeable, and waterproof. They are easy to clean, and can be deflated to facilitate transfers or during emergencies.
- **Alternating air-filled overlays** consist of a configuration of chambers through which air is pumped at regular intervals to provide inflation and deflation. They constantly change pressure points on the skin and create pressure gradients that enhance skin blood flow. They are easy to clean and can be deflated to facilitate transfers or during emergencies. However, in

some patients, the inflation and deflation may bother them or disturb their sleep.

II. Dynamic mattresses

- **Alternating pressure-point mattresses** consist of a series of vinyl tubes or cells, which are connected to a pump in such a way that when one cell or tube is inflated, an adjacent cell or tube is deflated. Its air cells tend to collapse under high local pressure, and lying directly on the plastic can increase discomfort, body heat, and perspiration, hence making the skin prone to maceration.
- **Rolling mattress (Cloud 9)** consists essentially of two long interconnected sausage-like air sacs. One sac alternately inflates and deflates, so that the other sac responds reciprocally, hence the patient is rolled from side to side while supported on an air cushion. This seems to be more comfortable and more effective in reducing tissue pressure than the alternating pressure-point mattress. It may, however, make some patients nauseous.

c. ***Static replacement mattresses*** are designed for use on an existing bed frame without an underlying mattress. They reduce staff time and are easy to clean; however, they have a high initial cost, may not control moisture, and lose effectiveness over time. They require at least 4 inches (10.2 cm) of foam to protect the greater trochanter. Although they may reduce pressures below those of a standard bed mattress, these pressures can be raised by spasm, postural change, and muscle contraction.

4. **Pressure-relieving specialty beds** reduce pressure consistently below capillary closing pressure of 32 mmHg. They are used to promote healing of pressure ulcers as well as to prevent the development of new pressure ulcers in patients with large stage III or stage IV pressure ulcers on multiple turning surfaces. In rehabilitation, they are generally used for short periods of time because they are not practical or are too expensive for home use. Pressure-relieving specialty beds use air flotation for pressure relief. They are comfortable, keep the skin dry (hence decreasing maceration), and promote healing. They are, however, noisy, heavy, costly, and the sensation of floating can cause motion sickness or disorientation.

a. ***Air-fluidized bed (Clinitron)*** uses a process in which a high volume of warm compressed air is forced through a diffuser into a medium of silicone beads to simulate a high-density fluid environment. The glass granules are enclosed in a woven polyester filter sheet, which prevents the beads from escaping but permits air to pass easily through it. The patient lying on top of the polyester sheet has the sensation of lying on a water bed, and it is claimed that no point in the body exceeds a pressure of 20 mmHg. The temperature of the air is usually kept at 31°C for optimal comfort with minimal perspiration. Air-fluidized beds are used for patients with stage III or IV pressure ulcers or in patients with skin grafts. They are also bactericidal by the sequestration and dessication of microorganisms by the silicone beads. To position a patient in a seated or semi-Fowler's position, foam cushions are required.

The adverse effects of air-fluidized beds are preventable. They include fluid loss, dehydration, and dry, scaly skin caused by the continuous flow of warm, dry air through the filter sheet. This is prevented by extra fluid intake and the use of skin moisturizers. The low relative humidity of the bed environment causes drying of the nasal mucosa, which can potentially result in epistaxis. This is prevented by regular spraying of the nasal mucous with saline nasal spray; but with chronic use, hypernatremia may occur. Moreover, with prolonged periods in a "weightless" environment, hypophosphatemia and hypocalcemia may occur. As much as medically possible, the patient should be placed in the seated, semi-Fowler, or standing position, and laboratory work-ups should be performed regularly. Although turning and repositioning may be difficult in air-fluidized beds, they should be performed regularly, otherwise new pressure ulcers may develop, especially at the heels. As a result of the lack of a firm back support, the patient's cough mechanism may be rendered ineffective, and thick pulmonary secretions can develop. Pulmonary hygiene is, therefore, essential. Leakage of the silicone beads may cause eye injury to the patient and caregivers; therefore, the filter sheet should be inspected frequently for tears and, if necessary, replaced.

b. ***Low-air-loss bed (Alamo, Kin-air, Medicus)*** consists of air-filled sacs that leak air slowly. A pump keeps the pillows filled to the desired firmness. It uses separate air-permeable sacs that are individually monitored to keep the pressure below 32 mmHg in the area of bony prominences. Compared to air-fluidized beds, the low-air-loss bed requires less volume of air to support the patient, which considerably reduces the noise and size of the blower unit and cost. It needs skilled set-up, and, if adjusted properly, its pressures can be equivalent to those of air-fluidized beds. The bed temperature can be easily regulated, and there is the additional advantage of allowing the patient to recline, or assume a semi-Fowler's position, thus making it useful for patients requiring both plastic surgery and rehabilitation for skin grafting, pressure ulcers, and burns.

5. **Systemic treatment of predisposing factors** can help prevent pressure ulcers (see treatment under section VII.A).

VII. Treatment

A. SYSTEMIC TREATMENT OF PREDISPOSING FACTORS

1. **Restoration of nutrition** is necessary for wound healing, especially in patients with nutritional deficiencies. On a tissue level, the critical local factor that causes skin breakdown is prolonged pressure. On a cellular level, however, the cells break down because they are unable to sustain metabolism because of poor delivery of nutrients and poor elimination of waste products. Fluid containing protein, vitamins, and minerals is lost continuously through the open surface of the pressure ulcer. Patients with pressure ulcers, therefore, should receive supplements of proteins, vitamins, and minerals, in addition to their basic nutritional requirements. Adequate calories should also be provided to promote anabolism. Fluid intake must be increased (240 mL every 2 hours or at least 1 liter/day) unless medically restricted.

a. ***Protein*** must be available for wound granulation to occur. If pressure ulcers are present, the patient's protein requirements may rise to between 1.5 and 2.0 g/kg of ideal body weight to maintain a positive nitrogen balance and promote protein synthesis for healing. Fever, infection, or wound drainage can increase protein demands. The patient's serum protein should be maintained above 6 mg/dL. If the patient's serum albumin drops below 3.1 g/dL, aggressive protein feeding must begin. Protein is given by mouth in the form of nutritionally complete food, but oral supplements or tube feedings may be used. Total parenteral nutrition is sometimes required. If the patient develops diarrhea because of the high-protein and high-calorie diet, the diet may be given every third meal to lessen gastrointestinal side-effects.

b. ***Vitamin C*** promotes collagen synthesis and should be supplemented orally at 1 g/day in divided doses. Excess vitamin C is excreted by the kidneys, and patients may be at risk for stone formation.

c. ***Zinc*** is necessary for protein synthesis and repair. Zinc levels should be checked and supplemented only if deficient because excess zinc (more than 400 mg/dL) can interfere with macrophage function. The recommended daily allowance

(RDA) for zinc is 15 mg. For zinc deficiencies, give 135–150 mg (9 to 10 times RDA) of elemental zinc daily, e.g., Zinkaps-220, 220 mg (containing 50 mg zinc), one tab, po, tid.

d. ***Vitamin and mineral deficiencies*** related to anemia must be treated (see section VII.A.2).

2. **Treatment of anemia** is important because low hemoglobin levels cause a lower blood oxygen content and, therefore, a decrease in oxygen delivery to the tissues. Patients with pressure ulcers often have hemoglobin levels of 10 g/dL or less because of decreased appetite, loss of serum and electrolytes from the ulcer, infection, and generalized debilitation. Malformation of red blood cells because of various nutritional deficiencies can further aggravate the problem. Non-nutritional-related anemia, such as blood loss through oozing of blood from the wound or from surgical debridement, may be treated with blood transfusion. When laboratory work-up shows anemia caused by the following nutritional deficiencies, they must be treated accordingly:

a. ***Iron deficiency:*** Ferrous sulfate, 325 mg, po, tid.

b. ***Folate deficiency:*** Folic acid, 1 mg, po, qd.

c. ***Vitamin B_{12} deficiency (nonpernicious anemia).*** 30–100 mg of cyanocobalamin (vitamin B_{12}), intramuscular/subcutaneous daily for 5–10 days depending on the severity of deficiency, followed by 100–200 mg/month or prn.

d. ***Vitamin B_6 deficiency:*** 10–20 mg of vitamin B_6 either by mouth, intramuscularly, or intravenously daily for 3 weeks, then 2–5 mg daily as a supplement to a proper diet.

3. **Relief of spasticity or spasm** is important because these involuntary movements may cause skin breakdown as the body part rubs against bed sheets, clothing, bedrails, or adaptive equipment. Spasticity can also cause contractures that preclude proper positioning. Treatments include oral medications, positioning, physical modalities (e.g., cold), splints and orthoses, muscle or nerve blocks, and selective rhizotomy. Refer to Chapter 5.4 for details on treatment of spasticity.

4. **Systemic antibiotics** are only given if there is evidence of systemic infection or in ulcers with surrounding cellulitis. Antibiotic treatment should be combined with surgical debridement in soft tissue infection or with osteotomy if there is osteomyelitis. Parenteral antibiotics for osteomyelitis are usually given for at least 6–8 weeks.

5. **Incontinence care** (see Chapter 5.7, section IV for bladder care, Chapter 5.8, section VI.A for bowel care) should be provided to prevent wound infection and skin maceration. Skin protection with barrier ointments or thick protective creams should be used. Incontinent patients should be checked frequently and urine or fecal materials should be cleaned immediately. High-absorbency diapers may be used but should not replace frequent skin checks and cleaning. For male patients, an external (Texas) condom catheter may be used. For stage III or IV ulcers, an indwelling catheter (especially for female patients) or fecal collector may be used. In extreme cases, the patient may need diversion procedures for stool (e.g., colostomy or ileostomy) or urine (e.g., urostomy).

B. **PRESSURE-REDUCTION AND PRESSURE-RELIEVING DEVICES** as outlined under section VI.B should be used. For guidelines on the selection of pressure-reducing support surfaces for patients with pressure ulcers, refer to Table 5.2-2.

C. **CONSERVATIVE WOUND CARE**

1. **Local wound care** of pressure ulcers involves proper wound cleaning, debridement of eschar and necrotic tissue, and wound dressing. Any pressure on the wound should be reduced or relieved by proper positioning and use of pressure-reducing surfaces. When cleaning the wound with gauze, cloth, or sponge, use the minimum mechanical force possible. Instead of antiseptic agents, normal

saline or wound cleansers should be used. If the ulcer has large amounts of exudates and necrotic tissue, hydrotherapy using whirlpool or Hubbard tanks (see Chapter 4.1, section III) should be considered. When using dressings, the ulcer bed should be kept continuously moist while the surrounding intact skin is kept dry. Pressure ulcer cavities should be loosely filled (not overpacked) with dressing materials to eliminate dead space.

a. ***Stage I*** skin erythema heralds skin ulceration. Preventive measures outlined above (see section VI) should be strictly enforced. If there is skin induration, ice may be applied in the first 24 hours to decrease metabolic rate, decrease oxygen demand, and decrease inflammation.

b. ***Stage II*** pressure ulcer can either be a blister or an open wound. Blisters should be kept dry and pressure-free. When it breaks, it should be debrided (by sharp or surgical debridement method) and treated as a second-degree burn (e.g., silvadene dressing). If there is a dry superficial scab on the skin, leave it alone and just debride around the periphery.

c. ***Stage III and Stage IV*** pressure ulcer. If there is compromised skin temperature and moisture control, a low-air-loss or air-fluidized bed may be needed for pressure relief. Surgery should be considered.

2. **Periwound skin care.** Periwound skin tissue injury may occur from mechanical stripping, shearing, or maceration of otherwise healthy tissue from prolonged exposure to moisture. Topical management approaches preclude aggressive adhesives on tissue with cutaneous atrophy because removal may result in stripping injuries. An effective approach for wounds with minimal atrophy of periwound skin would be to use a hydrogel in the wound bed with a secondary dressing and a nonadhesive dressing wrap, such as Coban self-adherent wrap. If drainage is significant, however, the periwound skin becomes macerated. A polyurethane foam dressing may be indicated at this point. It is easy to apply and may be secured with a nonadhesive wrap. Selection of a dressing that does not shift or become dislodged from the wound is particularly important for areas of maximum activity and irregular contour. Skin sealants (e.g., Skin Prep), solid form skin barriers (e.g., Stomahesive), or petrolatum ointments protect periwound skin from exudate or solutions used in wound care. These precautions are typically necessary when the wound is being packed with gauze. Maceration of the periwound skin when semipermeable dressings are used is an indication that exudate control is not effective. Absorption products, therefore, can be used in conjunction with hydrocolloids or other dressings.

3. **Electrical stimulation,** specifically high-voltage monophasic pulsed current (see discussion in Chapter 4.1, section V.A.3.I.2) has been shown by randomized controlled clinical trials to accelerate the healing rate of pressure ulcers in animals and humans. It can be used in conjunction with standard wound care interventions to promote closure of stage III or IV pressure ulcers.

4. **Adjuvant wound-care modalities** may be used in conjunction with other wound therapies. They are not first-line interventions because of the lack of research evidence on their efficacies and the problems with availability and reimbursement.

a. ***Growth factors*** are currently being investigated for use in pressure ulcer healing. They include epidermal growth factors, fibroblast growth factors, transforming growth factor-β1, extracts of autologous human platelets, i.e., platelet-derived growth factors, and others.

b. ***Hyperbaric oxygenation*** is the systemic (*not* local), intermittent administration of 100% oxygen while physically exposed to a chamber (either monoplace or multiplace) with atmospheric pressure of 2.0–2.4 ATA or 14.7–17.6 lb/inch^2 gauge pressure (psig). This raises the oxygen tension 10–13 times higher than breathing oxygen at ambient pressure, thus enhancing oxygen delivery to compromised tissues. Treatment is usually given for 90 minutes, 5–7 times a week for a total of 40–60 treatments. Side-effects or complications include claustrophobia, tympanic hemorrhage or rupture because of aural barotraumas or "ear squeeze"; sinus hemorrhage because of sinus barotraumas or "sinus squeeze", visual acuity change (e.g., worsening myopia), pneumothorax, and seizure. Absolute contraindications include untreated pneumothorax (diagnosed by chest X-ray) and intake of bleomycin (because of the increased oxygen toxicity risk), cis-platinum, sulfamylon, and disulfiram. Relative contraindications include pregnancy, known malignancy, emphysema, pneumonia, bronchitis, and hyperthermia. Although controlled clinical studies about its effectiveness are lacking, hyperbaric oxygenation may be used as a "last ditch" adjunct therapy in lower extremity pressure ulcers (e.g., heel ulcers) with hypoxic component (e.g., post-surgery with compromised skin grafts and/or flaps) when it is known that these wounds may not heal.

c. ***Sub-atmospheric or negative pressure wound therapy (NPWT), or vacuum-assisted closure (VAC)*** uses open-cell foam sponge inserted into an open wound, sealed with an adhesive drape, then, with the use of a computerized suction pump, subatmosperic (negative) pressure (75–125 mmHg) is applied via an evacuation tube. This negative pressure (applied intermittently or continuously) can help evacuate wound fluid, stimulate granulation tissue formation, and reduce bacterial colonization counts. Contraindications include nonviable tissue within the wound bed (thus, necrotic tissues must be thoroughly debrided before using NPWT or VAC to help granulation formation), untreated osteomyelitis, and malignancy in the wound margin. It must be used with caution in active bleeding, anticoagulant therapy, or when vital organs are exposed. Analgesics are usually prescribed because of pain triggered by the suction pump or during dressing change. Although controlled clinical studies about its effectiveness are lacking, NPWT or VAC may be used in stage III and IV pressure ulcers (e.g., to reduce wound size to prepare for surgical closure) or after surgical graft or flap (to help drainage and healing), if other measures have failed.

D. SURGICAL CARE of pressure ulcers is applicable to stage III or stage IV pressure ulcers. The goals of surgery are to reduce protein loss through the wound, prevent progressive osteomyelitis and sepsis, avoid progressive secondary amyloidosis and renal failure, reduce rehabilitation costs, improve patient hygiene and appearance, and avert future Marjolin's ulcer (a rare malignant degeneration of a chronic pressure ulcer present for more than 20 years). In general, stage III and IV ulcers heal faster and generate less scar tissue when treated surgically. Although elderly patients are poor candidates for major surgery, they are unable to tolerate large, open pressure ulcers; therefore, simple rhomboid or bilobe flaps may be used in the elderly patient because sensation is intact.

1. **Preoperative care**. Pressure ulcer surgery should not be performed until the patient's condition has stabilized, nutritional deficiencies have been corrected, and the pressure ulcer shows signs of improvement (i.e., all necrotic tissues are gone; evidence of healthy granulation tissue is present; and the ulcer is decreasing in size or shows re-epithelization). Before surgery, the patient must be well-hydrated and have a hematocrit above 30. If necessary, packed red blood cells may be transfused. Any infections such as urinary tract infections should be treated. Immediately before surgery, all patients should be given antibiotics and maintained on them postoperatively until the drains are out (at least 2 weeks in uncomplicated cases).
2. **Surgical closures**. Surgery usually involves total excision of the ulcer, surrounding scar, and underlying bursae and soft tissue calcification. All

infected bones should be completely removed, and bony prominences should be recontoured. The wound defect is then closed using one of the following methods:

a. ***Primary (direct) closure*** consists of excision of the ulcer margin to convert it into an ellipse. The skin margins are then sutured to obliterate the dead space. Direct closure can usually be completed as an outpatient procedure in a day surgery unit. It is inappropriate for large ulcers because paucity of soft tissue coverage can lead to excessive wound tension and poor healing. In this case, tissue expanders may be used to provide more skin surface and to facilitate closure. After direct closure, the patient must keep pressure off the area for 2 weeks. If there is good healing, the patient may be allowed to put short minimal pressure (e.g., sitting) on it after the second week. The sutures are removed on the third week. With this form of treatment, the patient loses a minimum of time and can remain reasonably active.

b. ***Skin grafts*** are skin segments separated from their blood supply and transplanted from the donor site to the surface of the wound. They provide only a skin barrier and when applied directly to granulating bone, they quickly erode, precluding healing. The transplanted skin is never as "tough" as the original skin.

I. **Partial thickness or split-thickness skin graft (STSG)** consists of the epidermis and only a portion of the underlying dermis. The STSG is more likely to survive than full-thickness skin graft (FTSG) because STSG can tolerate a longer phase of plasmatic absorption and, therefore, can survive longer before vascularization occurs. A STSG is the method of choice for shallow defects without exposed bone in sensate patients (e.g., shallow sacral ulcers). It is not indicated for ischial and trochanteric ulcers. The graft site needs to be continually lubricated because it does not contain dermal appendages (i.e., sweat glands and hair follicles).

II. **Full-thickness skin graft** consists of the epidermis and all of the dermis, and is less likely to survive than STSG.

c. ***Skin flap*** is used when the wound is too extensive for primary closure and loss of tissue mass precludes grafting. It consists of a "tongue" of skin and subcutaneous tissues detached from its surrounding tissue except for a pedicle or base, through which blood supply is maintained. Usually, patients need to be hospitalized for 4–6 weeks. Skin flaps are used to cover ischial, trochanteric, or sacral ulcers.

d. ***Myocutaneous flaps*** consist of a composite of skin, subcutaneous tissue, and underlying muscle, detached from its surrounding tissue with the major blood supply (which enters the proximal undersurface of the muscle) kept intact. It helps eliminate dead space in a deep wound, enhances perfusion and tissue coaptation, and provides a temporary pad for wider dispersion of residual pressure. It can also help heal osteomyelitis, and limit the damage caused by shearing, friction, and pressure. It is the procedure of choice for nonambulatory patients with spinal cord injury or when loss of muscle function (of the muscle being flapped) does not contribute to comorbidity. In ambulatory patients, the sacrifice of functional muscle units must be weighed against the need for good wound healing. Myocutaneous flaps can be used for sacral, ischial, and trochanteric ulcers. The most commonly used myocutaneous flaps are tensor fascia lata, posterior hamstring, and gluteal flaps. When the myocutaneous flap is placed over a bony prominence not normally covered by muscle, it eventually atrophies. The pressure ulcer may recur as early as 9.3 months in 61% of pressure ulcers treated.

e. ***Free flaps*** are muscle-type flaps (usually from the latissimus dorsi muscle) in which the vein and artery are disconnected at the donor site and reanastomosed to the vessels at the recipient site by microsurgical techniques. It is used as an end-stage salvage procedure for recurrent deep ulcers (e.g., ischial ulcers).

f. ***Amputation and fillet procedures*** are reserved for those patients who have extensive or combined ulcerations, with or without underlying osteomyelitis, and those who cannot be treated successfully with any of the procedures previously described. The amputation (unilateral or bilateral) can be transfemoral (above-knee) with removal (fillet) of the femur and use of the entire thigh for flap coverage. A more extensive procedure comprises amputation at the level of the ankle and fillet of the entire leg to provide the largest possible amount of muscle and subcutaneous tissue to cover the defects. These patients should be referred for psychological counseling when faced with the consequences of amputation.

3. **Surgical procedure selection**

a. ***Sacral pressure ulcers*** are best managed with myocutaneous flaps using the gluteus maximus muscle. If the ulcer is shallow (without bone exposure and with good sensation), it can be treated with skin grafting.

b. ***Ischial pressure ulcers*** have high rates of recurrence in the seated position and are usually associated with osteomyelitis. Skin graft is not indicated. A local myocutaneous flap using gluteus maximus combined with partial ischiectomy is appropriate for first treatment of deep ischial ulcers. Distant flaps using gracilis muscles, tensor fascia lata (TFL) muscle, or hamstring (biceps femoris) may also be used. As end-stage salvage procedure for recurrent deep ischial ulcers, free flaps can be brought from distant sites to provide additional padding.

c. ***Trochanteric ulcers*** are best managed with myocutaneous flaps. The local TFL flap is most useful for uncomplicated medium-sized ulcers, while the local vastus lateralis muscle flap or the distant gluteal thigh flaps are used for larger, deeper ulcers. Skin grafts should not be used for trochanter ulcers.

d. ***Multiple pressure ulcers or combined pressure ulcers*** have large soft tissue defects and are usually associated with osteomyelitis. A myocutaneous flap using the TFL may be used to cover trochanteric and ischial ulcers. If the ulcer is extensive, and all other procedures have failed, then the amputation and fillet procedure may be done.

4. **Postoperative care**. Suction drains (used to prevent hemostasis) are usually left for at least 2 weeks and removed when output is less than 30 mL/24 hours. Drains should be frequently stripped to prevent blockage. After surgery, the patient is usually kept prone for 2–4 weeks. If the patient is unable to tolerate the prone position (e.g., because of poor pulmonary reserve), an air-flotation bed (air-fluidized or low-air loss) may be used to allow placement in the supine position. To decrease the need for turning the patient and to prevent soiling and contamination of the surgical site, an indwelling catheter or a fecal incontinence bag is recommended until all drains are removed. Custom padding and scrotal supports, which are prepared preoperatively, are used to help prevent iatrogenic pressure ulcers. Oral feeding and bowel feeding are restarted 3 days postoperatively. Antibiotics given preoperatively are adjusted according to the intraoperative cultures and biopsies. For uncomplicated cases, antibiotics are used for 2 weeks. If there is evidence of osteomyelitis, they are used for 6–8 weeks. The dressing from the operating room should be removed on the third postoperative day, and the wound should be allowed to remain open to the drying effects of the air. Only the drain sites or skin grafts need a protective dressing. Sutures are usually left in place for 3 weeks. Antispasmodic and antispasticity drugs are used to decrease the risk of bleeding and hematoma formation caused by involuntary movements. Patients are usually kept on bed rest 2, 3, or 6 weeks depending on wound healing. Then gradual mobilization is started.

5. **Postsurgical complications**

a. ***Immediate postoperative complications*** include hematoma, seroma, infection, and wound separation caused by tension – all of which can lead to flap necrosis. These can be prevented by good surgical techniques, proper hemostasis procedures (e.g., surgical drain for 2 weeks after surgery and fibrin sealant), and adequate antibiotics.

b. ***Long-term postoperative complications*** include ulcer recurrence (in 40–50% of cases) caused by persistent osteomyelitis, inadequate osteotomy, a large surgical scar, and a persistent sinus tract. When identified early, these complications can be corrected by appropriate secondary procedures (e.g., more extensive osteotomy and sinus tract resection). Another common cause of recurrence is excessive pressure on the surgical site, which should be prevented by educating the patient and caretaker to strictly comply with the preventive measures outlined in section VI.

Further reading

Bergstrom N, Bennett MA, Carlson CE, *et al.*: *Treatment of pressure ulcers*, Clinical Practice Guideline Number 14. AHCPR Publication No. 95-0642, Rockville, MD, 1994, Agency for Health Care Policy and Research, US Dept of Health and Human Services.

Bergstrom N and the Panel for the Prediction and Prevention of Pressure Ulcers in Adults: *Pressure ulcers in adults: prediction and prevention*, Clinical Practice Guideline Number 3. AHCPR Publication No. 92-0047. Rockville, MD, 1992, Agency for Health Care Policy and Research, US Dept of Health and Human Services.

Bryant R, editor: *Acute and chronic wounds: nursing management*, ed 2, St Louis, 2000, Mosby.

Consortium for Spinal Cord Medicine: Pressure ulcer prevention and treatment following spinal cord injury: A clinical practice guideline for health care professionals. *J Spinal Cord Med* 24 (suppl 1):S39–S101, 2001.

Constantian MB: *Pressure ulcers: principles and techniques of management*, Boston, 1980, Little, Brown.

Kosiak M: Etiology of decubitus ulcers. *Arch Phys Med Rehabil* 42:19–28, 1961.

Krasner D: *Chronic wound care: a clinical source book for health care professionals*, King of Prussia, 1990, Health Management Publications, pp. 74–77, 152–156.

O'Connor K: Pressure ulcers. In DeLisa JA, Gans BM, Walsh NE, *et al.*, editors: *Physical medicine and rehabilitation: principles and practice*, ed 4, Philadelphia, 2005, Lippincott, Williams & Wilkins, pp. 1605–1618.

Salcido R, Goldman R: Prevention and management of pressure ulcers and other chronic wounds. In Braddom RL, editor: *Physical medicine and rehabilitation*, ed 2, Philadelphia, 2000, WB Saunders, pp. 645–664.

Yarkony GM: Pressure ulcers: a review. *Arch Phys Med Rehabil* 75:908–917, 1994.

CHAPTER 5.3
Venous thromboembolism

Venous thromboembolism (VTE) is a common occurrence in PM&R patients, particularly in those with limited mobility. It can involve the superficial or deep veins of the limbs. Superficial thrombophlebitis poses little risk for embolism and is generally controlled by supportive measures (i.e., local heat, elevation of the affected limb, rest, and, if needed, anti-inflammatory agents such as aspirin). On the other hand, deep vein thrombosis (DVT) presents a more difficult diagnostic and therapeutic problem and is associated with a significant risk of pulmonary embolism (PE). This chapter deals mainly with DVT and its major complication, PE.

I. Pathophysiology

The calf veins are the earliest and most frequent sites for DVT. The initial lesion begins (intimal lesion is not necessary) as a platelet nidus in the pocket behind a valve cusp of the vein (usually caused by venous stasis). There is activation of thrombin through the coagulation cascade, leading to irreversible platelet aggregation and thrombus formation. The subsequent fate of the thrombus depends on the continued formation of fibrin, the degree of local fibrinolytic activity, and the blood flow rate. It organizes and becomes adherent to the vein wall in 7–10 days then resolves through fibrinolysis. Occasionally the thrombus may dislodge and form a PE. In rehabilitation the following three factors (Virchow's triad) increase the risk of DVT:

A. **VENOUS STASIS** is the principal factor contributing to DVT formation in the lower limbs. It can be caused by bed rest; immobility [increased risk in paralyzed limbs of patients with stroke or spinal cord injury (SCI)]; general anesthesia exceeding 30 minutes (blood flow velocity decreases by 50% in the external iliac and popliteal veins); surgery (possibly as a result of vein compression during recumbency, use of a tourniquet, or mechanical trauma to femoral or iliac veins); medical problems such as obesity, hypotension, diabetes mellitus, stasis dermatitis, varicosities, circulatory compromise because of congestive heart failure, sepsis, prior DVT (risk is increased two- to three-fold if previous DVT is confirmed by objective test); and age (risk to those over 40 years is moderate to high, but for those over 50 years, it increases exponentially).

B. **ENDOTHELIAL INJURY TO THE VESSEL WALL** includes direct trauma, surgery (e.g., during total hip or knee replacement, surgery can cause kinking of vein; scissoring of the femoral vein between the internally rotated femur and pubis; and manipulation and traction of the anterior hip structures especially in anterior dislocation approach), tissue hypoxia, previous venous thrombosis, infection, and labor trauma (this probably accounts for the increased risk in the postpartum period compared to normal risk during pregnancy).

C. **INCREASED COAGULABILITY** is caused by altered blood elements; dehydration; increase of platelet aggregation (in SCI); increased fibrinogen during acute inflammatory response; acquired deficiencies including postoperative decrease in antithrombin III; medical problems such as diabetes mellitus, malignancy (particularly adenocarcinoma of the lung, breast, and viscera), and inflammatory bowel disease; and use of oral contraceptives. A rare cause of hypercoagulability is a congenital defect in coagulant inhibitors (e.g., deficiencies in protein C, protein S, and antithrombin III).

Table 5.3-1 Incidence of deep vein thrombosis (DVT) and pulmonary embolism (PE) and their effective prophylactic methods classified by level of risk (based on published data) as recommended by the 7th American College of Chest Physicians (ACCP) Consensus Conference on Antithrombotic Therapy (2004)

Level of risk	Calf DVT (%)	Proximal DVT (%)	Clinical PE (%)	Fatal PE (%)	Effective DVT/PE prophylaxis
Low risk (minor surgery in patients <40 years with no additional risk factors)	2	0.4	0.2	0.002	No specific prophylaxis; early and aggressive mobilization
Moderate risk (minor surgery in patients with additional risk factors; surgery in patients 40–60 years with no additional risk factors)	10–20	2–4	1–2	0.1–0.4	1. LDUH (5000 IU SQ q12h) or 2. LMWH (≤3400 IU* SQ daily) or 3. CS or 4. IPC
High risk [surgery in patients >60 or aged 40–60 years with additional risk factors (prior VTE, cancer, molecular hypercoagulability)]	20–40	4–8	2–4	0.4–1.0	1. LDUH (5000 IU SQ q8h) or 2. LMWH (≥3400 IU* SQ daily) or 3. IPC
Highest risk [surgery in patients with multiple risk factors (age >40 years, cancer, prior VTE); hip or knee arthoplasty; hip fracture surgery; major trauma; spinal cord injury]	40–80	10–20	4–10	0.2–5	1. LMWH (≥3400 IU* SQ daily) or 2. Fondaparinux (2.5 mg SQ daily) or 3. Warfarin (INR, 2–3) or 4. IPC or CS plus LDUH or LMWH

VTE = venous thromboembolism; CS = compressive stockings; IPC = intermittent pneumatic compression; LDUH = low-dose unfractionated heparin; LMWH = low molecular-weight heparin; INR = international normalized ratio.

** Refers to international units of antifactor Xa. In the US, the available LMWHs for DVT prophylaxis are enoxaparin (Lovenox, 30 mg, SQ, qd) and dalteparin (Fragmin, 2500 IU, SQ, qd) where one mg of enoxaparin = 100 IU of antifactor Xa.*

From: Geerts WH, Graham FP, Heit JA, et al.: *Prevention of venous thromboembolism. The Seventh ACCP Conference on Antithrombotic and Thrombolytic Therapy.* Chest *Suppl 126(3):341S, 2004, with permission.*

II. Epidemiology of DVT (see Geerts *et al.*, 2004)

In the absence of DVT prophylaxis, the incidence of objectively confirmed, hospital-acquired DVT is approximately 10–40% among medical or general surgical patients and 40–60% following major orthopedic surgery. Approximately one-quarter to one-third of these thrombi involve the proximal deep veins, which are much more likely to produce symptoms and to result in PE.

III. Diagnosis of DVT

A. CLINICAL EVALUATION for the diagnosis of DVT is insensitive and nonspecific. The majority of patients with DVT are clinically silent (probably because the vein is not totally obstructed and because of collateral circulation). Physical examination fails to detect 50–90% of DVTs. In more than 50% of patients with a clinical diagnosis of DVT, venography is unable to definitely confirm it. Clinical findings often associated with DVT include pain and tenderness (vague and nonspecific; located at the calf, popliteal fossa, posterior thigh; aggravated by ankle movement); leg swelling (may be localized or pitting; aggravated by prolonged sitting or early ambulation; usually subsides after the leg is elevated); Homan's sign (calf or popliteal pain with forced dorsiflexion of the ankle; an insensitive and nonspecific clinical test for DVT, which is present only with complete occlusion, and even then it is present in only 70% of such cases; Homan's test is discouraged because if a DVT is present, the thrombus may be dislodged and may embolize); palpable cord (in the groin, popliteal fossa, or upper calf); superficial venous distension (around the knee, groin, or anterior abdominal wall; relieved by leg elevation); and fever (usually low-grade).

Differential diagnoses for suspected DVT include: musculoskeletal disorders (lower extremity muscle strain, tear, or hematoma; Achilles tendinitis; knee or ankle arthritis, including gout; heterotopic ossification; sarcoma); vascular disorders (acute post-thrombotic syndrome, chronic venous insufficiency, superficial venous thrombosis, superficial thrombophlebitis in a varicose vein, peripheral arterial disease, femoral or popliteal artery aneurysm); dermatological disorders (cellulitis; dermatitis, erythema nodosum); focal collections (Baker's cyst, hematoma, abscess, pelvic mass resulting in venous compression); neurological disorders (leg swelling as a result of lower extremity paralysis, nerve root irritation, complex regional pain syndromes); drug-induced swelling (calcium-channel blockers; corticosteroid); and lymphedema.

B. DIAGNOSTIC TESTS. More definitive diagnostic tests (invasive or noninvasive) must be carried out if DVT (or PE) is suspected because of the unreliability of clinical diagnosis of DVT (see diagnostic algorithm for suspected DVT in Fig. 5.3-1).

1. **Noninvasive tests** (see Chapter 2.2, section III). Duplex scanning (using color-flow Doppler scanning) and impedance plethysmography (IPG) are considered ideal for monitoring patients who are at risk for DVT because they are highly sensitive and are safe to perform serially. The IPG test is the most cost-effective in DVT diagnosis especially in symptomatic patients. Formal studies on the cost-effectiveness of duplex scanning are not available; however, there is greater cost with duplex scanning (equipment costs $100 000 to $200 000 vs. about $15 000 for an IPG unit, and operating costs are higher for duplex scanning). If the IPG or duplex scan study is negative in a symptomatic patient (i.e., patients with clinical features suggestive of DVT), then it is safe to withhold anticoagulant therapy. This is because the diagnosis of thrombosis of the proximal vein (i.e., popliteal, femoral, and iliac vein) is virtually excluded if the IPG or duplex scan is negative. Even if a calf thrombus remains undetected (because IPG and duplex scanning are insensitive for detection of calf thrombi), they rarely embolize while confined to the calf. The initial negative IPG or duplex scan in a symptomatic patient with high suspicion of DVT should either be confirmed by venography or the noninvasive test (either IPG or duplex scanning) repeated serially several times during the next 10–14 days. If the results of the noninvasive test are equivocal, venography should be performed. On the other hand, if the IPG or duplex scan becomes positive, prompt anticoagulation is warranted. In

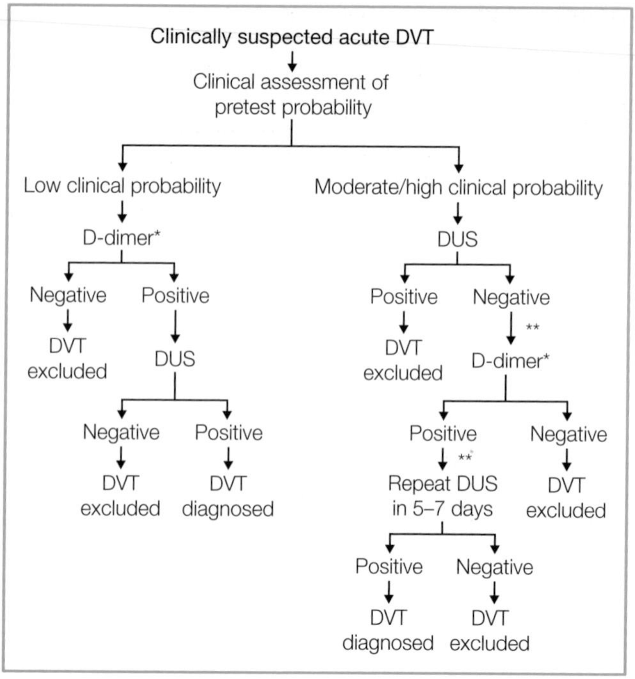

Figure 5.3-1 Diagnostic algorithm for suspected acute DVT using clinical probability, D-dimer testing, and duplex ultrasonography (DUS). * This applies to a sensitive D-dimer assay that has been well validated in the diagnosis of DVT. ** An alternative option would be to obtain a contrast venogram if clinical probability is high. (From Geerts WH, Selby R: Investigation of suspected deep vein thrombosis. In Dalen JE, editor: *Venous thromboembolism*, New York, 2003, Marcel Dekker, p. 103, with permission.)

patients with no DVT symptoms, the available noninvasive tests are unsatisfactory for DVT screening because of low sensitivity.

a. ***Venous duplex ultrasonography scanning*** is a form of vascular ultrasonography (see Chapter 2.2, section III.E.2.b) that combines pulsed-wave Doppler (for detection and localization of abnormal blood flow) with high-resolution, real-time, B-mode ultrasound imaging (for morphologic confirmation of the venous thrombosis). The venous Doppler uses the following compressive technique for detection of DVT: (a) a Doppler sensor is placed over the femoral vein with a background signal elicited (the S sound), which fluctuates significantly with respiration (i.e., venous flow increased with expiration or decreased with inspiration); (b) the thigh vein is then compressed gently at several distal points (e.g., mid-thigh) via external pressure from the hand-held ultrasound transducer, and the normal response is an augmented tone (the A sound); and (c) this process is then repeated with the sensor placed over the popliteal and posterior tibial veins, and the compression is applied distally at the calf and foot respectively. In the presence of DVT, the A sound is absent (i.e., there is failure of signal augmentation) or the S sound does not fluctuate significantly with respiration or the vein is noncompressible (i.e., the vein does not collapse under a force sufficient to distort the artery). The thrombus can be visualized either directly using the B-mode, grayscale, or indirectly by the lack of color in the lumen using **color-flow duplex scanning**. When the thrombi are visible, their echo characteristics may help determine their age and distinguish acute from chronic venous occlusion.

Duplex scanning is highly accurate in detecting occluded proximal DVT but is less accurate in detecting calf DVT (because the calf vein is difficult to compress) or nonobstructing proximal DVTs. In symptomatic patients, the high sensitivity (97%) and specificity (97%) of duplex scanning are slightly better than those of IPG; however, in nonsymptomatic patients, the sensitivity drops to 59%. In symptomatic patients, duplex scanning in itself is sufficient in confirming or disproving suspected cases of DVT, as long as a negative examination is followed by repeated noninvasive testing to detect proximal extension. In patients with clinical suspicion of isolated calf vein thrombosis, a venogram is recommended or the duplex scanning may be repeated every 2–3 days for 10–14 days to document possible progression of a suspected thrombosis. Duplex scanning is not as convenient as IPG (although some equipment may be transported to the bedside, they are not as easy to handle as an IPG unit).

b. ***Magnetic resonance venography*** appears to be as accurate as contrast venography in diagnosing acute DVT and may be more accurate than duplex ultrasonography, especially for pelvic and calf DVT. It may be used as an adjunct to MR angiography of the pulmonary arteries in diagnosing suspected PE. It has high sensitivity (87–100%) and specificity (97%) but is generally unavailable because of its cost.

c. ***Plethysmography*** (see Chapter 2.2, section IV.B)

I. **Impedance plethysmography (IPG)** assesses limb volume by detecting changes in the electrical impedance between two electrodes wrapped around the calf. A thigh cuff is inflated to obstruct venous flow and increase limb volume. Once the cuff is deflated, the limb volume returns to normal size within 3–4 seconds. If there is a venous obstruction proximal to the electrodes, the return to baseline is delayed when the cuff is deflated. In symptomatic patients, IPG has high sensitivity (92%) and specificity (95%) comparable to duplex scanning in the diagnosis of proximal DVT. False-negative results occur in patients with distal (calf) thrombi, small nonocclusive proximal thrombi, or when there are sufficient collateral veins. Hence the sensitivity of IPG drops to as low as 22% in nonsymptomatic patients, many of whom have nonoccluding thrombi. False-positive IPG tests may occur in patients with congestive cardiac (right heart) failure, excessive leg muscle tension, severe peripheral vascular disease, postoperative lower limb swelling, enlarged pelvic lymph nodes, in patients receiving mechanical ventilation, and in pregnant patients. When these conditions are present, either duplex scanning or venography may be used. In symptomatic patients, if serial IPG is persistently negative, then it is safe to withhold anticoagulation.

II. **Phleborheography** is a sophisticated form of whole-leg plethysmography using multiple air-filled cuffs to detect volume changes. Early studies show that its sensitivity and specificity are comparable to those of IPG; however, it is not widely used because it is time consuming and its interpretation is subjective.

2. **Invasive tests** (see Chapter 2.3, section II.A)

a. ***Contrast venography (phlebography) of the lower limb*** is accepted as the final diagnostic test for determining proximal DVT and distal DVT. It is not used routinely or serially because it is costly, painful, and can cause local venous or skin injury, secondary thrombophlebitis (in 2–3% of patients), and hypersensitivity reactions to the contrast medium. Its use is justified when the diagnosis of DVT requires confirmation in symptomatic patients (e.g., clinical suspicion of isolated calf DVT), when recurrent DVT is suspected, or when patients who have undergone hip operations require screening for postoperative DVT, but less invasive methods lack sensitivity. In such cases, the cost of venography is substantially less than the cost of hospitalization and the treatment for an incorrectly diagnosed illness. A positive venogram warrants prompt anticoagulation. However, a negative venogram does not guarantee that the patient will not develop a late PE even if the chance is extremely small.

b. ***Contrast computed tomography venography*** may be used to image the deep veins from the iliac crest to the proximal calf in patients who have an inadequate proximal duplex ultrasonography. Its limitations include flow artifacts, poor opacification of the deep veins, difficulties distinguishing acute from chronic DVT, and interobserver variability. It is also associated with moderate additional radiation.

c. ***Radionuclide venography*** can be used to detect proximal DVT. A labeled sample of the patient's platelets, proteins, or red cells is used to highlight the veins of the lower limbs for imaging. The label can either be a radioactive marker or a radiopharmaceutical solution injected into a vein in the foot. Radionuclide venography is still in the developmental stage.

d. ***Radioiodine-labeled fibrinogen,*** once widely used, has been withdrawn from the US market because it uses blood products and carries the risk of virus transmission (e.g., hepatitis).

C. **LABORATORY WORK-UPS** such as protein S, protein C, fibrinogen, antithrombin III levels, lupus anticoagulant, and anticardiolipin antibodies are indicated (prior to anticoagulation) in young patients with DVT, patients with recurrent DVT without obvious causes, and those with a family history of thrombotic disease. **D-dimer** (a marker of fibrin degradation), which can be tested using enzyme linked immunosorbent assay or latex agglutination tests, has emerged as a definite aid in the diagnosis of DVT or PE in the outpatient setting (i.e., a negative D-dimer test may be used to safely rule out DVT or PE in outpatients with low or at least nonhigh clinical probability).

IV. DVT prophylaxis

DVT prophylaxis in patients at risk is highly recommended for the following reasons. (a) The incidence of DVT and PE remains too high for a condition that is preventable (see Table 5.3-1). (b) DVT and PE are clinically silent with few specific clinical manifestations; moreover, clinical diagnosis for DVT is insensitive and unreliable. (c) Use of serial surveillance (e.g., IPG and duplex scanning) is expensive and has only moderate sensitivity and moderate positive predictive value when used in nonsymptomatic high-risk patients. (d) To rely on the diagnosis and treatment of established DVT may expose susceptible patients to unacceptable risk; although anticoagulant therapy is highly effective in treating DVTs, most patients who die of PE do so within 30 minutes of the acute event, too soon for the anticoagulant to be effective. (e) Unrecognized and untreated DVTs may lead to long-term morbidity from postphlebitic syndrome and predispose patients to future episodes of recurrent DVT. (f) Although there is legitimate concern about bleeding (e.g., hematoma in surgical patients, which can result in wound infection, dehiscence, or infection of the implanted prosthetic device), studies have shown that there is no significant increase in major bleeding with low-dose unfractionated heparin or low molecular weight heparin: besides, alternative mechanical methods of effective DVT prophylaxis that carry no bleeding risk (e.g., intermittent pneumatic leg compression) are available. (g) Studies have shown that broad application of DVT prophylaxis is cost-effective.

Effective DVT prophylaxis methods for different levels of DVT risk are summarized in Table 5.3-1. Methods of DVT prophylaxis for specific conditions commonly

Table 5.3-2	DVT prophylaxis in common PM&R conditions as recommended by the Seventh American College of Chest Physicians (ACCP) Conference on Antithrombotic and Thrombolytic Therapy (2004)
PM&R conditions	**ACCP recommendation for DVT prophylaxis**
Elective total hip replacement	1. LMWH [at a usual high-risk dose (⩾3400 IU SQ daily) started 12 h before surgery, or 12–24 h after surgery, or 4–6 h after surgery at half the usual high-risk dose and then increasing to the usual high-risk dose the following day], or 2. Fondaparinux (2.5 mg SQ daily started 6–8 h after surgery), or 3. Warfarin [started the evening before surgery or the evening after surgery (INR target, 2.5; INR range, 2.0–3.0)] Note: The use of aspirin, dextran, LDUH, CS, IPC, or VFP as the sole method of DVT prophylaxis is *not* recommended.
Elective total knee replacement	1. LMWH [at a usual high-risk dose (⩾3400 IU SQ daily)], or 2. Fondaparinux, or 3. Warfarin (INR target, 2.5; INR range, 2.0–3.0) Note: IPC may be used as an in-hospital adjunct to anticoagulant prophylaxis in the presence of multiple risk factors for postoperative VTE. The use of aspirin, LDUH, or VFP as the sole method of DVT prophylaxis is *not* recommended.
Knee arthroscopy	Except for early mobilization, routine DVT prophylaxis is *not* recommended.
Hip fracture surgery (HFS)	1. Fondaparinux, or 2. LMWH [at a usual high-risk dose (⩾3400 IU SQ daily)], or 3. Warfarin (INR target, 2.5; INR range, 2.0–3.0), or 4. LDUH Note: If surgery will likely be delayed, use either LDUH or LMWH during the time between hospital admission and surgery. If anticoagulant prophylaxis is contraindicated because of a high risk of bleeding, use CS and/or IPC. Aspirin alone is *not* recommended.
Intracranial neurosurgery	1. IPC with or without CS; or 2. LDUH or postoperative LMWH Note: In high-risk patients, use CS and/or IPC combined with LDUH or LMWH.
Acute ischemic stroke (AIS)	1. SQ LDUH, or LMWH, or danaparoid* is recommended for routine use 2. IPC or CS may be used if anticoagulant prophylaxis is contraindicated
Acute intracerebral hematoma	1. IPC is initially used 2. If stable, subcutaneous LDUH may be started as soon as 2nd day after hemorrhage onset
Acute spinal cord injury (SCI)	1. LMWH (to be started once primary hemostasis is evident), or 2. Combination of IPC and either LDUH or LMWH Note: During the rehabilitation phase following acute SCI, continue LMWH prophylaxis or convert to warfarin (INR target, 2.5; INR range, 2.0–3.0). Note: The following are *not* recommended: the use of an IVCF as primary prophylaxis against PE; and the use of LDUH, CS, or IPC as sole DVT prophylaxis.

(*Continued*)

Table 5.3-2 *(Continued)*

Major trauma	1. LMWH should be started as soon as it is considered safe to do so 2. Use IPC, or possibly CS alone if LMWH prophylaxis will be delayed or is contraindicated because of concerns about bleeding risk Note: Duplex ultrasonography scanning should be done in patients at high risk for VTE (e.g., the presence of SCI, lower extremity or pelvic fracture, major head injury, or an indwelling femoral venous line), and who have suboptimal or no DVT prophylaxis. Note: The use of IVCFs as primary DVT prophylaxis is *not* recommended.

VTE = venous thromboembolism; LDUH = low-dose unfractionated heparin; LMWH = low molecular-weight heparin; IPC = intermittent pneumatic compression; CS = compressive stockings; INR = international normalized ratio; PE = pulmonary embolism; VFP = venous foot pump; IVCF = inferior vena caval filter; SQ = subcutaneous.

** For DVT prophylaxis in AIS, danaparoid (see Chapter 4.8, section VII.A.5) can be initially given as IV bolus of up to 1000 IU, then 750 IU SQ q12 h (or using body weight: <90 kg = 750 IU q8 h; >90 kg = 1250 IU q12 h) for 14 days.*

Data tabulated from: Geerts WH, Graham FP, Heit JA, et al.: *Prevention of venous thromboembolism. The Seventh ACCP Conference on Antithrombotic and Thrombolytic Therapy.* Chest *Suppl 126(3): 338S–400S, 2004, with permission; and Albers GW, Amarenco P, Easton JD,* et al.: *Antithrombotic and thrombolytic therapy for ischemic stroke. The Seventh ACCP Conference on Antithrombotic and Thrombolytic Therapy.* Chest *Suppl 126(3): 483S–512S, 2004, with permission.*

encountered in PM&R are shown in Table 5.3-2. Despite prophylaxis, nonsymptomatic DVT and PE may still develop. Although there are sufficient data to make recommendations for the type of DVT prophylaxis, the decision on when to stop DVT prophylaxis remains uncertain. Extended out-of-hospital prophylaxis (e.g., using LMWH) beyond 7 to 10 days after surgery is recommended at least for high risk patients (see Table 5.3-1 for risk stratification). For elective total hip replacement (THR), total knee replacement (TKR), and hip fracture surgery (HFS), the American College of Chest Physicians (ACCP) recommends at least 10 days of prophylaxis after surgery, regardless of hospital length of stay, with extended prophylaxis for up to 28 to 35 days after surgery in THR or HFS patients. For acute nonambulatory SCI patients, the ACCP recommends at least 3 months of DVT prophylaxis (or at least until the completion of the inpatient rehabilitation phase). For the other conditions listed in Table 5.3-2, the clinical data are insufficient to make a definite recommendation about duration of prophylaxis. It is very likely that the risk of DVT is not uniform but varies according to the presence of other risk factors. Most studies report that more severe weakness is associated with a higher risk of DVT, and that more venous thromboembolic events occur in nonambulatory patients. These observations suggest that the risk of late DVT in stroke has a strong relationship to persisting leg weakness and nonambulatory status, and might not be a simple function of time. The evidence supports the value of continuing DVT prophylaxis into the postacute rehabilitation phase until the risk of DVT is low. The best assessment of risk is made on clinical grounds, including consideration of degree of leg weakness and ambulatory status.

A. **MECHANICAL OR PHYSICAL METHODS OF DVT PROPHYLAXIS** are generally less efficacious than anticoagulant drugs in DVT prophylaxis. Their main advantage is their lack of bleeding potential. Hence, they are recommended in patients who are at high risk of bleeding. They can also be used in combination with anticoagulant prophylaxis (either LMWH or LDUH) to improve efficacy. When used, they must be applied properly, removed for only a short period of time each day, and must not impede ambulation. The devices most commonly used in DVT prophylaxis are the intermittent pneumatic leg compression, venous foot pump, and compression stockings.

1. **Intermittent pneumatic compression (IPC) devices** consist of an inflatable garment for the leg or foot and an electrical pneumatic pump that fills the garment with compressed air. The garment is intermittently inflated and deflated to increase venous return and, possibly, stimulate intrinsic fibrinolysis. Although effective in preventing distal DVT formation, they have the same effect as placebo in preventing proximal DVT formation. They are most effective when applied either intraoperatively or immediately postoperatively, and are worn continuously at least until the patient is fully ambulatory. Their use is limited by the patient's poor compliance, improper use of the devices, intolerance, and inability to continue prophylaxis after hospital discharge. Because duration of daily compression is believed to be an important factor in determining their effectiveness, they may not be as effective in a rehabilitation setting where patients spend considerable time out of bed in therapeutic and recreational activities.

   According to the ACCP, intermittent pneumatic compression devices are recommended for DVT prophylaxis in moderate-, high-, and very-high-risk patients (see Table 5.3-1). They are not recommended as the sole device of DVT prophylaxis unless there is a bleeding potential (e.g., intracranial neurosurgery or acute intracerebral hematoma) or there is contraindication to the use of anticoagulants (e.g., hip fracture surgery, acite ischemic stroke, or major trauma). They are effective when combined with other prophylactic agents (either LDUH or LMWH) in high-risk patients undergoing intracranial neurosurgery and also in patients with acute SCI.

   a. ***Intermittent pneumatic leg compression devices*** consist of a double-lined stocking that contains a bladder that intermittently and segmentally inflates at a pressure of 35–40 mmHg lasting 10 seconds/min for each compression.

   b. ***Venous foot pump or plantar foot pump devices*** are designed to simulate the compression of the large venous plexus in the sole of the foot observed during the weight-bearing phase of normal ambulation when the plantar arch is flattened and stretched. They consist of a foot-shaped bladder, which is rapidly inflated (e.g., 0.4 second) at a pressure of 50–200 mmHg (usually around 125 mmHg is optimal). The inflation is then held for 1 to 3 seconds, followed by 20 seconds of deflation for complete refilling of the plexus. They are not recommended for use as the sole method of DVT prophylaxis in patients undergoing THR or TKR.

2. **Compression stockings (antiembolic stockings, thromboembolytic disease hose)** are graded compression elastic stockings (with pressure of 30–40 mmHg at ankle), either knee- or thigh-high, available in different standard sizes. They must be applied evenly (without being rolled) so that circulation to the legs is not obstructed. They can control leg edema and reduce the risk of leg DVT, but their effectiveness on proximal DVT prophylaxis remains to be proved. They can provide adequate DVT prophylaxis in patients with moderate risk of DVT. When used alone they may be effective for DVT prophylaxis in patients in whom anticoagulants are contraindicated (e.g., patients with hip fracture surgery, acute ischemic stroke, or major trauma). Compression stockings are effective when combined with other prophylactic agents (either LDUH or LMWH) in high-risk patients undergoing intracranial neurosurgery. They are not recommended as the sole method of DVT prophylaxis in patients with THR, TKR, or acute SCI.

   In patients who cannot tolerate CS, Ace bandages are an alternative; however, unless the Ace bandage is wrapped properly around the legs (i.e., with adequate pressure to provide decreasing compression from distal to proximal) and maintained throughout the day, they are probably less effective than CS for DVT prophylaxis. Most studies on DVT prophylaxis used CS instead of Ace wrap because CS are more convenient to apply and easier to standardize.

3. **Mobilization (exercises and ambulation)** can help improve peripheral venous flow in the legs and reduce venous stasis; however, they are not adequate in and of themselves for DVT prophylaxis. They include active range-of-motion (ROM) exercises, for example, active contraction of the calf muscle (ankle pumps), passive ROM exercises, use of continuous passive motion machines (their effectiveness in DVT prophylaxis after THR or TKR remains controversial), leg elevation to help reduce leg swelling, and early ambulation (although there are no data available, most physiatrists use ambulation distance as a guide in terminating DVT prophylaxis, especially in postsurgical patients).
4. **Functional electrical stimulation** has been tried for DVT prophylaxis in patients with acute SCI and stroke. It supposedly increases fibrinolytic activity and causes a mild to moderate increase in venous flow thus reducing the incidence of DVT; however, it has the problem of poor compliance because of discomfort and blister formation. Its effectiveness remains to be proven.

B. PHARMACOLOGICAL DVT PROPHYLAXIS (see Tables 5.3-1 and 5.3-2) is generally recommended to be given for at least 10 days in patients undergoing THR, TKA, or HFS. It can be extended for up to 28 to 35 days after THR or HFS.

1. Anticoagulant drugs

a. ***Warfarin (Coumadin, Panwarfin)*** (see Chapter 4.8, section VII.A.1) is an oral vitamin K antagonist used for DVT prophylaxis in the highest-risk patients (see Table 5.3-1), specifically in patients undergoing THR (effective when given the evening before surgery or the evening after surgery), TKR, or HFS, as well as during rehabilitation phase of SCI patients. Due to hemorrhagic complications, it is not recommended for DVT prophylaxis in patients with acute ischemic stroke, acute intracerebral hematoma, or intracranial neurosurgery. It must be monitored regularly to maintain the international normalized ratio (INR) at 2.0 to 3.0. If the INR is above the therapeutic range, refer to the ACCP guidelines in Table 5.3-3. Unexpected fluctuations in dose response could be attributed to changes in diet (e.g., high vitamin K diet) or undisclosed drug use (see Table 4.8-11 for drug and food interactions), inaccuracy of prothrombin time testing, poor patient compliance, surreptitious self-medication, or intermittent alcohol consumption.

b. ***Unfractionated heparin*** (previously referred to as **heparin**) (see Chapter 4.8, section VII.A)

I. **Low-dose unfractionated heparin** can be given subcutaneously in a fixed dose of 5000 IU q8 or 12 h for the prevention of DVT in moderate-, high-, and highest risk patients (see Table 5.3-1). In the highest risk patients, it may be used effectively with IPC or CS. Specific conditions include: HFS, intracranial surgery (may be combined with CS and/or IPC in high-risk patients), acute ischemic stroke, acute intracerebral hematoma (LDUH may be started as soon as the second day after hemorrhage onset if the patient is stable), and acute SCI (must be combined with IPC). It is not recommended in THR and TKR. Low-dose unfractionated heparin does not require activated partial thromboplastin time (aPTT) monitoring.

II. **Adjusted-dose unfractionated heparin (ADUH)**, given subcutaneously or intravenously, is currently not recommended by the ACCP for use in DVT prophylaxis (although it is still recommended for use in treating acute DVT and PE).

c. ***Low molecular weight heparin*** **(e.g., Enoxaparin [Lovenox]; Dalteparin [Fragmin])** (see Chapter 4.8, section VII.A.3 for details) can be given

Table 5.3-3	Management of elevated INRs or bleeding in patients receiving warfarin as recommended by the Seventh American College of Chest Physicians (ACCP) Conference on Antithrombotic and Thrombolytic Therapy (2004)	
INR	**Symptoms**	**ACCP recommendation**
Above therapeutic range but <5	No significant bleeding	• Lower or omit warfarin dose; • Check INR more frequently (e.g., q6 hr); and • Resume at lower dose when INR is therapeutic Note: If the INR is only minimally above the therapeutic range, dose reduction may *not* be needed.
≥5 to <9	No significant bleeding	• Omit the next 1 or 2 warfarin doses; • Check INR more frequently (e.g., q6 hr); and • Resume at lower dose when INR is in therapeutic range Note: Alternatively, if the patient is at increased risk of bleeding, omit warfarin dose and give oral vitamin K_1* (≤5 mg); or if more rapid reversal is needed because the patient needs urgent surgery, give 2–4 mg or oral vitamin K_1* with expectation of INR reduction in 24 hrs (if the INR is still high after 24 hrs, give additional 1–2 mg of oral vitamin K_1*).
≥9 to 20	No significant bleeding	• Hold warfarin dose and give oral vitamin K_1* at higher doses (5–10 mg) with expectation of substantial INR reduction in 24–48 hrs; • Check INR more frequently (e.g., q6 hr); and • Use additional oral vitamin K_1* if necessary (when INR returns to the therapeutic range, resume warfarin at a lower dose)
Any INR elevation	Serious bleeding	• Hold warfarin dose and give 10 mg of vitamin K_1* by slow IV infusion; supplemented with transfusion of fresh frozen plasma (FFP), 2–4 units, or prothrombin complex concentrate (or alternatively, recombinant factor VIIa), depending on the urgency of the situation; and • Check INR and, if needed, repeat IV vitamin K_1* q12 hr
	Life-threatening bleeding	• Hold warfarin and transfuse prothrombin complex concentrates (or alternatively, recombinant factor VIIa), supplemented with 10 mg of vitamin K_1* by slow IV infusion; and • Check INR and, if needed, repeat IV vitamin K_1*

INR = international normalized ratio.

** Vitamin K_1 or phytonadione is available as Mephyton tablets or AquaMephyton injection. If given by IV route it should be diluted and slowly infused over 20–30 min. If warfarin therapy needs to be resumed after high doses of vitamin K_1 (e.g., 10–15 mg which may cause resistance to warfarin for up to a week), then heparin can be given until the effects of vitamin K_1 have been reversed and the patient becomes responsive to warfarin.*

Table adapted from: Ansell J, Hirsh J, Poller L, et al.: The pharmacology and management of the vitamin K antagonists. The Seventh ACCP Conference on Antithrombotic and Thrombolytic Therapy. Chest *Suppl 126(3): 204S–233S, 2004, with permission.*

subcutaneously at ≤3400 IU daily in moderate-risk patients and ≥3400 IU daily in high-, and highest risk patients (see Table 5.3-2). It is recommended at ≥3400 IU daily in THR (started 12 h before surgery, or 12–24 h after surgery provided hemostasis has been established), TKR, and HFS patients. In intracranial neurosurgery, it is recommended postoperatively and may be combined with CS and/or IPC in high-risk patients. It can also be used for acute ischemic stroke and in acute SCI (once primary hemostasis is evident; may also be combined with IPC). It may be continued during rehabilitation phase of SCI until conversion to warfarin. In major trauma, it should be started as soon as it is considered safe. LMWH does not require aPTT monitoring. The duration of treatment (about 7–14 days) remains uncertain.

d. ***Fondaparinux (Arixtra)*** (see Chapter 4.8, section VII.A.4 for details), a new drug that indirectly inhibits factor Xa, can be administered at 2.5 mg SQ once daily, with the initial dose given 6–8 hours after surgery (after establishing hemostasis) for DVT prophylaxis in the highest risk patients (see Table 5.3-1), specifically in THR, TKR, and HFS patients. It is contraindicated in patients with severe renal impairment.

2. **Antiplatelet drugs** (see Chapter 4.8, section VII.B) including aspirin, dipyridamole, and dextran, are not recommended for use as the sole method of DVT prophylaxis.

C. INFERIOR VENA CAVAL FILTER (IVCF)

1. **Permanent IVCF (e.g., Greenfield filter, Venatech filter, Nitinol filter, TrapEase filter, bird's nest filter)** is the permanent use of an umbrella-like filter device that can be inserted percutaneously (with fluoroscopic guidance) through the femoral vein to the inferior vena cava to prevent PE. Permanent IVCF as primary prevention may be used in selected patients with very high risk for developing DVT and PE (e.g., those with multiple lower limb fractures, spinal cord injury, severe head injury, or indwelling femoral venous catheters) but in whom anticoagulation therapy is contraindicated or has failed or led to complications. Permanent IVCFs are mainly used as secondary prophylaxis in patients with DVT or recurrent DVT (see section V.C), in patients with "free-floating" or major clots in the iliac veins or vena cava, or in patients *in extremis* from PE (i.e., patients with massive PE resulting in sustained hypotension, right heart failure, and hypoxemia are candidates based upon the concept that they would not tolerate another embolic insult). Complications of permanent IVCF (although infrequent) include filter misplacement or migration, thrombosis at the insertion site or vena cava, occlusion of the filter, or perforation of the caval wall.

2. **Nonpermanent IVCF** can be placed during the period of highest risk and then removed when that period has passed or when alternative therapies can be safely used. It can either be temporary (i.e., removed after a fixed period of time, usually <14 days) or retrievable (i.e., removed after a short period, but with the option of remaining permanently in place if clinically indicated). They are still in the experimental stages.

D. DVT SURVEILLANCE (DUPLEX SCANNING or IPG) in high-risk patients is an attractive alternative in DVT prophylaxis; however, both IPG and duplex scanning are expensive and are shown to have only moderate sensitivity and positive predictive value when applied to nonsymptomatic high-risk patients. The DVT surveillance may be used effectively in high-risk patients (e.g., multiple trauma) in whom standard methods of DVT prophylaxis are not feasible or are shown to have uncertain efficacy. The IPG or duplex scanning for screening DVT in high-risk patients admitted to the rehabilitation service may be done (based on the physician's clinical judgment) in those not already on prophylaxis, those with clinical signs of DVT, and those who are nonambulatory because of severe leg weakness. There are insufficient data, however, to indicate whether all patients should be screened on admission to the rehabilitation unit. For patients already on DVT prophylaxis, there is continued risk of developing DVT extension or PE especially in patients with severe leg weakness or with limited or no ability to ambulate (or both). In such cases, serial IPG or duplex scanning may be justified on a case-to-case basis.

V. Management of DVT

DVT management is ultimately aimed at preventing PE by limiting thrombus extension and preventing thrombus recurrence. This is achieved primarily through anticoagulation therapy using SQ LMWH (or alternatively, SQ ADUH or IV ADUH) initially and then converted to oral warfarin for long term treatment. If warfarin is contraindicated (e.g., in pregnancy), or impractical, or in patients with concurrent cancer for whom LMWH regimens have been shown to be more effective and safer, then SQ LMWH or alternatively SQ ADUH may be used. In patients with suspected or confirmed DVT, the management as recommended by the ACCP is shown in Table 5.3-4.

Table 5.3-4 Management of suspected and confirmed deep venous thrombosis (DVT) or pulmonary embolism (PE) as recommended by the Seventh American College of Chest Physicians (ACCP) Conference on Antithrombotic and Thrombolytic Therapy (2004)

DVT or PE	Guidelines
High clinical suspicion of DVT or PE	1. Obtain baseline prothrombin time, aPTT, CBC and order diagnostic tests (see section III.B) 2. While awaiting study outcome, start one of the following treatments (i.e., if there is no contraindication): • SQ LMWH adjusted to total body weight (enoxaparin, 1 mg/kg/day not to exceed 180 mg or dalteparin, 200 IU/kg/day not to exceed 18 000 IU), or • IV ADUH (given either 5000 IU by IV bolus followed by a continuous infusion of at least 30 000 U for the first 24 hr or a weight-adjusted regimen of 80 IU/kg by IV bolus followed by 18 IU/kg, then dose adjusted according to Table 5.3-5), or • For DVT suspicion only, SQ ADUH may be given as IV bolus of 5000 IU, followed by SC dose of 17 500 IU q12 h on the first day, then adjusted to aPTT of 1.5–2.5
Objectively confirmed DVT or PE	1. If total body weight-adjusted SQ LMWH is used, continue it for at least 5 days, or if IV ADUH is used, adjust subsequent IV doses according Table 5.3-5 and continue for at least 5 days. If SQ ADUH is used for confirmed DVT (not for PE), the SQ dose should be adjusted with a target aPTT of 1.5–2.5 X control. In patients given ADUH or LMWH, platelet should be checked for thrombocytopenia within 3–5 days 2. Start warfarin (either 5 or 10 mg, depending on bleeding risk) together with LMWH or ADUH on the first treatment day, and discontinue LMWH or ADUH when INR is stable (range of 2.0–3.0), which is usually after 5–7 days 3. Continue warfarin for at least 3 months in patients with a first episode of DVT secondary to a transient (reversible) risk factor and for at least 6–12 months in patients with first episode of idiopathic DVT. Consider indefinite use of warfarin in patients with recurrent venous thrombosis or with continuing risk factor. Maintain INR between 2.0–3.0 for all duration of treatment

aPTT = activated partial thromboplastin time; CBC = complete blood count; SQ = subcutaneous; IV = intravenous; LMWH = low molecular weight heparin; ADUH = adjusted dose unfractionated heparin; INR = international normalized ratio.
Data from: Buller HR, Agnelli G, Hull RD, et al.: *Antithrombotic therapy for venous thromboembolic disease. The Seventh ACCP Conference on Antithrombotic and Thrombolytic Therapy.* Chest *Suppl 126(3): 401S–428S, 2004, with permission.*

A. ANTICOAGULATION THERAPY

1. **Low-molecular-weight heparin [LMWH; e.g., enoxaparin (Lovenox); dalteparin (Fragmin)]** is the preferred anticoagulant for treating suspected or confirmed DVT because, unlike unfractionated heparin, LMWH has more predictable pharmacokinetics, a greater bioavailability, and can also be given (even as an outpatient) without laboratory monitoring. For DVT treatment, LMWH can be administered SQ once or twice daily for at least 5 days using total body weight (TBW)-adjusted doses (i.e., enoxaparin, 1 mg/kg/day not to exceed 180 mg or dalteparin, 200 IU/kg/day not to exceed 18 000 IU) instead of fixed doses. In certain clinical situations (e.g., severe renal failure or pregnancy) LMWH dose might need to be adjusted (or if possible, IV ADUH should be used instead of LMWH) and its dose monitored by plasma anti-Xa assay (with a target range of 0.6–1.0 IU/mL) done 4 hrs after administration of LMWH.
2. **Adjusted-dose unfractionated heparin** (**ADUH**; see Chapter 4.8, section VII.A), particularly IV ADUH was previously the preferred initial treatment of DVT, but because of its unpredictable dose response and narrow therapeutic window (thereby making aPTT monitoring essential), it has been replaced by LMWH. If used, ADUH should be given for at least 5 days.

a. ***IV Adjusted-dose unfractionated heparin (IV ADUH),*** if used, can be started at either 5000 IU by IV bolus followed by a continuous infusion of at least 30 000 U for the first 24 h or a weight-adjusted regimen of 80 IU/kg by IV bolus followed by 18 IU/kg. Upon DVT confirmation, subsequent IV doses are then adjusted using the guidelines shown on Table 5.3-5.

b. ***SQ adjusted-dose unfractionated heparin (SQ ADUH)*** is at least as safe as IV ADUH and when given twice daily appeared to be more effective than IV ADUH for the initial treatment of DVT. The usual regimen includes an initial IV bolus of 5000 IU, followed by SC dose of 17 500 IU q12 h on the first day. The aPTT is drawn at 6 h after the morning administration and the dose is then adjusted to achieve a 1.5–2.5 prolongation of aPTT.

Table 5.3-5 Guidelines for adjusting dose of IV unfractionated heparin using body weight as recommended by the Seventh American College of Chest Physicians (ACCP) Conference on Antithrombotic and Thrombolytic Therapy (2004)

aPTT after initial dose*	Dose adjustment
<35 s (<1.2 × control)	Rebolus 80 IU/kg, then increase rate by 4 IU/kg/h
35–45 s (1.2–1.5 × control)	Rebolus 40 IU/kg, then increase rate 2 IU/kg/h
46–70 s (1.5–2.3 × control)†	Therapeutic range; no change
71–90 s (2.3–3 × control)	Decrease rate by 2 IU/kg/h
>90 s (>3 × control)	Hold infusion 1 h, then decrease rate by 3 IU/kg/h

aPTT = activated partial thromboplastin time.
** Note: Use full-strength unfractionated heparin concentration of 25 000 IU in 250 mL D_5W (i.e., 100 IU/mL). Initial loading dose is 80 IU/kg bolus followed by 18 IU/kg/h maintenance dose. The aPTT must be checked q6 h until therapeutic range is reached (i.e., aPTT of 46–70 s or 1.5–2.3 × control). Once reached, check aPTT q6 h for another 24 h. Thereafter, monitor aPTT once every morning unless it is outside the therapeutic range.*
† Therapeutic range of 46–70 s should correspond to anti-factor Xa assay of 0.3–0.7 IU/mL. In heparin-resistant patients requiring large daily doses of unfractionated heparin, anti-Xa assay for dose guidance is recommended.
Adapted from: Hirsh J, Raschke R: Heparin and low molecular weight heparin. The Seventh ACCP Conference on Antithrombotic and Thrombolytic Therapy. Chest Suppl 126(3):192S, 2004, with permission.

3. **Warfarin (Coumadin, Panwarfin**; see Chapter 4.8, section VII.A.1) should be started at a dose of 5 mg or 10 mg (depending on bleeding risk) together with LMWH or ADUH on the first day of DVT treatment and overlapped with LMWH or ADUH treatment until a stable target INR of 2.0–3.0 is reached (when this occurs, usually after 5 to 7 days of LMWH or ADUH therapy, then the LMWH or ADUH can be discontinued). Warfarin is given for at least 3 months in patients with a first episode of DVT secondary to a transient (reversible) risk factor and for at least 6 to 12 months in patients with first episode of idiopathic DVT. The indefinite use of warfarin should be considered in patients with recurrent venous thrombosis or a continuing risk factor, such as antithrombin III deficiency, protein C or S deficiency, lupus anticoagulant, or malignancy. For all treatment duration, the INR should be maintained at 2.5 (with INR range between 2.0–3.0). If INR is above therapeutic range, refer to ACCP guidelines in Table 5.3-3. Reasons for unexpected fluctuations in warfarin dose response are given in section IV.B.1.a.

B. THROMBOLYTIC THERAPY [e.g., STREPTOKINASE, UROKINASE, TISSUE PLASMINOGEN ACTIVATOR or tPA (ALTEPLASE)], given intravenously, may theoretically accelerate thrombus dissolution, resulting in a reduction in the incidence of postphlebitic syndrome. It may be indicated in select patients with proximal DVT or PE; however, because of uncertain long-term benefits and the increased risk of hemorrhagic complications, it is not recommended for routine use in patients with acute DVT. Thrombolytic therapy is contraindicated in patients with active bleeding, intracranial hemorrhage, recent surgery, severe trauma, and any hemorrhagic disease.

C. INFERIOR VENA CAVAL FILTER (**IVCF**, see section IV.C for its description and complications) is not recommended for routine use in most patients with DVT receiving anticoagulants. Although the use of IVCF in DVT patients had lowered the incident of PE at day 12, the incidence of recurrent DVT at 1 year was higher in patients with IVCF compared to those with no IVCF. IVCF is indicated when there is a contraindication or failure or complication of anticoagulant therapy in an individual with, or at high risk for, proximal vein thrombosis or PE. It is also recommended for recurrent thromboembolism that occurs despite adequate anticoagulation, in the presence of "free-floating" or major clots in the iliac veins or vena cava, in the patient with chronic recurrent embolism with pulmonary hypertension, during the concurrent performance of surgical pulmonary embolectomy or pulmonary endarterectomy, or in patients *in extremis* from PE (i.e., patients with massive PE resulting in sustained hypotension, right heart failure, and hypoxemia are candidates based upon the concept that they would not tolerate another embolic insult). Whenever possible, anticoagulants should be given following placement of a vena caval filter in a patient with proximal DVT of the lower limb.

D. MOBILIZATION of the affected limb and gait training have traditionally been prohibited for several days in patients with DVT receiving anticoagulation to avoid thrombi from breaking off and causing PE. With the use of SQ LMWHs in the initial treatment DVT, studies have shown that bed rest in addition to anticoagulation does not reduce the incidence of silent PE as detected by lung scanning and that early ambulation may increase the rate of resolution of pain and swelling. Hence, when SQ LMWH is used, patients with DVT should ambulate as tolerated. However, in patients with DVT using IV ADUH, activities should be restricted until the patient attains at least 1–2 days of therapeutic aPTT range while on IV heparin therapy. During this bed-rest regimen, the affected limb is elevated and the patient is prohibited from moving it and from walking; however, other rehabilitation measures (e.g., nursing-care measures, upper limb therapy, certain activities of daily living, communication, education, and counseling) may be continued at the bedside. The length of the bed-rest regimen may be up to 7–10 days for patients with proximal DVTs or a few days for patients with distal DVT, depending on the time it takes for the patient to attain therapeutic aPTT range. Based on its natural history, thrombus resolution by the fibrinolytic system occurs within a few days and organization of the thrombus in 10–14 days.

VI. Complications of DVT

A. **PULMONARY EMBOLISM** is the most serious and fatal complication of DVT. If the calf thrombus embolizes, it is usually small, and the resulting PE is not likely to be fatal. However, about 20% of calf thrombi progress and extend proximally into the popliteal and thigh veins. Half of these proximal thrombi embolize, and some are large and cause massive PE. In about 20% of cases with clinical features of PE, the event is fatal (see Table 5.3-1 for incidence of PE).

1. **Pathophysiology**. PE is caused by the dislodgment of a DVT into the pulmonary arterial system causing complete or partial obstruction of the distal lung. This leads to increased intrapulmonary dead space (ventilated without perfusion); air-space constriction in the affected lung; atelectasis because of loss of surfactant with decreased alveolar stability; loss of pulmonary vascular capacity with increased resistance to flow (pulmonary hypertension, right ventricular failure); and subsequent development of bronchial collateral arterial circulation. If the PE is massive (i.e., 60% or more of the pulmonary circulation obstructed), the patient can develop right-sided heart failure, which may progress to cardiovascular collapse leading to hypotension, coma, and death.

2. **Diagnosis of PE**

a. ***Clinical diagnosis***. Half of all PEs are clinically silent and are not suspected or diagnosed ante-mortem. Only 30% of patients with PE have clinical features of DVT, even though in about 70% of these patients DVT can be demonstrated by venography. As with DVT, the clinical diagnosis of PE is insensitive and nonspecific.

   I. **Submassive PE** can have clinical features that include tachypnea, tachycardia, and the signs of pulmonary infarction (i.e., pulmonary consolidation, rales, hemoptysis, pleuritic chest pain, pleural friction rub, pleural effusion, and fever). However, only a few of these usually present clinically. Sometimes the patient may only complain of malaise or fever.

   II. **Massive PE** can be fatal within 30 minutes of the acute event. The typical clinical features consist of an abrupt onset of tachypnea, tachycardia, cyanosis, raised jugular venous pressure, and altered mental status.

b. ***Diagnostic tests*** must be done to confirm or disprove a PE suspicion because of the unreliability of the clinical features associated with PE.

   I. **Arterial blood gas (ABG)** values are not helpful diagnostically because up to 15% of patients with PE are not hypoxic, and abnormal gas values occur in many respiratory disorders. Changes in ABG, however, may be used as a simple screening test. If PaO_2 is above 90 mmHg, significant PE is not likely.

   II. **Chest imaging**

   - **Chest radiogram** is often the first chest imaging study performed in patients with suspected PE. Its findings may be suggestive of or compatible with a diagnosis of PE, but at least 25% of patients with symptoms of PE have negative chest radiographs. The main value of a routine chest film is to rule out an alternative diagnosis such as a pneumothorax or pulmonary edema.

- **Lung scintigraphy or radionuclide ventilation–perfusion lung scan (V/Q scan)** (see Chapter 2.3, section I.D) is usually the second diagnostic imaging study performed following chest radiogram. It combines a perfusion lung scan (which is very sensitive in detecting PE, but is not specific) with a ventilation scan (which reveals pulmonary disorders in which there is impairment of both ventilation and perfusion). The ability of the lung scan alone to predict PE (as confirmed by angiography) is 88% for high-probability scans, 33% for intermediate-probability scans, 16% for low-probability scans, and 9% for normal or near-normal scans. In a patient with a high clinical suspicion of PE, however, a high-probability lung scan has a 96% likelihood of predicting PE. Patients with high clinical suspicion of PE but low- or intermediate-probability V/Q scan should undergo pulmonary angiography.
- **Pulmonary arteriography or angiography** is the most definitive study for the diagnosis of PE. It may be required in 40–60% of patients who have high clinical suspicion of PE but in whom the results of a V/Q scan are inconclusive. The need for pulmonary angiography can be reduced by performing leg venograms. Although a venogram is negative in up to 30% of patients with PE, if venography (or IPG or duplex scanning) is positive in a patient with a high clinical suspicion of PE, then pulmonary angiography would not be required, because full anticoagulation would be needed in any case.
- **Spiral or helical chest computed tomography (CT) with contrast** scans from the top of the aortic arch to below the inferior pulmonary veins. It may be used as an initial imaging technique in the setting of an abnormal chest radiogram, when there is a higher likelihood of nondiagnostic V/Q results, or following nondiagnostic V/Q scans, when V/Q scan findings are discordant with clinical suspicion, or in lieu of V/Q scans. Compared to pulmonary arteriography, spiral CT is usually readily available and does not require a skilled radiologist to perform. However, it often misses relatively small (subsegmental) PE.
- **Magnetic resonance imaging (MRI) and/or magnetic resonance angiography (MRA) of the chest** has sensitivity and accuracy that appear to be no better than, or perhaps inferior to spiral CT. It may be used in the setting of an abnormal chest radiogram, when a V/Q scan would be expected to be nondiagnostic and contraindication to contrast precludes the use of spiral CT. A new technique, **V/Q MRI** in which 100% oxygen is used for ventilation enhancement, is being developed.
- **Chest ultrasonography** has limited use in the direct diagnosis of PE itself because only peripheral signs, such as parenchymal or pleural changes, are analyzable and interference from bone and air may skew findings.

3. **Treatment for suspected and confirmed PE** is achieved primarily through anticoagulation therapy using SQ LMWH (or, alternatively, IV ADUH) initially and then converted to oral warfarin for long-term treatment. The recommendations for the use of SQ LMWH, IV ADUH, and warfarin in treating PE are similar that for DVT treatment (see section V and Table 5.3-4). However, compared to patients who are treated for DVT, those patients treated for PE are almost four times more likely (1.5% vs. 0.4%) to die of recurrent VTE in the next year. For most patients with PE who have no contraindication to receiving anticoagulation therapy, the routine use of the following are not recommended by the ACCP: local or systemic thrombolytic therapy, catheter-extraction or fragmentation of PE, pulmonary embolectomy, and IVCF. The indications for use of IVCF in patients with PE is similar to that for DVT (see section V.C). Because PE can be fatal, it is imperative to prevent it through DVT prophylactic measures.

B. **RECURRENCE OF DVT** is high after the initial treatment of DVT with short-term LMWH or ADUH, the risk being greatest in the first month and then diminishing over the next 6 months. Hence anticoagulation with warfarin (INR 2.0–3.0) for 3–6 months (probably indefinitely) is essential for secondary DVT prophylaxis. In patients refractory to warfarin (usually patients with underlying malignancy or other predisposition to thrombosis), chronic anticoagulation with SQ LMWH or SQ ADUH may be required.

C. POSTPHLEBITIC SYNDROME is a late complication of DVT and is associated with venous insufficiency. There is distal venous hypertension caused by residual obstruction to venous outflow from the limb and incompetent valves in the deep veins. The most frequent clinical feature is leg swelling, which may develop following an acute DVT and then persist to give a chronically swollen limb. In other patients the swelling may not be prominent until later, when patients begin to sit or stand with the limb dependent for long periods of time. The patient with postphlebitic syndrome may also have exercise-induced pain that is relieved with rest and elevation of the leg. About 23% of patients with long-standing venous insufficiency developed pigmentation of the legs, while 5% developed increased ulceration. The early detection and treatment of DVT limits the extent of proximal progression of a thrombus and minimizes the degree of overall venous obstruction that can lead to late postphlebitic syndrome. The use of DVT prophylaxis has decreased the incidence of postphlebitic syndrome, especially in its severe form. The ACCP recommends the use of an elastic CS with a pressure of 30–40 mmHg at the ankle during 2 years after an episode of DVT to prevent postphlebitic syndrome. In postphlebitic patients with mild edema, rutosides (e.g., Betarutin, 250–500 mg, po, qd) or CS may be used; whereas those with severe edema may benefit from a course of IPC.

Further reading

Albers GW, Amarenco P, Easton JD, *et al.*: Antithrombotic and thrombolytic therapy for ischemic stroke. The Seventh ACCP Conference on Antithrombotic and Thrombolytic Therapy. *Chest Suppl* 126(3):483S–512S, 2004.

Brandstater ME, Roth EJ, Siebens HC: Venous thromboembolism in stroke: literature review and implications for clinical practice. *Arch Phys Med Rehabil Suppl* 73:379–391, 1992.

Buller HR, Agnelli G, Hull RD, *et al.*: Antithrombotic therapy for venous thromboembolic disease. The Seventh ACCP Conference on Antithrombotic and Thrombolytic Therapy. *Chest Suppl* 126(3):401S–428S, 2004.

Clagett GP, Anderson Jr FA, Heit J, *et al.*: Prevention of venous thromboembolism. *Chest Suppl* 108(4):312–334, 1995.

Dalen J: Pulmonary embolism: what have we learned since Virchow?: Natural history, pathophysiology, and diagnosis. *Chest* 122:1440–1456, 2002.

Dalen J, editor: *Venous thromboembolism*, New York, 2003, Marcel Dekker.

Ferri FF: *Practical guide to the care of the medical patient*, ed 5, St Louis, 2001, Mosby.

Geerts WH, Graham FP, Heit JA, *et al.*: Prevention of venous thromboembolism. The Seventh ACCP Conference on Antithrombotic and Thrombolytic Therapy. *Chest Suppl* 126(3):338S–400S, 2004.

Imperiale TF, Speroff T: A meta-analysis of methods to prevent venous thromboembolism following total hip replacement. *JAMA* 271:1780–1785, 1994.

Interchange forum: developments in prophylactic therapy or venous thromboembolic disease. *Orthop Rev Suppl* 23(3A):1–56, 1994.

Physicians' desk reference, ed 58, Montvale, NJ, 2004, Thomson PDR.

Weinmann EA, Salzman EW: Deep vein thrombosis. *N Engl J Med* 331(24):1630–1641, 1994.

CHAPTER 5.4
Spasticity

Spasticity is a component of the upper motor neuron syndrome characterized by a velocity-dependent increase in muscle tone with exaggerated tendon jerks resulting from hyperexcitability of the stretch reflex. Common PM&R conditions associated with spasticity include spinal cord injury (SCI), demyelinating disease [e.g., multiple sclerosis (MS)], stroke, traumatic brain injury (TBI), and cerebral palsy (CP). Spasticity has to be distinguished from *spasms*, which refer to spontaneous uncontrolled movements, which may be the result of spasticity (e.g., painful flexor or extensor spasms), or to other hyperactive spinal reflexes such as cramps, dystonia, rigidity (decerebrate, decorticate, or parkinsonian), stiff-man syndrome, and metabolic contractures (e.g., McArdle's disease). The terms *spasticity* and *spasms* should also be differentiated from *muscle spasms*, which typically refer to focal areas of increased muscle activity associated with tenderness and splinting of the painful part occurring in the setting of nerve or muscle (or myofascial) injury (see also Chapter 4.8, section II).

I. Pathophysiology

A. NEURAL MECHANISM for spasticity can possibly be explained by the following.

1. Selective increase in motor neuronal excitability because of enhanced excitatory synaptic input, reduced inhibitory synaptic input, and/or changes in intrinsic electrical properties of the neuron.
2. Increase in stretch-evoked synaptic excitation of motor neurons as a result of gamma efferent hyperactivity and/or increased sensitivity of excitatory neurons to muscle afferent (e.g., collateral sprouting, denervation hypersensitivity, and decrease in presynaptic inhibition).

B. SUPRASPINAL MECHANISM for spasticity can possibly be caused by changes in the balance of the descending pathway activity, that is, increased excitation of the motor neurons innervating antigravity muscles (extensors in the legs and flexors in the arms) or loss of inhibition from the descending tracts.

II. Clinical evaluation

The clinical evaluation of spasticity should include quantification of spasticity and its functional effects so that effective comparisons and justifications can be made following treatment. After treatment, it should be kept in mind that decreasing spasticity in one area may precipitate changes in other unexpected areas.

A. PHYSICAL EXAMINATION OF SPASTICITY. The limb is placed in a relaxed state (as much as possible), then suddenly flexed or extended to check for hypertonia. Spasticity is velocity-dependent whereas spasms, contracture, capsule tightness, or other states of hypertonia are not. Spasticity usually involves the flexors of the upper limbs and extensors of the lower limbs. It occurs at the early range of joint motion and is characterized by a sudden relaxation (as in a clasp-knife release) of the limb when a static force is applied persistently to a spastic limb. Other associated features of spasticity include clonus (a cyclical hyperactivity of antagonistic muscles in response to stretch) and spasms (e.g., painful flexor or extensor spasms). Spasticity is one component in the assessment of upper motor neuron (UMN) lesions (cortical, subcortical, or spinal cord level). Abnormal symptoms of UMN lesions include positive cutaneomuscular reflex (e.g., Babinski's or Chaddock's response of the toes and Hoffman's response of the fingers), hyperreflexia, and loss of precise autonomic control below the level of the spinal cord lesion.

B. QUALITATIVE AND QUANTITATIVE ASSESSMENT OF SPASTICITY

1. **Modified Ashworth spasticity scale** (Table 5.4-1) is a qualitative scale which is commonly used in the assessment of spasticity. Assess all involved limbs and use consistent body and joint positions.
2. **Bilateral adductor tone score** is carried out for patients with increased hip adductor tone (0 = no increase in tone; 1 = increased tone; hips are easily abducted to 45° by one person; 2 = hips are abducted to 45° by one person with mild effort; 3 = hips are abducted to 45° by one person with moderate effort; 4 = two people are required to abduct the hips to 45°). Hip adductor spasticity may interfere with sexual function, perineal hygiene, and catheter care for both men and women.
3. **Spasm frequency score** is used to assess all muscle groups presenting with spasms (0 = no spasms; 1 = one or fewer spasms; 2 = between one and five spasms; 3 = between five and nine spasms; 4 = ten or more spasms or continuous contraction).
4. **Visual analog scale** for assessment of global pain may be used to assess the effects of spasticity. The patient is asked to rate the total amount of pain he or she had in the last 24 hours in the (affected part) using a 10-cm horizontal line with "no pain" written on the left end and "maximal pain" on the other end (Chapter 5.10, section IV.C.2.a.1).
5. **Other methods** of evaluating or quantifying spasticity include dynamic multichannel electromyogram (EMG), computerized gait analysis, the pendulum test, temporary anesthetic nerve blocks, and electrophysiologic testing (e.g., H reflex, H/M ratio, F waves, tonic vibration reflex, cutaneomuscular or flexor withdrawal response, and lumbosacral spinal evoked responses). Most of these tests are time-consuming, involve expensive equipment, or are used mainly

Table 5.4-1 Modified Ashworth scale for clinical grading of muscle spasticity

Spasticity grade	Definition
0	No increase in tone
1	Slight increase in muscle tone, manifested by a catch and release or by minimal resistance at the end of the range of motion (ROM) when the affected part(s) is moved in flexion or extension
1+	Slight increase in muscle tone, manifested by a catch, followed by minimal resistance throughout the remainder (<50%) of the ROM
2	More marked increase in muscle tone through most of the ROM; affected part(s) easily moved
3	Considerable increase in muscle tone; passive movement is difficult
4	Affected part(s) rigid in flexion or extension

From: Bohannon RW, Smith MB: Interrater reliability on modified Ashworth scale of muscle spasticity. Phys Ther *67:207, 1987, with permission of the American Physical Therapy Association.*

in research. Electrophysiological studies are not very useful because they study the patient at rest ignoring the biomechanic and neurophysiologic features of movement.

C. **FUNCTIONAL EVALUATION OF SPASTICITY**. Functionally, the performance deficits (negative symptoms) of UMN lesions include decreased dexterity, weakness, paralysis, synergy (i.e., loss of isolated voluntary activation), and increased fatigability. During examination, the adverse functional impact of spasticity must be determined.

1. **Activities of daily living (ADL)**: Assess all basic and instrumental ADLs (Chapter 4.5, sections II.A and II.B). Also note assistive devices used and amount of assistance required.
2. **Transfer abilities**: Assess the type, amount of assistance, and difficulties and safety for all forms of transfers, i.e., tub, chair, bed, toilet, and car.
3. **Resting positions**: Measure the joint resting angles in sitting, standing, and following ambulation. Note any deviations, difficulties, and adaptations with positioning for bed, chair, and wheelchair.
4. **Range of motion (ROM)**: Assess active and passive ROMs of the involved limbs.
5. **Balance skills**: Note sitting, standing, and walking balance.
6. **Endurance**: Determine how much endurance is lost because of the energy expended to overcome spasticity.
7. **Orthoses**: Assess existing splints or orthoses by noting fit, function, and joint position.
8. **Sleeping patterns**: Assess the effects of spasticity on sleep, e.g., the number of times per night the patient is awakened by spasms or spasticity, and the remedy or assistance required to resume sleep.
9. **Observational gait analysis** (Chapter 2.5, section VI.A): Determine gait patterns, compensations, and deviations. Also evaluate how the patient's gait and walking balance are affected by the arm position and swing.

III. Step-care for spasticity

Step-care for spasticity starts from the most conservative care with the least side-effects. If this is unsuccessful, then it progresses to higher steps of care which, although more effective, are more aggressive (invasive), more irreversible, and have more side-effects. Before starting any treatment, the functional impairment of spasticity must be carefully assessed. Not all spasticity should be treated because it may help in the patient's function, for example, mild to moderate extensor spasticity of the legs may provide a bracing function and assist in standing and ambulation activities. However, if spasticity is severe (e.g., awakening patient at night) or interferes with function (e.g., hip adductor spasticity, which causes "scissoring" of gait, limits effective ambulation, makes catheterization difficult, or makes transfers and positioning difficult), then it must be treated. By limiting the effects of spasticity, deformity and contractures can be prevented, nursing care can be improved, bracing will be better tolerated, and function will be enhanced. The treatment of spasticity should not be based solely on the decisions of the professionals, but should take into consideration the goals of the patient and the patient's family or significant others.

A. **STEP 1 CARE**

1. **Prevention of noxious stimuli** that can exacerbate spasticity, such as urinary tract infection, bowel impaction, pressure ulcers, fractures, paronychia, and the acute abdomen. The tendency to develop pressure ulcers is increased in spasticity because involuntary spastic movements may rub the body against bedsheets, clothing, bedrails, or adaptive equipment.

2. **Patient education** is geared towards decreasing the adverse effects of spasticity and improving patient function despite spasticity. It includes the use of slow movements and techniques on how to trigger useful extensor or flexor spasms during transfers or bed mobility. Patients should be taught how to use foot protection devices and remove heel-loop bolts from wheelchair footrests to prevent skin breakdown. In severe spasticity, waist or chest straps or contact guarding from another person may be needed. After giving a treatment that reduces spasticity, the patient should be taught to avoid previous substitutions or patterns that reinforce spasticity (e.g., cradling the upper limb in a flexed position or extending the lower limbs) and to use proper body mechanics for lifting, pushing, and pulling to help prevent future injury.

B. **STEP 2 CARE** includes the following which should be taught to both the patient and the patient's caretaker.

1. **Proper positioning and handling** of the patient in the bed, chair, and wheelchair to prevent or minimize spasticity, contractures, or pressure ulcers;
2. **Daily ROM and stretching exercise program** including static muscle stretch (e.g., standing activities) to prevent contracture and capsule tightness, reduce stretch reflex hyperactivity, and improve motor control.

C. **STEP 3 CARE**

1. **Physical modalities**

a. ***Muscle cooling*** (15 minutes or more) using ice, ice pack, or topical anesthesia reduces phasic stretch reflex activity and clonus. It can also be used with static stretch to overcome hyperactive stretch reflexes.

b. ***Heat (e.g., hot packs or ultrasound)*** may be effective in relaxing the spastic muscles in some patients.

c. ***Therapeutic exercises*** include techniques to facilitate or strengthen agonist voluntary movement and to inhibit antagonist spasticity. Underutilized mechano- and proprioceptors may be stimulated with weight bearing, joint compression, tendon vibration, and other techniques (e.g., proprioceptive neuromuscular facilitation) for improving tone and movement control described in Chapter 4.2, section IV.B. Muscle re-education should be taught to facilitate balance and equilibrium.

d. ***Biofeedback*** using either EMG or joint position sensors, and providing auditory or visual feedback have been tried.

e. ***Peripheral electrical stimulation*** of muscle or nerve for 15 minutes reduces spasticity and clonus for hours, but functional gains have not been demonstrated. Transcutaneous electrical nerve stimulation (TENS) has also been used.

2. **Splints (static or dynamic), serial casts, or orthoses** are used to provide prolonged static stretching (to reduce spasticity while slowly increasing ROM or flexibility) and to limit further deformities. However, surface electromyography (EMG) has not been able to demonstrate decreased muscle activity when using upper-limb splints (e.g., resting splints) or serial casts. Although lower-limb resting splints may improve ankle ROM and facilitate motor neuron activity as a result of cutaneous stimulation, they do not alleviate spasticity. Ankle–foot orthoses (AFOs) are used to control spastic equinus deformities at the ankle (e.g., using posterior leaf spring). Medial and lateral T-straps or anterior flare can be used to control varus or valgus deformities.

D. **STEP 4 CARE**

1. **Antispasticity medications** reduce tone, but their dosages have to be titrated so they do not limit the patient's function. Because the drugs act at different sites, they may be combined in dosages low enough to avoid major side-effects. The effects of the drugs are nonselective and systemic. They have adverse effects especially in large dosages. Some clinicians believe that drug therapy should

only be tried if chemical nerve blockade (section III.D.2), specifically motor point and peripheral nerve blocks, have failed.

a. ***Baclofen (Lioresal),*** an analog of γ-aminobutyric acid (GABA), binds to GABA receptors in the spinal cord and is probably the drug of choice in spinal forms of spasticity (e.g., painful flexor spasms in SCI or MS patients). It is less sedating than diazepam and, although used in clinical practice off-label, probably plays a questionable role in spasticity of cerebral origin (e.g., stroke or CP). Common side-effects are weakness, sedation, dizziness, gastrointestinal symptoms, tremor, insomnia, headache, and hypotension. Hepatic dysfunction may occur. Serious side-effects include personality disturbance and hallucinations. Epilepsy is a relative contraindication to its use. Alcohol use should be limited. Baclofen should not be withdrawn suddenly as this may lead to seizures and hallucinations. The half-life of baclofen is 3.5 hours. It is available in 10- and 20-mg tablets. For adults, start with 5 mg, po, bid, then increase by 5 mg as tolerated every 3 days to 30–80 mg daily in divided doses (tid or qid). Although the Food and Drug Administration (FDA)-recommended maximum dose is 80 mg/day, higher and more therapeutic doses (up to 100–120 mg) have been well-tolerated. For children, start with 2.5–5.0 mg, po, qd; then slowly titrate up to 30 mg (for children less than 8 years old) or 60 mg (for those over 8 years old) per day in divided doses. However, in children under 12 years old, it is generally not recommended because its safety has not been established.

b. ***Dantrolene sodium (Dantrium)*** acts at the level of intra- and extrafusal muscle fibers resulting in decreased release of calcium from the sarcoplasmic reticulum, therefore reducing the force produced by excitation–contraction coupling. It is preferred for spasticity of cerebral origins (e.g., stroke or CP) and can be a useful adjunct to the treatment of spasticity of spinal origin (especially in wheelchair-bound paraplegics). It produces benefit in proportion to an increasing degree of weakness, but when properly titrated, it usually does not impair motor performance. Its sedative effects are only mild to moderate. Side-effects include generalized weakness, fatigue, diarrhea, lethargy, and hepatotoxicity. The hepatotoxic effects may have been overstated because it occurs only in about 1% of patients (usually in women over 30 years old at a dosage of over 300 mg/day for more than 2 months). Liver function tests [aspartate aminotransferase (AST or SGOT) and alanine aminotransferase (ALT or SGPT)] and blood counts must be monitored during treatment. In patients with pre-existing liver disease, it is contraindicated. Although dantrolene has little effect on smooth and cardiac muscles, the manufacturer recommends caution when used in patients with severe cardiac or pulmonary disease. The half-life of dantrolene is 8.7 hours. It is available in 25-, 50-, and 100-mg capsules. For adults, start with 0.5 mg/kg/day or 25 mg, po, qd/bid, and titrate up to a maximum of 400 mg daily over a 1-month period. For children, start with 0.5 mg/kg, po, bid, slowly increase by 0.5 mg/kg to tid/qid up to a maximum of 3 mg/kg qid or 100 mg qid. Its long-term safety has not been established in children under 5 years old.

c. ***Diazepam (Valium)*** acts at both the brainstem reticular activating system and spinal cord. It facilitates the postsynaptic effects of GABA, although it has no direct GABA-mimetic effect. It is useful for spasticity (e.g., painful flexor spasms) caused by SCI and is generally unsuitable in patients with brain injury. It can cause sedation, urinary retention, ataxia, and drug dependence. Long-term side-effects include paradoxical insomnia, anxiety, and hostility. Sudden withdrawal may cause seizures. It is contraindicated in patients with narrow-angle glaucoma. It must be used with caution by patients taking alcohol or anticoagulation drugs. The half-life of diazepam is 27–37 hours (longer for active metabolites). Diazepam is available in 2-, 5-, and 10-mg tablets. For adults, start with 2–4 mg, po, qd/bid, and titrate up to 60 mg daily in divided doses (there is no absolute maximum dosage). For children, give 0.12–0.8 mg/kg, po, daily in divided doses.

d. ***Clonidine (Catapres)***, which is an α_2-adrenergic agonist and α_1-adrenergic blocker, has been fairly successful in treating spasticity caused by SCI. Side-effects include hypotension, syncope, nausea, depression, sedation, and dry mouth. For more details about its adverse drug reactions, contraindications, and precautions, see Chapter 4.8, section V.F. The half-life of oral clonidine is 12–16 hours. It is available in 0.1-, 0.2-, and 0.3-mg strengths in either tablet or patch (transdermal therapeutic system or TTS) form. Start with 0.05 mg, po, bid, and increase up to 0.2–0.4 mg/day. The adhesive patch form (Catapres-TTS) begins with a 0.1-mg patch and titrates up to a 0.3-mg patch every week. The dose and rate of titration is based on the patient's tolerance of the side-effects (especially hypotension).

e. ***Tizanidine (Zanaflex)***, is a centrally acting α_2-adrenergic agonist, which is chemically related to clonidine. It has been approved by the FDA for use in the acute and intermittent management of spasticity (particularly in patients with MS, SCI, or stroke). Tizanidine presumably acts by increasing presynaptic inhibition of motor neurons. Its antispastic effectiveness in patients with MS or stroke is comparable with that of baclofen and diazepam. Moreover, it produces less muscle weakness than baclofen, less sedation than diazepam, and fewer cardiovascular effects (e.g., hypotension) than clonidine. Common adverse effects include dry mouth, sedation, asthenia (tiredness), dizziness, hypotension, bradycardia, and possibly increased muscle tone. Although uncommon, hallucination and psychotic-like symptoms as well as liver injury have been reported. Tizanidine has no specific contraindication except in patients with known hypersensitivity to tizanidine or its ingredients. It must be used with caution in patients receiving concurrent antihypertensives or other sedatives, and in those with impaired liver function. Monitoring of liver function tests is recommended during the first 6 months of treatment (e.g., baseline, 1, 3, and 6 months) and periodically thereafter. Tizanidine is available in 2-, 4- and 6-mg tablets and may be started at 4 mg then gradually titrated by 2- to 4-mg steps to optimum control of spasticity up to 8 mg, po, tid (not to exceed a maximum of 36 mg/day).

f. ***Other oral drugs*** used for spasticity when the patient does not respond to the aforementioned drugs include a combination of 300 mg/day of **phenytoin (Dilantin)** and 300 mg/day of **chlorpromazine (Thorazine); ketazomal** (a benzodiazepine which is used in Europe but is not FDA-approved for use in the United States); **cannabinoids; progabide; threonine; clonopin; clorazepate; tetrazepam (Myolastan)**; and **vigabatrin.**

2. **Chemical nerve blockades** reduce localized spasticity with neurochemical agents (e.g., local anesthetics such as lidocaine, or neurolytic agents such as phenol) or neurotoxins (e.g., botulin) on individual nerves. Their potential benefits include increased ROM, decreased clonus (clonus may interfere with ADL), increased speed and dexterity of movement (because of blockade of inappropriately firing antagonists), improved crawling, sitting, and standing in children, and even diminished spasticity in the contralateral limbs. They also help prevent joint contractures and deformities; improve function (positioning and/or gait), thus facilitating other therapies; promote better tolerance of orthoses (e.g., serial casting) or positioning devices; buy time to allow rehabilitation to continue while awaiting spontaneous improvement (e.g., in TBI or SCI); allow better timing of surgical procedures in children (e.g., after growth spurt); and evaluate surgical results (by mimicking tendon lengthening).

a. ***Chemical agents used for nerve blockade in spasticity***

I. **Local anesthetics** (e.g., lidocaine and marcaine) can block nerve conduction for hours by interfering with the increase in permeability of sodium ions that normally occurs when the membrane is depolarized. It can be used to determine if a decreased ROM is the result of contracture or tone and to assess the potential effects of a longer-acting nerve block or surgical procedure.

II. **Chemical neurolytic agents** such as aqueous phenol (2–6% in water, saline, or glycerol) or absolute ethyl alcohol (45–50%) can block spasticity for 6–12 months or longer. Usually after 4–6 months (less for motor point blocks), the effect is lost because of distal axonal regeneration from the site of injection. Phenol or alcohol may then be repeated once or twice, after which little significant change is seen. Phenol has a higher incidence of skin sloughs and, unlike alcohol, which has no systemic effect when injected intravascularly, phenol can cause severe systemic reactions when injected intravascularly.

III. **Neurotoxin** such as botulinal type-A toxin (available as Botox in the United States and Dysport in Europe) is claimed to be more effective than phenol or alcohol for neurolysis of motor points (i.e., the terminal branches of motor nerves) because Botox diffuses through muscle membranes, causing a "leaking" of the neuromuscular effect, thus blocking motor points at multiple sites. Botox inhibits the release of acetylcholine at the neuromuscular junction and interferes with the uptake of cytoplasmic acetylcholine. Botox injections can be carried out with a typical electromyography machine and do not require exact needle placement in the neuromuscular junction as in phenol injections. Unlike phenol motor point blocks, Botox injection is directed toward the muscle belly rather than the nerve in the neuromuscular junction.

The FDA has currently approved Botox for use in blepharospasm and strabismus (associated with dystonia), cervical dystonia (spasmodic torticollis), and temporary improvement of glabellar lines (using Botox Cosmetic). However, Botox has been used in PM&R for treating spasticity limited to a "functional unit" (e.g., thigh adductors, plantar flexors, or neck extensors), movement disorders (e.g., focal dystonias, tremors), facial disorders (oromandibular dystonia, hemifacial spasm), painful conditions caused by prolonged muscle spasm and contractures, chronic pain (e.g., postoperative back pain), myofascial pain, thoracic outlet syndrome associated with spasm of the scalene musculature (to improve peripheral blood flow), and detrusor sphincter dyssynergia. The FDA statement of efficacy does not include young children (less than 12 years old); however, clinicians have used Botox in children (most common indication being abnormal tone as a result of CP). Botox is contraindicated in patients receiving aminoglycoside or spectinomycin antibiotics, known sensitivity to botulin, myasthenia gravis, Lambert–Eaton myasthenic syndrome, motor neuron disease, upper eyelid apraxia, and ptosis. Its safety during pregnancy and lactation has not been established yet.

b. ***Chemical nerve blockade procedures***

I. **Motor point blocks (MPBs)** are applied to distal motor nerve branches to reduce clonus and velocity-dependent increase in the stretch reflex response in a spastic muscle. However, they are less effective for the more incapacitating manifestations of spasticity, that is, nonvelocity-dependent tone, flexor spasms, rigidity, and dystonia. If spasticity is generalized, MPB is generally ineffective; but, if focal muscle groups can be identified as the primary generator of a diffuse spastic reaction or for cases in which individual muscle groups are explicitly involved in function and hygiene, MPB may be helpful. Advantages of MPB include no need for general anesthesia (except when the patient is very young or uncooperative, or when severe spasticity complicates positioning); high acceptance compared to systemic medications; no sensory side-effects compared to nerve block; and no apparent tolerance to repeated injections (however, localization in repeat MPB may be more difficult). The use of alcohol and phenol needs precise localization of motor points and is not as effective clinically because it is time consuming to locate the multiple number of motor points within a muscle. On the other hand, botulin (as described above) can diffuse into the muscle and is, therefore, less time consuming and does not need as precise localization as alcohol or phenol for MPB.

- **Botulin preparation**. Botulin for clinical use is marketed by Allergan Pharmaceuticals as Botox. It is supplied in a highly purified, freeze-dried state in vials of 100 units, stored in a styrofoam container at −5°C. It is reconstituted by adding 2 mL of preservative-free normal (0.9%) saline to get a final dilution of 5 units per 0.1 mL (if 1 mL of saline is added, the final dilution is 10 units/0.1 mL; if 4 mL of saline is added, the final dilution is 2.5 units/0.1 mL). The saline from the prefilled syringe should be sucked into the vacuum-sealed vial without having to push the plunger. If this does not occur, the unused vial should be returned to the manufacturer. Once reconstituted, the vial should not be agitated and should be stored at 2–4°C until use. It remains effective for about 4 hours at room temperature. As a result of its high cost, it is advisable to schedule more than one patient at a time so that any medication left over from one patient can be given to the next.
- **Selection of patient and muscle for Botox MPB** is crucial for its success. Patients should be informed of possible complications (especially weakness), the variability of outcome, and the possibility of recurrence. If they are on nonsteroidal drugs or are taking anticoagulants, they should be warned of the possibility of increased bruising at the injection site. The joint where the spastic muscle crosses should have no fixed deformity. Botox MPB, which causes weakening of the spastic limb, should not further compromise residual function (including gait). The muscles (e.g., antagonist) to be blocked should be spastic enough that they interfere with normal movement of the opposite (e.g., agonist) muscles. Prior to blocking the spastic muscle (e.g., antagonist), determine if the opposite muscle (e.g., agonist) is capable of hypertrophy and strengthening if allowed to perform through the appropriate ROM. Determine also if induction of partial or complete paralysis (i.e., flaccidity) of one or more muscles improves the overall function of the patient.
- **Botox MPB injection** can be given with or without EMG guidance. For superficial muscles, a 1.0-mL tuberculin-type syringe with a 25-gauge, 5/8-inch (1.6-cm) needle may be used. For deeper muscles and for treatment of conditions in which the identification of the hyperactive muscles is difficult, EMG guidance may be necessary. A hypodermic (cannulated) monopolar needle cathode, through which the Botox can be injected, is used. For small muscles (e.g., facial), a 30-gauge, 1-inch (2.5 cm) needle is used, but for large muscles (e.g., hamstrings), a 26-gauge, 1- or 1.5-inch needle is used. The cannulated needle cathode, insulated with Teflon except at the tip, is inserted into the selected muscle. A surface anode (reference) and ground electrode are then placed near the cathodal needle. The patient should be as relaxed as possible and the joint should be positioned so that the muscles that are contracting are not doing so in a normal postural response to their current positioning. Once the motor point is located, Botox is injected intramuscularly after aspirating to prevent intravascular administration of the drug. If alcohol is used to cleanse the skin, it should be allowed to dry to prevent toxin deactivation.
  - **For dystonic spastic muscles** associated with hemiplegia or other central nervous system pathology, the motor point is located by inserting the

needle into the muscle and looking for the classic burst of rhythmic dystonic firing pattern of the muscle group involved on EMG. If dystonic firing is not evident after needle placement, the patient should assume body posture or movements that normally trigger the dystonia. It is frequently helpful to needle muscles that are not obviously involved from the clinical examination alone. If dystonia is demonstrated on EMG, these muscles may also be injected.

- **For nondystonic spastic muscles**, the motor point is located by connecting the hub of the cathodal needle to a stimulator that is found in most standard EMG machines. The clinician stimulates the muscle by delivering a square pulse of approximately 0.1 ms once or twice per second at 5 mA intensity through the needle and watches for a brisk visible twitch in the desired muscle. The needle is then gradually moved until only the minimal current (approximately 1 mA) is necessary to obtain a maximal twitch in the desired muscle(s). This site is the motor point.

- **Dosage of Botox**. Exact dosages of Botox for specific diagnoses have not been clearly established. Based on the recommendation of the WE MOVE Spasticity Study Group (2002), the adult dosing guidelines for the management of spasticity using Botox-A are shown in Table 5.4-2. In general, the Botox dose may be decreased in patients with low body weight, chronic therapy, very small muscle bulk, many muscles being injected simultaneously, low Ashworth score, high concern that treatment may result in excess weakness (including swallowing problems), and too much weakness from previous therapy. However, in patients with high body weight, acute therapy, very large muscle bulk, few numbers of muscles being injected simultaneously, very high Ashworth scale, low concern that treatment may result in excess weakness (including swallowing problems), and inadequate response to previous therapy, the Botox dose may be increased.

  It is preferable to underdose an individual with Botox during the first treatment (e.g., 200 units at the first session). If the desired effect is not achieved, a booster dose (e.g., 100 units) may be given (usually in 1–3 weeks) until the desired clinical effect is obtained. The dose of Botox injected is typically divided between two to four sites per muscle, with higher doses reserved for larger muscles. When injecting regional muscles in combination (e.g., wrist flexors, finger flexors, and biceps), the dose per muscle should be reduced so that the maximum volume per site is 0.5–1.0 mL and the combined maximum dose is ≤400 units per person per treatment session every 3 months (although a total dose of up to 600 units has also been used in the clinical setting without adverse effect). The onset of the Botox effect occurs within 24–72 hours, peaks at 4–6 weeks, and lasts for 3–6 months. Although the effect of Botox on individual nerve terminals is effectively irreversible, recovery of neuromuscular control occurs because of new terminal formation and nerve sprouting.

- **Nonresponse to Botox MPB** can either be primary (i.e., no response to initial injection of Botox) or secondary (i.e., a relative or complete loss of efficacy at subsequent visit). Factors that might contribute to nonresponse include underdosage, poor injection techniques (may require EMG guidance), inappropriate reconstitution or storage of toxin, weakness or atrophy present on examination with no functional benefit, change in pattern of muscle involvement during treatment, and presence of neutralizing antibodies (confirmed by assay). To avoid resistance because of antibody formation, wait as long as possible between injections (at least 3 months), avoid booster injections (given 1–3 weeks after the initial treatment session), and use the smallest clinically effective dose. A patient should only be classified

Table 5.4-2 Botox-A (Botox®) adult dosing guidelines for the management of spasticity as recommended by WE MOVE Spasticity Study Group (2002)

Clinical pattern	Potential muscles involved	Average starting dose/units	Botox® dose units/visit	Number of injection sites
Upper limbs				
Adducted/ internally rotated shoulder	Pectoralis complex	100	75–150	2–4
	Latissimus dorsi	100	50–150	3–4
	Teres major	50	25–100	1–2
	Subscapularis	75	50–100	1–2
Flexed elbow	Brachioradialis	60	25–100	1–3
	Biceps	100	75–200	2–4
	Brachialis	60	40–100	2
Pronated forearm	Pronator quadratus	25	10–50	1
	Pronator teres	40	25–75	1–2
Flexed wrist	Flexor carpi radialis	50	25–100	2
	Flexor carpi ulnaris	40	20–70	2
Thumb-in-palm	Flexor pollicis longus	20	10–30	1
	Adductor pollicis	10	5–25	1
	Flexor pollicis brevis/opponens	10	5–25	1
Clenched fist	Flexor digitorum superficialis (per fascicle)	20	20–40	1
	Flexor digitorum profundus (per fascicle)	20	20–40	1
Intrinsic plus hand	Lumbricales/ interossei (per lumbrical)	10	5–10	1
Lower limbs				
Flexed hip	Iliopsoas*	150	50–200	2
	Psoas	100	50–200	2
	Rectus femoris	100	75–200	3
Flexed knee	Medial hamstrings	100	50–200	3
	Gastrocnemius (as knee flexor)	150	50–150	4
	Lateral hamstrings	100	100–200	3
Adducted thighs	Adductor longus/brevis/ magnus	200/leg	75–300	6/leg
Stiff (extended) knee	Quadriceps mechanism	100	50–200	6
Equinovarus foot	Gastrocnemius medial/lateral	100	50–250	4
	Soleus	100	50–200	2
	Tibialis posterior	75	50–150	2
	Tibialis anterior	75	50–150	2–3
	Flexor digitorum longus	75	50–100	3

(*Continued*)

Table 5.4-2 (*Continued*)

Clinical pattern	Potential muscles involved	Average starting dose/units	Botox® dose units/visit	Number of injection sites
	Flexor digitorum brevis	25	20–40	1
	Flexor hallucis longus	50	25–75	2
Striatal toe	Extensor hallucis longus	50	20–100	2
Head and neck				
	Sternocleidomastoid (SCM)†	40	25–100	3
	Scalenus complex	30	15–50	3
	Splenius capitis	60	50–150	3
	Semispinalis capitis	60	50–150	3
	Longissimus capitis	60	50–150	3
	Trapezius	60	50–150	3
	Levator scapulae	80	25–100	3
	Masseter	40/side	20–60/side	2/side
	Temporalis	20/side	20–40/side	1–2/side

*Note: * Use fluoroscopy or ultrasound to localize psoas.*
† Reduce dose by 50% if both SCM muscles are injected.
From: Movement Disorder Virtual University (MDVU). *Botox-A Adult Dosing Guidelines.* Edition 2.0, Revised April 2001. Available at: http://www.mdvu.org/library/dosingtables/btxa_adg.html. Accessed November 9, 2004.

as unresponsive to Botox therapy if they do not exhibit any reduction in muscle tone 4–6 weeks after one or more injections.

- **Side-effects of Botox** are usually temporary and well-tolerated by the patient. Most of them result from diffusion of the toxin into adjacent structures and are site-specific. They include unwanted weakness in injected and neighboring muscles, temporary change in posturing or pain because of realignment of nerve–muscle–bone relationships, and subjective symptoms of weakness and fatigue ("flu-like" syndrome with headache and nausea), which usually last less than 4 days. No anaphylactic reactions have been reported.
- **Postinjection care and follow-up**. Pain after Botox MPB is similar to that of a standard EMG examination. Muscle relaxants or acetaminophen may be given to patients after Botox MPB if any discomfort occurs over the next 24–48 hours. Stronger analgesics are rarely required. A follow-up appointment in 2–3 weeks after the initial treatment is helpful in determining if an adequate dosage was given. Treatments are repeated as necessary based on individual patient needs. Botox treatment should be combined with modifications in the physical and occupational therapy programs to increase range of motion, strength, and functional use of treated muscles.

II. **Peripheral nerve blocks** refer to the application of local anesthetics (e.g., lidocaine or marcaine) or neurolytic agents (e.g., phenol or alcohol) to disrupt peripheral nerve functions. Peripheral nerve blocks may be quite effective and may last 3–6 months or more. Compared to oral medications, they are relatively selective and have rare systemic side-effects. They are easier and safer to perform compared to surgery.

- **Peripheral nerve block procedure** is performed using EMG guidance and a Teflon-coated needle similar to that used for nondystonic spastic muscle

MPBs (section III.D.2.b.1.c). If needed, light general inhalation anesthesia may be given.

- **Indications for specific peripheral nerve blocks**. In the upper limbs, median and ulnar blocks are generally avoided because of the high risk of sensory complications.
  - **Lumbar spinal nerves** may be blocked paravertebrally to reduce hip flexor spasticity. Special caution should be observed because of the proximity of important visceral and vascular structures.
  - **Obturator nerves (anterior and posterior branches)** may be blocked to reduce adductor tone, diminish lower limb scissoring during gait, facilitate hip abduction to ease personal hygiene, and promote passive abduction as a means of protecting hip joint integrity.
  - **Femoral nerves** may be blocked inferior to the inguinal ligament and lateral to the femoral pulse to diminish severe spastic genu recurvatum in CP patients, and midstance recurvatum in gait unresponsive to AFO dorsiflexion. Branches to individual components of the quadriceps may be locally blocked.
  - **Perineal nerves** may be blocked to significantly reduce postvoid residual volumes when the external urethral sphincter is very spastic.
  - **Sciatic nerves (e.g., branch to the medial hamstrings)** may be blocked to diminish crouch gait and internal rotation deformities.
  - **Tibial nerves (e.g., tibial branch to the heads of the gastrocnemius)** may be blocked to diminish severe equinovarus ankle posturing (because of increased plantar flexion tone) or painful clawing of the toes, thus allowing better tolerance of AFOs.
  - **Musculocutaneous nerves** may be blocked at the medial upper arm near insertion of the pectoralis tendon to promote elbow extension and facilitate reach. It is helpful in the hemiplegic patient with severe elbow flexion contracture or in the C5 tetraplegic patient with flexor contractures as a result of loss of triceps function. Elbow flexion is preserved through the action of the brachioradialis muscle which is innervated by the radial nerve.
  - **Median nerves** are usually avoided but may be blocked to help relax the tightly flexed wrist and fingers of hemiplegic patients.
- **Side-effects**. Nerve blockade to a major nerve trunk containing a significant number of cutaneous nerve fibers (e.g., tibial, median, and ulnar nerves) can produce 10–30% risk of dysesthesia and causalgia (with symptoms of burning sensation and discomfort). Severe persistent dysesthesias may be treated with oral steroids, transcutaneous nerve stimulation, or repetition of the nerve block. To presumably reduce the incidence of dysesthesia, an open procedure may be performed by a surgeon. The selected motor trunk is exposed surgically and phenol or alcohol is injected at the site where the motor nerve enters the muscle bulk, thus leaving the cutaneous sensory fibers unharmed.

  Muscle weakness after nerve blockade is usually temporary, that is, lasting for hours or days. Occasionally permanent weakness may occur, which leads to deformity (e.g., tibial block can cause weakness or paralysis of all posterior compartment muscles resulting in unopposed dorsiflexion and eversion, i.e., calcaneovalgus foot). Overdosage with phenol can cause convulsions, central nervous system depression, and cardiovascular collapse. However, the usual dosages of phenol (e.g., 20 mL of 5 or 6% phenol) are well below its lethal range (at least 8.5 g). Another complication of phenol nerve block is venous thromboses.

III. **Spinal block** is the intrathecal or epidural administration of local anesthetic (e.g., lidocaine or marcaine) or neurolytic agents (e.g., absolute alcohol, which has more permanent effects than phenol) to reduce severe spasticity of the lower limbs. Patients are immobilized to allow layering of the neurolytic material so that damage is limited to the desired spinal roots. However, control over affected fibers is imprecise and complications arise in 1–10%, which includes urinary and bowel incontinence, loss of sexual function, paresis, paresthesias, and even death.

E. STEP 5 CARE

1. Intrathecal medications

a. ***Intrathecal baclofen (IT-B)*** allows delivery of baclofen directly to the cerebrospinal fluid (CSF) so that higher effective dosages can be attained at the receptor sites in the spinal cord than with oral administration. This is because baclofen has low lipid solubility and does not effectively cross the blood–brain barrier; hence, in some patients, the effective dose cannot be reached with oral baclofen, or side-effects become intolerable at the effective oral dose. A typical intrathecal dose of baclofen is 0.3–0.5% of the oral dose, because an oral dose of 60 mg baclofen per day gives 24 μg/L of lumbar concentration of baclofen, while intrathecal infusion of 600 μg/day gives a lumbar concentration of 1240 μg/L.

Intrathecal baclofen can be administered via a pump implanted subcutaneously in the abdominal wall, with a catheter surgically placed into the subarachnoid space. The two types of pumps available are the Infusaid pump (a gas-powered bellows device, which is purely mechanical and has no battery, can only infuse drug at a constant rate, and the dosage can only be adjusted at the time of refill) and Medtronic SynchroMed pump (an electronic battery-operated pump, which can be programmed to deliver precise drug dosage several times daily through an onboard computer so spasticity may be reduced or increased at certain times of the day; its battery lasts about 4–5 years). The cost of the pump alone is about $7000 plus another $3000/year for the drug itself plus surgical costs. The IT-B is used if spasticity is multisegmental and diffuse. It may be used in conjunction with Botox MPB. It is effective for spasticity related to spinal cord dysfunction (e.g., SCI or MS) and to CP with some preserved function below the level of the lesion allowing the patient to be ambulatory.

I. **Patient selection for IT-B**. Possible candidates for IT-B should be free of active infection and pressure ulcers, have an anterior abdominal wall site suitable for pump placement (any abdominal procedures, e.g., colostomies, ileal conduits, and feeding tubes must be separated from the pump site), and have no block in CSF flow (myelography may be needed to ensure communication between the proposed site of infusion and the source of spasticity). Candidates must also live in a place that has access to magnetic resonance imaging (MRI) centers (in case of complications) as well as to clinicians experienced with IT-B maintenance. Prior to implanting the IT-B pump, the patient is admitted to the hospital and injected intrathecally with a trial dose of baclofen (starting at 50 μg, then increasing to 75–100 μg) via lumbar puncture or spinal catheter. Effects of baclofen are observed 2–8 hours after each dose. If there is a significant decrease in muscle tone, frequency, or severity of spasms, the patient is scheduled for IT-B.

II. **Surgical phase of IT-B**. The patient is placed under intravenous deep sedation or general anesthesia. The pump is implanted in a subcutaneous abdominal pocket, the site of which is selected with consideration of the patient's belt lines, wheelchair arms, and physical activities. The pump's catheter is tunneled, using a 15- or 16-gauge Tuohy needle, to the midline lumbar area, where it is inserted into the intrathecal space at L3–L4, then advanced up a minimum of 10 cm (with the catheter tip at T10 to T12 level). Intraoperative fluoroscopy is performed to confirm catheter placement into the intrathecal sac with no twisting or coiling. This surgical procedure is usually not difficult and takes 1–2 hours.

III. **Drug adjustment of IT-B.** On the first day postimplantation, the pump is programmed to begin continuous infusion of 500 μg/mL of baclofen at a rate of about twice the bolus responsive trial dose (given presurgically) or less if the patient had a prolonged effect (more than 12 hours) from the trial dose. The patient is observed for any untoward effects during the first 24 hours. Then, the dose is increased 10–15% every 24 hours. Once a clinical response becomes evident, the patient is discharged from the hospital and followed for gradual dose adjustments every 1–4 weeks until an optimal effect is achieved (i.e., muscle tone as close to normal as possible without weakness; and minimal frequency and severity of spasms without intolerable side-effects). If a sudden change in spasticity occurs, causes (e.g., urinary tract infection, or inadequate bowel or bladder regime) should be corrected before changing dosage. Dose is adjusted in the office using a portable computer-based programming device through a telemetry head. Usual infusion rate is 0.004 mL/h to 0.90 mL/h or 300–800 μg/day (i.e., average of 600 μg/day or lumbar concentration of 1240 μg/L).

Intrathecal baclofen has a half-life of 1.5 hours in the CSF. The ratio of lumbar to cervical concentration of intrathecal baclofen is about 4 to 1, which is important for patients with spasticity in their lower limbs as it allows relief of spasticity without causing intolerable supraspinal side-effects. If the Medtronic SynchroMed pump is used, the drug delivery mode may be changed, during follow-up visits, from continuous to either continuous-complex (drug delivered continuously in a series of 2–10 steps for specified times, e.g., at night-time for patients who have increased spasms at night) or bolus-delay (drug delivered intermittently at a prescribed dose and at specified intervals, e.g., the flow rate can be programmed to change 2 hours before the time of desired clinical effect).

IV. **Maintenance phase of IT-B.** Depending upon the dose, the pump is refilled percutaneously every 4–12 weeks (baclofen is stable in the pump for up to 90 days). The pump alarm should be set to alert the patient of a low reservoir. It is important that patients keep their appointment for refill to avoid an empty pump which may lead to withdrawal symptoms (i.e., return of spasticity, agitation, fever, and tachycardia). After the refill procedure, the patient should be monitored for any unusual reactions (e.g., swelling around the pump site, which may indicate a pocket infusion due to missed reservoir port).

V. **Side-effects and complications of IT-B.** The most common side-effects (i.e., drowsiness, dizziness, nausea, hypotension, headache, and weakness) are dose-related and usually subside by reducing the dosage by 10–20%. The IT-B can decrease the detrusor reflex, but can also depress the pelvic floor reflex, hence resulting in a bladder with low pressure, which empties less effectively (an undesirable effect in tetraplegic patients). Complications from IT-B include tube dysfunction (dislodgment, disconnection, kinkage, and blockage), pump failure, infection, and baclofen overdosage (because of programming error or too rapid increase in dosage). The signs and symptoms of overdose include drowsiness, lightheadedness, nausea, bradycardia, weakness, fatigue, somnolence, seizures, respiratory depression, rostral progression of hypotonia, and loss of consciousness progressing to reversible coma. The anticholinesterase, physostigmine (Antilirium), 2 mg, IV, may be given to reverse the respiratory depression caused by baclofen overdose.

b. ***Intrathecal morphine*** (1–2 mg) may be used instead of IT-B to reduce spasticity in patients with SCI. Although it can be effective (long-term follow-up shows that patients do not seem to develop drug tolerance), it is currently rarely used.

2. **Rhizotomy**, the sectioning of the spinal roots or rootlets, may be categorized as open (requiring laminectomy) or closed (percutaneous), complete or selective, or anterior or posterior. Anterior rhizotomy is associated with severe denervation-type atrophy of all innervated muscles and is seldom done.

a. ***Selective dorsal (or posterior) rhizotomy (SDR)*** refers to the neurosurgical sectioning of a particular proportion of selected dorsal segmental roots or rootlets to modulate afferent sensory input and reset muscle spindles so that there is less spasticity. Posterior rhizotomy is easier to perform than anterior rhizotomy and does not result in denervation muscle atrophy. Although SDR disrupts spinal reflex arcs, it does not abolish spasticity mediated by suprasegmental pathways. There are reports of improvement in tone, range, posture, and functional status in about 85% of candidates. Early gait analysis studies show improvement in stride length and hip and knee ROM in children with CP. Objective randomized studies on gains in the range of functional motor performance deficits, however, remain to be seen.

I. **Patient selection for SDR**. Selective dorsal rhizotomy is indicated in young children (3–8 years old) with spastic CP (usually spastic diplegic) and for treatment of spasticity and pain in the hemiplegic upper limb. For CP patients, the favorable selection criteria for SDR include pure spasticity (absent or very mild dystonia, athetosis, ataxia, rigidity); function limited primarily by spasticity and not significantly affected by primitive reflexes or movement patterns; no severe underlying weakness; selective motor control (e.g., some degree of spontaneous forward locomotion and adequate truncal balance and righting responses); minimal joint contractures or spine deformity; adequate cognitive ability to participate in intensive physical therapy after surgery; no significant motivational or behavioral problems; and a supportive and interactive family. It is contraindicated in neurodegenerative disorders, beneficial pattern of spasticity, and multiple fixed or orthopedic deformities.

II. **Surgical procedure of SDR**. The dorsal aspect of the thecal sac is exposed by multilevel laminectomy (e.g., L1 or L2 to S1) with the facet joints left intact. The dorsal roots are identified and stimulated with an insulated bipolar stimulator at frequencies of 1–50 Hz. The responses are recorded on a multichannel EMG (surface or intramuscular) from the ipsilateral and contralateral muscles of various myotomes. The dorsal afferent rootlets that cause reflex "spastic" responses in muscles are chosen for SDR (specific criteria for determining this choice remain controversial). The selected dorsal rootlets are only partially sectioned (25–80%) as complete sectioning may cause complete loss of sensation. Selective dorsal rhizotomy is most frequently performed at L5 and S1 roots. The S2–S4 dorsal roots are avoided to prevent bowel and bladder dysfunction.

III. **Post-SDR care**. Postlaminectomy precautions are observed for 6 weeks (i.e., no passive trunk rotation, no straight leg raising, no hip flexion above 90°, and no hamstring stretching). Intensive physical therapy for up to a year is required to maximize long-term functional changes. These include gentle stretching, neurodevelopmental techniques, proprioceptive neuromuscular facilitation techniques, muscle re-education prior to controlled ambulation training, use of adaptive equipment (e.g., tricycle), and use of less restrictive hinged AFOs with or without single lateral uprights with pelvic band and free hips and knees to control any residual internal rotation.

IV. **Complications of SDR** are most commonly hypotonia (usually temporary) and weakness. Other complications include sensory changes (25% with transient dysesthesias), bladder dysfunction, bronchospasm and pneumonia, hip subluxation and dislocation, ataxia, and recurrence of spasticity. There is also a questionable potential of spinal stenosis in later life because of multilevel laminectomy.

b. ***Percutaneous (closed) radiofrequency rhizotomies*** are performed under fluoroscopic guidance using a radiofrequency needle to destroy nerve tissue. They are effective in reducing spasticity in the lower limbs with minimal morbidity; however, the effects are not permanent.

F. STEP 6 CARE

1. **Orthopedic surgeries (e.g., tenotomy, tendon lengthening, tendon transfers, myotomy, arthrodesis, and neurectomy)** are performed to increase function (e.g., ambulation, grasp, and dressing), to increase ROM (e.g., to facilitate self-care or nursing care), to correct deformity, reduce pain, or for cosmesis. They have been used successfully in spastic patients whose voluntary movements are preserved (e.g., patients with CP, stroke, TBI, spina bifida, and SCI). Surgery should only be done when the recovery has more or less plateaued (i.e., at least 6 months after a stroke and up to 12–24 months after TBI). Patients must be informed that the original deformity may recur after tenotomies or tendon-lengthening procedures because the number of sarcomeres in the muscle decreases, or an alternate deformity may develop from overcorrection.

A careful physical examination must be carried out to make sure that the weakness is the result of upper-motor neuron insult and not undiscovered lower-motor neuron injury (e.g., brachial plexopathy or peripheral nerve injury). Static deformities (i.e., fixed contractures that are present both at rest and with movement) must be differentiated from dynamic deformities (i.e., dysfunction that appears with movement) by physical examination or by a diagnostic block with short-acting anesthetic (e.g., lidocaine). For example, if after median nerve block at the elbow, deformity of the finger and wrist flexion persists, it is most likely the result of a fixed contracture. Preoperative radiograph and bone scans may be done to rule out fractures, dislocations, arthritis, and heterotopic ossification. For the upper limb, sensory input is vital and can be assessed with a variety of tools (e.g., two-point discrimination). To assess the residual motor function in the upper limb, the degree of remaining trunk and shoulder stability must be determined also. For the lower limb, gait analysis with multichannel electromyography is frequently used as an adjunct in planning procedures in the lower limb. The following classification and description of orthopedic surgery for spastic limbs are primarily from Keenan, Kozin, and Berlet's Manual of Orthopedic Surgery for Spasticity (see Further reading section).

a. ***Orthopedic surgery for the spastic lower limb***

I. **Static contractures** are corrected to reduce pain; improve perineal hygiene; prevent skin maceration and breakdown; facilitate lower-limb dressing, positioning, and transfers; and improve cosmesis. Correcting static contractures also helps increase gait efficiency.

- **Hip adduction contracture** is corrected by releasing the adductor longus, adductor brevis, and gracilis muscles. Adductor magnus is not released because it is also a hip extensor. This is followed by 4 weeks of forced abduction with casts (using an abduction bar) or an abduction pillow splint.
- **Hip flexion contracture** is corrected by releasing the sartorius, rectus femoris, iliopsoas, and pectineus muscles. If involved, tensor fascia lata and the anterior part of the gluteus medius may also be released. The hip-joint capsule is left undisturbed. Postoperative care includes the prone position

three times per day for increasing periods, followed by gentle stretching exercises. Patients may sit in a wheelchair for short periods.

- **Hip extension contracture** is corrected by releasing the origins of medial and lateral hamstring muscles. Postoperative care includes gentle hip ROM and sitting activities (e.g., in a wheelchair).
- **Knee flexion contracture** is corrected by releasing the distal hamstring (biceps femoris, semitendinosus, and semimembranosus), gracilis, and sartorius muscles. The posterior knee capsule is left undisturbed to prevent posterior tibial subluxation. Transfer of the distal hamstring insertion has also been used. Only 50% of the contracture is corrected during surgery to prevent excessive tension on the contracted neurovascular bundle. Postoperative care includes long leg casting with the knees extended maximally (forced extension is avoided as it may cause limb ischemia and necrosis). The cast is changed weekly until full extension is achieved. This is followed by 4 weeks of nightly splinting to maintain extension. Transfers and gait training (weight bearing as tolerated) are started once the cast is applied.
- **Knee extension contracture** is corrected by quadriceps V-Y lengthening, i.e., an inverted-V portion of the distal rectus femoris tendon is harvested, then the knee is flexed to 90° and the rectus tendon is sutured to complete the V-Y lengthening on the flexed knee (V-Y refers to the shapes of the proximal and distal ends of the tendon after a V-shaped incision). Postoperative care includes knee casting in 90° of flexion for 3 weeks. Continuous passive motion and gait training (weight bearing as tolerated) are started once the cast is removed.
- **Fixed equinovarus contracture** is treated similarly as in dynamic equinovarus deformity (section III.F.1.a.2.e). In addition, a release of the plantar fascia or triple arthrodesis of the ankle, or both may be done.
- **Fixed equinus contracture** is treated similarly as in dynamic equinus deformity (section III.F.1.a.2.f).
- **Fixed toe curling contracture** is treated similarly as in dynamic toe-curling deformity (section III.F.1.a.2.g).

II. Dynamic deformities of the lower limb are corrected to primarily make gait and transfers more efficient and less energy consuming.

- **Lower-limb scissoring** with narrow-based gait results from spastic hip adductors. A preoperative obturator nerve block is performed to rule out static hip adduction contracture, which if present is treated as described in section III.D.2.b.2.b.2. If there is no hip adduction contracture, obturator neurectomy of the anterior branch is performed. Complete obturator neurectomy is not carried out as it may lead to adductor paralysis and an inability to walk (because both the anterior and posterior branches of the obturator nerve supply the adductor magnus). Postoperative care includes early gait training with weight bearing as tolerated. No immobilization or abduction splinting is needed.
- **Crouched gait** results from spastic hip flexors and is associated with compensatory knee flexion and lumbar hyperlordosis. The spastic iliopsoas tendon is released from the lesser trochanter while maintaining its capsular attachments, hence weakening iliopsoas pull and allowing it to recess proximally (i.e., become attached more proximally). Postoperative care includes early hip ROM (active and passive) and gait training (weight bearing as tolerated). There is no need for postoperative immobilization. Knee flexion contracture may also be corrected (section III.F.1.a.1.d.) to improve the crouched gait.
- **Stiff-knee (stiff-legged) gait** with inadequate knee flexion during swing phase results from inappropriate firing of the quadriceps muscle (75%

involve all four heads whereas 25% involve either rectus femoris or vastus intermedius or both). Lower limb clearance is achieved by hip-hiking gait or by circumduction gait. The spastic heads of the quadriceps are selectively released after they are identified preoperatively by EMG during dynamic gait analysis. Postoperative care includes a posterior knee splint applied for 5 days to control pain. Gait training (weight bearing as tolerated) is allowed on the first postoperative day. ROM and quadriceps strengthening exercises are performed on the 5th postoperative day.

- **Dynamic knee flexion deformity** results from hamstring spasticity which prevents adequate knee extension during the stance phase. Fractional lengthening of the biceps femoris, semimembranosus, and sartorius is done at the myotendinous junction. The semitendinosus and gracilis are transected. The posterior knee capsule is left undisturbed to prevent posterior tibial subluxation. Postoperative care is the same as that for static knee flexion contracture (section III.F.1.a.1.d).
- **Dynamic equinovarus deformity** is the most common deformity in the lower limb. The ankle is plantar flexed (because of spastic gastrocnemius and soleus) and the foot is turned-in and supinated (because of spastic tibialis anterior). Often, the toes are curled (because of spastic extrinsic and intrinsic toe flexors). The spastic muscles are identified preoperatively by EMG during dynamic gait analysis. The split anterior tibialis tendon transfer (SPLATT) procedure is carried out by splitting the tibialis anterior tendon along its length, then tunneling the distal end of the lateral half of the tibialis anterior into the cuboid and sometimes the third cuneiform bones. This creates an eversion force that counteracts the varus pull of the remaining medial portion of the tibialis anterior, so rebalancing the forefoot deformity. The SPLATT is usually carried out in combination with tendo-Achilles lengthening and release of the toe flexors. If the posterior tibialis is spastic, it may be transferred through the interosseous membrane to the foot dorsum, or it may be sectioned. Postoperative care includes a short-leg walking cast with the foot in neutral for 6 weeks followed by a rigid molded AFO for an additional 4.5 months. Transfers and gait training (weight bearing as tolerated) are started once the cast is applied on the first postoperative day.
- **Dynamic equinus deformity** as a result of spastic gastrocnemius and soleus hinders both swing and stance phases of ambulation by making limb clearance difficult and preventing initial heel contact. Tendo-Achilles lengthening using a step-cut (Z-plasty) lengthening procedure is done. Postoperative care is similar to that for equinovarus deformity (section III.F.1.a.2.e).
- **Dynamic toe-curling deformity** because of spasticity of the extrinsic and intrinsic toe flexor muscles causes pain, callosities on the dorsum of the toes, and difficulty with shoe wear. All intrinsic and extrinsic toe flexors at the base of each toe (metatarsophalangeal level) are released. Postoperative care includes a soft dressing to maintain the toes in the corrected position. If SPLATT, tendo-Achilles lengthening, or both are performed, the short-leg walking cast with toe-plate is used (section III.F.1.a.2.e).
- **Dynamic foot valgus or pronation deformity** results from the spastic peroneus longus muscle during stance phase and is usually associated with an equinovarus deformity (i.e., "combination foot deformity") seen during the swing phase. It is corrected by the release and transfer of the peroneus longus across the dorsum of the foot into the navicular bone. The equinovarus deformity correction and postoperative care are similar to that for equinovarus deformity (section III.F.1.a.2.e).

b. Orthopedic surgery for spastic upper limb

I. **Static contractures of the upper limbs** are corrected mainly for cosmetic reasons in a nonfunctional spastic upper limb. Correction can also reduce pain, improve axillary hygiene, reduce skin maceration and breakdown, and facilitate upper limb dressing, positioning, and transfers.

- **Adduction and internal rotation contracture of the shoulder** is corrected by releasing the humeral insertion of the pectoralis major, subscapularis, teres major, and latissimus dorsi muscles. The shoulder capsule is left undisturbed to prevent shoulder instability and capsular adhesion. Postoperative care includes aggressive mobilization and a passive stretching program after wound healing. Recurrence is prevented by positioning (e.g., using sling, splint, or pillows) the shoulder in abduction and external rotation for several months. In the paretic shoulder, inferior subluxation is a frequent problem. When the sling gives inadequate symptomatic or functional relief, the biceps tendon can be looped over the coracoid process of the shoulder to serve as a static sling.
- **Flexion contracture of the elbow** (usually associated with ulnar nerve compression at the elbow) is corrected by releasing the brachioradialis and biceps tendon at the elbow, and by fractional (or myotendinous) lengthening of the brachialis muscles. Brachialis muscle release is only performed in severe contractures present for several years. The anterior capsule is left undisturbed to prevent postoperative adhesions. Only 50% of the contracture is corrected during surgery to prevent excessive tension on the contracted neurovascular bundle. Postoperative care includes serial casting every week to obtain further extension.
- **Wrist flexion contracture** (usually associated with median nerve compression at the transverse carpal ligament) is corrected by releasing the wrist flexor tendons (palmaris longus, flexor carpi ulnaris, and radialis). Often there are concomitant finger flexion contractures, which can be corrected by fractional (or myotendinous) lengthening of the finger flexors, or a superficialis to profundus tendon transfer (STP). If carpal tunnel syndrome is present, the medial nerve is decompressed. Postoperative care includes short arm casts for 3 weeks to immobilize the wrist, followed by nightly volar splinting for an additional 3 weeks to maintain the correction. After the cast is removed, gentle ROM exercise is started. If there is severe wrist flexion contracture, wrist arthrodesis may be performed. Postoperative care for wrist arthrodesis includes a long arm splint, which should be elevated until swelling subsides. Then a short arm cast is applied for 6–8 weeks until fusion is seen on a radiograph.
- **Clenched-fist contracture** is corrected by STP, which provides sufficient flexor tendon lengthening with preservation of a passive tether to prevent a hyperextension deformity. Neurectomy of the motor branch of the ulnar nerve in the Guyon's canal is routinely done because intrinsic spasticity, which is always present, may cause intrinsic-plus hand deformity after surgery. Transection of the flexor tendon is not recommended as it may lead to hyperextension deformity as a result of unopposed extensor muscles. The associated wrist flexion deformity is corrected as described in section III.F.1.b.2.c. Postoperative care includes immobilization for 4 weeks in a short arm cast extended to the fingertips followed by ROM exercises after the cast is removed.
- **Intrinsic-plus hand contracture** results in flexed metacarpophalangeal (MCP) and extended interphalangeal (IP) joints and is often associated with boutonnière or swan-neck deformities of the fingers. It is corrected by releasing the lateral band and oblique fibers of the extensor hood. A concomitant

neurectomy of the motor branch of the ulnar nerve in the Guyon's canal is advisable to prevent a recurrence of intrinsic-plus hand deformity. Postoperative care includes hand immobilization in a bulky dressing for 1 week followed by passive ROM exercises.

II. **Dynamic deformities of the upper limbs** are corrected to improve upper limb function and provide cosmesis. The efficacy of correcting dynamic deformities in hemiplegic patients is unclear because the patient frequently continues to carry out most activities with the uninvolved upper limb.

- **Dynamic elbow flexion deformity** as a result of elbow flexor spasticity is associated with a cog-wheel type of motion during attempted elbow extension, while elbow flexion is relatively normal. It is corrected by myotomy of the proximal brachioradialis, tenotomy of the brachialis tendon, step-cut (Z-plasty) lengthening of the biceps tendon, and fractional (or myotendinous) lengthening of the brachialis muscle. Postoperative care includes a long arm cast with the elbow in 45° of flexion for 4 weeks. After the cast is removed, active ROM exercises are started, and night splints are used for an additional 4 weeks to protect the biceps tendon repair.
- **Dynamic elbow extension deformity** as a result of triceps spasticity rarely occurs. It is corrected by V-Y lengthening of the triceps. In severe cases, triceps release may be necessary.
- **Dynamic wrist and finger flexion deformity** due to wrist and finger flexor spasticity is corrected by fractional (or myotendinous) step-cut (Z-plasty) lengthening of flexor digitorum superficialis (FDS) and flexor digitorum profundus (FDP) combined with step-cut (Z-plasty) lengthening of the flexor pollicis longus and overlengthening of the flexor carpi radialis and flexor carpi ulnaris. The palmaris longus tendon is also released if tight. Postoperative care includes 3 weeks in a short arm cast, which includes thumb and fingers with the wrist held in 20° of extension, the MCP joint in 60° of flexion, and the IP joint extended. After the cast is removed, active ROM exercises are started and resting splints are worn at night for an additional 3 weeks to protect the tendon from inadvertent stretching. Because overlengthening of the finger flexors can result in a loss of grip strength, a flexor–pronator origin release may be done for patients with voluntary control but overpowering flexors.
- **Dynamic thumb-in-palm deformity** causes the thumb to be flexed and adducted within the palm because of spastic adductor pollicis and thenar muscles. The flexor pollicis longus and the first dorsal interosseous (DI) commonly contribute to the deformity. It is corrected by proximal myotomy at the origin of all thenar muscles. Distal releases are avoided as they may cause hyperextension deformity of the thumb MCP joint. Flexion deformity of the IP thumb joint is corrected by either fractional or Z-plasty lengthening of the flexor pollicis in the forearm. The IP joint can also be stabilized by percutaneous arthrodesis. If the first DI is contracted, it is released. If the web space is contracted, a Z-plasty of the thumb web space is necessary. Postoperative care includes a thumb spica cast for 4 weeks followed by active ROM exercises after cast removal.
- **Dynamic intrinsic-plus hand deformity** results in flexed MCP and extended IP joints and is often associated with boutonnière or swan-neck deformities of the fingers. It is corrected by blocking the motor branch of the ulnar nerve in the Guyon's canal either by neurectomy for permanent ablation or by injection of phenol into the exposed nerve under direct vision. Usually, 5% phenol in glycerine is used because the glycerine allows the phenol to be released more slowly thus prolonging its effects (up to

6 months). Postoperative care includes soft dressing applied to the hand with ROM exercises (active and passive) started on the first day after surgery.

2. **Peripheral neurectomy** is the sectioning of peripheral nerves to relieve spasticity. For example, anterior obturator neurectomies are used to relieve hip adductor spasticity and improve scissoring of gait in CP patients; neurectomy of the motor branch of the ulnar nerve is carried out to prevent intrinsic-plus hand deformity. See section III.D.2.b.2.b for other nerves used in neurectomies.

a. ***Complete peripheral neurectomy*** abolishes all muscle tone and voluntary movements. It is associated with profound muscular atrophy and sensory loss.

b. ***Selective peripheral neurectomy*** refers to the partial sectioning of the nerve using microsurgical techniques and intraoperative electrical stimulation, thus preserving some voluntary muscle activity, lessening atrophy, and preserving cutaneous sensory branches.

3. **Central electrical stimulations**, including **epidural (dorsal column) electrical stimulation** and **cerebellar stimulation** have been tried to reduce spasticity, but their long-term objective efficacy and functional gains under blinded conditions have not been shown.

G. **STEP 7 CARE**. Myelotomy, cordotomy, and cordectomy are rarely performed because they can lead to severe muscle atrophy, loss of bowel and bladder functions, and loss of erectile function. They are contraindicated when useful voluntary motor control is preserved or when motor recovery is possible.

1. **Myelotomy** involves severing of the tracts in the spinal cord.
2. **Cordotomy** involves sectioning and **cordectomy** involves excision of portions of the cord.

Further reading

Glen MB. Nerve blocks for treatment of spasticity. *Phys Med Rehabil State Art Rev* 8(3): 481–505, 1994.

Katz RT, Campagnolo DI. Pharmacological management of spasticity. *Phys Med Rehabil State Art Rev* 8(3):473–480, 1994.

Katz RT, Dewald JPA, Schmit BD: Spasticity. In Braddom RL, editor: *Physical medicine and rehabilitation*, ed 2, Philadelphia, 2000, WB Saunders, pp. 592–615.

Keenan MA, Kozin S, Berlet A: *Manual of orthopedic surgery for spasticity*, New York, 1993, Raven Press.

Little JW, Massagli TL: Spasticity and associated abnormalities of muscle tone. In DeLisa JA, Gans BM, editors: *Rehabilitation medicine: Principles and practice*, ed 3, Philadelphia, 1998, JB Lippincott-Raven, pp. 997–1013.

MacDonald CM: Selective dorsal rhizotomy: Patient selection, intraoperative electrophysiologic monitoring and clinical outcome. *Phys Med Rehabil State Art Rev* 8(3):579–604, 1994.

Mayer NH, Simpson DM, editors: *Spasticity: Etiology, evaluation, management, and the role of Botulinum Toxin Type A*, New York, We MOVE, 2002.

Merritt JL: Management of spasticity in spinal cord injury. *Mayo Clin Proc* 56:614–622, 1981.

O'Brien C, Yablon S, editors: *Management of spasticity with botulinum toxin: a clinical monograph*, Littleton, 1995, Postgraduate Institute of Medicine.

Schwartz RG: Botulinum toxin injections for neurologic conditions. In Lennard TA, editor: *Pain procedures in clinical practice*, Philadelphia, 2000, Hanley & Belfus, pp. 203–212.

Worldwide Education and Awareness for Movement Disorders (WE MOVE): *Spasticity: diagnosis and treatment*, Mount Sinai Medical Center, New York, 1995, WE MOVE publication.

Young RR, editor: Role of tizanidine in the treatment of spasticity. *Neurology* 44(suppl 9):S1–S80, 1994.

CHAPTER 5.5
Neurogenic communication disorders

This chapter deals only with acquired neurogenic communication disorders in adults encompassing the following dimensions of human communication: language, cognition, attention and perception, speech, voice, fluency, and hearing. It does not include developmental communication problems (e.g., developmental stuttering) or non-neurogenic voice or hearing disorders (e.g., laryngeal cancer and cholesteatoma), as these are beyond the scope of PM&R.

I. Language impairments

Language impairment can result from focal injury of the dominant (usually left) hemisphere (e.g., aphasia because of a stroke or neurosurgical procedure) or it may result from a more diffuse axonal injury (e.g., cognitive-communication impairments because of closed head injury). Although mild language impairment may be associated with right hemisphere communication impairments (RHCI), RHCI is discussed separately in section II because its underlying pathomechanism is non-linguistic in origin (i.e., attentional and perceptual disorders).

A. APHASIA (DYSPHASIA) is an acquired focal neurologic disorder (e.g., brain damage as a result of stroke) resulting in impairment of the processing for receptive language (i.e., auditory and reading comprehension) or expressive language (i.e., expressive speech, intonation, gestures, and written expression) or both receptive and expressive languages. The multimodal loss or reduction in language is disproportional to the impairment of other intellectual functions and cannot be attributed to dementia, sensory loss, or motor dysfunction. Aphasia is characteristically seen in lesions of the dominant hemisphere, which in 85% of all individuals is the left hemisphere. In the United States alone, there are more than a million people who suffer from aphasia, and each day almost 300 new cases are added to the list.

Aphasia must be differentiated from other cortical and subcortical speech and language disorders such as (a) *agnosia* in which, unlike the multimodal aphasia, the disorder tends to be confined to only one input or output modality despite intact end-organ function (e.g., auditory agnosia in which hearing is compromised despite normal hearing threshold, but visual modalities such as reading remain intact); (b) speech disorders (e.g., *apraxia of speech* or *dysarthria*, both described in section III); (c) *dementia*, which is primarily the result of cognitive deficits (involving orientation, judgment, memory, attention, and visual–perceptual skills) caused by Alzheimer's disease or multiple infarct dementia, which have a progressively deteriorating course (hence prognosis is less favorable than that for aphasia); and (d) *confusion*, which is characterized by reduced recognition, reduced understanding of and responsiveness to the environment, faulty memory, unclear thinking, and disorientation. Unlike dementia, confusion is associated with head trauma, is generally not progressive, and has a more favorable outcome. Both dementia and confusion have cognitive deficits that extend beyond the communication seen in aphasic patients.

1. **Classification of aphasia:** The algorithm for screening and classifying aphasia (using the Boston classification) is shown in Fig. 5.5-1. Standardized screening tests (see section I.A.2) may be used. Informal bedside screening may be carried out as follows. (a) Determine the patient's verbal fluency (fluent vs.

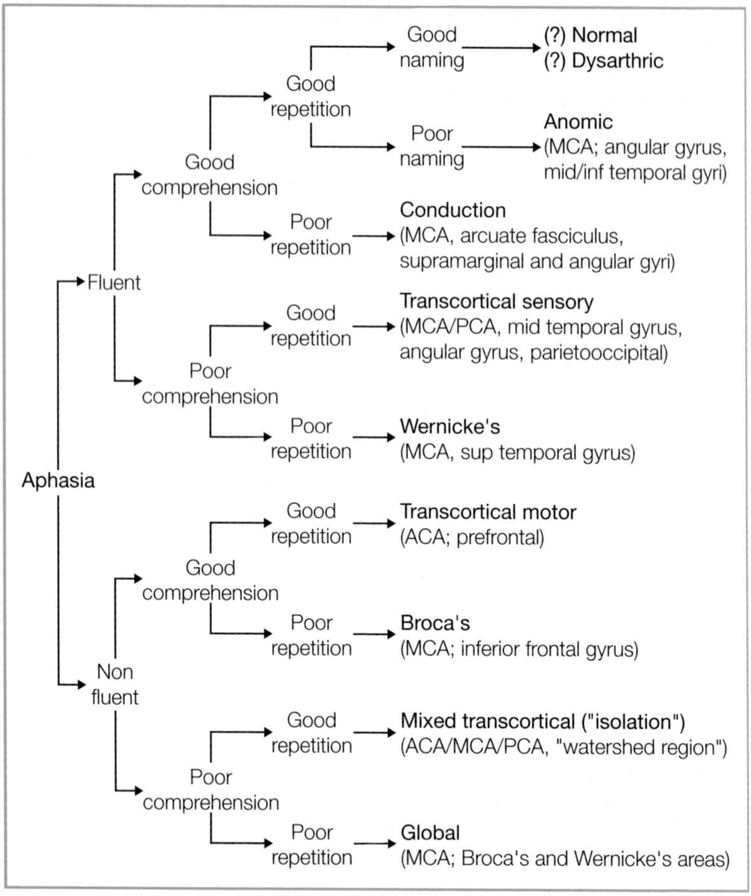

Figure 5.5-1 Algorithm for screening and classifying aphasia (using the Boston Aphasia Research Center classification). Listed in parentheses are the main sites of pathology and the blood vessels involved, usually located on the left or dominant hemisphere. See text for explanation of informal bedside screening of aphasia. MCA = middle cerebral artery; ACA = anterior cerebral artery; PCA = posterior cerebral artery; mid = middle; inf = inferior; sup = superior.

nonfluent characteristics are described in sections I.A.1.a and b) by asking the patient, "Tell me what happened today" or "Tell me about your family" or by asking the patient to say as many words within 1 minute beginning with the letter *A* or *S* (most normal people can list at least 12 words in 1 minute). (b) Check for comprehension by asking the patient to follow one-, two-, or three-step commands (e.g., "Point your right thumb to your left ear, then to the door, then to your bed."). (c) Have the patient repeat verbally after you using one random number at a time (e.g., "two," "eighteen," "twenty-nine," and so on) or one word at a time (e.g., "apple," "school," "chocolate," and so on), or simple sentences (e.g., "The cat ate the fish"); the sentences can be made progressively more complicated by increasing the length and raising the grammatical complexity (e.g., "When the busy doctor went to the cafeteria he found that all the seats were occupied by medical students"). (d) Evaluate confrontation naming ability by showing the patient a common object (e.g., pencil or tie) and ask for its name. Naming is severely impaired in patients with anomic or global aphasia.

The following subtypes of aphasia (based on the Boston classification) are caused by cortical lesions. Subcortical lesions, however, may also cause aphasias, for example, *anterior subcortical aphasia*, which involves the internal capsule limb and the putamen (aphasia characteristics are sparse verbal output with severely impaired articulation and hypophonic speech), and *posterior subcortical aphasia*, which involves the thalamus or neighboring white matter [resulting in aphasia that is fluent, with intact comprehension and repetition skills but with major difficulty in word finding and paraphasia (defined in section I.A.1.a)].

a. ***Fluent aphasia*** is associated with cerebral lesions posterior to the rolandic fissure, often in the temporoparietal region of the dominant (left) hemisphere. It is relatively normal in the following aspects: word output is 100 to 200 words per minute (wpm); speech production is easy and without effort; articulation is good; phrase length is more than five to eight words/phrase; and prosodic quality is acceptable. (*Prosody* refers to the speech rate, rhythm, pitch, loudness, and intonation, which can convey additional meaning such as joy, anger, or sadness.) The speech content, however, lacks substance ("empty speech") and is characterized by *circumlocution* (i.e., attempts at word retrieval, which end in descriptions or associations related to the intended word), and frequent *paraphasia* (i.e., substitution of an incorrect or unintended word for a correct one, e.g., pen for pencil). This mostly incomprehensible but well-articulated speech output is called *jargon*. Fluent aphasics tend to pause and seem to have word-finding difficulty when semantically meaningful and picturable action words are needed. If asked "What did you have for lunch?" The answer might be, "Lunch. Yes, I have great lunches everyday. I love to munch. I would never miss munching for anything in the world. Yum, Yum. I love munching. My lunch I love lunch. I just love it. Everyday of the week is really super." Although verbose, this "fluent" answer lacks substance.

I. **Major fluent aphasia**

- **Wernicke's aphasia** (also known as "posterior", "receptive", "sensory", "acoustic", or "syntactic" aphasia) is associated with lesions of the posterior region of the superior temporal gyrus (i.e., Wernicke's area; supplied by the middle cerebral artery). It is predominantly a "receptive" aphasia, that is, comprehension (auditory and reading) skills are impaired. The well-articulated ("fluent") speech is characterized by paragrammatism (i.e., incorrect use of grammatical words), paraphasia (defined in section I.A.1.a), circumlocution (defined in section I.A.1.a), and neologism (i.e., typically made-up words, or "new" fabricated words). Patients with Wernicke's aphasia are unaware that their verbalization does not make sense, and they seem to have an irrepressible desire to continue in their incomprehensible monologue (i.e., "press for speech"). Their repetition and writing skills are also impaired. Moreover, naming ability is poor (i.e., confrontational naming and word finding, especially for substantive words). They also tend to show paranoid behaviors, probably because of consistent confusion or neglect from their listener.
- **Conduction aphasia** ("afferent-motor" or "central" aphasia) is associated with perisylvian lesions involving the arcuate fasciculus (i.e., part of the superior longitudinal fasciculus that interconnects Wernicke's area with Broca's area), supramarginal gyrus, angular gyrus, primary auditory cortex, insula, and portion of the surrounding association cortex (all of which are supplied by the middle cerebral artery). Its most discriminating feature is the significant impairment in repetition (which is more evident on repetition of phrases, short sentences, polysyllabic words, and unfamiliar phrases). While repetition difficulties may also be seen in other aphasias (e.g., Broca's,

Wernicke's, or global), patients with conduction aphasia have relatively intact "fluency" and comprehension (auditory comprehension may be slightly impaired but is functional) which are disproportionate to their repetition impairment. Although considered "fluent", their speech (which may be limited to short bursts of fluency) may be interspersed with long pauses and expressive struggles because of naming (i.e., word-finding) difficulties. In addition, writing is impaired while reading skills remain relatively intact.

II. **Minor fluent aphasia**

- **Transcortical sensory (TCS) aphasia** (or "Wernicke's aphasia type II") is a rare syndrome associated with lesions in the posterior sector of the middle temporal gyrus and in the angular gyrus (which are supplied by the middle cerebral artery) as well as parieto-occipital cortex (which is supplied by the posterior cerebral artery). Like Wernicke's aphasia, the speech is fluent but comprehension (auditory and reading) is poor. Unlike Wernicke's aphasia, however, repetition skill is intact and may be echolalic (i.e., accurate repetition of a preceding utterance when repetition is not required during conversational speech). Naming (including word-finding abilities) and writing skills are also impaired.
- **Anomic aphasia** (also known as "semantic", "nominal", or "amnesic" aphasia) can be caused by lesions in multiple brain areas, including the angular gyrus, the middle or inferior temporal gyrus, and dorsolateral frontal cortex (these are supplied by the middle cerebral artery). It can also be caused by a thalamic lesion. It is a "milder" form of fluent aphasia whose major feature is word-finding difficulty, both orally and in writing. Unlike other fluent aphasias with word-finding difficulties (e.g., Wernicke's, conduction, and TCS aphasias), patients with anomic aphasia have relatively good comprehension (reading and listening skills are at least functional) and good-to-normal repetition skills. Their fluent, grammatically well-formed speech tends to be circumlocutory and may seem empty, as the content words tend to be omitted.

b. ***Nonfluent aphasia*** is associated with cerebral lesions anterior to the rolandic fissure, often in the frontal region of the dominant (left) hemisphere. It is characterized by the following: word output is sparse (i.e., less than 50 wpm); speech production is effortful (e.g., slow speech accompanied by facial grimacing and groping for words); articulation is poor; phrase length is short (one or two words per phrase); and speech is dysprosodic (i.e., unmelodic, dysrhythmic, and incompetently inflected). Paraphasia is rare, however, and speech is packed with substantive words (i.e., nouns, action verbs, or descriptive adjectives) but is significantly lacking in syntactical words. The sparsely worded speech tends to be "telegraphic" and may be characterized by agrammatism (i.e., devoid of any grammatical structure). If asked "What did you have for lunch?" The answer might be, "Uh . . . salad . . . uh . . . chicken . . . fried . . . good." Although the answer is choppy, telegraphic, and agrammatic, it is packed with information.

I. **Major nonfluent aphasia**

- **Broca's aphasia** (also known as "anterior", "nonfluent", "expressive", "motor", "verbal-efferent", "motor-expressive", or "cortical-motor" aphasia) is the most common type of aphasia in patients receiving comprehensive rehabilitation. It is associated with lesions in the opercular and triangular sections of the inferior frontal gyrus (i.e., Broca's area; supplied by the middle cerebral artery). It is predominantly an "expressive" aphasia (featuring all the nonfluent characteristics described above) with relatively intact and often functional auditory and reading comprehension (i.e., patients with Broca's aphasia are able to follow most everyday conversation and communicate through yes and no questions or multiple choices, but they may have trouble following complex grammatical statements). Repetition and naming skills are often moderately to severely impaired. Their writing output also tends to be as "nonfluent" as their speech. As a result of their awareness of their inability to express themselves, they tend to show varying degrees of frustration when they make errors (in contrast, patients with Wernicke's aphasia often show little frustration or awareness of error).

- **Global aphasia** is associated with lesions involving the Broca's and Wernicke's areas (both supplied by the middle cerebral artery). Language comprehension (both auditory and reading) and expression (including naming repetition, and writing) are severely impaired. Global aphasics may be able to utter automatic (stereotyped) words and phrases, but they are rarely able to use them in the appropriate context. They may compensate for their lack of verbal skills by using nonverbal means of communication (e.g., primitive gestures). As comprehension improves, patients with gloabal aphasia may transition into and resemble Broca's aphasia.

II. **Minor nonfluent aphasia**

- **Transcortical motor (TCM) aphasia** is associated with lesions in the prefrontal or supplemental speech area (which is supplied by the anterior cerebral artery). Like Broca's aphasia, the speech is nonfluent (writing is also impaired) and comprehension (auditory and reading) is relatively intact and functional. Unlike Broca's aphasia however, repetition skill is intact (and may be echolalic). The naming ability of TCM aphasics, which is usually fairly good, may be slightly abnormal in some patients, for example during confrontation naming, perseveration may be noted (i.e., patient may continue to give a past answer for a new stimulus). Moreover, unlike Broca's aphasics, patients with TCM aphasia have occasional breakthroughs of grammatical and well-articulated speech with little to no paraphasia. Another feature of TCM aphasia is adynamia (i.e., difficulty in initiating speech or one-word factual responses; marked reduction in initiation and organization; and either akinetic or bradykinetic movements).
- **Mixed transcortical aphasia** ("isolation of speech", "mixed nonfluent", or "sensorimotor aphasia") is a rare syndrome associated with lesions similar to those of TCM and TCS aphasias (the anterior, middle, and posterior cerebral arteries at the vascular watershed zone may be involved). Like global aphasia, the speech is nonfluent (writing is also impaired) and comprehension (auditory and reading) is poor. Unlike global aphasia, however, repetition skill is intact and may be echolalic. Unlike TCM aphasia, naming skills are impaired.

2. **Assessment tools** for aphasia can be used clinically to identify the nature and severity of the aphasia and its specific deficits, classify aphasia into subtypes, assess functional communication skills, establish prognosis and determine treatment necessity, guide in the treatment planning, and monitor treatment progress. They are commonly administered by speech–language pathologists (formerly called speech pathologists or speech therapists). The interpretation of quantitative assessment tools must be performed with caution because they may not always reflect "real-life" communication skills. Likewise, a "mild" impairment rating may be considered "severe" for that individual, especially when one considers occupation.

Screening tests for aphasia may be done informally (using the bedside screening method for classifying aphasia as described in section I.A.1) or formally (using standardized screening tests). Standardized screening tests for aphasia include: Aphasia Language Performance Scale (ALPS), Frenchay Aphasia Screening Test (FAST), Bedside Evaluation Screening Test–second edition (BEST-2), Quick Assessment for Aphasia, Aphasia Screening Test (AST), Sklar Aphasia

Scale (SAS), Sheffield Screening Test for Acquired Language Disorder, Aphasia Screening Test, and Acute Aphasia Screening Protocol (AASP). Most of these can be administered at the bedside within 30 minutes (the FAST taking only 3–10 minutes). The following section describes the more popular aphasia test batteries used to evaluate comprehensive language, functional communication skills, and other related language modalities. Currently, the two most frequently used standardized aphasia examinations are the Boston Diagnostic Aphasia Examination (BDAE) and the Western Aphasia Battery (WAB).

a. ***Comprehensive language tests***

I. **The Boston Diagnostic Aphasia Examination (BDAE)** contains 27 subtests and an additional group of nonlanguage subtests to evaluate parietal lobe dysfunction. It evaluates auditory comprehension, oral expression, understanding of written language, and writing. It is useful in classifying patients into the subtypes of aphasia (based on the Boston classification), assessing therapeutic progress, and in guiding treatment programs. It does not provide, however, prognostic information or a specific treatment plan. It may take several hours to administer. It has good internal validity, but reliability has not been clearly shown.

II. **Western Aphasia Battery (WAB)** is a modification and expansion of BDAE. It measures oral language abilities (i.e., fluency and information content of spontaneous speech, comprehension, repetition, and naming) and auditory verbal comprehension. Both the auditory and expressive modalities yield an aphasia quotient (AQ). An AQ below 93.8 is consistent with aphasia. Like BDAE, it is useful in classifying patients into the subtypes of aphasia (based on the Boston classification). It has high reliability and is highly correlated with Neurosensory Center Comprehensive Examination for Aphasia (NCCEA) scores. It requires 1–2 hours to administer (much less than that for the BDAE) and is widely used as a clinical and research tool.

III. **Porch Index of Communicative Ability (PICA)** has 18 subtests and uses 10 common objects to elicit patient responses. Every response is scored by a specially trained tester according to a unique 16-point multidimensional system based on accuracy, completeness, promptness, and responsiveness. Results are reported in percentiles and can be compared with scores of other patients with bilateral and left hemisphere damage. It is useful in determining prognosis, assessing therapeutic progress, and in planning programmed treatment and research. It assesses a narrow range of verbal functions and is not sensitive to patients with mild or severe linguistic deficits. It provides the most detailed qualitative record of response and takes 1 hour to administer and score. It has high reliability and has concurrent validity with BDAE, Functional Communication Profile (FCP), and Communicative Abilities in Daily Living (CADL) tests.

IV. **Minnesota Test for Differential Diagnosis of Aphasia (MTDDA)** consists of 47 subtests which focus on five areas of disorders: auditory disturbances, visual and reading disturbances, speech and language disturbances, visuomotor and writing disturbances, and disturbances of numerical relationships and arithmetic processes. It is most useful for recognizing and classifying deficits of auditory comprehension, for classifying patients into aphasia type (on which prognosis for recovery is based), and for treatment planning. The test takes about 3 hours and is given in multiple sessions. Its reliability and validity are not as well documented as for the BDAE or WAB.

V. **Neurosensory Center Comprehensive Examination for Aphasia (NCCEA)** contains 20 language subtests (to assess the level of comprehension and expression, the ability to retain verbally presented material, and the ability to make functional use of reading and writing skills) and four control tests (to assess visual and tactile functions). It compares the patient's specific deficits with the performance of normal adults and has been tested on adult aphasics and on nonaphasic adults with brain damage. It also has norms for children as young as 6 years old. It can measure severity of aphasia and can distinguish the patient's specific areas of strength and weakness; therefore, it can be used to monitor recovery. However, it does not assess spontaneous speech, does not specify aphasia classification, and does not specify treatment plan. It takes 90 minutes to administer. Its reliability is satisfactory, and has concurrent validity with WAB and FCP tests.

b. ***Functional communication tests***

I. **Functional Communication Profile (FCP)** consists of 45 communication behaviors divided into five major groups: movement (gesture), speaking, understanding, reading, and others (e.g., handling of money). Data are collected in a nonstructured, conversational situation as the rater informally interacts with the patient. An overall percentage score reflects the patient's functional communication skills after the injury or disease and compares it to his or her own premorbid norm, which is inferred from the patient's education, personality, etc. It takes 20–30 minutes to administer by an experienced clinician. Although rating is subjective, it has high interrater reliability. The FCP can be used to follow recovery and predict outcome.

II. **Communicative Abilities in Daily Living (CADL)** consists of 68 easily administered items incorporating 10 categories of everyday language activities presented in interview and role-playing situations. It provides information about the functional communication skills of aphasic patients in everyday situations and is used in patients whose PICA scores have plateaued. It has high reliability and has high concurrent validity with the PICA, FCP, and BDAE tests.

III. **Communication Effectiveness Index (CETI)** is a more recent functional communication assessment tool that focuses on communicative need and assesses communication for social needs, life skills, basic needs, and health threats. It is based on direct observation (carried out by the patient's spouse or significant other) of the patient's ability to perform 16 communicative skills relative to premorbid abilities in those skill areas.

IV **American Speech and Hearing Association–Functional Assessment of Communication Skills (ASHA–FACS)** consists of 43 items that measure adult functional communication across four assessment domains (i.e., social communication; communication of basic needs; reading, writing, and number concepts; and daily planning) and four qualitative dimensions (i.e., adequacy, appropriateness, promptness, and communication sharing). It has high intra- and intertester reliability and takes about 20 minutes to administer. It has been tested on 131 adult aphasics with left hemisphere stroke (with good correlation with WAB) and 54 adults with cognitive-communication impairments as a result of traumatic brain injury (TBI) [with good correlation with the Scale of Cognitive Abilities for Traumatic Brain Injury (SCATBI); see section I.B.2.c].

c. ***Specialized aphasia tests*** include the Token Test, which measures subtle mild auditory comprehension deficit (in which the patient is asked to manipulate 20 tokens of two sizes, big and small, two shapes, square and round, and five colors through nonredundant language of increasing length and complexity); Reporter's Test, a variation of the Token Test, in which the examiner moves the token and the patient describes the movements to another person who has not seen them; Reading Comprehension Battery, which assesses reading skills in greater detail than most aphasia batteries; Auditory Comprehension Test for Sentences (ACTS), which examines auditory comprehension, may be used in mildly impaired patients; Boston Assessment of Severe Aphasia (BASA), which is used in patients with severe or global aphasia for whom other tests are too difficult; Peabody Picture Vocabulary Test (PPVT), which is used to test naming ability. Multilingual tests of aphasia include the Multilingual Aphasia Examination (MAE) and the Bilingual Aphasia Test (BAT).

3. **Prognosis** for speech recovery in aphasic patients may be determined by using one of the comprehensive language tests (i.e., WAB, PICA, or MTDDA). In general, the following characteristics of aphasia tend to have poorer prognosis: severe auditory comprehension deficits, the presence of perseveration, the inability to match objects, unreliable yes and no responses, and the use of jargon and empty speech without self-correction. Among the four types of prognostic variables listed below, the medical and speech and language variables are more potent. However, there is no single variable that exerts such strong negative influence that it precludes a trial of speech therapy.

a. ***Medical variables*** include

I. **Etiologic factors**. Aphasia of vascular etiology has a poorer outcome than aphasia as a result of trauma. Aphasia caused by tumor has a variable prognosis (but is often poor).

II. **Site and extent of lesion**. In general, the larger the dominant-hemisphere lesion, the poorer the prognosis; small lesions, if multiple, have a poorer outcome; left-side lesions have a poorer prognosis than right-side lesions; and bilateral lesions, even when small, have a poorer prognosis. However, despite poor prognosis because of the site and extent of the lesion, there are case reports of good recovery. A trial of speech therapy, therefore, should at least be considered.

III. **Coexisting medical problems**, if present, contribute to poor outcome.

b. ***Speech and language variables***

I. **Severity of disorder**. Middle cerebral artery deficits frequently result in severe aphasia. Patients with severely impaired initial ability to speak or with severe impairment in auditory recognition and comprehension have a poorer prognosis. Likewise, the longer the length of their hospital stay, the poorer the outcome (probably because of coexisting medical problems in addition to severe impairments).

II. **Auditory process**. Patients with peripheral hearing loss or impaired central auditory processes have a poorer outcome.

III. **Classification and type of disorder**. Broca's and Wernicke's aphasias have similar prognoses whereas global aphasia has a notably poorer prognosis. The poor auditory comprehension in Wernicke's aphasia makes it less amenable to treatment than other aphasias. Conduction aphasias generally have the greatest gains. The prognosis for TCM or TCS aphasia is generally good. In mixed transcortical aphasia, the prognosis is relatively good but is generally poorer than that for TCM or TCS aphasia.

IV. **Nonlanguage cognitive defects**, for example, major perceptual defects, visual or auditory, or memory and attentional deficits (if any of these are present, the outcome is poorer); coexisting communicative impairment, for example, apraxia (if present, treatment efficacy may be limited).

c. ***Patient variables***

I. **Age at onset**. Younger patients possibly have better outcomes (controversial).

II. **Education, premorbid intelligence, and communication skills**. Patients with higher level of premorbid education tend to respond better probably due to richer vocabularies, higher intelligence, and better communication skills. In illiterates, aphasia is less severe, probably because of more bilateral representation of language.

III. **Handedness.** Reports that left-handed patients have better outcome are controversial (studies seem to indicate that handedness is probably not related to hemispheric dominance, i.e., many left-handed people are left-brain dominant with left-sided language representation).

IV. **Multilinguals (polyglots).** Both the Ribot's rule and Pitre's law are not shown to be consistently true. The Ribot's rule states that in a multilingual aphasic, the language best recovered would be the mother tongue; however, the Pitre's law states that the language that the multilingual aphasic was consistently using at the onset of the aphasia will be the first to be recovered even though it is not the first learned. Currently, there is no simple or steadfast rule of language recovery that can be consistently applied to the multilingual aphasics. There are reports that indicate that probably the language milieu during recovery determines the first language to be recovered. There are also reports of more frequent crossed aphasics in right-handers who are multilingual, suggesting greater right-hemisphere participation. Most clinical evidence seems to indicate that the degree of control the left hemisphere has on the first and subsequent languages is probably the same.

V. **Gender** is probably unrelated to prognosis. Data favoring recovery in either sex have been reported.

d. Other variables

I. **Months after onset.** The longer the time elapsed, the poorer the prognosis.

II. **Motivation.** Poorly motivated patients have poorer outcome.

III. **Environment and attitude of support system.** Patients whose family or significant others are supportive have better outcomes.

4. **Treatment** of aphasia is a dynamic, organized process tailored to all the personal, neuropsychological, and linguistic factors affecting each patient. Although aphasia therapy is individualized, group therapy with peers can be beneficial in some patients as it can provide a comfortable atmosphere in which patients can vent feelings, meet new friends, gain feedback on their impairment and their progress, and practice functional communication skills. Aphasia therapy mainly uses the language intervention strategies described below. Pharmacological treatment (e.g., bromocriptine, L-dopa, amphetamine, and piracetam) has been reported in a few studies, but its efficacy remains doubtful. The general goals of aphasia treatment are (a) to stimulate the disrupted process and to promote functional reorganization; (b) to teach the use of residual abilities as compensatory strategies for communication; (c) to provide education and counseling and to promote adjustment of the patient and family; (d) to eliminate "bad habits" that interfere with successful communication; (e) to promote a suitable communication environment; and (f) to provide psychological support and improve the patient's attitude, morale, and other significant social factors (i.e., speech therapy can be used to channel attention and energies toward constructive ends, thus reducing depression). The ultimate goal of treatment is to progress toward successful "real-life" communication, outside the professional program, within the limits of the brain damage.

There are two stages of language recovery: first, an initial spontaneous recovery (reflecting resolution of edema, hemorrhage, and other cellular damage), which starts within a few days of onset and lasts about 1 month (or even longer) after onset; and second, a long-term recovery, which takes place for months or even years (reflecting reorganization of language function in the brain, possibly from increased participation of uninjured parts of the brain or from relearning). Ideally, intensive aphasia treatment should be started and maintained as soon as the patient is medically and neurologically stable (although, even with delay of up to 6 months postonset, therapy has been shown to be beneficial). Speech therapy should be directed to the patient and the patient's family or significant others. If available, it should ideally be given three to five times per week for 2–3 months during which time the patient is periodically re-evaluated, such as in the first month and again after the 2nd or 3rd month. When the treatment progress has plateaued, the treatment may be gradually discontinued (abrupt cessation may be psychologically harmful) by reducing it to once or twice per week, then every 1–2 months, with re-evaluation at the 6th and 10th months. Strategies commonly used for aphasic therapy are described below. For specific treatment of different types of fluent and nonfluent aphasia, the reader is referred to LaPointe's *Aphasia and related neurogenic language disorders*, and Chapey's *Language intervention strategies in adult aphasia* (see Further reading section).

Speech therapy (individual or group) for aphasia is generally reported to be beneficial and not harmful in patients with nonprogressive etiologies (e.g., stroke or excised brain tumor). The traditional belief is that significant spontaneous recovery is completed by 3–6 months postonset. However, a study on the evolution of severe aphasia in the first 2 years postonset noted significant improvements in communicative functions for up to 18 months, with the greatest improvement occurring in the first 6 months (Nicholas *et al.*, 1993). There is some justification, therefore, for continuing speech therapy longer than 6 months in selected cases.

a. ***Language intervention strategies*** are based on two schools of thought. The first school believes that language in the damaged brain is not "erased", but that its access is impaired. The brain, therefore, needs to be retrained to retrieve its individual language units (i.e., use a *retraining approach* to build the lost or inhibited language processes). The second school believes that the language function subserved by the damaged brain is not recoverable; therefore, the patient must compensate for what is lost (i.e., use a *compensatory approach* to learn alternate ways of communicating, which may be nonverbal). Cueing strategies commonly used include varying the speed and means of presentation of an item, providing additional information about an item or providing phonemic or semantic starters. For clinical use, a multimodal (holistic) approach, that is, combining the retraining and compensatory approaches, is probably most effective.

I. **Retraining approach** (or "restorative" approach) attempts to activate any essential verbal behavior and facilitate language recovery through repetitive stimulation, primarily of the auditory system, which is believed to be the primary mode of language acquisition as well as the feedback system that processes and controls the information. Another system frequently stimulated is the visual system. The stimulation is constantly repeated as repetition is essential for organization, storage, and retrieval of information in the brain.

- **Stimulation techniques** emphasize effective verbal communication through stimulation of input modalities to improve spoken and written language, without putting too much emphasis on personal relevancy of lexicon or grammar. It is exemplified by the Stimulation–Facilitation Therapy, which typically has the following features: the clinician generally assumes the role of stimulator or facilitator and initiates and directs language-based exchanges; auditory stimulations, as well as pictorial and printed stimuli, are used to improve propositional word retrieval and to increase length and completeness of utterances; convergent confrontative strategies are used to increase available vocabulary; and treatments, which are given in an individual clinical setting, are based on the analysis of the individual patient's profiles of language strengths and deficits derived from assessment tools. Other examples include the Sentence-Level Auditory Comprehension Treatment Program (SLAC), which is designed to improve auditory comprehension using controlled auditory stimulation, and Language Enrichment

Therapy (LET), which uses a pedagogical language training approach (applied by clinicians as well as trained relatives) in an attempt to improve functional communication.

- **Programmed learning (behavior modification) techniques** involve the use of a methodical framework in which each program contains a defined success criterion, and the course of therapy is planned and conducted in small steps with a hierarchy of difficulties. Examples include Respondent–Contingent Small-Step Treatment (RCSST), Audio-Visual Stimulation and Direct-Production Treatment, Filmed Language Instruction, Sentence Repetition, "Loose" training (which facilitates responses by allowing patients to use their own creative language rather than demanding specific target responses), and group therapy.
- **Symptom-specific techniques** involve the use of specific types of linguistic deficits as specific communicative goals in therapy (e.g., therapy to improve word retrieval or spontaneous speech). Examples include self-cueing, which uses linguistic cues or microcomputers to improve word retrieval or improve spontaneous speech; Treatment of Aphasic Perseveration (TAP), which uses inhibitory techniques to treat perseveration; and the Preventative Method, which is used to prevent secondary symptoms, (e.g., telegraphic speech) from developing.
- **Language-oriented (psycho- or neurolinguistic) techniques** involve the use of a programmed instruction approach addressing the actual deficit and progressing from lower levels of functioning to higher linguistic levels according to predetermined steps.

  - **Structure-based techniques** emphasize the relearning of linguistics units through repeated performances (resembling a didactical grammar exercise). Examples include Sentence Construction Board (SCB), Systematic Therapy for Auditory Comprehension Disorders, Training Formal Structure of Language, and Mapping Thematic Relations.
  - **Deblocking techniques** systematically pair weak with strong modalities to "deblock" impaired performances, for example, Helm-elicited Language Program for Syntax Stimulation (HELPSS) program used in patients with agrammatism, which involves the use of proper cues to remove blocks that interfere with the accessing process of syntactic information.
  - **Voluntary Control of Involuntary Utterances (VCIU)** is a recently used method that attempts to develop a functional vocabulary from the spontaneous utterances of patients with global aphasia.

II. **Compensatory approach** (or "substitutive retraining") assumes that, despite a certain amount of neural plasticity in adult brains, other areas of the brain cannot relearn what the damaged area subserved. Hence, rather than retraining lost or inhibited language functions, patients are taught how to compensate using whatever residual function they have (e.g., using gestures or melodic stimulation) to attain communication, of which language is an important, but not the only, means.

- **Functional communication (pragmatic) techniques** focus on effective verbal communication, stressing the pragmatic approach (i.e., the context-based use of social rules of communication) rather than on the grammatical aspects of language. Functional communication strategies need not replace but instead may be viewed as an extension of language retraining methods. Although patients may benefit by maximally improving the lexical and syntactic aspects of the language, the learned language should also be tested and used in various functional contexts. The pragmatic approach is exemplified by the Functional Communication Therapy (FCT), which focuses on the following: (a) the clinician alternates as listener and speaker by creating situations requiring equal participation from the patient, (b) patient comprehension and response are maximized by enriching the context of natural conversation with writing, gestures, use of situational cues, and interrogative probes, (c) the environment of the treatment setting (e.g., in a group setting) is made as natural as possible, and (d) when contrived situations are used, the situation should simulate real-life scenes and context and must stress functional communication content (e.g., stimuli such as menus, road maps, calendars may be used in FCT to create role-playing situations).

Other examples of the pragmatic approach are Visual Action Therapy (VAT) in which the patient creates symbolic or representational gestures to represent visually absent objects; Promoting Aphasics' Communicative Effectiveness (PACE) Therapy, which involves getting a message across by any means possible, whether it be via language, drawing, gesture, tone of voice, or any of a variety of other expressive methods; Response Elaboration Training (RET), which is based on the "loose training" concept described in section I.A.4.a.1.b; Visual Communication Therapy (VIC), which was designed for global aphasics and which uses an artificial language consisting of arbitrary symbols representing syntactic and lexical components of language that the patient learns to manipulate; Computer-Aided Visual Communication (C-VIC) System, which is a computerized adaptation of VIC; Communicative Strategies, which includes asking other people to speak slower or to simplify their complicated messages; Conversational Coaching, which involves coaching of the patient by the clinician in different settings as the patient uses a scripted short monologue; and Behavioral Modification to Train Requesting in which the patient is prompted by the clinician to ask for information on chosen topics.

- **Right hemisphere (or minor hemisphere) mediation techniques** use minor (nondominant, usually right) hemisphere abilities to mediate (facilitate) communication through the use of imagery, contextually rich stimuli, novel stimuli, drawing (e.g., Back to Drawing Board or BDB), melody (e.g., melodic intonation therapy or MIT, which uses natural melody patterns to facilitate speech in nonfluent aphasics with good comprehension), or humor (e.g., laughter therapy).
- **Nonverbal communication techniques** substitute spoken words with visual symbols or gestures. They may be augmented or supplemented by Augmentative and Alternative Communication Aids ranging from pointing tools (e.g., communication board, which the patient can use to convey messages by pointing to the board's printed letters, numbers, words, or pictures, using a finger, head pointer, or foot) to computer-based systems (e.g., using a computerized scanning system through which the patient can indicate his or her chosen message displayed on the computer screen by either typing or inputting other signals such as infrared beams transmitted through head nods, eye blink, etc.). Nonverbal techniques differ from previously mentioned methods (e.g., VAT or VIC) in the greater degree of stress they place on nonverbal means of communication. Examples include Blissymbolics, which uses line-drawn symbols to represent basic nouns, verbs, adjective, or function words; sign language such as those used by the deaf; Amer-Ind Code treatment, which uses gestural communication consisting of nearly 250 iconic gestural signals (modified from American Indian sign language) to facilitate oral speech production.

b. Speech therapy aids

I. **Social-context aids** are used to improve the patient's social interaction abilities and promote understanding of the aphasic syndrome in both the patient and the patient's immediate social support system. Examples include family therapy, which encourages the aphasic patient and their family members to act out the emotional feelings connected with the trauma to improve family communication skills and avoid emotional problems and psychological deterioration, and linguistic role playing to stimulate residual language and develop compensatory communicative abilities.

II. **Affective-context aids** are aimed at helping the patient cope with the affective aspects such as depression, anxiety, and frustration. Examples include hypnotherapy to sharpen memory and integrate skills learned during therapy; and laughter therapy (see section I.A.4.a.2.b) to relax the patient and improve the mood of the therapy session.

c. ***Interdisciplinary team approach*** emphasizes that everyone caring for the aphasic patient (professionals and nonprofessionals) should be actively involved in the speech rehabilitation of the patient. Almost all patients with aphasia have some degree of difficulty in comprehending spoken language, and the patient's auditory comprehension varies greatly, depending on the context and complexity of the task at hand. In communicating with aphasic patients, the following guidelines are suggested:

- Use short and simple sentences.
- Speak a little more slowly and give the patient enough time to process the information and formulate a response.
- Ask unequivocal choice questions that can be answered with "yes" or "no" or another single word (e.g., "did you have cereal or bagel?").
- Use physical assistive cues to facilitate the patient's comprehension (e.g., gestures, facial expression, and voice inflection).
- Be aware that aphasic patients often find it easier to respond to whole body or axial commands (e.g., "stand up") than distal commands (e.g., "pick up").
- Be consistent in giving instructions and, if needed, repeat the instruction or rephrase it and supplement speech with body language gestures or written instructions.
- If the patient becomes visibly frustrated, remain calm and try again later.
- Encourage patients to produce single-word repetitive speech that coincides with physical movements (this supplements the patient's speech practice).
- Do not make demands that are beyond the patient's level of preserved communicative skill (this can be determined by consulting with the speech–language pathologists).

B. COGNITIVE-COMMUNICATION IMPAIRMENT (CCI) or cognitive-linguistic impairment is a nonaphasic language impairment, which occurs following diffuse brain damage caused by a nonpenetrating TBI, in particular a closed head injury (CHI) in which the primary traumatic force is a sudden acceleration or deceleration of the brain within the skull (e.g., motor vehicular crash, fall, or head blow with a blunt object). Aside from diffuse axonal injury, the pathophysiology of the CHI can also include focal lesions, ischemia, and neurochemical changes, all of which interact with the severity of the CHI and the patient's premorbid status to produce heterogeneous patterns of neurobehavioral deficits. The language impairment in CCI is differentiated from aphasia in that its deficit (involving attention, information processing, and cognition) is more discernible on tasks with greater cognitive demands than those discerned in conventional measures used for aphasia. Moreover, the conceptual framework used to explain CCI focuses on how one uses language (e.g., in discourse), not simply on how one performs isolated linguistic measures.

1. **Classification** of communication deficits associated with CCI.

a. ***Aphasic language deficits*** include anomia (the most common aphasic language deficit in CCI), reduced word fluency, impaired comprehension of complex oral commands, verbal paraphasic errors (especially in complex tasks, e.g., picture-description task and use of antonyms, synonyms, and metaphor), impairments of reading and writing, impaired sentence repetition, disruption in flow of language (i.e., slowed rate of speech, hesitations, and repetition of words or phrases), and perseveration.

b. ***Nonaphasic language deficits*** have also been referred to as "cognitive linguistic deficits", "subclinical aphasic disorder", "high-level language deficits", "global disorganization of language", "confused thought content", "impaired language processing", and "fragmented and tangential conversation". These deficits, which become evident during discourse, include difficulties in topic management (in both appropriate selection and maintenance of conversational topic); noncoherent topic changes; ambiguous, unrelated, and incomplete ideational units; and unrelated responses. Grammatical or syntactic errors (e.g., omission of the subject or the main verb) occur less frequently but seem to be more than those committed by normal subjects. Although traditional naming ability is commonly disrupted in CCI patients, it does not appear to have a direct association with discourse function.

c. ***General cognitive deficits***

I. **Attention deficits** include impulsivity (in which the patient cannot sustain concentration long enough to monitor the quality of ongoing behavior), inappropriate social judgment, lack of insight, literal interpretations, perseveration, stimulus boundedness, disinhibition, and comprehension difficulties.

II. **Information processing deficits** refer to impairments involving areas of language, visual perceptual skills, motor skills, and memory (i.e., analysis and synthesis of information in sequential steps). Specifically, they may include aphasia, alexia (reading disorder), agraphia (writing disorder), acalculia (calculation disorder), agnosia (defined in section I.A), apraxia of speech (see section III.A), amnesia, and memory impairments. Perceptual disturbance (e.g., unilateral spatial neglect), associated with CCI, can also be considered an information-processing deficit because it reflects failure of the brain to adequately process stimuli to the point of meaningfulness.

III. **Cognition deficits** include disorders in perception, discrimination, organization, recall, orientation, judgment, and problem solving, all of which may be difficult to separate from language disorders or from attention or information-processing deficits.

2. Assessment

a. ***Aphasia language batteries*** (see section I.A.2) may be used to identify certain linguistic deficits in CCI. However, because they measure language primarily at the word and sentence levels, they may be relatively insensitive to the nonaphasic language deficits (e.g., poor discourse and poor cognitive abilities) seen in CCI. One functional communication test that has been validated for CCI is the ASHA-FACS (see section I.A.2.b.4). The ASHA-FACS has a good correlation (0.78) with the Scale of Cognitive Abilities for Traumatic Brain Injury (SCATBI; see section I.B.2.c).

b. ***Nonaphasia language (discourse) tests*** focus on narrative, procedural, descriptive, and conversational discourse. They measure informational content, cohesive ties, story and topic production, sequential organization of information, informativity, and semantic coherence at either a global level (i.e., relevance of information to a unifying theme or topic of the conversation) or a local level (i.e., connectivity between sentences as marked by cohesive devices, e.g., reference and connectors).

c. ***General cognitive tests*** for CCI include tests of perception, discrimination, organization, recall, convergent thinking, deductive reasoning, inductive reasoning, divergent thinking, and problem solving. Examples include Scale of Cognitive Abilities for Traumatic Brain Injury (SCATBI), Wechsler Memory Scale, Benton Visual Retention Test, Woodcock–Johnson Test of Cognitive Abilities, Detroit Test of Learning Abilities (DTLA), Test of Problem Solving, and Ross Information Processing Assessment (RIPA). Neuropsychologic tests (see Chapter 2.9) may also be used to assess cognitive skills [e.g., Halstead–Reitan Neuropsychological Battery (HRNB) and Luria–Nebraska Neuropsychological Battery (LNNB)].

3. **Prognosis** for CCI recovery is most favorable for younger patients, patients who spend less than 3 months in a coma, patients with support network, and patients who are highly motivated and goal-oriented. While age is important in determining recovery, age alone cannot predict recovery. The severity of diffuse cerebral insult (as reflected by duration of coma) is the major determinant of language competence 1 year after severe head injury. The course of language recovery in CHI is generally manifested initially by a collapse of the language system, followed by gradual recovery (typically within 6 months) until "normal speech" is attained, as measured by conventional aphasia language tests. In fact, about two-thirds of CHI patients with aphasia in the acute stage show overall improvement in aphasic linguistic abilities. Certain aspects of language, however, have been reported to remain impaired years after injury, such as, naming or word finding, word fluency, and comprehension of multistage commands. Nonaphasic linguistic deficits at the discourse level generally have a less favorable prognosis following CHI.

4. **Treatment** of CCI is ultimately aimed at developing in the patient the ability to practice, to learn from that practice, to use feedback purposely, and to encourage relearning of daily skills, which will then enhance functional living. It may include some of the techniques (and principles) used for aphasia with greater emphasis placed on the cognitive aspects and on discourse. During the earlier stage of recovery the treatment may include environmental intervention, structured activities, and cognitive-communication activities. As recovery progresses, the patient is taught compensatory strategies, memory organization, and problem solving. The interdisciplinary approach provides consistency, feedback, and reinforcement to the patient. Family involvement at the start of the program cannot be overemphasized.

   The treatment program must be individualized although it may be given in a group setting. Group therapy can provide opportunities for the patient to increase social interaction and self-monitoring skills in a communication environment, which is more natural than the individual therapy setting; increase self-esteem and self-motivation; increase ability to develop short- and long-term goals that are meaningful; and allow the patient to share feelings and needs with peers as well as to provide and receive peer review of behaviors. Computers may also be used for CCI rehabilitation to provide a controlled, consistent presentation of task stimuli with objective feedback. However, improvement in computer tasks does not necessarily generalize to other, more meaningful, areas of the patient's life. Computerized systems that train attention, visual scanning, and concentration seems to hold the greatest promise for generalizing to "real-life" activities. Neuropharmacologic agents (described below) may also be used to improve attention, memory, and learning. At present, there are no definitive studies available to suggest what works and does not work in CCI rehabilitation.

a. ***Aphasic language rehabilitation*** includes both retraining and compensatory strategies used for aphasia (see section I.A.4.a). Specific strategies used for anomia (the most common aphasic language deficit, which may persist beyond

6 months of recovery) include word retrieval techniques (confrontational naming, confrontational naming with prestimulation, sentence completion, cueing hierarchies, and word focus), generalization (e.g., picture description, prepared monologue, story retelling, story elaboration, referential communication, and role playing), and compensatory strategies (e.g., develop patient's use of generated cues, gestures, and drawing).

b. ***Nonaphasic language rehabilitation***, specifically on discourse, concentrates on the close interaction of cognition and linguistics. Patients are trained through a feedback and cueing system in a different setting to improve sequential organization of information, increase informativity, increase global cohesiveness (i.e., relationship of a response or sentence to the topic of conversation), increase local cohesiveness (i.e., connectivity between adjacent sentences as marked by cohesive devices, e.g., references and connectors), increase cognitive organization of information in the narrative discourse (avoid incomplete episodes), and to decrease use of repetitions and revisions.

c. ***Cognitive remediation*** is usually administered by neuropsychologists (or specially trained speech–language pathologists). It is quite controversial and seems to be of benefit only to mild or moderate CCI. The treatment has a three-stage hierarchy consisting of arousal and alerting, operant retraining, and a community-oriented, self-reliant treatment program. Computers are usually used in cognitive remediation, although their long-term benefit and generalizability to "real-life" situations remains unproved.

I. **Attention-focusing techniques** include techniques for focusing attention (e.g., using the starter phrase "are you ready?" or waiting for eye contact before initiating a task with the patient); reducing environmental distractions (which can be added gradually as attention improves); techniques to make the session interesting (e.g., varying the treatment concept, time, rates, and sequences); and sensory stimulation to activate any response to a stimulus and to gradually increase the frequency, type, and duration of the response.

II. **Information processing techniques**, specifically on improving memory, which include techniques to facilitate short-term memory storage (e.g., using meaningful verbal information); facilitate short-term to long-term memory storage (by analyzing, organizing, and rehearsing information); decrease reliance on feedback for memory (by gradually weaning the patient from memory cues); and determine the best method of processing information for each patient. The usefulness of rote repetition in improving memory is unclear. Patients with severe deficits can often use external memory aids (e.g., calendars, bulletin boards, message machines, and small notebooks), while patients with more subtle deficits may use internal aids such as mnemonic strategies [i.e., letter strategies, which use acronyms and acrostics; keyword strategies, which associate new information to keywords already encoded in the memory; or pegword strategies, which use rhyming words to represent a number or order (e.g., "tree" to represent "three")], "chunking" (i.e., memorizing in smaller segments such as 263-925-424 instead of 263925424), or verbal rehearsal.

III. **Cognitive retraining methods** vary from simple low-technology interventions to complex computerized interventions. The selected interventions should match the patient's home and work environment as closely as possible. They include techniques for improving perception (e.g., tracking, sound recognition, shape recognition, and work recognition); discrimination, (e.g., color discrimination, matching objects, pointing to objects, visual matching picture to sentence, and auditory discrimination between words or sentences); organization [e.g., categorization and closure (identification of geometric forms with sections missing), and sequencing]; recall [e.g., verbal description, visual imagery, chunking activities, categorization of information, rehearsal, association, temporal spatial ordering, primacy and recency benefits (first and last items are accented visually or auditorily), PQRST approach (preview, question, read, state, and test), and mnemonic devices]; and problem solving (e.g., convergent thinking, deductive reasoning, inductive reasoning, divergent thinking, and multiprocess reasoning).

d. ***Psychopharmacological interventions*** seem to be beneficial in CCI patients with deficits in attention, memory, or learning. They must be used judiciously, however, and their dosages monitored as their "therapeutic windows" are often narrow. The drugs commonly used to improve attention and concentration (which in turn are supposed to improve memory and learning) are central nervous system stimulants (i.e., catecholamine agonists). They include dextroamphetamine (Dexedrine), 2.5–5 mg, po, bid (given in the morning and at midday; may be increased to 30–60 mg/day; available in 5- and 10-mg tabs and 5 mg/5 mL elixir); methylphenidate (Ritalin), 0.30 mg/kg, po, bid or 5–10 mg, po, bid/tid (available in 5-, 10-, and 20-mg tabs); and Pemoline (Cylert), 37.5 mg, po, every morning (may increase by 18.75 mg at 1-week intervals up to 75–112.5 mg/day; the effective daily dose is 56.25–75 mg; available in 18.75-, 37.5-, and 75-mg tabs). Drugs shown to improve cognitive function (memory and learning) by anticholinesterase inhibition include donepezil (Aricept, 5 or 10 mg, po, hs), rivastigmine (Exelon, 3–6 mg, po, bid) and galantamine (Reminyl, start at 4 mg, po, bid for 4 weeks, then maintain at 8 mg, po, bid). Older anticholinesterase inhibitor such as Tacrine (Cognex) is no longer used due to hepatotoxicity. Memantine (Namenda, 10 mg, po, bid after 3 week titration of 5 mg increments) is an antagonist of N-methyl-D-aspartate (NMDA), which can also increase cognitive function. Experimental drugs that are used to improve cognitive function include physostigmine (a short-acting cholinergic agonist available only in oral form for experimental use) and pramiracetam ([Neupramir, Pramistar], considered a "nootropic" or "cognitive activator"). For details on the drugs, see Chapter 4.8, section V.E.

II. Right hemisphere communication impairment (RHCI)

RHCI is an acquired disturbance of the attentional and perceptual mechanisms of the right (nondominant) hemisphere (e.g., as a result of stroke, TBI, or tumor), which results in impaired reception and expression of contextually based communication. Patients with RHCI may appear linguistically adequate (unlike aphasics, they have no apparent difficulty with laboratory language and speech tasks), but they communicate inefficiently because they are neither able to appreciate nor interpret the context of incoming visual and auditory information, e.g., emotion conveyed in another's voice.

A. CLASSIFICATION of communication deficits associated with RHCI

1. Extralinguistic deficits reflect a failure to adequately interpret cues and organize or express information in an efficient manner. They are actually considered to be the result of processing deficits in the nonlinguistic area.

a. ***Receptive deficits*** may result in difficulty in organizing information because of failure to make use of contextual or emotional cues.

I. **Context-cue interpretation difficulties** can lead to failure to recognize the implicit or implied meaning whether in verbal exchange or in pictures and ongoing events. Specifically, the RHCI patient has difficulty in distinguishing relevant from irrelevant information, grasping figurative meaning (i.e., they are literal minded), and recognizing humor and metaphorical language structures.

II. **Emotional-cue interpretation difficulties** include the inability to interpret the tone of voice, prosody, facial expression, and situational context. The emotional impairment is in its superficial expression and comprehension rather than its actual experience.

b. ***Expressive deficits*** can make turn-taking during conversation difficult because of the inability to maintain a conversational topic.

I. **Emotional expression difficulties** can result in flat affect and monotonous speech (i.e., lack of facial expression while speaking, failure to maintain eye contact, failure to use gesture, and a lack of vocal inflection or emotional overlay), or it may occasionally manifest inappropriately as hypereuphoric or jocular speech.

II. **Impulsive responses** to complex questions are given with no apparent thought or regard for the listener's reaction. The responses given immediately are usually shallow, inaccurate, or inappropriate, and they reflect the RHCI patient's refusal to admit their uncertainty or lack of knowledge.

III. **Interpretive-response difficulties** result in a tendency to use more explicit (i.e., excessive irrelevant details because of a failure to distinguish significant from insignificant information) rather than interpretive concepts in the response (e.g., "the young woman in her mid-twenties breastfeeding the baby" rather than interpreting it as the "mother breastfeeding the baby").

IV. **Overpersonalized responses** (i.e., excessive reliance on personal or internal associations) are given because it is easier to reminisce than to interact when one is uncertain about the nature of the conversation or unsure of how to organize an opinion or explanation.

2. **Nonlinguistic deficits** comprise the underlying pathomechanism of RHCI and are usually manifested in the extralinguistic aspects of communication. In the rehabilitation setting, the nonlinguistic deficits (i.e., attentional and perceptual disorders) can make ambulation and activities of daily living (ADL) training more difficult and can lead to multiple accidents and falls.

a. ***Attentional disorders*** have recently been shown to involve space in general, rather than being limited only to the contralateral (left) side. Attentional disorders involve the inability to focus attention as well as difficulty deciding which features require attention. Specifically, they include the inability to recognize the boundaries of relevant space, to recognize significant features within that space, and to act upon those features.

I. **Unilateral spatial neglect (USN) (left-sided neglect)** is the inability to register and to integrate stimuli and perceptions from the one side (usually left side) of the body and environment. Patients with pure USN (i.e., without homonymous hemianopsia) have intact vision but seem unaware of the problem and do not attempt to compensate spontaneously by turning their head. In contrast, patients with left homonymous hemianopia have actual loss of vision from the left visual field of both eyes and may be aware of the problem and automatically compensate by turning their head. An extreme case of USN is *anosognosia,* in which the patient not only completely neglects the left paralyzed side (and the left environment), but they may even deny that the left limbs belong to them.

- **Sensory neglect** can lead to disrupted input of sensory stimulation from the left side (e.g., failure to read the left side of a book page), hence decreased ability to integrate concrete sensory and perhaps even abstract information. Tests include the visual field cut test to rule out coexisting homonymous hemianopsia and the cortical sensory extinction using simultaneous bilateral stimulation in the visual, auditory, and tactile modalities.

- **Motor neglect** can lead to impairment in the interaction with and the exploration or manipulation of the left-sided external space (e.g., impaired use of left-sided margins and punctuation in writing). Constructional abilities and scanning (e.g., visual scanning or tracking) can also be impaired.

II. **Confusion** can result from impaired contextual processing and impaired visual associations. It can lead to an inability to attend adequately to environmental cues resulting in *reduplicative paramnesia* (i.e., geographic disorientation in which the patient is convinced he or she is in another location), *prosopagnosia* (i.e., inability to recognize familiar faces), or topographical disorientation (i.e., inability to get to the destination).

b. ***Perceptual disorders (visuospatial perceptual deficits)*** can lead to impairment in the rapid recognition and synthesis of features into a form that is more than the sum of its parts (i.e., bits of information are seen but not integrated).

3. **Linguistic deficits** in RHCI, if present, are usually mild. They include problems in word finding (e.g., confrontation naming, body-part naming, and word fluency), auditory comprehension of complex material, oral sentence reading, and writing (e.g., dysgraphia, which manifests as substitutions, repetitions, and omissions of words). Their speech also tends to be monotonous.

B. **ASSESSMENT**. The only formal assessment tool for RHCI is the Rehabilitation Institute of Chicago Evaluation of Communication Problems in Right Hemisphere Dysfunction (RIC-ECPRHD), which provides a check list and rating scale for pragmatic functions (e.g., eye contact and facial gestures), interpretation of metaphorical language, memory skills, writing, visual scanning and tracking, and an analysis of conversation including topic maintenance, verbosity, and reference. The screening battery for assessing cognition in patients with right-sided stroke is an informal tool that screens basic language skills; analyzes single word responses to part–whole tasks, oral opposites, written opposites, oral analogies, and printed analogies; evaluates interpretation of idioms, proverbs, effects of imagery; and evaluates the ability to appreciate humor. Other related tests include tests for visual perception (e.g., Spatial Orientation Memory Test and the Hooper Test of Visual Organization), tests of verbal or nonverbal relationships (e.g., subtests of Detroit Test of Learning Aptitude and Woodcock–Johnson Psycho-Educational Battery respectively); tests of language function (e.g., standard aphasia battery and "Cookie Theft" picture subtest from Boston Diagnostic Aphasia Examination), and cognitive test batteries (e.g., mathematics subtest to assess mathematics skills, which can be impaired in patients with RHCI).

1. **Extralinguistic tests** assess interpretative skills that measure ability to distinguish relevant from irrelevant information (e.g., "Cookie Theft" picture description and story interpretation; Woodcock–Johnson Psycho-Educational Battery to determine nonverbal ability to see relationship; Detroit Test of Learning Aptitude to assess verbal relationship using analogy tests), organizational skills (e.g., ask patient for opinion on topic of current interest), pragmatic skills (e.g., RIC-ECPRHD to rate pragmatic functions such as facial gestures during conversation), emotional responsiveness (e.g., explain emotional content in pictures and stories), and prosodic skills (e.g., read aloud sentences in a happy, sad, or angry tone).

2. **Nonlinguistic testings** include neuropsychological examinations for motor neglect (e.g., spontaneous drawing and copy drawing of symmetrical objects to determine left vs. right details; line bisection tasks to establish sense of midline; and cancellation tests such as uncrossing of lines to determine severity of neglect), sensory neglect (e.g., visual field cuts and cortical extinction), visual perception (e.g., Hooper Test of Visual Organization and the Spatial Orientation Memory Test), attention (i.e., short and immediate memory, e.g., digit span and

story retelling), and confusion (e.g., orientation to place and recognition of familiar faces).

3. **Linguistic tests** include the standard aphasia battery or its subtests, the standard reading battery, and the test of writing skills. Even if language appears normal, standardized language tests (to assess visual confrontational naming, word fluency, auditory and written paragraph comprehension, and reading and writing skills) are useful.

C. **PROGNOSIS** for recovery from RHCI, as in aphasia, is affected by the site and size of the lesion, age, and degree of lateralization. Neglect symptoms in stroke patients usually subside 6 months after the stroke onset. If neglect persists beyond the first few months, the prognosis for improvement seems to be poor.

D. **TREATMENT** for extralinguistic deficits should not only be focused on compensatory strategies but should also incorporate treatments for the underlying nonlinguistic problems. Nonlinguistic deficits can be approached through patient education and through feedback paradigms. The patient is trained to increase awareness of the neglected side by initially presenting stimuli (especially those specialized for the right hemisphere, e.g., shapes or blocks) on the intact side, gradually shifting the stimuli to the midline then to the neglected side. The patient is given training on anchoring visual attention to a certain starting point, systematic scanning (e.g., left-to-right visual scanning), slowing down their performance, recognizing errors and stimulus load via feedback, and manipulating the complexity of the task. He or she is also taught to position the head and eye toward the involved field. During physical therapy, weight bearing (after proper splinting) of the affected side and stimulation of the proprioceptors of the affected joints may provide effective feedback to improve limb perception. Aside from awareness skills, techniques to facilitate recovery of deficits in perception and attention (e.g., "edgeness" and "bookness") may also be used. For linguistic deficits, an aphasia treatment regimen may be used. The following techniques are used in RHCI patients with nonlinguistic and extralinguistic deficits.

1. **Perception- and attention-recovery techniques**

a. ***"Edgeness" technique*** requires the patient to detect (using both visual and tactile tracing methods) the boundaries of relevant space (e.g., a grid) and to explore within the boundaries (e.g., by asking the patient to find colored cubes placed in varying locations on the grid). After practicing with the grid, the patient progresses to the perimeter of any surface (e.g., lapboard or table) on which they are working.

b. ***"Bookness" technique*** is an extension of the "edgeness" technique. The patient is asked to use the eyes to trace the outline of the book and to describe what he or she sees. This is done on every reading session, first with the book closed then with the book opened. It also includes reading tasks that involve matching stimuli on the left page with those on the right page. Initial stimuli include shapes that progress to letters, words, and, finally, sentences. In the "bookness" technique, the concept of reading is treated as a whole instead of a left-to-right scanning task.

2. **Compensatory strategies** involve teaching the RHCI patient to use unimpaired language capabilities (e.g., auditory or visual) to compensate for the impaired visuomotor skills. The patient is given tasks that help him or her to pay attention to the contextual and pragmatic cues (e.g., facial expression and tone); to reduce verbosity; to improve the ability to maintain a conversational topic; to retell stories in a fashion that highlights the relevant points; and to produce language that follows a logical sequence. Feedback may be given to the patient in individual (e.g., by cueing from the clinician and playing back taped conversations) or group sessions.

3. **Interdisciplinary team approach** emphasizes active involvement of the entire rehabilitation team. The patient's family or significant others (as well as the rest of the rehabilitation team) are not only counseled on the impact of RHCI on the patient and their own perception of the patient's personality, but they are instructed in a consistent approach for treatment. For example, the whole team should be involved in providing feedback cues on pragmatic skills and in listing step-by-step the approach to accomplishing transfers, ambulation, or other activities of daily living.

III. Speech disorders

A. **APRAXIA OF SPEECH (AOS)** is a nondysarthric, nonaphasic sensorimotor disorder of articulation and prosody (prosody is defined in section I.A.1.a). Apraxia of speech is similar to other kinds of motor apraxia in that it involves the person's inability to initiate and execute learned voluntary movements (e.g., speech articulation) in the absence of actual paralysis, incoordination, sensory loss, or incomprehension of or inattention to commands. The person hears and understands the requested task, and knows that he is physically capable of performing this task, but when he attempts to do it, he cannot execute the movements or series of movements needed to complete the task. In patients with AOS, most vegetative and reflexive actions (e.g., coughing or chewing) are intact; however, higher cortical functions are disrupted, specifically the brain's ability to program the positioning of the speech musculature and to sequence the movements for volitional production of speech.

The lesion of AOS is typically in the left frontal lobe adjacent to Broca's area. This has led to controversy as to whether AOS is a separate entity or part of aphasia. Although AOS can coexist with aphasia and dysarthia, AOS has unique features (e.g., relatively normal pronunciation of serial or automatic speech, absence of significant motor control problems, inconsistent articulatory errors, and rare involvement of the respiratory or phonatory subsystems) that distinguishes it from both disorders. The linguistic hallmarks of AOS include (a) articulatory errors (i.e., omissions, substitution, distortions, additions, and repetition of speech sounds) that are highly inconsistent on repeated productions of the same utterance and that vary with the complexity of the sound patterns and length of target words; moreover, the errors are increased when using less frequently articulated words and decreased with successive repetition of the word; (b) difficulty with initial consonants and in initiating an utterance; (c) effortful, trial-and-error groping for the proper articulatory position or sequence of positions; although the speaker is often aware of errors, he or she is usually unable to anticipate, modify, or correct them; attempts to monitor and anticipate errors often leads to a slowed speech rate; (d) automatic-spontaneous speech (e.g., counting 1 to 10) is usually intact while volitional-purposeful speech (e.g., counting backwards from 10 to 1) is impaired; and (e) dysprosody unrelieved by extended periods of normal rhythm, stress, and intonation.

1. **Assessment**

a. ***Language screening tests*** are similar to those used in aphasia (see section I.A.2) and are performed routinely because AOS almost always coexists with aphasia. Aphasia tests for patients with AOS show relatively intact auditory and reading comprehension skills, and better writing than speaking skills.

b. ***Speech production tests*** are used to elicit simple and progressively more complex volitional utterances under varying conditions (e.g., by imitation, oral reading, or spontaneous speech).

2. **Treatment** for AOS is usually concomitant with treatment for coexisting aphasia or dysarthria. If accompanied by moderate to severe aphasia, there is poor prognosis for AOS recovery. The treatment goals for AOS are to improve volitional control of the oral musculature for speech purposes and to teach communication strategies that get the message across in the most efficient and effective manner possible. There are some studies that show the beneficial effects of speech therapy even in patients with severe AOS. Long-term recovery of AOS (up to 10 years) has been reported in case studies. As with aphasia treatment, AOS treatment can be categorized into the retraining approach and the compensatory approach.

a. ***Retraining approaches*** involve teaching patients with AOS how to program sound patterns to shift from one sound to another and to use preserved melodic and rhythmic patterns to improve their articulation and speech. They are given articulation drills, which start at simple tasks and proceed to exercises of increasing complexity under constant supervision and correction. The drills that are designed to improve phonetic placement accuracy typically use imitation, stress, and progressive approximation. The cues used for retraining include auditory (i.e., rhythm), visual (i.e., spatial), and kinesthetic (i.e., movement) cues. The AOS patients begin with nonoral imitation, followed by sounds, utterances, words, and finally phrases. They are advanced from limited, automatic reactive speech to appropriate, volitional-purposeful communication to progressively meaningful speech sound sequencing. Based on AOS severity, the following specific strategies are recommended: expanded contrastive stress for mild AOS; inter- and intrasystemic facilitators for moderate AOS; and contrastive stress drills, imitation of contrasts, and segmental/syllabic level imitation for severe AOS.

   I. **Rate and melodic (rhythmic) flow training** emphasizes stress and intonation in which the patient generates the rhythm to facilitate articulation accuracy. Examples include intersystemic facilitators (e.g., tapping foot, tapping leg, finger-counting, and finger-tapping), intrasystemic facilitators (e.g., pacing board), and expanded contrastive stress drills.

   II. **Kinesthetic awareness (movement units) plus rate-and-melody flow training**, for example, contrastive stress drills, which consist of repetitive practice of contrasting words (e.g., pin–bin and day–may) to promote kinesthetic awareness of speech units and facilitate articulation accuracy.

   III. **Postural shaping (spatial targeting) plus kinesthetic awareness training**, for example, imitation of contrasts technique.

   IV. **Postural shaping training**, for example, segmental/syllabic level imitation (with imitation, phonetic placement, phonetic derivation, derivation and placement, and key word techniques).

b. ***Compensatory approaches*** focus on using residual function (e.g., nonverbal means rather than language-based drills) for communication. Examples include **melodic intonation therapy (MIT)**, which uses natural melody patterns (a right hemisphere function) to facilitate speech in nonfluent aphasics with good comprehension; and Amer-Ind code training, which uses gestures modified from the American Indian sign language to facilitate speech; and eight-step task continuum with integral stimulation in which the clinician elicits a patient response (utterance) by using cues ranging from spoken words, to mime, written words, and role playing.

B. **DYSARTHRIA** is strictly a problem with the motor control of speech, affecting articulation (e.g., in stroke patients with upper motor neuron lesions resulting in weakness, spasticity, and slowness of motor speech). Patients with pure dysarthria have intact language function (i.e., they are able to retrieve words and comprehend and express both written and spoken language). The layman's term *slurred speech* is inaccurate as it refers to only one component of dysarthria. The three features of dysarthria that distinguish it from AOS are: impairment of the automatic (i.e., nonspeech) movements, highly consistent articulatory errors, and involvement of all speech subsystems (including respiration and phonation). In contrast, AOS has intact automatic movements, inconsistent articulatory errors, and rare involvement of respiratory or phonatory subsystems.

1. **Classification of dysarthria (Mayo Clinic classification)**

a. ***Flaccid dysarthria*** is characterized by a breathy voice (reduced speech volume and audible exhalation), hypernasality (with nasal emission of air during speech), and imprecise articulation of consonants and vowels. It is caused by hypotonia, muscular weakness (e.g., of the tongue and lips), and failure to generate sufficient intraoral breath pressure because of velopharyngeal incompetence. It is seen in patients with bulbar palsy, facial palsy, poliomyelitis, myasthenia gravis, stroke, tumor, trauma, or infection of the lower motor neurons.

b. ***Spastic dysarthria*** is characterized by slow and labored speech, imprecise consonant articulation, low and monotonous pitch, a harsh quality to the voice (strained-strangled voice), and hypernasality. It is caused by hypertonia leading to slow, weak movements with reduced range. It is seen in patients with pseudobulbar palsy, spastic cerebral palsy, encephalitis, and stroke, tumor, trauma, or infection involving the upper motor neurons.

c. ***Ataxic dysarthria*** is characterized by irregular, imprecise consonant articulation, distorted vowel production, excessive loudness variation, "excess and equal" pattern of syllable stress, and an occasionally harsh voice. It is caused by hypotonia and slow movement with inaccurate range, timing, and direction. It occurs in patients with Friedreich's ataxia, ataxic cerebral palsy, alcohol intoxication, multiple sclerosis, and stroke, tumor, trauma, or infection involving the cerebellar system.

d. ***Hypokinetic dysarthria*** is characterized by monotonous pitch and loudness, reduced speech stress, short rushes of speech with inappropriate silences, reduced speech volume and rate, blurring of consonant articulation, and difficulty in initiating articulation (with repetition of initial sounds). It is caused by slow movements with limited range, rigidity, paucity of movement, loss of automatic aspects of movement, resting tremor, and variable speed of repetitive movements. It is seen in patients with Parkinson's disease or drug-induced (e.g., reserpine or phenothiazine) disorders of the extrapyramidal system.

e. ***Hyperkinetic dysarthria*** occurs in patients with excessive motor activity as a result of extrapyramidal system (EPS) disorders.

I. **Predominantly quick pattern** is caused by quick, unsustained, random, involuntary movements (e.g., tics and myoclonic jerks) with variable muscle tone. These result in an altered breathing cycle, which causes sudden exhalatory gusts of breath, bursts of loudness, elevations of pitch, imprecise consonants, distorted vowels, abnormally prolonged, variable speaking rate, monopitch, inappropriate silences, harsh voice quality, and overall increase in loudness. It is seen in patients with chorea, myoclonus, Tourette's syndrome, or ballism.

II. **Predominantly slow pattern** is caused by involuntary body and facial movements (sustained, distorted twisting and writhing movements and postures, slowness, and hypertonus), which leads to unpredictable voice stoppages, imprecise consonant articulation, prolonged and distorted vowels, excessive loudness variation, a harsh voice (strained and strangled quality), monotonous pitch and loudness, and irregular articulatory breakdowns. It is seen in patients with dystonia, dyskinesia (e.g., torticollis and tardive dyskinesia), athetosis (or choreoathetosis), stroke, tumor, infection, or drug-induced (e.g., tranquilizers) disorders of the EPS.

f. ***Mixed dysarthria*** pattern has components of different dysarthric types and occurs in patients with extensive neurologic involvement. It can be spastic-flaccid (amyotrophic lateral sclerosis, stroke, head trauma), spastic-ataxic hypokinetic (Wilson's disease), or spastic-ataxic-flaccid or variable (multiple sclerosis).

2. Dysarthria assessment

a. ***Speech impairment assessment techniques*** includes perceptual tools (which rely on the trained eyes and ears of the clinician) and the use of instruments (to measure acoustic, aerodynamic movement, or myoelectric aspects of speech). They systematically evaluate the different subsystems along the vocal tract where speech activities occur. The following have rating scales that indicate the severity of the impairment of each subsystem.

I. **Respiratory subsystem measurements** include perceptual tools (i.e., ratings of the number of words per breath, loudness of samples of connected speech, and visual observation of clavicular breathing) and instrumental tools (i.e., respiratory inductive plethysmography to measure movement of the rib cage and abdomen during breathing and speech; acoustic measure of vocal intensity and utterance durations; and aerodynamic measurement of subglottal air pressure).

II. **Phonatory or laryngeal subsystem measurements** include perceptual tools that rate pitch characteristics (pitch level, pitch breaks, monopitch, voice tremor), loudness (monoloudness, excess loudness, variation of volume), and voice quality (harsh voice, hoarseness, wet voice, breathiness, strained and strangled voice). It also includes instrumental tools, that is, acoustic measures of frequency and intensity, and aerodynamic measures of laryngeal resistance.

III. **Velopharyngeal subsystem measurements** include perceptual tools (i.e., judgment of hypernasality or occurrence of nasal air emission) and instrumental tools (i.e., acoustic measurement of nasalization; aerodynamic measures of air pressure and air flow during selected speech samples; and cineradiographic techniques to measure velopharyngeal movement).

IV. **Oral articulation subsystem measurements** include perceptual tools (i.e., rating of consonant and vowel precision) and instrumental tools (i.e., the use of cineradiographic and electromyographic recordings).

b. ***Speech functional disability assessment techniques*** include measurements of speech intelligibility, rate, and naturalness to determine severity of disability, monitor progress over time, and measure the effectiveness of specific interventional techniques. Among these, intelligibility tests (e.g., standardized tools to measure single word and sentence intelligibility) are most commonly used to assess the index of overall speech adequacy.

3. Treatment of dysarthria in nonprogressive disorders focuses mainly on maximizing speech intelligibility. Unfortunately, this is not always a realistic goal, especially in patients who are unable to communicate verbally because of severe impairment in intelligibility; therefore, alternative means of communication and augmentative communication devices may be used. In patients with progressive disorders (e.g., Parkinson's disease, multiple sclerosis, and amyotrophic lateral sclerosis), the patients are initially encouraged to maximize the functional communication level by addressing the speech volume [an example is the Lee Silverman Voice Treatment (LSVT) for patients with PD, which focuses exclusively on vocal loudness and involves calibration of the patient's sense of vocal effort and loudness] and articulatory precision. Subsequently the patients need to modify speaking patterns by controlling rate, consonant emphasis, and reducing the number of words per breath. In severe cases, a communication augmentation system may be considered.

a. ***Techniques that maximize speech intelligibility*** can be enhanced through breathing exercises (to facilitate control of pitch, phonation, and volume), or exercises of the tongue, mouth, and facial muscles (to help improve control of oral musculature), or exercises that strengthen the soft palate and adjacent muscles (to counteract hypernasality). The efficacy of oromotor exercises, however, is controversial.

I. **Rate control**, that is, slowing the rate of speech, is often used in patients with coordination problems (e.g., ataxic dysarthria) and patients with Parkinson's disease. Techniques include pacing boards, alphabet supplementation, rhythmic cueing (computerized or clinician-controlled), delayed auditory feedback, and the use of an oscilloscope (for visual feedback).

II. **Precision training** involves techniques that emphasize speech sounds in the final position of words, controls the number of words per breath, and stresses important words in a sentence. Techniques used include articulatory drills and natural stress patterning. Exercises involving the tongue, mouth, and facial muscles help improve control of oral musculature.

III. **Palatal lift fitting** uses a dental retainer to elevate the soft palate to the height necessary to reduce hypernasality and nasal emission. When fitted properly, it allows certain dysarthric speakers to better produce speech sounds that require the build up of oral air pressure (e.g., /p/, /t/, and /d/).

b. ***Functional speech training*** includes exercises in the production of sounds, melodic flow of speech, or coordination of respiration and speaking.

c. ***Augmentative and alternative communication systems*** are used in patients who are unable to communicate verbally to augment, supplement, or replace verbal and/or written communication. They include communication boards, books, or computer-based systems, which employ speech synthesis and printed output.

IV. Voice disorders

Voice disorders exist when the quality, pitch, or loudness of the voice differs from that of other persons of similar age, sex, cultural background, and geographic location. A common defining feature of a voice disorder is when a given voice draws attention to the speaker. Disorders range from aphonia (no voice) to various dysphonias (disorders of sound quality). In PM&R, voice disorders of neurological origins are commonly encountered. They may be the result of unilateral or bilateral vocal cord paralysis (e.g., after intubation or in tracheostomized patients). Patients with cords fixed in an adducted position usually require a tracheostomy (see Chapter 5.12, section V.A.2) to maintain a functional airway. Voice disorders of psychosocial origin may require psychological intervention in concert with the speech-therapy voice regimen.

A. ASSESSMENT. Voice disorders must be referred to an otolaryngologist [ear, nose, and throat (ENT) specialist] to rule out organic (e.g., laryngitis; laryngeal ulcers, nodules, polyps, or cancer; and laryngeal paralysis) or functional (e.g., psychogenic or hysterical) causes. If there is no need for further medical or surgical intervention, the patient is referred to a speech–language pathologist for voice assessment, which typically includes an extensive interview, oral peripheral examination, voice analysis (including respiration, phonation, resonance, and prosody), as well as an objective voice analysis using instrumentation. The purpose is to uncover the factors contributing to the vocal problem (e.g., voice misuse or abuse, smoking, and alcohol use); to determine the patient's stimulability to achieve an improved vocal cord approximation; to gauge the degree of the patient's understanding of the disorder; and, finally, to assess the patient's willingness to participate in a remediation program.

B. TREATMENT for dysphonia typically involves a systematic step-by-step patient education and implementation regimen attempting to identify misuse or abuse, describe the effects of the patterns of misuse or abuse, define the specific instances or circumstances of abuse or misuse, modify the behavior, and monitor vocal change. The regimen may include periods of voice rest and often includes counseling to reduce or eliminate substance abuse. Management of the vocal components basically involves re-establishing the proper coordination of respiration, phonation, resonance, and prosody and determining appropriate pitch, quality, and intensity.

1. Speaking options

a. ***Nontracheostomized patients with laryngectomy.*** Speaking options include the use of electrolarynx prosthesis (e.g., a neck type or intraoral type, which must be coordinated in placement and timing with articulated speech), artificial larynx (to generate sound for speech production purposes), esophageal voice (produced by oral injection of air into the esophagus followed by a rapid vibrating expulsion), and tracheoesophageal shunt (a one-way valve prosthesis, which permits air to pass from the trachea into the esophagus, producing an "esophageal sound" within the esophagus).

b. ***Tracheostomized patients.*** Speaking options include the allowing of air leakage into the larynx [e.g., by using uncuffed tracheostomy tubes (TT), cuff-deflated fenestrated or unfenestrated TT, smaller size TT, tracheal buttons, or tracheal plugs]; the use of talking tracheostomy tubes (e.g., Portex "Talk" tube, Communi-trach); and the use of one-way speaking valves (e.g., Passy-Muir Speaking Valve, Olympic Trach-talk). These are discussed in Chapter 5.12, sections V.A.2.b.4 and 5.

2. Nonspeaking options include the use of writing, complex and simple gestures, communication boards, or portable personal computers.

V. Fluency disorders (stuttering)

Fluency disorders are defined as the phenomenon of gaps, prolongations, or involuntary repetitions of a sound or syllable that occur during speech production. The most common type of stuttering is developmental and is beyond the scope of physiatry. The acquired type is fairly rare (only 2% of cases estimated after the age of 10 years) but is occasionally encountered by the physiatrist; therefore, only this type is discussed. Acquired stuttering is primarily the result of brain injury and is thus also called neurogenic or cortical stuttering. Non-neurogenic stuttering (i.e., psychogenic and malingering) is extremely rare.

A. CLASSIFICATION of neurogenic stuttering can be subdivided into dysarthric (poor motor speech control), dyspraxic (poor volitional vocal control because of impaired motor programming), and dysnomic (word-finding problem).

B. ASSESSMENT of neurogenic stuttering should include a detailed history relating to its onset; an oral peripheral examination; a voice, speech, language, and cognitive screen; and an extensive speech sample that includes imitation, oral reading, narrative discourse, conversation, and singing. Differential diagnoses of neurogenic stuttering include palalalia (a paroxysmal speech characterized by sudden involuntary vocalizations such as rhythmic repetitions of syllables, words, and phrases; the words or phrase repetition gets faster and faster with each repetition and may or may not become more unintelligible); multiple self-corrections (may be seen in fluent aphasics); psychogenic stuttering (caused by emotional trauma); or malingering stuttering (faked for some secondary gain).

C. TREATMENT of neurogenic stuttering has been reported to be effective for all three subtypes. This includes patient education and counseling; breathing exercises to control phonation; the use of masking noise to distract speakers from their own speech; the use of delayed auditory feedback forcing the speaker to reduce speech rate; and use of pacing strategies such as finger- or foot-tapping.

VI. Hearing impairment

Hearing impairment interferes with the patient's quality of life by hampering free and easy communication. It most commonly leads to depression and social isolation. In patients with severe hearing loss, paranoid behaviors have been reported. In the United States, 20 million Americans, or one in 10, have some degree of hearing loss. About 12 million Americans have serious hearing impairment, and 2 million are either totally deaf or lack sufficient hearing to understand speech. Any PM&R patients with hearing loss should be referred to an otologist (for diagnosis and management of medical and surgical hearing problems) and to an audiologist (for audiologic testing and management). The physiatrist should be able to detect basic hearing problems and know the available tests and treatment options.

A. CLASSIFICATION. Hearing impairment can be categorized as temporary, progressive, or permanent; unilateral or bilateral; and partial (i.e., hard of hearing) or complete (i.e., deaf).

The following classification of hearing impairment is by site of structural damage (using audiograms):

1. **Conductive hearing impairment** results from involvement of the outer and middle ear systems. Possible causes include external blockage, perforated ear drum, otitis media, and otosclerosis.
2. **Sensorineural hearing impairment** stems from damage to the inner ear or neural fibers of the eighth cranial nerve. Possible causes include presbycusis, hereditary hearing loss, trauma, tumors, noise, viral and bacterial illness, or Ménière's disease.
3. **Mixed hearing impairment** comprises both conductive and sensorineural components. Possible causes are the same as for sensorineural hearing impairment.
4. **Central hearing impairment** influences one's ability to comprehend spoken language and is related to damage in the auditory pathways of the brain. Possible causes include trauma, tumors, and vascular damage.

B. ASSESSMENT

1. **Pure tone audiometry** is used to classify hearing impairment.

a. ***Air conduction audiometry*** provides information on the degree of hearing impairment as well as the configuration of the hearing loss. It measures each ear separately using earphones. A hearing impairment can be the result of a disorder anywhere in the auditory system from external auditory canal to the brain.

b. ***Bone conduction audiometry*** uses a small vibrator placed on the mastoid process to bypass the outer and middle ear, thus reflecting only the sensitivity of the sensorineural system. A masking noise in the nontest ear ensures that bone conduction is not perceived by the nontest ear.

2. **Speech audiometry** tests the patient's ability to discriminate (i.e., recognize or understand) speech. It augments the findings of pure tone audiometry and helps determine the extent of a patient's hearing loss and tolerance. It is used in hearing aid evaluations. Speech audiometry tests are usually presented through earphones in either ear (monoaurally) or in both ears simultaneously (biaurally).

Other less common modes of testing are through a bone-conduction vibrator or in the sound field through a loudspeaker. The patient is then asked to repeat back each word heard.

a. ***Speech threshold testing*** measures the speech reception threshold (SRT), which is the softest intensity level at which 50% of spondees (i.e., familiar two-syllable words pronounced with equal stress and effort such as "hotdog" or "baseball") are correctly repeated. Normally, the SRT should agree within +10 dB of the pure tone average (PTA) threshold levels at 500, 1000, and 2000 Hz. Otherwise, hearing loss is suspected.

b. ***Word discrimination (WD) test (or speech discrimination test)*** analyzes the patient's ability to understand words and is not a threshold or sensitivity test. It measures the word discrimination score (WDS), which is the percentage of words correctly repeated. The words, which are phonetically balanced (e.g., darn or art), are presented at comfortably loud levels to the patient from a standardized list of 25 or 50 single-syllable words. The WDS interpretations are as follows: 90–100% (normal limits); 75–90% (slight difficulty in discrimination); 60–75% (moderate difficulty in discrimination); 50–60% (poor discrimination, i.e., marked difficulty in following conversation); and less than 50% (very poor discrimination, probably unable to follow running speech).

3. **Auditory tests for site-of-lesion** are special tests indicated for patients with asymmetric sensorineural or clinical suspicion of eighth nerve or central auditory involvement. They include the loudness recruitment tests (to measure the growth of loudness in the pathological ear as compared to normal subjects); differential intensity discrimination tests (to determine the smallest change in intensity that can be recognized as a change in loudness); threshold tone decay tests (to determine the rates at which tones fade away from audibility); Bekesy audiometry (to determine the ability to detect the presence of transient changes in intensity); measurements of impedance (static and dynamic impedance tests) and compliance in the plane of the tympanic membrane (tympanometry); brainstem auditory evoked potentials audiometry (the electrophysiologic analysis of brainstem auditory evoked potentials, which is sensitive for diagnosing cochlear tumors); and electrocochleography (which measures electrophysiologic signals from the cochlea).

C. TREATMENT

1. **Hearing aid** is a miniature amplifier that amplifies sound intensity for the hearing-impaired ear. It is indicated for patients with hearing loss above 40 dB because of difficulty in understanding normal speech. For its successful use, patients must accept their hearing difficulties and express their desire to improve, be motivated, have positive attitudes, and have a good support system. Aside from being easy to use, affordable, and cosmetically appealing, the ideal hearing aid should provide the lowest SRT, the highest WDS, a most comfortable loudness level close to the level of normal conversation, a broad range of comfortable loudness, and the least amount of noise and background interference.

a. ***Body- or pocket-hearing aids*** are housed in a case worn at chest level. Although powerful and durable, they are larger than other hearing aids and are uncosmetic. They are indicated for patients who have severe or profound hearing loss, as well as those with poor manual dexterity who are unable to manipulate smaller hearing aids.

b. ***Eyeglass hearing aids*** are housed in an eyeglass frame. They are seldom used because wearers find them annoying.

c. ***Behind-the-ear (BTE) aids*** fit into a curved base that rests behind the ear. They are indicated for severe as well as mild and moderate hearing loss patients. They have a power equivalent to most body-hearing aids.

d. ***In-the-ear (ITE) hearing aids*** are custom-fitted into the ear concha. They are cosmetically appealing and easier to use than behind-the-ear aids.
e. ***In-the-canal (ITC) or custom-canal hearing aids*** are custom-molded to fit within the ear canal. Because of their extremely small size, they can only provide adequate amplification for patients with mild-to-moderate hearing loss. They are highly appealing cosmetically and are expensive.
f. ***Contralateral-routing-of-signals (CROS) hearing aids*** are indicated for patients with unilateral severe or profound hearing loss but with a normal contralateral ear. A microphone on the hearing-impaired ear transmits radio waves to a receiver unit attached to the normal ear. This permits the wearer to "hear" people speaking on their hearing-impaired ear side. A variation is the bi-CROS hearing aid, which is used in patients with bilateral hearing loss but whose poorer ear is not suitable for amplification.
g. ***Digital and programmable hearing aids*** use microchips to provide users with the following options: advanced signal processing (to automatically adjust the volume to incoming sounds); multichannel capability (to respond differently to low- and high-pitched sounds); multimemory capability (to allow the user to choose situation-specific computer programs for use in a variety of listening situations, i.e., quiet, small groups, large groups, telephone, listening to music, attending meetings, going to restaurants, etc.); multimicrophone capability (to allow the user to pick up sound either from a broad area or from a narrower listening range); and noise-reduction capability. They are operated by the user using a remote control, which can be hidden in a pocket or purse (this is in contrast to traditional hearing aids, which have a limited number of control options that are preset or manually adjusted). They can be reprogrammed if hearing changes. They can cost up to three to four times more than traditional hearing aids.

2. **Assistive listening devices (ALDs)** are designed to reduce the level of noise and background interferences in adverse listening situations. One form of ALD transmits sound directly from the source to the hearing-impaired listener through an infrared, audio loop, FM radio system, or direct audio input to the hearing aid. Other forms of ALDs include amplified telephones, low-frequency doorbells and telephone ringers, and closed-caption TV decoders. Visual cues (e.g., flashing alarm clocks, flashing smoke detectors, and use of typed messages via telephone modem) and vibration cues (e.g., alarm bed vibrators) may be used instead of sound to alert the hearing-impaired person.
3. **Speech-reading and auditory training** combines visual input and auditory input for understanding speech. Speech-reading teaches the patient how to interpret visual cues (e.g., facial expression, body movements, or gestures); however, only about one-third of English speech sounds are clearly visible. Hence, auditory training needs to be supplemented to teach the patient how to make the most effective use of the minimal auditory cues imposed by the hearing loss.
4. **Cochlear implants** are internal electrode wires surgically placed into the cochlea. They are connected to an external microphone and signal converter. Sound waves are converted into electrical impulses and are delivered directly to the cochlea. Cochlear implants are indicated for patients with profound sensorineural hearing loss. Although sound or speech can be detected (hence increasing the patient's environmental awareness), the patient is unable to understand or discriminate the speech.
5. **Tactile aids** convert sound into vibrations to provide the patient with awareness of sound. They are indicated in profoundly deaf patients who are not candidates for any of the aforementioned treatments.

Further reading

Adamovich BB, Henderson JA, Auerbach S: *Cognitive rehabilitation of closed head injury patients*, San Diego, 1985, College-Hill Press.

Benson DF, Ardila A: *Aphasia: a clinical perspective*, New York, 1996, Oxford University.

Cardenas DD, McLean Jr. A: Psychopharmacologic management of traumatic brain injury. *Phys Med Rehabil Clin North Am*, 3(2):273–290, 1992.

Chapey R, editor: *Language intervention strategies in aphasia and related neurogenic communication disorders*, ed 4, Philadelphia, 2001, Lippincott, Williams & Wilkins.

Chapman SB, Levin HS, Culhane KA: Language impairment in closed head injury. In Kirshner JS, editor: *Handbook of neurological speech and language disorders*, New York, 1995, Marcel Dekker, pp. 387–414.

Damasio AR: Aphasia. *N Engl J Med*, 326(8):531–539, 1992.

Frattali CM, Thompson CK, Holland AL, *et al.*: *American Speech and Hearing Association (ASHA): Functional assessment of communication skills for adults*, Rockville, MD, 1995, ASHA.

Kerman-Lerner P: Communication disorders. In Goodgold J, editor: *Rehabilitation medicine*, St Louis, 1988, Mosby-Year Book, pp. 787–814.

Kirk A, Kertesz: Assessment of aphasia. *Phys Med Rehabil State Art Rev* 6(3):433–450, 1992.

LaPointe L, editor: *Aphasia and related neurogenic language disorders*, New York, 1990, Thieme Medical Publisher.

Methe S, Huber W, Paradis M: Inventory and classification of rehabilitation methods. In Paradis M, editor: *Foundations of aphasia rehabilitation*, Oxford, 1993, Pergamon Press, pp. 3–60.

Miller RM, Groher ME, Yorkston KM, *et al.*: Speech, language, swallowing, and auditory rehabilitation. In DeLisa JA, Gans BM, Walsh NE, *et al.*, editors: *Physical medicine and rehabilitation: principles and practice*, ed 4, Philadelphia, 2005, Lippincott, Williams & Wilkins, pp. 1025–1050.

Nicholas ML, Helm-Estabrook N, Ward-Lonergan J, *et al.*: Evolution of severe aphasia in the first two years post onset. *Arch Phys Med Rehabil* 74:830–836, 1993.

Porcelli J: Aphasia assessment and treatment. *Phys Med Rehabil Clin North Am*, 2(3):487–500, 1991.

Rao PR: Adult communication disorders. In Braddom R, editor: *Physical medicine and rehabilitation*, Philadelphia, 1996, WB Saunders, pp. 49–65.

Sarno MT, editor: *Acquired aphasia*, ed 3, San Diego, CA, 1998, Academic Press.

Sarno MT: Neurogenic disorders of speech and language. In O'Sullivan SB, Schmitz TJ, editors: *Physical rehabilitation: assessment and treatment*, ed 4, Philadelphia, 2001, FA Davis, pp. 1001–1024.

Yorkston KM, Beukelman DR: Speech and language disorders. In Kottke FJ, Stillwell G, Lehmann JF, editors: *Krusen's handbook of physical medicine and rehabilitation*, ed 4, Philadelphia, 1990, WB Saunders, pp. 126–152.

Wertz RT, LaPointe LL, Rosenbeck JC: *Apraxia of speech in adults*, New York, 1984, Grune & Stratton.

CHAPTER 5.6
Dysphagia

Swallowing disorders of neurologic origin (which usually involve the oral or pharyngeal stage or both) are commonly managed by physiatrists in a multidisciplinary inpatient setting [involving the patient, family or significant others, swallowing therapist (usually a speech–language pathologist, in some clinics an occupational therapist), nutritionist or dietitian, rehabilitation nurse, home health attendant, respiratory care practitioner, radiologist, etc.]. In addition to neurogenic dysphagia, physiatrists also deal with non-neurogenic dysphagias such as those as a result of rheumatologic conditions (e.g., scleroderma, Sjögren's syndrome, systemic lupus erythematosus, mixed connective tissue disease, and rheumatoid arthritis) or foreign devices (e.g., tracheostomy tube). Although this chapter deals specifically with neurogenic dysphagia, most of the diagnostic and treatment strategies presented here can also be applied to dysphagia of non-neurogenic origin. For a discussion on assistive and adaptive equipment and strategies for oral feeding (i.e., food preparation and mechanisms for bringing food to the mouth), refer to Chapter 4.5, section II.A.3.a.

I. Pathophysiology

The pathophysiology of swallowing can be divided into four overlapping phases (see Logeman, 1998 for details and reference citations):

A. ORAL PREPARATORY PHASE involves food manipulation and, if needed, food mastication in the mouth, reducing it to a consistency ready to swallow. In this phase, the larynx and pharynx are at rest. Before oral preparatory movements can be initiated, sensory recognition of food approaching the mouth and being placed in the mouth is critical. To prevent spillage of food or liquid, intact labial musculature is needed to maintain a labial seal. The individual also has to have open nasal airway for nasal breathing. If there is no active chewing, the soft palate is pulled down and forward, sealing off the oral cavity from the pharynx. The individual may hold the food between the midline of the tongue and hard palate with the tongue tip elevated and contacting the anterior alveolar ridge ("tipper" position) or the food may be held on the floor of the mouth in front of the tongue ("dipper" position). For material requiring mastication, a rotary lateral movement of the mandible and tongue is needed. After chewing, the tongue pulls the food into a semicohesive bolus before the oral phase of swallow is initiated. Regardless of age, high masticatory performance was maintained in normal individuals with complete, or almost complete, dentition. Poor dentition or dentures is generally associated with more chewing strokes (Feldman *et al.*, 1980). Oral preparatory phase pathologies include:

- Decreased labial seal leading to anterior spillage and inability to remove food from utensil
- Tongue and buccal weakness (e.g., reduced range of tongue movement laterally during mastication, reduced range of tongue movement vertically, reduced tongue movement to form the bolus, reduced range and coordination of tongue movement to hold the bolus, reduced ability to hold the bolus in normal position; reduced buccal tension; buccal scarring) leading to difficulty in forming the bolus resulting in pooling or pocketing of food

between the cheeks and teeth, difficulty in retaining the bolus resulting in drooling, and difficulty in moving food to the back of the mouth

- Jaw weakness (e.g., reduced range of mandibular movement laterally) resulting in chewing difficulty
- Reduced oral sensitivity.

B. ORAL PHASE starts when the tongue propels the bolus posteriorly and ends when the pharyngeal swallow is triggered. It requires intact lingual musculature to propel the bolus posteriorly and intact buccal musculature to ensure the material does not fall into the lateral sulci. Bolus held in the dipper position is moved forward by the tongue and lifted onto the tongue into the tipper position. The midline of the tongue sequentially squeezes the bolus posteriorly against the hard palate. A central groove is then formed in the tongue, acting as a ramp or chute for the bolus to pass through as it moves posteriorly. The oral phase, which typically takes <1–1.5 seconds to complete, increases slightly as the viscosity of the bolus increases. More viscous foods also require greater lingual muscle activity. Older individuals tend to hold food using the dipper position with slightly longer oral phase of swallowing (Dodds *et al.*, 1989). The "normal" delay in the triggering of the pharyngeal swallow is also slightly longer. Oral phase pathologies include:

- Poor tongue coordination, i.e., slow diodochokinetic rate; disorganized patterns of anterior–posterior tongue movement (such as multiple anterior–posterior tongue movements or tongue pumping before swallow)
- Tongue thrust, i.e., tongue is pushed anteriorly against the central incisors to initiate swallow
- Reduced tongue strength, reduced anterior-posterior tongue movement, reduced tongue elevation
- Scarred tongue contour
- Problems with oral sequencing (e.g., delayed or absent triggering of the pharyngeal swallow) and swallowing apraxia, which results in aspiration before the swallow.

C. PHARYNGEAL PHASE is initiated as the leading edge of the bolus passes any point between the anterior faucial arches and the point where the tongue base crosses the lower rim of the mandible. Sensory receptors in the oropharynx and tongue itself (particularly deep propioceptive receptors) are stimulated, sending sensory information to the cortex and brainstem via cranial nerves (CN) V, VII, IX, and X. It is hypothesized that a sensory recognition center in the medulla in the nucleus tractus solitarus decodes the incoming sensory information and sends this information to the nucleus ambiguous, where either swallowing or a gag reflex is triggered. When the swallowing reflex is triggered, output is passed from the medulla to the nuclei of CN V, VII, IX, X, and XII and subsequently to the muscles they innervate.

This results in the triggering of the following pharyngeal swallowing reflex responses: (1) velopharyngeal closure, which occurs almost simultaneously with elevation and anterior movement of the hyoid and larynx; (2) closure of the larynx, which begins essentially simultaneously with cricopharyngeal opening; (3) ramping of the base of the tongue to deliver the bolus to the pharynx followed by tongue base retraction to contact the anteriorly bulging posterior pharyngeal wall; and (6) progressive top to bottom contraction in the pharyngeal constrictors (strictly speaking, this is not peristalsis because the pharynx is not a muscular tube). The function of the epiglottis seems to be directing of the bolus around the airway rather than over the top of the airway. During the pharyngeal phase, inspiration and expiration are inhibited to prevent aspiration. Pharyngeal transit time is typically ≤1 second. When it is over, very little residual food is left in the pharynx, even in older individuals. If pharyngeal swallow is not triggered, the bolus propelled by the tongue into the pharynx may be deposited in the valleculae or pyriform sinus. If the material is liquid, it may splash into the pharynx and into the open airway.

The strength of pharyngeal contraction is reduced as adults reach 70 years and beyond, resulting in some need to swallow a second time to clear residual material from the pharynx after the swallow. Although the penetration of material into the laryngeal vestibule is reported as increasing with frequency with age, there is no increase in aspiration in older adults (Robbins *et al.*, 1992). After cricopharyngeal opening was attained, hyoid and laryngeal elevation continued in young men but remained stable in old men, indicating that old men have reduced neuromuscular reserve. Moreover, old men have reduced flexibility in cricopharyngeal opening, that is, less change as volume increases. Both the reduction in reserve and in flexibility puts older individuals at increased risk for developing swallowing problems if they become physically weak as a result of any illness, even if it is not in the head and neck region.

Disorders affecting the pharyngeal stage of the swallow include:

- Pharyngeal dysfunction (e.g., bilateral reduction in pharyngeal contraction, unilateral pharyngeal paralysis, and scarred pharyngeal wall)
- Cervical osteophyte
- Pseudoepiglottis at the base of the tongue in total laryngectomees
- Cricopharyngeal dysfunction (e.g., failure of cricopharyngeal muscular portion of the cricopharyngeal or upper esophageal sphincter to relax adequately, thereby keeping the larynx from lifting and moving forward; reduced laryngeal motion up and forward; and/or poor pressure to drive the bolus through the sphincter and widen the opening)
- Laryngeal dysfunction (e.g., reduced laryngeal elevation, reduced laryngeal closure at the airway entrance, and reduced laryngeal closure at the vocal folds).

D. **ESOPHAGEAL PHASE** begins from the point where the bolus enters the esophagus at the cricopharyngeal juncture. Esophageal peristalsis then carries the bolus through the cervical and thoracic esophagus. The esophageal phase ends when the bolus passes into the stomach at the gastroesophageal juncture. Esophageal transit is typically from 8–20 seconds. In older adults, esophageal transit and clearance are slower and less efficient. Esophageal stage pathologies include esophageal pain and obstruction (e.g., stricture, tumor, web, spasms, and dysmotility) and gastroesophageal (GE) reflux.

II. Epidemiology

The overall incidence and prevalence of dysphagia is difficult to quantify as they vary according to the patient's stage of recovery from the underlying cause. Some of the reported incidences for dysphagia caused by specific neurologic disorders are stroke (up to 30–45%; 28% of all left hemispheric strokes; 21% of all right hemispheric strokes; up to 67% of brainstem strokes), traumatic brain injury (up to 27%), cerebral palsy (40%), parkinsonism (50–70%), myasthenia gravis (15–63%), and postpolio syndrome (18%).

III. Dysphagia evaluation

Evaluation of dysphagia is performed to screen for the presence or absence of a swallowing impairment; establish a possible local anatomic and physiologic cause for the dysphagia; assess the patient's ability to protect the airway (i.e., aspiration risk);

determine the practicality of oral feeding and/or recommend alternative methods for nutritional management; determine the need for additional specific diagnostic tests, studies, or referrals; and collect baseline clinical data, which can be used to chart changes in swallowing function of patients. Clinical (bedside) evaluation tends to underestimate aspiration occurrence in patients who are elderly, have expressive aphasia, and in whom more than 30 days have elapsed since the onset of injury. In most cases, because of the patient's altered mental status or severely impaired speech, information may be obtained from a health-care attendant, family member, or medical records. The swallowing evaluation is usually performed by the speech–language pathologist or occupational therapist with the radiologist, if necessary.

A. HISTORY

1. History of present illness

a. ***Dysphagia symptoms*** including duration, frequency (intermittent vs. constant), factors exacerbating or relieving the symptoms, influence of food texture (solids, semi-solids, and liquids; influence of hot and cold foods), and course of symptoms.

b. ***Associated symptoms*** including sensation of obstruction while swallowing, a "globus sensation" or foreign-body feeling, intermittent obstruction, mouth or throat pain (odynophagia), nasal regurgitation, foul mouth odor, choking or coughing while swallowing, change in speech and voice (e.g., wet voice), history of pneumonia, other respiratory symptoms (chronic cough, dyspnea, asthmatic episodes), GE reflux (sensation of heartburn, globus sensation, hiccups, a sour taste, dry throat, or pain in the throat or tongue), and chest pain (can be related to diffuse esophageal spasm).

c. ***Ancillary symptoms*** including weight loss, change in eating habits (e.g., avoidance of certain foods, such as lettuce, because of pharyngeal weakness; increase in eating time; decrease in usual meal size; increase in fluid intake with meals), decrease in appetite, change in taste, dry mouth, thickening of saliva consistency (e.g., as a result of chronic dehydration from impaired swallowing of liquids or related to mouth breathing, salivary gland dysfunction, or medications), change in speech or voice (hoarseness or temporary loss of voice, slurred or clumsy speech), and sleep disturbance (e.g., because of GE reflux).

2. Past history including neurologic conditions (e.g., stroke, traumatic brain injury, central nervous system infection, demyelinating disease, and motor neuron disease), previous swallowing examinations, neck problems (e.g., cervical spondylosis or ankylosis), dental disorders, presence of dentures, radiation therapy to the head and neck or mediastinum, cardiopulmonary disease (e.g., chronic obstructive pulmonary disease, congestive heart failure, and recurrent pneumonia), psychiatric and psychologic history (e.g., dementia), and surgery of the head, neck, or gastrointestinal tract.

3. Family history, for example, muscular dystrophy or myopathy.

4. Current medications that may contribute to dysphagia including sedatives (can cause disorientation and confusion), antispastics (can cause oropharyngeal muscle weakness), anticholinergics (can cause mucosal drying), antidepressants with anticholinergic effects, diuretics (can cause dehydration with drying of the mouth), antipsychotics or neuroleptics (can cause extrapyramidal symptoms, which may affect feeding and swallowing, such as tardive dyskinesia, dystonia, and pseudoparkinsonism), topical mouth anesthetics or denture powders with anesthetics, and any drugs that may decrease appetite. In addition, β-adrenergic drugs, theophylline, alcohol, and tobacco have been reported to lower or overcome esophageal sphincter tone and promote GE reflux.

B. PHYSICAL EXAMINATION

1. General inspection including current feeding methods [e.g., oral route vs. extraoral route, such as through nasogastric tube (NGT), surgically placed gastrostomy, percutaneous endoscopic gastrostomy (PEG), or percutaneous endoscopic jejunostomy (PEJ)], presence of tracheostomy (note the type and size of tube and the status of the cuff, i.e., inflated, partially inflated, or deflated), nutrition and hydration status, and presence or absence of drooling.

2. **Oropharyngeal status** including lip protrusion or closure, lip and mandibular tone, range of motion (ROM), strength, and sensation of the lips, tongue, and mandible; abnormal oropharyngeal reflexes; teeth condition (e.g., dental plates, false dentures, and malocclusion); and oropharyngeal mucosa condition (e.g., dryness, tenacious mucus, sores, odor, and presence of pocketed food).
3. **Pulmonary system** including rate and depth of breathing (too rapid and shallow breathing can affect timing of swallowing), cough reflex (voluntary and involuntary cough, cough strength, measurement of vital capacity to predict cough effectiveness), and chest auscultation to rule out pneumonia or chronic obstructive pulmonary disease.
4. **Musculoskeletal system** including posture, deformity, muscle tone (spasticity, flaccidity, rigidity, dystonia), and ROM, strength and coordination of the neck and limbs.
5. **Neurologic system**

a. ***Mental status*** including level of consciousness, cognition (i.e., alertness, orientation, attention, judgment, memory, ability to cooperate and follow instructions), behavioral characteristics (e.g., agitation and impulsivity), and perception (e.g., unilateral neglect).

b. ***Language ability***, such as receptive and expressive aphasia, to determine the ability to communicate and follow instructions.

c. ***Speech and voice*** including quality and strength of voice (e.g., a hoarse voice may indicate reduced laryngeal closure; a wet or gurgly voice, extreme breathiness, or loss of voice may indicate pooling of saliva or secretions at the laryngeal level and possible acute aspiration); phonation (e.g., hypernasality may suggest impaired palatopharyngeal function; hyponasality may imply filling of the nasopharynx or occlusion of the nasal passages); and speed and precision of articulation (e.g., oral diadochokinetic tasks, i.e., forced rapid alternating movements using consonant–vowel combinations to determine the integrity of the oral motor system). If the dysphagic patient has unimpaired voice and speech, the swallowing problem may possibly be related to the late pharyngeal stage (cricopharyngeal function) or to esophageal function.

d. ***Cranial nerves (CN)*** including CN V (biting, side-to-side jaw grinding, sensation of forehead, face, and jaw), CN VII (facial expression, cheek puffing, lip sealing, taste in the anterior two-thirds of the tongue), CN IX and CN X (phonation, position of uvula, palatal elevation, gag reflex, swallowing, taste in the posterior third of the tongue), CN XI (head movement), and CN XII (tongue movement).

e. ***Reflexes***

I. **Swallowing reflex**, which can be palpated by placing a finger on the thyroid notch between the hyoid bone and the larynx and feeling the larynx move up and forward during swallowing. Failure to detect laryngeal elevation may indicate weak swallowing muscles or an inadequate swallowing reflex, which leaves the airway unprotected. The swallowing reflex can be clinically tested on the right and left sides by the following.

- **Tactile and taste stimulation**, for example, rubbing a lemon glycerin swab (that has been squeezed out) to the lips, teeth, gums, and tongue to stimulate a pharyngeal swallow and to determine the ability to taste (which in turn can stimulate salivary flow and, eventually, swallowing).
- **Thermal stimulation**, for example, tapping an ice-cold laryngoscopic mirror (size 00) or small metal spoon to the base of the anterior fauces to facilitate a pharyngeal swallow (either with or without verbal cueing).

II. **Gag reflex**, which is highly variable even among healthy persons, should be elicited from both sides (the right and left sides should also be compared). A diminished or absent gag does not automatically mean that the patient is unable to swallow or protect the airway although it may give information about both cranial nerve function and the ability to achieve laryngeal closure. A diminished gag reflex is probably significant only when found in patients who have evidence of weakened or paralyzed pharyngeal palatine musculature, an asymmetric gag reflex, or other signs of cranial nerve dysfunction.

III. **Cough reflex**, which is the final protective mechanism to prevent aspiration, is in itself not an indication that the patient is experiencing tracheal aspiration. In fact, oral feeding should not be started unless the patient has an adequate cough reflex (as patients with inadequate cough reflex may silently aspirate without this protective mechanism). The cough reflex can be assessed by having the patient swallow 3 fl oz of water. Coughing during the swallow may indicate reduced vocal cord closure while coughing elicited within 1 minute after the pharyngeal swallow may indicate decreased laryngeal elevation, reduced pharyngeal peristalsis, or upper esophageal sphincter deficits. Likewise, if the patient develops a wet, hoarse voice or cough after the swallow, or if the patient experiences some choking or respiratory distress that is not immediately relieved by coughing, then probably some aspiration has taken place.

IV. **Pathological reflexes** including suck, bite, tongue thrust, suck–swallow, asymmetric tonic neck, and tonic labyrinthine reflexes.

f. ***Motor control*** including coordination (e.g., finger-to-nose test, rapid alternating hand movements, tongue wiggling, and finger wiggling), involuntary movements (e.g., tremors, chorea, athetosis, ballismus, dystonia, myoclonus, asterixis, tics, and tardive dyskinesia), and motor planning ability (e.g., feeding apraxia).

C. DIAGNOSTIC TESTS

1. Swallowing tests

a. ***Clinical (or bedside) swallowing studies (CSS)*** are not as reliable as videofluoroscopic swallowing studies (VFSS) (see section III.C.1.b), which remain the "gold standard" in determining the safety of oral feeding. Unlike VFSS, CSS is incapable of detecting "silent" (or coughless) aspiration and can only provide limited information about either structure or function of the swallowing mechanism. However, CSSs are still carried out because patients who are able to swallow safely during VFSS may have different functional skills at the bedside because of problems with endurance, insight, judgment, and planning during mealtime. Also, CSS may be used to screen for the need for VFSS, except in patients with high risk for aspiration (in which case, VFSS should be performed prior to CSS). Patients undergoing CSS must have an intact cough reflex to protect the airway in case of aspiration. They should also have adequate hydration and moist mucosa, and must be able to follow directions. Any CSS should be carried out during the mealtime (if possible) with the patient in an upright position (i.e., seated at 90° or reclining backward at a 45° angle or more) and the head tilted slightly forward. If the patient is hemiplegic, the weaker side should be elevated above the stronger side. During CSS, the following feeding behaviors are observed: impulsivity (which can affect the rate and size of the bolus), attention and distractibility during the meal, abnormal head and body positions, rate of intake, bolus size, and drooling or oral spillage of liquids or the bolus.

The best food consistency to be used during CSS is selected based on the patient's history, oral control, as well as laryngeal and pharyngeal control. According to Logemann (1998), patients with poor oral control will generally do best with thickened liquid first, followed by materials of thin consistency;

patients with a delayed pharyngeal swallow will generally do best with materials of a thicker consistency, e.g., apple sauce or mashed potatoes; patients with reduced tongue base or pharyngeal wall contraction will generally do best with liquids; patients with reduced laryngeal elevation or reduced upper esophageal sphincter opening will generally do better with liquids; and patients with reduced closure of the laryngeal entrance will generally do best with materials of a thicker consistency.

For each selected food consistency, laryngeal elevation is determined by observing the elevation of the hyoid and thyroid cartilages. The time delay should be about 1 second from the initiation of lingual movement after bolus formation to the elevation of the larynx, indicating triggering of the pharyngeal swallow and laryngeal protection of the airway. A stethoscope may be placed against the patient's neck during the swallow to listen for the occurrence of the swallow and also to detect possible aspiration. For each selected food presentation, the following are noted: the average number of swallows required per bolus (i.e., repeated swallows, which may indicate possible pooling in the pharyngeal area or reduced pharyngeal peristalsis); chewing difficulties (for solid or semisolid foods); fatigue during chewing or swallowing (swallowing or chewing can be performed successively to elicit fatigue if the patient has subjective complaints suggestive of fatigue); the location of any discomfort/pain during swallowing; occurrence of the cough reflex (see section III.B.5.e.3) during or after the swallow; presence of excessive secretions; and nasal regurgitation (especially when testing with liquids).

After each swallow, the following are noted: any changes in the patient's color (a possible sign of choking), any changes in phonation and vocal quality (see section III.B.5.c), and presence of food pocketing, i.e., retention of food in the oral cavity, which may indicate reduced bolus formation and/or sensory loss (e.g., pocketing of food on the neglected side of parietal stroke patients). To reduce the risk of aspiration of any residual food in the oropharynx, the patient must be seated upright for at least 30 minutes after the CSS. Also, monitor the patient for any changes in his or her respiratory or medical status over a 24-hour period (e.g., increased temperature or increased amount of secretions). If the patient does not exhibit any signs of aspiration, a trial oral feeding program may be initiated. If needed, a VFSS can be used to confirm the results of the CSS and to help determine appropriate compensatory head postures and swallowing techniques that may be necessary for safe swallowing.

I. **Nontracheostomized patients** are initially evaluated by presenting them with a small ice-chip from a spoon and observing lip function, tongue propulsion, any chewing ability, and the initiation of the pharyngeal swallow (by palpating for laryngeal elevation). Ice-chips are initially used because they are relatively safe if partially aspirated; they provide a good medium for eliciting the chewing reflex (because of their solid texture and stimulatory effect on the cold receptors in the gums); and they help facilitate a pharyngeal swallowing reflex (probably because of cold stimulation). If the patient appears to have difficulty with ice-chips, there must be extra caution in completing the swallowing evaluation. If there is adequate laryngeal elevation and a cough reflex, the patient may be tested with food of different textures and consistencies (e.g., pureed foods, thick liquids, ground solids, chopped solids, regular solids, and thin liquids; see section V.A.2.b.1 for description and examples of different food textures) unless contraindicated by medical or behavioral problems.

   The sequence of presentation of different food consistencies is based on the patient's history, his or her medical status, prior observations of the patient, and suspected areas of difficulty. If a delayed pharyngeal swallow is suspected during ice-chip testing, then pureed foods and thick liquids should be presented before thin liquids to reduce the possibility of aspiration. However, if upper esophageal sphincter dysfunction or esophageal stricture is suspected (e.g., complaints of discomfort), then thin liquids should be presented first because they can easily pass through the esophagus. If the patient does not voluntarily initiate chewing, the lateral side of the tongue may be rubbed with a soft solid food to facilitate a chewing response. It is safest to begin with small amounts (e.g., ¼ teaspoon) and gradually increase the amount of each presentation up to 1 to 2 teaspoons of each consistency. In a patient with a nasogastric tube (NGT), the tube should be removed prior to testing as it may potentially interfere with normal swallowing because of altered pharyngeal sensations and deflection of the bolus. Patients with NGT may need to be properly hydrated because they tend to mouth breathe, thus causing dry oral mucosa, which can interfere with swallowing.

II. **Tracheostomized patients** rarely have dysphagia that can be directly attributed to the tracheostomy tube itself. However, the presence of the tracheostomy tube may predispose these patients to tracheal aspiration for the following reasons: (a) the tracheostomy cannula has a tendency to tether the larynx anteriorly (to the trachea) thus restricting normal laryngeal elevation and resulting in reduced glottal closure and increased laryngeal penetration; (b) the lack of movement of the laryngeal muscles, together with restricted movement of the pretracheal strap muscles, can interfere with laryngeal elevation and cricopharyngeal relaxation; and (c) the cannula in the trachea may desensitize the airway, thus raising the threshold for coughing and throat-clearing activities, which are necessary to expel any material from the airway.

To test swallowing in tracheostomized patients, a blue food coloring (e.g., Evans blue or methylene blue dye) is used so that the aspirated material can be distinguished from other possible tracheal secretions. The blue dye is initially applied to the tongue, and the trachea is suctioned to detect the dye's presence. If the test is negative (i.e., dye is absent in the trachea), the patient is presented with small amounts (e.g., ¼ teaspoon) of food or liquid colored by the blue dye. The tracheostomy is momentarily occluded with a finger to establish near-normal tracheal pressure. Laryngeal elevation is observed as well as signs of swallowing difficulties such as coughing, gurgling, or leakage of blue substance around the tracheostomy site. If difficulty is noted, the patient is suctioned immediately to see if any blue-tinged solution shows up in the trachea. If not, the amount of food or liquid is increased to 1 to 2 teaspoons, followed by tracheal suctioning to detect any blue-tinged secretions. Before proceeding to a new consistency, the patient is suctioned thoroughly to help differentiate the specific consistencies with which the patient is having difficulty. If a very small amount of blue-tinged secretion is detected in the tracheostoma several minutes after a test swallow, it does not necessarily indicate impaired swallowing (as this is a common finding because of the tendency of the color-contrast solutions to coat the entire oropharyngeal mucosa). In tracheostomized patients with negative dye tests, a trial oral feeding program may be initiated.

- **Occluded vs. unoccluded tracheostomy**. Before testing the swallow, the tracheostomy tube should be plugged for several seconds to assess the patient's ability to breathe through the larynx, and the voluntary laryngeal cough. When the tracheostomy tube is not occluded, the risk of aspiration may increase because of the patient's inability to expel air to clear the larynx of foreign materials.

- **Inflated vs. deflated tracheostomy cuffs**. Inflated tracheostomy cuffs do not guarantee safety as they can cause swallowing difficulties because of increased compression of the bolus material around the cuff into the tracheal area, tracheal irritation, restriction of laryngeal elevation, and prevention of the exhalation of pulmonary air that normally clears the larynx. Cuff deflation, therefore, is usually recommended during the CSS (a deflated cuff also makes it easier to immediately detect any signs of aspiration). If the cuff cannot be deflated for medical reasons (e.g., in ventilator-dependent patients, who need the cuff inflated to maintain adequate ventilation), then oral feeding may be premature. Prior to cuff deflation, the trachea above the cuff should be suctioned to prevent aspiration of any residual food above the inflated cuff. The cuff is then deflated slowly and the patient suctioned again. If the patient has been given blue-tinged food, the amount and quality of the secretion is observed for any traces of food coloring.

b. ***Videofluoroscopic swallowing study*** (**VFSS**) is the "gold standard" for evaluating swallowing disorders. For most patients, it is carried out after the CSS to confirm the results of the CSS and to help determine appropriate compensatory head postures and swallowing maneuvers that may be necessary for safe swallowing. If the patient is at high risk for aspiration, however, VFSS is recommended prior to CSS. In VFSS, the patient is tested in an upright position to reflect normal eating and drinking (this is unlike an esophagram, i.e., a contrast study of the esophagus, which is conducted in the horizontal position to eliminate the effect of gravity on esophageal contraction). Controlled amounts (e.g., using a teaspoon, tablespoon, cup, or straw) of barium-impregnated food and liquid substances of different textures (e.g., thin liquid, thick liquid, pureed food, mechanical soft food, or solid food such as cookies; see section V.A.2.b.1 for description and examples of different food textures) are administered to the patient by a swallowing therapist (usually a speech–language pathologist). As the patient chews (if necessary) and swallows the bolus, a videorecording is made of the fluoroscopic radiogram (usually a lateral view; see Fig. 5.6-1) of the oral, pharyngeal, and esophageal stages of swallowing. The videotape can then be subsequently played at a slow speed for swallowing analysis.

   Qualitative swallowing pathologies (e.g., "silent" or coughless aspiration, laryngeal penetration, pharyngeal pooling, and delayed oral stage) and quantitative swallowing pathologies (e.g., abnormal pharyngeal transit time over 2 seconds) can be identified from the VFSS to determine the quantity and texture of food or liquid that the patient can tolerate safely. Treatment strategies are introduced during VFSS, in the following order: (1) use of postural techniques (see section V.B.1); (2) introduction of techniques to increase oral sensation, when appropriate (see section V.B.2); (3) swallowing maneuvers (see section V.C.1.c); and (4) diet or food consistency changes (see section V.B.5). Based upon these treatment strategies, feeding and swallowing recommendations can be formulated. However, the clinician must be aware that patients who are able to swallow safely during VFSS may have poor functional skills at the bedside as a result of problems with endurance, insight, judgment, and planning during mealtime. A VFSS is contraindicated if the patient has a low level of consciousness or is unable to cooperate or follow commands. Although the radiation exposure to the patient is generally small (especially in a well-planned VFSS session), the patient or family must be informed about it and, if the patient is a female of childbearing age, the patient should be screened for pregnancy (if pregnant, appropriate protection, such as a lead apron, should then be provided).

c. ***Swallowing ultrasound*** is useful in studying the oral stage of swallowing, in particular tongue motions. In itself, it is not useful in studying the pharyngeal

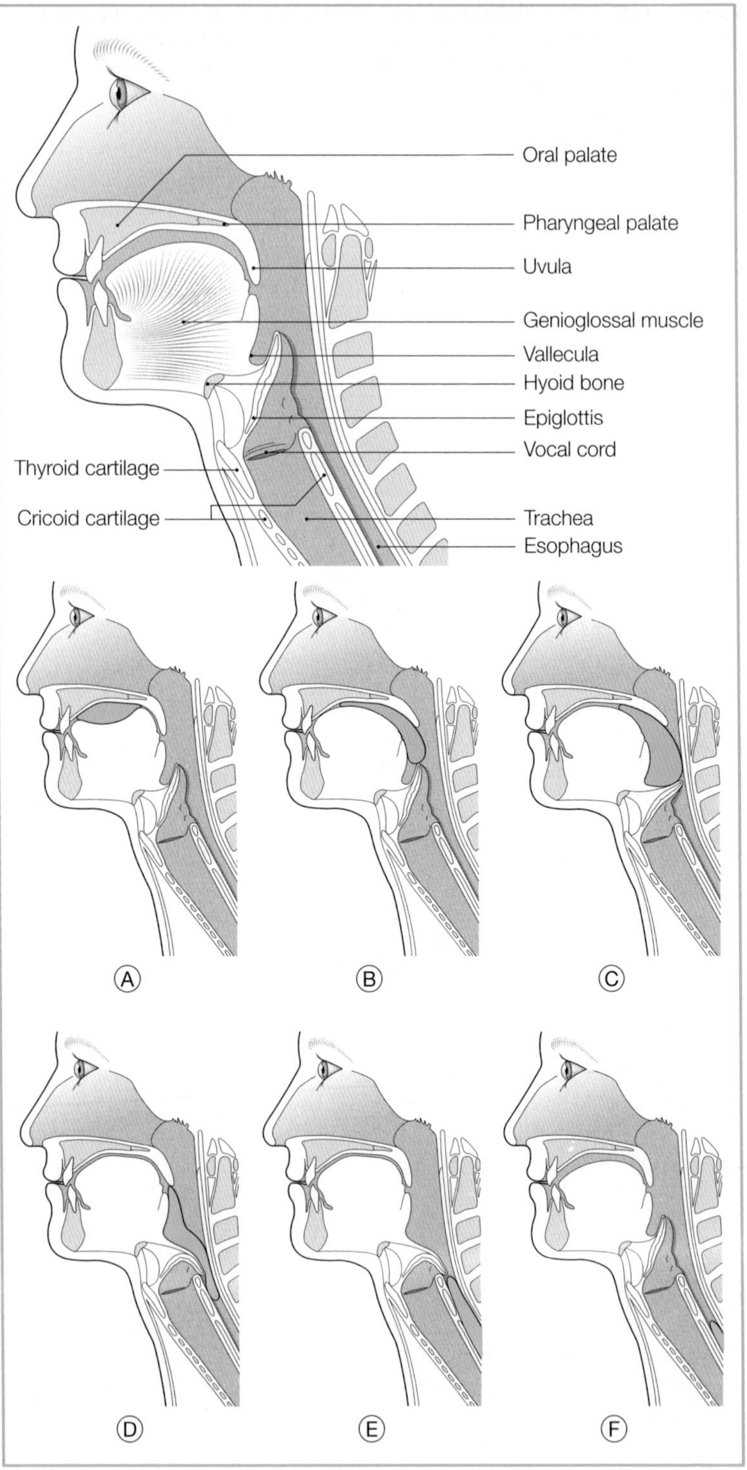
Oral palate
Pharyngeal palate
Uvula
Genioglossal muscle
Vallecula
Hyoid bone
Epiglottis
Vocal cord
Thyroid cartilage
Cricoid cartilage
Trachea
Esophagus
A
B
C
D
E
F

Figure 5.6-1 Lateral videofluoroscopic view of oropharyngeal swallow of large liquid bolus in an adult. **A.** Bolus preparation in the oral cavity (the velum is approximated with the tongue; nasal respiration can continue). **B.** Bolus is transported by the tongue to the anterior faucial arch where the pharyngeal swallow reflex is triggered (the velum is displaced upward and backward and is approximated by a protrusion on the posterior pharyngeal wall). **C.** The bolus is propelled to the laryngopharnyx (the epiglottis is folded downward; the hyoid and larynx are fully displaced upward and forward; the vocal cord adducts to protect the trachea from food aspiration; contraction waves descend in the constrictor wall). **D.** The bolus penetrates the opened pharyngoesophageal segment (contraction waves descend further; the upper part of the palatopharyngeal isthmus reopens). **E.** The bolus has nearly traversed the pharynx (contraction waves reach the hypopharynx; the oropharynx is beginning to reopen). **F.** The mouth (now empty) and the pharynx return to their usual position. (From: Donner MW, Bosma JF, Robertson D: Anatomy and physiology of the pharynx. *Gastrointestinal Radiology* 10: 196, 205, 1985, copyright © 1985, Springer-Verlag, with permission.)

stage of swallowing. When combined with VFSS, however, it may be used to document aspiration and to further evaluate esophageal function.

d. ***Swallowing surface electromyography*** uses surface electrodes to determine laryngeal movement during swallowing to screen the risk for aspiration and serve as a bedside biofeedback tool for teaching compensatory swallowing maneuvers. However, further research needs to be done before it can be recommended clinically.

e. ***Swallowing scintigraphy***, that is, radionuclide imaging of the swallowed bolus mixed with radioisotopes (e.g., technetium-99 sulfur colloid), can be used to quantify aspiration and to evaluate esophageal motility disorders and GE reflux.

f. ***Fiberoptic videoendoscopic swallow study*** may be used to directly visualize the upper aerodigestive structures to rule out aspiration and to determine appropriate compensatory head postures and swallowing maneuvers that may be necessary for safe swallowing. A flexible endoscope is introduced through the nose and a laryngopharyngeal sensory testing is first done. Then a bolus transport assessment is done by having the patient swallow food with different consistencies at increasing larger bolus, in which a green food coloring is mixed to enhance visualization on the television monitor. The oral transit time, timeliness of swallow initiation, movement of the tongue base, laryngeal elevation, spillage, residue, strength and coordination of the swallow, laryngeal closure, reflux, penetration, and aspiration can be evaluated, but the oral phase of the swallow is not directly assessed.

2. **Laryngoscopy (mirror or fiberoptic)**, done by an otolaryngologist, can detect premature spillage, laryngeal penetration, tracheal aspiration, and pharyngeal residue in patients who are too ill to undergo VFSS or unable to tolerate any risk of aspiration, or in patients with a weak or absent cough or with an altered vocal quality (e.g., hoarse or breathy).
3. **Imaging studies** include chest radiograph to determine pulmonary infiltrates (this may raise the suspicion but is not pathognomonic of aspiration pneumonia) and computed tomography or magnetic resonance imaging scan to identify and stage masses in the upper digestive tract or diagnose a central or peripheral nervous system mass, which could explain the swallowing disorder. A magnetic resonance imaging scan is superior to computed tomography for this purpose.
4. **Esophageal manometry** uses a multilumen catheter system to evaluate esophageal motor disorders; however, it is time consuming and uncomfortable.

5. **Nutritional work-up** includes serum total protein, prealbumin (a better indicator than serum albumin for determining the patient's current visceral protein stores and protein status change over time), cholesterol, triglycerides, creatinine, blood urea nitrogen (to determine protein catabolism), electrolytes, and glucose; caloric counting; and serial weighing.

IV. Classification by causative factors

A. NEUROGENIC DISORDERS

1. **Upper motor neuron and cortical disorders**
   a. ***Vascular:*** stroke, intracranial hemorrhage, cerebral palsy.
   b. ***Degenerative and extrapyramidal:*** parkinsonism, spinocerebellar degeneration, olivopontocerebellar atrophy, progressive supranuclear palsy, Huntington's disease, Alzheimer's disease, adrenoleukodystrophy, dystonia, tardive dyskinesia, dementia.
   c. ***Demyelinating:*** multiple sclerosis.
   d. ***Infectious:*** encephalitis, meningitis, Creutzfeldt–Jakob disease, acquired immune deficiency syndrome.
   e. ***Structural:*** neoplasm, Arnold–Chiari malformation, syringomyelia, and syringobulbia.
   f. ***Exogenous:*** traumatic brain injury, cervical spinal cord injuries, drug-induced causes.
   g. ***Other cortical etiologies:*** mental retardation.
2. **Combined upper and lower motor neuron disorders:** amyotrophic lateral sclerosis, progressive muscular atrophy, progressive bulbar palsy, primary lateral sclerosis.
3. **Lower motor neuron disorders**
   a. ***Motor neuron:*** spinal muscular atrophy, poliomyelitis, postpolio syndrome.
   b. ***Peripheral nervous system:*** Guillain–Barré syndrome, sarcoidosis, porphyria.
   c. ***Neuromuscular junction:*** myasthenia gravis, Eaton–Lambert syndrome, botulism.
   d. ***Muscles:*** inflammatory myopathies (e.g., polymyositis and dermatomyositis), metabolic myopathies (e.g., mitochondrial and thyroid myopathies), myotonic dystrophy, oculopharyngeal dystrophy, Duchenne's muscular dystrophy (late phase).

B. NON-NEUROGENIC DISORDERS: **rheumatologic disorders** (e.g., scleroderma, Sjögren's syndrome, systemic lupus erythematosus, mixed connective tissue disease, and rheumatoid arthritis); **metabolic disorders** (e.g., hypercalcemia and diabetes mellitus); **structural disorders** [e.g., cervical osteophytes, goiters, neoplasm, scarring (especially as a result of tuberculosis); tracheoesophageal fistula, foreign bodies, congenital anomalies (such as cleft palate); vascular aneurysm or anomalies; hypertonic cricopharyngeus muscle; fixation of larynx; Zenker's diverticulum; esophageal stricture, tumor, or web; Schatzki's ring; and severe dental anomalies]; **esophageal dysmotility disorders** (e.g., GE reflux, achalasia, diffuse esophageal spasm, and "Nutcracker" esophagus); **gastrointestinal diseases** (e.g., Crohn's disease, ulcerative colitis, and amyloidosis); **infectious diseases** (e.g., caused by *Candida*, cytomegalovirus, herpesvirus, and human immunodeficiency virus); **psychiatric disorders** (e.g., globus hystericus); **skin diseases** (e.g., mucus membrane pemphigoid, epidermolysis bullosa dystrophica, lichen planus, psoriasis, Stevens–Johnson syndrome, and chronic graft-vs.-host disease); **treatment-related etiologies** [e.g., postoperative head and neck radiation, foreign devices (such as tracheostomy and NGT), and postchemotherapy mucositis].

V. Nonsurgical management of dysphagia

Nonsurgical management of dysphagia has the following general goals: to minimize the risk of aspiration and to advance the difficulty and variety of oral intake, both for the nutrition and for the enjoyment of the patient. Feeding route, oral vs. extra-oral, can be determined by the swallowing tests. If oral intake is inadequate, it may be supplemented by extra-oral feedings using an NGT, PEG (see section VI.D), or PEJ (see section VI.D). Calorie counts, which are done by nutritionists or dietitians, are used to determine the patient's nutritional status and need for feeding supplementation. In severe dysphagia, an NGT may be temporarily used to provide full or supplemental nutrition to the patient. An NGT should not be used for more than 2–3 weeks as it is uncomfortable, may cause erosion of the nasopharynx, and does not prevent aspiration. If a prolonged extra-oral feeding route is required, a PEG or PEJ is indicated as it is more comfortable and provides lesser (but not absent) aspiration risk than an NGT.

Patients with extra-oral feeding sources can be progressed as follows: as the patient recovers swallowing abilities, he or she receives therapeutic feedings by his or her caregiver under the supervision of an allied health personnel. When the amount of intake increases and safe feeding behaviors are noted, the patient is permitted to eat under the supervision of the trained caregiver or allied health personnel. As intake improves and calories are consistently sufficient, the extra-oral feeding source may be used only for hydration and medication intake. Eventually, if the patient continues to improve, he or she will become able to drink enough fluid and take medication so that the extra-oral feeding source can be removed. It is important that throughout this process the patient be weighed at regular intervals and be monitored for signs of dehydration or malnutrition.

Progression of swallowing treatment should be made based on individual performance with appropriate assessment based on sophisticated techniques (e.g., VFSS) or on quantification of clinical outcomes, such as, decreases in pharyngeal swallow time, increases in the frequency of spontaneous swallows, advancements to oral feedings, upgrades in food or liquid textures, reductions in the degree of required supervision, improved nutritional status, and decreases in the time required to eat a meal safely.

In addition to specific swallowing treatment presented below, oral hygiene, such as cleaning the dentition and mucosa after meals, is recommended to reduce the risk of aspiration pneumonia. Therapeutic interventions focusing on postural and limb control as well as cognitive, behavioral, and perceptual remediation, if necessary, should be done. **Biofeedback techniques** may be used to assist swallowing therapy. Taped VFSS or ultrasonography may be used to promote lingual bolus control and coordinated tongue movement during the oral stage of swallowing. Electromyography and esophageal manometry may be repeated over the course of treatment and used to demonstrate progress towards the goals of increasing strength and pressure exerted by the tongue and the pharynx during swallowing. For teaching laryngeal valving maneuvers, fiberoptic videoendoscopy may be used as a biofeedback tool by allowing visualization of laryngeal valving during compensatory breath holding strategies.

Feeding adaptations (see Chapter 4.5, section II.A.3.a.) may be needed in dysphagic patients due to decreased upper-limb function (such as limited grasp, incoordination, decreased ROM, hemiparesis, and hemiplegia). They include the use of adapted feeding utensils, such as small-bowled utensils to decrease bolus size and covered cups with small openings or pinching the straw to limit amount of liquids. In dysphagic patients with problems in judgment, attention, or motor planning, **feeding environment adaptations**, such as feeding in a quiet, distraction-free environment, may be needed. Table 5.6-1 shows the factors to be considered in

Table 5.6-1 Factors to consider in prescribing nonsurgical management of dysphagia

Factors	Comments
Oral vs. nonoral (e.g., NGT, PEG, PEJ)	• If >10% of every bolus is aspirated, regardless of consistency of food, do not feed orally • If it takes >10 s for oral and pharyngeal transit time to swallow every consistency of food attempted, but there is no aspiration, the patient may feed by mouth but will need nonoral feeding as supplement • If it appears that it will take more than 3–4 weeks to improve the swallowing, a PEG or PEJ may be needed
Diagnosis	Consider the speed and potential for recovery, for example: • In non-complicated stroke likely to recover in 1–2 weeks, only compensatory techniques are needed • In patients with motor neuron disease, active exercises may cause fatigue • In patients with dementia, any therapy needing direction following is not appropriate
Prognosis	• If recovery of full or partial oral intake is possible, swallowing therapy is appropriate • In patients with degenerative process, a course of therapy may be appropriate initially depending upon goals. As the disease progresses, swallowing therapy may no longer be effective due to significant loss of neuromotor control
Reaction to compensatory strategies	• If symptoms of dysphagia (e.g., aspiration) are eliminated by compensatory strategies, such that the patient can take full oral intake safely and sufficiently, then swallowing therapy is not needed Re-evaluate in 3–4 weeks to determine need for active exercises
Dysphagia severity	• If dysphagia is too severe and cannot be ameliorated with compensatory techniques, then do indirect therapy with no food or liquid
Ability to follow directions	• Swallow maneuvers need complex direction following. • Compensatory techniques, which are largely under the control of the caregiver, involve little if any need to follow directions
Respiratory function	• Normal swallowing needs airway closure for 0.3 to 0.6 s for liquids, 3 to 5 s or more during continuous cup drinking. Hence, it the respiratory function is poor, the swallowing maneuvers are inappropriate
Availability of caregiver support	• Must be available to ensure regular practice of therapy procedures
Patient motivation and interest	• Most patients will be motivated to do swallowing therapy, but some will prefer non-oral feeding

Tabulated from Logeman JA: Evaluation and treatment of swallowing disorders, *ed 2, Austin, Texas, 1998, Pro-Ed Publishers, pp. 191–250.*

determining the feeding route, the necessity of the swallowing therapy, and the type of swallowing therapy to be prescribed. Nonsurgical treatment options for a few selected swallowing disorders are shown in Table 5.6-2. For comprehensive listing and specific detail on the nonsurgical management of swallowing disorders affecting each phase of swallow, as well as citations of multiple studies supporting the treatment techniques, refer to Logeman (1998).

A. COGNITIVE STIMULATION TECHNIQUES

1. **Dysphagia education** including the nature of the swallowing disorder, safety precautions, nutritional requirements, diet modifications, and the rationale for treatment methods, are given not only to the patient but also to the family or caregiver(s) and other interdisciplinary team members.
2. **Verbal cueing,** such as telling the patient with cognitive deficits to close the lips, move the tongue, and "think" swallow, are more effective than simply telling the patient to "swallow" after placing the bolus in the mouth.

B. COMPENSATORY STRATEGIES are treatment procedures designed to control the flow of food and eliminate the patient's symptoms (e.g., aspiration). However, they do not necessarily change the physiology of the patient's swallow. These procedures can be used with patients of all ages and cognitive levels because they are largely under the control of the caregiver or clinician. They generally involve less muscle effort or work for the patient and thus do not fatigue the patient as quickly as some swallow exercises. They are usually introduced first in the diagnostic procedure (e.g., during VFSS).

1. **Postural techniques (feeding positions or postures)** redirect food flow and change pharyngeal dimensions in systematic ways. They are usually used temporarily until the patient's swallow recovers or direct therapy procedures take effect to improve oropharyngeal motor function. Occasionally, some patients may use it permanently (e.g., those with severe neurologic or structural damage) to eliminate aspiration and facilitate swallowing efficiency. It should be combined with other measures such as controlling bolus volumes, modifying bolus textures, slowing feeding rates, cognitive stimulation techniques, and compensatory airway protective maneuvers. Their effectiveness can be objectively tested using the VFSS. After feeding, patients should remain upright for at least 30 minutes to decrease the risk of aspiration and GE reflux.

a. ***Sitting position at a 90° angle*** with the trunk erect, the head in the midline, and the neck slightly flexed forward (at 45° angle), is considered by some clinicians as the optimal feeding position that achieves maximum airway protection in most patients with neurogenic dysphagia.

b. ***Head position***

I. **Chin-tuck (chin-down) posture** can reduce the opening to the airway, draw the tongue forward, and widen the vallecular space, thus preventing or minimizing premature entry of the bolus into the pharynx and open larynx. The open laryngeal vestibule is also drawn forward and is somewhat channeled under the tongue base, thereby making it less vulnerable to penetration due to the additional protection from the tongue. Chin-tuck is an effective airway protective position in appropriate patients who present with delayed initiation of the pharyngeal swallow; however, it must not be used for all types of dysphagia as it can promote aspiration in some cases. For example, in patients whose pharyngeal swallow is so delayed that it is not initiated until the bolus reaches the pyriform sinuses and in whom there is also delay in laryngeal elevation and closure, the chin-tuck posture may facilitate the anterior diversion of the hesitated bolus in the pyriform sinus into the airway during laryngeal elevation. In patients with sensorimotor impairment of the lips and tongue, the chin-tuck may also cause inefficient oral bolus containment, control, and transport. Also, if the chin-tuck is not combined with bolus volume control, the large thin liquid bolus can fill the valleculae causing an overflow into the pharynx and into the laryngeal inlet.

II. **Chin-up posture** (i.e., head tilted backward) is used in patients with reduced tongue control to drain food from the oral cavity using gravity. If there is concern about airway protection, swallowing maneuvers (e.g., supraglottic maneuver described in section V.C.1.c.1) may be used.

III. **Head-rotation posture** is used in patients with unilateral pharyngeal wall impairment to help pharyngeal clearance. The head is turned toward the weaker side to close the damaged side of the pharynx and to direct food down the stronger or normal side of the pharynx. It can also be used in patients with a unilateral vocal fold weakness because head rotation to the weak side pushes the damaged side toward midline, thus improving adduction.

IV. **Chin-down and head rotation postures** may be combined to increase airway protection in selected patients.

V. **Head-tilt posture** is used in patients with both a unilateral oral impairment and a unilateral pharyngeal impairment on the same side. The head is always tilted to the stronger side so gravity can help drain food down the stronger side, where there is better control.

c. ***Recumbent posture***

I. **Supine position** may eliminate the aspiration if the patient has bilateral reduction in pharyngeal wall contraction or reduced laryngeal elevation, resulting in residue in the pharynx that is aspirated after the swallow. In this position, straw drinking is the only way to take liquids efficiently. If there is a buildup of residue in the pharynx with successive swallows, the supine position for feeding should not be used. If the patient has gastroesophageal reflux, their upper body may need to be elevated 15° to 30° to prevent reflux but still eliminate aspiration.

II. **Side-lying position** can reduce hypopharyngeal pooling in selected patients by eliminating gravitational effect on pharyngeal residues. It is used in patients with reduced pharyngeal contraction with residue spread throughout the pharynx.

2. **Oral sensory–motor enhancement techniques** done prior to swallow are generally recommended for patients with swallow apraxia, tactile agnosia for food, delayed onset of the oral swallow, reduced oral sensation, or delayed triggering of the pharyngeal swallow. Their function is to alert the central nervous system and lower the threshold of the swallowing center. They are considered compensatory strategies (e.g., in patients with Alzheimer's disease, motor neuron disease, and other degenerative process) because they are under the control of the caregiver and do not change the motor control of the swallow. However, in other patients with diseases (e.g., stroke, TBI) from which recovery is anticipated, sensory enhancement techniques could be considered a therapy procedure (see section V.C) because they can change the timing of swallow by reducing both oral onset time and pharyngeal delay time. Sensory enhancement techniques include:

a. ***Tactile and pressure stimulation,*** which consist of downward pressure of the empty spoon against anterior third of the tongue as the bolus is delivered into the mouth.

b. ***Presentation of a bolus with increased sensory characteristics,*** such as cold bolus or a textured bolus (e.g., rice pudding) or a bolus with strong flavor (e.g., sour bolus with 50% lemon juice and 50% barium). Carbonated beverages have been used in dysphagic patients to enhance patient awareness of the liquid during pharyngeal swallowing via the carbon dioxide bubbles (Bulow *et al.*, 2003).

c. ***Presentation of a bolus requiring chewing*** so that the mastication can provide preliminary oral stimulation.

d. ***Presentation of a larger volume bolus*** (e.g., 3 mL or more).

e. ***Thermal–tactile stimulation and suck–swallow.*** The thermal–tactile stimulation is designed to heighten oral awareness and provide an alerting sensory stimulus to the cortex and brainstem such that, when the patient initiates the oral stage of swallow, the pharyngeal swallow will trigger more rapidly and reduce the delay of several swallows thereafter. An exaggerated suck–swallow, using increased vertical tongue–jaw sucking movements with the lips closed, can help facilitate the triggering of the pharyngeal swallow. This technique also draws saliva to the back of the mouth, which is helpful for patients with poor saliva control. Both thermal–tactile stimulation and suck-swallow techniques are most commonly used to improve triggering of the pharyngeal swallow.

For thermal–tactile stimulation, a laryngeal mirror (size 00) is placed in ice for approximately 10 seconds and then placed along the area of the anterior faucial arch (bilaterally or alternating between the right and left sides) and rubbed or tapped 4–5 times. After this icing procedure, the patient is asked to swallow food or, if oral feeding is not allowed, to perform a dry swallow. Cold stimulation is performed for short periods (i.e., stop after 5 minutes, or if fatigue occurs as evidenced by increased time before initiation or coughing) and several times throughout the day as well as before mealtimes.

3. **Modification of bolus volume** involves the use of smaller volumes to prevent or minimize the degree of aspiration that may occur. Recommended bolus volumes, as determined during the VFSS are 2 mL (½ teaspoon), 5 mL (1 teaspoon), 10 mL (small sip or by straw), and 20 mL (average bolus in normal adults; by filled tablespoon or by cup).
4. **Modification of timing of food presentation** can help control bolus volume. There should be at least a 30-second delay between bolus presentations to avoid overloading the mouth in patients with problems in oral preparation and oral phases of swallow.
5. **Modification of food consistency (diet)** are individually determined for each patient during CSS or VFSS. It involves the gradual progression of the patient's diet through food of different texture or consistency with the goal of returning to a regular diet. In general, food of thinner consistencies (e.g., thin liquids) are more difficult to control and have a higher risk for aspiration because they can leak into the pharynx before swallowing is triggered. Hence, thickened liquids and soft cohesive solids are generally the safest consistencies. By increasing the viscosity or thickness of the food or liquid bolus in patients with oral sensory or motor deficits, there is reduced tendency for the material to escape from the oral cavity, fall into the laryngeal inlet, or penetrate the incompletely sealed larynx during the delay before pharyngeal swallow initiation. Also, more viscous materials may increase tongue movements and enhance mechanoreceptor displacement thus facilitating more timely initiation of the pharyngeal swallow. However, if the patient has a delayed pharyngeal swallow and is unable to significantly clear the pharynx of viscous materials, then the use of thick or viscous materials will not improve swallowing safety. Moreover, liquid thickening can adversely affect the patient's hydration (if necessary, these patients should be hydrated intravenously or through the feeding tube).

a. ***Dysphagia NPO (non per os or nothing by mouth)*** is indicated in patients with high risk for aspiration because of reduced alertness, reduced responsiveness to stimulation, absent swallow, absent protective cough, and difficulty handling secretions as evidenced by excessive coughing and choking, copious secretions, and a wet gurgly voice quality; or significant reductions in the range and strength of oral pharyngeal and laryngeal movements. Even if indicated for aspiration prevention, NPO is disadvantageous to treating dysphagia because swallowing itself is the best exercise for its recovery. Hence, although a patient may remain NPO, treatment may be recommended to improve prefeeding skills such as oral-pharyngeal sensorimotor functioning or alertness and responsiveness. If indicated, single food items may be used in NPO patients for trial feeding purposes. Patients on NPO can be given intravenous (IV) hydration, total parenteral nutrition (central or peripheral), or can be fed through an NGT, PEG, or PEJ.

b. ***Dysphagia mechanical soft (semisolid) diets*** require little chewing and are easy to control in the mouth. Examples include minced food (e.g., ground meats with gravy and meatloaf) and soft food (e.g., bananas). In these patients, liquids are not allowed.

c. ***Dysphagia pureed diets*** are smooth, soft, moist, blenderized foods that do not require chewing (e.g., apple sauce and whipped potatoes). They are indicated for patients with chewing difficulty or who are unable to form a cohesive bolus because of decreased tongue function. In these patients, liquids are not allowed.

d. ***Thick liquids,*** which are liquids that have body, are easier to control in the mouth than thin liquids because they have less tendency to leak from the base of the tongue before swallowing is triggered. They should be introduced gradually under supervision in conjunction with the dysphagia pureed or dysphagia mechanical soft diet.

   I. **Honey-thick (full-thick or spoon-thick) liquids** are made of very thick, yet pourable, consistency, such as honey, thickened cream soups, pudding, and cooked cereal. They need to be spooned up instead of drunk.

   II. **Nectar-thick (medium-thick) liquids** are used as a transition from honey-thick to thin liquids. They include tomato juice, sherbet, eggnogs, milkshakes, regular or strained cream soups, and nectars (e.g., peach, pear, or apricot). Thin liquids can be thickened to a nectar-thick consistency using food thickeners.

e. ***Thin liquids*** are clear with little or no body (e.g., water, tea, fruit juice, coffee, and milk). Ice cream and Jello are also considered thin liquids because they melt in the mouth. Thin liquids are only recommended when nectar-thick liquids are tolerated and should be introduced gradually under supervision in conjunction with the dysphagia pureed or dysphagia mechanical soft diet.

f. ***Regular diets*** have no texture restrictions and are allowed if the patient can safely tolerate pureed or semisolid foods as well as thick or thin liquids. Solid foods used in the regular diet may be chopped or cut to the size of a fingernail or smaller.

6. **Intra-oral prosthetic devices,** e.g., palatal augmentation or reshaping prostheses, can be used to lower the palatal vault to enhance tongue-to-palate contact and to potentially improve the pharyngeal phase of swallow (i.e., by improving pharyngeal transit time). Use of palatal augmentation prostheses requires training regarding optimum oral bolus positioning and compensatory tongue placements for articulation; therefore, the patient must be motivated to tolerate and adapt to the prosthesis during speech and swallowing. Palatal augmentation prostheses are effective in patients with significant tongue resections or bilateral tongue paralysis. Other intra-oral prosthetics include palatal lift prosthesis (which lifts the soft palate into an elevated or closed position in patients with velar paralysis) and palatal obturator (which is used in cancer patients with significant resection of the soft palate).

C. **THERAPY PROCEDURES** are designed to change the physiology of swallow, in contrast to compensatory strategies, which are designed to eliminate symptoms. Therapy procedures are generally used to improve range of motion (ROM) of oral or pharyngeal structures, to improve sensory input prior to the swallow, or to take voluntary control over the timing or coordination of selected oropharyngeal movements during swallow. Moreover, therapy procedures, generally, but not always, require the patient to follow directions and practice independently of the clinician to get best effect. Any of the therapy described below can be done indirectly or directly.

1. **Indirect therapy** involves exercise programs or swallows of saliva, but no food or liquid is given. It is recommended in patients who are unsafe for any oral intake because they aspirate on all food consistencies and volumes. In general, if

the patient is aspirating more than 10% of each bolus swallowed, and therapeutic techniques applied at the time are unable to reduce this aspiration, the patient will function better if therapy focuses on improving the control of muscle needed for swallowing rather than working directly on swallowing by using food or liquid (Griffin, 1974).

a. ***Oral sensory-motor enhancement techniques*** discussed under the section V.B.2 as a compensatory procedure, can also be considered a therapy procedure, particularly in patients with stroke, head injury, head and neck cancer treatment, or other procedures from which some recovery is anticipated. As a therapy procedure, they are designed to regularly improve and maintain an improved onset of the oral swallow and the triggering of the pharyngeal swallow. In general, they are appropriate for patients with reduced recognition of food in the mouth or a very slowed oral transit because of an apraxic component or a delay in triggering of the pharyngeal swallow. The therapy techniques used are the same as those used under compensatory procedures (see section V.B.2). If feasible, the patient should be given the spoon containing the desired bolus and allowed to place the food in the mouth themselves or with assistance by the caregiver, as needed. This arm-and-hand action of the feeding act itself may provide the patient with additional preliminary sensory input, alerting the cortex and brainstem that food is coming to the mouth.

b. ***Therapeutic exercises*** are used to facilitate oral motor ROM, strength, and coordination. Patients must be able to follow instructions (one-step or more) and be able to imitate isolated orofacial movements. All exercises must be written down for the patient and his or her family or caregiver. Unless stated otherwise, they should be repeated 5–10 times per set during the session, which is then repeated 5–10 times per day.

   I. **Active range of motion (AROM) exercises** for patients with oropharyngeal swallowing impairments are preferred over passive ROM exercises.

   - **Jaw AROM exercises** are used to facilitate jaw opening and closure as well as rotary and lateral movements to help maintain any bolus within the oral cavity. Exercises include opening the mouth as wide as possible; moving the jaw from side to side; alternating left to right jaw extensions; chewing a soft piece of chewing gum wrapped in gauze and tied to a string that is held by the clinician; chewing lightly against the tip of a soft-sponged toothette held firmly by the clinician; and biting against a block made of soft material of different widths applied interdentally between the central incisors to facilitate a gradual increase in the distance between the upper and lower teeth (using a mirror, the patient later attempts to match the opening width without the use of the bite block device). In patients with an exaggerated bite response, systematic desensitization techniques should be used (i.e., the jaw is pushed closed and held firmly for a few seconds, then the pressure is released and the jaw is allowed to relax) rather than trying to pry the mouth open.
   - **Lip AROM exercises** are used to help prevent food or liquid from leaking out of the oral cavity. These include opening the mouth wide; smiling, grinning, or sneering; repeating "pa, pa, pa, ba, ba, ba"; and blowing through a straw or blowing bubbles. Any exercise that is directed toward increasing mandibular elevation can also improve the approximation of the upper and lower lips. Patients can also be taught to imitate lateral and medial labial movements to prevent lip stiffening and enhance mobility for speech, swallowing, and better physical appearance. On each trial, the patient is instructed to hold the targeted lip posture for a few seconds before returning to the rest position.
   - **Tongue AROM exercises** are used to improve tongue lateralization during chewing, tongue elevation to the hard palate, and anterior-posterior movement of the midline of the tongue (which is needed in the initiation of the

voluntary or oral stage of the swallow). With mouth wide open, the patient is instructed to: move the tongue to the left and right side, elevate the tongue in the front, elevate the back of the tongue, and extend and pull back the tongue straight out and into the mouth. The tongue position is held for one second at the end range of each tongue ROM exercise, then released.

- **Pharyngeal AROM exercises** are done if postural techniques see section V.B.1) and swallowing maneuvers (see section V.C.1.c) are not able to correct the pharyngeal problem. In patients with cardiac conditions (e.g., hypertension, arrhythmia, or coronary artery disease), Valsalva effects involving breath holding and bearing down, should either be avoided or used cautiously.

– **Airway entrance closure exercises**. While seated, the patient is told to hold his or her breath and to bear down for one second, then let go. The patient may either push down or pull up on the chair with both hands. If Valsalva maneuver is contraindicated, the alternative is to have the patient say "ah" as described below.

– **Vocal fold adduction exercises** are performed as an attempt to strengthen weak cords and approximate them to prevent aspiration. While seated the patient is asked to bear down against the chair with one hand (rather than two) and to repeat "ah" 5 times, with each set repeated 3 times for 5–10 times a day. If swallowing is not improved after one week, then he or she is asked to repeat the exercises by bearing down with two hands (rather than one) and prolonging the "ah" by saying it for 5–10 seconds. Then, if after 1–2 weeks, the swallowing is still not improved, the patient is asked to take a breath, hold it, and cough as strongly as possible. The above exercises will generally improve the patient's swallowing within 2–3 weeks; but it may take longer (up to 6–8 months) in patients who had supraglottic laryngectomy or other extensive laryngeal damage.

– **Tongue base retraction exercises**. The patient is asked to pull back the tongue base by pretending to gurgle (or yawn) as hard as possible, then relax. Another exercise for tongue base retraction is to do the effortful swallow maneuver described in section V.C.1.c.3.

– **Laryngeal elevation exercises (the falsetto exercise)**. The patient is asked to slide up the pitch scale as high as possible to a high squeaky voice, then hold the high note for several seconds with as much effort as possible. The patient may do a manual assist by using his or her hand to gently pull up on the larynx during the exercise.

II. **Strengthening exercises** are indicated for nonprogressive or recovering dysphagic patients with weakness of the striated muscles of the oral cavity, pharynx, and larynx. They are not indicated for patients with progressive neurologic diseases. Any AROM exercises described in section V.C.1.b.1 for the lips, tongue, or jaw can be modified into strengthening exercise by applying manual resistance.

- **Jaw strengthening exercises** are the same as jaw AROM exercises with the addition of manual resistance.
- **Lip strengthening exercises** are used to improve the integrity of the lip seal to maintain foods and liquids in the oral cavity. The patient is asked to purse the lips, holding them tightly together for about 5 seconds, followed by a slow release. To further increase lip strength, an intervening tongue blade or soft-sponged swab may be pulled by the clinician from the patient's lips as the patient purses his or her lips against it.
- **Tongue strengthening exercises** can help control the bolus and propel it to the pharynx. Exercises include manual depression of the top, side, and back of the tongue with a tongue blade and asking the patient to displace the

tongue against the blade. The patient may also be asked to use the tongue to cup an oral stimulus while the clinician attempts to remove it. Examples of oral stimuli include a moistened, soft-sponged toothette, flavored suckers, popsicles, or rolled pieces of flavored gauze held at one end by the clinician.

- **Soft palate (i.e., levator veli palatini muscle) strengthening exercises** can help seal the back of the tongue to prevent premature spillage of bolus into the pharynx and to prevent misdirection of foods or liquids into the nasal cavity. However, the application of resistive activities to the levator muscle is difficult. Hence patients with flaccid or surgically altered soft palates are typically managed by fitting them with palatal augmentation prostheses (see section V.B.6).
- **Respiratory strengthening exercises** are needed so that the patient can hold respiration while swallowing and can also clear penetrated or aspirated material from the airway. They include inhaling deeply and exhaling slowly; repeating "ah, ah, ah" as long as possible; blowing through a straw or onto a windmill; and reading poems or singing songs. Patients with a weak cough should also be taught assisted-coughing (see Chapter 5.12, section IV.B.1.b.1.c), which involves having the supine patient take a deep breath, followed by coughing effort done in synchrony with the clinician (or assisting person) pushing on the patient's abdomen and lower ribs. This can help achieve normal cough airflow velocity despite paralysis and can also help clear the tracheobronchial tree of secretions and aspirated materials.

III. **Bolus control and propulsion exercises** are used to improve lingual control of the bolus without asking the patient to swallow.

- **Exercise to improve gross manipulaton of bolus material**. The patient is asked to hold a rolled 4 × 4 inch gauze pad (or a flexible licorice whip) between his or her tongue and palate and to move it from one side to the other and to slide it forward and backward in the mouth. During exercise, the other end of the bolus material is held by the clinician to prevent the patient from choking. When the patient is able to move the gauze or licorice whip in three directions in one second without losing control, the bolus material is progressed to a lifesaver candy tied to a thread held by a clinician, then to a thin cloth tape soaked in small amount of orange or cranberry juice, then finally to a chewing gum without the clinician's control.
- **Exercises to hold a cohesive bolus**. The patient is asked to cup the tongue around the bolus and move it around the mouth without losing it or allowing it to spread out around the mouth. After the exercise, the bolus is spat out. About ⅓ teaspoonful of paste bolus is used, which can be progressed by increasing the bolus size, then subsequently to ⅓ teaspoonful of liquid bolus as the patient improves.
- **Exercises to improve posterior propulsion of the bolus**. The patient is asked to push his or her tongue upward and backward against a 4 inch long, narrow roll of gauze soaked in orange or cranberry juice and to squeeze the liquid out of the gauze to stimulate a swallow. During exercise, one end of the gauze is held by the clinician to prevent the patient from choking. In patients with decreased vertical ROM of the tongue, the diameter of the roll of gauze can be made larger by placing two or three 4 × 4 inch gauze pads on top of one another and then rolling them. The rolled gauze (dipped in small amout of liquid) is placed between the tongue and hard palate so the patient can practice pushing the tongue upward and backward against the hard palate. The thickness of the gauze roll can be decreased as the tongue vertical ROM improves.

IV. **Shaker exercise** is an exercise directed to the cervical muscles to open the upper esophageal sphincter by pulling the hyoid and larynx up and forward.

In the supine position (with no pillow), the patient is asked to look at his or her toes by lifting only the head about 4 inches (make sure that the shoulders are not lifted). In the extended Shaker exercise, this head-lift is held for 1 minute, rested for 1 minute, then repeated three times. In the repetitive Shaker exercise, the head-lift is held for 1 second, lowered, then lifted again 30 times.

c. ***Swallow maneuvers*** are designed to place specific aspects of pharyngeal swallow physiology under voluntary control. The patient must be able to understand the rationale for the maneuver, follow two- to three-step instructions, concentrate on the execution of the maneuver, and retain instructions over time. Because they require increased muscular effort, they are not appropriate if patient fatigues easily. Usually, they are used temporarily as the patient's swallow recovers and are then discontinued as the swallow physiology returns to normal. The efficacy of the swallow maneuvers can be confirmed by VFSS or by fiberoptic video endoscopy.

   I. **Supraglottic swallow** is designed to voluntarily close the airway at the level of the true vocal folds before and during the swallow to clear potential residue, primarily from the laryngeal vestibule and pyriform sinuses. It is indicated in patients with reduced or late laryngeal closure, delayed initiation of the pharyngeal swallow, incomplete supraglottic valving, and incomplete pharyngeal clearance. It consists of taking a deep breath and holding the breath, placing the bolus in the mouth, swallowing (2–3 times or more) while still holding the breath, then followed immediately by coughing to clear the throat. The patient should only re-establish breathing after the sequence to prevent inhalation of pharyngeal residue. Instead of coughing, the patient may be told to clear the throat "out" because most patients will attempt to inhale before a coughing. To make sure that the vocal fold is closed during breath holding, the patient may be told to "inhale then exhale slightly" followed by breath holding.

   II. **Super-supraglottic swallow** is designed to voluntarily close the airway at its entrance by tilting the arytenoids cartilage anteriorly to the base of the epiglottis before and during the swallow and closing the false cords tightly. It is used to improve the rate of laryngeal elevation at the beginning of the swallow in patients who underwent supraglottic laryngectomy or a full course of radiotherapy to the neck. It can also be used to improve tongue base retraction in patients with normal anatomy. It consists of taking a deep breath and holding the breath tightly as the patient bears down (by pushing on a table or pressing both hands together to create a Valsalva effect), placing the bolus in the mouth, swallowing (2–3 times or more) while still holding the breath, then followed immediately by coughing to clear the throat. Due to the Valsalva effect, it should be avoided (or used cautiously) in cardiac patients.

   III. **Effortful (or hard) swallow** is designed to increase posterior motion of the tongue base during the pharyngeal swallow to help improve clearance of the bolus from the valleculae. The patient is instructed to swallow and "squeeze hard with all of your muscles" to increase the pressure exerted by the tongue at all points along the palate and at the tongue base, thus increasing backward motion of the tongue base. This maneuver can improve the strength of the tongue base retraction and the pharyngeal wall contraction, which are both needed to complete pharyngeal clearance.

   IV. **Mendelsohn maneuver** is designed to hold the larynx up and forward and thereby increase the opening duration of the upper esophageal (cricopharyngeal) sphincter. It can also help improve the overall coordination of the swallow. The patient is instructed as follows: "Swallow your saliva several times and pay attention to your neck as you swallow. Tell me if you can feel that something (your Adam's apple or voice box) lifts and lowers as you swallow. Now this time, when you swallow and you feel something lift as you swallow, don't let your Adams's apple drop. Hold it up with your muscles for several seconds." Or alternatively, the patient is instructed that "as you swallow, can you feel that everything squeezes together in the middle of the swallow? When you can feel this, swallow and hold the squeeze." By "holding the squeeze," there is prolongation of the duration of laryngeal elevation and tongue base retraction.

2. **Direct therapy** involves the presentation of food or liquid to the patient and asking him or her to swallow it while following specified instructions. The patient must be alert, have adequate communicative and cognitive abilities, be medically stable, and have good endurance and pulmonary function. It may involve positioning of the head or body to eliminate aspiration or following a sequence of instructions (as many as seven steps) to improve his or her swallowing. All instructions should be written and provided to the patient and the patient's family or caregiver. Before proceeding to swallows of liquid or food, the patient should first practice dry swallows. If food or liquid is provided for practice swallows, only small amounts should be given. Whenever needed, the patient should be encouraged to cough to clear the airway.

VI. Surgical procedures

A. Tracheostomy (see Chapter 5.12, section V.A.2) can be used for short-term protection of the airway from aspiration. However, tracheostomy can also possibly increase aspiration risk because of impaired laryngeal elevation caused by tethering of the tracheostomy tube to the larynx and trachea. If an inflated tracheostomy cuff is used (see section III.C.1.a.2.b), careful suctioning is needed prior to deflation because food that accumulates above the cuff may be aspirated on cuff deflation. The treatment of dysphagia in patients with tracheostomy tubes is controversial. Oral intake for either evaluation or treatment should probably be postponed if the patient's tracheostomy tube is a Jackson size 5 or larger or if the patient's respiratory status necessitates an inflated cuff.

In tracheostomized patients, treatment should be directed toward decannulation, which can be accomplished by gradual reduction in the size of the tracheostomy tube; removal of the cuff; introduction of a fenestrated tube; gradually increasing the period of time that the patient tolerates occlusion for uncuffed or fenestrated tubes; and the use of a one-way valve (e.g., Passy–Muir Speaking Valve and Olympic Trach-talk; see Chapter 5.12, section V.A.2.b.4.b). A one-way valve opens on inhalation and closes on exhalation thus forcing expired air through the larynx and upper glottis. This helps blow out any food residue in the trachea (which might otherwise penetrate more deeply into the airway) and restore phonation. Swallowing evaluation and treatment may proceed in conjunction with decannulation for patients who demonstrate limited success with oral intake as swallowing treatment may improve the patient's ability to handle his or her secretions (thus facilitating decannulation). A patient with a cuffed tracheostomy tube can be decannulated by drinking 4 fl oz of blue-dyed water (e.g., with methylene blue) at intervals of 15 minutes for an hour and thoroughly suctioning the trachea to note any blue-tinged secretions. If this test is negative, the cuff is deflated for meals and at other times, with close supervision for 24 hours. Although a positive test result suggests aspiration, decannulation may still proceed if the patient shows adequate swallowing during meals with the cuff deflated.

B. **CRICOPHARYNGEAL MYOTOMY**, which is used in patients with Zenker's diverticulum and cricopharyngeal achalasia, can also be effectively performed in patients with generalized dysphagia because of neuromuscular disease.

C. **LARYNGEAL PROTECTION PROCEDURES**, for example, vocal cord augmentation for mild aspiration and laryngeal diversion for more severe and chronic aspirations, may be used.

D. **SURGICAL FEEDING TUBE INSERTION** (e.g., surgically placed gastrostomy, PEG, or PEJ) may be used for nutritional purposes in patients with high risk for aspiration (NGT may initially be used temporarily for less than 2–3 weeks). Surgically placed gastrostomy or PEG does not necessarily protect the patient from aspiration as the patient may aspirate his or her saliva or gastric contents, which reach the pharynx by reflux. However, PEJ (wherein a thin tube is deposited in the distal duodenum or proximal jejunum through a mature PEG tract) may possibly reduce the risk of aspiration.

VII. Complications

A. **ASPIRATION PNEUMONIA** usually occurs at the time of eating although it may occur even during sleep. It can be prevented by elevating the head of the bed, using H_2-blockers or antacids to increase the gastric pH above 2.5, and decreasing food intake before sleep. In patients with recurrent aspiration, a PEG or PEJ tube may be inserted.

1. **Chemical pneumonitis** is caused by gastric reflux and aspiration of a sufficient quantity of stomach acid with pH below 2.5. Clinical features include acute dyspnea, hypoxemia, tachypnea, tachycardia with or without cyanosis, bronchospasm, and fever. Sputum may be pink and frothy. Radiographs may show infiltrates in one or both lower lobes. The clinical course is variable, ranging from rapid improvement within 5 days to a fulminant course, which may lead to death. Treatment is supportive and includes positive-pressure breathing, IV fluids, and tracheal suction as needed. The benefit of corticosteroids and antibiotics remains controversial.
2. **Bacterial infection** is usually caused by aspiration of oropharyngeal bacteria (usually anaerobes in community-acquired pneumonias and *Staphylococcus aureus* in hospital-acquired pneumonias). Onset is usually insidious. Symptoms include cough, fever, and purulent sputum. The radiograph shows infiltrates involving the dependent pulmonary segments or lobes with or without cavitation. Treatment is antibiotics given empirically or based on sputum culture.
3. **Mechanical airway obstruction** results from aspiration of particulate matters (e.g., food) or inert fluids and usually involves the right main-stem bronchus territory. Symptoms include wheezing, coughing, choking, and respiratory distress (e.g., acute dyspnea and cyanosis with or without apnea). Depending on the level of obstruction and the size of the particle aspirated, the patient may develop an irritating chronic cough (with or without recurrent infections) or develop acute apnea leading to rapid death. Treatment is extraction of the particulate matter (e.g., by the Heimlich maneuver) or, if inert fluids are present, tracheal suction and intermittent positive-pressure breathing with oxygen and isoproterenol as needed. If there is a superimposed bacterial infection (as a result of obstruction of normal pulmonary drainage), antibiotics may be given.

B. **MALNUTRITION** is an imbalance between nutrient intake and bodily requirements. It is significant if the patient has a recent weight loss of more than 10–15%; weight below 90% of ideal body weight (IBW) (see Table 5.6-2 for IBW computation); or serum albumin below 3.5 g/dL. In malnutrition, the daily

Table 5.6-2	Quick calculation for ideal body weights (IBW)	
Body condition	**Male IBW**	**Female IBW**
Medium-built	Allow 106 lb for the first 5 feet, plus 6 lb for each additional inch	Allow 100 lb for the first 5 feet, plus 5 lb for each additional inch
Small-built	Subtract 10% of IBW	Subtract 10% of IBW
Large-built	Add 10% of IBW	Add 10% of IBW
Para- or tetraplegia	Subtract 5–10% of IBW	Subtract 5–10% of IBW
Amputations		
Foot	Subtract 1.8% of IBW	Subtract 1.8% of IBW
Below knee	Subtract 6.0% of IBW	Subtract 6.0% of IBW
Above knee	Subtract 15.0% of IBW	Subtract 15.0% of IBW
Entire unilateral LE	Subtract 18.5% of IBW	Subtract 18.5% of IBW
Hand	Subtract 1.0% of IBW	Subtract 1.0% of IBW
Below elbow	Subtract 3.0% of IBW	Subtract 3.0% of IBW
Entire unilateral UE	Subtract 6.5% of IBW	Subtract 6.5% of IBW

1 lb = 0.454 kg; 1 foot = 30.5 cm; 1 inch = 2.54 cm.
LE = lower extremity; UE = upper extremity
Tabulated from the IBW formulae used by the nutrition departments of the New York University Medical Center, New York, NY and Goldwater Memorial Hospital, Roosevelt Island, NY. Data adapted from: Peiffer SC, Blust P, Leyson JFJ: Nutritional assessment of the spinal cord injured patient. J Am Dietetics Assoc *78:501–505, 1981; and Le Veau B: Williams and Lissner: Biomechanics of human motion, ed 2, Philadelphia, 1977, WB Saunders, pp. 205–215.*

caloric needs can be determined by the Harris–Benedict formula for basal energy expenditure (BEE; where wt is weight and ht is height):

- Male: BEE in kcal/day = 66 + (13.7 × wt in kg) + (5 × ht in cm) – (6.8 × age in years)
- Female: BEE in kcal/day = 655 + (9.6 × wt in kg) + (1.8 × ht in cm) – (4.7 × age in years)

The caloric needs of general hospital patients are about 120% of BEE, but if there is a major medical stress, caloric requirements can be as high as 150–200% of BEE. Caloric need (i.e., kcal per kg) for sedentary activity is 20 to 30 × IBW; for light activity, 25 to 35 × IBW; for moderate activity, 30 to 40 × IBW; and for heavy activity, 45 to 50 × IBW. The protein requirement for healthy adults is 0.8 g/kg/day, but for hospitalized patients, it is about 1.0–1.5 g/kg/day (higher in catabolic state and lower in renal or liver disease). Fluid requirement is approximately 30–35 mL/kg. Enteral feeding (e.g., NGT feeding) may be used if nutritional needs are not met by oral feeding (e.g., as a result of recurrent aspiration). For prolonged enteral feeding, a PEG or PEJ is preferred over NGTs. In the PM&R setting, intermittent or bolus feeding in the daytime is preferred so that the patient can participate in rehabilitation activities.

In patients with chronic pulmonary disease (especially chronic obstructive pulmonary disease), there is increased energy cost of breathing even at rest; therefore, the result of the above BEE computation needs to be adjusted by multiplying it by a correction factor of 1.2 to 1.5 (the higher factor is used for emaciated patients). If the patient is not confined in bed, the adjusted BEE is further adjusted by multiplying it by a factor of 1.06. In using IBW to determine the status of patients with chronic pulmonary disease, cut-off values of less than 90% or as low as less than 70–85% IBW may be justifiable (as discussed in Chapter 5.12, section IV.A.1.b). For further discussion about the pulmonary relationship, effects, and management of malnutrition in patients with chronic pulmonary problems, refer to Chapter 5.12, section IV.A.1.b.

Further reading

Bartlett JG: Aspiration pneumonia. In Baum GL, Wolinsky E, editors: *Textbook of pulmonary diseases*, ed 5, vol 1, Boston, 1994, Little, Brown, p. 593.

Bülow M, Olsson R, Ekberg O: Videoradiographic analysis of how carbonated thin liquids and thickened liquids affect the physiology of swallowing in subjects with aspiration on thin liquids. *Acta Radiol* 44: 366–372, 2003.

Cherney LR: *Rehabilitation Institute of Chicago: clinical management of dysphagia in adults and children*, ed 2, Gaithersburg, MD, 1994, Aspen.

Dodds WJ, Taylor AJ, Stewart ET, *et al.*: Tipper and dipper types of oral swallows. *Am J Roentgenol* 153:1197–1199, 1989.

Feldman R, Kapur K, Alman J, *et al.*: Aging and mastication: Changes in performance and in the swallowing threshold with natural dentition. *Am Geriat Soc* 28:97–103, 1980.

Greenbaum DM: Decannulation of the tracheostomized patient. *Heart Lung* 5:119–123, 1976.

Griffin K: Swallowing training for dysphagic patients. *Arch Phys Med Rehabil* 55:467–470, 1974.

Groher M, editor: *Dysphagia: diagnosis and management*, ed 3, Boston, 1997, Butterworth-Heinemann.

Johnson R, McKenzie S, Rosenquist C, *et al.*: Dysphagia following stroke: quantitative evaluation of pharyngeal transit times. *Arch Phys Med Rehabil* 73:419–423, 1992.

Langmore SE, Miller RM: Behavioral treatment for adults with oropharyngeal dysphagia. *Arch Phys Med Rehabil* 75:1154–1160, 1994.

Logemann JA: *Evaluation and treatment of swallowing disorders*, ed 2, Austin, TX, 1998, Pro-Ed Publishers.

Miller RM, Langmore SE: Treatment efficacy for adults with oropharyngeal dysphagia. *Arch Phys Med Rehabil* 75:1256–1262, 1994.

Noll SF, Bender CE, Nelson MC, *et al.*: Rehabilitation of patients with swallowing disorders. In Braddom RL, editor: *Physical Medicine and Rehabilitation*, ed 2, Philadelphia, 2000, WB Saunders, pp. 535–560.

Nutrition and Food Service: *Goldwater Memorial Hospital pocketbook of diet manual*, New York, 1993, Goldwater Memorial Hospital.

Robbins J, Hamilton JW, Lof GL, *et al.*: Oropharyngeal swallowing in normal adults of different ages. *Gastroenterology* 103:823–829, 1992.

Shaker R, Kern M, Bardan E, *et al.*: Effect of isotonic/isometric head lift exercise on hypopharyngeal intrabolus pressure. *Dysphagia* 12:107, 1997.

Stefans V, Gray RP, Sowell T: Pediatric and adult swallowing videofluoroscopy. In Lennard TA, editor: *Physiatric procedures in clinical practice*, ed 2, Philadelphia, 2000, Hanley & Belfus, pp. 56–65.

CHAPTER 5.7
Voiding dysfunctions

Aside from urinary tract infections, voiding disorder is the most common urinary problem managed by physiatrists in the inpatient rehabilitation setting. This chapter concentrates mainly on voiding dysfunctions of neurourologic origin.

I. Neuroanatomy and neurophysiology of voiding

A. PERIPHERAL PATHWAYS

1. Efferent fibers

a. Autonomic efferents

I. **Parasympathetic efferents** from the **S2–S4** segments of the spinal cord (i.e., the conus medullaris) travel through the pelvic nerves (also called pelvic splanchnic nerves or nervi erigentes) to the parasympathetic (cholinergic muscarinic M2 and M3) receptors distributed throughout the detrusor muscle (more in the body of the bladder than at the base). Among muscarinic receptors, the M3 receptors are believed to be responsible for bladder contraction (i.e., emptying).

II. **Sympathetic efferents** from the **T11–L2** segments of the spinal cord travel through the hypogastric plexi to sympathetic (α and β_2 adrenergic) receptors. Stimulation of β_2 receptors located primarily in the body of the bladder causes bladder relaxation (urine storage). Stimulation of α (mainly α_{1A}) receptors, which are located primarily at the base of the bladder, causes closing of the internal urethral sphincter (IUS) at the bladder outlet (formed by smooth muscle fibers), promoting urine storage.

b. ***Somatic efferents*** from the **S2–S4** segments of the spinal cord travel through the pudendal nerves to innervate the striated muscles of the external urethral sphincter (EUS). The EUS is marginally closed with its normal tone (thus preventing urine emptying or leakage) during the collecting phase of the urinary bladder and is opened passively by forceful urinary flow with contraction of the detrusor and the abdominal muscles. Voluntary contractions of the EUS and the pelvic floor muscles can hold the urine in the bladder for a limited period of time, while the detrusor muscle is contracting involuntarily.

2. **Afferent fiber** signals travel through the pudendal and pelvic nerves to the conus medullaris, and through the hypogastric plexi to the thoracolumbar spinal cord. They originate from the detrusor muscle stretch receptors, and from sensory nerve endings in the proximal urethra. Filling of the bladder up to a threshold level activates the stretch receptors in the bladder and stimulates the sensory nerve endings in the proximal urethra, sending impulses through the afferent nerves (i.e., probably through the hypogastric, pudendal, and pelvic nerves; exact physiology is unknown) to the conus medullaris and to the frontal lobes, and then descending signals to the brainstem and to the conus, hence resulting in reflect detrusor contractions, opening of sphincters, and emptying of the bladder.

B. CENTRAL AND PERIPHERAL PATHWAYS ("VOIDING CENTERS")

1. **Loop I** consists of a circuit between the anteromedial portion of the frontal lobe and the brainstem detrusor nucleus. A lesion above the pontine micturition

center [e.g., stroke, traumatic brain injury (TBI), hydrocephalus, brain tumor, and Parkinson's disease] can result in loss of micturition control of the cerebral cortex; therefore, low threshold detrusor reflex [or neurogenically overactivate detrusor (formerly called hyper-reflexic detrusor)] with small bladder capacity (i.e., urinary incontinence) results. Since the pontine micturition center, the spinal cord, the sacral micturition center, and the peripheral system remain intact, there would be no sphincter dyssenergia.

2. **Loop II** begins at the pontine micturition center, and consists of a spinal cord component (ascending and descending tracts) and a peripheral component (proprioceptive sensory axon from the detrusor muscles and pre- and post-ganglionic pelvic motor nerve fibers). A lesion at or below the pontine micturition center and above the sacral cord [e.g., traumatic spinal cord injury (SCI), transverse myelitis, multiple sclerosis (MS) involving the cord, syringomyelia, and intrinsic or extrinsic spinal cord tumor] would have both neurogenic detrusor overactivity (formerly called detrusor hyper-reflexia) and external sphincter spasticity (sphincter–detrusor dyssynergia) with reflex voiding pattern and no sensory feedback mechanism. This type of neurogenic bladder may lead to urinary retention, vesicourecteral reflux, or hydronephrosis.
3. **Loop III** consists of proprioceptive sensory axons from the detrusor muscle terminating in the pudendal nuclei in the sacral micturition center. It is responsible for maintaining normal tone of the pelvic floor muscles and the EUS during the collecting phase of the urinary bladder. A lesion involving the scaral micturition center or below [e.g., conus and cauda equina injuries, lumbar disc herniation, tumor, myelodysplasias, arteriovenous (AV) malformation, lumbar stenosis, and inflammatory process such as arachnoiditis] or peripheral nerves (e.g., diabetic neuropathy and pelvic trauma) can result in a lower motor neurogenic bladder with outlet incompetence as well as detrusor areflexia.
4. **Loop IV** includes the segmental pudendal nerve innervation as well as the spinal cord (posterior columns and corticospinal tracts) and the frontal lobes. It is responsible for the voluntary control of the external urethral sphincter.

II. Evaluation

A. **UROLOGIC HISTORY** includes voiding complaints (urgency, frequency, hesitancy, dysuria, and incontinence), voiding history, previous surgery (abdominal, pelvic, and transurethral), medications (sedatives, hypnotics, anticholinergics, antidepressants, antipsychotics, antihistamines, antispasmodics, opiates, sympathetic blockers, diuretics, and calcium-channel blockers), other medical problems [stroke, cognitive disorders, endocrine disorders such as diabetes mellitus, recurrent urinary tract infections (UTIs), restricted mobility, and stool impaction or incontinence], fluid intake and output over several 24-hour periods, activities of daily living (hand function, ability to perform transfers, and ability to dress and undress), availability of support system (e.g., family and home health aides), life-style, and sexuality. The mnemonic for the reversible (transient) causes of incontinence in the elderly that must be ruled out in history-taking is **DIAPPERS** – **D**elirium or confusional state, **I**nfection (urinary, symptomatic), **A**trophic vaginitis and/or urethritis, **P**harmaceuticals (sedatives or hypnotics, especially long-acting agents; anticholinergic agents; loop diuretics; α-adrenergic agonists and antagonists; calcium-channel blockers), **P**sychological disorders (depression), **E**ndocrine disorders (hyperglycemia or hypercalcemia), **R**educed mobility, and **S**tool impaction.

B. **PHYSICAL EXAMINATION** includes assessment of motor level, sensory level (sacral sensation), deep tendon reflexes, pathological reflexes (e.g., Babinski), anal wink (S1–S4), bulbocavernosus reflex (S2–S4), ice-water test (instill 50–100 mL of ice water into the bladder through a catheter; if the bladder contracts and expels the catheter as well as water, it signifies that patients with upper motor lesions are out of the spinal-shock stage), prostate examination in men, and degree of vaginal support and estrogenization in women.

C. DIAGNOSTIC TESTS

1. Upper urinary tract studies

a. ***Intravenous pyelogram (IVP) or excretory urogram*** is used to visualize the size, shape, and function of the whole urinary tracts (kidneys, ureters, and bladder) and to detect hydronephrosis, pyelonephritis, calculi, tumor, and renovascular hypertension. A radio-opaque substance is injected intravenously, and a series of radiographs are taken 3, 5, 10, 15, and 20 minutes after dye injection. At the end of the test, the patient voids and another radiograph is taken to visualize the residual dye in the bladder. The major disadvantage of IVP is the patient's potential allergic reactions to the dye, radiation exposure, and patient inconvenience (patient should be *non per os* and take laxatives). It can cause contrast nephropathy in patients with compromised renal function (especially in patients with insulin-dependent diabetes mellitus or creatinine greater than 1.5 mg/dL).

b. ***Renal ultrasound*** is useful for detecting hydronephrosis and kidney stones. Unlike IVP, it does not subject the patient to radiation; however, it is operator-dependent, and it does not give information on kidney function.

c. ***Plain radiogram of kidneys, ureter, and bladder (KUB)*** is used with renal ultrasound to identify possible radio-opaque calculi missed by ultrasound.

d. ***Quantitative renal scan*** monitors renal function and drainage.

I. **Technetium-99 m (^{99m}Tc)** scan using ^{99m}Tc-dimercaptosuccinic acid (DMSA) is used for both differential function and evaluation of the functioning areas of the renal cortex. ^{99m}Tc-mercaptoacetyltriglycine (MAG3) is used to assess urinary tract drainage as well as differential function.

II. **Hippuran ^{131}I scan** is used to monitor renal perfusion and determine glomerular filtration rate and excretory renal plasma flow.

e. ***Twenty-four hour urine creatinine clearance*** may be used to follow quantitative renal function; however, creatinine clearance may remain normal despite moderate to severe renal deterioration.

2. Lower urinary tract studies

a. ***Urinalysis and urine culture and sensitivity*** are used to detect UTI. Pyuria accompanied by a bacterial colony count of 100 000/mL or more organisms of a single microbial species indicates the presence of a UTI. The antibiotic sensitivity of the cultured bacteria is used to guide the choice of antibiotic therapy.

b. ***Postvoid residual (PVR)*** involves transurethral catheterization to measure residual urine volume in the bladder immediately after voiding to determine the ability of the bladder to empty and to gauge the effectiveness of any therapeutic interventions for the bladder. A large PVR must be interpreted with caution because it may not have been taken immediately after voiding or the patient may not have understood the instruction to void completely. Consistently low PVR may rule out outlet obstruction, but incontinence does not rule out urinary retention. A "balanced bladder" in men with SCI had less than 100 mL PVR with reflex voiding.

c. ***Voiding cystourethrography*** is a radiologic study that provides structural and dynamic measures of bladder function. Contrast dye is introduced into the bladder via a catheter, and a radiograph of the bladder is taken. The catheter is removed and the patient is asked to void. During voiding, another radiograph, which includes the urethra, is taken. These radiographs are taken to demonstrate the size and shape of the bladder, the function of the sphincter (i.e., open or closed), contrast in the urethra, and presence or absence of vesicoureteral reflux. This study can also detect a peno-scrotal diverticulum, diverticuli of the bladder wall, fistula, extravasation in the prostate, tumor, and a rupture of the bladder.

d. ***Cystoscopy*** is a procedure for direct visualization of the bladder wall and urethra. It is also used for a tissue biopsy and for removal of stones and debris from the distal ureter, bladder, or urethra. Clinical indications include hematuria, recurrent symptomatic UTIs, and outlet obstruction with urinary retention. It can also be used to rule out bladder carcinoma.

e. ***Urodynamics*** including **cystometrogram (CMG)** documents the intravesical pressure, the activity of the external urinary sphincter [via perineal surface electromyograph (EMG) electrodes], and the patient's subjective sensation of voiding as the bladder is progressively filled transurethrally with either normal saline or carbon dioxide (CO_2). Although normal saline is more physiologic, it takes a longer time to fill the bladder. In the office or bedside setting, CO_2 is commonly used because it fills the bladder fast; however, the voiding phase of micturition cannot be evaluated with CO_2. Recently, video urodynamics has become popular in assessing morphology and function of the bladder and urethra. Urodynamic studies are indicated for evaluation of voiding dysfunction (i.e., urinary frequency, incontinence, and retention) and occasionally for evaluation of effects of neurourologic drugs.

I. **Filling-phase study**. As the bladder volume increases, there is a slow rise in intravesical pressure due to the contractile property of the bladder, while normal tone of the EUS shown on EMG prevents urine leakage. At around 100–200 mL, the first sensation of bladder filling normally occurs. At around 300–400 mL, a mild desire to void usually occurs. As the bladder fills to around 400–500 mL, there is a strong desire to void (urgency). A full normal bladder during the filling phase (maximum capacity of 400 to 750 mL in adults) has intravesical pressures of 0 to 6 cm H_2O, which should not rise above 15 cm H_2O. In patients with neurogenic detrusor overactivity caused by upper motor neuron lesions, the bladder contracts and empties at low volumes. Patients with atonic (areflexic) bladders due to a lower motor neuron lesion, however, have a large capacity without showing an increase in the intravesical pressure despite the introduction of large volumes of fluid or CO_2.

II. **Voiding-phase study** is used to determine the functional relationship between the bladder and the EUS during micturition. During normal voiding, there is a sudden silence of sphincter EMG activity as well as a drop in proximal urethral pressure (due to inhibition of the sympathetic α-adrenergic receptors). The bladder (detrusor) then contracts, and a voiding occurs. The detrusor muscle contraction results from the sacral parasympathetic outflow to the bladder via the pelvic nerve in addition to the suppression of sympathetic β_2 adrenergic influence on the detrusor muscle. Contractions of the detrusor muscle and opening of the sphincters (internal and external) are coordinated by the "pontine and sacral micturition centers." After voiding, the EMG of the EUS demonstrates return of normal sphincter tone. This coordination is lost in patients with detrusor–sphincter dyssynergia. The detrusor pressure is below 30 cm H_2O in women and between 30 and 50 cm H_2O in men during voiding. The flow rate is between 15 and 20 mL H_2O for men if there is at least 150 mL of urine in the bladder. The urethral sphincter EMG should remain silent throughout voiding.

III. Classifications of voiding dysfunctions

Classifications have been based on neurologic lesions (e.g., Bors–Comarr or Bradley), functional classification (Wein), urodynamic findings (e.g., Lapides or Krane–Siroky),

Table 5.7-1 Functional classification of voiding dysfunctions and their treatment options

Functional classification	Treatment options
I. Incontinence (failure to store)	
A. Due to neurogenic detrusor overactivity (e.g., suprapontine lesions such as stroke, TBI, MS, neoplasm, hydrocephalus, PD)	1. Behavioral: timed voids, fluid restrictions 2. Collecting devices: diaper, catheter (condom or indwelling) 3. Clean intermittent catheterization 4. Drugs: anticholinergics, musculotropics, tricyclic antidepressant, intrathecal baclofen*, prostaglandin inhibitors*, intravesical capsaicin* 5. Surgery: augmentation, continent diversion, denervation procedures*, neurostimulation*
B. Due to outlet or sphincter incompetence (e.g., children with myelodysplasia; stress incontinence in women with infrasacral lesion and denervated pelvic floor; or rarely, men with complete denervation)	1. Behavioral: timed voids, pelvic floor exercises, biofeedback, fluid restrictions 2. Collecting devices: diaper, catheter (condom or indwelling) 3. Drugs: α-adrenergic agonists, imipramine, estrogen cream 4. Surgery: collagen injection, fascial sling, artificial sphincter, Teflon injection*, neurostimulation*
II. Retention (failure to empty)	
A. Due to bladder areflexia (e.g., spinal shock in SCI; MS; peripheral neuropathies; sacral lesions such as spinal trauma, herniated lumbar disk, spinal tumors, myelodysplasia, arteriovenous malformation, lumbar stenosis, arachnoiditis)	1. Behavioral: timed voids, bladder stimulation (suprapubic jabbing; transurethral electrical bladder stimulation), Valsalva's and Credé's maneuvers 2. Collecting devices: indwelling catheter 3. Clean intermittent catheterization 4. Drugs: cholinergic agonists, intravesical prostaglandins*, narcotic antagonists* 5. Surgery: neurostimulation*
B. Due to outlet or sphincter dyssynergia (e.g., suprasacral traumatic SCI)	1. Behavioral: anal stretch void, suprapubic tapping, biofeedback 2. Collecting devices: indwelling catheters 3. Clean intermittent catheterization 4. Drugs: α-adrenergic blockers, oral striated muscle relaxant (baclofen, diazepam, dantrolene), intrathecal baclofen* 5. Surgery: sphincterotomy incision, bladder neck incision, prostate resection, pudendal neurectomy*, stent, sphincterotomy*
III. Failure of storage and emptying with nonusable urethra	Surgery: suprapubic catheter $\pm$ bladder neck closure, ileal conduit, continent diversion

MS, multiple sclerosis; PD, Parkinson's disease; SCI, spinal cord injury; TBI, traumatic brain injury

** indicates experimental or nonstandard treatment.*

Adapted from: Linsenmeyer TA, Stone JM: Neurogenic bladder and bowel dysfunction. In DeLisa JA and Gans BM, editors: Rehabilitation medicine: principles and practice, *ed 3, Philadelphia, 1998, Lippincott-Raven, p. 1086; and Cardenas DD, Mayo ME: Management of bladder dysfunction. In Braddom RL, editor:* Physical medicine and rehabilitation, *ed 2, Philadelphia, 2000, WB Saunders, p. 569.*

or a combination of bladder and urethral function based on urodynamics (e.g., International Continence Society). In the PM&R setting, the functional classification by Wein (determined by urodynamics) is useful for deciding on treatment options (see Table 5.7-1). Classification terms such as *neurogenic bladder* should not be used when referring to nonbladder (e.g., outlet or sphincter) dysfunction.

IV. Treatment

Treatment goals are to decrease or prevent lower tract complications (e.g., by maintaining continence), to preserve the upper tracts (e.g., by avoiding persistently high intravesical pressure, which may cause vesicoureteral reflux), and to implement a realistic bladder management program.

A. BEHAVIORAL MANAGEMENT

1. **Timed (scheduled) voiding** before the bladder reaches full capacity to prevent urine leakage as a result of high intravesical pressure. Individuals with dementia need constant reminding.
2. **Bladder training** is done by progressively increasing the time between voiding by 10–15 minutes every 2–5 days until a reasonable interval between voidings is attained (regular voiding of at least every 3 hours). The patient is made fully responsible for adhering to a drinking, voiding, and catheterization schedule. The drinking schedule usually consists of a well-timed fluid intake of 1800 mL per day (400 mL at mealtimes and 200 mL at 10 a.m., 2 p.m., and 4 p.m.). The patient attempts to void at least every 3 hours while awake by using specific techniques that were found to give the best response during urodynamics. The intermittent catheterization schedule is adjusted in accordance with the residual urine volume. The following records are made by the patient: fluid intake, intentional voiding (amount in milliliters), unintentional voiding (in relative degrees), and the amount of residual urine volume obtained by straight urinary catheterization after a trial of self-voiding. These day-to-day data are then represented in graph form and kept on a clipboard at the bedside to determine the efficiency of voiding. Bladder training is most effective in patients who are recovering from an insult in the CNS (e.g., stroke or TBI) and in patients who suffer from atonic myogenic detrusor insufficiency (underactive bladder and normoactive outlet). Bladder retraining may be contraindicated in patients with decompensating renal function, especially when accompanied by incompetent vesicoureteral junctions. It is also contraindicated in patients with severe cystitis, bladder calculi, or major structural changes of either the bladder or the urethra; in patients who cannot adhere to the necessary training procedures and record keeping; in the very young; in debilitated elderly patients; in unmotivated or undisciplined patients; and in patients who are unable to do the necessary activities for voiding, such as transferring to the toilet or dressing and undressing.
3. **Bladder stimulation**
   a. ***Suprapubic jabbing***, that is, by pressing deep over the bladder to mechanically stretch its wall, is more effective than suprapubic tapping (rapid, yet light tapping at a place where the highest degree of reflex response is obtained) or stroking or pinching of the perineal skin. However, suprapubic jabbing is contraindicated in hyperreflexic detrusor–external sphincter dyssynergia with vesicoureteral reflux.
   b. ***Transurethral electrical bladder stimulation*** has recently been tried experimentally to activate mechanoreceptor afferents, which perceive the sensation of bladder filling, and in turn, activate efferent nerves, resulting in detrusor muscle contractions.
4. **Valsalva's maneuver** increases intravesical pressure by increasing intra-abdominal pressure. It involves sitting and resting the abdomen forward on the thighs for both men and women. During straining in this position, hugging of the knees and legs may prevent any bulging of the abdomen. In this manner, all of the increase in intra-abdominal pressure is transferred to the bladder and the pelvic floor. Adverse effects include exacerbation of hemorrhoids, rectal prolapse, or hernia. In patients with vesicoureteral reflux, it is contraindicated.

5. **Credé's maneuvers** increase intravesical pressure by manually pushing down on the bladder. This technique has the same adverse effects and contraindications as Valsalva's maneuver.

a. ***The open-hand Credé's method*** involves placing the thumb of each hand over the area of the left and right anterosuperior iliac spine and the digits over the suprapubic area with slight overlapping of the tips. The slightly overlapped digits are then pressed into the abdomen. When they are well behind the symphysis, the pressure is directed downward to compress the fundus of the bladder. Both hands are then pressed as deeply as possible downward into the pelvic cavity.

b. ***Closed-hand Credé's method*** compresses the bladder by using the closed fist of one hand or a rolled-up towel.

6. **Anal stretch voiding** involves relaxation of the pelvic floor by first stretching the anal sphincter and then evacuating by Valsalva's maneuver. It can be used in paraplegic patients with no anal sensation who are able to transfer to a toilet and perform Valsalva's maneuver.

7. **Pelvic floor exercises or Kegel exercises** (see also Chapter 5.8, section VI.A.6.b.1) are effective only in women with mild to moderate stress incontinence because of a hypotonic sphincter. Patients need to be highly motivated as it may take 4–8 weeks before any effect is noted.

8. **Biofeedback** (see also Chapter 4.1, section VI) may be used in conjunction with Kegel exercise. It may also be used in patients (often children) who voluntarily tighten their sphincters during voiding.

B. URINE COLLECTION DEVICES

1. **External condom catheters** are used in men with neurogenic detrusor overactivity (e.g., SCI) or with normal unobstructed bladder function with incontinence because of immobility or dementia. Unlike diapers, it is changed usually once a day; however, the patient must wear a leg bag for urine collection, and there is a slight increased risk for UTI as well as a potential for penile skin breakdown and urethral damage. The condom catheter may also get dislodged, particularly during transfers.

2. **Indwelling urethral or suprapubic catheters** are used when other treatment options have failed or for the patient's convenience. Complications include bladder stones, hematuria, bacteremia (especially when catheter is obstructed), metal erosions, penile and scrotal fistulae, vesicovaginal fistula, epididymo-orchitis, urethral stricture, urethral diverticulum, and bladder carcinoma (with long-term use). To prevent or reduce complications, the indwelling catheter must be changed every 2 to 4 weeks; patients must orally take at least 2 L/day of fluids; the catheter must be taped up to the abdomen in men to prevent traction and risk for a penoscrotal fistula; the urethral meatus must be cleaned with soap and water; the collecting bag must be sterilized with bleach; anticholinergics should be given for neurogenic detrusor overactivity to prevent development of a contracted bladder; and the collecting bag must never be raised above the bladder level to prevent a reflux of urine into the bladder while in bed.

3. **Adult diapers and other protective garments** are a combination of high-absorbent gel-impregnated material that allows the lining against the patient's skin to stay dry. They are used for incontinence, e.g., in patients with dementia and adequate bladder emptying. They tend to be expensive, may be difficult to put on and off (in some patients, personal care by an aide may be required), and can potentially cause skin macerations or fungal infections if not changed within 2–4 hours of getting wet.

C. INTERMITTENT CATHETERIZATION (IC) is the method of choice for the management of urinary retention, particularly following SCI. Anticholinergic medications may be used in female patients with neurogenic detrusor overactivity. In an acute care setting (e.g., acute SCI centers), the sterile technique is recommended to prevent UTI; however, in outpatient or chronic care facility settings, a nonsterile but "clean" technique (called clean intermittent catheterization [CIC]) may be used. The use of concomitant bacteriostatic and acidifying medications for UTI prophylaxis remain controversial (e.g., methenamine salts such as Mandelamine, 1 g, po, qid, or Hiprex, 1 g, po, bid, or Vitamin C, 1–3 g, po, tid/qid).

Fluid intake should be restricted to 2 L per day, while undergoing intermittent catheterizations to keep residual urine volume below 400–500 mL. If the patient has an urge to void, additional catheterization may be needed. For a timed IC schedule, an easy mnemonic is the "1-2-3-4" system, i.e., for residual volume of 100 (±50) mL, catheterize once a day; 200 (±50) mL, twice a day; 300 (±50) mL, three times a day; 400 (±50) mL, four times a day). If the residual volume is consistently below 100 mL, the daily IC may no longer be necessary.

Relative contraindications to a self-IC program include significant leg adductor spasticity, PMH of urethral false passage, poor eye–hand coordination, poor cognition, and poor motivation. Complications of IC are symptomatic bacteriuria, urethral trauma, and bladder stone formations (hair or lint introduced during catheterization has been found to be the nidus for stone formation). If sphincter spasm or resistance is felt, extra lubrication and local anesthetic urethral gel (lidocaine 2%) or a curved-tip (coudé) catheter may be used. Repeated bleeding during IC may warrant use of indwelling catheter until the traumatic source (e.g., urethral mucosa trauma or urethral false passage) has resolved.

D. DRUGS (see Table 5.7-2 for drugs commonly used in treating voiding dysfunction):

1. Drugs used in incontinence caused by neurogenic detrusor overactivity act by relaxing the detrusor, hence increasing bladder capacity.

a. Anticholinergic drugs (see Table 5.7-2) are used to control neurogenic detrusor overactivity by blocking acetylcholine receptors competitively at the postganglionic cholinergic receptor sites. Adverse drug reactions (ADRs) include decreased secretion of tears, saliva, sweat, and milk; mydriasis, blurred vision, and increased intraocular pressure; tachycardia and palpitations; mental confusion, headache, dizziness, nervousness, drowsiness, insomnia, and weakness; nausea, vomiting, and decreased gastrointestinal mobility (i.e., paralytic ileus and constipation); impotence; and allergic reactions. Contraindications include glaucoma, urinary outlet obstruction (e.g., hypertrophic prostate), acute paralytic ileus, gastrointestinal obstruction (e.g., pyloroduodenal stenosis), severe colitis, and myasthenia gravis.

I. **Propantheline bromide (Pro-Banthine)** is a muscarinic receptor antagonist that decreases the frequency and amplitude of uninhibited bladder contractions and, therefore, increases total bladder capacity.

II. **Oxybutynin (Ditropan)** exerts a direct antispasmodic effect on the smooth muscle cell membrane (musculotropic effect) and, to a lesser extent, inhibits the muscarinic action of acetylcholine on smooth muscles. It increases bladder capacity; decreases the frequency of uninhibited bladder contractions; and decreases urgency, frequency, and urge incontinence. It can also decrease dysuria because of its local anesthetic effects on the bladder. Aside from the oral route, it may be instilled intravesically during IC by dissolving a 5-mg tablet in sterile water. This reportedly has fewer ADRs than when given orally. It is available in extended release (Ditropan XL) and transdermal (Oxytrol) preparations.

III. **Hyoscyamine (Levsin)** inhibits acetylcholine receptors of the postganglionic cholinergic nerves, hence relaxing the neurogenically overactive

Table 5.7-2 Drugs commonly used in treating voiding dysfunction

Generic	Brand-name (partial list)	Available preparations (mg)	Dosage (mg), route, frequency	MDD (mg)
I. Anticholinergics				
Trospium	Sanctura	Tab 20	20 po bid (may be adjusted to qd) 1 h ac	40
Tolterodine	Detrol; Detrol LA	Tab 1, 2; LA caps 4	2 po bid initially (may be adjusted to 1 po bid); LA: 4 po qd	4
Oxybutinin	Ditropan; Ditropan XL; Oxytrol Transdermal	Tab 5; elix 5/5 mL; XL 5,10,15; TD 3.9 per day	5 po bid/tid/qid; Peds: 5 po bid/tid; XL: 5 po qd (may increase by 5-mg interval weekly); TD 1 patch q3–4 days	20; XL:30
Propantheline	ProBanthine	Tab 7.5, 15	7.5–15 po 30 min ac tid and 30 qhs	75
Hyoscyamine	Levsin; Nulev; Levsinex Timecaps	Tab 0.125; elix/drops 0.125/5 mL; Timecaps 0.375	0.125–0.25 po/sl Tid/qid; Timecaps: 0.375 po bid	1.5
Imipramine	Tofranil	Tab 10, 25, 50	50–150 po qhs; pediatric use (>6 yr): 25 po qhs; ↑ to 50 (6–12 yr); ↑ to 75 (>12 yr)	100–150; pediatric: 2.5/kg/day
Amitriptyline	Elavil; Endep	Tab 10, 25, 50, 75, 100, 150	10–25 po tid; or 20–75 po qhs	75
II. Cholinergics				
Bethanechol	Urecholine	Tab 5, 10, 25, 50	10–50 mg po tid/qid	200
III. α-adrenergic agonists*				
Pseudoephedrine*	Sudafed;*	Tab 30,60; elix 30/5 mL	30–60 po q4–6h	240
IV. α-adrenergic blockers				
Prazosin	Minipress	Cap 1,2,5	Start 0.5 po bid/tid up to 2 po bid	4
Terazosin	Hytrin	Tab 1,2,5,10	1 po qhs; ↑ stepwise to 2, 5, 10, 20 qhs	20
Doxazosin	Cardura	Tab 1,2,4,8	Start 1 po qd up to 8 po qd	8
Tamsulosin	Flomax	Tab 0.4	0.4–0.8 po qd	0.8

** Available in combination with antitussive, bronchodilators, nasal decongestant, or antihistamines.*
MDD, maximum daily dose.

bladder. It is available in extended release (Levsinex Timecaps) and sublingual (Nulev) preparations.

IV. **Tolterodine (Detrol)** is a competitive muscarinic receptor antagonist, which acts on the lower urinary tract. It decreases detrusor pressure, leading to an increased bladder capacity. It is as effective as oxybutinin but with fewer side-effects from dry mouth and constipation. It is available in an extended release form (Detrol LA).

V. **Sanctura (trospium chloride)** is a direct selective antagonist of muscarinic receptors, which can relax the detrusor muscle. It is equally as effective as oxybutinin but, unlike oxybutinin, it does not cross the blood–brain barrier, thus causing fewer side-effects than oxybutinin.

b. ***Tricyclic antidepressants*** are known to cause urinary retention because of their anticholinergic effects. They are also thought to assist in the closing of the internal sphincter by potentiating adrenergic responses (via inhibition of norepinephrine reuptake). They may be used alone or in combination with anticholinergics (e.g., oxybutinin or propantheline). For details about the mechanism of action, ADRs, contraindications and precautions, and drug administration guidelines of tricyclic antidepressants, see Chapter 4.8, section V.A.1.

I. **Imipramine (Tofranil)** is mainly indicated for children with nocturnal enuresis (nonorganic etiology).

II. **Amitriptyline (Elavil, Endep)** may cause urinary retention because of its anticholinergic effects. Its effects are potentiated by cimetidine and other anticholinergic drugs.

c. ***Experimental drugs*** include **terodilene** (a calcium-channel blocker that relaxes the detrusor but has been withdrawn because of cardiac arrhythmias), **prostaglandin inhibitors** (e.g., nonsteroidal anti-inflammatory drugs such as **flurbiprofen**), **propiverine** (a muscarinic receptor antagonist and calcium-channel blocker; undergoing clinical trial), **darifenacin** (a muscarinic receptor antagonist; undergoing clinical trial), and **intrathecal baclofen**. Intrathecal baclofen decreases the detrusor reflex but also depresses the pelvic floor reflex with the net result of low intravesical pressure, which empties less effectively.

2. **Drugs used in incontinence caused by outlet or sphincter incompetence** act primarily by stimulating α-adrenergic receptors or potentiating adrenergic effects via inhibition of norepinephrine reuptake, hence enhancing the closure of the internal urethral sphincter (IUS) at the bladder outlet and promoting urine storage. β-Adrenergic agonists and antagonists are not used because they clinically have little effect on bladder functions.

a. ***α-Adrenergic agonists*** may be tried for improving mild to moderate stress incontinence because of incompetance the internal sphincter. Potential side-effects include anxiety, insomnia, headache, increased blood pressure, sweating, and palpitations. Contraindications include hypertension, cardiovascular disease, and hyperthyroidism. Their oral forms are usually available in combination with decongestants, bronchodilators, antitussives, and/or antihistamine.

I. **Ephedrine** directly stimulates the α- and β-adrenoceptors and causes release of norepinephrine. It has anecdotally been used in enuretic children with myelodysplasia at 15–50 mg, po, qhs. It is rarely used in adults.

II. **Phenylpropanolamine** is similar to ephedrine but has less CNS side effects, and is usually found in many cold remedies.

III. **Pseudoephedrine** (e.g., **Sudafed**) works well with oxybutinin in women with SCI who tend to develop reflexogenic incontinence in between intermittent catheterizations.

b. ***Premarin (conjugated estrogen) vaginal cream*** is helpful in postmenopausal women with stress incontinence caused by atrophy of the urethral epithelium or irritative symptoms from atrophic urethritis. It probably increases the sensitivity or increases the number of α-adrenergic receptors. To be effective, the pelvic floor musculatures have to be at least partially innervated. Dosage is 2–4 g (0.625 mg/g) applied intravaginally daily. If used for short duration (4–6 weeks), the risk for endometrial carcinoma, thrombosis, or withdrawal bleeding is negligible. It is contraindicated in women with breast cancer, pregnancy, genital bleeding, or thromboembolic disease.

c. ***Tricyclic antidepressants*** (see section IV.D.1.b)

3. **Drugs used in retention caused by bladder areflexia** (see Table 5.7-2)

a. ***Bethanechol (Urecholine)*** is a cholinergic agent that stimulates the release of acetylcholine. It is also resistant to rapid hydrolysis by acetylcholinesterase. It increases detrusor tension but probably does not stimulate physiologic bladder contraction. At an oral dose that is tolerated by patients, its effectiveness has been controversial; however, it may be used to augment mechanical stimulation of the detrusor by administration 45 minutes before voiding maneuvers (e.g., Credé's). Contraindications include ileus, bladder outlet obstruction, spastic sphincter detrusor dyssynergia, asthma, peptic ulcer, cardiac arrhythmia, coronary artery disease, and hyperthyroidism. Adverse drug reactions include flushing, salivation, nausea, vomiting, diarrhea, gastrointestinal cramps, bronchospasms, sweating, lacrimation, miosis, difficulty with visual accommodation, headache, malaise, bradycardia, and hypotension with reflex tachycardia.

b. ***Experimental drugs*** include narcotic antagonists (to block enkephalins, which are thought to inhibit the sacral micturition reflex) and intravesical prostaglandin F_{2a} to increase detrusor pressure.

4. **Drugs used in retention caused by internal sphincter closure or benign prostatic hyperplasia** (Table 5.7-2)

a. ***α-adrenergic blockers*** may improve bladder emptying in patients with sphincter–detrusor dyssynergia (e.g., in SCI), hyporeflexic bladder, or prostate outlet obstruction (because prostate smooth muscle is also mediated by α-adrenoceptors). The α-blocker is theoretically useful for modifying symptoms of autonomic dysreflexia (AD) associated with bladder distention. Its daytime use, when prescribed, should be avoided in patients with episodes of orthostatic hypotension. Common ADRs include dizziness, headache, orthostatic hypotension, palpitation, fatigue or malaise, weakness, nausea, edema, dyspnea, and nasal congestion. Less common ADRs include vertigo, rash, arthralgia, myalgia, paresthesia, ataxia, dry mouth, flushing, abnormal vision, eye pain, tinnitus, somnolence, nervousness, depression, insomnia, sexual dysfunction, diarrhea, constipation, polyuria, and chest pain.

I. **Doxazosin (Cardura)** is a blocker of α_1 adrenoceptor. It is available in once-a-day doses at bedtime.

II. **Terazosin (Hytrin)** is a blocker of α_1 adrenoceptor, and is used for urinary retention due to benign prostatic hyperplasia.

III. **Prazosin (Minipress)** is a postsynaptic blocker of α-adrenoceptors.

IV. **Tamsulosin (Flomax)** is a selective blocker of α-1 adrenoceptors in the bladder neck and in the prostate. Unlike aforementioned α-1 adrenoceptor blockers, a dose titration is not necessary.

b. ***Oral striated muscle relaxants (baclofen, diazepam, and dantrolene)*** may be used to promote relaxation of the striated muscles of the external urethral sphincter muscles. They are discussed in Chapter 5.4, section III.D.1.

E. **INVASIVE PROCEDURES (INJECTIONS OR SURGERY)** to improve voiding are used only if conservative treatment methods have failed.

1. **Bladder augmentation (augmentation cystoplasty)** can be considered to increase bladder capacity and to reduce intravesical pressure, especially in women with SCI. It is indicated for a contracted bladder with neurogenic detrusor overactivity or with reduced bladder compliance that failed nonsurgical

treatment options. The distal ileum is usually used for bladder augmentation. Postoperatively, long-term IC is required due to inefficient bladder emptying. Immediate postoperative complications in tetraplegic patients include autonomic dysreflexia, prolonged intestinal ileus, anastomotic leak with peritonitis, adhesions, wound infection, and pulmonary complications (pneumonia and emboli). Increased mucus secretion in the augmented bladder, which can be annoying in the first three postoperative months, may be modified by daily CIC with bladder irrigation. Long-term sequelae could include chronic bacteriuria and possible diarrhea or malabsorption from a shortened gut or decreased intestinal transit time. Its theoretical risk of neoplastic change as well as hyperchloremic acidaemia (due to absorption of urine with secondary mobilization of skeletal calcium as a buffer), remain controversial.

2. **Continent diversion** uses bowel not just to increase bladder capacity, but also to form a continent catheterizable channel which opens into the abdominal wall. It is useful in women who have difficulty with IC through the urethra (e.g., leg adductor spasticity, severe urethral incontinence, and obesity) or men who are unable to do IC because of strictures, false passages, or fistulas. Compliance with daily IC is mandatory, otherwise an overdistended bowel may rupture internally.
3. **Denervation procedures** may be considered for selective patients with neurogenic overactive bladder. They can be done at the root (e.g., sacral rhizotomies), peripheral nerve (e.g., unilateral pudendal nerve block or neurectomy), or at the perivesical area (i.e., gangliectomy). They can cause bladder areflexia.
4. **Implantation of an electrical neurostimulator** for selective stimulation of the detrusor muscle with areflexia can be applied in patients with cauda equina injury, but its use remains experimental and controversial.
5. **Bladder outlet procedures**

a. ***Injection therapy***. The injection of Teflon for urinary incontinence is currently not used because of the danger of particle migration. Injections of autologous fat and bovine collagen have low potential side-effects and are especially suitable for elderly and poor surgical candidates. Botulinum toxin type A (Botox) may be injected into the spastic striated sphincter in male patients with detrusor dyssynergia to enhance spontaneous voiding. Pudendal nerve block may also be done for the management of symptoms associated with external sphincter spasticity in patients with SCI.

b. ***External compressive surgical procedures***

I. **Fascial sling procedure**. A fascial strip is taken from the anterior abdominal rectus or tensor fascia lata, then wrapped around the bladder neck as a sling for the management of severe outlet incompetence. Patients must have a compliant low-pressure bladder and must agree to do self-IC for as long as medically and urologically necessary.

II. **Artificial urinary sphincter (AUS) implant** consists of a cuff implanted around the bladder neck, a pressure regulating balloon, and a control pump (implanted in the labia or scrotum to allow the patient to open and close the cuff for voiding). Problems of AUS include mechanical failure, cuff erosions, and infection. An advantage is that patients can do Valsalva's maneuver to void and do not need an IC program. About 10% of patients with myelodysplasia may show uncontrolled bladder overactivity in the first year after implantation and may probably need bladder augmentation. An AUS is not used in SCI patients with high intravesical pressure because of potential damage to the upper urinary tract (i.e., vesicoureteral reflux). There is also an increased risk of prosthesis infection or erosion of the cuff because of frequent bacteriuria. It may be used in patients with conus medullaris dysfunction who can be relied upon to empty their bladder every 4–6 hours daily. It is wise to delay the AUS implantation at least 6–12 months following an injury to the conus medullaris or to the cauda equina in order to ascertain that there is no clinical evidence of further neurological recovery.

c. ***Sphincterotomy*** is the ablation (usually by incision) of the striated sphincter muscle with severe spasticity. It is applied to decrease outflow resistance in patients with low volume bladder (less than 200 mL) and adequate detrusor contraction (less than 20 seconds rise time of contraction with more than 50 cm H_2O amplitude, and duration of at least 2 minutes), e.g., male SCI patients with frequent episodes of autonomic dysreflexia due to hyperreflexic detrusor–external sphincter dyssynergia despite pharmacological measures and IC. Other indications include vesicoureteral reflux and frequent urinary tract infections associated with external sphincter spasticity and high residual volumes. Postoperatively, it requires close observation for autonomic dysreflexia, bleeding, clot obstruction of an indwelling catheter (during the first few days after surgery), and constipation. Long-term complications include recurrent obstruction from stricture (scar formation). The procedure is irreversible, and the patient must wear a leg bag for life.

d. ***Stainless inert stent*** can be implanted to keep the outlet open. However, the urethra, where the stent was implanted, may become stenotic again.

6. **Urinary diversions** using the small bowels or a portion of large bowel can be done in certain SCI patients (especially female), when intermittent catheterization or indwelling catheterization (transurethral or suprapubic) is not considered as the method of choice for managing urinary retention or incontinence.

V. Complications of voiding dysfunctions

A. **URINARY TRACT INFECTION (UTI)** is the most common complication of voiding dysfunctions. It is not recommended to treat asymptomatic bacteriuria with no evidence of tissue invasion. The short-term use of an indwelling urinary catheter is not uncommon in the hospital setting, and does not require prophylactic antibiotics. Bacteriuria in SCI patients should be treated if the patient is symptomatic (e.g., fever, urine leakage around the Foley catheter, increased spasticity, and AD) or if urinalysis (UA) reveals WBC/hpf of >10. Common urine pathogens in uncomplicated UTI are *Enterococcus* species and *Escherichia coli;* and in patients with catheter-associated UTI there is usually a mixture of organisms, including *Proteus, Klebsiella, Pseudomonas, Serratia, Providencia, Escherichia coli, Enterococci,* and *Staphylococcus epidermides.*

Proper antibiotic treatment is chosen based on urine culture and sensitivity (urine C/S). If unavailable, empirical treatment should be started immediately after UA and urine C/S were sent to the laboratory. **Trimethoprim-sulfamethoxazole (Bactrim, Septra)**, one tab, po, bid (double strength 160/800 mg or single strength 80/400 mg), may be given but does not cover *Pseudomonas aeruginosa.* Oral quinolones are currently recommended for treatment of UTIs because they may also cover *P. aeruginosa.* Examples are **ciprofloxacin (Cipro)**, 250 to 750 mg, po, bid or **levofloxacin (Levaquin)**, 250 to 750 mg, po, qd. For more seriously ill patients, IV antibiotics may be needed. Antibiotics should be given for at least 7–14 days depending on the severity of UTI. In recurrent UTIs or severe UTIs, further diagnostic work-ups (e.g., urodynamic evaluation, excretory urogram, cystogram) should be done to identify an underlying etiology.

B. **STONES**

1. **Bladder stones** are usually associated with an indwelling Foley catheter or prolonged urinary retention. It can occasionally be caused by foreign body introduction (public hair or retained portion of the Foley balloon). It predisposes the

patient to hematuria, persistent UTI, autonomic dysreflexia or occasionally obstruction of the urethra; however, it does not cause renal deterioration. Treatment of choice is removal of bladder calculi, which can be done by cystolitholopaxy or, less frequently, by lithotripsy.

2. **Kidney stones** are seen in 1–2% of SCI patients of all follow-up visits. If left untreated, it can lead to urosepsis or even death. In 98% of urinary calculi, the stone is made up of magnesium ammonium phosphate (struvite) and calcium phosphate because of alkaline urine from urease producing bacteria. Treatment of choice is extracorporeal shock wave lithotripsy (ESWL) for stones less than 3 cm in diameter and the percutaneous approach for stones above 3 cm in diameter.

C. **VESICOURETERAL REFLUX (VUR)** is often associated with hyperreflexic detrusor–external sphincter dyssynergia (i.e., neurogenic detrusor overactivity and spastic external urinary sphincter) and high pressure voiding, or it could be congenital. It can lead to renal deterioration, especially in the presence of bacteria. Patients with bilateral reflux may have 30% less creatinine clearance than those without reflux.

D. **PYELONEPHRITIS**, often associated with VUR, kidney stones and outlet obstruction, can lead to renal deterioration. In SCI patients, anatomy and function of the upper urinary tracts are evaluated with KUB, IVP or excretory urogram, renal US, CT or MRI, quantitative renal scan, or 24-hour urine creatinine clearance.

E. **BLADDER CANCER** (usually squamous cell carcinoma) is more prevalent in patients with long-term indwelling catheters. These patients should be periodically monitored with cystoscopy. If a suspicious lesion is found, a biopsy should be performed.

F. **AUTONOMIC DYSREFLEXIA (AD)**, which is observed in patients with SCI at or above the T6 level, is characterized by exaggerated autonomic response to noxious stimuli from a source below the level of inury (e.g., bladder distension, which is the most common cause of AD). Its symptoms include severe pounding headache, sweating and skin flushing in the forehead, neck, and upper trunk, blurred vision, nasal obstruction, piloerection, paresthesia, and anxiety. Clinical signs of AD, in addition to cutaneous manifestation, include paroxysmal hypertension (generally speaking, the systolic BP of a patient with SCI above T6 in a stable condition is 90–110 mmHg), bradycardia (asystole is often noted in tetraplegic patients during the very acute stage), and nonspecific ST-T changes on EKG. It is precipitated by acute bladder distension, and can also be caused by fecal impaction, hemorrhoids, ingrown toenail, urinary stones, and acute abdomen. AD can occur in female patients with SCI or during sexual intercourse or during surgery. Of most concern is the potentially dangerous elevation in BP. Immediate management of AD includes:

1. Sitting up the patient in bed, and removing tight clothing and constrictive devices.
2. Checking vital signs.
3. Identifying and removing the source of noxious stimuli (e.g., start bladder catheterization; examination of indwelling catheter and replacement of the catheter if it is blocked). When the source of AD is identified and removed, its symptoms and signs resolve usually without medication.
4. Consideration of the following pharmacological agents (see chapter 5.8, section, VI.B.3.), particularly when the systolic BP is elevated above 160 mmHg:

a. ***Nitropaste,*** 1 inch, above the level of the SCI. If the systolic BP drops below 100 mmHg, the Nitropaste should be discontinued.

b. ***Nifedipine,*** 10 mg, using the immediate-release form (i.e., bite-and-swallow).

c. ***Others,*** such as **central α_2-adrenergic agonist** (e.g., clonidine; see Chapter 4.8, section IX.A.1.); **ganglionic blocking agents** (e.g., mecanylamine); and direct arterial vasodilator (e.g., hydralazine, diazoxide) may be used with proper monitoring.

Further reading

Agency for Health Care Policy and Research Clinical Guideline Panel for Urinary Incontinence: *Acute and chronic urinary incontinence in adults*, Rockville, MD, 1996, Department of Health and Human Services.

Bradley WE: Innervation of the male urinary bladder. *Urol Clin North Am* 5(2):279–293, 1978.

Cardenas DD, Mayo ME: Management of bladder dysfunction. In Braddom RL, editor: *Physical medicine and rehabilitation*, ed 2, Philadelphia, 2000, WB Saunders, pp. 561–578.

Chancellor MB: Urodynamic evaluation after spinal cord injury. *Phys Med Rehabil Clin North Am* 4(2):273–298, 1993.

Chapple CR, Yamanishi T, Chess-Williams R: Muscarinic receptor subtypes and management of the overactive bladder. *Urology* 60 (Suppl 5A): 82–89, 2002.

Consortium for Spinal Cord Medicine: Clinical practice guideline: acute management of autonomic dysreflexia. *J Spinal Cord Med* 20:284–311, 1997.

Doughty DB, editor: *Urinary and fecal incontinence: nursing management*, ed 2, St Louis, 2000, Mosby.

Lisenmeyer TA, Stone JM, Steins SA: Neurogenic bladder and bowel dysfunction. In DeLisa JA, Gans BM, Walsh NE, *et al.*, editors: *Physical medicine and rehabilitation: principles and practice*, ed 4, Philadelphia, 2005, Lippincott, Williams & Wilkins, pp. 1619–1654.

Perkash I: Urologic diagnostic testing. In Lennard TA, editor: *Pain procedures in clinical practice*, ed 2, Philadelphia, 2000, Hanley & Belfus, pp. 66–74.

Resnick NM, Yalla SV: Management of urinary incontinence in the elderly. *N Engl Med J* 313:800–805, 1985.

Stover SL, DeLisa JA, Whiteneck GG: *Spinal cord injury clinical outcomes from the model systems*, New York, 1995, Aspen.

Wein AJ: Lower urinary tract function and pharmacologic management of lower urinary tract dysfunction. *Urol Clin North Am* 14(2):273–296, 1987.

Wein AJ, Rovner ES: Definition and epidemiology of overactive bladder. *Urology* 60 (Suppl 5A): 7–12, 2002.

CHAPTER 5.8
Bowel dysfunction

This chapter deals with bowel dysfunction, which is commonly encountered in PM&R, with special emphasis on neurogenic bowel dysfunction. Neurogenic bowel dysfunction is the loss of voluntary control of defecation caused by impairment of the extrinsic (sympathetic, parasympathetic, or somatic) nervous control of the bowel and anorectal mechanisms, resulting in fecal incontinence (FI) or difficulty with evacuation (DWE). In neurogenic bowel dysfunction [e.g., caused by spinal cord injury (SCI), stroke, traumatic brain injury, multiple sclerosis, diabetic neuropathy, or myelomeningocele], the rehabilitation goal is not necessarily to restore normal defecation (as this may not always be feasible) but rather to attain "social continence", i.e., predictable scheduled adequate defecation without incontinence at socially unacceptable times.

I. Neuroanatomy and neurophysiology

A. EFFERENT FIBERS

1. **Autonomic efferents** modulate the enteric nervous system (ENS) rather than directly control the smooth muscles of the gastrointestinal (GI) tract. The intrinsic **enteric nervous system** (ENS) of the GI tract is a collection of highly organized neurons in two primary layers, i.e., the submucosal (Meissner's) and myenteric (Auerbach's) plexi. The ENS is located along the bowel wall from the esophagus to the internal anal sphincter (IAS) and forms the final common pathway to control the bowel wall smooth muscle. The autonomic efferents inhibit the ENS, which in turn directly inhibits the GI tract peristalsis (i.e., the continuous, distal-moving phasic contractions produced by the inherent electromechanical automaticity of the GI tract smooth muscles). Ablation of all ENS activity by neurotoxin (e.g., tetrodotoxin) causes uninhibited GI tract contraction (from esophagus to IAS).

a. ***Parasympathetic efferents*** inhibit the inhibitory influences of the ENS, hence increasing GI tract motility. The upper or right colon (i.e., ascending and proximal transverse colons) is innervated by the **vagus nerve (cranial nerve X)** from the medulla, while the lower (or left) GI tract, i.e., distal transverse colon, descending colon, rectum, and IAS, is supplied by the pelvic nerves (also called pelvic splanchnic nerves or nervi erigentes) from **S2** to **S4**. Injury to the S2–S4 (e.g., conus medullaris or cauda equina lesion) or the pelvic nerves can lead to flaccidity of the lower GI tract, which often leads to DWE, including fecal impactions and functional obstructions. In impacted patients, liquid stool (which accumulates as a result of the decreased absorption capacity of the lower colon) may flow past a bolus of solid feces and may erroneously be diagnosed as fecal incontinence.

b. ***Sympathetic efferents*** promote the storage function by enhancing anal tone and inhibiting colonic contractions. Sympathetic stimulation leads to adynamic ileus and decreased bowel activity. But bilateral sympathectomy only causes minor clinical deficits. Sympathetic efferents from **T11** to **L2** travel through the pelvic ganglion and hypogastric plexi to increase contraction of the IAS. In the resting state, the tonic contraction of the IAS, which accounts for about 80% of resting sphincter pressure, maintains fecal continence. Sympathetic efferents from **L1** to **L2** travel through the inferior mesenteric ganglion to inhibit contractions of the lower (or left) GI tract.

2. **Somatic efferents** are not affected by the ENS or the parasympathetic efferents but are under sympathetic efferent and voluntary (cortical) control. They consist of α-motor neurons, which directly innervate the external anal sphincter (EAS) and puborectalis muscles. Both of these voluntary striated skeletal muscles are normally in continuous tonic contraction (even during sleep), hence maintaining continence. Tonic contraction of the circular EAS (which surrounds the IAS and extends distally to the subcutaneous tissue surrounding the anus) closes the anal canal while tonic contraction of the puborectalis (which extends from the pubic arch and loops around the posterior part of the rectum and back to the pubic arch) draws the rectum forward, producing an angulation between the axis of the rectum and the axis of the anal canal of about 90°, which is most crucial for maintaining solid continence. This 90° anorectal angle maintains solid continence by: occluding the lumen; providing a sharp curve, which makes it difficult for the stool bolus to pass through; and making it likely that increases in intra-abdominal pressure result in compression of the anterior wall of the rectum against the posterior wall, further occluding the lumen.

   The EAS is innervated by the **S2–S4 roots** through the pudendal nerves, and the puborectalis is innervated by **direct sacral root branches from S1 to S5 roots** (mainly S3–S4). In an isolated pudendal injury (e.g., "stretch neuropathy" during childbirth, injury caused by anorectal surgery, and chronic straining), fecal transit time is normal, but there is predominant fecal incontinence because of EAS flaccid paralysis. Likewise, injury to the sacral roots innervating the puborectalis muscle (e.g., polyneuropathy or cauda equina lesions), causes a predominant fecal incontinence with normal fecal transit time. In women over 50 years old, there is a significant decline in EAS function (thus predisposing to incontinence) compared with that of younger women. This decline is not seen in men and is probably because of previous childbirth or hormonal changes affecting the pelvic floor muscles after menopause.

B. **AFFERENT FIBERS** originate from the sensory receptors of the GI tract. The intestine and rectal mucosa are sensitive only to distension (most people can differentiate distension caused by solid, liquid, or gas in the rectum), while the epithelium of the anal canal is sensitive to pain, touch, and temperature. Afferent impulses are processed in three centers: the central nervous system (CNS) (through the vagus nerve through cell bodies in the nodose ganglia or through the sympathetic nerves through cell bodies in the dorsal root ganglia); the prevertebral sympathetic ganglia; and the interneurons within the GI tract wall. Afferent impulses to the CNS and the prevertebral sympathetic ganglia interact with each other and influence the GI tract interneurons; however, afferent impulses going to the GI tract interneurons can interact directly with the efferent fibers. All these afferent impulses ultimately modulate the autonomic efferents (which also control the ENS) but not the somatic efferents. Loss of afferent (sensory) input results in a lack of awareness of rectal filling and may contribute to constipation and eventually to fecal impaction.

II. Phases of bowel evacuation

A. **COLONIC PHASE** is a continuous process of phasic colonic contractions, which propels the feces into the rectum but is not sufficient to overcome EAS tonic contraction. Colonic contents of the ascending and transverse colon are constantly stirred and mixed so they can be exposed to the colon wall for further reabsorption. Typically, the colonic walls reabsorb up to 30 L of fluids per day (with only 100 mL water loss in feces) and up to 90% of the 7–10 L of gas produced by bacterial fermentation. Stool transit time in the colon is also affected by the time of day, and even the person's surroundings. Normally, the fecal transit time from cecum to anus is 12–48 hours with giant migratory contractions (GMCs) of the colon occurring up to twice a day in a normal colon or approximately four times per day in a fasting colon. The GMCs are associated with mass movement of the feces (to as far as one-third the length of the colon) and can increase in the first 30–60 minutes after a meal (because of the gastrocolic reflex) leading to shortened fecal transit time. The fecal transit time can also be shortened or decreased (i.e., GMCs and defecation frequency are increased) by the type of diet (e.g., fiber supplements, which increase stool bulk) and by physical exercise. Patients with SCI have prolonged fecal transit time, reduced frequency of GMCs, and less GMC facilitation by defecation, exercise, or food ingestion, all of which predispose them to chronic constipation and fecal impaction. Specifically, the fecal transit time for patients with upper motor neuron (UMN) lesions is more than 72 hours while for patients with lower motor neuron (LMN) lesions, it is more than 6 days (especially of the left colon).

B. VOLUNTARY DEFECATION PHASE (see Fig. 5.8-1)

1. **Holding phase** starts upon the delivery of feces of an appropriate consistency into the rectum. The amount, consistency, and rate at which feces enter the rectum is controlled by the proximal bowel. The feces are initially retained in the sigmoid colon and are intermittently propelled to the rectum at about 100 g of solid stool per day through a rectorectal reflex (i.e., bowel proximal to the stool contracts as the distal bowel relaxes; the exact mechanism underlying this process is unclear). As the feces enter the rectum, there is a decrease in intraluminal pressure proportional to the distending volume because of rectal accommodation and partial relaxation of the IAS; therefore, the rectum, which does not actively contract, serves as an accommodating and compliant reservoir of feces. Continence in the holding phase is maintained by the tonic contraction

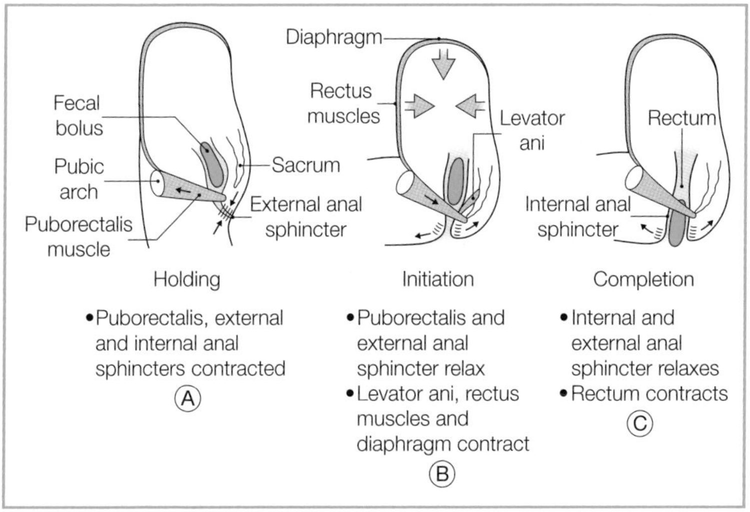

Figure 5.8-1 Voluntary defecation phases. (Adapted from Schiller LR: Fecal incontinence. In Sleisenger MH, Fordtran JS, editors: *Gastrointestinal disease: pathophysiology, diagnosis, management,* ed 4, Philadelphia, 1989, WB Saunders, p. 322.)

of the puborectalis and EAS muscles (see discussion under section I.A.2), which are normally reinforced by cortical control until defecation is socially acceptable. Moreover, as the feces come in contact with the upper anal canal, there is reflex contraction of the EAS. Continence can be maintained for both solid and liquid stools, unless there are voluminous phasic flows of liquid stool, which overwhelms the continence mechanism leading to urgency and incontinence. In patients with supraconus disease processes, from SCI (i.e., UMN lesions) to dementia, the cortical modulation is lost and spontaneous defecation may occur reflexively even in socially unacceptable situations. In patients with combination UMN lesions with posterior rhizotomy or in patients with LMN lesions, reflex defecation is absent.

2. **Initiation phase** starts with the sensation of rectal distension (which is perceived at volumes as low as 10 mL). When the rectal volume reaches at least 100–150 mL (i.e., intrarectal pressure reaches at least 100 cmH_2O), the urge to defecate becomes strongly felt, but the urge may dissipate as accommodation occurs (i.e., the initial rise in intrarectal pressure soon drops back to its original level as the compliant rectum relaxes and accommodates the fecal mass) or the urge may be cortically suppressed. The ability to sense the urge to defecate is decreased in patients with UMN lesions caused by impaired spinal–cortical pathways (although in 43% of these patients, there is a vague sense of abdominal distension or discomfort probably mediated by afferent fibers bypassing the zone of cord injury in sympathetic nerves). Compared to normal, the rectal distension studies of patients with UMN lesions show elevated rectosigmoid pressures, especially when higher or continuous filling rates are used. The elevated rectosigmoid pressure is probably associated with increased EAS pressure because of sacral reflexes (rather than being associated with true decreased colonic compliance as seen in patients with ischemic or postinflammatory rectal bowel wall caused by fibrosis).

   When the person decides to defecate, he or she voluntarily contracts the levator ani (to reflexively open the proximal anal canal) and voluntarily relaxes the EAS and puborectalis muscles. Puborectalis relaxation in combination with the sitting or squatting position makes the anorectal angle straighter thus facilitating stool passage. Stool passage is propelled distally with the aid of Valsalva's maneuver, that is, closure of glottis and contraction of the abdominal muscles to increase intra-abdominal pressure (IAP) by at least 100 cmH_2O. The inability to perform Valsalva's maneuver because of paralyzed abdominal muscles (e.g., patients with C5–C6 level SCI who can rarely generate more than 10 cmH_2O of IAP) contributes significantly to DWE. During Valsalva's maneuver (see section VI.B.1.c.2), the EAS pressure increases (so-called protective vesicoanal reflex) to prevent incontinence; however, this protective vesicoanal reflex can be overcame by coordinated voluntary relaxation of the EAS during defecation. In patients with UMN lesions, the protective vesicoanal reflex is present (because of intact or increased anal sphincter tone), but in patients with denervation and atrophy of the EAS (e.g., in patients with LMN lesions or in patients with a combination of UMN lesion and posterior rhizotomy), the protective vesicoanal reflex is absent. The loss of the protective vesicoanal reflex can result in fecal incontinence (caused by the increased abdominal pressures associated with daily activities) and in excessive perineal descent and even rectal prolapse during Valsalva's maneuver.

3. **Completion phase** occurs as the IAS and EAS continue to relax, and the rectal propulsive contractions (in conjunction with the forces described in the initiation phase) expel the bolus through the open canal. Once evacuation is initiated, the entire left colon may empty by mass peristaltic action, or the fecal bolus may be passed bit by bit. In the American norm, approximately 100 g of

solid feces is expelled daily or less frequently. The major factor in determining the pattern of defecation is probably the consistency of the stool. In SCI patients, IAS and EAS relaxation occurs upon rectal distension (resulting in expulsion of the fecal bolus) as in normal subjects.

III. Epidemiology

The prevalence of fecal incontinence (FI) and fecal impaction ranges from 0.3 to 5.0% in the general population. Fecal incontinence in the elderly is often caused by local factors (most commonly undetected fecal impaction) rather than from cerebral deterioration, and it decreases the return-to-home rates for stroke patients. The 1983 cost for the care of fecally incontinent institutionalized patients in the United States was 8 billion dollars. The prevalence of DWE ranges from 10 to 50% among hospitalized or institutionalized elderly. In SCI patients, 43% have chronic complaints of vague abdominal distension and discomfort, which eases with bowel evacuation. In outpatient SCI patients, the prevalence of bowel disturbances is 29%, especially in those with more than 5 years of complete SCI.

IV. Diagnosis

A. HISTORY

1. **History of present illness**. A bowel function diary for 1–2 weeks may be needed to determine current bowel patterns.

a. ***Current and premorbid bowel function,*** such as defecation frequency and duration; typical time(s) of the day for defecation; associated predefecatory activities (e.g., effect of body position, eating, trigger foods, bowel-care medications and techniques, and urinary function); presence of GI sensations or pain, warning sensations for defecation, sense of urgency, and ability to prevent stool loss during Valsalva activities (e.g., laughing, sneezing, coughing, or transfers); stool consistency; onset of bowel symptoms and the events that occur around that time (e.g., change in living situation); and functional impact of bowel function on ability to work, travel, interact with others, and carry out activities of daily living.

b. ***Associated symptoms,*** such as autonomic dysreflexia, abdominal wall spasticity, fever, weight change, and rectal bleeding.

2. **Past medical history,** such as number of pregnancies or deliveries, history of traumatic deliveries, history of anorectal surgery or GI surgery, trauma to the perineum, trauma to the spinal cord, neurologic disease, diabetes, radiation therapy, neurogenic bladder, impotence, and other illness (premorbid GI disease).
3. **Medication history**. Past and present use of medications that can cause diarrhea (see section V.A.2.c) or constipation (see section V.B.2.c).
4. **Diet history,** such as intake of fluids, dietary bulks and fibers, and dietary irritants.
5. **Personal history,** such as physical activity and emotional status.

B. PHYSICAL EXAMINATION

1. **Anal inspection.** Anal–buttock contour (normal in patients with UMN lesions or combination UMN lesions with posterior rhizotomy; flattened, fanned-out, or "scalloped" in patients with LMN lesions because of loss of EAS muscle bulk), perianal soiling or excoriations (caused by fecal incontinence), anal opening (e.g., patulous gaping orifice because of overdistension or trauma), and perineal descent during Valsalva's maneuver (i.e., bulging of the anus below the ischial tuberosities in excessive descent or prolapse of the perineum).

2. **Digital examination of the anus and rectum**. Assess rectal vault for fecal impaction; sphincter tone (which should normally be in a state of contraction at rest); length of anus (i.e., 2.5–4.5 cm long from anal opening to anorectal junction where finger senses a decrease in rectal pressure; a shortened length of anal pressure zone suggests EAS muscle atrophy, e.g., in LMN lesions); puborectalis muscular sling (palpated as a ridge along the posterior wall, 1.5–2.5 cm from the anal verge; absence of the ridge suggests puborectalis atrophy or dysfunction such as in LMN lesions); volitional EAS and puborectalis tone and control (by asking the patient to volitionally squeeze the anus; patients with SCI are unable to do this); bulbocavernosus reflex, that is, anal contraction elicited by rapid tapping or squeezing of the clitoris or glans penis, and anocutaneous reflex or "anal wink", that is, visible anal sphincter contraction elicited by sharp stimulation to the perianal skin (both bulbocavernosus and anocutaneous reflexes are present or increased in UMN lesions; and absent or decreased in LMN lesions or in combination UMN lesion with posterior rhizotomy); and anal closing reflex (which is normally brisk when the finger is withdrawn).
3. **Transabdominal palpation** to detect hard stool in the colon (this should not be present in the ascending colon at the right side of the abdomen).
4. **Musculoskeletal system**. Assess patient's gait, the time required for position change and ambulation, use of assistive devices, and the patient's ability to manipulate clothing rapidly in preparation for toileting.

C. **DIAGNOSTIC TESTS** may be helpful when the cause of FI or DWE is obscure, conservative interventions have failed, or surgical intervention is contemplated.

1. **Laboratory studies** may be needed if disease or disorder of the intestinal tract is suspected, for example, acute diarrhea of undetermined origin. They include complete blood count, serum electrolytes and biochemistry, stool culture and sensitivity tests, stool analysis for ova and parasites, and stool assay for *Clostridium difficile* toxin.
2. **Morphological studies** are used to identify anatomical lesions or causes of GI obstruction; however, they are of limited benefit in assessing bowel function.

a. ***Endoscopy,*** for example colonoscopy, rectosigmoidoscopy, and anoscopy, are used to directly visualize the lower GI tract.

b. ***Anatomical radiologic studies,*** that is radiographs (e.g., barium enema studies), computed tomography scans, or magnetic resonance imaging studies, may be used for further anatomical investigation of diseases or disorders of the GI tract.

c. ***Biopsy,*** for instance rectal biopsy, may be used for histopathologic diagnosis.

3. **Functional studies**

a. ***Sensory function studies***

I. **Sensory electromyography (EMG)** is used to assess sensory pelvic afferents (by nerve conduction studies), or somatosensory evoked potentials. It can also be used to assess the bulbocavernosus reflex (e.g., **sacral evoked response study** described in Chapter 5.9, section III.D.1.a).

II. **Intrarectal balloon distension test** is used to determine the rectal sensory threshold (i.e., normally the smallest volume of rectal **distension** sensed by the patient is 15 mL within less than 2 seconds).

b. ***Motor function studies***

I. **Motor EMG** using needle or wire electrodes can be used to assess volitional motor control of the puborectalis, anococcygeus, levator ani, and EAS; however, abnormal potentials may be difficult to detect because the EAS is an atypical striated muscle (i.e., it maintains tonus even when it is not voluntarily contracted). Motor EMG may help identify the location of the EAS when the normal anatomy has been disrupted (e.g., because of congenital anomaly or trauma). Single-fiber EMG may be used to identify muscle denervation and give an estimate of its degree.

II. **Anorectal pressure and sphincter function studies**

- **Anorectal catheter manometry** uses an intra-anal pressure-sensitive catheter balloon probe, which is connected to a transducer and a recorder or computer. It measures the pressures and resting tone of the IAS, the contractility of the EAS, and the functional length of the anal canal. The parameters measured are anal canal pressures (both resting pressure and maximum squeeze pressure) and the rectoanal or rectosphincteric reflex (i.e., relaxation of the internal sphincter and contraction of the external sphincter in response to balloon distension of the rectum). Manometric resting and contractile pressures are decreased in cases of sphincter laceration or denervation and during a reflex reaction to rectal distension (e.g., because of fecal impaction). These pressures are increased in cases of anal fissure and in some patients with hemorrhoids.
- **Balloon sphincterography or kymography** is a simpler method than manometry and is used to evaluate the EAS mechanism of anal canal closure and the production of the anorectal angle by the puborectalis. It uses an intrarectal cylindrical balloon connected by tubing to a bag of radio-opaque dye (the pressure in the balloon corresponds to the height of the fluid in the bag and can be measured or controlled by raising or lowering the bag). Plain radiograph, fluoroscopy, or ultrasound is used to visualize the shape of the dye-filled balloon within the anal canal and rectum during voluntary contraction and relaxation of the external sphincter and puborectalis. The parameters measured include the resting and maximum squeeze pressures, the length of the anal canal, and the degree of perineal descent. The accuracy and reliability of this method have recently been questioned.

III. **Rectodynamics** is a combination of anorectal pressure studies and motor EMG. A concentric EMG needle is placed in the EAS to measure resistive forces of bowel evacuation and a triple-lumen balloon catheter is inserted through the anus to measure expulsive forces of bowel evacuation (i.e., intra-abdominal pressure, colorectal contraction, and rectal compliance). The catheter is positioned so that the first lumen measures the rectal pressure and the second lumen measures the pressure of the anal canal. The third lumen is used to fill a balloon located in the rectum. Rectal and anal pressures, as well as EMG of EAS, are measured at rest and during stimulation of the anorectum by digital stimulation, Valsalva's maneuver, rapid rectal distension (i.e., rapid injection and removal of air from the rectal balloon to elicit the rectoanal inhibitory reflex), and slow, continuous filling of the rectal balloon at a constant rate of 20 mL/min. Rectodynamics can help in the management of patients with neurogenic bowel by identifying the following patterns of bowel evacuation: anorectal dyssynergia (i.e., loss of coordination between the rectal pressure and anal relaxation) vs. insufficient expulsive forces to overcome normal anal sphincter tone (i.e., rectal volumes over 500 mL, instead of the normal 100–150 mL, are needed to trigger anal relaxation; seen in patients with long-standing cervical cord injuries, often with associated megacolon and megarectum).

IV. **Functional radiographic studies** may be used to examine anal continence mechanisms, colonic transit time, and defecation mechanism.

- **Defecography** is used to visualize the kinesiology of defecation and evaluate the pelvic floor muscles. The rectum is filled with a barium suspension and the patient is placed on a radiolucent chair and asked to alternately defecate and contract the sphincter while sequential lateral radiographic films are taken. The anorectal angle, the length of the anal canal, and perineal descent (if present) can be demonstrated.

- **Serial radiographs of tiny radio-opaque plastic beads** ingested with food are used to evaluate colonic transit time. This is useful in confirming constipation history and in identifying dysfunctional bowel segments (for planning colostomy level).

V. **Anal continence studies**

- **Saline continence test** is used to objectively assess the degree or severity of FI. A saline solution is run into the rectum through a length of polyethylene tubing at the rate of 60 mL/min for 25 minutes. In normally continent individuals, 1500 mL can be retained before the first leakage of over 10 mL occurs (as measured via a funnel connected to a graduated cylinder placed beneath the seat of a toilet). In patients with incontinence, however, the first leakage almost invariably occurs when approximately 500 mL have been instilled. The result varies with the strength of the EAS, degree of rectal compliance, and the patient's motivation.
- **Solid-sphere continence test** measures maximal anal resistance to the active and passive passage of solid spheres of standard sizes, which are attached to a string and inserted into the rectum.
- **Functional radiographic studies** (see section IV.C.3.b.4) may be used to examine anal continence.

c. ***Rectal accommodation*** (i.e., reservoir function) ***studies***

I. **Rectal capacity and compliance test** uses a large capacity balloon (or condom) inserted into the rectum. The balloon is tied to a polyethylene tubing, which is connected to a three-way stopcock and a 50-mL syringe. Rectal accommodation is determined by inflating the balloon in 50-mL increments.

II. **Colon capacity and motility test**, for example, using colonoscopy, barium enema, or both.

V. Classification by causative factors

A. FAILURE TO STORE (FECAL INCONTINENCE AND DIARRHEA)

1. Neurogenic causes

a. ***UMN and/or cortical lesions that cause constipation*** (see section V.B.1.a) can lead to unrecognized fecal impaction with overflow incontinence (i.e., seepage of watery stool around the obstructing fecal mass; or stool leakage because of loss of normal rectal tone caused by chronic constipation thus resulting in loss of sensation of rectal fullness and loss of voluntary contraction of the external sphincter). Also, patients who are demented, sedated, mentally retarded, or with cognitive deficits may be fecally incontinent (although not diarrheic).

b. ***LMN lesions,*** such as isolated pudendal nerve injury with EAS denervation (e.g., because of childbirth, anorectal surgery, or chronic straining), injury to the sacral roots with puborectalis denervation (e.g., polyneuropathy or cauda equina lesions), LMN myelomeningocele, or Guillain–Barré syndrome (may have occasional transient FI).

2. Non-neurogenic causes

a. ***Medical diseases***

I. **Gastroenteritis**, which can be caused by viruses, bacteria (e.g., *Clostridium difficile, Shigella, Salmonella, Mycobacterium avium intracellulare*, or invasive *Escherichia coli*), parasites (e.g., *Giardia* or amoeba), or fungus (e.g., intestinal candidiasis caused by aggressive antibiotic therapy that destroys normal intestinal flora). Patients prone to gastroenteritis are immunocompromised patients (e.g., patients receiving cancer treatment or steroids, malnourished patients, or patients with the human immunodeficiency virus) and patients who are receiving organ and bone marrow transplants (because of graft-vs.-host disease or immunosuppresive drugs).

II. **Bowel diseases**, such as celiac disease, malabsorption conditions, inflammatory bowel disease, or chronic intestinal conditions that result in motility change (e.g., radiation injury to the bowel).

b. ***Dietary factors,*** such as caffeine, alcohol (in large quantities), artificial sweeteners or additives (e.g., fructose, sorbitol, mannitol, and nutmeg), any food to which the person is intolerant (e.g., milk products, meat, potatoes, or wheat), fruit juices, cruciferous vegetables, fatty food, or enteral feedings (especially if the patient is severely malnourished or has received nothing by mouth for several days).

c. ***Medications causing diarrhea,*** such as antacids (e.g., those containing magnesium), antibiotics, cardiac medications (e.g., digitalis or quinidine), antihypertensives (e.g., hydralazine, methyldopa, propranolol, or guanethidine), potassium supplements, cholinergic agents (e.g., bethanechol), diuretics, anticoagulants, sulfasalazine, indomethacin, colchicine, theophylline, cholestyramine, chenodeoxycholic acid, stool softeners, or laxatives (see section VI.B.3.a).

d. ***Others causes,*** such as women over 50 years old (men are not affected) because of significant decline in EAS function probably caused by previous childbirths or hormonal changes affecting the pelvic floor muscles after menopause; and any unrecognized fecal impaction (e.g., because of poor bowel hygiene or other non-neurogenic causes), which can lead to overflow incontinence.

B. FAILURE TO ELIMINATE (i.e., CONSTIPATION OR DWE)

1. Neurogenic causes

a. ***UMN or cortical lesions,*** which cause constipation because of loss (complete or partial) of voluntary control of defecation, loss or decrease in the ability to sense the urge to defecate, prolonged colonic transit time, reduced frequency of GMC, or increased EAS tone. Their causes can be vascular (e.g., stroke or intracranial hemorrhage); degenerative and/or extrapyramidal (e.g., parkinsonism, Alzheimer's disease, or dementia), demyelinating (e.g., multiple sclerosis), structural (e.g., neoplasm or UMN myelomeningocele), exogenous (e.g., traumatic brain injury, supraconus SCI, or drug-induced lesions), or others (e.g., mental retardation).

b. ***LMN lesions,*** for example neuropathy involving the parasympathetic nerves (which can lead to constipation because of prolonged colonic transit time) caused by diabetes, tumor, trauma (e.g., from childbirth, pelvic surgery, or chronic straining), or lesions of the conus medullaris, cauda equina, or nervi erigentes.

2. Non-neurogenic causes

a. ***Medical diseases***

I. **Metabolic causes**, such as diabetic acidosis or neuropathy, porphyria, uremia, amyloidosis, or electrolyte abnormalities (e.g., hypokalemia).

II. **Endocrine causes**, such as hypercalcemia, hyperparathyroidism, hypothyroidism, pheochromocytoma, or panhypopituitarism.

III. **Large intestinal causes**, such as obstruction to flow in the ileal and colonic area (e.g., malignant carcinoma or benign conditions such as polyp, abscess, adhesion, diverticular stricture, or ischemic stricture), anal abnormalities (e.g., paradoxical puborectalis contraction, rectoanal intussusception, rectocele, fibrosis, or abscess), Hirschprung disease (or aganglionic megacolon), pelvic floor abnormalities, or muscular diseases (e.g., scleroderma or dermatomyositis).

IV. **Other disorders** that cause pain on defecation, such as thrombosed external hemorrhoids, anal fissures, or anal strictures.

b. ***Dietary factors,*** such as inadequate intake of fluids and dietary bulk.

c. ***Medications causing constipation,*** such as analgesics (e.g., opiates or non-steroidal anti-inflammatory drugs), anesthetic agents, antacids (e.g., cimetidine, ranitidine, or aluminum compounds), anticholinergics (e.g., oxybutinin or propantheline), anticonvulsants (e.g., carbamazepine, phenytoin, or valproic acid), antidepressants (e.g., amitriptyline, desipramine, doxepin, imipramine, or nortriptyline), barium sulfate, bismuth, ganglionic blockers, hematinics (especially dietary iron supplements), hypotensives (e.g., diltiazem, nifedipine, or verapamil), laxative or enema abuse, loop-diuretics (producing electrolyte abnormalities such as hypokalemia), monoamine oxidase inhibitors, metallic intoxication (e.g., arsenic, lead, mercury, or phosphorus), muscle paralyzers, parkinsonism medications (e.g., amantadine, benztropine, biperiden, or procyclidine), psychotherapeutic drugs, smooth-muscle relaxants, or tranquilizers.

d. ***Others,*** such as reduced peristaltic activity because of aging or inactivity (e.g., chronically ill, immobilized, or postoperative patients), poor bowel hygiene (e.g., prolonged failure to defecate), or impaired diaphragmatic and abdominal wall function.

VI. Nonsurgical management

Nonsurgical management involves the determination and correction of the underlying reasons for diarrhea or constipation, as well as the use of general symptomatic control measures. The treatment of non-neurogenic medical bowel diseases (except for diarrhea caused by *Clostridium difficile*) is beyond the scope of this book.

A. FAILURE TO STORE (FECAL INCONTINENCE AND DIARRHEA)

1. **Dietary measures** that help thicken stool consistency by absorbing fluid from the stool or by forming stool bulk.

a. ***Constipating diet,*** which increases fluid absorption from the colon, such as rice, bananas, apples or unfiltered apple juice, yogurt, cheese, marshmallows, or some wheat products.

b. ***High-fiber (bulk-forming) diet:*** See section VI.B.2.

c. ***Avoidance of diarrheic diet,*** as partially listed in section V.A.2.b.

d. ***Fluid and electrolyte replacement,*** given orally or intravenously, may be needed to prevent fluid-volume deficit caused by diarrhea. Oral fluid replacements include electrolyte drinks (developed for athletes and ostomy patients) or a homemade electrolyte solution (e.g., mix 1 tablespoon salt, 1 tablespoon baking soda, 1 tablespoon corn syrup, 6 oz (180 mL) of orange juice concentrate, and add water to make one quart (0.946 L) of liquid). If possible, replace fluid volume lost through diarrhea with an equivalent volume of solution or if unable to estimate fluid loss, replace with 8 oz (240 mL) of solution for every bowel movement. If unable to tolerate oral fluids, the patient may be temporarily placed on nothing by mouth and intravenous fluids may be given if needed.

e. ***Modification of enteral feeding.*** Although the diarrhea during enteral feeding is usually attributed to the formula itself, it is more commonly caused by an underlying malnutrition (i.e., albumin level of less than 2.8/100 mL) that results in edema of the gut wall and malabsorption (may be associated with atrophy of the intestinal villi). Enteral feeding modification includes the use of isotonic formula with bulk agents and with antidiarrheals, and gradual increase in feeding rate (starting at 50 mL/hour). Short-term use of antiperistaltic drugs [e.g., loperamide (Imodium) or diphenoylate with atrophine (Lomotil)] may be warranted in refractory cases.

f. ***Bacterial cultures*** may be ingested to normalize the intestinal flora for cases of diarrhea caused by antibiotics. Examples are *Lactobacillus* products (Lactinex) or dairy products that contain bacterial cultures (e.g., buttermilk or yogurt). These should not be used by patients with high fever or by children under 3 years old.

2. **Drug therapy**

a. ***Antidiarrheal drugs*** are used either to achieve appropriate stool consistency or to reduce intestinal peristalsis and stool frequency. They are nonspecific and tend to be overused. In most acute diarrhea they are not necessary, and in chronic cases, they must not be used as a substitute for treatment of the underlying illnesses. Prior to giving antidiarrheal drugs, any drug causing diarrhea (see section V.A.2.c) should be discontinued if possible.

I. **Antiperistaltic drugs** should only be used after fecal impaction is ruled out. They may precipitate toxic megacolon in patients with invasive bacterial infection. Most of them contain opium or its derivative and have potential for abuse. They should be used with caution by patients with asthma, chronic lung disease, benign prostatic hypertrophy, and acute angle-closure glaucoma. Of the following drugs, only loperamide (Imodium) and Lomotil have been scientifically assessed for effectiveness in controlling diarrhea:

- **Loperamide (Imodium)**, a synthetic opioid, is the drug of choice for antiperistalsis because it acts directly on the smooth and circular muscles to decrease peristalsis and prolong transit time. It also increases the basal anal sphincter tone. It must be used with caution in patients with acute ulcerative colitis, antibiotic-induced pseudomembranous colitis, hepatic dysfunction, and dehydration with electrolyte imbalance. It is contraindicated in acute dysentery. Adverse drug reactions (ADRs) include nausea, vomiting, skin rash, dry mouth, drowsiness, bloating, and GI distress. It is available in 2 mg capsules or 1 mg/5 mL elixir. Oral dosage is 4 mg initially, then 2 mg, prn (after each loose bowel movement), to a maximum of 16 mg/day. If ineffective, discontinue after 48 hours.
- **Diphenoxylate with atropine (Lomotil)** is a combination of opioid (meperidine congener) and anticholinergic agents, which acts on smooth muscle to inhibit motility and propulsion. The ADRs are uncommon although nausea, vomiting, sedation, paralytic ileus, and headache have been reported. Its use is contraindicated in pseudomembranous enterocolitis, obstructive jaundice, electrolyte imbalance, and glaucoma. It must be used with caution by patients with dehydration, acute ulcerative colitis, and advanced hepatic or renal disease, and drug abusers. It is available in tablet or liquid forms (i.e., 2.5 mg of diphenoxylate with 0.025 mg of atropine per tablet or per 5 mL). Oral dosage is 2 tablets or 10 mL, qid, until initial control of diarrhea is achieved, followed by the lowest effective dose.
- **Cholinergic blockers** act locally on the gut to inhibit intestinal secretions and motility and reduce GI tract spasms. The ADRs include dry mouth; blurred vision; dizziness; headache; dry, flushed skin; drowsiness; tinnitus; vertigo; changes in affect and behavior; and vitamin B deficiency. Its use is contraindicated in patients with glaucoma, unstable cardiovascular status, paralytic ileus, chronic lung disease, asthma, pyloric stenosis, liver damage, pregnancy, renal insufficiency, and convulsive disorders. Examples are atropine (see Lomotil described above) and belladonna (e.g., combination of 25 mg powdered opium and 15 mg belladona, one capsule, po, tid or qid, prn).
- **Other opium derivatives** act on the smooth muscle of the large bowel to increase tone and decrease motility. The ADRs include addiction as well as sodium and potassium loss. Examples include paregoric (camphorated tincture of opium), 4–8 mL, po [diluted in 3 oz (90 mL) of water to ensure

stomach absorption], qid or after each liquid stool, not to exceed 32 mL/day; or deodorized tincture of opium, 0.3–1.0 mL, po, qid, prn up to a maximum of 6 mL/day; or codeine, 30–60 mg, po, bid to qid, prn.

II. **Absorption agents**

- **Kaolin and pectin (Kaopectate)** act as protectants and demulcents. They are contraindicated in pseudomembranous colitis. Oral dosage is 60–120 mL of regular strength or 45–90 mL of concentrate after each loose bowel movement.
- **Attapulgite (Parepectolin; Donnagel)** acts as an absorbent. It is available in 600 mg/15 mL suspension and as a 600-mg chewable tablet. The oral dosage is 30 mL or two chewable tablets after each loose bowel movement for a maximum of seven liquid doses or 14 tablets per 24 hours for 2 days.
- **Activated charcoal** may be used to absorb water to firm the stool. No adverse effects have been reported. For treating diarrhea, combination agents may be used, e.g., Flatulex, which has 250 mg of activated charcoal with 80 mg of simethicone, given 1 tablet, po, qid (after meals and at bedtime) for a maximum of 6 tablets per day.

III. **Astringent and coating agents**

- **Bismuth subsalicylate (Pepto-Bismol)** acts by coating and astringent effects. It may decrease the effects of anticoagulants and interfere with abdominal radiographs. It is useful in cases of traveler's diarrhea. It is available in tablets (262 mg) and suspension (262 and 524 mg/5 mL). Oral dosage is two tablets or 30 mL, every hour for each loose bowel movement up to 8 doses/day.
- **Aluminum hydroxide (Alternagel; Amphojel)** produces a barrier coating between the intestinal contents and intestinal wall. The ADRs include constipation, nausea, vomiting, and phosphate deficiency with prolonged use. It is contraindicated in patients on low-sodium diets, tetracycline, or anticoagulants. It is available in tablets (300 and 600 mg) and suspension (320 and 600 mg/5 mL). Oral dosage is 500–1500 mg up to six times daily.

b. ***Antibacterials*** for *Clostridium difficile* diarrhea are commonly prescribed in the rehabilitation ward because of frequent use of broad-spectrum antibiotic therapy (e.g., for treatment of infections of the urinary tract and wound), which can alter the normal intestinal flora and cause proliferation of the anaerobic *C. difficile*. If untreated, the toxin of *C. difficile* can cause pseudomembranous colitis. *Clostridium difficile* diarrhea is clinically presumed in patients who develop watery diarrhea during or after an antibiotic (for as long as 1–3 weeks after cessation of antibiotics). This can be confirmed by assaying the *C. difficile* toxin. Treatment consists of discontinuation of the antimicrobial therapy (if possible), avoidance of antiperistaltic drugs, and use of oral metronidazole or vancomycin.

I. **Metronidazole (Flagyl)** is available as capsules (250 and 500 mg). Oral dosage is 500 mg, bid or tid, for 7–10 days.

II. **Vancomycin (Vancocin)** is available as capsules (125 and 250 mg) or as powder for oral solution (1 and 10 g). Oral dosage is 125 mg, qid, for 7–10 days.

3. **Stool containment** measures provide skin protection, improve patient comfort, reduce nursing time, and provide an accurate measurement of fluid losses.

a. ***External collection devices*** consist of a drainable pouch attached to a synthetic, adhesive skin barrier, which conforms to the perianal area and buttocks. These devices adhere to the skin for an average of 24 hours. They are most effective when applied to clean, dry skin that is free of skin breakdown (any skin breakdown must be treated, e.g., with a skin barrier powder, before the pouch is applied).

b. ***Internal drainage systems*** may be used on a short-term basis if external devices are not feasible (e.g., because of skin breakdown or lack of adherence). They consist of a large-bore catheter (e.g., French size 30 catheter) inserted into the anorectal junction and connected to a bedside drainage bag. The catheter balloon may be inflated to prevent catheter slippage, but this carries the risk of bowel wall necrosis (unless the balloon is regularly deflated). Internal drainage systems are contraindicated in patients with rectal disease or neutropenia, or those who are immunocompromised.

c. ***Incontinence pants*** may be used by patients with severe diarrhea that cannot be managed with external collection devices; however, contact dermatitis and odor may limit the use of incontinence pants.

d. ***Anal plugs*** made from soft foams (e.g., Peristeen anal plug) may be used to create an effective plug in the anus to prevent undesirable fecal discharges and odor as well as problems with skin irritation.

4. **Skin care**

a. ***Routine skin care*** includes gentle cleansing of the perianal area after each bowel movement or incontinent episode followed by protection of intact skin with a moisture barrier cream or ointment (most with petrolatum base) or a skin sealant (e.g., copolymer film product). Tepid water, pH-balanced soaps, commercial formulas designed for incontinence care, or mineral oil may be used for cleansing.

b. ***Skin-breakdown care*** (see Chapter 5.2 for details) includes application of a skin barrier powder (above which a moisture barrier may be applied), premixed ointments and pastes, or hydrocolloid wafer dressings.

c. ***Fungal rash care*** includes nystatin (Mycostatin) applied bid or tid for *Candida albicans* and the more broad-spectrum antifungal imidazoles, for example clotrimazole (Lotrimin, Mycelex), econazole (Spectazole), ketoconazole (Nizoral), miconazole (Monistat), or oxiconazole (Oxistat), each applied bid. If available, the powder form (over which a sealant or moisture barrier cream may be applied) is preferred over the ointment or cream forms, which appear to lengthen the time required for healing because of the retention of moisture at the skin surface.

5. **Odor control,** such as pouch deodorants (if perianal pouch is used), deodorizing skin cleansers, and effective room-deodorizing sprays.

6. **Behavioral management** for patients with fecal incontinence because of cognitive dysfunction and alterations in sensory awareness or sphincter control.

a. ***Timed (scheduled) bowel movements*** can decrease incontinence between bowel movements (because of less stool accumulation between desired defecation times) and can enhance stool elimination (the establishment of regular, soft, bulky stools is discussed in section VI.B.2).

b. ***Anal-sphincter retraining*** involves training the patient to voluntarily contract the EAS when the rectal vault fills to prevent stool leakage. It is indicated if the patient has a weak but contractable EAS and if anatomic defects are minimal or absent, that is, no large amount of scar tissue (from episiotomy or surgical procedure) or severe congenital defects.

   I. **Pelvic floor exercises** involve repeated tightening of the pelvic floor muscles to increase their muscle tone to help prevent stool leakage. The correct muscle is identified by squeezing as tightly as possible around a finger placed in the anal canal or vagina, or by instructing the patient to stop urine flow in midstream and concentrate on the muscle used. Once identified, the muscle is squeezed for 10 seconds followed by a 10-second relaxation, for a total of 20–25 times, three times per day. This exercise can be done while standing, sitting, or lying down, and even incorporated into the patient's daily lifestyle. When done in combination with biofeedback techniques, this exercise seems to be more effective in reducing incontinence.

II. **Anorectal biofeedback therapy** (see Chapter 4.1, section VI) can help restore not just social continence but normal defecatory control. It is indicated in motivated individuals with incomplete neurogenic bowel deficits (i.e., with some residual degree of anorectal sensation and volitional EAS activation). It involves the use of a sensing device inserted into the rectum to record the baseline resting pressure as well as the squeeze pressure. Two common anorectal biofeedback methods include (a) the use of a manometric device with three balloons to provide feedback on a recording apparatus, and (b) the use of a rectal plug to provide feedback from an EMG or a computer monitor. The patient is then taught how to squeeze the EAS around the balloon or plug. A video monitor or a strip recording provides immediate visual or auditory (or both) feedback on any changes in the squeeze pressure. Additional EMG readings may also be taken from the abdominal and puborectalis muscle to prevent any inappropriate contractions of the abdominal muscles and to provide visual correlation between contractions of the EAS and the puborectalis. All these feedback signals are used to reinforce the patient's anorectal squeeze sensation as well as squeeze efforts. The biofeedback sessions last from 30 minutes to 2 hours and take an average of one to three sessions to learn.

B. FAILURE TO ELIMINATE (CONSTIPATION, DWE) is difficult to objectively define because the patient's perception of "normal" bowel habits varies widely. In 94% of unimpaired persons, the average bowel movement is at least three times per week. Frequent bowel evacuation (e.g., every other day or more frequently) can decrease stool accumulation and hardening. The general treatment goal is to prevent long-term complications by minimizing anorectal overdistension, anal trauma, and chronic use of oral laxative stimulants. The key to success in any bowel program is consistency, adequate follow-up, modifications as necessary, and ongoing support. A step-care system for sequential nonsurgical management of constipation or DWE in non-neurogenic and neurogenic patients is provided in Table 5.8-1.

1. Behavioral management is indicated if the patient is willing to alter prior bowel habits.

a. ***Timed (scheduled) bowel movements*** must be done at a consistent time that is convenient for the patient (or caregiver) at a frequency of every other day or more frequently. An adequate time for evacuation (10–15 minutes for non-neurogenic patients and longer for neurogenic patients) should be set aside for evacuation at periods of high colonic motility (e.g., after waking up in the morning or 20–40 minutes after regularly scheduled meals). Failure to produce a bowel movement at that specific time should not discourage the patient as evacuation can be attempted again at another time in the day. It may take several weeks of training to establish a consistent time for bowel movements.

b. ***Exercises*** include getting out of bed, exercises in the upright position, walking (e.g., shortly after breakfast), abdominal training (e.g., pelvic tilt or modified sit-ups), and aerobic exercises, if appropriate. For patients with rectal sensory deficits, rectal sensory re-education may be carried out. This technique involves the inflation of a rectal balloon catheter to an initial sensory threshold level (i.e., when pressure sensation is first felt) followed by patient training (with or without biofeedback) to sense progressively less degree of inflation (until the sensory threshold is within normal limits of 15–30 mL). For patients with anal sphincter motor deficits, anal sphincter training (i.e., Kegel exercise and biofeedback training, described in sections VI.A.6.b.1 and VI.A.6.b.2) may be used to improve defecation.

c. ***Defecation techniques*** include

I. **Proper defecation position,** that is, approximation of squatting position to achieve the proper angle between the rectum and the anal canal (if needed, a footstool may be used), or if unable to sit, a left side-lying position is best.

II. **Valsalva's maneuver** involves having the patient "bear down", that is, lean forward, close the glottis, hold the breath, and contract the diaphragm and the abdominal muscles to increase IAP and pelvic muscle tone. The increase in IAP is transferred to the pelvic floor and rectum to facilitate defecation. This should not be done by patients with rectal prolapse, hernias, hemorrhoids, or vesicoureteral reflux.

Table 5.8-1 Step-care system for sequential nonsurgical management of constipation

Step	Sequential recommendations for constipation*
I	Behavioral training, e.g., time schedule, diet modification (i.e., high-fiber diet), regular exercise, Valsalva's maneuver, proper defecation position, digital rectal stimulation
II	Bulk-forming agents or high-fiber supplements
III	For non-neurogenic bowel (with refractory constipation) 1. Oral stool softeners (i.e., docusates; avoid those combined with stimulant laxatives) or, if with high colonic constipation, oral mineral oil lubricants (unless contraindicated). 2. a. Oral hyperosmotic agents (e.g., lactulose or sorbitol); or b. Sparing use of hyperosmotic suppositories (e.g., glycerin, which may be combined with digital stimulation 20 min after suppository insertion). 3. Sparing use of mini-enemas (e.g., Enemeez) or enemas (e.g., tap-water enemas, mineral oil retention enemas, or sodium phosphate enemas). 4. Intermittent and sparing use of rectal stimulant laxatives or enemas (e.g., bisacodyl suppository or enema) for refractory constipation. Avoid oral stimulant laxatives. For neurogenic bowel (bowel habituation program) 1. Bowel clean-out at the start of the bowel training program (e.g., using multiple saline or bisacodyl enemas if stool is present at the rectal vault; or using oral mineral oil if stool is palpable proximal to the descending colon). 2. Hyperosmotic suppository (e.g., glycerin) 20–30 min after meal and 10 min later on toilet. Suppositories must be placed against rectal wall and not into fecal mass. a. If no defecation 20 minutes after suppository insertion, digital stimulation is performed and repeated once every 5 minutes up to three times. b. If defecation occurs in less than 10 minutes after suppository insertion, wean off suppository and only use digital stimulation to trigger defecations at desired time. If liquid glycerin with docusate is used (e.g., Enemeez mini-enema), a faster response time is anticipated as it does not have to wait for the solid suppository to melt. 3. Same as 2 but stimulant suppository (e.g., bisacodyl) is used instead of glycerin. 4. Oral stimulant laxatives, e.g., casanthranol-docusate sodium combination (e.g., Peri-Colace), senna (e.g., Senokot), bisacodyl (e.g., Dulcolax) given 6–10 hours before anticipated bowel movement schedule (time can be adjusted so that defecation would otherwise result 30 min to 1 hour after the scheduled bowel triggering with suppository and/or digital stimulation).

**Note: Steps I and II should be implemented vigorously in younger patients (below 50 years old). Each new step or substep should only be implemented if the previous step or substep has failed after a consistent trial for a reasonable period (e.g., 2 weeks). Details are described in the text.*

d. ***Manual bowel stimulation*** is most effective when the patient is sitting or squatting.

I. **Digital bowel (or digital-rectal) stimulation** is favored over manual disimpaction. It is done by inserting a gloved, lubricated finger into the anal canal and gently moving the finger in a circular motion (with the finger continually maintaining contact with the mucosa) until the IAS relaxes and the rectum dilates. It is performed for 30 seconds to 2 minutes and repeated every 5 minutes up to three times or it may be done continuously without interruption until defecation occurs or for a maximum period of 20 minutes. A suppository or enema is usually applied prior to digital bowel stimulation.

II. **Manual disimpaction** of feces should be done only if digital stimulation has failed. It is performed gently to prevent inadvertent overstretching of the anal sphincter (especially in insensate patients) or traumatic anorectal injury (e.g., ulceration or perforation, which can lead to bacterial sepsis). In patients predisposed to autonomic dysreflexia because of fecal impaction (e.g., patients with T6 or higher SCI), lubrication with lidocaine gel (see section VI.B.3.e) may help decrease nociceptive sensory input.

2. Dietary measures

a. ***High-fiber (bulk-forming) diet*** is the cornerstone in the prevention and treatment of constipation. It has hydrophilic properties that increase the stool's weight, bulks and fluidity; decrease the colonic transit time (hence increasing stool frequency); and enhance colonic bacterial load (hence increasing colonic fecal mass). For the high-fiber diet to be effective (and prevent further constipation), the person must have adequate oral fluid intake (i.e., 2.0–3.5 liters per day of any fluid except those containing alcohol, caffeine, or other diuretic agents). The standard formula used to estimate the fluid needs of the general public is 40 mL/kg body weight, but for patients with spinal cord injury, 500 mL/day should be added. Costs can be minimized by promoting dietary changes (i.e., increasing intake of fruits, vegetables, and cereals) rather than by addition of dietary fiber supplements. Dietary fiber should be increased gradually, as rapid and sudden increases can result in flatulence, eructation (belching), diarrhea, and abdominal bloating.

Daily recommended dietary fiber varies from 14.4 g to 20–35 g (usually 20–30 g). The ingestion of water-soluble fibers (i.e., mucilages and pectin such as those found in oats, barley, peas, dried beans, potatoes, seeds, apples, oranges, and grapefruits) has the additional benefit of decreasing levels of serum cholesterol and lipids. The effect of a high-fiber diet in decreasing bowel malignancy is controversial. The use of a high-fiber diet and bulk-forming agents is contraindicated in patients with intestinal obstruction (as documented by radiologic or endoscopic procedures), with allergic reactions (e.g., urticaria and bronchial asthma) either to the bulk-forming agent or to substances contained in the preparations, and who are under strict fluid restriction for medical reasons (e.g., hyponatremia).

I. **Natural high-fiber foods**

- **Cereals**, such as bran, shredded wheat, wheatgerm, oats, and barley. The recommended dosage for bran is one to two tablespoons taken once or twice a day with subsequent doses titrated based on individual response. Although an increase in stool frequency and flatus may occur during the first 2–3 weeks of bran therapy, bowel regularity is usually established within 1 month.
- **Vegetables**, such as Brussels sprouts, peas, artichokes, pumpkins, lima beans, and potatoes.

- **Fruits**, such as dates, avocados, raisins, blackberries, blueberries, apples, oranges, and grapefruits.

II. **Commercial fiber supplements** (see section VI.B.3.a.1). The bulk-forming laxative with the highest fiber content is psyllium.

b. ***Fruit juices,*** such as 4 oz (120 mL) of prune, fig, or pear juices can provide mild defecation stimulus when given 30 minutes to 1 hour before the established time of defecation.

3. Drug therapy

a. ***Laxatives*** are used either to achieve appropriate stool consistency or to increase intestinal peristalsis and stool frequency. They are available for oral or rectal use (enemas are also discussed in section VI.B.3.b), and most of them can be obtained over the counter. When suppositories are used, they must be applied against the rectal wall and not into the fecal mass. They are contraindicated in patients with intestinal obstruction (partial or complete).

I. **Bulk-forming agents** thicken the stool by absorbing fluid in the bowel and forming stool bulk. They also provide dietary fiber (especially psyllium seed derivatives which can also lower serum cholesterol with chronic use) and as with fiber intake, fluid intake of 2.0–3.5 L/day (see section VI.B.2.a for computation) are necessary (otherwise, further constipation and dehydration may ensue). Their effectiveness generally occurs within 12–24 hours (or may take several days depending upon transit times). The dosage is based upon individual patient response (usually one or two doses every 12–24 hours is sufficient).

The ADRs of bulk-forming agents (e.g., diarrhea, bloating, abdominal distress, and possible appetite reduction) can be decreased by reducing their doses or by using gradual dose titration. Bulk-forming agents must be used with caution by patients taking loop diuretics (as hypokalemia may occur) and by patients taking cardiac glycosides, nitrofurantoin, salicylates, and coumadin (because intestinal absorption of these drugs may be decreased). The adverse effect on serum electrolyte or blood urea levels in dialysis patients remains controversial. For diabetic patients, a sugar substitute may be used (nonabsorbable sugar substitutes may also help promote catharsis by an osmotic mechanism). Contraindications to the use of bulk-forming agents are similar to those noted previously for high-fiber diets (see section V.B.2.a).

Commercial preparations are supplied as individual packets, bulk packages, capsules, pills, or wafers. The manufacturer's recommended dosage is usually one teaspoon, tablespoon, pill, capsules or wafer to be taken one to three times daily with water or juice. Examples include psyllium or plantago seed derivatives (Konsyl, Metamucil, Modane-Bulk, Mucilose, Fiberall, Effersyllium, Hydrocil instant, Sarake, Syllact, Siblin, Naturacil, Nuggets), methylcellulose (Cologel, Citrucel, Hydrolose), polycarbophil (Mitrolan, Fibercon, Equalactin), malt soup extract (Maltsupex), plant gum, and guar. They are also available in combination with other laxatives, for example psyllium with senna (Perdiem), plant gums with mineral oil (Kondremul), or plant gums with docusate sodium (Gentlax-B). Isphagula husk, a natural nonwheat source of fiber, is not indicated as it may cause serious allergic reactions.

II. **Emollient (or surfactant) laxatives** soften the stool without adding bulk, increasing peristalsis, or causing any sense of urgency. They act primarily as surfactants that facilitate the mixture of aqueous and fatty substances in the fecal mass to soften it. The prototype is docusate (active ingredient is dioctyl sodium sulfosuccinate), which is supplied as either a sodium, potassium, or calcium salt. They are nonhabit-forming and are indicated for hard stools or for short-term use when straining at stools is to be avoided (e.g., postmyocardial infarct and postanorectal surgery). They are primarily not absorbed, but they may increase the absorption of other agents administered concurrently. In fact, this is suspected to be the mechanism of hepatotoxicity when combined with danthron (see section VI.B.3.a.5.b.3) and the mechanism of foreign-body reactions in lymphoid tissues when combined with mineral oil (see section VI.B.3.a.3). They may be safe, however, when used concomitantly with bulk-forming agents. Docusate sodium has been reported to be associated with periportal hepatitis but not with chronic active hepatitis.

The oral daily dose (taken with adequate fluid intake) for docusate sodium is 50–500 mg; docusate calcium is 240 mg; and docusate potassium is 100–300 mg. They are supplied as: docusate sodium capsule (50, 100, 240, 250 mg), oral liquid (200 mg/5 mL, 150 mg/15 mL), or tablet (100 mg); docusate calcium capsule (240 mg); and docusate potassium capsule (100 and 240 mg). Examples include docusate sodium (Afko-lube, Colace, Coloctyl, Comfolax, Correctol, Dio-Medicone, Diosate, Diosul, Doctate, Doxinate, Kasof, Modane-Soft, Regul-Aid, Regutol, Softenex), docusate potassium (Dialose), and docusate calcium (Surfak). They are available in combination with other laxatives, for example, docusate sodium with casanthranol (Peri-Colace, Constiban, D-S-S plus) or with cascara (Stimulax) or with danthron (Doctate, Dorbantyl, Unilax) or with senna (Senokot-S, Gentlax-S); and docusate potassium with casanthranol (Dialose plus). Docusate sodium is also available for rectal use, for example, as one of the ingredients in the Enemeez mini-enema (see section VI.B.3.b). Oral docusate is indicated in situations in which straining must be avoided, for example, in patients with angina, painful hemorrhoids, or who are prone to autonomic dysreflexia.

III. **Lubricant laxatives** promote defecation by facilitating the movement of stool. The prototype for lubricant laxatives is mineral oil, which consists of aliphatic hydrocarbons, which coat and penetrate the fecal material thus decreasing colonic absorption of water and allowing easier passage of oil-coated feces. It is given in doses of 5–45 mL either orally or as enemas (see enemas in section VI.B.3.c) for short-term management of constipation (especially if there are formed stools in the transverse colon or higher as detected by radiographs). The ADRs include pruritus ani, leakage of mineral oil from the anus (in some patients with poor sphincter tone), lipoid aspiration pneumonia, foreign-body reactions in lymphoid tissues (especially when combined with docusates), inhibition of absorption of fat-soluble vitamins (i.e., vitamines A, D, Es and K) in chronic use, and anal stenosis in long-term use. It is contraindicated in elderly patients and in patients prone to gastroesophageal reflux or aspiration (e.g., poststroke). Also, it should not be ingested at bedtime or when lying down (because of aspiration risk) nor should it be combined with docusates. Commercial preparations of mineral oil include Milkinol, Neo-Cultrol, Petrogalar, Fleet Mineral Oil Retention Enema, and Saf-tip Oil Retention Enema. It is also available in combination with other laxatives, such as mineral oil with magnesium hydroxide (Haley's M-O, Milk of Magnesia–Mineral Oil Emulsion), or with bulk-forming agents (Agoral Plain, Kondremul). Other lubricant laxatives include liquid paraffin and seed oils, such as croton and arachis oils.

IV. **Osmotic laxatives** are relatively nonabsorbable salts or carbohydrates that osmotically retain water in the lumen of the colon. They are indicated for immediate evacuation of bowel contents (e.g., at the start of the bowel training program or for preparing the bowel for endoscopy, surgery, or radiologic studies) and should not be used chronically.

- **Saline laxatives.** Magnesium salts and sodium phosphates must be used with caution in patients with renal impairment, heart disease, or pre-existing electrolyte imbalance.
  - **Magnesium salt** usually has an effect within 3–4 hours and is most effective when given on an empty stomach. It can cause hypermagnesemia (which may manifest as hypotension and muscle weakness) in patients with renal failure. Examples include magnesium citrate (Citrate of Magnesia, Citroma, Citronesia, Evac-Q-Mag), 200 mL or 11–18 g in 10 oz (300 mL), po; magnesium hydroxide (Milk of Magnesia), 15–30 mL or 2.4–4.8 g, po; and magnesium sulfate (Phillip's Milk of Magnesia), 10–30 g, po.
  - **Sodium phosphates** can be given orally (e.g., Fleet Phosphosoda, 20–45 mL, po) or as enemas (e.g., Fleet Phosphate Enema or Saf-Tip Phosphate Enema). They should not be used in patients with congestive heart failure as they may cause hypernatremic dehydration.
  - **Polyethylene glycol** with salts in colonic lavage solutions (Colyte, GoLytely, Nulytely; Miralax) are effective for rapid bowel cleansing (dose of 4–6 L, po, over 3–4 hours which may be ingested at 8 oz (240 mL) every 10 minutes) or for chronic constipation [oral dose of 224–448 g or 8–16 oz (240–480 mL) per day]. Polyethylene glycol does not cause either electrolyte imbalance or mucosal irritation, although some patients may be allergic to it.
- **Hyperosmotic laxatives**
  - **Glycerin** should be applied rectally as it is well-absorbed when given orally. It softens the fecal material and lubricates the anus and rectum, causing bowel evacuation within 30 minutes. Recommended rectal dose is 3 g. Chronic or daily use is not recommended as it may cause rectal irritation. It is available as Fleet Glycerin, Fleet Babylax, or generically as glycerin suppository. It is also one of the ingredients in Enemeez mini-enema (see section VI.B.3.b).
  - **Lactulose** is a nonabsorbable synthetic disaccharide, which exerts an osmotic effect when unmetabolized. When metabolized by colonic bacteria into lactate, it has both an osmotic and a stimulant effect. It is commonly used in elderly patients with constipation. The ADRs include GI complaints (e.g., flatulence, cramps, diarrhea, nausea, and vomiting) and electrolyte imbalance. Serum electrolytes need to be monitored in long-term use. It is contraindicated in patients on galactose-restricted diets and should be avoided when concomitant antacid is taken. Daily oral dose is 15–30 mL (maximum of 60 mL/day), qd or bid. To prevent ADRs, it may be started at 5 mL, po, qid and increased as necessary. Examples include Constulose, Enulose, Cephulac, Cholac, Chronulac, Constilac, and Duphalac.
  - **Other carbohydrates**, such as sorbitol and lactilol may be used as hyperosmotic laxatives. Sorbitol (30–70%, 30 mL, po, qd) is shown to be as effective as lactulose but is not widely used because of its limited commercial availability. Yogurt modified with lactilol, wheat bran, and guar may be given as snacks to elderly patients with chronic constipation.

V. **Stimulant (irritant or contact) laxatives** stimulate peristalsis by promoting water and electrolyte movement into the gut and inhibiting their absorption. They should be used sparingly and intermittently only if other laxative methods have failed. Local rectal stimulant suppositories and enemas carry less risk than oral stimulant medications and do not appear to lead to chronic inflammatory changes of the rectal mucosa. The chronic abuse of oral laxative stimulants can lead to atonic "cathartic bowel" syndrome caused by dysfunction or damage to the ENS. This is specially true for the chronic use of anthroquinone stimulant laxatives in patients with non-neurogenic bowel dysfunction (however, it remains unestablished for patients with neurogenic bowel dysfunction, e.g., because of SCI). Stimulant laxatives can cause autonomic dysreflexia as a result of hyperperistalsis in SCI patients with T6 lesions or higher (in these patients, senna, which is a mild stimulant, may be used if necessary). In nauseous patients, stimulant laxatives may cause vomiting because of reverse peristalsis.

- **Diphenylmethane derivatives**
  - **Phenolphthalein** stimulates colon motility and inhibits the absorption of sodium and glucose (which causes accumulation of intraluminal fluid). It was withdrawn from the market by the United States FDA because animal studies indicate a potential cancer risk to people, especially if used excessively. Laxatives previously containing phenolphthalein had been replaced with bisacodyl (e.g., Correctol and Feen-a-Mint) or senna (e.g., Ex-Lax).
  - **Bisacodyl**, a congener of phenolphthalein, stimulates the mucosal nerve plexus of the colon, producing contractions of the entire colon and inhibiting water absorption in the small and large bowel. Unlike phenolphthalein, it does not require absorption and subsequent metabolism before being effective. Rather, it is readily converted to its active desactyl metabolite by intestinal enzymes, both bacterial and mucosal. Its laxative effect occurs within 6–12 hours after oral administration or 15–60 minutes after rectal administration. It must be taken at least 1 hour before milk or antacids are given. The usual dose is 10–15 mg (0.3 mg/kg), po or pr, as needed. It is available in 5-mg enteric-coated tablets, 10-mg suppositories, or 10-mg/30 mL rectal enemas. The ADRs include abdominal cramps and laxative dependence. Examples are Dulcolax, Fleet Bisacodyl Enema, Carter's Little Pills Correctol, Feen-a-Mint, and Theralax.
  - **Oxyphenisatin** is no longer available because of its association with chronic active hepatitis.
- **Anthraquinone derivatives** stimulate colonic motility via Auerbach's plexus. They need to be metabolized by colonic bacteria when orally administered and need approximately 6–10 hours for the laxative effect to occur. The ADRs include melanosis coli (when used in large amounts over long periods; reversible upon cessation; benign) and acute nephritis (when ingested in large doses). Because metabolites of the anthraquinones are found in breast milk, urine, and saliva, toxic quantities of these secretions can have laxative effects in the infants of nursing mothers.
  - **Senna** is the mildest of the anthraquinone derivatives and may be used safely even in tetraplegic patients. Oral administration of senna results in poor initial absorption from the small intestine. More significant absorption occurs after metabolism by colonic bacteria. These agents produce primarily a colonic effect, which accounts for the 6–10 hours usually required for its laxative action to occur. It is available in 8.6-mg tablets, 15-mg granules, and in 8.8-mg/5 mL syrup. Daily oral dose is one or two tablets, one teaspoon of granules, or 10–15 mL, po, qhs or bid. Examples include Senokot, Dosaflex, Fletcher's Castoria, Ex-Lax and Nytilax. It is also available in combination with docusate sodium (Gentlax-S).
  - **Cascara** usually requires 6–10 hours for its laxative action to occur. Dosage varies from 2 to 6 mL, po, qhs because of the variable amounts of cascara in the commercial preparations. Examples include Cas-Evac and Extract of Cascara. It is also available in combination forms, for example, cascara with milk of magnesia (also called "black and white", an effective laxative after barium swallow) or with docusate sodium (Stimulax).
  - **Danthron** is given at a dose of 75–150 mg orally. Examples include Dorbane and Tonelax. It is also available in combination with emollient laxatives, for example, danthron with docusate sodium (Doctate, Dorbantyl, Unilax).

This combination, however, has been shown to cause hepatotoxicity similar to chronic active hepatitis.

- **Casanthranol** is given at a dose of 30 mg orally. Examples include Black Draught and Lanes Pills. It is also available in combination with emollient laxatives, such as, casanthranol with docusate sodium (Constiban, D-S-S plus, Peri-Colace), or with docusate potassium (Dialose plus).
- **Other anthraquinones** include *Cassia alata* from Thailand and mulberry extract used primarily in China. Their effectiveness and mechanism of action have not been well studied in the West.

- **Castor oil** is metabolized into ricinoleic acid, which promotes intestinal peristalsis and reduces the absorption of fluid and electrolytes. It acts within 2–6 hours and can result in a complete bowel evacuation. It is given at 15–45 mL, po, qhs or up to 60 mL if used for bowel preparation for radiologic or endoscopic procedures. However, it has a disagreeable odor and taste and is seldom prescribed for constipation as it can cause painful cramps, watery bowel movements, malabsorption, electrolyte abnormalities, and dehydration. Examples include Fleet Flavored Castor Oil Emulsion, Neoloid, and Purge Evacuant.

VI. **Carbon dioxide suppository (e.g., Ceo-Two)** releases carbon dioxide as it melts into the rectum causing rectal distension, a reflex colonic peristalsis, and subsequent mechanical expulsion of stool. It may be used during bowel training for low-level SCI patients with loss of anorectal reflex; however, it is expensive and may cause autonomic dysreflexia in SCI patients with T6 lesions or higher.

b. ***Mini-enemas,*** so named because they contain a small volume of fluid (4 mL), can help improve rectal evacuation by increasing the response time. They produce a bowel movement within 15 minutes because, unlike a solid suppository, they do not need a waiting period for melting. An example is Enemeez mini-enema, which contains docusate sodium in a soap base of glycerin and polyethylene glycol. Some variants also contain benzocaine, an anesthetic. Enemeez mini-enema triggers reflex-mediated colonic peristalsis by acting as a mucosal stimulus, and provides lubrication by penetrating the stool and softening it by the action of the docusate. It is commonly used in SCI patients, especially those with T6 or higher lesions because it reduces nociceptive stimuli that might precipitate autonomic dysreflexia. It is packaged in a single-use, ready-to-squeeze container with applicator tip. The tip should be punctured and *not* cut (to prevent sharp edges which could injure the anal sphincter, especially in insensate SCI patients).

c. ***Enemas*** are usually used as purgatives for bowel cleansing in preparing the patient for surgery or X-ray or endoscopic procedures. They may also be used in selected patients to help maintain regular bowel function and prevent skin breakdown (e.g., elderly patients with chronic constipation in whom rehabilitation is not feasible and who do not respond well to lesser stimuli, such as suppositories). Enemas must be used sparingly and intermittently because of their potential to cause enema-dependency bowel, rectoanal trauma, bowel perforation, electrolyte disturbances, bacteremia, colonic infections, and autonomic dysreflexia. They should only be used when more conservative bowel-care procedures (e.g., use of suppositories and digital bowel stimulation) have failed. In the elderly or insensate patients, enemas should be administered using a cone tip (such as the tip used for colostomy irrigations) or using the nipple of a baby bottle fitted around the tip of the catheter to prevent backflow. If the enema is prepackaged in ready-to-use plastic squeeze bottles with applicator tips, the tip should not be cut to prevent sharp edges.

I. **Enemas containing laxative drugs** include saline osmotic enemas (see sodium phosphates described in section VI.B.3.a.4.a), mineral oil enemas (see section VI.B.3.a.3), stimulant enemas (see bisacodyl described in section VI.B.3.a.5), and lactulose enemas (which generate the release of carbon dioxide and hydrogen to break up impacted feces).

II. **Tap-water enema** is benign and may be used to break up impacted stool. It is safer than a soap-suds enema, which can also be used to break up fat in the stool. The soap-suds enema is popular among the elderly but has been reported to cause acute colitis (the mechanisms of action are unknown; probably caused by long-chain fatty acid toxicity). Although the colitis is usually benign, there have been reports of anaphylaxis, rectal gangrene, excessive fluid loss, and death attributed to the use of soap-suds enemas.

III. **Nontraditional enemas** containing coffee, herbal laxative additives, wheat grass, or hydrogen peroxide have been used not just for relief of constipation but as part of alternative medicine (e.g., for cancer treatment, increasing sexual potency, or total-body cleansing). These claims, however, have little scientific basis.

d. ***Other peristaltic drugs***

I. **Prokinetic agents**

- **Cisapride (Propulsid)**, a prokinetic and noncholinergic agent that stimulates colonic smooth muscle, was withdrawn by the manufacturer because of reports of cardiac arrhythmias and deaths.
- **Metoclopramide (Reglan)** is an antiemetic agent that also promotes gastric emptying, probably by sensitizing tissues to acetylcholine. Although it has no direct effect on the colon, it can help resolve ileus after SCI. In high-dose or long-term use, it can cause dystonic reactions and other extrapyramidal side-effects. It can be given at a dosage of 5–20 mg, po, tid or qid.
- **Erythromycin** is a macrolide antibiotic that stimulates gastric, small bowel, and colon motor activity, thus accelerating colonic transit and increasing stool frequency. It has been effective at a dosage of 500 mg, po, qid in selective SCI patients with refractory constipation because of ileus.

e. ***Viscous 2% lidocaine***, applied topically, may be beneficial if rectodynamic studies show anorectal dyssynergia. It may also be used during manual disimpaction (see section VI.B.1.d.2) in SCI patients with T6 or higher lesions who are predisposed to autonomic dysreflexia.

VII. Surgery

Surgery to improve defecation is used only if conservative treatment methods have failed.

A. SURGERY FOR FI PATIENTS to improve sphincter mechanism

1. **Anal sphincter repair** involves direct apposition or the overlapping of the EAS muscle. It is indicated for patients who have a deficient EAS with no neurologic damage (e.g., aging).
2. **Muscle transplant** involves the transposition of innervated muscles (e.g., gracilis, adductor longus, or gluteus maximus) or free muscle graft (e.g., palmaris longus) to replace puborectalis, levator ani, or EAS functions in patients with sacral nerve deficits. Chronic electrical stimulation may be used with these transplants.
3. **Artificial anal sphincters** involve the use of a subcutaneous pump mechanism that controls defecation by manually deflating a cuff placed around the EAS, which automatically reinflates over a period of 10 minutes to provide

continence. It is indicated only for patients who have failed other surgery because of high complication rates and poor outcomes.

B. SURGERY FOR PATIENTS WITH DWE

1. **Myotomy** involves IAS or partial EAS incision to improve incomplete EAS relaxation during defecation (e.g., in anorectal dyssynergia). Although it relieves constipation in 62% of patients, it causes FI in 16%.
2. **Transrectal (Brindley) stimulation** of anterior (parasympathetic) roots of S2–S4 is used in complete SCI patients to stimulate the distal colon and increase defecation frequency; however, electrodefecation results are unpredictable.

C. SURGERY FOR PATIENTS WITH FI OR DWE

1. **Fecal diversion (e.g., colostomy or ileostomy)** can be used in patients with fecal incontinence (to attain social continence in intractable FI), chronic DWE or impaction (for reducing bowel care time and relieving abdominal distension), intrinsic bowel deficits (e.g., Hirschsprung's disease or atonic "cathartic colon"), pressure ulcers or other skin lesions that cannot be effectively healed because of frequent soiling, or frequent urinary tract infections caused by seeding from frequent fecal impactions. Aside from the surgical risks, problems include cosmetic difficulties and embarrassing leakage of stool (e.g., loosening of ostomy bag). However, because of the improvement in quality of life it provides (i.e., simplification of bowel care), many patients with neurogenic bowel have refused to have their fecal diversion reversed (e.g., after healing of pressure ulcers).
2. **Antegrade continence enema (ACE) procedure or appendicocecostomy** can be used in chronic refractory neurogenic bowel with FI or DWE (e.g., spina bifida children) when there is sufficient rectal tone to allow the use of rectal enemas. The appendix (or part of the cecum) is used to make a fistula between the cecum and the skin (with a stoma on the abdominal wall). Enema fluid (e.g., saline solution or phosphate enema) can then be introduced through the stoma via a catheter into the bowel to push the feces out through the anus (called "washout") 30 minutes later. Complications include narrowing of the stoma and infection. An alternative to the ACE procedure is the **cecostomy button**, which uses a plastic device (instead of the fistula made of appendix or cecum) to connect the cecum to the skin.
3. **Bowel resection** may be performed on diseased bowel that contributes to FI or DWE.

VIII. Bowel complications

A. FECAL IMPACTION has a morbidity range between 0% and 6% in the normal population (being higher in the cognitively impaired elderly). It is the most common bowel complication of chronic SCI patients (i.e., seen in at least 80% of the 27% of SCI patients who, 5 years after injury, develop significant bowel complications despite previous satisfactory bowel management). It is a common and potentially dangerous cause of autonomic dysreflexia in SCI patients with lesions at or above T6 because of the substantial time that may be required for its clearance. It can also lead to perforation or even death. Treatments include manual disimpaction (see section VI.B.1.d.2) in conjunction with laxatives or enemas, disimpaction by hydraulic lithotripsy, or by surgical decompression. Preventive measures are described above (see the step-care system in Table 5.8-1).

B. HEMORRHOIDS are frequently (i.e., in over 90% of Americans or over 70% of SCI cases) caused by high pressures in the anorectal marginal veins associated with DWE. They can cause pain as well as rectal bleeding. They can be prevented by adequate softening of stool (see under diet in section VI.B.2 and medications in section VI.B.3) without causing incontinence. Topical anti-inflammatory (hydrocortisone) creams or suppositories (e.g., Anusol HC cream or suppository) may be used. Hemorrhoid surgery (e.g., by rubber-band ligation or operative hemorrhoidectomy) may be carried out if there is bleeding (i.e., blood dripping into the commode or passage of clots), mucus soilage, or difficulty with anal hygiene.

C. RECTAL PROLAPSE can be associated with an overstretched patulous non-competent sphincter because of the passage of very large hard stools through a weakened or atonic anorectal mechanism (e.g., because of lower motor neurogenic bowel). Treatment includes avoidance of straining and stretching of atonic bowel (e.g., softening of stool by diet or medications and avoidance of Valsalva's maneuver). If manual disimpaction is used, it must be performed gently to avoid trauma to the denervated structures. A temporary colostomy (see section VII.C for indication) may allow the overdistended bowel to regain tone.

D. RECTAL BLEEDING (i.e., streaks of blood on the glove or stool) after SCI is most commonly caused by traumatic superficial circumferential mucosal erosion (which can be treated conservatively). In patients over 45 years old, a flexible sigmoidoscopy may be done followed by a full colonoscopy if polyps or tumors are seen.

E. BLOATING, ABDOMINAL DISTENSION, AND FLATULENCE can be especially severe in those with anorectal dyssynergia (i.e., hyperactive EAS in response to rectal distension). Treatment includes increasing the frequency of the bowel program, avoidance of foods that produce excessive gas (e.g., beans), digital release of flatus, and antiflatulent medications (e.g., those containing simethicone).

F. ACQUIRED MEGACOLON and/or **MEGARECTUM** denotes colonic or rectal dilatation that is not caused by mechanical obstruction. Acquired megacolon has a 3% risk of spontaneous perforation. Megarectum is characterized by increased rectal compliance and reduced sensitivity to rectal distension, thus the rectum is unable to contract and empty effectively. In megarectum, the anus may gape open secondary to the dysfunction of the internal sphincter mechanism, thus the patient may present with factitious diarrhea secondary to overflow incontinence. In the absence of perforation, acute treatment includes fecal disimpaction (see section VI.B.1.d.2), evacuation by enemas and suppositories (see section VI.B.3.c), removal of the underlying cause (e.g., narcotics, anticholinergic agents, calcium-channel blockers), decompression using nasogastric tubes as well as rectal tubes, and if the dilatation persists or worsens, colonoscopic decompression can be tried (however, dilatation usually recurs). In stable patients, the recommended regimen includes a bowel habituation program and use of bulking agents (see step-care system in Table 5.8-1). Surgical options include total abdominal colectomy with ileorectal anastomosis (the operation of choice for megacolon with normal-sized rectum), total proctocolectomy with ileostomy, and total proctocolectomy with ileoanal anastomosis, depending on the site of the colon affected.

G. OTHER BOWEL COMPLICATIONS (e.g., PREMATURE DIVERTICULOSIS, COLONIC CANCER).

Further reading

Banwell JG, Creaswey GH, Aggarwal AM, *et al.*: Management of the neurogenic bowel in patients with spinal cord injury. *Urol Clin North Am* 20:517–526, 1993.

Consortium for Spinal Cord Medicine: Clinical practice guideline: neurogenic bowel management in adults with spinal cord injury. *J Spinal Cord Med* 21:248–293, 1998.

Doughty DB, editor: *Urinary and fecal incontinence: nursing management*, ed 2, St Louis, 2000, Mosby.

Hasler W: Motility of the small intestine and colon. In Yamada T, editor: *Textbook of gastroenterology*, vol 1, ed 4, Philadelphia, 2003, Lippincott, Williams & Wilkins, pp. 220–247.
King JC, Stiens SA: Neurogenic bowel: dysfunction and management. In Braddom RL, editor: *Physical medicine and rehabilitation*, ed 2, Philadelphia, 2000, WB Saunders, pp. 579–591.
Lennard-Jones, JE: Constipation. In Feldman M, Scharschmidt BF, Sleisinger MH, editors: *Sleisenger and Fordtran's gastrointestinal and liver disease: pathophysiology/diagnosis/management*, vol 1, ed 6, Philadelphia, 1998, WB Saunders, pp. 174–197.
Lisenmeyer TA, Stone JM, Steins SA: Neurogenic bladder and bowel dysfunction. In DeLisa JA, Gans BM, Walsh *et al.*, editors: *Physical medicine and rehabilitation: principles and practice*, 2005, Lippincott, Williams & Wilkins, pp. 1619–1654.
Schiller LR: Fecal incontinence. In Feldman M, Scharschmidt BF, Sleisinger MH, editors: *Sleisenger and Fordtran's gastrointestinal and liver disease: pathophysiology/diagnosis/management*, vol 1, ed 6, Philadelphia, 1998, WB Saunders, pp. 160–173.
Stiens SA, Bergman SB, Goetz LL: Neurogenic bowel dysfunction after spinal cord injury: clinical evaluation and rehabilitative management. *Arch Phys Med Rehabil* 78 (3-S):S86–S102, 1997.
Tedesco FJ, Di Piro JT: American College of Gastroenterology's committee on FDA-related matters: laxative use in constipation. *Am J Gastroenterol* 80:303, 1985.
Wexner SD, Bartolo DCC: *Constipation: etiology, evaluation and management*, Oxford, 1995, Butterworth-Heinemann.

Supplemental references

Stiens SA, Braunschweig C, Cowel F, *et al.*: *Neurogenic bowel: What you should know. A guide for people with spinal cord injury*, Washington, DC, 1999, Consortium for Spinal Cord Medicine, p. 53.
Stiens SA, Pidde T, Veland B, *et al.*: *Accidents Stink! or Bowel Care 202* (videocassette), Seattle, 2003, VA Puget Sound Health Care System (available from Concepts in Confidence, tel. 1-800-822-4050).

CHAPTER 5.9
Problems in human sexuality

The impact of disability on the patient's sexuality and sexual function is a common concern of PM&R patients. Although sex is considered one of the basic activities of daily living, it is often neglected because the sex drive does not have immediate consequences for survival and most health-care providers are uncomfortable with the subject. As experts in the rehabilitation of the whole patient, physiatrists must be knowledgeable in dealing with sexual issues considering that 80% of sexual complaints can be successfully managed in the office setting. This chapter deals with the physiological, mechanical, and psychosocial issues of sexual dysfunction and related sexual issues, such as fertility, contraception, pregnancy, labor, and lactation. For other important issues, such as sexually transmitted diseases (STD), the reader is referred to any standard medical textbook.

I. Definitions

A. **SEX DRIVE (LIBIDO)** is a primary drive similar to hunger, thirst, and avoidance of pain. The conscious or unconscious decline in sexual drive or desire (e.g., because of anxiety, pain, malaise, stress, or fatigue) is referred to as *decreased libido*. Sex drive is not abolished by physical disability.

B. **SEX ACTS (OR "SEX")** are human behaviors that result in pleasurable sensations through contact with one's own or another person's body, usually, but not necessarily, involving erogenous zones. *Sexual activity*, such as *intercourse*, which is an example of a sex act, should not be limited to *coitus* (penetration of erect penis into the vagina). In PM&R, *sexual activity* refers to communication involving sexual self-expression and associated pleasuring, with or without genital involvement.

C. **SEXUALITY** refers to the expression of one's sex drive within the context of the sexual identity of the person. It integrates the physical, emotional, intellectual, and social aspects of an individual's personality, and expresses maleness or femaleness. It is a dynamic process grounded in developmental learning experiences involving the individual's self-concept, relationships with others, and specific repertoire of sexual behaviors. Interactions with others, personal hygiene, dress, speech, and expressions of affection are all important parts of sexuality. Sexuality is not completely determined by physical characteristics, and persons with physical disabilities do not lose their sexuality.

D. **INTIMACY** should not be equated with sexuality as it does not always involve sexuality. Intimacy is a special state of mutual understanding, trust, and acceptance. The need and capacity for intimacy remains although physical disability may interfere with sex drive and sex acts.

E. **SEXUAL DYSFUNCTION** (see Table 5.9-1 for classification), according to the American Psychiatric Association DSM-IV (2000), is characterized by disturbance in male or female sexual desire and in the psychophysiological changes that characterize the sexual response cycle and cause marked distress and interpersonal difficulty. This definition was specifically limited to psychiatric disorders and was not intended to be used for classification of organic causes of female sexual dysfunctions. The interdisciplinary panel of the International Consensus

Table 5.9-1 Classification of sexual dysfunction based on the *Diagnostic and Statistical Manual of Mental Disorders* (DSM-IV) of the American Psychiatric Association and on the Report of the International Consensus Development Conference of Female Sexual Dysfunction (ICDCFSD)

Classification	M	F	Definition
I. Sexual desire disorders			
1. Hypoactive sexual desire disorder	√	√	**D:** *Deficiency or absence of sexual fantasies and desire for sexual acitivity **C:** Persistent or recurrent deficiency (or absence) of sexual fantasies/thoughts, and/or desire for or receptivity to sexual activity, which causes personal distress†
2. Sexual aversion disorder	√	√	**D:** *Aversion to and active avoidance of genital sexual contact with a sexual partner
		√	**C:** Persistent or recurrent phobic aversion to and avoidance of sexual contact with a sexual partner, which causes personal distress†
II. Sexual arousal disorder			
1. Female sexual arousal disorder		√	**D:** * A persistent or recurrent inability to attain, or to maintain until completion of the sexual activity, an adequate lubrication-swelling response of sexual excitement
		√	**C:** Persistent or recurrent inability to attain or maintain sufficient sexual excitement, causing personal distress†, which may be expressed as a lack of subjective excitement, or genital (lubrication/swelling) or other somatic responses
2. Male erectile dysfunction	√		**D:** * A persistent or recurrent inability to attain, or to maintain until completion of the sexual activity, an adequate erection
III. Orgasmic disorders			
1. Female orgasmic disorder		√	**D:** * A persistent or recurrent delay in, or absence of, orgasm following a normal sexual excitement phase. The diagnosis is based on the clinician's judgment that the woman's orgasmic capacity is less than would be reasonable for her age, sexual experience, and the adequacy of sexual stimulation she receives
		√	**C:** Persistent or recurrent difficulty, delay in, or absence of attaining orgasm following sufficient sexual stimulation and arousal, which causes personal distress†
2. Male orgasmic disorder	√		**D:** * A persistent or recurrent delay in, or absence of, orgasm following a normal sexual excitement phase. In judging whether the stimulation is delayed, the clinician should consider the person's age and whether the stimulation is adequate in focus, intensity, and duration

(*Continued*)

Table 5.9-1 (*Continued*)

Classification	M	F	Definition
3. Premature ejaculation	√		**D:** *A persistent or recurrent onset of orgasm and ejaculation with minimal sexual stimulation before, on, or shortly after penetration and before the person wishes it. The clinician must consider factors that affect duration of the excitement phase, such as age, novelty of the sexual partner or situation, and recent frequency of sexual activity. The premature ejaculation is not due exclusively to the direct effects of a substance (e.g., withdrawal from opioids)
IV. Sexual pain disorder (not due to a general medical condition)			
1. Dyspareunia	√	√	**D:** *Genital pain associated with sexual intercourse (may occur before or after intercourse), not caused exclusively by vaginismus or lack of lubrication and not due exclusively to the direct physiological effects of a substance (e.g., a drug of abuse, a medication) or a general medical condition
		√	**C:** Recurrent or persistent genital pain associated with sexual intercourse
2. Vaginismus		√	**D:** *Recurrent or persistent involuntary contraction of the perineal muscles surrounding the outer third of the vagina when vaginal penetration with penis, finger, tampon, or speculum is attempted. It is not due exclusively to the direct physiological effects of a general medical condition
		√	**C:** Recurrent or persistent involuntary spasm of the musculature of the outer third of the vagina that interferes with vaginal penetration, which causes personal distress†
3. ‡Other sexual pain disorders including noncoital sexual pain disorder		√	**C:** Noncoital sexual pain disorder is recurrent or persistent genital pain induced by noncoital sexual stimulation, who would not be included in the categories of dyspareunia or vaginismus

D = DSM-IV; C = ICDCFSD; M = male; F = female.

**In addition, the disturbance must cause marked distress or interpersonal difficulty and is not better accounted for by another Axis I disorder.*

† Personal distress, which is essential (according to the ICDCFSD) can be assessed by clinical interview or standardized questionnaire. The diagnosis of a particular sexual dysfunction cannot be given unless the patient has personal distress. Although the distress of the patient's partner is not sufficient to make the diagnosis, this is still a cause of concern and counseling is recommended.

‡ This new category of sexual pain disorder (including noncoital sexual pain) was added by the ICDCFSD.

Data from: American Psychiatric Association: DSM-IV-TR: Diagnostic and Statistical Manual of Mental Disorders, Test revision, *ed 4, Washington, DC, 2000, American Psychiatric Association Press, pp. 535–582; and Basson R, Berman J, Burnett A,* et al.: *Report of the International Consensus Development Conference of Female Sexual Dysfunction: definitions and classifications.* J Urol *163: 888–893, 2000.*

Development Conference of Female Sexual Dysfunction (ICDCFSD; see Basson *et al.*, 2000), reported that female sexual dysfunction is a multicausal and multidimensional problem combining biological, psychological, and interpersonal determinants. Hence, the panel of the ICDCFSD revised the existing DSM-IV definitions, added a new sexual dysfunction category (i.e., noncoital sexual pain disorder), and put emphasis on personal distress criterion for most of the diagnostic categories of female sexual dysfunction (see Table 5.9-1).

F. SEXUAL ADJUSTMENT refers to the intimate communication involving a mutually pleasurable and practical repertoire of behavior, which may or may not emphasize genital behavior. Its adequacy is solely determined by the patient and partner.

II. The phases of sexual response

The physiology of the sexual response is presented below and is classified in four phases (based on Masters and Johnson's classification of sexual response).

A. EXCITEMENT OR AROUSAL PHASE, which lasts several minutes to hours, occurs in response to sexual stimulation either because of touch (reflexogenic) or imagination (psychogenic). In men, the penis becomes erect, the scrotum contracts, and the testes are brought close to the body. In women, there is vaginal lubrication (with vasocongestion leading to a transudate of fluid), swelling of the labia, clitoral erection, expansion of the inner two-thirds of the vagina, and elevation of the uterine body, cervix, and labia majora. The vascular mechanism of erection occurs because of vasocongestion of the erectile tissues of the genitals resulting from arteriolar and sinusoidal dilation, which passively occludes venous outflow. Both sexes have increased muscle tension, blood pressure, and heart rate. In elderly men, the following changes may be noted: erections occur two or three times slower than with younger men; tactile stimulation may be necessary; erection which is not as firm approaches full rigidity only seconds before ejaculation. In elderly women, the arousal phase is also delayed and there is less voluminous vaginal secretion with delayed and reduced vaginal expansion.

1. **Reflexogenic excitement** can be elicited by direct genital stimulation (e.g., stroking, oral stimulation, vibration, pulling pubic hair, or a full bladder) independent of erotic stimuli or thoughts. The sensory impulse travels through the dorsal afferent nerve to the sacral cord through the pudendal nerve. From the sacral cord, parasympathetic efferents originate from the anterior division of S2–S4 and travel via the cauda equina through the pelvic nerves (also called pelvic splanchnic nerves or nervi erigentes) to the cavernosal nerves and into the corporal trabeculae. The parasympathetic efferent stimuli cause vasodilation, which leads to vasocongestion of the genitalia. Hence, interruption of the S2–S4 parasympathetic reflex arc (e.g., in complete lower motor neuron lesions) leads to loss of reflexogenic excitement; but, if the sacral reflex activity (i.e., bulbocavernosus reflex) is intact (e.g., in upper motor neuron lesion), reflexogenic excitement can occur.
2. **Psychogenic excitement** is believed to originate in the cerebral cortex through the different senses, such as audio-visual stimuli (e.g., erotic movies or pictures) or through erotic fantasies. The stimulating psychogenic impulses travel through the hypothalamic and thalamic centers to the thoracolumbar (sympathetic) cord. Hence, even if reflexogenic excitement is lost because of an abolished S2–S4 parasympathetic reflex arc (e.g., in patients with complete lower motor neuron lesions), psychogenic excitement may still occur as long as the

thoracolumbar (sympathetic) cord is intact. In SCI patients with incomplete upper motor neuron lesion above T10 (i.e., intact sympathetic cord), psychogenic as well as reflexogenic excitement is possible. The sympathetic efferents originate from T11–L2 and travel to the genitalia through the hypogastric plexi. Thus, the greater the preservation of sensory function in this area, the greater the likelihood of retained psychogenic genital vasocongestion. In the nonexcited state, tonic sympathetic discharge (probably through postsynaptic α-receptors) causes contraction of the genital arterioles and sinusoids thus keeping the blood from entering the erectile tissues of the genitals. During excitement, it is theorized that norepinephrine acts on the postsynaptic β-receptors resulting in smooth muscle relaxation and vasodilation of the genital arterioles and sinusoids, which leads to vasocongestion of the genitalia.

B. PLATEAU PHASE, which can last from seconds to minutes, consists of the high levels of sexual arousal that precede the threshold levels required to trigger orgasm. It involves maximal vasocongestion of the sexual organs with additional increases in heart rate and blood pressure. In men, vasocongestion continues; the penis enlarges further and can deepen in color. The testes elevate and rotate anteriorly, coming to rest against the perineum. In women, the processes of vaginal expansion and clitoral and nipple engorgement continue. A "sex flush" may spread over the abdomen, breasts, and chest wall. In both sexes, there is tachypnea, tachycardia, elevated blood pressure, and generalized myotonia. In elderly men, the plateau phase is prolonged, and there is a poorly defined sense of impending orgasm whereas in elderly women, there is less discernible nipple swelling and erection. Patients who have anorgasmy do not progress further than the plateau stage.

C. ORGASM PHASE involves rhythmic contractions of the penis and prostate in men (i.e., ejaculation). In women, there are rhythmic contractions of the uterus and outer one-third of the vagina. In both sexes, there is sometimes rhythmic contraction of the perineal muscles and other more diffuse responses (e.g., peripheral muscular contractions).

Although orgasm in men is usually associated with ejaculation, it is not a prerequisite (likewise, erection is not a prerequisite of ejaculation, which is reflexive). Men with transurethral prostatectomy (TURP) may still experience orgasm despite 90% incidence of ejaculatory failure (with 50–60% incidence of retrograde ejaculation). In elderly men, there is reduced volume of the seminal fluid, and the ejaculatory event is shorter with fewer and less forceful expulsive contractions of the urethra (i.e., seepage may occur instead of forceful ejaculation). In women, it is uncertain whether ejaculation occurs. The nature of female ejaculate remains controversial (it has been reported to consist of vaginal transudate, which accumulates throughout the arousal process). Women who have had a hysterectomy or clitoridectomy may still experience orgasm. During menopause, there is a decrease in the frequency of vaginal and uterine contraction during orgasm because of a relative estrogen deficit.

In both sexes, orgasms occur post-SCI (Sipski *et al.*, 2001). Although approximately 50% of men and women with complete and incomplete SCIs report the ability to achieve orgasm, the subset of persons with complete lower motor neuron injuries affecting the sacral segments was shown to be relatively anorgasmic. Thus, orgasm is believed to be a reflex response of the autonomic nervous system that can be inhibited or facilitated by cognitive inputs. Of note, the descriptions of orgasms of persons with SCIs are indistinguishable from those of the able-bodied. Likewise, blood pressure and heart rate changes are similar. However, latency to orgasm is generally greater post-SCI.

D. RESOLUTION PHASE, which usually occurs over a period of 5–15 minutes, involves the return of the body to its normal resting state. Sympathetic tonic discharge resumes in the genitals, resulting in contraction of the smooth muscles around the sinusoids and arterioles. Arterial blood flow is decreased and venous channels are reopened. In men, there is a refractory period immediately after ejaculation in which further ejaculation cannot occur (although erection may occur). In contrast, women do not experience a refractory period and have the potential to experience several successive orgasms. In elderly men, detumescence is more rapid and the refractory period is longer (i.e., about 12–24 hours in those over 55 years old).

III. Sexual assessment

Sexual assessment should be initiated by the physiatrist and, ideally, it should be performed in a multidisciplinary fashion (to identify psychological factors). History and physical examination can be incorporated with sexual counseling by using the ENIGMA model (i.e., Engage, Normalize, Inform, Guide, Maximize, and Assess) described in section V.B.

A. HISTORY should be open-ended and nonjudgmental (see Table 5.9-2 for sample format). It should include general and specific current and premorbid sexual functioning (e.g., ability to obtain reflex and psychogenic erections, ability to lubricate, and sexual positioning difficulties), current medications (see Table 5.9-3), recreational drugs (e.g., alcohol, opioids, marijuana, and tobacco can all cause erectile dysfunction and probably decrease libido), associated injuries (e.g., pelvic fracture or prior pelvic surgery), the patient's and the partner's psychological adjustment to injury, the patient's sexual orientation, relationship, and family status, and the patient's need for additional services concerning sexuality.

B. PHYSICAL EXAMINATION sessions should be used as an opportunity to check the patient's knowledge of sexually transmitted diseases (STDs). All patients who are sexually active in nonexclusive relationships without STD precautions (i.e., condoms used consistently) should be screened for infection. Most patients, female and male, are neither aware of the signs or symptoms of STDs, nor are they aware of the fact that a significant portion of the infected population is without signs or symptoms.

1. **General**. Demeanor, posture, clothing, and grooming.
2. **Skin.** Scars, rashes, open wounds, pressure ulcers, and skin lesions.
3. **Mental health**

a. ***Cognition***. Competence in consenting to sexual activity; judgment to make safe decisions about high-risk sexual activity and contraception.

b. ***Mood***. Depressed, abusive.

4. **Neurologic**. Educate about possible new erotic areas (insensate–sensate border); instruct patient that masturbation can still lead to orgasm despite a lack of surface sensation (but it may take longer); instruct patient that learning how their body functions and educating their partner is important; if patient has dysesthesia, teach techniques for desensitization or position to avoid stimulating dysesthetic areas.

a. ***Sensation***. Sensory distribution; potential for touching, caressing, receiving touch; erogenous zones (identified by patient or believed to be important by physician, e.g., dermatomal levels just above anesthetic area); areas of dysesthesia. In post-SCI patients, determine whether sensation is preserved between T11 and L2 (the greater the preservation of sensation in this area, the greater the capacity for psychogenic genital vasocongestion).

b. ***Strength***. Paralysis or paresis.

c. ***Communication***. Aphasia, dysarthria, visual and hearing disorders.

Table 5.9-2 Sample interview format

Category	Question or statement
Introduction	• I'd like to discuss with you your present sexual functioning. (Assure patient of confidentiality)
Current sexual functioning (general)	• Are you sexually active at present? Have you ever been sexually active? • Are you satisfied with your current sexual relationship(s)? With your current sexual adjustment? • How has your illness or injury affected your enjoyment of or ability to engage in sexual relations? (Frequency, quality, course of adjustment) • What is your sexual repertoire? Or what type of sexual and affectionate behavior do you engage in? Is self-stimulation or masturbation one of the options that you choose? • Do you have any concerns or questions about your sexual functioning? [Stop interview here if no questions or concerns]
Current sexual functioning (specific)	• (Men) Are you able to have and maintain an erection sufficient for coitus? Is this a problem for you or your partner? Under what circumstances do you have difficulty? • (Women) Are you able to reach orgasm? From intercourse, or by means of other stimulation? In what situations do you have difficulty?
Partner satisfaction and relationship history	• Are you able to have sexual relations without pain or discomfort? Are you sufficiently lubricating? Under what circumstances? • Are you able to stimulate and satisfy your partner? Does your partner know what pleases you? Are you able to communicate effectively about sex? About other aspects of the relationship? • How long have you been in your present relationship? Have you been able to work out a compatible adjustment? What difficulties have you encountered, and how did you resolve them successfully? How has having children/not having children affected your relationship?
Other effects on the relationship	• How stable is your health at present? What is expected in the future? • Do you take any prescription medication? • What method of contraception do you use? Are you satisfied with it? • Do you use alcohol or other drugs? How often? How does this affect your relationship? Your sexual relationship? • Have you had any negative or traumatic sexual experiences?
Follow-up	• Would you be interested in speaking with a specialist in sexual functioning about the questions or problems that you've raised in this interview?

From: Ducharme S, Gill KM, Biener-Bergman S, et al.: *Sexual functioning: medical and psychological aspects. In DeLisa JA and Gans BM, editors:* Rehabilitation medicine: principles and practice, *ed 2, Philadelphia, 1993, JB Lippincot, p. 767, with permission.*

5. **Breast.** Gynecomastia; teach female patients how to do breast self-examination (or arrange to have their breasts examined at least every 3 months).
6. **Musculoskeletal**

a. ***Contractures***. Arthritic deformities, patient's knowledge of stretching, need for surgery.

b. ***Spasticity***. Spasticity in men and women may interfere with sexual activity.

Table 5.9-3 Partial list of prescription medications that can cause sexual dysfunction

Drug classification	Decreased libido (M/F)	Erectile dysfunction (M)	Impaired ejaculation (M)	Comments
A. Anticholinergics		+	(+)	Decrease vaginal lubrication; dry mouth may affect oral sex
B. Antihypertensives	(+)	+	(+)	Decreased penile perfusion because of decreased blood pressure
C. Antiseizure	(+)	(+)		Can lower testosterone and estrogen; sedation
D. Antispasmodics				
1. Baclofen		+	+	
2. Dantrolene		+		
3. Diazepam	+	(+)		Sedation; menstrual changes
E. Diuretics	(+)	+	(+)	Menstrual changes
F. Estrogen	+	(+)		Menstrual changes
G. H_2-blockers	(+)	+		Dry mouth may affect oral sex
H. Psychotherapeutics (TCA; MAOI, SRI)	(+)	+	(+)	Sedation, anticholinergic
I. Recreational drugs (alcohol, cocaine, opioids, marijuana, tobacco)	(+)	(+)	(+)	Relationship problems; alcohol may suppress libido
J. Steroids (anabolic)	(+)	(+)		High dose can suppress hypothalamic–pituitary–adrenal axis and spermatogenesis; menses changes

Note: + indicates that the sexual dysfunction is listed for that drug or most of the drugs in that classification in the Physicians' desk reference; *whereas (+) indicates that the sexual dysfunction has been reported for that drug or most of the drug in that classification in the medical literature (but not in the* Physicians' desk reference*). TCA = tricyclic antidepressants; MAOI = monoamine oxidase inhibitor; SRI = serotonin reuptake inhibitors; M = male; F = female.*

7. **Genitalia**

a. ***Hygiene.*** Odors or yeast infection, need for attendant care.

b. **Neurologic findings.** Determine the type of neurologic injury affecting the S3–S5 segments, e.g., those persons with complete LMN injury in this area are significantly less likely to achieve orgasm.

c. ***General.*** Genital anatomy; open lesions; STDs (condyloma, herpes); in females, pelvic examination (may need to be done in a modified position).

8. **Urologic.** Continence (if incontinent, check for skin breakdown; if with indwelling catheter, check for scrotal fistula; if with external catheter, check if there is a good seal); epididymitis.

9. **Gastrointestinal examination** provides an opportunity to instruct patients about reflexogenic erection or lubrication.
a. ***General.*** Check for any ostomy sites or equipment.
b. ***Rectal.*** Anal wink, sphincter tone, voluntary control, bulbocavernosus reflex (in both male and female), open lesions.
10. **Vascular**. Diabetes mellitus and peripheral vascular disease (both may contribute to erectile or lubrication problems because of vascular sclerosis).
11. **Cardiac**. Blood pressure (prolonged hypertension may lead to vascular sclerosis), pulse rate, arrhythmias, heaves, rubs, murmur.
12. **Pulmonary**. Cough, rales, shortness of breath, consolidation, signs of chronic obstructive pulmonary disease.

C. **LABORATORIES**. Electrolytes and glucose, hormonal assays (e.g., prolactin, luteinizing hormone, follicle-stimulating hormone, testosterone, and estrogen), thyroid work-up, diabetes work-up.

D. **DIAGNOSTIC TESTS** can be used to determine organic vs. psychogenic sexual dysfunctions. Neurophysiological studies are used in patients with sexual dysfunction to confirm the presence, location, and nature of a previously diagnosed neurological lesion (e.g., early polysensory neuropathies). They include:

1. **Sacral evoked response (SER) study**, which is used to determine the integrity of the bulbocavernosus reflex, i.e., the afferent dorsal nerve pathway, the S2–S4 cord, and the efferent pudendal nerve pathway. It confirms the presence, the anatomical location (peripheral, sacral, and suprasacral lesions), the side (left or right), and the nature (motor or sensory) of the neurological lesion associated with the sexual dysfunction (e.g., erectile dysfunction). A stimulus is applied to the skin pudendal sensory nerve through electrodes applied to the penis or clitoris. The motor response is recorded through an electromyography (EMG) needle electrode from the bulbocavernosus muscle, from the external urethral sphincter, or from the external anal sphincter. Normal SER has a stable mean latency of 35 (±5) ms. The SER is prolonged if patients with abnormal bulbocavernosus reflex (e.g., sacral cord or cauda equina lesions).
2. **Nocturnal penile tumescence (NPT) studies** is an indirect test of cavernous efferent neurointegrity. It can be performed in a sleep laboratory with monitoring of sleep electroencephalogram (EEG), electrooculogram, or EMG. A normal NPT done in a sleep laboratory shows erections lasting 15–30 minutes and occurring 3 to 5 times per night during rapid eye movement sleep. The NPT can also be done at home (without formal sleep monitoring) using a portable unit (e.g., RigiScan). A normal NPT using RigiScan shows erections lasting an average of 10–15 minutes and occurring 3 to 6 times per 8-hour sleep session. In addition to NPT, the RigiScan also determines penile compressibility by measuring the tightening of the loops placed around the penis and determining the penile resistance to compression. Compressibility should not be confused, however, with rigidity, which can be determined by awakening the patient during maximal tumescence and measuring the force sufficient to buckle the penile shaft. The minimum buckling resistance required for coital penetration is 500–550 g.

E. **QUESTIONNAIRE ASSESSMENTS** may be used to determine factors affecting sexuality and relationships. They include the IIEF (International Index of Erectile Function), the FSFI (Female Sexual Function Index), and the FSDS (Female Sexual Distress Scale), which document status of sexual functioning. The Female Spinal Sexual Function Classification (FSSFC), recently described for women with SCI provides a means to document the presence or absence of sexual dysfunction and the anticipated effects of SCI on female sexual response. Others include the Psychological Adjustment to Illness Scale (PAIS), which focuses on sexuality and relationships; Dyadic Adjustment Inventory (DAI), which determines relationship satisfaction or quality of a marital relationship; Sexual

Interaction Inventory (SII), which measures sexual adjustment and satisfaction in couples; Derogatis Sexual Functioning Inventory (DSFI), which measures current sexual functioning; Sex-role Inventory (SRI), which measures gender role definition; Sexual Knowledge and Attitude Test (SKAT), which measures sexual attitudes, knowledge, demography, and experiences.

IV. Classification and management of sexual dysfunction in PM&R

A. PHYSIOLOGIC DYSFUNCTION is often caused by a lesion in the neural pathways.

1. **Erectile dysfunction (ED)** (preferred term instead of impotence) is defined as the inability to achieve an erect penis as part of the overall multifaceted process of male sexual function (not necessarily for coitus). Organic causes are vasculogenic (most common), neurogenic, endocrine, and iatrogenic (medications are estimated to cause 25% of ED; sphincterotomy or TURP can also cause ED). Psychogenic causes are discussed under section IV.C. In PM&R, the most commonly encountered organic ED is neurogenic in origin, such as SCI, multiple sclerosis, diabetic neuropathy, or, rarely, stroke. In general, erection may be achieved by reflexogenic means (e.g., manual stimulation of the genital area or by rubbing the genitals on clothing or bed linen) or by psychogenic means (e.g., fantasizing, videos, magazines, or books). However, it is often difficult to maintain an erection for successful coitus (i.e., intromission and intravaginally sustained erection long enough to satisfy the partner) because once stimulation has been removed, the erection may subside. The following are mainly used for neurogenic-based ED:

a. ***Noninvasive techniques***

I. **Education.** Patients should be counseled that they can also satisfy their sexual partners even without penile erection (e.g., using a vibrator, or through oral or digital sex). Likewise they could satisfy themselves or learn what their sexual potential is through masturbation using manual or vibratory techniques. In many patients, it may be sufficient just to be aware what their sexual potential is and that there are treatment options for their ED. There is no evidence to support the belief that patients will interpret sexuality education as an endorsement and thus increase the frequency of sexual behavior.

II. **Vibrator stimulation** can induce erection when applied to the glans, frenulum, shaft, or base of the penis; however, the erection may not be sufficient for coitus.

III. **"Stuffing"** refers to the insertion of the semi-erect penis into the vagina and through the "milking activity" of the vaginal muscles, blood flow into the penis may be improved long enough for successful coitus.

IV. **Artificial penis (dildo)** can be strapped on the groin to simulate a natural erection.

V. **Vacuum tumescence constriction therapy** (VTCT) has been reported to achieve an erection rigid enough for coitus in up to 90% of men. Although it can maintain the erection for up to 30 minutes, it does not change the patient's ability to ejaculate or achieve orgasm. The sequence of VTCT is the flaccid penis is inserted in a rigid plastic cylinder; a manual or battery-operated pump is operated to create negative pressure (i.e., vacuum) in the cylinder, which draws blood into the penile corpora causing it to become erect; and finally, a constricting band (made of rubber) is guided through the cylinder and placed at the base of the penis to maintain the erection, after which the cylinder is removed. When erection is not desired, the band is removed and detumescence follows rapidly. Common side-effects include pain; penile hematoma, ecchymosis, or petechiae; penile numbness; "cold" penis; pulling of scrotal tissue into the cylinder; pivoting of penis (because of lack of erection at the band); and blocked antegrade ejaculation (may be painful). In patients with upper-limb dysfunction and poor hand function, their partners can be trained in its use or a battery-operated unit may be used. Patients must remove the constricting band after 30 minutes to prevent penile ischemia and necrosis. VTCT is contraindicated in patients receiving anticoagulant medications or with bleeding disorders.

VI. **Oral or topical erectogenic medications** should ideally be effective, useful "on demand", free of toxicity and side-effects, and affordable; however, there is currently no such universal drug. Three oral drugs approved by the Food and Drug Administration (FDA) in 1998 [Sildenafil (Viagra)], 2001 [Valdenafil (Levitra)], and 2003 [Tadalafil (Cialis)] are generally safe and effective. They act by increasing the concentration of cyclic guanosine monophosphate (cGMP) through selective inhibition of cGMP-specific PDE-5 (phosphodiesterase-5 is responsible for cGMP degradation). The cGMP, which is formed by nitrous oxide (NO) during sexual excitement, relaxes the corpus cavernosal smooth muscle cells and dilates the arteries, arterioles, and sinusoids of the corpus cavernosum, thus leading to erection. Unlike Sildenafil, Valdenafil, and Tadalafil most erectogenic drugs (e.g., cantharidin or Spanish fly) are based on anecdotal information or poorly designed studies. Some of the promising erectogenic drugs reported in the medical literature are included below. They probably act on the central mechanism of erection and have very limited peripheral activities. They are given orally unless stated otherwise.

- **Adrenergic receptor antagonists**. Yohimbine (a controversial "aphrodisiac" available as Yocon, Yohimex, Aphrodyne, Erex, or Yovital); some studies did not show it to be more effective than a placebo; others show it to be effective in psychogenic ED; it can be given at 5.4 mg, po, tid (up to 20–30 mg/day) in patients without coronary disease or moderate-to-severe hypertension, who are unwilling to try other treatment options. Major side-effects include angina exacerbation, central nervous system excitation with increased pulse rate and blood pressure, anxiety, fine tremors, dizziness, or nausea. Buccal phentolamine (20–40 mg applied through a strip of filter paper to the oral mucosa 15 minutes before coitus) required further studies; and delquamine is a new selective α_2-adrenergic antagonist.
- **Nitric oxide (NO) vasodilators**. Sildenafil (Viagra) and Valdenafil (Levitra) are taken orally an hour before sexual activity; whereas Tadalafil (Cialis) can be taken orally up to 36 hours before sexual activity. They do not trigger an automatic erection (as injections do). Hence, sexual stimulation is required. Erection can last up to 4 hours (if longer than 4 hours and painful, i.e., priapism, see section IV.A.1.b.1 for treatment). The recommended dose for Viagra is 50 mg, which may be adjusted to 100 mg or 25 mg, depending on its efficacy and side-effects. The recommended dose for Levitra and Cialis is 10 mg, which may be adjusted to 20 mg or 5 mg (or 2.5 mg for Levitra) depending on their efficacy and side-effects. Neither Viagra nor Levitra nor Cialis should be used more than once a day. Frequent side-effects of Viagra, Levitra, and Cialis include headache, flushing, dyspepsia, and nasal congestion. Cialis can also cause back pain and muscle ache. They are all contraindicated in men taking nitrates. Men taking α-blockers are also contraindicated from taking Levitra and Cialis. They should all be used with caution in men who have had a heart attack, stroke, or life-threatening arrhythmia within the past 6 months; have resting blood pressure of <90/50

or >170/110 mmHg; have a history of cardiac failure or coronary artery disease causing unstable angina; have severe liver impairment; or have a history of retinitis pigmentosa. A cardiac work-up, including exercise treadmill testing, should be considered in patients with heart disease, suspected heart disease, and/or risk factors for heart disease.

Other NO vasodilators include: L-arginine (precursor of NO), given at 2800 mg, po, daily (it has no reported side-effects, but further studies are needed); and nitroglycerine paste (2 cm of 2% paste) applied directly to the penis or to the perineum in an attempt to avoid partner contamination. Nitroglycerine paste can stimulate an erection rigid enough for coitus in only 25% of patients. Its frequent side-effects include hypotension and headaches, which may manifest in the contaminated partner.

- **Hormones.** Testosterone (for patients with hypogonadism; may cause liver damage) and bromocriptine (for patients with hyperprolactinemia).

b. Invasive techniques

I. **Intracavernous injection of vasoactive substances** can produce an erection in patients with neurogenic-based ED but whose vasculature is intact. These medications do not affect the man's ability to ejaculate or have orgasm; however, partner satisfaction is high. The vasoactive agents are injected (by the man or his partner, using a 26- to 30-gauge needle and a 1-mL insulin syringe) with a sterile technique without aspiration into the posterolateral aspect of the base of the penile shaft (3 or 9 o'clock position), avoiding midline neurovascular structures. The dose is carefully titrated by a physician because of the risk of priapism (prolonged painful erection lasting over 4 hours, because of lack of drainage of the corpus cavernosum). Men with neurogenic-based ED are more prone to sustain erections lasting more than 6 hours and can develop priapism even with small doses. The dose is typically titrated upward until an erection adequate for coitus lasting 30–60 minutes is attained.

Complications of intracavernous injection of vasoactive agents include pain (common at the injection site); minor hematoma or ecchymosis at the injection site (which can be prevented by compressing the injection site for 2–5 minutes); liver function abnormalities (common but clinically insignificant); vasovagal episodes (e.g., dizziness and hypotension, usually self-limited, rare); infection (rare); corporal fibrosis or penile plaque formation, rarely with subsequent penile angulation, occurs in 2–5% of patients after at least 1 year of use (chance of plaque formation can be reduced by injecting alternate sides of the penis and by limiting injections to twice a week); and priapism in 3–10% of patients.

Patients with priapism can take oral terbutaline (Bricanyl or Brethine tablets), 5 mg, which can be repeated every 15 minutes until detumescence occurs (for a maximum of 15 mg or three doses). If priapism persists (over 4 hours), the old blood may be aspirated from the side of the corpus cavernosum using a 19-gauge scalp vein needle. This is followed by slow intracavernosal injection of an α-adrenergic drug, such as phenylephrine solution, 0.5–1.0 mL (made by mixing 0.5 mL from a 10 mg/mL phenylephrine vial with 9.5 mL of saline to make a total of 10 mL phenylephrine solution), which may be reinjected after 15–20 minutes if erection persists, or NeoSynephrine, 200 mg, given every 5 minutes until detumescence occurs. After the intracavernosal injection, the penis is wrapped in a compression bandage for several hours.

The following vasoactive agents are commonly used for intracavernosal injections in patients with ED (except for alprostadil, these agents are not

FDA approved and, therefore, the patient must sign an informed consent form):

- **Single therapy agents**
  - **Papaverine** is a nonspecific smooth muscle relaxant, which decreases resistance to arterial inflow and increases resistance to venous outflow. As the sinusoids fill up, venous outflow is also passively obstructed. In neurogenic ED, a starting dose of 3 mg (0.1 mL of 30 mg/mL vial) is used, which can be increased at 3-mg increments. Typically, less than 12 mg is required to attain an adequate erection, although doses as high as 80–120 mg have been used with erections lasting up to 18 hours. Because repeated injections can cause corporal fibrotic nodules, papaverine use as monotherapy has declined. Instead it is usually combined with other agents.
  - **Prostaglandin E_1 (PGE_1)**, also called alprostadil (Prostin; Caverject), is currently the most commonly used monotherapy agent because of its superior pharmacologic profile (i.e., a powerful smooth muscle relaxant with very low incidence of fibrosis). It is approved by the FDA for the treatment of neurogenic ED. It is used in doses ranging from 1 to 40 mg (patients with SCI may respond to as little as 1–2 mg). Adverse effects include penile pain at injection site (a common complaint) and development of hypotension. One way of alleviating the penile pain is to add 20 mg of procaine to the PGE_1.

    Instead of injection, a prefilled applicator can be used to deliver a pellet of alprostadil (marketed as Muse) about an inch deep into the urethra. Erection usually begins within 8–10 minutes and may last 30–60 minutes. The most common side-effects of Muse include aching in the penis, testicles, and perineum; warmth or burning sensation in the urethra; redness from increased blood flow to the penis; and minor urethral bleeding or spotting.
- **Combination therapy agents**
  - **Duo-mix (papaverine + phentolamine)** is made by aspirating 1 mL of papaverine solution from 300-mg/10-mL vial and injecting it into a 5-mg vial of phentolamine (Regitine) powder. The powder is shaken until dissolved, then the mixture is aspirated and reinjected into the original papaverine vial to create a 10 mL solution containing 30 mg/mL of papaverine and 0.5 mg/mL of phentolamine. In patients with neurogenic impotence (e.g., SCI), a low dose of 0.1–0.2 mL of duo-mix is injected into one of the corpora cavernosa. If no erection occurs within 20 minutes, another injection is given which can be repeated up to a total of 1 mL of the duo-mix. The erection usually lasts 1–2 hours and should subside in 4 hours. Phentolamine produces an α-adrenergic blockade, which reduces arterial resistance; however, it does not increase resistance to venous outflow and is less effective than papaverine.
  - **Tri-mix (papaverine + phentolamine + prostaglandin E_1)** is made as follows: 0.2 mL (100 mg) of PGE_1 is added to a vial of papaverine (300 mg/10 mL); two 5-mg vials of phentolamine are reconstituted as described above for duo-mix; both solutions are then added to 6.8 mL of injectable normal saline to yield a total volume of 17 mL consisting of 17.6 mg/mL of papaverine, 0.58 mg/mL of phentolamine, and 5.9 mg/mL of PGE_1. The protocol and dose for injection is similar to that of the duo-mix. The use of a low dose of PGE_1 in tri-mix reduces penile pain at the injection site.

II. **Implantable penile prostheses** can either be semi-rigid (hinged, malleable, or articulating) or inflatable (self-contained or multicomponent). Semi-rigid prostheses consist of two flexible silicone or polyurethane rods implanted into both corpora cavernosa to provide a permanent partial erection, which may not be noticeable if the patient is sitting in a wheelchair but may be embarrassing in ambulatory patients. Inflatable prostheses consist of a pair of inflatable tubes, which are implanted adjacent to the corpora cavernosa, and which can be inflated to full erection using fluid from an abdominal wall reservoir by means of a pump located in the scrotum or deflated by opening a valve. Some of the manufacturers of penile prostheses include: American Medical System (AMS), Mentor, Dacomed, Jonas, and Small-Carrion. Penile prostheses must only be considered when other options have failed because patients with implants are often not able to benefit from other options because of the disruption of the normal anatomy. There has been a recent decline in the use of penile prostheses because of their complications (e.g., postoperative infection, urethral or corporal erosion and perforation, extrusion of the device, mechanical failure, and cosmetic deformity because of inadequate sizing) and the availability of other simpler, safer, cost-effective, nonsurgical methods of attaining erection (see above).

2. **Ejaculation or emission failures** are seen in 30% of men with incomplete lower motor neuron lesions, 99% of men with complete upper motor neuron lesions, and 90% of men with TURP. Psychological reasons may also contribute to this problem. Emission, or secretion of seminal fluid into the posterior urethra, should be distinguished from actual ejaculation, that is, expulsion of fluid from the urethra to the outside (antegrade ejaculation) or back towards the bladder (retrograde ejaculation). Retrograde ejaculation can be caused by failure of closure of the internal sphincter or the use of a constriction band in VTCT. Vibroejaculation and electroejaculation have been used to induce ejaculation for procreative purposes (see section VI.A). They may also be helpful in improving sexual pleasure (however, further study is needed in this area). Patients with ejaculation or emission dysfunction need counseling. They should also be told that orgasm or other pleasurable feelings can occur without ejaculation or emission and that sometimes after neurologic injury significantly greater stimulation is needed to ejaculate. Awareness of mind and of other bodily changes can sometimes enhance the patient's sensation of pleasure.
3. **Lubrication dysfunction** in women may be caused by similar events, which cause ED in men. In women with SCI, regardless of the level of injury, the greater the ability to perceive pinprick and light touch in the T11–L2 dermatomes, the greater the likelihood of vaginal lubrication. Inadequate lubrication can lead to dyspareunia (i.e., painful coitus) and may be associated with difficulty achieving orgasm. Its psychological ramifications (e.g., doubting of one's attractiveness or femininity) may affect relationships or potential relationships. As with male erection, similar reflexogenic and psychogenic means can be used to elicit lubrication. If needed, vaginal lubricants such as saliva, Astroglide, Aqualube, Replens, or K-Y jelly may be used. Patients should also be reminded that they can satisfy their sexual partners even without coitus (e.g., using a vibrator or through oral or digital sex). Likewise they could satisfy themselves through masturbation using manual or vibratory techniques but it may take longer than prior to injury.
4. **Difficulty in attaining orgasm** may be caused by physical dysfunction (e.g., sensory deficits, lubrication dysfunction, or SCI) or by psychological reasons. In able-bodied females, approximately 10% have never achieved orgasm and up to 75% do not routinely achieve orgasm with penile thrusting alone. In men, orgasm may be attained without ejaculation or emission. Recent research has shown that the only group of persons with SCIs that are unable to achieve orgasm are those persons with complete lower motor neuron injuries affecting their S2–S5 segments. In all other persons with SCI, about 50% report orgasmic capacity. Based upon laboratory analysis, the preferred method to achieve orgasm is through genital stimulation. Subjective descriptions of orgasms are similar between able-bodied and SCI subjects; likewise blood pressure and heart

rate response are similar. However, the latency to orgasm is significantly greater post SCI.

B. MECHANICAL DYSFUNCTIONS that interfere with sexual activity may result from problems related to bladder or bowel care or problems in positioning (e.g., because of pain, weakness, limited range of motion, or spasticity). If a comfortable position for coitus cannot be attained, masturbation or mutual masturbation may be considered.

1. Positioning difficulties may be the result of the following.

a. ***Spasticity*** can be reduced by movements that inhibit spasticity (e.g., performing sexual motions slowly, slow rocking motions; gentle shaking, or slow stroking); by using heat or cold modalities; by using antispasticity agents (see Chapter 5.4, section III.D.1); or by experimenting with different sexual positioning that lessens spasticity (e.g., positioning a bolster between the knees may decrease adduction spasticity or scissoring of the hips).

b. ***Weakness*** can be alleviated by using physical support (e.g., pillows, towels, or even bolsters) to prop up body parts, or if pelvic thrusting is difficult (e.g., in patients with poor arm or leg function), the down position with the partner on top may be tried.

c. ***Decreased range of motion*** can be accommodated with rear entry or side-lying sexual positions (e.g., in patients with arthritis or hip flexion contractures).

d. ***Pain*** can be reduced with side-lying or partner-on-top positions (to reduce stress on the joints), by scheduling sexual activities when pain is diminished (e.g., after taking pain medications), or after taking a warm bath.

e. ***Low endurance*** can be accommodated by assuming positions in which sexual performance takes less energy (usual positions with the same partner are least stressful; positions that do not restrict breathing; consider masturbation as it requires less energy than coitus) and timing of sex when there is most energy or after resting (e.g., upon waking up).

2. Bladder and bowel problems, especially incontinence during sex, are of high concern in both disabled men and women. To avoid embarrassing reflex loss of urine during intercourse, patients are advised to limit fluid intake during the hours preceding sexual activity and to empty their bladder prior to having intercourse (e.g., self-catheterization or suprapubic tapping to elicit a bladder contraction). Likewise, patients with bowel incontinence should avoid heavy meals and should empty their bowels (e.g., using an enema) prior to sexual activities. In men with indwelling catheters, the catheter may be folded on itself (if needed, taped to the side of the penis) and covered with a condom. In the disabled woman, the indwelling catheter tube may be taped to the abdomen and ignored. If so desired, the catheter may be removed just prior to intercourse and then replaced afterward. Patients with SCI lesions above T6 should be counseled on how to recognize and acutely manage autonomic dysreflexia (see Chapter 5.7, section V.F) as it may be triggered by a distended bladder or orgasm. After sexual activities, patients are advised to void or to catheterize themselves to lessen the chances of urinary tract infection.

C. IATROGENIC CAUSES that may affect sexual response include medications that are often taken by persons with disabilities such as antispasticity drugs, antidepressants, and narcotics. Adjustments of dosage of these medications can help alleviate sexual dysfunctions.

D. PSYCHOSOCIAL DYSFUNCTIONS that may play a role in sexual dysfunction, include social isolation (e.g., from poor sexual–social skills to attract a partner), altered body image and self-concept, inability of the disabled person or partner to accept changes in sexual functioning because of the disability (e.g., role changes of patient and partner), unhealthy attitudes and perceptions of the patient by others, poor judgment, egocentricity, emotional lability, disinhibition, low tolerance for delayed gratification, and poor memory. They may result in sexual desire disorders (hypoactive or hyperactive sexual desires), sexual aversion disorders, sexual arousal disorders (female sexual arousal disorder, male erectile disorder), orgasm disorder (inhibited female orgasm, inhibited male orgasm, premature ejaculation), sexual pain disorder (dyspareunias and vaginismus), and other sexual dysfunction.

Treatment of sexual problems because of psychosocial dysfunction is more intensive than the sexual rehabilitation counseling given by clinicians within the context of the patient's other rehabilitation problems. It involves sex therapy in which sex is assumed to be the highest priority at the time of treatment. Sex therapy may be in the form of prolonged and intensive psychotherapy (integrating psychodynamic, systems, behavioral, and cognitive approaches), which often involves intrapersonal and psychological issues and relationship counseling. It may also include behavioral modification and intensive symptom-oriented sex therapy. It may be done in an individual setting or it may involve family or couple therapy. Group therapy settings may also be used. For a free list of a specially trained professional sexual therapists in each state, the clinician should send a self-addressed, self-stamped business envelope to the American Association of Sex Educators, Counselors, and Therapists (AASECT), PO Box 5488, Richmond, VA 23220-0488 (website: *www.aasect.org*).

V. Sexual rehabilitation counseling

Counseling for sexual rehabilitation can be approached using one of the following models:

A. PLISSIT (OR P-LI-SS-IT) COUNSELING MODEL, which was developed by Annon and Robinson (1980), refers to three levels of brief counseling (i.e., Permission, Limited Information, and Specific Suggestions) and a fourth level of Intensive Therapy. All physiatrists should be skilled in the first two levels of counseling, permission and limited information. Some may have further training and develop the skills needed to intervene at the third level, specific suggestions. Patients needing intensive therapy because of psychosocial or organic dysfunction should be referred to appropriate sources (see section IV.C). General information about sex may be obtained from the Sex Information and Education Council of the United States (SIECUS), 130 W. 42nd St., Suite 350, New York, NY 10036-7802, tel. (212) 819-9770, website: *http://www.siecus.org*; Through the Looking Glass, 2198 6th St., Suite 100, Berkeley, CA 94710-2204, tel. (510) 848-4445, (800) 644-2666, website: *http://lookingglass.org*; and United Cerebral Palsy Associates, 1660 L St., NW, Suite 700, Washington, DC 20036, tel. (800) USA-5UCP, website: *http://www.ucpa.org*.

1. **P – permission** is the first and most basic level of sexual counseling. The clinician generates an attitude in which the patient with sexual concerns senses permission and feels comfortable to ask questions, seek advice, and experiment about sexual issues. This can be done by asking leading questions, initiating talk about sensitive subjects (do not expect the patient to initiate the discussion), or simply by listening to the spoken or body language of the patient or making observations about physical manifestations such as reflex erections in SCI men. The mere taking of a sexual history usually produces a therapeutic effect by giving the patient permission to be sexual, filling knowledge gaps, and providing reality-based feedback. Patients are reassured that their sexual concerns are neither unique nor unusual and that sexuality is a legitimate concern in the rehabilitation process. Permission is directed toward their thoughts, fantasies, feelings, and sexual activities that do not carry the risk of being dangerous or

illegal. To develop proficiency on this level, the clinician should read general textbooks and review articles about sexuality (see examples under Supplemental references).

2. **LI – limited information** entails provision of specific limited information for general problem solving of a specific sexual concern, either by the clinician or by way of educational materials. This limited information is typically educational and nonpersonal and deals with the disability and its implications on sexual health in a general sense (for cardiac patients, see Table 5.13-2). It gives factual information, which serves to dispel general sexual myths relating to breast and genital size, masturbation, oral–genital contact, anal intercourse, sexual frequency, etc. The disabled persons may also be given information about alternative methods of giving and receiving sexual pleasure (e.g., to seek out new areas of hypersensitivity or erogenous zones or to increase level of stimulation), changes in sexual response secondary to disease or medications, and fertility. The overall goal is to change relevant attitudes and behavior. The limited information should be provided during history taking or after physical examination when the patient is fully clothed (see section III.B). Limited information should be given to the family and significant others as well (see examples of pamphlets or educational handouts listed under Supplemental references).
3. **SS – specific suggestions** is the third and final level of brief counseling. It involves providing specific suggestions about sexual concerns and dysfunctions, e.g., sensate focus exercises. The clinician takes a limited history about the sexual problem, including a description of the problem, its onset and course, the patient's concept of cause and maintenance of the problem, past treatment, and current expectations and goals of treatment. Specific suggestions tailored to the patient's sexual concerns and dysfunctions are then provided. These interventions are usually simple, have a behavioral focus, and need to be practiced either alone or with a partner at home. Specific techniques (see also section IV.A.1.a) include sexual positioning for comfortable love-making, sensual ways of undressing, exploration of erogenous zones, foreplay techniques, the use of erotic fantasy, use of available sexual mechanical devices, and ways of dealing with urinary or bowel problems. Peer counseling may also be helpful. Examples of books with specific suggestions (e.g., different love-making options) for patients with sexual dysfunction are listed under Supplemental references.
4. **IT – intensive therapy** is indicated for patients whose sexual dysfunction is caused by deep-seated psychosocial dysfunctions (see section IV.D) or for patients requiring medical or surgical management of their sexual problems.

B. **ENIGMA COUNSELING MODEL** is part of the process of assessment and recommendation for sexual satisfaction (PARSS), the main goal being to minimize sexual dysfunction and maximize sexual satisfaction by enabling patients to express their concerns openly and to offer them counseling and education, whenever possible. It encompasses the first three levels of brief counseling in the PLISSIT model (i.e., P-LI-SS) and includes specific strategies for the physician to initiate discussions related to sexual concerns (e.g., incorporating sexual counseling and education with physical examination; see section III.B). The ENIGMA model is open-ended and allows the patient to make sexual issues an ongoing subject for subsequent doctor's visits.

1. **E – engage** the patient in conversation, which provides opportunities to discuss topics that may not be directly sexual, such as history of surgery or other significant medical conditions. In this step, the clinician can determine the patient's interpersonal skills for expression of need, as well as the status of the patient's current relationships. Although the first contact may be solely with the patient, the patient's partner should be included as soon as the patient gives permission.

2. **N – normalize** and legitimize the patient's sexual interest and activity. In a matter-of-fact open discussion, acknowledge individual variations; clarify sexual concerns, preferences, interests, experiences, values; and clarify satisfaction with sexual functioning and the existence and nature of any problem with sexual functioning. The goal is to help patients gain self-acceptance and to validate their sexual interests.
3. **I – inform** the patient and partner about sexual physiology and anatomy thus answering their questions in a more natural fashion. This step includes a thorough, frank but sensitive education of function and response, both physical and emotional, of the disabling condition and its effects on motor and sensory function, communication, cognition, and fertility, a discussion on health issues relevant to patient's sexual behavior (e.g., risk factors for human immunodeficiency virus), re-education about masturbation, and discussion about health issues relevant to the patient's medications.
4. **G – guide** the patient and his or her partner by responding in the same language the patient uses (may be vernacular) and metaphors, rather than in medical terminology (e.g., "hard-on" for erection and "come" for experiencing orgasm). Problems such as pain, spasticity, decreased endurance, and bowel and bladder function may also be introduced by the clinician.
5. **M – maximize** their problem-solving ability by encouraging experimentation, reading, and peer counseling. This step includes discussion of experimentation with masturbation, sexual aids (e.g., vibrators), or couple-play and provision of a list of reading materials (medical and lay) or educational videos about sexual issues (see examples of reading materials listed under the PLISSIT section in the Supplemental references).
6. **A – assess** and reassess the sexual issues at subsequent visits and make it an ongoing subject, not a one-time thing. At each visit, briefly review a checklist through the ENIGMA model to monitor progress, hang-ups or anxiety, and acceptance of each area. This step may include patient reassurance about their anxieties and misconceptions (e.g., on issues about sex after heart attack – see Table 5.13-2 – hysterectomy, stroke, or life-altering medical conditions), discussion about the patient's sexual experience since the onset of the disability, and assessment of interpersonal and psychosocial factors that may enhance or interfere with sexual relationships.

VI. Related sexual issues

Related sexual issues, including fertility, contraception, pregnancy, delivery, and lactation, may not be the primary domain of physiatry; however, if proper sexual counseling and education are to be given to the patient, the physiatrist should at least be knowledgeable about these issues. An excellent resource is Haseltine FP, Cole SS, Gray DB: *Reproductive issues for persons with physical disabilities*, Baltimore, 1993, Paul H. Brooks.

A. MALE FERTILITY is retained in most types of physical disabilities; however, in men with SCI, infertility may occur. The spontaneous fertility rate in men with complete and incomplete SCI is less than 10%. In general, men with incomplete lesions are more likely to be fertile than those with complete lesions. Among patients with incomplete SCI, those with lower motor neuron lesions are more likely to be fertile than those with upper motor neuron lesions. Possible reasons for infertility causing poor semen quality include stasis of prostatic fluid, testicular hyperthermia (which can be caused by the life-style of sitting in a wheelchair with thighs together or crossed, not shifting position frequently, or wearing tight clothes; some studies have shown that lowering the testicular temperature can reverse the maturation arrest caused by the increased temperature), repeated urinary tract infections (UTIs), abnormal testicular histology (decreased spermatogenesis and interstitial sclerosis; testicular atrophy, which is commonly associated with weakness and marked debility), sperm contact with urine (e.g., in retrograde ejaculation), possible changes in the hypothalamic–pituitary–testicular axis (although most studies seem to indicate close to normal levels of testosterone and gonadotropin with an intact hypothalamus–pituitary–testicular axis), possible anti-sperm antibodies (because of blockage of ductal tracts and UTIs), and long-term use of various medications (e.g., nitrofurantoin can cause temporary spermatogenesis arrest in rats). Other reasons for male infertility may arise from ejaculatory failure, obstruction of genital passages, impairment of spermatogenesis, or a combination of the above. Methods of collecting sperm (which can be kept in a sperm bank and used for *in vivo* or *in vitro* fertilization) include the following:

1. **Electroejaculation** involves transrectal electrical stimulation (using 5–30 V, 200–500 mA, 60 Hz current) of the myelinated preganglionic efferent sympathetic fibers of the hypogastric plexi to obtain seminal emission into the posterior urethra, from where the semen can be obtained by milking the urethral bulb and by catheterization. Its effectiveness is unrelated to the duration of injury (it may be used successfully within the first 6 months postinjury) or to the level of injury as long as T10–L1 spinal segments are intact. It may be successful even in patients with conus or caudal lesions. The sperm collected by electroejaculation appears to have decreased motility, with normal fertility seen in only 25% (probably because of the use of an electric current and aqueous jelly and changes in semen osmolarity). Electroejaculation must be done in an office or hospital setting because of the need to monitor for autonomic dysreflexia and to perform anoscopy to evaluate the rectal mucosa. Pretreatment with sublingual nifedipine (10 mg) for patients with lesions above T6 has decreased the risk of autonomic dysreflexia. Patients with incomplete lesions may need anesthesia because of pain.
2. **Vibroejaculation (VEJ)** involves the use of a vibrator (e.g., Ferticare, Ling, or Relax vibrator) applied to glans, frenulum, shaft, or base of the penis of patients with lesions above T10 or intact conus and cauda equina (i.e., intact lumbosacral reflexes, e.g., reflex hip flexion after stroking the bottom of the foot and positive bulbocavernosus reflex). Suggested vibratory parameters are 2.5 mm peak-to-peak amplitude at a frequency of 100 Hz applied for 3 minutes (may be repeated for six consecutive times after 1–2 minutes of rest in between stimulations). Its advantages include noninvasiveness, possible home use, possibility of "natural" fertilization, less likely occurrence of retrograde ejaculation, and overall better quality semen (fertility rate is about 50% of SCI males). With weekly use of vibroejaculation, the quantity and quality of sperm seems to improve. The main disadvantage of vibroejaculation is the unpredictability of response in many patients and the high risk of autonomic dysreflexia in patients with lesions above T6 (pretreatment of 10 mg of sublingual nifedipine can be given). Moreover, unlike electroejaculation, it does not work during the spinal shock period (which may occur within the first 6 months up to a year postinjury). Adjunctive use of neostigmine (Prostigmine) is not recommended as it can lead to greater risk of autonomic dysreflexia and even death.
3. **Direct extraction of sperm** can be attempted through cannulation of the vas deferens when the other methods have failed.
4. **Surgery** may be performed to release obstructed passages of the vas deferens, epididymis, and seminiferous tubules, all of which can be the result of repeated UTIs.

B. FEMALE FERTILITY is usually not affected by most disabilities. In women with SCI, menses may continue without interruption or they may temporarily cease, returning to normal within about 6 months or up to a year. Once their menstrual

Table 5.9-4 Contraceptive failure rates in the United State during the first year of use (Data from the 1995 National Survey of Family Growth conducted by the National Center for Health Statistics of the Centers for Disease Control and Prevention)

Method	Women with pregnancy (%) Lowest expected*	Typical†
No method	85.0%	85.0%
Natural methods		
Periodic abstinence		20.5
Calendar or Rhythm	9.0	
Cervical mucus or ovulation	3.0	
Symptothermal	2.0	
Withdrawal	4.0	23.6
Barrier methods		
Condom – male	3.0	13.9
Condom – female	5.0	21.0
Spermicides (nonoxynol-9)	6.0	25.7
Diaphragm and spermicides	6.0	12.1
Intravaginal sponge (spermicidal)		
nulliparous women	9.0	20.0
parous women	20.0	40.0
Cervical cap		
nulliparous women	9.0	20.0
parous women	20.0	40.0
Hormonal contraceptives		
Oral progestin–estrogen pill	0.1	7.6
Oral progestin-only pill	0.5	3.0
Implant (Levonorgestrel)	0.05	0.2
Injectable (Depo-Provera)	0.3	3.1
Intrauterine devices (IUDs)		
Progesterone IUD	1.5	2.0
Levonorgestrel IUD	0.1	0.1
Copper T 380A	0.6	0.8
Sterilization – male (vasectomy)	0.1	0.15
Sterilization – female (tubal ligation)	0.05	0.05

** Lowest expected failure rate = failure of the method despite correct use, as determined in clinical trials where the combination of highly motivated subjects and frequent support from the study personnel yields the best results.*
† Typical failure rates = failure of the method in typical or usual use.
Adapted from Speroff L, Darney P: A clinical guide for contraception, *ed 3, Baltimore, 2001, Lippincott, Williams & Wilkins, p. 5.*

periods return, fertility returns to preinjury levels. Because their first few ovulation cycles may be unpredictable, SCI women engaging in sexual activities must consider contraception (see next section) from the beginning.

C. **CONTRACEPTION METHODS** with the lowest expected failure rates (<1%) in able-bodied women are oral hormonal contraceptives, subdermal Norplant, Levonorgestrel or Copper T 380A intrauterine devices (IUDs), injectable steroid contraceptives, and sterilization (male or female). Contraceptive failure rates during the first year of use in the United States are shown in Table 5.9-4.

1. **Barrier methods** either kill spermatozoa or block their entry into the cervix. They are reversible and are among the safest methods (if properly used); however, patients need to be highly motivated to use them with each coitus. In patients with poor hand dexterity, adaptive applicators may be used or the partner may help in putting them on/in.

a. ***Condom*** for men consists of a cylindrical sheath (usually made of latex; also available in polyurethane, silicone rubber, and lamb's intestine) applied to the erect penis; while the condom for women consists of a polyurethane pouch which lines the vagina and partially covers the perineum. Both male and female condoms are readily available, do not need a prescription, are relatively inexpensive, and have the additional advantage of being the only contraceptive method that offers protection against STDs, including human immunodeficiency virus. They must be reapplied for each act of coitus. Female condoms have recently been available commercially (e.g., Reality) but are not as popular as male condoms because they are relatively more expensive and more cumbersome to use. The lowest expected failure rate of the female condom is 5%, but its typical failure rate is 21%.

The following discussions are about male condoms. The tip of the penile condom should extend beyond the end of the erect penis by about ½ inch (1.25 cm) to collect the ejaculate. They are available as nonlubricated or lubricated (may contain spermicides). If the condom needs to be lubricated (e.g., to protect indwelling catheter), a water-based lubricant (e.g., Aqua-Lube, Astroglide, and K-Y jelly) should be used to preserve the integrity of the condom latex. Oil-based lubricants, e.g., Vaseline, should not be used as they weaken the latex. For patients with allergy to latex, nonlatex condoms (e.g., lamb's intestine) are available, although they may not offer the same protection against STDs as latex condoms. The taste of the condom may be offensive for oral sex.

b. ***Spermicides (nonoxynol-9)***, which must be applied within 10–30 minutes before coitus, are available as an intravaginal sponge, foam, foaming tablet, jelly, cream, gel, suppository, or film. Among the vehicles of spermicide application, the intravaginal sponge (e.g., Today Sponge) is the most popular because it is effective for 24 hours and does not have to be reinserted into the vagina before each coitus. Spermicides are readily available and do not require prescription. Side-effects include toxic shock syndrome (incidence is slightly higher in users of the sponge) and allergy to the spermicide.

c. ***Diaphragm*** is a shallow, dome-shaped rubber cup with flexible rim, which is inserted between the posterior vaginal wall and the recess behind the pubic arch. It must be initially fitted by a health-care professional, after which the user must be taught how to insert and remove it. Patients with weakened pelvic muscles may not be able to hold the diaphragm in place. Spermicide cream or jelly must be applied to the diaphragm and added intravaginally each time coitus is repeated, especially more than 8 hours after diaphragm insertion. After coitus, the diaphragm must be left in place for at least 8 hours but not more than 24 hours. Using it for more than 24 hours increases the risks for UTI (because of mechanical obstruction of urine outflow) and vaginal ulceration.

d. ***Cervical cap*** is a deep, soft rubber cup with a firm round rim. It is commonly used in Europe and is available in the United States as Prentif cavity-rim cervical cap. As with the diaphragm, it is initially fitted onto the cervix by a health professional, after which the patient is taught how to insert and remove it and to place spermicide inside the cap before each use. It can be left in place for up to 48 hours (longer use may cause ulceration, unpleasant odor, or infection). Users are advised to have a Pap smear done every 3 months to detect any abnormal cervical cytology.

2. **IUDs** consist of a flexible, usually plastic device inserted by a physician into the patient's uterus. To increase their contraceptive effectiveness, metal or hormones (e.g., progesterone; levonorgestrel) may be added. The most commonly used metal is copper (e.g., copper T-380A), which interferes with the effects of estrogen or progesterone on the endometrium. The IUD produces a local sterile inflammatory response caused by the presence of a foreign body in the uterus, which causes lysis of the blastocyst and sperm and the prevention of implantation. It also has deleterious effects on spermatozoa as they pass through the

uterus. Adverse effects of the IUD include pelvic inflammatory disease (PID) and abnormal uterine bleeding patterns. Contraindications include cervicitis, vaginitis, endometritis, PID, a nonmonogamous sexual relationship, history of STD, or ectopic pregnancy. Manual dexterity is needed to regularly check for its placement.

3. **Hormonal contraception** works by altering the cervical mucus, thus inhibiting sperm transport; by inhibiting ovulation; and by causing atrophy of the endometrium, thus inhibiting implantation. Contraindications include active thromboembolic disease, undiagnosed vaginal bleeding, breast cancer, and acute liver disease.

a. ***Oral steroid contraceptives***

I. **Progestin–estrogen contraceptives** ("**birth control pill**" or "**the pill**") are the most effective type of oral contraceptives because they consistently inhibit the mid-cycle gonadotropin surge and thus prevent ovulation. However, they carry the risk of venous thromboembolism (especially in SCI patients) and are associated with cardiovascular, cerebrovascular, and thrombophlebitic disease. They are strongly contraindicated in smokers over age 35, and in women with severe headaches, hypertension, diabetes, long leg casts or with major surgery to the legs, anticipated elective surgery within 4 weeks, and sickle cell disease. There are multiple brands available. The brand name contains the number of the dose of both progestin and estrogen. Triphasic pills change the dosing of the components throughout the cycle and can be identified by "tri-" in the name or by the use of three numbers instead of two.

The FDA recommends using the least amount of estrogen (e.g., 35 mg or less of ethinyl estradiol) and progestin (1 mg or less of norethindrone) that is compatible with a low failure rate and the need of the individual patient, such as Ortho-Novum 1/35, Ovcon 35, Norinyl 1 + 35, Loestrin 1.5/30, or Tri-Norinyl. The combination pill is given daily for 3 out of every 4 weeks (e.g., started on the Sunday after a period begins). If estrogen-related or progesterone-related side-effects occur with one formulation, a different agent with less estrogenic or progesterogenic activity can be given. For example, if symptoms of estrogen excess occur (e.g., weight gain or breast tenderness), change to a lower estrogen concentration (e.g., 30 mg) or instead of using norethindrone, change to a progestin with less estrogenic effect such as norgestrel (Lo/Ovral), norgestimate (Ortho-Tri-Cyclen), or levonorgestrel (Levlen, Tri-Levlen, or Triphasil); if symptoms of androgen excess occur (e.g., nausea, dizziness, acne, hirsutism, and pruritus), change to a progestin with fewer androgenic effects such as ethynodiol diacetate (Demulen); if menses are missed and patient is not pregnant, it is probably because of estrogen deficiency, which can be treated by increasing the estrogen (e.g., 50 mg).

II. **Progestin-only pills (POPs) or "the minipill"** may be used by women who must avoid estrogens. Although POPs [e.g., norethindrone (Micronol, NorQD), 0.35 mg, given daily, every day of the year, starting on the first day of menstruation] have a lower incidence of adverse metabolic effects, they cause a high frequency of abnormal uterine bleeding patterns.

III. **Estrogen compounds** are used as postcoital oral emergency contraception (see section VI.C.6 below).

b. ***Injectable long-acting steroid contraceptives*** include the commonly used depo-medroxyprogesterone (DMPA) (Depo-Provera), given at 150 mg, intramuscularly, every 3 months, and other agents such as norethindrone enanthate given at 200 mg, intramuscularly, every 2 months, and other once-a-month injections of combinations of different progestins and estrogens. DMPA is highly efficacious and requires no motivation after injection; however, users may experience intermittent spotting, and 50% become amenorrheic at the end of 1 year of use. There are variable rates of return of fertility, controversy over carcinogenicity, and occurrence of progesterone side-effects (e.g., headache, weight gain, and depression).

c. ***Levonorgestrel implant (Norplant)*** consists of six Silastic capsules, each containing 36 mg of levonorgestrel, which are implanted into the forearm (for 5 years). Once inserted, this method requires no motivation for use. When removed, there is rapid return of fertility. Side-effects include frequent irregular menstrual bleeding and progesterone-related side-effects (e.g., headaches, weight gain, depression, and psychic symptoms similar to menopause or premenstrual syndrome). It is a good option for women who do not desire children for a period of years and has the added benefit of reducing or totally eliminating menstrual bleeding, which can facilitate hygiene. Unlike estrogenic agents, it has not been shown to produce thromboembolic, cerebrovascular, or cardiovascular disease; however, patients need to be monitored for hypertension and thrombophlebitis. Its effectiveness in SCI women needs to be studied.

4. **Natural family planning** involves periodic abstinence during the days of the menstrual cycle when the ovum can be fertilized. It includes the **calendar** (or **rhythm**) method, **basal body temperature** method, **cervical mucus** (or **ovulation** or **Billings**) methods, and **symptothermal** method (combination of the calendar, temperature, and cervical mucus methods; more effective but more difficult to learn). It requires training, strong motivation, and can only be used in women with regular cycles. It has a relatively high failure rates. In women with SCI, the basal body temperature method is extremely unreliable because of poor temperature control.
5. **Sterilization** includes bilateral tubal ligation in women or vasectomy in men. Sterilization is generally not reversible.
6. **Emergency postcoital contraception ("morning after" treatment)**, which should be started within 72 hours after intercourse, may be considered when a condom breaks, if diaphragms or cervical caps dislodge, or with the lapsed use of any method. It has a high rate of side-effects and is intended to be a one-time protection. Oral emergency postcoital contraceptives include **estrogen compounds** given for 5 days (e.g., diethylstilbestrol, 25–50 mg/day; ethynyl estradiol, 5 mg/day; and conjugated estrogens, 30 mg/day); high-dose **progestin** [e.g., Levonorgestrel (Plan B) at 0.75 mg given twice, 12 hours apart]; combination **estrogen–progestin** (e.g., Preven); or **mifepristone** (RU486 or Mifeprex) in a single dose of 600 mg. Because a high dose of estrogens is used in emergency contraception, it should not be used in women with either a personal or close family history (parent or sibling) of idiopathic thrombotic disease. A nonoral emergency postcoital contraceptive is the insertion of a **copper IUD** up to 5 days after unprotected intercourse.
7. **Induced abortion** (medical or surgical) is controversial. The patient (preferably with the patient's partner) should receive proper counseling.
8. **Experimental methods** for women include the vaginal contraceptive pill, and contraceptive vaccine. For men, they include the contraceptive pill, contraceptive implant system, injectable contraception, and contraceptive vaccine.

D. **PREGNANCY** once attained usually progresses without difficulty in a disabled woman. Possible problems include UTIs (acidification of urine and hydration may help; see Chapter 5.7, section V.A), anemia (the hematocrit should be monitored; iron supplements should be given and, if needed, blood transfusion), constipation (suppositories and stool softeners may be used; see Chapter 5.8, section VI.B.3), altered balance because of the expanding uterus [wheelchair-bound patients may need seating system modifications (see Chapter 4.7); ambulatory patients may need assistive devices to prevent falls and possible fractures (see

Chapter 4.6)], thrombophlebitis (see Chapter 5.3), pressure ulcers (see Chapter 5.2), deconditioning (see Chapter 5.1), osteoporosis (may be as a result of immobility; treat with calcium-rich diet), premature labor, small-for-date infants, and toxemia of pregnancy (especially in patients with repeated UTIs). However, there is no increase in the number of spontaneous abortions. As with able-bodied women, disabled women should receive regular prenatal care with an obstetrician–gynecologist who is knowledgeable about disabled women. The role of the physiatrist is to educate both the patient and other physicians concerning disability-related issues, e.g., on the recognition and management of autonomic dysreflexia in women with a lesion above T6 (see Chapter 5.7, section V.F).

E. LABOR takes place normally in most disabled patients because the uterus retains its ability to contract, despite denervation, because of hormonal influences. As a result of paralysis of the abdominal muscles, however, the expulsive force may be ineffective, hence forceps delivery or episiotomy (because patient may not sense tears during delivery as a result of perineal insensitivity) may be necessary. In most women with an SCI, the discomfort of labor is felt as in able-bodied women, and the onset of labor is typically detected as a different sensation. Labor contractions may be stronger, more prolonged, and more frequent, but the duration of labor is shorter than for able-bodied women. Women with complete SCI lesions above T10 will not appreciate uterine contractions or fetal movement; therefore, they need to be admitted to the maternity ward about 10 days before their estimated date of birth to prevent a precipitous, unsupervised birth because of their inability to feel the onset of labor. SCI *per se* is not an indication for Caesarean section (except in women with lesions at T10–T11 as the uterus is deprived of all reflex function), and it should only be performed when indicated (as with able-bodied women).

In women with lesions above T6, autonomic dysreflexia occurring during labor should be distinguished from eclampsia or pre-eclampsia. In autonomic dysreflexia, blood pressure rises with contractions, and falls between contractions; there is headache, piloerection, and tachycardia or reflex bradycardia; and it does not respond to magnesium sulfate. While in toxemia of pregnancy, there is hypertension, proteinuria, edema, and the blood pressure increase is not episodic and is not associated with uterine contractions or bowel or bladder distension. The treatment of choice for autonomic dysreflexia during labor is epidural anesthesia, which can be administered continuously. Other alternatives include oral antihypertensives (e.g., premedication with Arfonad) or immediate delivery if the blood pressure cannot be controlled by any other means. Postpartum, there is a high incidence of UTI and venous thrombosis.

F. LACTATION (BREASTFEEDING) can be successfully administered by disabled mothers (although it may require adaptation of wheelchairs or assistance from others). As in all nursing mothers, any medication that is not absolutely necessary for the mother's health should be discontinued. Women with lesions above T6 usually experience a decrease in milk production after 6 weeks (possibly because of lack of nipple sensation). For contraception in lactating women, the following "**Rule of 3's**" applies:

- For women giving FULL breastfeeding, a contraceptive method should be used at the beginning of the third postpartum *month*;
- For women giving PARTIAL breastfeeding or NO breastfeeding, a contraceptive method should begin during the third postpartum *week*.

Further reading

Annon JS, Robinson CH: Treatment of common male and female sexual concerns. In Ferguson JM, Taylor CB, editors: *The comprehensive handbook of behavioral medicine*, vol 1, New York, 1980, SP Medical & Scientific Books, pp. 273–296.

Baker ER, Cardenas DD: Pregnancy in spinal cord injured women. *Arch Phys Med Rehabil* 77:501–507, 1996.

Baum N, Rhodes D: A practical approach to the evaluation and treatment of erectile dysfunction: a private practitioner's viewpoint. *Urol Clin North Am* 22(4):865–878, 1995.

Boone TB: Evaluation and management of impotence in physically disabled men. *Phys Med Rehabil State Art Rev* 9(2):523–537, 1995.

Cheadle MJ: The screening sexual history: getting to the problem. *Clin Geriatr Med* 7:9–13, 1991.

Cole TM, Cole SS. Rehabilitation of problems of sexuality in physical disability. In Kottke FJ, Stillwell G, Lehmann JF, editors: *Krusen's handbook of physical medicine and rehabilitation*, ed 4, Philadelphia, 1990, WB Saunders, pp. 988–1008.

Derogatis LR: Psychological assessment of psychosexual functions. *Psych Clin North Am* 3(1):113–131, 1980.

Ducharme SH: Sexual aspects of physical disability. In Grabois M, Garrison SJ, Hart KA, *et al.*, editors: *Physical medicine and rehabilitation: the complete approach*, Malden, MA, 2000, Blackwell Science, pp. 966–980.

Gilbert DM: Sexuality issues in persons with disabilities. In Braddom RL, editor: *Physical medicine and rehabilitation*, ed 2, Philadelphia, 2000, WB Saunders, pp. 616–644.

Hatcher RA, Trussel J, Stewart F, *et al.*: *Contraceptive technology*, ed 17, New York, 2004, Arcent Media.

Hirshkowitz M, Ware JC: Studies of nocturnal penile tumescence and rigidity. In Singer C, Weiner WJ, editors: *Sexual dysfunction: a neuro-medical approach*, Armonk, NY, 1994, Futura, pp. 77–99.

Masters WH, Johnson VE, Kolodny RC: *Human sexuality*, ed 5, Boston, 1995, Addison-Wesley.

Mishell DR: Overview of contraception. In Wallach EE, Zacur HA, editors: *Reproductive medicine and surgery*, St Louis, 1995, Mosby-Year Book, pp. 289–316.

Morales A, Heaton JPW, Johnston B, *et al.*: Oral and topical treatment of erectile dysfunction: present and future. *Urol Clin North Am* 22(4):879–886, 1995.

Ohl DA, Menge AC, Sonksen J: Penile vibratory stimulation in spinal cord injured men: optimized vibration parameters and prognostic factors. *Arch Phys Med Rehabil* 77:903–905, 1996.

O'Keefe M, Hunt DK: Assessment and treatment of impotence. *Med Clin North Am* 79(2):415–434, 1995.

Padma-Nathan H: Neurophysiological studies of sexual dysfunction. In Singer C, Weiner WJ, editors: *Sexual dysfunction: a neuro-medical approach*, Armonk, NY, 1994, Futura, pp. 101–115.

Physicians' desk reference, ed 58, Montvale, NJ, 2004, Thomson PDR.

Rohe DE: Sexuality and disability. In Sinaki M, editor: *Basic clinical rehabilitation medicine*, St Louis, 1994, Mosby-Year Book, pp. 425–432.

Sipski ML, Alexander CJ: *Sexual function in people with disability and chronic illness: a health professional's guide*. Gathersburg, MD, 1997, Aspen Publishers.

Sipski ML, Alexander CJ, Rosen R: Sexual arousal and orgasm in women: effects of spinal cord injury. *Ann Neurol* 49:35–44, 2001.

Sipski ML, Alexander CJ, Sherman A: Sexuality and disability. In DeLisa JA, Gans BM, Walsh NE, *et al.*, editors: *Physical medicine and rehabilitation: principles and practice*, ed 4, Philadelphia, 2005, Lippincott, Williams & Wilkins, pp. 1583–1603.

Sipski ML, Alexander CJ, Rosen RC: Orgasm in women with spinal cord injuries: a laboratory-based assessment. *Arch Phys Med Rehabil* 76:1097–1102, 1995.

Smith EM, Bodner DR: Sexual dysfunction after spinal cord injury. *Urol Clin North Am* 20(3):535–541, 1993.

Speroff L, Darney P: *A clinical guide for contraception*, ed 3, Baltimore, 2001, Lippincott, Williams & Wilkins.

Yarkony GM, Chen D: Sexuality in patients with spinal cord injury. *Phys Med Rehabil State Art Rev* 9(2):325–344, 1995.

Supplemental reading

General references about sexuality

Brecher EM, and the Editors of Consumer Report Books: *Love, sex, and aging*, Boston, 1984, Little, Brown.

Butler RN, Lewis MI: *The new love and sex after 60*, rev ed, New York, 2002, Ballantine.

Comfort A: *Sexual consequences of disability*, Philadelphia, 1978, GF Stickley.

Croft LH: *Sexuality in later life: a counseling guide for physicians*, Boston, 1982, John Wright.

Hite S: *The Hite report: a nationwide study of female sexuality*, ed 2, New York, 2004, Seven Stories Press.

Hite S: *The Hite report on male sexuality*, New York, 1987, Ballantine.
Kaplan HS: *The evaluation of sexual disorders: psychological and medical aspects*, New York, 1983, Brunner-Mazel.
Kennedy E: *Sexual counseling: a practical guide for those who help others*, New York, 1989, Continuum Publishing Co.
Kroll K, Klein E: *Enabling romance: a guide to love, sex, and relationships for people with disabilities (and the people who care about them)*, Horsham, PA, 1992, No Limits Communications.
Lief HI, editor: *Sexual problems in medical practice*, Monroe, WI, 1981, American Medical Association.
Masters WH, Johnson VE, Kolodny RC: *Masters and Johnson on sex and human loving*, Boston, 1988, Little, Brown.
Munjack DJ, Oziel LJ: *Sexual medicine and counseling in office practice: a comprehensive treatment guide*, Boston, 1980, Little, Brown.
Neidstadt ME, Feida M: *Choices: a guide to sex counseling with physically disabled adults*, Malabar, FL, 1987, Krieger.
Reinisch JM: *The Kinsey Institute new report on sex: what you must know to be sexually literate*, New York, 1990, St Martin's Press.
Sandowski C: *Sexual concern when illness or disability strikes*, Springfield, 1989, Charles C Thomas.
Schover LR, Jensen JB: *Sexuality and chronic illness: a comprehensive approach*, New York, 1988, Guilford Press.
Silverburg C, Kaufman M, Odette F: *The ultimate guide to sex and disability: for all of us who live with disabilities, chronic pain and illness*, San Francisco, CA, 2003, Cleis Press.
Yoselle H: *Sexuality in later years*, Rockville, MD, 1981, Aspen Systems.

Books or articles with specific suggestions for patients with sexual dysfunction.

Barrett M: *Sexuality and multiple sclerosis*, ed 3, Toronto, Canada, 1999, Multiple Sclerosis Society of Canada.
Bregman S: *Sexuality and the spinal cord injured woman*, Minneapolis, 1975, Sister Kenny Foundation.
Cole SS, Hossler CJ: Intimacy and chronic lung disease. In Fishman AP, editor: *Pulmonary rehabilitation*, New York, 1996, Marcel Dekker, pp. 251–287.
Comfort A, editor: *The joy of sex: a gourmet guide to lovemaking*, New York, 1972, Simon & Schuster.
Ducharme SH, Gill KM: *Sexuality after spinal cord injury: answers to your questions*, Baltimore, 1997, Brookes Publishing Company.
Gregory MF: *Sexual adjustment: a guide for the spinal cord injured*, Bloomington, IL, 1993, Accent on Living.
Griffith ER, Lemberg S: *Sexuality and the person with traumatic brain injury: a guide for families*, Philadelphia, 1993, FA Davis.
Herbert L: *Sex and back pain*, Bloomington, MN, 1987, Educational Opportunities.
Leyson JF: *Sexual rehabilitation of the spinal-cord-injured patient*, Totowa, 1991, Humana Press.
McCormick GP, Riffer DJ, Thompson MM: Coital positioning for stroke afflicted couples. *Rehabil Nurs* 11:17–19, 1986.
Mooney TO, Cole TM, Chilgren RA: *Sexual options for paraplegics and quadriplegics*, Boston, 1975, Little, Brown.
Rabin BJ: *The sensuous wheeler*, Long Beach, CA, 1980, Barry J Rabin.

Pamphlets and educational handouts about sexuality for the disabled.

Arthritis Foundation: Guide to intimacy with arthritis, 06/28/2002 (tel. (800) 283-7800; website: *http://www.arthritis.org/resources/relationships/intimacy/intimacy_home.asp*).
National Spinal Cord Injury Association: *Male reproductive function after spinal cord injury: fact sheet No. 10*, 1995–1998 (tel. (800) 962-9629; website: *http://www.makoa.org/nscia/fact10.html*).
National Spinal Cord Injury Association: *Sexuality after spinal cord injury: fact sheet No. 3*, 1995–1998 (tel. (800) 962-9629; website: *http://www.makoa.org/nscia/fact03.html*).

CHAPTER 5.10
Acute and chronic pain

Pain, as defined by the International Association for the Study of Pain, is "an unpleasant sensory and emotional experience usually associated with actual or potential tissue damage, or described in terms of such damage". In 2001, the Joint Commission on Accreditation of Healthcare Organization (JCAHO) recommended pain as the fifth vital sign (in addition to patient's temperature, blood pressure, heart rate, and respiratory rate). In the medical, as well as PM&R, settings, pain is one of the most common reasons for patients seeking care. In North America, the estimated costs of chronic pain, including direct medical expenses, lost income, lost productivity, compensation payments, and legal charges, are approximately $90 billion a year. This chapter deals with acute and chronic pain affecting the neuromuscular and musculoskeletal systems.

I. Neuroanatomy and neurophysiology

Peripheral pain receptors (i.e., free-nerve endings called nociceptors) are found in virtually every cutaneous, deep somatic, or visceral structure of the body (including skin, fat pads, muscles, ligaments, fascia, joint capsules, periosteum, subchondral bone, and blood vessel walls). In the presence of noxious or potentially noxious stimuli, the nociceptors release endogenous chemicals, which peripherally transduce these stimuli to pain (or nociceptive) impulses via unknown mechanisms. The three types of endogenous chemical mediators of pain include: (a) those that produce direct local pain (e.g., bradykinin, histamine, acetylcholine, and potassium); (b) those that facilitate pain by sensitization of nociceptors without stimulating it (e.g., prostaglandins, leukotrienes, interleukins, and thromboxanes); and (c) those that produce extravasation of neuropeptides (e.g., substance P and calcitonin gene-related peptide). The excessive release of substance P and other neuropeptides may exert proinflammatory effects in tissues (i.e., "wheal-and-flare"-type reaction mediated, in part, by mast cells) and may lead to "neurogenic inflammation", which can contribute to chronic pain syndromes (see section V.B).

The pain impulses are then transmitted to the dorsal horn of the spinal cord via the following afferent fibers: (a) the large (diameter 1–4 mm), fast (velocity 12–30 m/s), myelinated A-δ fibers, which transmit sharp, localized pain; (b) the small (diameter 0.1–1.0 mm), slow (velocity 1–2 m/s), unmyelinated C fibers, which transmit diffuse, burning, throbbing, and aching pain; and (c) the A-α (diameter 12–20 mm; velocity 70–120 m/s) and A-β (diameter 5–12 mm; velocity 30–70 m/s) fibers, both of which transmit episodic, sharp, and stabbing pain, which are difficult to control [because they can become involved through recruitment and plasticity in the injured nervous system, and their input does not undergo the same checks and balances as does that of the A-δ and C fibers in the central nervous system (CNS)]. Different function-specific cell layers for A-δ, C, A-α, or A-β fibers are found in the substantia gelatinosa of the dorsal horn, and they serve as relay stations for the pain impulses.

From the spinal cord, pain impulses ascend through the contralateral spinothalamic tracts to the lateral and medial thalamic nuclei and via the spinoreticular tracts to the brainstem. The myelinated (A-δ) fibers relay painful stimuli to the neothalamus and somatosensory cortex where the pain quality can be discriminated and its position can be localized so that the person can promptly withdraw from the noxious stimulus. On the other hand, the unmyelinated C fibers establish numerous synaptic contacts within the brainstem, midbrain nuclei, and cortical limbic system. Because of their persistent nature, the C fibers are primarily responsible for conditioned behavior and learned avoidance. On a teleological level such behavior serves to avoid further injury and promote wound healing; however, other less desirable affective responses can also be produced such as profound suffering, increased anxiety, and release of stress hormones and catecholamines.

Pain impulses also stimulate the sympathetic nervous system, which in turn can contribute to pain [e.g., in sympathetically maintained pain, complex regional pain syndrome (CRPS) type I (previously called reflex sympathetic dystrophy) with sympathetically maintained pain features]. The increase in sympathetic tone produces peripheral vasoconstriction (which causes peripheral ischemia, which in turn can aggravate pain) presumably by repeated incoming afferent C-fiber nociceptive impulses causing hypersensitivity in the dorsal horn of the spinal cord. It has been hypothesized that following trauma (e.g., peripheral nerve injuries, fractures, soft tissue traumas, myocardial infarctions, or strokes), norepinephrine is released from peripheral sympathetic terminals to activate nociceptors and there is a change in the residual (and intact) sensory nerves so that nerves that were previously unresponsive to sympathetic stimulation can be excited by such stimulation. It remains unclear whether sympathetic–adrenergic interactions are mediated via the α_1- or α_2-adrenoceptor; however, it is clear that drugs or procedures that cause sympathetic blockade at either receptor can relieve pain under the correct circumstances. Persistent peripheral pain input (e.g., if pain is left untreated) may induce changes in the spinal cord neurons that enhance responsiveness to the same stimuli and increase the receptive field, thus possibly contributing to chronic pain syndromes (see section V.B).

Pain impulses can be inhibited by both pre- and postsynaptic stimulation of the opioid receptors (see Chapter 4.8, section I.B), e.g., through exogenous sources such as opioid or nonopioid analgesics or through endogenous sources such as β-endorphins and enkephalins. Pain impulses can also be modulated by many substances including serotonin (5-hydroxytryptamine) and norepinephrine, which inhibit the response of dorsal horn neurons to noxious stimuli. Substance P, which is one of the endogenous chemical mediators of pain, can be inhibited by endogenous opioid peptides (e.g., β-endorphin, enkephalins, and dynorphins) in the CNS and periphery. In addition, descending circuits from many levels of the CNS can also modify the transmission and processing of pain impulses. These descending modulation systems can be triggered by drugs or by hypnosis and can be modified by behavioral mechanisms (e.g., operant conditioning in which good consequences produce increased frequency of the behavior and bad consequences produce decreased frequency of the behavior). Examples of behavioral modifiers that can possibly reinforce loss of function in chronic pain patients include worker's compensation or social security paying the patient for not working, significant others giving attention in response to illness behavior, and pain occurring in association with physical activity.

II. Physiologic effects

As the pain input reaches the CNS, it triggers the following reflex responses: (a) segmental spinal reflexes, which result in muscle spasm and vasoconstriction; (b) suprasegmental reflex responses, which are the result of noxious input from a number of spinal segments accumulating to cause the release of catecholamines, steroids, and renin–angiotensin, all of which result in metabolic and physiologic effects; and (c) cortical reaction to the seemingly inescapable pain (i.e., what the patient thinks and believes about the pain can strongly influence the effectiveness of the other therapy provided). The physiologic effects resulting from the summation of the spinal, suprasegmental, and cortical responses can either be beneficial [e.g., maintenance of blood pressure, maintenance of cerebral perfusion, maintenance of cardiac output, maintenance of intravenous volume, enhanced hemostasis, substrate mobilization, enhanced energy production, immobilization (to minimize further tissue injury), and learned avoidance] or it can be detrimental to the body (e.g., overstressing of one physiologic system in an already compromised, critically ill patient can result in multisystem organ failure).

A. PHYSICAL EFFECTS include cardiovascular (tachycardia, hypertension, increased cardiac work, increased myocardial oxygen demand), pulmonary [hypoxia, hypercarbia, atelectasis, perfusion/ventilation (V/Q) mismatch, decreased cough, decreased vital capacity, decreased functional residual capacity], gastrointestinal (nausea, vomiting, ileus, intolerance for oral intake), renal (oliguria, urinary retention), musculoskeletal (spasm, limited mobility), vascular (thromboembolism), endocrine (excessive adrenergic activity, vagal inhibition, catabolic metabolism, increased oxygen consumption, negative nitrogen balance, hyperglycemia), CNS (sedation, fatigue), and immunologic (inhibited cellular immunity, possible increased risk of infection and impaired wound healing).

B. PSYCHOPHYSIOLOGIC EFFECTS include general arousal (mediated by the sympathetic nervous system); sleep disturbance; reduced activity [including overall level of work, social and recreational activity, as well as activities of daily living (ADL)], which leads to a vicious pain cycle (i.e., inactivity, fatigue, and muscle weakness further increase pain, which promotes inactivity, fatigue, and muscle weakness); impaired behavioral and cognitive responses (including concentration, problem-solving, memory, and ability to make decisions); negative emotional reactions (e.g., fear, anxiety, depression, anger, and frustration); and negative family and social responses (e.g., fear, confusion, and helplessness or overprotectiveness).

III. Psychosocial factors

Psychosocial factors have recently been found to affect pain in addition to traditionally known factors, such as the type, location, and extent of tissue involvement, and the physical state of the patient. Factors that lower pain threshold (and increase pain perception) include discomfort, insomnia, fatigue, anxiety, fear, anger, sadness, depression, mental isolation, introversion, and past experience. Factors that raise the pain threshold (and decrease pain perception) include relief of symptoms (e.g., analgesics), anxiolytics, sleep, rest, sympathy, understanding, diversion, and elevation of mood (e.g., antidepressants).

A. INTERNAL (i.e., INDIVIDUAL DIFFERENCE) FACTORS

1. **The specific meaning** attributed to pain varies according to the patient's personal history (e.g., in a patient with a history of physical or sexual abuse, the current pain may reactivate disruptive but previously repressed memories), prior learning about pain (i.e., early childhood pain experiences and observation of how parents or role models respond to pain), environmental factors (e.g., secondary gain, dysfunctional family support of pain behavior, or interpersonal conflict with the caregivers), cultural factors (i.e., racial, religious, and ethnic groups), and the character of the illness or injury and the circumstances surrounding them.
2. **Pre-existing levels of problem-solving skills,** i.e., patients with positive problem-solving skills in the major arenas of life (e.g., education, work, family,

and social interaction) tend to have more productive problem-solving behaviors and positive attitudes toward pain.

3. **Coping style,** which is an internalized way of balancing personal emotional reactions with externally oriented, problem-solving behavior.

a. ***Coping strategies,*** that is, use of active coping or problem-focused coping (e.g., by seeking out information and taking specific action) tends to decrease pain perception especially in a situation in which one's own efforts can reduce pain. The use of avoidant coping or emotion-focused coping (e.g., efforts toward suppressing or dealing with emotional reactions such as by relaxation, denial, or avoidance) can also be effective under certain circumstances (e.g., in dealing with short-term situations, especially if there is little ability to control aspects of the situation).

b. ***Locus of control*** refers to whether one perceives that control over one's environment and over the outcome of events (such as pain) lies within oneself (internal locus of control) or with powerful others (external locus of control). In general, patients with an internal locus of control are more likely to cope actively and report less severe pain than those with an external locus of control.

c. ***Negative thinking and catastrophizing*** are consistently ineffective in helping cope with pain.

4. **Emotional age** reflects the emotional fluctuations (i.e., regression) often generated by the stress of acute pain. Pervasive regression may represent a character-disordered patient.

5. **Hypnotic capacity** reflects the capacity to assume a natural state of focused attention similar to that of daydreaming. This can be an asset or a liability depending on whether these states occur spontaneously and unwittingly or are purposefully elicited. For example, patients with hypnotic capacity who are prone to negativity and catastrophizing can unwittingly aggravate their pain experience through negative self-suggestion. If hypnotic capacity is purposefully elicited and directed (e.g., by training), however, it can help alleviate pain.

B. **PROCESS FACTORS**

1. **Affective and cognitive principles** governing the awareness of pain include pain beliefs and "meaning" attributed to pain (e.g., childbirth pain is generally perceived as more tolerable than is cancer pain) and emotional arousal (i.e., negative emotional arousal caused by anxiety, fear, depression, anger, irritability, and frustration can lead to increased awareness of pain). The meaning of pain can be altered by primary and secondary gain factors.

2. **Perceived control,** i.e., patients with an increase in perceived control are more likely to exhibit self-initiated pain management and increased cooperation with treatment. Situational factors such as predictability and familiarity of events also increase one's perceived control and may increase pain tolerance. Patients who actually have a degree of control (e.g., use of patient-controlled analgesic pumps) typically report adequate pain management and actually use less pain medication than patients receiving conventional methods of postoperative injections.

3. **"Recovery" status** of patient, that is for pain treatment to be successful, patients must progress from "victim of injury" to "manager of recovery" and must move through the grieving process (i.e., from shock to denial to anger to bargaining to mourning, and finally, to acceptance) and not be arrested in one grief stage.

IV. Assessment

Assessment of pain is difficult to objectify because its perception is subjective. Despite its subjectivity, however, all pain complaints must be assumed to be real.

A. HISTORY includes pain description (i.e., quality; location, extension, or radiation, intensity, onset, duration, frequency, pattern of involvement, progression, aggravating or relieving factors, previous tests results and treatment effects, and other associated manifestations), mechanism of the injury (if present), presence of chronic medical problems (including chronic pain syndromes and other preexisting conditions that may affect the physical consequences or physiologic reserve of the patient), personal and psychosocial history (i.e., current and past social situation, including vocational, family, and interpersonal stresses), current medications, functional limitations in ADL, dependence on adaptive equipment, litigation status, and other aspects of potential secondary gain which may impede recovery.

B. PHYSICAL EXAMINATION is generally directed to neuromuscular and joint examination. Observe the patient walking, sitting, and moving in situations when being directed and when patient is unaware of being observed. Identify the painful structures and document variations from the normal, which may interfere with function. Seek alterations in muscle strength, sensation, and deep tendon reflexes. Search carefully for dermatomal or root level dysfunction of sensory and reflex systems. Examine joint structures for effusion, decreased range of motion (ROM), and deformity. Palpate tendons and ligamentous structures. Palpate muscles to evaluate for trigger areas or tight bands of muscle that, when deeply palpated, cause referred pain. Instruct the patient to perform specific maneuvers such as a straight leg raising test (patient supine, leg raised from horizontal), Tinel's sign (tap over median nerves of wrist), or the Finkelstein test (thumb wrapped up in fist, wrist ulnar deviated) to aid in the clinical confirmation of the suspected diagnosis. Vital signs do not necessarily correlate with the intensity or the seriousness of the pain. Observation for signs of distress, body posturing, and the cooperation with verbal responses is important. In addition, the area of injury and the associated physiologic systems must also be evaluated.

C. PAIN MEASUREMENT TOOLS attempt to measure pain "objectively". In patients with chronic pain, psychosocial factors play an important role.

1. Physical and psychophysiologic assessment

a. ***Pressure algometry (dolorimetry)*** uses hand-held mechanical instruments (Pressure Threshold Meter, Tissue Compliance Meter) to measure the amount of force (pressure), which induces pain or discomfort. These devices consist of a rubber disk tip (with 1 cm^2 surface) attached to an analog force gauge, which measures pressure ranging from 0.1 kg to 5 or 10 kg. They can be used to quantify pain because of trigger points (taut and fibrotic bands), tender spots, muscle spasm, edema, hematomas, and other soft tissue pathologies. They have good reliability (intratester reliability is higher than intertester reliability) in trained examiners. They are valid in terms of pressure measurement, but they must be used with caution because pain perception varies in different persons under various conditions, psychological states, and levels of motivation.

b. ***Surface EMG biofeedback*** records muscular electrical activities, which are assumed to correlate with the patient's underlying pain syndrome; however, this area remains controversial.

2. Pain scales (see Fig. 5.10-1 for algorithm on selection of pain measurement instruments)

a. ***Unidimensional pain scales*** are simple subjective pain measurements designed to assess a single dimension of pain such as intensity, location, or degree of relief. It is clear and simple and can be used with children and elderly populations of various cognitive levels. Administration and scoring are simple and straightforward. Although it supposedly measures only a single dimension such as pain intensity, it is actually influenced by other factors such as the emotional state of the patient.

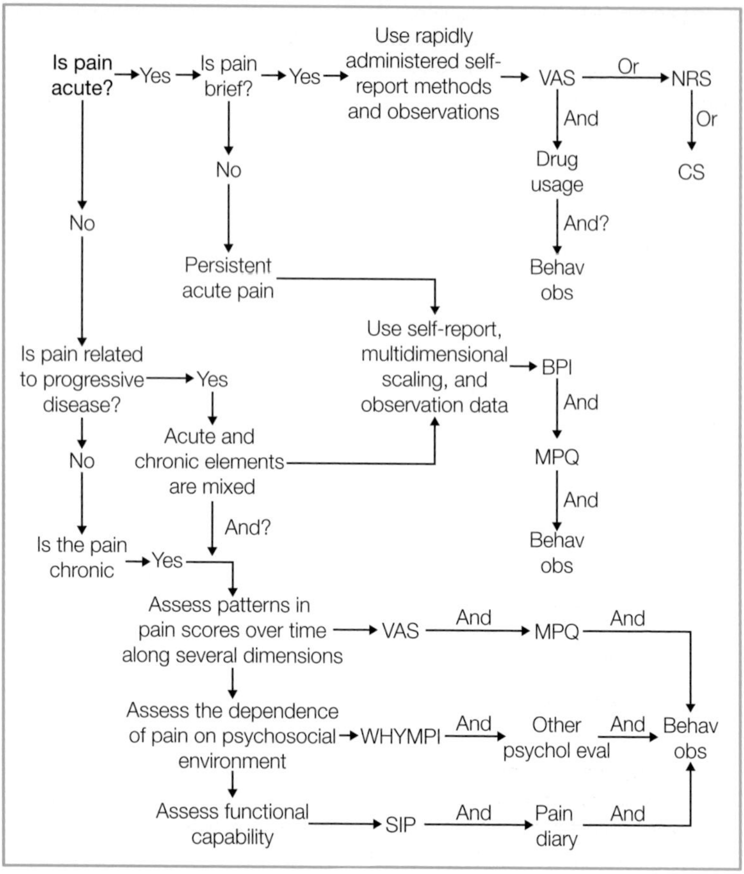

Figure 5.10-1 Algorithm for selection of pain measurement instruments, including functional status scales. BPI = Brief pain inventory; Behav obs = Behavioral observation; CS = Category scale; MPQ = McGill Pain Questionnaire; NRS = Numerical rating scale; Other psychol eval = Other psychological evaluations; SIP = Sickness impact profile; VAS = Visual analog scale; WHYMPI = West Haven–Yale Multidimensional Pain Inventory. (Adapted from: Chapman CR, Syrjala KL: Measurement of pain. In Loeser JD, editor: *Bonica's management of pain,* ed 3, Philadelphia, 2001, Lippincott, Williams & Wilkins, p. 325.)

I. **Visual analog scale (VAS)** (see Fig. 5.10-2) is the most commonly used pain scale. It consists of a 10 cm (100 mm) unmarked line, either vertical or horizontal with verbal or pictorial anchors indicating a continuum from "no pain" at one end to "severe pain" ("pain as bad as it could be") at the other end. There is no descriptor along the length of the line. The patient is asked to mark on the line the pain he or she is experiencing (e.g., how bad is your pain?). This mark is then measured with a ruler and expressed in cm (or mm), with 10 cm (100 mm) representing severe pain. The advantages of VAS include: simple to use, information is quickly obtained, sensitive (i.e., a high number of response options, so that it is sensitive to changes in pain intensity; also with good sensitivity to treatment effects), reproducible results, positive association with other self-report measures, and useful in a wide range of clinical and research conditions. Also, it can be used to reassess pain

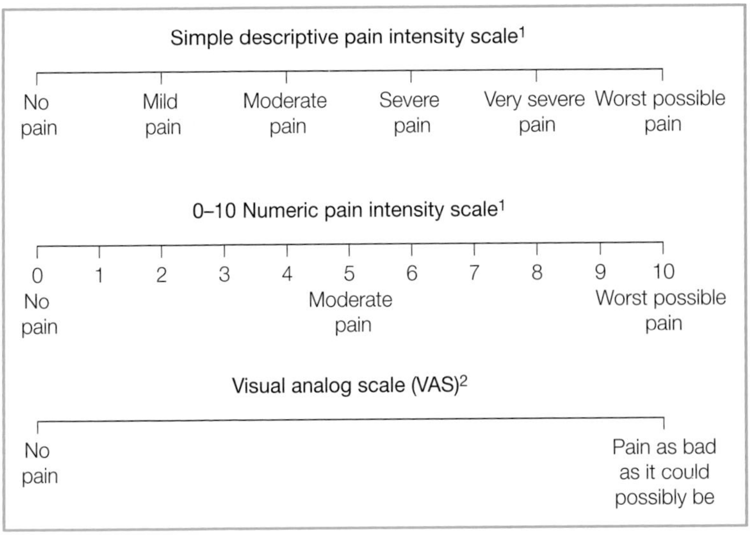

Figure 5.10-2 Three commonly used self-report pain intensity scales. [1]If used as a graphic rating scale, a 10-cm baseline is recommended. [2]A 10-cm baseline is recommended for VAS scale. (From Jacox A, Carr PR, Payne R, *et al.*: *Management of cancer pain: clinical practical guideline No. 9.* AHCPR Publication No. 94-0592, Rockville, MD, March 1994, Agency for Health Care Policy and Research, US Department of Health and Human Services, p. 26, with permission.)

in the same patient at different times. The disadvantages of VAS include a lack of quantification of pain between the end-points; the need for a certain level of cognitive functioning to cooperate with it; patients must be at least 8 years old; and the linear measurement of the patient's response, which adds time and a potential source of error.

II. **Numerical rating system (NRS)** (see Fig. 5.10-2) uses a number span (e.g., 0–5, 0–10, 1–100, or 0–100%) to reflect increasing degrees of pain. Some patients find it easier to assign a monetary value to their pain, perhaps because it offers a slightly more concrete image of the 0 to 100 scale. The patient is asked, "If 0 = no pain and $1.00 = the worst pain imaginable, how much is your pain worth?" The numerical scale is discrete and not continuous. Although simple it is not as sensitive as the VAS. The advantages of numerical scales include their being easy to score and administer, the high number of response categories possible, good patient cooperation, and support for their validity. The disadvantages relate to the weak statistical basis of the data and the low treatment sensitivity. Additionally, like the VAS, numerical scales demand a requisite level of mental functioning and abstract thinking to be usable.

III. **Verbal scales** involve asking the patient to pick a descriptive word that reflects the intensity of his or her pain from a list of words or from words spaced along a horizontal or vertical line (see Fig. 5.10-2). A patient's self-report is probably the best verbal test, but this option may be severely limited in the intensive-care unit patient. Verbal scales can be used to assess not only the intensity of pain or symptom but also the relief of pain or symptom after treatment, depending on the grouping of words chosen. The advantages of verbal scales are that they are easy to administer and score and that there is good evidence of their validity. The disadvantages include the

McGill–Melzack pain questionnaire

Patient's name ______________ Date ________ Time ________ am/pm

Analgesic(s) __________ Dosage __________ Time given ______ am/pm

__________ Dosage __________ Time given ______ am/pm

Analgesic time difference (hours): +4 +1 +2 +3

PRI: S_____ (1–10) A_____ (11–15) E_____ (16) M(S)_____ (17–19) M(AE)_____ (20) M(T)_____ (17–20) PRI(T)_____ (1–20)

1 Flickering ☐ Quivering ☐ Pulsing ☐ Beating ☐ Pounding ☐

2 Jumping ☐ Flashing ☐ Shooting ☐

3 Pricking ☐ Boring ☐ Drilling ☐ Stabbing ☐ Lancinating ☐

4 Sharp ☐ Cutting ☐ Lacerating ☐

5 Pinching ☐ Pressing ☐ Gnawing ☐ Cramping ☐ Crushing ☐

6 Tugging ☐ Pulling ☐ Wrenching ☐

7 Hot ☐ Burning ☐ Scalding ☐ Searing ☐

8 Tingling ☐ Itchy ☐ Smarting ☐ Stinging ☐

9 Dull ☐ Sore ☐ Hurting ☐ Aching ☐ Heavy ☐

10 Tender ☐ Taut ☐ Rasping ☐ Splitting ☐

11 Tiring ☐ Exhausting ☐

12 Sickening ☐ Suffocating ☐

13 Fearful ☐ Frightful ☐ Terrifying ☐

14 Punishing ☐ Grueling ☐ Cruel ☐ Vicious ☐ Killing ☐

15 Wretched ☐ Blinding ☐

16 Annoying ☐ Troublesome ☐ Miserable ☐ Intense ☐ Unbearable ☐

17 Spreading ☐ Radiating ☐ Penetrating ☐ Piercing ☐

18 Tight ☐ Numb ☐ Drawing ☐ Squeezing ☐ Tearing ☐

19 Cool ☐ Cold ☐ Freezing ☐

20 Nagging ☐ Nauseating ☐ Agonizing ☐ Dreadful ☐ Torturing ☐

PPI
0 No pain ☐
1 Mild ☐
2 Discomforting ☐
3 Distressing ☐
4 Horrible ☐
5 Excruciating ☐

PPI __________ Comments:

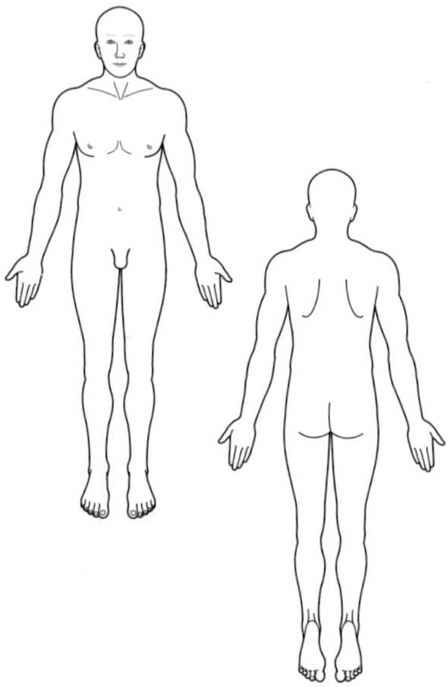

Constant ☐ Periodic ☐ Brief ☐

Accompanying symptoms: Nausea ☐ Headache ☐ Dizziness ☐ Drowsiness ☐ Constipation ☐ Diarrhea ☐

Comments:

Sleep: Good ☐ Fitful ☐ Can't sleep ☐

Comments:

Food intake: Good ☐ Some ☐ Little ☐ None ☐

Comments:

Activity: Good ☐ Some ☐ Little ☐ None ☐

Comments:

Figure 5.10-3 McGill–Melzack Pain Questionnaire (MPQ). (Used with permission of Ronald Melzack, PhD, McGill University.)

Mark the areas on your body where you feel the described sensations.
Use the appropriate symbol. Mark areas of radiation.
Include all affected areas.

Numbness	——	INC Sensitivity	0000
Constant	xxx	Sharp twinge	////
Throbbing ache	xxx		

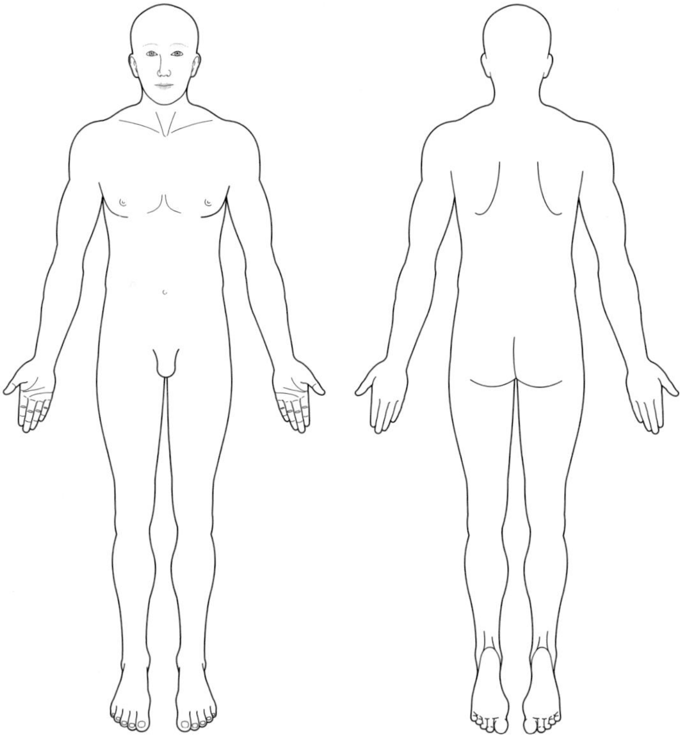

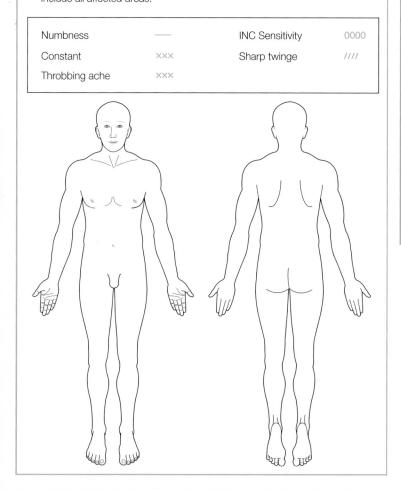

Figure 5.10-4 Pain drawing. (From Bigos SJ, Bowyer OR, Braen GR, *et al.*: Acute low back problems in adults: Clinical practice guideline No. 14. AHCPR Publication No. 95-0642, Rockville, MD, December 1994, Agency for Health Care Policy and Research, US Department of Health and Human Services, p. 146, with permission.)

demand on the patient to choose a word that may not be exactly descriptive of the pain, the need for education to understand the words and the concept, there being only as many response categories as there are words, and the fact that the data are only somewhat amenable to statistical review. An example is the *Patient Assessment Inventory and Narrative* from the University of Virginia, which became the basis for the *McGill–Melzack Pain Questionnaire* (see section IV.C.2.b.1; Fig. 5.10-3).

IV. **Pain drawings** (see Fig. 5.10-4) on body figures is a technique that provides more data about the location of pain than other pain scales. In general, the more widespread the drawing of the pain, the more intense, frequent, and disruptive the pain is. This pain scale requires coordination, visual integrity, and, depending on the task given, a variable level of cognitive functioning.

V. **Category rating scale or graphic rating scale** consists of a series of words along a continuum of increasing values (absent, mild, moderate, severe pain). In children, pictures of faces expressing varying amounts of distress (e.g., **Face Scale, Oucher Scale**) or colors, and poker chips representing "pieces of hurt" (**Poker Chip Tool**) may be used. Category rating scales are nonspecific, not very sensitive, and not consistently reproducible. A variation is the pain-relief scale with the following descriptors of pain relief: none, slight, moderate, good relief.

b. ***Multidimensional or complex pain scales*** measure not only the intensity but also the quality of pain and its resultant effects on other psychological and social variables, as well as ADL. They are not practical for most acutely injured or critically ill patients.

I. **McGill–Melzack Pain Questionnaire (MPQ)** is the most thoroughly researched multidimensional pain scale (see Fig. 5.10-3). It consists of 20 category scales of pain adjective descriptors, which can be grouped into four major dimensions of the pain experience: sensory (scales 1–11), affective (scales 12–15), evaluative or intensity (scale 16), and miscellaneous (scales 17–20). It provides three measures: pain rating index, which is the sum of the rank value for each descriptor based on its position in the word set; present pain intensity, which is based on a scale of 0 (no pain) to 5 (excruciating pain); and number of words chosen. The MPQ is a consistent, useful, easy, and rapid way of measuring pain; however, it takes both time and education (i.e., greater vocabulary base to understand the pain adjective descriptors) and can be influenced by repeat testing, past experience, and unrelated events. The reported ability of the MPQ to differentiate among various pain syndromes (e.g., neuralgia, arthritis, CRPS type 1, and radiculopathy) as well as its reliability remain controversial.

II. **West Haven–Yale Multidimensional Pain Inventory (WHYMPI)** is a 52-item inventory that is divided into three parts: (a) general dimensions of the experience of pain and suffering, interference with normal family and work functioning, and social support; (b) patient's perceptions of the responses of others to displays of pain and suffering; and (c) frequency of engagement in common daily activities. It can be completed in 10–15 minutes and has a broader approach than the MPQ in that it includes assessment of the impact of the pain problem on the patient's general functioning.

III. **Brief Pain Inventory (BPI)** is a quick, multidimensional pain measurement tool used in patients with cancer pain and other chronic pain to assess the severity of pain, impact of pain on daily function (i.e., general activity, mood, ability to walk, normal work, socializing with others, enjoyment of life, and sleep), location of pain, pain medications, and amount of pain relief in the past 24 hours or the past week. It uses simple numeric rating scales from 0 to10 that are easy to understand and easy to translate into other languages. On the BPI, mild pain is defined as a worst pain score of 1–4, moderate pain is defined as a worst pain score of 5 or 6, and severe pain is defined as a worst pain score of 7–10. The BPI is available in long form (56 questions; can be completed in 10 minutes) and short form (15 questions; can be completed 5 minutes), see Fig. 5.10-5. It responds to both behavioral and pharmacological pain interventions. It is reliable (0.77 to 0.91) and has been validated in at least 12 different languages.

IV. **Emory University Pain Estimate Chart** evaluates four pain factors: overall physical findings, neurologic examination, radiological findings, and laboratory results. Each factor is assigned a numerical value from 0 (normal) to

Study ID#: ______________ Hospital#: ______________

Do not write above this line

Brief pain inventory (short form)

Date: ___/___/___ Time: __________

Name: ______________ ______________ ______________
Last First Middle initial

1. Throughout our lives, most of us have had pain from time to time (such as minor headaches, sprains and toothaches). Have you had pain other than these kinds of everyday pain today?

   1. Yes 2. No

2. On the diagram, shade in the areas where you feel pain. Put an X on the area that hurts the most.

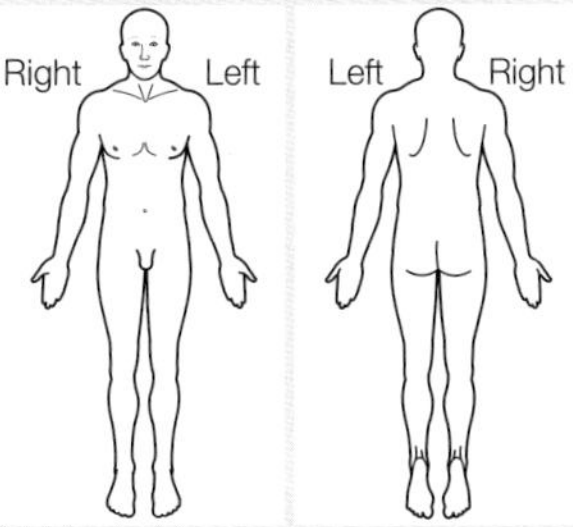

3. Please rate your pain by circling the one number that best describes your pain at its **worst** in the last 24 hours.

0	1	2	3	4	5	6	7	8	9	10
No pain										Pain as bad as you can imagine

4. Please rate your pain by circling the one number that best describes your pain at its **least** in the last 24 hours.

0	1	2	3	4	5	6	7	8	9	10
No pain										Pain as bad as you can imagine

5. Please rate your pain by circling the one number that best describes your pain on the **average.**

0	1	2	3	4	5	6	7	8	9	10
No pain										Pain as bad as you can imagine

6. Please rate your pain by circling the one number that tells how much pain you have **right now.**

0	1	2	3	4	5	6	7	8	9	10
No pain										Pain as bad as you can imagine

7. What treatments or medications are you recieving for your pain?

____

8. In the last 24 hours, how much relief have pain treatments or medications provided? Please circle the one percentage that most shows how much **relief** you have recieved.

0%	10%	20%	30%	40%	50%	60%	70%	80%	90%	100%
No relief										Complete relief

9. Circle the one number that describes how, during the past 24 hours, pain has interfered with your:

   A. **General activity**

0	1	2	3	4	5	6	7	8	9	10
Does not interfere										Completely interferes

   B. **Mood**

0	1	2	3	4	5	6	7	8	9	10
Does not interfere										Completely interferes

(Continued)

C. Walking Ability

0	1	2	3	4	5	6	7	8	9	10
Does not interfere										Completely interferes

D. Normal Work (includes both work outside the home and housework)

0	1	2	3	4	5	6	7	8	9	10
Does not interfere										Completely interferes

E. Relations with other people

0	1	2	3	4	5	6	7	8	9	10
Does not interfere										Completely interferes

F. Steep

0	1	2	3	4	5	6	7	8	9	10
Does not interfere										Completely interferes

G. Enjoyment of life

0	1	2	3	4	5	6	7	8	9	10
Does not interfere										Completely interferes

Figure 5.10-5 Brief pain inventory (short form). (From: Cleeland CS, Ryan KM: Pain assessment: global use of the Brief Pain Inventory. *Ann Acad Med Sing* 23:129–138, 1994, with permission.)

2.5 (maximum pathology). Other specific measures of pain behavior (verbalization, activity, drug use, and psychological dysfunctions) are also scaled. A score below 5 is low and a score above 5 is high for any given category. Patients are divided into four classes, which aids in quantifying impairment, choosing treatment, and in prognostication of pain. Class I is low in pain pathology but high in pain behavior. Class II is low in both categories, and class III is high in both categories. Class IV is high in pain pathology but low in pain behavior.

D. BEHAVIORAL ASSESSMENT includes the psychosocial ramifications (i.e., impact on patient's attitudes, behavior, life-style, and functional abilities, be they physical or psychological); perceived consequences of the pain; patient's understanding and degree of acceptance of his or her situation, attitudes, and the premorbid emotional status of the patient; signs of depression (e.g., irritability, decreased energy, poor concentration, and decreased appetite); and issues of loss of control as a result of hospitalization. Behavioral tests are commonly used in chronic pain patients because: (a) these patients are likely to develop comorbid psychiatric symptoms; and (b) the presence of major psychopathology is indicative of a poor prognosis in the treatment of chronic pain and disability. Commonly used behavioral assessments include:

1. Functional status (life-style impact) scales (see Fig. 5.10-1 for algorithm on selection of pain measurement instruments, including functional status scales).

a. Sickness impact profile (see Chapter 2.8, section IV.B) is a 136-item self-report or interviewer-administered measure yielding 12 subscale scores: mobility, ambulation, domestic affairs, social interaction, behavior, communications, recreation, eating, work, sleep, emotions, and self-care. Its scores (range of 0–100%) discriminate between psychosocial and physical dysfunction. It has satisfactory internal consistency, good test–retest reliability, and construct validity.

b. ***Activity diaries*** are self-reports of hourly activities in sitting, standing, walking, and reclining positions, as well as type and amount of medications taken and pain ratings on a 0 to 10 scale of severity, recorded in 1–2 weeks. Weekly total sitting and standing times of under 80 hours (normal is about 112 hours) suggest considerable functional impairment. The validity and reliability of activity diaries remain to be established.

2. **Tests of general psychopathology** involving structured tests and questionnaires, include the following.

a. ***Personality tests***

I. **Minnesota Multiphasic Personality Inventory-2 (MMPI-2)** (see Chapter 2.9.I.A) is the most widely used test of psychopathology applied to chronic pain. Despite the problem of not being able to distinguish premorbid from comorbid expressions, it remains the most effective at delineating psychiatric disorders and symptomatology in chronic pain patients.

II. **Millon Behavioral Health Inventory (MBHI)** (see Chapter 2.9.I.C) is used to identify patients' attitudes towards health and health-care providers. It can be used to understand how health attitudes and personality factors are likely to influence the chronic pain patient's participation in the rehabilitation process.

b. ***Mood assessment scales***

I. **Beck Depression Inventory (BDI)** (see Chapter 2.9.VII.A) is commonly used as a measure of improvement in the treatment of chronic pain patients.

II. **Spielberger State–Trait Anxiety Inventory (STAI)** (see Chapter 2.9.VII.C) is used to measure anxiety in adults. It can differentiate between the temporary condition of "state anxiety" and the more general and long-standing quality of "trait anxiety". Trait anxiety levels are expected to remain relatively stable across conditions, including those imposed by chronic pain; whereas state anxiety is expected to show a greater degree of variability and, therefore, may be more useful in evaluating treatment outcomes.

c. ***Symptom Checklist 90-revised (SCL-90-R)*** is a 90-item problem checklist that allows the patient to rate symptoms of physical and emotional distress on a five-point scale (from "not at all" to "extremely"). It scores nine symptom dimensions (somatization, obsessiveness, interpersonal sensitivity, depression, anxiety, hostility, phobic anxiety, paranoid ideation, and psychoticism) and three global indices of distress (global severity index, positive symptom distress index, and positive symptom total). It takes 15–30 minutes to complete and is reliable. Its generalizability to pain patients is questionable because it was standardized using psychiatric patients. It can be used as a screening device to evaluate psychologic distress that may need to be a focus of treatment in chronic pain patients.

E. **DIAGNOSTIC TESTS** include radiographs or computed tomography scans to identify fractures and other bone and joint pathologies; magnetic resonance imaging to identify muscle, tendon, and ligament abnormalities; electrodiagnostic testing to evaluate the neuromuscular system and nerve entrapments; radiculopathies, myopathies, or CNS reactivation; measures of specific organ system function (e.g., vital capacity, functional residual capacity, and liver function tests); physical quantitative testing (e.g., exercise stress test); laboratory tests (e.g., diagnosis-specific tests, such as rheumatoid factor, antinuclear antibodies, and creatine phosphokinase, or stress-response tests, such as corticosteroid levels, renin–angiotensin–aldosterone release, negative nitrogen balance, and sodium/water retention); in addition to diagnostic blocks (see Chapter 4.10, section I).

It must be emphasized, however, that negative diagnostic results do not always mean that there is no "real" pain or that psychopathology is dominant.

V. Pain classification by duration

A. ACUTE PAIN is usually linked to a precipitating event (e.g., trauma or surgery). The pain symptom is physiologically useful as it can provoke an escape or protection reaction to potentially dangerous tissue damage. Acute pain may be accompanied by anxiety, anger, and temporary life-style adjustments. Its evaluation and treatment usually takes less time because of its short, self-limiting course (usually less than 3 months) and its high rate of successful cure. Acute pain may be superimposed on a chronic pain (e.g., surgery in a cancer patient) or an acute exacerbation may occur in a chronic pain patient (e.g., pathological fracture of long bones in a cancer patient or acute exacerbation of rheumatoid arthritis during cold weather). The differential diagnosis of acute pain is discussed in Chapter 3.1.

B. CHRONIC PAIN can be caused by persistence of organic pathology (e.g., cancer) or it can be caused by persistence of pain despite the resolution of the original tissue damage with excessive loss of function (i.e., noncancer chronic pain, also referred to as "nonmalignant chronic pain", "benign chronic pain", or "chronic pain syndrome"). In noncancer chronic pain (NCP), the pain has lost its physiologic adaptive value, and the persistent pain has become a disease in itself (with morphologic changes in the nervous system, the exact mechanism of which is unknown; see section I). NCP is accompanied by physical deconditioning (as a result of inactivity), frustration and depression, and major changes in behavior, productivity, life-style, and attitudes toward becoming healthy. Its course is prolonged (over 3–6 months), and its evaluation and treatment are time-consuming. The treatment goal is aimed at helping the patient control or cope with the residual pain (rather than in curing it as in acute pain). Examples of NCP include chronic neuropathic pain [e.g., painful polyneuropathy, painful mononeuropathy, phantom pain, central pain, postherpetic neuralgia, avulsion of nerve plexus, sympathetic mediated pain syndromes, and CRPS type I (reflex sympathetic dystrophy) and CRPS type II (causalgia)], and chronic musculoskeletal pain (e.g., fibromyalgia, myofascial pain syndrome, chronic low back pain, and chronic arthritic and bone pain). The differential diagnosis for acute and chronic pain is discussed in Chapter 3.1, section I.A. Treatment options for musculoskeletal pain are shown in Table 5.10-1, while Tables 5.10-2, 5.10-3, and 5.10-4 show the treatment options for neuropathic pain.

VI. Management

Management of pain begins with the assumptions that all pain complaints are real until proved otherwise and that almost all pain has a psychosocial component (see psychosocial factors affecting pain in section III). Pain is best approached by treating its underlying etiology, although this is not always present or easy to identify. Timely treatment of pain is not only humane but can also help in increasing the patient's cooperation with his or her rehabilitative program, restoring the patient's normal activity, shortening the patient's hospital stay, and reducing health-care costs. In postoperative patients, additional benefits of adequate analgesia include improvement in postoperative pulmonary function; decreased length of postoperative ventilation and intensive-care unit stay; decreased mortality in patients with traumatic thoracic injuries; attenuation of the stress response to surgery; associated

Table 5.10-1 Pain treatment options for acute and chronic musculoskeletal pain. The following treatments have been tried but have not been definitely proven

Musculoskeletal pain	Pain treatment options
I. Acute*	**PM&R:** RICE (**R**est, **I**ce, **C**ompression, **E**levation); sensory modulation (e.g., TENS; acupuncture); patient education†; **Drugs:** NSAIDS, opioids, muscle relaxants, and possibly benzodiazepines
II. Chronic*	
1. Chronic low back pain	**PM&R:** sensory modulation (e.g., TENS; acupuncture); exercise (e.g., conditioning; strengthening; aerobic); patient education†; short-term bracing, manipulation, or passive modalities (heat, cold, and massage) in conjunction with active exercises; trigger point injections; **Drugs:** NSAIDs; opioids on selected patients; adjuvants (e.g., tricyclic antidepressants, anticonvulsants, baclofen); pain cocktails; **Nerve blocks:** epidural steroid injections in selected patients; **Surgery:** spinal fusion
2. "Non-inflammatory" arthritis (e.g., osteoarthritis)	**PM&R:** reduce the stress on the joints (e.g., rest, cane, strengthening exercises, weight reduction); sensory modulation (e.g., TENS; acupuncture); helium-neon laser (?); patient education†; **Drugs:** acetaminophen; judicious and short-term use of NSAIDS, topical analgesics (e.g., capsaicin); antidepressants, anticonvulsants, intra- and peri-articular injections (corticosteroids); opioids for severe pain; **Surgery:** total joint replacement; synovectomy; arthrodesis
3. Inflammatory arthritis (e.g., rheumatoid arthritis)	**PM&R:** rest, splinting, exercise, orthotics; heat/cold; sensory modulation (e.g., TENS); cold laser (?); patient education†; **Drugs:** NSAIDS (with acetaminophen); antidepressants; anticonvulsants; corticosteroids; disease-modifying antirheumatic drugs (e.g., gold, D-penicillamine, methotrexate); opioids for severe pain; **Surgery:** total joint replacement; synovectomy; arthrodesis
4. Fibromyalgia	**PM&R:** exercise (especially aerobic); patient education†; biofeedback; short-term manipulation; sensory modulation (e.g., TENS); **Drugs:** amitriptyline; cyclobenzapine, alprazolam, NSAIDs in selected cases; corticosteroids are ineffective
5. Myofascial pain syndrome	**PM&R:** stretch and spray; cold; trigger point injection (with or without steroids); exercise (especially aerobic); patient education†; sensory modulation (e.g., TENS, acupuncture); cold laser (?); **Drugs:** short-term NSAIDs or opioids; antispastics (e.g., baclofen); antidepressants

** Psychosocial interventions (e.g., cognitive-behavioral modification, psychotherapy, hypnotherapy, relaxation) and vocational counseling (if appropriate) should be included especially in chronic cases.*
† Patient education including joint conservation, lifting techniques, and other biomechanic and ergonomic principles.

improvement in the metabolic response to injury; maintenance of immunocompetence; earlier mobilization, which may lead to a decreased incidence of thrombotic sequelae; and overall hastening of recovery. Hence, delay in pain treatment and undermedication of pain (especially acute pain) are medically unacceptable.

Because of marked individual variations in pain response, pain treatment protocols should be individualized and flexible. There should also be favorable interaction

Table 5.10-2 Pain treatment options for neuropathic pain of predominantly "central" process. The following treatments have been tried but have not been definitely proven

"Central" pain	Pain treatment options
I. Deafferentation	
1. Phantom pain	**PM&R:** prosthesis; sensory modulation (e.g., TENS); exercise; biofeedback; **Drugs:** adjuvant analgesics (e.g., calcitonin, antidepressants, anticonvulsants, propranolol); opioids; tramadol; **Anesthetic:** local anesthetic injection into stump or into hyperalgesic contralateral limb; sympathetic blockade; **Surgery:** dorsal root entry zone (DREZ) lesion; "pre-emptive analgesia" prior to amputation; cordotomy; neurectomy; rhizotomy; **Psychosocial interventions***
2. Avulsion of nerve plexus	**PM&R:** splinting; exercise; TENS; vocational retraining; **Drugs:** adjuvant analgesics (e.g., anticonvulsants); opioids; tramadol; **Anesthetic:** sympathetic blockade; **Surgery:** DREZ lesion; **Psychosocial interventions***
3. Postherpetic neuralgia	**PM&R:** sensory modulation (e.g., TENS); exercise; helium-neon laser; **Drugs:** adjuvant analgesics including topical agents (e.g., 5% lidocaine, EMLA, capsaicin); antidepressants (e.g., amitriptyline, desipramine, maprotiline); combination of tricyclic antidepressants with neuroleptics (e.g., phenothiazines); anticonvulsants (e.g., gabapentin, carbamazepine, clonazepam, phenytoin, valproate); clonidine; NSAIDs; tramadol; opioids; **Anesthetic:** skin infiltration with local anesthetic, or local anesthetic and steroids; IV local anesthetic; temporary or permanent blocks of peripheral nerves or nerve roots; sympathetic blocks, epidural steroid, use of cryoprobe to painful scar; **Surgery:** DREZ lesion; neurectomy, rhizotomy, sympathectomy, trigeminal tractotomy, cordotomy, thalamotomy, mesencephalotomy, mesencephalothalamotomy; **Psychosocial interventions***
4. Central pain	**PM&R:** sensory modulation (e.g., TENS), exercise; **Drugs:** adjuvant analgesics [e.g., tricyclic antidepressants (especially amitriptyline), anticonvulsants (e.g., carbamazepine), naloxone infusion, local anesthetics (e.g., mexiletene), antihistamines, neuroleptics, propranolol]; tramadol; opioids; **Anesthetic:** temporary somatic nerve block with local anesthetic; sympathetic block; **Surgery:** dorsal column stimulation, deep brain stimulation; DREZ lesion; **Psychosocial interventions***
II. Sympathetic maintained pain (e.g., SMP subtypes of complex regional pain syndrome type I: reflex sympathetic dystrophy or type II: causalgia)	**PM&R:** sensory modulation (e.g., TENS, acupuncture); exercise; biofeedback; contrast baths; **Drugs:** adjuvant analgesics [e.g., calcitonin; nifedipine; propranolol; clonidine; oral sympatholytic agents (prazosin; phenoxybenzamine); antidepressant; anticonvulsants (gabapentin); local anesthetic antiarrhythmic (oral mexiletine; topical lidocaine patch; IV lidocaine infusion); pulsed oral corticosteroid]; opioids; tramadol; **Anesthetic:** sympathetic blockade; **Surgery:** sympathectomy; percutaneous electrical stimulation, dorsal column stimulation, deep brain stimulation; intrathecal opioid therapy; **Psychosocial interventions***

** Psychosocial interventions include cognitive-behavioral modification, psychotherapy, hypnotherapy, relaxation, etc. If appropriate, vocational counseling should also be included.*

Table 5.10-3 Pain treatment options for neuropathic pain of predominantly "peripheral" process. The following treatments have been tried but have not been definitely proven

"Peripheral" pain	Pain treatment options
I. Painful polyneuropathies	**PM&R:** orthotics (e.g., shoe lift); bedsheet cradle at night; sensory modulation (e.g., TENS); exercise; **Drugs:** replacement of missing compounds; primary treatment of diabetes with hypoglycemics; use of aldose reductase inhibitors; adjuvant analgesics (e.g., tricyclic antidepressants, oral local anesthetics; topical capsaicin, anticonvulsants, propranolol); NSAIDs; opioids; tramadol; **Anesthetic:** sympathetic blockade; **Surgery:** surgical interruption of afferent neural pathways (no evidence of efficacy); **Psychosocial interventions***
II. Painful mononeuropathies	
1. Lancinating neuralgia	**PM&R:** sensory modulation (e.g., TENS); helium-neon laser; **Drugs:** adjuvant drugs [e.g., anticonvulsants (carbamazepine is first choice; phenytoin; valproate; clonazepam); baclofen; oral local anesthetics (mexiletine); tricyclic antidepressants; propranolol; pimozide, if refractory]; tramadol; **Anesthetic:** temporary or prolonged nerve blocks with local anesthetics; chemical neurolysis/rhizotomy; **Surgery:** neurectomy, microvascular decompression; percutaneous radiofrequency lesioning; rhizotomy; cryotherapy; gangliolysis; peripheral nerve avulsion; **Psychosocial interventions***
2. Nerve trauma, compression, inflammation, or neoplasm	**PM&R:** sensory modulation (e.g., TENS); exercise; **Drugs:** adjuvant drugs [e.g., antidepressants, anticonvulsants, topical analgesics (e.g., capsaicin), clonidine; others]; tramadol; opioids; short-term systemic steroids or epidural steroid (both controversial); **Anesthetic:** temporary or prolonged nerve blocks with local anesthetics; chemical neurolysis; cryoblock; **Surgical:** nerve decompression; excision of neuroma; neurectomy, rhizotomy, cordotomy, dorsal root entry zone (DREZ) lesion; **Psychosocial interventions***

** Psychosocial interventions include cognitive-behavioral modification, psychotherapy, hypnotherapy, relaxation, etc. If appropriate, vocational counseling should also be included.*

between the patient and physician (which has been demonstrated to enhance patient compliance). Treatment principles for acute pain include discontinuing the source of tissue damage, resting of the damaged part, pain-relieving physical modalities, informal (or minor) use of behavioral management, and short-term use of nonnarcotic analgesics [acetaminophen, nonsteroidal anti-inflammatory drugs (NSAIDs)] or adjuvant analgesics (e.g., "skeletal muscle relaxants" or diazepam) or, if indicated (i.e., in severe pain), the limited use of opioid analgesics. The use of the PRICE treatment approach (i.e., Protection, Relative rest, Ice, Compression, and Elevation) can be initially helpful in acute injuries. The three stages of recovery in acute pain are: stage one – pain relief through modalities; stage two – regaining of normal resting muscle length through ROM and flexibility exercises, and stage three – gradual muscle strengthening and aerobic exercises. Throughout treatment, the patient must be educated on preventive and ergonomic measures. It is imperative to prevent chronicity of pain because the longer pain persists (over 3–6 months), the less likely complete resolution becomes and the less likely the patient will return to a productive life. Patients with a tendency of developing chronic pain are those

Table 5.10-4 Pharmacological management of neuropathic pain based on the 2003 recommendations of the Fourth International Conference on the Mechanisms and Treatment of Neuropathic Pain

Neuropathic pain* treatment	Recommended medications†
First-line medications‡ (recommended with high degree of confidence because of multiple randomized controlled trials)	1. Gabapentin 2. Lidocaine 5% patch 3. Opioid analgesics: controlled-release and short-acting • Oxycodone hydrochloride monotherapy or in combination with hydrocodone and acetaminophen, aspirin, or ibuprofen • Morphine sulfate • Levorphanol • Transdermal fentanyl • Methadone hydrochloride 4. Tramadol 5. Tricyclic antidepressants (TCAs), such as: • Amitriptyline • Nortriptyline§ • Desipramine
Second-line medications (recommended with moderate confidence after failure of first-line medications, alone or in combination)	1. Other anticonvulsant medications • Lamotrigine • Carbamazepine¶ • Other second-generation anticonvulsants (i.e., levetiracetam, oxcarbazepine, topiramate, zonisamide) 2. Other antidepressant medications • Atypical antidepressant (i.e., Bupropion, Citalopram, and Venlafaxine) • Selective serotonin reuptake inhibitor or SSRI (i.e., Paroxetine) • TCA (i.e., Imipramine)
Beyond second-line medications (clinical trials results are inconsistent; may be occasionally effective in individual circumstance)	1. Capsaicin 2. Clonidine 3. Dextromethorphan 4. Mexiletine

** These recommendations may apply to complex regional pain syndrome type I, which is believed to be the result of nervous system dysfunction without permanent injury to a nerve trunk.*
† Pharmacological treatment is not a cure and should be an integral component of a more comprehensive treatment approach including all or part of the nonpharmacologic treatment outlined in section VI in the text.
‡ As a result of multiple pain mechanisms of neuropathic pain, patients who do not respond to one of the five first-line medications should be treated with another one. One or more first-line medications can be combined when patients have a partial response to a single drug or at the beginning of treatment, either to increase the likelihood of a beneficial response or when a medication that requires titration to reach an effective dosage is also being used. Combination therapy, however, may increase the risk of adverse effects.
§ In a randomized placebo-controlled trial of chronic radicular low back pain, it was found that patients responded best to nortriptyline, probably because of the contribution of the neuropathic component (in combination with the skeletal and myofascial components) to its pain mechanism.
¶ For trigeminal neuralgia (tic douloureux), carbamazepine (first-line drug), phenytoin, and baclofen are recommended.
Data from: Dworkin RH, Backonja M, Rowbotham MC, et al.: *Advances in neuropathic pain: diagnosis, mechanisms, and treatment recommendations.* Arch Neurol *60(11): 1524–1534, 2003.*

with significant psychosocial issues, secondary gain motives, or lack of insight. In patients with chronic pain, the principles of treatment emphasize mobilization of underused affected areas, the use of formal behavioral management (usually in an interdisciplinary setting), and avoidance of addicting medications (e.g., opioids).

A. PATIENT EDUCATION should be an integral part of the comprehensive clinical care of patients with acute or chronic musculoskeletal and neuropathic pain. It consists of a combination of planned learning experiences to empower the patients and make them active participants in their own treatment program by facilitating them to voluntarily adopt and maintain good health-conducive behaviors and to prevent relapse of disease-related behavior. Clinical evidence shows that patient education can enhance compliance to the therapeutic regimen, produce physiologic and immunologic changes in response to behavioral change, and result in clinically significant improvement in health outcomes. Contrary to popular beliefs, informing patients about possible side-effects of therapy does not increase the occurrence of side-effects or have other adverse effects.

To ensure successful patient education, the clinician should deal with the following patient issues: specific behaviors (e.g., appointment keeping, taking medications, performing exercises, changing diet, and managing stress), belief systems about the disease and efficacy of treatment, motivation and perceived self-efficacy, locus of control, skills and resources necessary to make behavioral changes (e.g., communication skills and skills to perform specific disease-related management tasks, such as exercises and self-medication), and reinforcing factors (e.g., from family members, members of the health-care team, and even fellow patients). Patient education can be classified into preoperative education, medication self-administration, outpatient education programs, discharge planning education, family education, peer education, cooperative care, early discharge education, home health education programs, and mutual aid and self-help groups. It may be given individually or in small groups (e.g., Back School, Neck School, or Stress School) (see Chapter 5.11, section VI.A.2). Educational techniques include:

- Using direct instruction during clinical visits with repetition and reinforcement of the instructions during subsequent visits
- Encouraging patients to take notes
- Having patients clarify instructions and repeat the instructions back
- Having patients set short-term goals
- Encouraging patients to self-monitor (e.g., checklists or diaries)
- Having patients sign a written contract specifying the duration, frequency, and quality of required behaviors (e.g., exercise)
- Using a variety of audiovisual aids when teaching (e.g., slides, audio- or videotapes, films, charts, and model skeletons)
- Providing the patient with tip sheets, pamphlets, newsletters, and other written instructions to supplement oral instructions
- Providing language translations and large-type versions of instructions when appropriate
- Including family members or significant others in patient education
- Telephoning patients a few days following office visits to follow-up, clarify, and reinforce instructions.

The emphasis of patient education should be focused not only on improving knowledge but also on changing attitudes, beliefs, and behaviors. The information should be presented more than once, and in more than one way because patients seek information from multiple sources. The general content of patient education includes the following.

1. **General overview**, that is, definition of pain (acute vs. chronic), anatomy and pathophysiology of pain, pain assessment scales, preventive approaches to pain control, the importance of reporting pain to doctors and nurses as active participants in their own care, emphasizing that almost all pain can be effectively managed, and the important role that the patient needs to play in pain control.
2. **Pharmacologic management**, that is, overview of drug management of pain, overcoming fears of addiction (i.e., use of opioid analgesics will not in itself lead to addiction), understanding drug tolerance (i.e., tolerance to opioid analgesics can be dealt with by upward dosage adjustment), understanding respiratory depression and the methods of controlling common side-effects of drugs, and emphasizing the importance of pain prevention by the use of regularly scheduled analgesics. It should also address fears that the pain cannot be effectively controlled without unacceptable consequences or that choices might have to be made between treating the disease or treating the pain and other misconceptions (e.g., pain medication should be saved for when pain is severe or it might not be effective).
3. **Nonpharmacological management**, that is, its importance; the use of nonpharmacologic modalities as adjuncts to analgesics, review of previous experience with nonpharmacologic modalities, peer support groups and pastoral counseling, and demonstration of heat, cold, massage, relaxation, imagery, and distraction. For patients with musculoskeletal pain, it should also include joint and energy conservation techniques (see Chapter 4.5, section I.B.3), lifting and carrying techniques (see Chapter 5.11, section VI.A.2.c.2), sitting and standing techniques (see Chapter 5.11, section VI.A.2.c.1), environmental or workplace modifications (see Chapter 4.5 section VI.A.2.d.1 and Chapter 5.11, section VI.A.2.d), and other biomechanic and ergonomic principles (see Chapter 5.11, section VI.A.2.d).

B. PHYSICAL MODALITIES for pain relief are discussed in Chapter 4.1. (All the following cross-references within this subsection are in Chapter 4.1.) They include therapeutic heat (i.e., superficial and deep heating agents; see section I), therapeutic cold (e.g., cold packs and vapocoolant sprays; see section II), hydrotheraphy (including pool therapy; see section III), electrotherapy [e.g., transcutaneous nerve stimulation (TENS) and high-voltage monophasic pulsed current; see section V], iontophoresis (see section V.A.1.a) or phonophoresis (see section I.B.1), low-power cold laser (see section IV.B), biofeedback (see section VI), traction (see section VII), mobilization and manipulation (see section VIII), massage (see section IX), and acupuncture (see section X). Because of their passive nature, these physical modalities must only be used in the acute phase in combination with more active exercises. The use of some of these physical modalities, which are considered to be sensory modulation modalities (e.g., TENS, acupuncture, alternating use of hot and cold, and massage including vibration and percussion), is based on the hypothesis that hyperstimulation of the nervous system will "drown out" pain messages to the CNS and, thereby, prevent the cascade of adverse physiologic consequences.

C. ORTHOSES (e.g., casts, splints, or braces), gait aids (e.g., cane, crutches, or walkers), and adaptive devices for ADLs may be used temporarily if a specific joint or limb must be rested or protected because of pain. See Chapter 4.3 for details of orthoses, Chapter 4.6 for details about gait aids, and Chapter 4.5 for details about adaptive devices for ADLs.

D. THERAPEUTIC EXERCISES (discussed in Chapter 4.2) are an important adjunct in pain therapy. In acute pain, rest (for 2–3 days or up to a week) may initially be necessary to allow healing of the acutely inflamed muscle or joint (e.g., in rheumatoid arthritis); however, complete immobility can rapidly lead to muscle weakness and joint contracture. Isometric exercise (in combination with heating or cold modalities), therefore, may be initiated even in the presence of acute joint inflammation, and, if the patient can tolerate, gentle ROM and flexibility exercises should be started as soon as the inflammation subsides. As the pain improves, strengthening and aerobic exercises can be started to prevent recurrences of the painful episodes. In the acute phase, ROM exercise may be done up to, but not past, the point of pain. Causing pain during the ROM of the joint may only restart the vicious cycle of pain and may delay tissue healing. In contrast, pain is not necessarily a good guideline for exercise in chronic pain patients (as the original tissue has already healed in most cases, and the pain is usually caused by immobilization and deconditioning). In fact, the quota system is more effective in the chronic pain patient (i.e., a goal is set within the patient's capability, and the patient is encouraged to attain that goal regardless of pain complaints). Aside from mobility, strengthening, and aerobic exercises (e.g., walking and swimming), the use of relaxation exercises is beneficial, especially in chronic pain patients.

E. ORAL AND PARENTERAL MEDICATIONS should not be considered as a cure. They should be an integral component of a more comprehensive approach to treatment including all or part of the nonpharmacologic treatment as outlined under section VI. Special dosage titration and monitoring is required in patients who are elderly; with a history of substance abuse; with depression; with cardiovascular disease, hepatic insufficiency, or renal insufficiency; and who are taking medications that have the potential for interaction with pain medications.

1. Analgesics should only be considered as one component of a multimodal approach to pain treatment (including physical and psychosocial measures and adjuvant drugs). The general principles in initiating and monitoring analgesic therapy are:

- Individualize analgesic therapy based on the severity and nature of the pain as well as underlying condition(s).
- Begin with a simple, single-entity agent, which is appropriate for the patient's pain and which produces the most benefit with the least adverse effect.
- If a single-entity analgesic agent is ineffective or produces intolerable adverse effects, combination therapy should be tried.
- If possible, give the analgesic on a scheduled basis with constant adjustment of doses (depending on pain control) rather than the traditional "prn" dosing, which is frequently ineffective for adequate pain control.
- Use the analgesic for an adequate period of time (avoiding long-term use if possible).
- Warn the patient about the drug's potential adverse effects and inform him or her that these adverse effects may gradually subside with time or that measures can be taken to reduce the severity of or eliminate a particular adverse effect.
- When using centrally acting analgesics (e.g., opioids), be aware of tolerance and dependence tendencies (especially in chronic pain patients with prior history of substance abuse or in patients with severe personality disorders).
- Monitor all patients for impending tolerance to centrally acting analgesics by slowly titrating the doses of these analgesics, spreading the interval of administration, avoiding excessive renewal of prescriptions, or switching to an alternative drug if dependence becomes apparent. If addiction is suspected, the drug should be slowly withdrawn or the patient should be referred to an addiction specialist.

a. Non-narcotic analgesics

I. **Acetaminophen** is a centrally acting analgesic with similar effectiveness to aspirin but unlike aspirin, it does not have anti-inflammatory or antiplatelet properties and does not cause gastric toxicity. Because of its low side-effect profile, it is the first-line drug for the relief of mild to moderate pain. It is available in an oral form either singly or in combination with NSAIDs or opioids. It is also available singly in suppository forms. For details, see Chapter 4.8, section I.A.1.

II. **Tramadol (Ultram**; **Ultracet**; see Chapter 4.8, section I.A.2) is an oral synthetic nonopioid drug, which probably causes analgesia by binding to the μ-opioid receptors and by inhibiting reuptake of norepinephrine and serotonin. It is used as an alternative to opioids for the relief of moderate to moderately severe pain and has a place in the second step of the World Health Organization analgesic ladder approach to pain management (see section VI.E.1.b). It is also considered one of the first-line drugs in neuropathic pain (see Table 5.10-4), especially in patients with painful diabetic neuropathy and in patients with polyneuropathy of various causes.

III. **NSAIDs** reduce inflammation by inhibiting the synthesis and release of prostaglandins (specifically PGE_2), but they are not prostaglandin antagonists. This implies that the previously existing prostaglandins need to be depleted before the NSAID can take effect. Thus, in patients with pre-existing tissue trauma (e.g., rheumatoid arthritis), the anti-inflammatory (and, indirectly, the analgesic) effect of the NSAID may not be felt until after several days of regular, repeated dosing. In fact, it has been reported that, in certain situations (e.g., patients with low risk for gastrointestinal bleeding), starting NSAIDs preoperatively is more effective than starting them postoperatively.

The anti-inflammatory effect of NSAIDs is not the most important factor in producing NSAID analgesia. This is shown in dental pain studies in which NSAIDs achieve analgesia exceeding that produced by corticosteroids even though the anti-inflammatory effect of corticosteroids is greater. Aside from reducing peripheral inflammation, therefore, NSAIDs probably produce analgesia by decreasing painful responses to peripheral chemical mediators as well as by acting centrally. The analgesic effect of NSAIDs (present even without a peripheral focus of inflammation) has a more rapid onset of less than 1 hour (i.e., 10 minutes for the injectable ketorolac Toradol and, generally, 30–60 minutes for most oral NSAIDs). For the oral NSAIDs, the limiting factor for onset is the rate of gastrointestinal absorption of the drug. Even for pro-drug NSAIDs, which must be metabolized in the liver to the active form [e.g., nabumetone (Relafen) and sulindac (Clinoril)], the onset is not significantly delayed because hepatic metabolism is rapid. The NSAID dosage needed to produce analgesia is two to four times lower than that required for the anti-inflammatory effect. The mechanism of action, indications, contraindications, adverse drug reactions (ADRs), chemical classification, and dosages of NSAIDs are described in Chapter 4.8, section I.A.3.

The NSAIDs have the following advantages over opioid analgesics: low abuse potential; fewer respiratory, cardiovascular, and CNS adverse effects; and ease of prescription and administration (i.e., absence of controlled substance restrictions and availability of multiple over-the-counter oral preparations such as aspirin, ibuprofen, and naproxen). The NSAIDs are indicated in the management of mild to moderate pain. For severe acute pain, NSAIDs are used to supplement a primary analgesic agent (e.g., morphine) to decrease the need for the opioid and to minimize the opioid side-effects. Topical NSAIDs are also available (see section VI.E.2.d.2).

b. ***Opioid (or narcotic) analgesics*** are discussed in detail in Chapter 4.8, section I.B. They inhibit afferent nociceptive impulses at the dorsal horn of the spinal cord and at supraspinal sites by interacting with opioid receptors (i.e., μ, κ, δ, and σ receptors). Opioids are relatively safe and effective in the short-term management of moderate to severe acute pain (e.g., postoperative or post-traumatic pain) and in the long-term management of chronic cancer pain. All pain, however, is not responsive to opioid analgesics alone. Opioid-resistant pain can be classified into (a) *pseudoresistant,* for example, underdosing, poor alimentary absorption (rare), poor alimentary intake because of vomiting, and ignoring of psychosocial aspects of care; (b) *semi-resistant,* that is, pain that is relieved by the concurrent use of an opioid, an adjuvant drug, and/or nondrug measures (examples of opioid semi-resistant pain include bone metastasis, activity-related pain, and some cases of neuropathic pain); and (c) *resistant,* that is, pain that is not relieved by opioids but is relieved by other drugs and/or nondrug measures (examples of opioid-resistant pain include muscle spasm and some cases of neuropathic pain).

The use of opioids has been recognized by the US Drug Enforcement Administration as appropriate in treating NCP. Hence, its use has become more accepted among pain specialists. In neuropathic pain, opioid therapy (i.e., oxycodone, morphine, levorphanol, transdermal fentanyl, and methadone) is considered one of the first-line treatments (see Table 5.10-4), especially in patients with postherpetic neuralgia, painful diabetic neuropathy, phantom limb pain, and a variety of other peripheral and central neuropathic pain syndromes. In NCP patients with non-neuropathic pain, opioid therapy may be initiated after all other reasonable analgesic therapies have been tried and failed. Because of the extreme heterogeneous nature of NCP patients, it is expected that some patients benefit while others deteriorate during opioid treatment.

Prior to using opioid therapy, the physician must be familiar with the proposed guideline in Table 5.10-5, which stresses a structured approach and ongoing monitoring of efficacy, adverse effects, functional outcomes, and the occurrence of aberrant drug-related behaviors. It must be clearly emphasized that opioid therapy would not be useful if it augmented pain-related disability or undermined the efficacy of rehabilitation efforts, regardless of its effects on the pain. In general, opioid therapy should only be used as a complement to, not as a substitute for, a comprehensive pain management approach, which incorporates psychosocial and rehabilitative therapies. The patient must agree in a contractual arrangement (which can be in the form of a written document) that opioids will be supplied for a limited term (i.e., time-contingent rather than pain-contingent) in exchange for meeting agreed goals such as increased mobilization, return to work, no unauthorized use of other opioids, and changes in unacceptable or nonproductive behaviors. The patient must also understand that there will be regular and random blood samples collected to ensure compliance with dosing schedule and that other opioid drugs are not being used.

For acute pain, some physicians are still reluctant to use opioid analgesics because of concerns about life-threatening side-effects and the potential for iatrogenic addiction. These concerns, while legitimate, are not supported by current scientific data and hence do not justify a delay in the initiation of opioid therapy, if otherwise indicated, or the withholding of therapy from those with long life expectancies (e.g., noncancer patients). Clinical evidence shows that life-threatening side-effects of opioids (e.g., respiratory depression) are extremely uncommon in patients who undergo gradual dose escalation. Even if it occurs, it can promptly be reversed by administering an opioid antagonist (naloxone). Likewise, studies have shown that mere exposure to an opioid, even for prolonged periods, does not produce the aberrant behaviors consistent with

Table 5.10-5 Proposed guidelines for the use of opioid therapy in non-cancer chronic pain

I. Pretreatment considerations

1. Consider opioid only after all other reasonable analgesic therapies have failed.
2. A single practitioner should take primary responsibility for treatment.
3. A history of substance abuse, severe character pathology, or chaotic home environment should be viewed as relative contraindications.
4. Informed consent (a written contract may be used) should include:
   (a) Recognition of the low risk of true addiction as an outcome;
   (b) Potential for cognitive impairment from the drug alone or from the combination of the drug with other centrally acting drugs;
   (c) Potential for other side-effects;
   (d) Likelihood that physical dependence will occur (abstinence syndrome possible with acute discontinuation);
   (e) Need for responsible drug-taking behavior (e.g., no unsanctioned dose escalation, no prescriptions from other physicians, and so on).

II. Drug administration

1. Oral route must be used (except in rare circumstances).
2. Long-acting opioids (e.g., controlled-release morphine or oxycodone) are preferred.
3. "Around the clock" dosing is preferable if with continuous or frequently recurring pain.
4. Allow patient to escalate dose transiently on days of increased pain by either method:
   (a) Prescription of an additional four to six "rescue" doses to be taken as needed during the month; or
   (b) Instruction that one or two extra doses may be taken on any day but must be followed by an equal reduction of dose on subsequent days.
5. Initial dose titration should be performed after the agreed period of several weeks.
6. Failure to achieve at least partial analgesia at relatively low initial doses in the patient with limited prior opioid consumption should raise questions about the potential treatability of the pain syndrome with opioids and lead to reassessment.
7. Exacerbations of pain not effectively treated by transient and small increases in dose are best managed in the hospital, where dose escalation, if appropriate, can be observed closely and return to baseline doses can be accomplished in a controlled environment.

III. Follow-up

1. Initially, patients must be seen and drugs must be prescribed at least monthly; when patient is stable, less frequent visits may be acceptable.
2. Follow-up visits should specifically address and document:
   (a) Comfort or degree of analgesia (may use self-report instruments);
   (b) Functional status (physical and psychosocial; may use self-report instruments);
   (c) Opioid-related side-effects; and
   (d) Existence of persistent aberrant drug-related behaviors during the course of therapy (see Table 5.10-6).
3. Determine if opioid therapy should be continued with rigid guidelines; or be tapered and discontinued; or if the patient needs to consult an addiction medicine specialist.

Adapted from: Portenoy RK: Opioid therapy for chronic nonmalignant pain: current status. In Fields HL, Liebeskind IC, editors: Progress in pain research and management: Vol 1: Pharmacological approaches to the treatment of chronic pain: New concepts and critical issues, *Seattle, 1994, IASP Press, pp. 274–275.*

addiction disorders. Other factors such as underlying personality, social environment, and availability of money are more strongly correlated with drug abuse. Unless the patient has a prior history of drug abuse, addiction appears to be extremely low (less than 0.1%) during chronic opioid therapy for cancer and noncancer pain. In addition to the opioids, nonopioid analgesics and adjuvant drugs should be used concurrently if indicated.

Addiction should not be equated with drug tolerance or physical dependence. Tolerance is a process defined by the occurrence of decreasing effects at a constant dose or the need for a higher dose to maintain an effect. With the exception of constipation and miosis, tolerance to the nonanalgesic adverse effects of opioids (e.g., nausea, somnolence, mental clouding, and respiratory depression) occurs more readily than tolerance to analgesia in patients whose pain is stable. This is clinically beneficial because it increases the likelihood that a favorable balance between analgesia and side-effects will be attained during dose escalation. Tolerance should not be assumed in patients with chronic diseases who experience diminishing analgesia after a period of stable dosing. Studies have shown that the main reason for increasing the dose is not tolerance but progression or recurrence of the disease or the development of new pathology. Should tolerance to analgesia develop, an upward adjustment of dose is all that is necessary to regain pain control.

Physical dependence, which refers to a physiologic phenomenon characterized by the development of an abstinence syndrome, does not indicate the presence or absence of the behaviors that define addiction. While addicted patients can be physically dependent, physically dependent patients are not necessarily addicted. Physical dependence can develop after as little as a few days of opioid therapy. When the opioid is suddenly withdrawn or when an opioid antagonist is administered in a physically dependent patient, abstinence syndromes (which are rarely life-threatening) can develop. Prevention and treatment of abstinence syndromes are discussed in Chapter 4.8, section I.B.

If the patient engages in aberrant drug-related behaviors (listed in Table 5.10-6), the clinician must assess whether the problem is transitory and impulsive (perhaps related to a flare of unrelieved symptoms) or more serious and abiding. Patients with drug-seeking behavior because of uncontrolled pain ("pseudoaddiction") must be distinguished from true addicts who compulsively seek the drug to experience its psychological effects and who continue drug use despite harm. In patients with pseudoaddiction, the aberrant behaviors can be eliminated by improving pain control, which is often achieved by escalation of the opioid dose. If opioid addiction is suspected, tapering and discontinuation of opioid therapy may be necessary or the patient should be referred to an addiction specialist.

General guidelines for opioid administration are discussed in Chapter 4.8, section I.B. For patients with cancer pain, the following additional guidelines must be considered: opioids should be given "by the mouth", "by the clock" (i.e., fixed intervals), "for the individual", "with an adjuvant analgesic", and "by the ladder" (i.e., analgesic ladder). Adjuvant analgesics are discussed in section VI.E.2. The three-step analgesic ladder approach, which was developed by a committee of the World Health Organization (WHO), is as follows:

Step 1. For mild to moderate cancer pain, use nonopioid drugs (e.g., acetaminophen, NSAIDs; see sections VI.E.1.a.1 and VI.E.1.a.3 respectively). If indicated, adjuvant drugs (see section VI.E.2) may be added for additional analgesia or for the treatment of a different symptom (either a side-effect of the analgesic or a coexisting symptom other than pain).

Step 2. If mild to moderate pain persists despite step 1, add a "weak" pure-agonist opioid drug to the nonopioid analgesic (see Table 4.8-4 for classification and initial dose of "weak" opioids). If indicated, add adjuvant drugs (as in step one). The pure-agonist opioid drugs, which are operationally (rather than pharmacologically) classified as "weak", include codeine, hydrocodone, dihydrocodeine, oxycodone (combined with aspirin or acetaminophen), propoxyphene, and, occasionally, meperidine. Although these opioids do not have a "ceiling" effect for analgesia, they are not indicated in the management

Table 5.10-6 Aberrant drug-related behaviors that raise concern about addiction potential

I. Behaviors more suggestive of an addiction disorder:
- Selling prescription drugs
- Prescription forgery
- Stealing or "borrowing" drugs from others
- Injecting oral formulations
- Obtaining prescription drugs from nonmedical sources
- Concurrent abuse of alcohol or illicit drugs
- Multiple dose escalations or other noncompliance with therapy despite warnings
- Multiple episodes of prescription "loss"
- Repeatedly seeking prescriptions from other clinicians or from emergency rooms without informing prescriber or after warnings to desist
- Evidence of deterioration in the ability to function at work, in the family, or socially that appears to be related to drug use
- Repeated resistance to changes in therapy despite clear evidence of adverse physical or psychological effects from the drug

II. Behaviors less suggestive of an addiction disorder:
- Aggressive complaining about the need for more drug
- Drug hoarding during periods of reduced symptoms
- Requesting specific drugs
- Openly acquiring similar drugs from other medical sources
- Unsanctioned dose escalation or other noncompliance with therapy on one or two occasions
- Unapproved use of the drug to treat another symptom
- Reporting psychic effects not intended by the clinician
- Resistance to a change in therapy associated with "tolerable" adverse effects, with expressions of anxiety related to the return of severe symptoms

From: Portenoy RK: Opioid therapy for chronic nonmalignant pain: current status. In Fields HL, and Lieberskind JC, editors: Progress in pain research and management, Vol 1: Pharmacological approaches to the treatment of chronic pain: New concepts and critical issues, *Seattle, 1994, IASP Press, p. 267, with permission.*

of more severe pain because of relatively increased toxicity at higher doses (particularly propoxyphene, meperidine, and codeine). Oxycodone, hydrocodone, and dihydrocodeine (all of which are given in combination with aspirin or acetaminophen) cannot be given in quantities that exceed the maximal safe amount of the nonopioid coanalgesics (e.g., 4–6 g acetaminophen per day). Another nonopioid alternative for "weak" opioids is tramadol.

Step 3. If pain is moderate to severe, or if pain persists despite step 2, then replace the "weak" pure-agonist opioids with "strong" pure-agonist opioids (see Table 4.8-4 for classification and initial dosing of "strong" opioids). The pure-agonist opioid drugs, which are operationally classified as "strong", include morphine (first-line drug), hydromorphone, methadone, fentanyl, and levorphanol. Hydromorphone is used in cases of morphine toxicity in patients with renal disease. If the "strong" opioids still do not achieve adequate pain control, then adjuvant analgesics (see next paragraph) may be added to maximize pain control and lower the required dosage of opioids.

The above WHO three-step analgesic ladder may not be routinely applicable to all chronic pain patients, hence it is not universally used by all physicians. Another approach (from the Fourth International Conference on the Mechanisms and Treatment of Neuropathic Pain; see Dworkin *et al.*, 2003) is to begin treatment with a short-acting opioid (e.g., oxycodone alone; or combination of hydrocodone or oxycodone with acetaminophen, aspirin, or ibuprofen) at dosages equianalgesic to the oral administration of morphine sulfate at 5–15 mg every 4 hours as needed. After 1–2 weeks of treatment, the patient's total daily dosage of a short-acting opioid analgesic can be converted to an equianalgesic daily dosage of one of the long-acting opioid analgesics (e.g., controlled-release morphine, controlled-release oxycodone, transdermal fentanyl, levorphanol, or methadone hydrochloride). Limited use of short-acting medication for breakthrough pain may be prescribed. It is expected that for the 1–2 weeks, there will be considerable dosage adjustment as the patient converts from short-acting to long-acting opioids. Once a stable dosage of a long-acting opioid is established, it must be tried for 4–6 weeks to assess both pain and function. If pain is reduced without improvement in function, then the treatment may need to be modified. When carefully titrated and monitored, there is no clear "ceiling" dosage of opioids. But if the morphine sulfate equianalgesic dosages exceed 120–180 mg/day, the patient should be referred to a pain specialist for evaluation because double-blind trials have not established their benefit above 180 mg/day.

2. **Adjuvant analgesics** are drugs primarily approved for the treatment of conditions other than pain but act as analgesics in selected circumstances. They have large interindividual and intraindividual variability, hence sequential trials (i.e., multiple series of trial and error) are usually needed before a therapeutic regimen is attained. Some groups of adjuvant drugs (e.g., antidepressants, neuroleptics, α_2-adrenergic agonists) are considered multipurpose adjuvant analgesics (i.e., they have established utility in different pain syndromes) and are potentially useful in the management of any chronic pain patients.

a. ***Antidepressants*** (see Chapter 4.8, section V.A) can produce analgesia independent of their antidepressant effect. They can enhance the availability of neurotransmitters (e.g., serotonin and norepinephrine) probably by inhibiting their reuptake at the neuronal membrane. Their multifactorial mechanism of analgesia probably includes raising the pain threshold, allowing improved sleep, altering the perception of pain, and possibly improving mood (although analgesia can occur independent of mood elevation because it is usually given at a dose lower than that needed for antidepression). Antidepressants also potentiate the analgesic effectiveness of concomitant use of opioids, NSAIDs, or both.

Antidepressants are multipurpose adjuvant analgesics used in patients with chronic neuropathic pain (except possibly pure lancinating neuropathic pain such as trigeminal neuralgia, which responds better to anticonvulsant therapy), chronic musculoskeletal pain (e.g., rheumatoid arthritis, osteoarthritis, fibromyalgia, or myofascial pain), chronic headache, chronic facial pain, cancer pain, post-traumatic encephalopathies, and psychogenic pain. They are rarely indicated in patients with acute pain (except when used in patients expected to have long-term pain problems) because it takes them 2–4 weeks to achieve effective analgesia. The average analgesic response rate to antidepressant medications is reported to be 62% (range of 44–70%). In general, antidepressants classified as tricyclic antidepressants (TCA; see Table 4.8-7 for side-effect profiles) should not be used by patients with recent myocardial infarction or cardiac conduction problems or by those who cannot tolerate anticholinergic effects such as symptomatic prostatic hypertrophy or narrow-angle glaucoma (TCAs with secondary amines, such as desipramine and nortriptyline, or nontricyclic antidepressants may be tried because of lesser anticholinergic effects). It is advisable to check the electrocardiogram (ECG) (especially when using TCAs) and laboratory tests (e.g., complete blood count, differential count, and liver and renal function tests) before starting treatment and periodically thereafter. For details about the pharmacology of antidepressants, see Chapter 4.8, section V.A.

TCAs, in particular **amitriptyline (Elavil)**, are the most common nonanalgesic medications used in the treatment of chronic pain. The TCAs considered as first-line treatment in the management of neuropathic pain include **amitriptyline, nortriptyline (Pamelor, Aventyl)**, and **desipramine (Norpramin)**. Cardiovascular monitoring in TCA use is discussed in Chapter 4.8, section V.A.

For chronic pain treatment, a trial of amitriptyline should be considered first, unless relatively contraindicated by its side-effect profile or if another antidepressant has been shown to be more clinically effective for that particular diagnosis. The usual starting dose for amitriptyline is 10 mg in the elderly or 25 mg in younger patients given as a single dose at bedtime to take advantage of its sedating effect and minimize daytime drowsiness (in some patients with late afternoon pain, the dose may need to be divided). The dose is then titrated every 3–7 days by 10–25 mg/day as tolerated (with the initial dosing increments being usually the same size as the starting dose). The dose needed for pain relief is generally believed to be lower than that required for the antidepressant effect, but there is no systematic evidence of this. Hence, it can be titrated to dosages of 75–150 mg/day as tolerated. At dosages of 100–150 mg, plasma drug concentration should be used to help guide dose titration for analgesia. If the plasma drug concentration is above 100–150 ng/mL of the active drug and its metabolite, the drug should be stopped (despite absence of adverse effects) because the likelihood of benefit is probably low and the risks of toxicity are increased.

If at dosages of 100–150 mg, the plasma drug concentration is <100 ng/mL of the active drug and its metabolite, then it can be further titrated up (as long as there are no intolerable side-effects) with monitoring of electrocardiogram and its plasma drug concentration (levels > 500 ng/mL are associated with toxicity). For an adequate trial, it should be taken for 6–8 weeks with at least 1–2 weeks at the maximum tolerated dosage (because analgesic effects usually occur within the next 4–7 days after reaching maximum tolerated dosage). To ensure drug compliance, the patient must be instructed that although sedation and other side-effects may occur within a week, the analgesic effect may require an average of 2–4 weeks to occur. The patient must also be told that side-effects may decrease after a few weeks as the patient develops tolerance. The duration of amitriptyline therapy for pain management is controversial. Once sustained analgesia is achieved for a period of months, the dose can be gradually reduced until the drug is discontinued if neither pain nor any other rebound effects occur.

If treatment with amitriptyline has failed or is not indicated because of concerns about side-effects, **desipramine (Norpramine)** or **nortriptyline (Pamelor, Aventyl)** are appropriate alternatives, given their good evidence of analgesia and favorable side-effect profiles (see Chapter 4.8, section V.A and Table 4.8-7). Among the TCAs, it is generally considered that desipramine has the least sedating effect while nortriptyline probably has lesser orthostatic hypotensive effect than desipramine. In a randomized placebo-controlled trial of chronic radicular low back pain, it was found that patients responded best to nortriptyline, probably because of the contribution of the neuropathic component (in combination with the skeletal and myofascial components) to its pain mechanism.

In refractory cases (especially in neuropathic pain), some of the recommended second-line treatments (see Table 5.10-4) include the following antidepressants: atypical antidepressants [i.e., **buproprion (Wellbutrin, Zyban)**, **citalopram (Celexa)**, and **venlafaxine (Effexor)**], selective serotonin reuptake inhibitor or SSRI [i.e., **paroxetine (Paxil)**], and TCA [i.e., **imipramine (Tofranil)**]. They may be tried sequentially because of variations in individual response. Another TCA, i.e., topical **doxepin**, is being investigated for its potential analgesic effect in patients with neuropathic pain.

b. ***Anticonvulsants*** (see Chapter 4.8, section IV) produce analgesia by an unknown mechanism, which probably involves blockade of sodium channels and/or calcium channels to stabilize the neuronal membrane and reduce neuronal hyperexcitability; inhibition of the release of excitatory amino acid (e.g., glutamate and aspartate); and/or enhancement of the effects of the inhibitory neurotransmitter, γ-aminobutyric acid (GABA). Their usefulness in pain control is usually limited by their ADRs (including bone marrow depression, hepatic dysfunction, nystagmus, diplopia, ataxia, nausea, lymphadenopathy, confusion, and vertigo). However, one of the second-generation anticonvulsants, i.e., **gabapentin (Neurontin)**, has minimal ADRs (nonlife-threatening) and has no documented long-term toxicity, active metabolites, hepatic enzyme induction, or major drug interactions. It was also shown to be effective in treating postherpetic neuralgia (this is FDA-approved) and other types of neuropathic pain (e.g., diabetic neuropathy, trigeminal neuralgia, complex regional pain syndrome, nerve trauma, brachial and lumbosacral plexus pain syndromes, phantom limb pain, Guillian–Barré syndrome, and acute and chronic pain from spinal cord injury). Hence, gabapentin has been considered one of the first-line drugs in the management of neuropathic pain (see Table 5.10-4).

To avoid or minimize ADRs, gabapentin can be initiated at 100–300 mg, po, qhs, on day one; 100–300 mg, po, bid, on day two; and 100–300 mg, po, tid, on day three. If needed, it can be further increased by 100–300 mg/day every 1–7 days as tolerated. Target doses for postherpetic neuralgia ranged from 1800 mg/day (600 mg, po, tid; this dose is FDA-approved) to 3600 mg/day (1200 mg, po, tid). The final dosage is determined either by achieving complete analgesia or by the development of unacceptable ADRs that do not resolve promptly. An adequate trial of gabapentin would include 3–8 weeks for titration (to allow the development of tolerance to the ADRs), plus 1–2 weeks at the maximum tolerated dosage.

There is great individual variation in the response to anticonvulsants, hence, trials with alternative drugs should be considered if the patient fails to respond or is unable to tolerate any particular anticonvulsant. In patients who have not responded to an adequate trial of gabapentin when treatment with an anticonvulsant is sought, then other anticonvulsants may be tried as second-line drugs in the management of neuropathic pain (see Table 5.10-4). They include **lamotrigine (Lamictal)**, **carbamazepine (Tegretol, Carbatrol)**, and other second-generation anticonvulsants (i.e., **levetiracetam [Keppra]**, **oxcarbazepine [Trileptal]**, **tiagabine [Gabitril]**, **topiramate [Topamax]**, **zonisamide [Zonegran]**) (see Chapter 4.8, section IV for details and Table 4.8-6 for recommended dosages). The off–label use of tiagabine (Gabitril) in patients with neuropathic pain has been discouraged by its manufacturer (Cephalon), because post-marketing reports have shown its use to be associated with new onset seizures and status epilepticus in patients without epilepsy.

Lamotrigine is effective in controlling pain in patients with human immunodeficiency virus (HIV) sensory neuropathy, painful diabetic neuropathy, central poststroke pain, and pain from incomplete spinal cord lesions. However, it is not considered a first-line drug because it requires slow and careful titration and it has also been reported to cause potentially life-threatening rashes, i.e., Stevens–Johnson syndrome and hypersensitivity syndrome, especially when used with valproic acid.

Carbamazepine is considered a first-line drug for trigeminal neuralgia (or tic douloureux), for which it has also been FDA-approved for use. Aside from carbamazepine, the two other anticonvulsants recommended for trigeminal neuralgia are phenytoin and baclofen. Carbamazepine is considered a second-line drug in other neuropathic pain because of its serious ADRs [e.g., blood dyscrasias, hepatotoxicity, inappropriate secretion of antidiuretic hormone, cardiovascular effects (e.g., congestive heart failure, arrhythmias, and orthostatic hypotension), hypersensitivity reactions (Stevens–Johnson syndrome), pancreatitis, and eye changes (cortical lens opacity, conjunctivitis)].

For reports on various uses of different drugs in the management of chronic neuropathic pain, refer to individual anticonvulsant drugs in Chapter 4.8, section IV.

c. ***Local anesthetics*** produce analgesia probably by stabilizing the neuronal membrane, blocking depolarization of the action potential, and suppressing aberrant electrical activity generated by central neurons, damaged peripheral axons, or both. Their ADRs, which are dose-dependent, include CNS effects (e.g., dizziness, sedation, perioral numbness and other paresthesias, tremor, progressive encephalopathy, and seizures), cardiovascular effects (e.g., bradycardia, hypotension, and cardiac arrest), allergic effects, and other effects (e.g., respiratory depression and vomiting). All local anesthetics should be avoided in patients with severe heart failure or cardiac rhythm disturbances and in those on antiarrhythmic drugs. Patients with other significant cardiac disease should be monitored with repeated electrocardiograms or consultation with a cardiologist prior to treatment. A trial of intravenous (IV) infusion of local anesthetic may be implemented prior to starting oral local anesthetic or vice versa. There are no data to support the belief that the patient's response to IV local anesthetics is predictive of the response to oral local anesthetics and vice versa. Hence oral local anesthetics are justified even if there is no response to the IV local anesthetic and vice versa.

I. **Intravenous local anesthetics** [e.g., **lidocaine (Xylocaine), procaine (Procan)**] can occasionally produce durable effects after a brief infusion but analgesia is usually not prolonged. An IV local anesthetic commonly used for pain management is **lidocaine (Xylocaine)**, given at 2–5 mg/kg infused over a period of 20–30 minutes.

II. **Oral local anesthetics** [e.g., **mexiletine (Mexitil), tocainamide (Tonacard), and flecainide (Tambocor)**] provide an opportunity for long-term pain management. The preferred agent is **mexiletine (Mexitil)** started at 150 mg/day, then gradually titrated up every 2–3 days to a maximum of 300 mg, po, tid. Additional ADRs of mexiletine include nausea and vomiting (which can be diminished by ingesting the drug with food) and rare but serious side-effects, including liver damage and blood dyscrasias. Hence, complete blood count and liver function tests should be performed periodically. Mexiletine is considered as a "beyond second-line" drug (see Table 5.10-4) in the management of neuropathic pain from continuous dysesthesias (e.g., diabetic peripheral neuropathy) refractory to antidepressants and patients with lancinating pains (e.g., trigeminal neuralgia) refractory to anticonvulsant drugs (e.g., carbamazepine, phenytoin) and baclofen.

III. **Topical local anesthetic preparations**

- **Topical lidocaine patch (Lidoderm 5% patch)** is considered one of the first-line drugs in the management of neuropathic pain (see Table 5.10-4) and has been FDA-approved for postherpetic neuralgia. Anecdotal evidence of its benefits in other types of neuropathic pain with allodynia has been published. It is comprised of a 10 × 14 cm adhesive patch containing 5% lidocaine. Each adhesive patch contains 700 mg of lidocaine (50 mg/g adhesive) in an aqueous base. The penetration of lidocaine into intact skin after application of a Lidoderm 5% patch is sufficient to produce an analgesic effect, but less than the amount necessary to produce loss of sensation or numbness. Reactions to the Lidoderm 5% patch are generally mild and transient, e.g., the skin at the treatment site may develop erythema, edema, or abnormal sensation. In patients with normal hepatic function, blood levels of the drug are minimal, and accumulation does not occur with a dosage schedule of 12 hours on, 12 hours off. Treatment with the 5% lidocaine patch consists of the application of no more than three patches daily for a maximum of 12 hours, with the patch applied directly to intact skin at the most painful area. Titration of the 5% lidocaine patch is not necessary, and an adequate trial would last 2 weeks. In debilitated patients, the patch may be cut into smaller sizes with scissors prior to removal of the release liner. Clothing may be worn over the area of application.

- **Topical lidocaine cream (e.g., EMLA, Ela-Max, or LMX cream)** produces an area of dense cutaneous anesthesia, presumably by blocking local nerve conduction or by activation of receptor organs at a peripheral level. EMLA cream consists of 2.5% lidocaine and 2.5% prilocaine. It is indicated as a local anesthetic analgesic on normal intact skin and has been used in patients with neuropathic pain (e.g., postherpetic neuralgia). Although systemic effects are unlikely, it should not be used in patients with congenital methemoglobinemia (because of rare reports of methemoglobinemia caused by the metabolites of the prilocaine). To produce an area of dense cutaneous anesthesia, a relatively thick application must remain in contact with the skin under an occlusive dressing for at least 1 hour. The occlusive dressing can be an ordinary plastic wrap for large areas or a synthetic occlusive dressing (e.g., Tegaderm) for smaller areas. This mode of administration, however, may be difficult if the area of pain is on the face or on a mobile area of the body.

d. ***Topical analgesic agents*** have generally been applied to neuropathic pain characterized by both a predominating peripheral mechanism and continuous dysesthesia. Their systemic absorption is minimal, making them useful for patients who are predisposed to side-effects from systemically administered drugs, such as the elderly or those with comorbid conditions such as dementia.

I. **Capsaicin (Zostrix)** is an alkaloid neurotoxin (found in hot peppers), which renders the skin and joints insensitive to pain by depleting and preventing reaccumulation of the principal chemical pain mediator, substance P, in peripheral sensory neurons (nociceptors). It is considered one of the "beyond second-line" medications in the management of neuropathic pain. Aside from its use in treating allodynia (i.e., pain produced by a normally nonpainful stimulus such as light touch, wind, and mild temperature changes), which occurs in postherpetic neuralgia, CRPS, painful diabetic neuropathy, traumatic mononeuropathies (e.g., postsurgical neuropathic pain in postmastectomy scar), cluster headaches, and other painful mono- and polyneuropathies, it is also indicated for treating pain as a result of rheumatoid arthritis and osteoarthritis. It has no known systemic side-effects or drug interactions, hence making it especially helpful for older patients taking systemic medications for concomitant diseases. Some patients complain of a local burning and stinging sensation, which is not related to tissue damage and appears to pose no risk to the patient. This is usually transitory, that is, disappearing with repeated administrations over days to weeks. If it is persistent, it may be preceded by application of a local anesthetic, ingestion of an analgesic, or the capsaicin may be discontinued. Capsaicin (Zostrix) is available in 0.025% and 0.075% creams. It is applied to the affected area three or four times daily. Before deciding on its ineffectiveness, the 0.075% cream given four times daily should be tried for at least 4 weeks. Nitroglycerin 2% ointment may be added to reduce the burning discomfort associated with capsaicin and to improve compliance. Nitroglycerin is also known to have an anti-inflammatory effect and may augment the analgesia from the capsaicin.

II. **Topical NSAID preparations** probably reduce tissue levels of prostaglandins, thereby diminishing the impact of prostaglandins on the peripheral activation of nociceptive primary afferent neurons. Various NSAIDs, such as flurbiprofen (5%), ketoprofen (1–10%), ibuprofen/ureagel (10%) can be used topically four times a day. Piroxicam (0.5%) can be combined with ibuprofen/urea gel or flurbiprofen (0.5%) for topical use once or twice a day. Other

NSAIDs (e.g., aspirin, indomethacin, and diclofenac) have been investigated for topical use in neuropathic pain (e.g., postherpetic neuralgia). Although topical NSAIDs appear to be safe (with minimal systemic absorption; although they may cause skin irritation or photosensitivity), their efficacy remains questionable.

III. **Topical lidocaine patch (Lidoderm 5% patch)** or **cream (EMLA, Ela-Max)** are described in section VI.E.2.c.3.

e. ***Neuroleptic drugs*** (see Chapter 4.8, section V.B) are multipurpose adjuvant analgesics with potential usefulness as second-line agents in the management of chronic neuropathic pain (e.g., continuous dysesthesias) or arthritic pain that is refractory to sequential trials of antidepressants, oral local anesthetics, and other drugs (e.g., anticonvulsants and baclofen). They are also useful in treating acute delirium and can occasionally be used for their sedative and anxiolytic effects. Some of their adverse effects include postural hypotension, excessive sedation, anticholinergic effects, and extrapyramidal reactions (e.g., tardive dyskinesia in long-term use). The use of lower initial doses, which can then be increased to these levels, is particularly important in the elderly. A trial of several weeks is reasonable, given experience with other adjuvant analgesics, and the failure to obtain a clear-cut analgesic response should be followed by discontinuation of the drug.

Only one neuroleptic drug, **methotrimeprazine (Levoprome)**, has been shown to have an unequivocal analgesic effect (its mechanism of action is unknown; probably involving the dopaminergic pathways or through α-adrenergic blockade). Methotrimeprazine is a phenothiazine, which also has antiemetic and anxiolytic effects. It is often considered for intermittent, short-term use in patients with refractory chronic pain (e.g., because of advanced cancer) who have some other indication for a neuroleptic (e.g., delirium), are largely bedridden, or in whom gastrointestinal disease (e.g., acute bowel obstruction) or pulmonary disease is sufficient to impede opioid use. A 15-mg dose of intramuscular (IM) methotrimeprazine is equianalgesic to 10 mg of IM morphine. Methotrimeprazine is initially given at 5 mg, IM, and titrated up to 10–20 mg, IM, q6h. It has prominent sedative side-effects and is not available in oral form.

Fluphenazine (Prolixin), a phenothiazine, has mild analgesic properties and can be used in combination with a tricyclic antidepressant (e.g., amitriptyline) to treat refractory neuropathic pain (e.g., postherpetic neuralgia). Evidence of efficacy is controversial. The doses recommended are between 1 and 3 mg a day (given orally or IM), starting with a low dose and slowly escalating to 3 mg in combination with 50–100 mg of amitriptyline. Because the antihistamines, such as hydroxyzine (Vistaril, Atarax; see section VI.E.2.f.2), often seem to be as effective as the phenothiazines when used by chronic pain patients, the long-term use of phenothiazines must be weighed against the potential risk of tardive dyskinesia.

The other nonphenothiazine neuroleptic drugs with potential usefulness in chronic pain management are haloperidol (a butyrophenone) and pimozide. **Haloperidol (Haldol)** has been suggested to have coanalgesic properties at low doses (0.5–1 mg titrated to no higher than 2–5 mg, po, bid/tid). **Pimozide (Orap)** at high dose (4–12 mg/day) has been shown to be effective for patients with refractory neuropathic pain characterized by lancinating or paroxysmal dysesthesia. However, pimozide also has a high incidence of physical and mental slowing, tremors, and slight parkinsonian symptoms.

f. ***Anxiolytics and sedatives***

I. **Benzodiazepines** (see Chapter 4.8, section V.C.1) are CNS depressants whose exact mechanism of action is unknown (they probably act by potentiating the inhibitory effects of GABA). By themselves, they generally do not have specific analgesic properties (except possibly for clonazepam) and do not produce additive effects when combined with another analgesics (e.g., opioids). Their roles as analgesics are probably limited to the following: **diazepam (Valium)**, 2–10 mg, po, tid/qid (see Chapter 4.8, section V.C.1.b.1), for use as a short-term "skeletal muscle relaxant" in patients with acute musculoskeletal pain; **clonazepam (Klonopin)**, 0.5 mg, po, tid, titrated up by 0.5–1 mg q3d to a maximum of 20 mg/day (see Chapter 4.8, section IV.D) for use in patients with refractory lancinating or paroxysmal neuropathic pain; and **alprazolam (Xanax)**, 0.25–0.5 mg, po, bid/tid, maximum of 4 mg/day (see Chapter 4.8, section V.C.1.a.3), for use in cancer patients with neuropathic pain or in patients with fibromyalgia. The benzodiazepines, however, play a significant role in the total management of acute or chronic pain patients with anxiety as the overriding clinical symptom (e.g., anxiety that is acute, severe, disabling, or lasting longer than 2 weeks).

Some pain specialists believe that benzodiazepines should not be used at all in chronic pain patients (except for very short-term treatment). Aside from their abuse potential (especially after prolonged use) and the possibility of hampering functional restoration, benzodiazepines (especially in prolonged use) are believed to be antianalgesic, that is, they may increase pain perception, probably by inhibiting serotonin release and inducing benzodiazepine receptor subsensitivity. Benzodiazepines may also cause an increase in anger and hostility when given over a period of 8 weeks.

II. **Hydroxyzine (Atarax, Vistaril)** is discussed in Chapter 4.8, section VI.A. It is an antihistaminic agent, which has anxiolytic and sedative effects as well as an analgesic effect (i.e., 100 mg of parenteral hydroxyzine is equianalgesic to 8 mg of morphine). When combined with morphine, it has additive analgesic effects, while the sedative effect is only slightly greater than that of morphine alone.

g. ***Skeletal muscle relaxants*** (see Chapter 4.8, section II) produce nonspecific analgesia but their precise mechanism of action remains unknown although it is probably related to their central depressant effects. The name "skeletal muscle relaxants" is misleading because (except perhaps for diazepam) they have little or no direct relaxation effect on the skeletal muscles of man. "Skeletal muscle relaxants" are indicated for short-term relief of acute musculoskeletal pains (with or without muscle spasm). They should be viewed as alternatives to the nonopioid and opioid analgesics or, in more severe cases, as potentially useful drugs to combine with these other analgesics (and help lessen the need for high doses of these other agents). Available data have shown that their analgesic efficacy in treating common acute musculoskeletal pains is superior to placebo, acetaminophen, or aspirin; however, there are no controlled studies comparing them to NSAIDs or opioids. Also, there are no data on the relative efficacy or side-effect profiles of different "skeletal muscle relaxants". Except for the use of **cyclobenzaprine (Flexeril)** (see Chapter 4.8, section II.A.1) in fibromyalgia, their use in the treatment of chronic pain is probably limited (there is report of abuse of these drugs in some patients with NCP). Also, their sedative effects can hamper rehabilitative efforts. "Skeletal muscle relaxants" are available orally in single formulations and in combination with other compounds (usually with aspirin or codeine). In some types of skeletal muscle relaxants, parenteral forms are also available. For details, see Chapter 4.8, section II.

h. ***Antispasticity drugs,*** including **baclofen (Lioresal)** and **diazepam (Valium)**, act as agonists of the inhibitory neurotransmitter GABA. Baclofen (see Chapter 5.4, section III.D.1.a) acts presynaptically, and diazepam (see above section VI.E.2.f.1; also Chapter 4.8, section V.C.1.b.1; Chapter 5.4, section III.D.1.c) acts postsynaptically. In addition, baclofen may also reduce the release of excitatory transmitters (possibly including substance P) from nociceptive afferent nerve endings. The analgesic efficacy of baclofen in trigeminal neuralgia has been established. Baclofen can also be used empirically in treating myofascial pain syndromes and other types of lancinating or paroxysmal neuropathic pains in which muscle spasm is contributing to the pain. It can be started at a dose of 5 mg, po, tid, which can be gradually titrated up until favorable effects occur or side-effects supervene. Common side-effects include nausea, confusion, drowsiness, dizziness, and hypotension. Baclofen should not be abruptly withdrawn as this may produce seizures and hallucinations.

i. ***Antihypertensive drugs***

I. **Clonidine (Catapres)**, an α_2-adrenergic agonist and α_1-adrenergic blocker, is a multipurpose adjuvant analgesic, which is beneficial in various neuropathic pain syndromes, including migraine, postoperative pain, painful diabetic neuropathy, postherpetic neuralgia, nocturnal leg pains, sympathetically maintained pain, and cancer pain. It is considered as a "beyond second-line" drug (see Table 5.10-4) in the management of neuropathic pain in patients refractory to trials of NSAIDs, antidepressants, and other drugs. The mechanism of action of its analgesic effect is probably related to its effects on norepinephrine as well as its inhibition of firing of dorsal horn nociceptors. Clonidine can be administered through the oral route (Catapres), transdermal route (Catapres TTS), or intrathecal route (Duraclon). Choice of either oral or transdermal route is based on patient preference. To avoid adverse effects (especially hypotension), the oral dose is started at 0.1 mg/day, po, then gradually increased until side-effects occur or a significant effect on blood pressure is noted (usual analgesic dose is 0.1–0.4 mg/day; maximum of 2.4 mg/day). See Chapter 4.8, section IX.A.1 and Chapter 5.4, section III.D.1.d for details about its ADRs, contraindications and precautions, and dosing administration guidelines.

When administered intrathecally (epidurally), it has an effect on the descending noradrenergic pathways, which produces analgesia (this effect is unfortunately not associated with oral administration). Intrathecal clonidine is approved for treatment of severe neuropathic pain in cancer patients that is not adequately relieved by opioid analgesics alone. The recommended starting dose of Duraclon for continuous epidural infusion is 30 μg/hour, which can be titrated either up (to 40 μg/hour) or down depending on pain relief and occurrence of adverse events. There has also been a report of the analgesic efficacy of long-term use of continuous intrathecal clonidine (at 50–75 μg/hour) in patients with chronic, intractable, noncancer pain using an implanted programmable pump.

II. **Prazosin (Minipress)** is a selective α_1-adrenergic blocker, which has anecdotally been reported to be effective for neuropathic pain, possibly from upregulation of α_1-adrenergic receptors in injured nerves. Its ADRs include hypotension, syncope, dizziness, headache, drowsiness, lack of energy, weakness, palpitations, and nausea. It can be started at 1 mg, po, qhs, then gradually titrated up to 4–12 mg/day (maximum daily dose is 20 mg in divided doses). It is available in 1-, 2-, and 5-mg capsule forms. See also Chapter 4.8, section IX.A.3.

III. **Phenoxybenzamine (Dibenzyline)**, an α_1- and α_2-adrenergic blocker primarily used in the management of hypertension in patients with pheochromocytoma, has been anecdotally reported to be effective in relieving pain by producing and maintaining "chemical sympathectomy" in selected cases of CRPS and possibly painful plexopathies. Because of unopposed β-adrenergic activity, there is exaggerated hypotension and tachycardia. If these side-effects are intolerable, a β-blocker (e.g., propranolol) may be used concomitantly.

Phenoxybenzamine is available in 10-mg capsules and can be given at 10 mg, po, q8h, gradually titrated up to 120 mg over a 6-week period.

IV. **Propranolol (Inderal)**, a nonselective β-blocker, has been used in patients with CRPS, trigeminal neuralgia, phantom pain, and diabetic neuropathy. It is described in Chapter 4.8, sections IX.A.5 and V.F.

V. **Nifedipine (Procardia, Adalat)**, a calcium-channel blocker (see Chapter 4.8, section IX.B), which induces vasodilation, can be used in patients with CRPS and Raynaud's phenomenon. The major ADRs include headache, hypotension, dizziness, flushing, weakness, nausea, muscle cramps, tremor, peripheral edema, nervousness, palpitation, dyspnea, and nasal congestion. It can be given at 10 mg, po, tid, and, if needed, increased weekly up to 30 mg, po, tid. If there is partial or complete improvement, the effective dose is continued for 2 weeks after which the dose is tapered and discontinued over several days.

VI. **Peripherally acting adrenergic blockers**, e.g., **guanethidine** and **reserpine**, can be used as ganglionic-blocking agents for IV regional sympathetic blocks in patients with CRPS. They appear to act on the sympathetic nervous tissue, displacing norepinephrine from presynaptic vesicles and preventing reuptake. Their ADRs include a burning pain upon injection, prolonged postural hypotension, vertigo, nausea, vomiting, somnolence, and facial flushing. Clinical trials have shown that IV regional guanethidine block appears to yield more consistent and more reliable response than blocks performed with reserpine. At present, the parenteral forms of guanethidine and reserpine are only available for experimental use.

j. ***Corticosteroids*** (see Chapter 4.8, section III) have been shown to have analgesic effects, probably as a result of their anti-inflammatory effects, antiedema effects, and possibly because of a direct influence on the electrical activity of injured nerves. Steroids have been used as an adjuvant analgesic in cancer patients, specifically in patients with metastatic bone pain, neuropathic pain (e.g., plexopathy) because of infiltration or compression by the tumor, acute spinal cord compression, superior vena cava syndrome, raised intracranial pressure, symptomatic lymphedema, and hepatic capsular distension. They have also been used in NCP, such as postherpetic neuralgia, CRPS, and lumbar disk disease, although patient response has been variable. For chronic pain treatment, dexamethasone is usually used because of its relatively low mineralocorticoid effects. The dose varies from 4 to 16 mg/day or higher (initial dose may be as high as 100 mg IV) depending on the clinical situation. The use of corticosteroids has to be balanced with the potentially serious side-effects (see Chapter 4.8, section III) especially in long-term use.

The analgesic benefit of corticosteroids in rheumatic and collagen disorders is probably related to their ability to modify the specific disease. Their analgesic role in acute neuropathy is controversial. High-dose oral steroids (e.g., prednisone, 60–80 mg, every morning) given for a short period (e.g., 5 days) has anecdotally been reported to have analgesic effects in patients with acute radiculopathy because inflammation in the nerve root is believed to cause the pain. Corticosteroid use for less than 1 week helps minimize adverse effects (e.g., there is no suppression of hypothalamic–pituitary–adrenal axis).

k. ***Psychostimulants,*** such as **dextroamphetamine (Dexedrine)** and **methylphenidate (Ritalin)**, may be used to counteract the unwanted sedative effects caused by other analgesics (e.g., opioids); however, they should be used with caution by patients receiving opioids with long half-lives (e.g., methadone). Moreover, sedation and respiratory depression masked during the day may manifest when the effect of the amphetamine has worn off and the patient goes to sleep. Caffeine is another psychostimulant, which is used in combination forms with opioids, NSAIDs, or "skeletal muscle relaxants" (see Chapter 4.8, section I.A.4; I.B.2). For details about psychostimulant drugs, see Chapter 4.8, section V.E.

l. ***Bone-pain drugs*** used in cancer patients include calcitonin (**Calcimar, Miacalcin**) (see Chapter 4.8, section VIII.A.3), bisphosphonates such as pamidronate (**Aredia**; see Chapter 4.8, section VIII.A.4), and bone-seeking radionuclides such as **strontium-99**. Calcitonin given at a starting dose of 25 IU daily titrated up to 100–150 IU once or twice daily may be used as a last resort in the treatment of refractory neuropathic pain including sympathetically maintained pain and phantom limb pain.

m. ***L-Tryptophan*** is the amino-acid precursor of serotonin, which may be used singly or in combination with antidepressants (e.g., TCAs or monoamine oxidase inhibitors) in treating patients with refractory neuropathic pain. Although the use of L-tryptophan is theoretically sensible, its analgesic efficacy has not yet been confirmed clinically; however, its use in refractory neuropathic pain may be justified because it is a relatively safe and well-tolerated drug. The alleged causal relationship of tryptophan supplements to eosinophilia–myalgia syndrome has reportedly been caused by a contaminant originating from supplements provided by a single Japanese manufacturer. L-Tryptophan can be started at a low dose (e.g., 1 g, po, bid) and then titrated up to 3–5 g/day. Side-effects, which appear to be dose-related, include sedation and nausea. The effect of L-tryptophan may be potentiated by adding a low-protein/high-carbohydrate diet with vitamin supplements (e.g., niacin and B_6) which probably ensures adequate entry of L-tryptophan into the brain for conversion to serotonin.

n. ***Glucosamine*** has been hypothesized to impede the breakdown of cartilage, help regenerate cartilage, and probably reduce inflammation. It can be used in treating osteoarthritic pain with cartilage erosion. Some of its common ADRs include gastrointestinal upset and rash. It is available over-the-counter as a food supplement. The preferred form is glucosamine sulfate, which is better absorbed in the gastrointestinal tract. Its recommended dose is 1500 mg/day (for body weight <180 lb or <82 kg) or 2000 mg/day (for body weight >180 lb or >82 kg). It must be taken for at least 4 weeks before any effects can be noticeable. Although relatively safe, it still needs long-term studies examining the implications of altering cartilage breakdown and formation in the body and possible associated toxicities.

o. ***N-methyl-D-aspartate (NMDA)-receptor antagonists (dextromethorphan, ketamine, amantadine, methadone)*** act by blocking excitatory, hyperalgesic pain stimuli induced by NMDA activation as a result of tissue and nerve damage. Their efficacy in treating patients with neuropathic pain are undergoing investigation. **Dextromethorphan** (readily available as an over-the-counter antitussive) is considered one of the "beyond second-line" drugs in the management of neuropathic pain (e.g., postherpetic neuralgia and painful diabetic neuropathy). However, effective dextromethorphan doses may be so high that unacceptable side-effects occur. A new dextromethorphan drug (**Neurodex**) is undergoing clinical trial in patients with painful diabetic neuropathy. **Ketamine (Ketanest; Ketalar)**, given IV or subcutaneously, has proven beneficial in the treatment of neuropathic pain (e.g., postherpetic neuralgia, chronic post-traumatic pain, and pain associated with CNS lesions), but its use has been limited by ADRs. Recent work suggested that subtherapeutic doses of ketamine may be used to potentiate the effect of opioids without undesirable side-effects. **Amantadine (Symmetrel**; see Chapter 4.8, sections V.E.4 and XIII.B), an antiviral and anti-Parkinsonian agent, is undergoing clinical trial to determine if its administration can significantly reduce surgical neuropathic pain in cancer patients.

p. ***Experimental drugs*** that may soon be available for the management of neuropathic pain include: **butyl-para-aminobensoate (Butamben)**, an ester local anesthetic, **bupivacaine microspheres; SNX-III**, a selective calcium-channel blocker. Nicotinic acetylcholine receptor agonists such as **ABT-594**, which may also prove efficacious, are in preliminary research stages. Animal studies have revealed the following as potential therapies in neuropathic pain: **civamine**, an orally bioavailable capsaicin analog; **levodopa**; intrathecal injection of **chromaffin cells;** intrathecal injection of **nitric oxide synthase inhibitor** L-*N*-G-**nitro arginine methyl ester** (L-NAME); intrathecal **neostigmine**; and use of **proglumide, a cholecystokinin antagonist.**

3. **Pain cocktail program** is a patient-blinded detoxification protocol used in chronic pain patients for reducing and eliminating excessive or abusive use of opioids, tranquilizers, and sedative-hypnotic medications. All parenteral medications are first switched into oral forms. The oral medications are then given on an as-needed ("prn") basis for 24–48 hours to obtain the typical 24-hour baseline requirement. No new or additional opioid, tranquilizer, or sedative-hypnotics are added during the entire program. For patients with opioid abuse, the pain cocktail can be made up of a long-acting opioid (e.g., methadone), in an equivalent dose equal to the currently used opioid, mixed in a masking vehicle (e.g., cherry syrup). The pain cocktail is given orally around the clock at an interval established for the patient. Over a 3–6-week period, the active ingredient (e.g., opioid) is gradually reduced (e.g., 5–20% reduction per day) with an equal increase in the masking vehicle. The decrements are made slowly so as not to elicit withdrawal syndromes. When the patient is receiving the masking vehicle only, the vehicle is maintained for 2–10 days prior to discontinuation. Before starting the pain cocktail program, the entire procedure is explained to the patient, except the time when the active ingredient will be reduced. This approach used for opioids can also be used for tranquilizer or sedative-hypnotic drugs. To ensure compliance, pain cocktail programs are usually incorporated as part of a structured in-hospital or day-hospital program (a chronic pain center treatment program is described in Chapter 5.11, section VI.B.4.). The pain cocktail is usually mixed and prepared by the pharmacist.

F. **PSYCHOSOCIAL AND SELF-REGULATION TECHNIQUES** give the patient a sense of control over postoperative and post-traumatic pain and its consequences, as well as demonstrating to the patient that his or her opinions and beliefs are important.

1. **Psychosocial support** refers to reassurance supplied through social and professional interactions with trained personnel as well as through individual psychotherapy and peer support groups.
2. **Procedural and sensory information** can be provided to the patient and the patient's family or support system. Procedural information is the specifics of the surgery or medical procedure, such as the time of the procedure, the risks associated with the anesthetic or surgery, and the sequence of events. Sensory information describes the sensory experiences the patient may confront such as aching, cramping, or burning pain at the incision. The methods of transmitting information include booklets, verbal presentations by staff, and audiotaped or videotaped presentations. The patient must have a good memory to remember information (or it may be repeated or given in written form). The clinician must be aware that for patients who use denial as a means to cope, the information may increase their anxiety.
3. **Coping-skills training** refers to teaching patients specific behaviors and strategies that may be used to cope with pain during the postoperative period or during the actual procedure (e.g., procedures in which the patient is awake).

a. ***Cognitive coping skills*** include distraction, calming self-statements, pleasant imagery, humor, music, reading, stress-inoculation training, brief psychotherapy, reinterpreting pain stimuli, and cognitive reappraisal of the event.

b. ***Relaxation training*** (see Chapter 4.2, section VI) includes alternative forms of self-regulation that are based on modifying a chosen physiologic parameter, such as heart rate, breathing, or muscle spasm, with progressive training. Relaxation training activity takes time and practice, so the patient must be alert, responsive, and interactive. Relaxation may be incorporated with **biofeedback** training (see Chapter 4.1, section VI).

c. ***Systemic desensitization*** includes procedures in which the steps or parts of an experience such as a painful procedure are enumerated in a hierarchical order from the least distressing or painful for the patient to the most distressing or painful. The patient is then gradually exposed (either in imagination or *in vivo*) to each step, while applying relaxation or cognitive coping strategies and given positive reinforcement for mastering each step.

d. ***Modeling and exposure*** involves the patient watching a videotape of another person who serves as a role model by showing successful techniques of coping with pain and anxiety in a situation similar to that experienced or to be experienced by the patient (e.g., preparation for surgery or other specific procedures).

e. ***Hypnosis*** is a general term for states of focused attention, which can be achieved by many individuals under various circumstances. Hypnosis involves training and practice and can be an effective analgesic and anxiolytic tool in patients with long-term problems. It includes hetero- and autohypnoses and may use complex hypnotic phenomena (e.g., dissociation, sensory alteration, and time distortion).

4. Intervention with family members who were trained to help the patient cope with painful procedures (e.g., by coaching the patient to use paced breathing and distraction techniques).

G. VOCATIONAL COUNSELING should be included as part of pain management if indicated.

H. INVASIVE TECHNIQUES should only be used if noninvasive techniques have failed, except in rare cases where the invasive procedure can correct the underlying pathology (e.g., surgical decompression of the nerve).

1. Joint and soft tissue injections using corticosteroid or mixtures of corticosteroid and local anesthetic agents are considered as adjunct treatments for the relief of pain and inflammation of the joint (e.g., synovitis) and soft tissues (e.g., bursitis, tendinitis, or tenosynovitis). They are described in detail in Chapter 4.9. Facet joint blocks, which may be indicated in patients with deep, dull, aching back pain without neurological abnormalities, have variable success rates.

2. Nerve blocks involve the administration of local anesthetics or a neurolytic agent (e.g., chemical agents such as phenol and absolute alcohol, cold agents such as cryoprobe, and heat agents such as radiofrequency coagulation) into a somatic nerve (see Chapter 4.10, section IV.A), a sympathetic ganglion (see Chapter 4.10, section IV.B), or a localized pain-sensitive trigger point or tender spot (see Chapter 4.11). Epidural blocks using steroids are discussed in Chapter 4.10, section IV.A.3.e.

3. Surgical interventions

a. ***Neurosurgical procedures*** for pain relief are generally reserved for refractory cases of chronic pain only after conservative measures fail. They have been associated with high morbidity and mortality in the past, but recent improvements in the understanding of the pathophysiology of pain and in the neurosurgical techniques have resulted in a high rate of success and a low incidence of complications. If patients are carefully selected, surgery performed by a skilled surgeon may provide dramatic relief. A significant number of patients, however, may have recurrence of some symptoms as early as 3–6 months after the procedure (probably as a result of nerve regeneration or scar formation). Procedures that are used to arrest nociceptive transmission include the following.

I. **Nondestructive techniques**, which attempt to correct the disordered physiology of nerves without creating a lesion, such as carpal tunnel release, thoracic outlet decompression, root decompression, and cranial nerve decompression.

II. **Destructive or interruptive techniques (neuroablation)**

- **Peripheral or primary afferent procedures** transect the primary afferent fibers at the level of the peripheral nerve, root, or ganglion. Examples include peripheral neurectomy, excision or relocation of neuromas, rhizotomy (cranial nerve or spinal), sympathetic gangliolysis or ganglionectomy, and trigeminal system procedures (i.e., retrogasserian radiofrequency thermal rhizotomy, percutaneous glycerol rhizolysis, balloon microcompression).
- **Spinal cord procedures** interrupt ascending sensory tracts in the spinal cord or brainstem. Cordotomy is the most effective and widely used, e.g., anterolateral cordotomy (spinal tractotomy) or high cervical cordotomy (C1–C2), which may be done percutaneously by radiofrequency under fluoroscopic guidance; and open laminectomy at the low cervical or upper thoracic spine. Other procedures include commissural (or midline) myelotomy (which disrupts pain conducting fibers as well as polysynaptic pain pathways that run through the center of the spinal cord), dorsal root ganglionectomy, dorsal rhizotomy, and dorsal root entry zone lesions (using radiofrequency).
- **Deep brain procedures** include stereotactically placed lesions of deep brain structures, such as stereotactic tractotomy (medulla, pons, thalamus, hypothalamus, or spinal thalamic or spinal reticular tracts) and psychosurgery (e.g., cingulotomy).
- **Pituitary destruction (hypophysectomy)**, i.e., anterior pituitary ablation.
- **Sympathetic nerve procedures** include thoracic or lumbar sympathectomy (in selected cases of sympathetically maintained pain) and cortical and subcortical ablation.

III. **Modulatory techniques**

- **Implantation of drug infusion systems** (e.g., morphine infusion). Epidural, spinal intrathecal, intraventricular.
- **Chronic stimulation (neuroaugmentation)** of the central or peripheral nervous system to stimulate an analgesia mechanism in the CNS (e.g., to alter the gate-control mechanism or to increase secretion of endogenous opioids). Examples include stimulation of the spinal cord (i.e., dorsal column), peripheral nerve [major extremity nerve (median, ulnar, radial, sciatic, peroneal, tibial), occipital nerve, peripheral trigeminal nerve, spinal nerve root], deep brain [periventricular-periaqueductal gray, lemniscal system (medial lemniscus, sensory thalamus, internal capsule)], and motor cortex.

b. ***Musculoskeletal procedures*** include total joint replacement, synovectomy, and curative excision or palliative debulking of a tumor.

4. **Radiation therapy** can be used for cancer patients to relieve metastatic pain as well as symptoms from local extension of the primary disease. Radiation therapy includes localized radiation therapy, wide-field radiation therapy, and radiopharmaceuticals (e.g., iodine-131 and strontium-99).

Further reading

Acute Pain Management Guideline Panel: *Clinical practice guideline: acute pain management.* AHCPR Publication No. 92-0032, Rockville, MD, Feb, 1992, Agency for Health Care Policy and Research.

Allegrante JP: Patient education. In Paget S, Gibofsky A, Beary III JF, editors: *Manual of rheumatology and outpatient orthopedic disorders*, ed 4, Philadelphia, 2000, Lippincott, Williams & Wilkins, pp. 48–51.

Aronoff GM, editor: *Evaluation and treatment of chronic pain*, Baltimore, 1992, Williams & Wilkins.

Bartlett EE: Which patient education strategies will pay off under prospective pricing? *Patient Educ Couns* 12:51, 1988.

Cleeland CS: Measurement of pain by subjective report. In Chapman CR, Loeser JD, editors: *Advances in pain research and therapy,* Vol 12: *Issues in pain measurement*, New York, 1989, Raven Press, pp. 391–403.

Dean BZ, Williams FH, King JC, *et al.*: Pain rehabilitation. 4. Therapeutic options in pain management. *Arch Phys Med Rehabil* Suppl 75:S21–S30, 1994.

Dworkin RH, Backonja M, Rowbotham MC, *et al.*: Advances in neuropathic pain: diagnosis, mechanisms, and treatment recommendations. *Arch Neurol* 60(11): 1524–34, 2003.

Erickson JJ, Braverman DL, Shah RV: Interventions in chronic pain management. 4. Medications in pain management. *Arch Phys Med Rehabil* Suppl 75:S50–S56, 2003.

Fordyce WE: *Behavioral methods for chronic pain and illness*, St Louis, 1978, Mosby-Year Book.

Grabois M: Chronic pain. In Garrison SJ, editor: *Handbook of physical medicine and rehabilitation; the basics*, ed 2, Philadelphia, 2003, Lippincott, Williams & Wilkins, pp. 105–126.

Hamill RJ, Rowlingson JC, editor: *Handbook of critical care pain management*, New York, 1994, McGraw-Hill.

Katz WA: Approach to the management of nonmalignant pain. *Am J Med* 101 (suppl 1A):54S–63S, 1996.

Loeser JD, editor: *Bonica's management of pain*, ed 3, Philadelphia, 2001, Lippincott, Williams & Wilkins.

Markenson JA: Mechanism of chronic pain. *Am J Med* 101 (suppl 1A):7S–18S, 1996.

Management of Cancer Pain Guideline Panel: *Clinical practice guideline: management of cancer pain.* AHCPR Publication No. 94-0592, Rockville, MD, March, 1992, Agency for Health Care Policy and Research.

Physicians' desk reference, ed 58, Montvale, NJ, 2004, Thomson PDR.

Portenoy RK, Kanner RM, editors: *Pain management: theory and practice*, Philadelphia, 1996, FA Davis.

Raj PP, editor: *Pain medicine: a comprehensive review*, ed 2, St Louis, 2003, Mosby.

Sinatra RS, Hord AH, Ginsberg B, *et al.*, editors: *Acute pain: mechanism and management*, St Louis, 1992, Mosby-Year Book.

Tollison CD, Satterthwaite JR, Tollison JW, editors: *Practical pain management*, ed 3, Philadelphia, 2002, Lippincott, Williams & Wilkins.

Turk DC, Michenbaum DM, Gemest M: *Pain and behavioral medicine: a cognitive-behavioral perspective*, New York, 1983, Guilford.

Wall PD, Melzack R, editors: *Textbook of pain*, ed 4, Edinburgh, 1999, Churchill Livingstone.

Warfield CA, editor: *Principles and practice of pain management*, New York, 1993, McGraw-Hill.

Warfield CA, Fausett HJ, editors: *Manual of pain management*, ed 2, Philadelphia, 2002, Lippincott, Williams & Wilkins.

World Health Organization: *Cancer pain relief and palliative care*, Geneva, 1990, World Health Organization.

CHAPTER 5.11
Work-related musculoskeletal problems

Work continues to pose considerable risk of musculoskeletal injury despite major advances in industrial safety and technology. This is costly to both the worker (because of lost wages) and to the industry (because of lost productivity and revenue). The two most important factors contributing to musculoskeletal injuries are: (a) increasing worker specialization, which has led to an increase in task repetitiveness (hence greater chance for musculoskeletal overexertion and boredom), and (b) the combination of open hiring policies and workers' compensation insurance, which promotes hiring of any applicants without regard to prior disability, if not job task related, resulting in greater likelihood that a worker will apply for and obtain employment that may not be physically suitable for him or her.

Physiatrists, because of their extensive training in neuromusculoskeletal disorders as well as their interdisciplinary team approach, play an important role in the evaluation, treatment, and rehabilitation of workers to help them recover and return to work. The goals of PM&R in work-related musculoskeletal injuries include pain reduction; enhancement of functional capabilities, work tolerance, and job safety; instruction in proper body mechanics and posture; prevention and reduction of work-related injuries and disabilities; and return of workers to significant gainful employment in an expedient and cost-effective manner.

I. Epidemiology

Epidemiological studies indicate that work injuries are certainly not unique to the United States but are world-wide. In 2002, the US Department of Labor's Bureau of Labor Statistics reported the following nonfatal injuries and illnesses statistics in private industry: a total of 4.7 million cases (resulting in a rate of 5.3 cases per 100 equivalent full-time workers); 1 436 200 days away from work (resulting in a rate of 1.6 cases per 100 equivalent full-time workers); 617 186 cases involving sprains, strains, tears; 345 294 cases of back injuries; and 272 988 cases of falls. These data cannot be compared with data for prior years because effective from January 1, 2002, the Occupational Safety and Health Administration (OSHA) changed its requirements for recording occupational injuries and illnesses. However, comparison of data from 1992 to 2001 shows a steady decline in the rate of nonfatal injury and illness cases per 100 full-time workers in private industry, i.e., from 8.9 to 5.7 for total recordable cases; and from 3.9 to 2.8 for lost workday cases. Although declining, musculoskeletal injuries continue to account for the majority of the cases that result in work losses.

II. Costs

Costs resulting from work-related injury are reflected in the direct costs (e.g., expenditures for medical care and compensation for lost wages) and the less tangible indirect costs (e.g., lost production, consumer cost increases, expenses of employee retraining or replacement, and litigation). Approximately two-thirds of the direct costs are payments for partial or permanent disability and one-third for medical expenses. According to the National Academy of Social Insurance, in 2001: the total workers' compensation benefit payment was $49.4 billion (3.5% higher than in 2000); the employer costs were $63.9 billion (8.0% higher than in 2000); and the percent of benefits paid for medical care was 44.9% (2.4% higher than in 2000). Based on the 1999–2000 National Workers Compensation Database Statistics (*http://nohsc.info.au.com*), the percentages of worker's compensation based on body parts affected were 28.5% for the trunk, 19.4% for lower limbs, 31.2% for upper limbs, 3% for the neck, 8.7% for the head, 4.9% for multiple locations, and 4.1% for systemic, nonphysical, and unspecified locations. The costs of medical care and disability benefits are greatest for persons with prolonged disability (it is estimated that 10% of claims account for approximately 80% of costs because of disability). In addition to the monetary costs, work-related disability results in inestimable human pain, suffering, and decreased quality of life for the individual and the worker's family. Often, workers with long-term, work-related disabilities become exceedingly depressed, have limited activity levels, and undergo interpersonal disruptions (e.g., divorce).

III. The Americans with Disabilities Act (ADA) of 1990

This Act provides persons with disabilities with civil rights protection in five areas: employment, public services, transportation, public accommodation, and telecommunication. Title I of the ADA (implemented on July 26, 1994 for employers with 15–24 employees) pertains to protection of the "qualified individuals with a disability" against discrimination from employers or labor organizations. A "qualified individual with a disability" is a disabled person who, with or without reasonable accommodation (see section III.B), can perform the essential functions of the job being sought. Aside from physical disability, a person with a psychiatric disorder can also qualify as being disabled; however, a person who is currently engaged in the illegal use of drugs is not considered a "qualified individual with a disability". The employer will decide essential job functions and is advised to develop a written detailed job description. Discrimination against disabled persons is outlawed in every aspect of the employment process, including pre-employment examination inquiries related to the disability, medical examinations to screen out workers, and the limiting or classifying of job applicants to adversely affect job opportunity. Ability to perform job-specific functions (as opposed to generic inquiries about physical, sense organ, or cognitive limitations) may, however, be considered in the hiring decision. Also, an employer may require a posthiring testing (i.e., preplacement testing), and may make the employment offer contingent on the results of that testing.

A. PREPLACEMENT TESTING may be carried out only after a job offer has been made to the prospective employee. All new employees for the same job must be examined with the same tests. The test must be job-specific (or related to "essential" job functions; factors determining job or task "essentiality" are described in section V.D.2.a) with the goal of ensuring that the employee is physically and emotionally capable of performing the job so as to not endanger himself or herself or other employees. If the employee is unable to successfully perform the testing because of some functional limitation, the industry is obliged to determine if reasonable accommodations (see below) could be implemented that would allow the successful performance of the required job tasks. All information obtained is collected confidentially.

B. "REASONABLE ACCOMMODATION" may include making physical facilities accessible (see Chapter 4.5, section II.B.2.e) for persons with disabilities; job restructuring; modifying work schedules; reassigning to a vacant position;

modifying or acquiring equipment or devices; modifying or adjusting examinations, training materials, or policies; providing reserved parking; and providing a person (e.g., an interpreter) to help an employee. The ADA, however, does not require "reasonable accommodation" if it causes "undue hardship" on the employer as determined on a case-by-case basis.

IV. Return to work (RTW) issues

The interdisciplinary rehabilitation team play significant roles in determining the patient's capability to return to work, in task analysis of the patient's job, as well as in adaptations of work tools and work environment (e.g., barrier-free architectural designs and modification of tools). First, the health status of the patient is determined by medical, physical, and psychosocial testing. The health status or restriction is then matched to the job profile, which includes an analysis of both the physical abilities required for performing the job and the working conditions at the workplace. Job profiles compiled from one workplace cannot be used at another place because job titles of the same name may not involve the same tasks. If the patient is able to match all the critical tasks identified in the job profile, then he or she can be recommended to return to full duty with no limitation. However, this is not always feasible. Most of the time, the patient may either return to work with some limitations (e.g., light duty with limitations or part time) or the employer may modify the job or workplace to suit the impairment. Returning a worker to modified duty has been shown to be cost-effective. If this is not possible, an alternative job may be found in the same company making use of the worker's residual skills; however, if alternative jobs cannot be found or if the patient has severe injuries, then retraining for a different vocation may be considered. Usually, this is the last resort because retraining is costly. In making legal determinations of disability and fitness to work, the classification of jobs in the United States based on levels of exertion (see Table 5.11-1) is commonly used. The following variables are associated with poor RTW:

A. **OCCUPATIONAL VARIABLES** including increased time off work (likelihood of RTW is about 50% if off 6 months, 25% if off 1 year, and less than 5% if off 2 years), poor job satisfaction (which also contributes to increased risk of injury, lost time, and delayed recovery), mismatch between the patient's physical capacities and demands of the job, and unavailability of job or unwillingness of the employer to make reasonable accommodations or to modify the job, or consider temporary light-duty work for the employee.

B. **PSYCHOSOCIAL VARIABLES** including poor language proficiency, a disabled spouse, anger or excessive fault finding at the system or employer (i.e., adversarial relationship between the employer and employee), pending litigation, and secondary gain (e.g., financial compensation, increased attention and support from family and friends, and use of the illness as a tool of control in the family and against the employer).

C. **MEDICAL VARIABLES** including history of previous injury, history of substance abuse (including prescription medication), poor cardiovascular fitness, and physical and psychological deconditioning.

V. Work assessment

Work assessment consists of an interview (to determine subjective information), direct measures of physical capacities [to objectively measure strength, range of motion (ROM), sensation, coordination, balance, functional mobility, and

Table 5.11-1 Physical demand characteristics of work for any jobs in the United States based on the US Department of Labor's *Dictionary of Occupational Titles* (see also Table 2.7-5 in Chapter 2.7 for correlation with the New York Heart Association Functional and Therapeutic Classification of cardiac or cardiopulmonary impairment/disability)

Physical demand level of work	Occasional load (1/3 of the time)	Frequent load (1/3 to 2/3 of the time)	Constant load (>2/3 of the time)	Typical energy required (METs)
Sedentary*	≤10 lb	Negligible	Negligible	1–2
Light	10–20 lb	≤10 lb†	Negligible‡	2–4
Medium	20–50 lb	10–25 lb	≤10 lb	4–6
Heavy	50–100 lb	25–50 lb	10–20 lb	7–8
Very heavy	>100 lb	>50 lb	>20 lb	>8

1 lb = 454 g.
** Sedentary work involves sitting most of the time, but may require occasional walking or standing or lifting/carrying (of papers, small tools, or file folders).*
† Even though the load is <10 lb, the job is classified as light if it requires a great deal of walking, standing, pushing, and/or pulling of arm or leg controls.
‡ Even though the load is negligible, the job is classified as light if it requires a great deal of pushing and/or pulling of arm or leg controls while seated.
Data adapted from: US Department of Labor Employment and Training Administration: Dictionary of Occupational Titles, *vol II, ed 4, revised, Washington, DC, 1991, US Government Printing Press, p. 1013.*

cardiovascular fitness and endurance], diagnostic tests, and functional capacity evaluation (including physical and work capacity evaluation). The duration of work assessment can range from 2 hours to 1 week. It is used to determine the worker's existing physical capacities following injury (based on the medical conditions, the individual's transferable skills, vocational interest, and aptitudes, interpersonal skills, and psychological and motivational status) and to compare them against given criteria to predict the worker's potential to engage in work. The criteria used for comparison may be job-specific (to determine if the injured worker may eventually return to that specific job) or it may be general (i.e., based on general classification of work levels as defined by the US Department of Labor in Table 5.11-1). Work assessment can also be used to formulate recommendations for intervention (e.g., work-hardening programs) with the ultimate goal of returning the injured patient to work.

Medical evaluation of the injured worker is important for determining the stability of the patient's medical condition. The physiatric evaluation may be in the form of pre-employment examination, postinjury assessment, recovery assessment after injury, physical impairment rating (or anatomic incapacity rating), Social Security disability evaluation, independent medical evaluation, and evaluation on compliance with regulations of the ADA. The insurance company (e.g., Worker's Compensation Board) may request that the physiatrist determine if the illness or injury is work-related, if the history of the illness or injury is consistent with the clinical findings and diagnosis, if there are any pre-existing conditions or nonoccupational factors that could account for the clinical problem, and if there is a clear cause-and-effect relationship between the work activities and the clinical presentation. In some states, the physiatrist may be asked to determine compensation awards by "rating" the physical impairment (e.g., limitation of ROM or muscle weakness) of the worker based on a standardized system (e.g., using the *American Medical Association's Guides to the Evaluation of Permanent Impairment*) and by determining if the patient has reached maximal medical improvement (i.e., patient's progress has reached a plateau and is not expected to change further). Physiatrists may also be asked to provide medical testimony as a factual or expert witness in ongoing work-related litigation.

A. HISTORY

1. History of present illness

a. ***Pain description,*** for example, pain quality, location, radiation, intensity, and timing; aggravating and alleviating factors; other associated manifestations; previous test results; effects of previous treatments such as active physical therapy, work conditioning, or work hardening.

b. ***Accident history,*** for example, position, posture, and footing at the time of the accident; time of day and day of week the accident occurred; nature of the job (i.e., is it a new task? or how long has the worker been on this specific job?); occurrence of similar incidents with other workers on that job; problems with the equipment used on the job; initial medical examination and treatment; and initial response of the employer to the injury.

2. Past history including general physical fitness; pre-existing problems that could have contributed to the accident or injury or will affect the recovery process (e.g., diabetes, arthritis, heart disease, pulmonary disease, and obesity); prior hospitalizations; past traumas and accidents; past surgeries and treatments (and their effectiveness); past minor and major psychiatric illnesses.

3. Current medications including all current prescription and nonprescription drugs.

4. Personal history including life-styles (e.g., a description of the patient's typical day; time spent in bed, in watching television, in getting out of the house, in hobbies and recreation, and in performing exercises), habits (e.g., use of recreational drugs, alcohol, and tobacco), and premorbid personality and emotional response to previous illnesses and injuries. (For example, is the worker passive and inactive or is there any attempt to stay active and productive or to return to work? Is there a positive or negative outlook for the future?)

5. Social history including marital status and history, home situation, and available support systems.

6. Vocational and economic history including educational and training history, work history (e.g., previous jobs and attempts to return to work), work environment (see Chapter 4.5, section II.B.2.e); current relationship with the employer (e.g., does the worker have a job to return to? Is the employer willing to accept the worker back on the job?), financial situation, insurance, and pending litigation (which often slows down recovery and limits the response to treatment).

B. PHYSICAL EXAMINATION should include all the pertinent systems (see Chapter 1.1, section II) with special emphasis on the neuromuscular and musculoskeletal systems as well as on nonorganic signs (seen in patients with symptom magnification syndromes). Pain measurement scales (e.g., Visual Analog Scale) and dolorimetry (see Chapter 5.10, section IV.C.2.a.1) may be used to assess pain.

1. Musculoskeletal system. ROM, joint stability, strength, pain behavior (e.g., marked grimacing, groans, and limping), tenderness (focal or widespread, trigger and/or tender points), muscle tightness and guarding, deformities, muscle atrophy (focal and localized or generalized), and deep pain (for the upper limb, hyperextend the small finger; for the lower limb, firmly compress the calf muscle or Achilles tendon).

a. ***Spine.*** Posture, straight leg raising, Spurling's test.

b. ***Upper limb.*** ROM (include cervical ROM), grip strength, tests that provoke symptoms (e.g., Tinel's, Phalen's wrist flexion test, and Finkelstein's test), tests for thoracic outlet syndrome, scapular winging, and pain pattern (is it produced at any point in the arc of motion?).

c. ***Lower limb.*** Patrick's test, Gaenslen test, Drawer's test, Lachman's test, pivot shift test, and leg-length inequalities.

2. **Neuromuscular system.** Motor functions, sensation (e.g., superficial and deep sensation, vibratory sensation, joint position or proprioception, and sensory distribution), reflexes (including hamstring and gastrocsoleus reflexes because more than 90% of lumbosacral radiculopathies involve S1 or L5 nerve roots), gait (e.g., assistive device used and type of gait), and functional activities (e.g., toe-walk, heel-walk, squat, touch toes, hop on one foot, and run in place).

3. **Nonorganic findings** are seen in patients with symptom magnification syndrome (usually with excessive complaints of pain with disproportionately low objective findings). In these patients, a psychologically or behaviorally based intervention may be warranted. Examples of nonorganic findings include "ratchety" (instead of smooth) quality of the "give-way" during muscle testing; right-to-left difference in vibratory sensation in a midline bone, such as the skull or sternum; a pain drawing chart showing extracorporeal pain markings, additional writings or comments, demarcating lines, and nonanatomic drawings; Waddell signs for nonorganic back pain (i.e., tenderness of the skin to light pinch over a widespread area; deep tenderness in a nonanatomical distribution; reproduction of back pain with axial loading by pressing down on the worker's head while he or she is standing; reproduction of back pain when the shoulders and pelvis are rotated together as a unit; inconsistent responses to straight-leg raising in the seated vs. the supine position; widespread, inconsistent, and/or nonanatomic weakness or sensory loss; and overreaction during examination (e.g., disproportionate verbalization, facial expression, slow exaggerated movements, muscle tension and tremor, collapsing, or sweating).

C. **DIAGNOSTIC TESTS** should not be used in "shotgun" fashion but should be used for specific indications. They include noninvasive imaging studies (see Chapter 2.2), invasive imaging studies (see Chapter 2.3), laboratory testing (see Chapter 2.1), electrodiagnostic testing (see Chapter 2.4), and diagnostic injections (see Chapter 4.10). Diagnostic tests are useless unless they are closely correlated with clinical findings.

D. **FUNCTIONAL CAPACITY EVALUATION (FCE)**, in the context of RTW programs, usually refers to a physical and work capacity evaluation. The FCE is typically performed by physical or occupational therapists. The information obtained from FCE can be used to establish maximal permissible limits for nonrepetitive activities and to delineate safe parameters for repetitive activities. Examples of commercially available FCEs are the Blankenship system and the EPIC system (which provides six modules that evaluate lift capacity: motor coordination, finger and hand dexterity, standing whole body ROM, balance while walking, carrying and climbing, and industrial pushing and pulling).

1. **Physical capacity evaluation (PCE)** typically assesses isolated parts of the body or functional units, such as lumbar region or upper limbs. Physical tests include gross physical capabilities (e.g., ROM, strength, endurance, lifting capacity, walking balance, carrying, and climbing), finger and hand dexterity skills [e.g., Purdue Pegboard, Crawford Small Parts, Minnesota Rate of Manipulation, Stromberg Dexterity, Bennet Hand Tool tests, and using equipment available from Baltimore Therapeutic Equipment (BTE), EPIC Functional Capacity Evaluation System, Isernhagen Work Systems, Key Functional Assessment, Lafayette Instruments, Valpar, Work Evaluation Systems Technology (WEST), and Work Recovery System], and movement accuracy (e.g., Employee Aptitude Survey #9, EPIC 2 Motor Coordination test, and the ERGOS Work Simulator). An example of a commercially available PCE is the Smith Physical Capacity Evaluation (which measures 154 performance items) and the Blankenship system.

2. **Work capacity evaluation (WCE)** is a comprehensive process that systematically uses work (real or simulated) to assess and measure an individual's capacity to work safely and efficiently in specific job tasks. In persons with disabilities, WCE can help determine if the person needs to change his type of employment (i.e., undergo vocational or prevocational rehabilitation) or to resume previous employment using adapted tools or methods. Primary factors measured by WCE include work feasibility (e.g., using the Feasibility Evaluation Checklist, which consists of 21 behavior-anchored rating scales for items such as the ability to accept supervision and work with others, safety in the workplace, and the quantity and quality of the patient's productivity), which is determined prior to assessing work tolerance (e.g., strength, energy reserve, flexibility, and the effect of pain and other limiting factors on task performance such as sitting and standing tolerance). Secondary factors measured by WCE include aptitudes, interests, and vocational skills. The WCE results are then compared with the demands of the job as listed by the US Department of Labor in the *Dictionary of Occupational Titles*. If there is a deficit that affects performance of the job, intervention (such as modified work hardening or a work conditioning program) may be recommended. During performance of the WCE it is helpful to learn from the worker the amount of energy and effort being expended by using the Rating of Perceived Exertion Scale (Borg Scale) described in Chapter 4.2, section III.A.3. The following discussion provides an overview of the four common categories of WCE tools that can be used independently or as part of a FCE:

a. ***Job analyses (on-the-job or worksite evaluations)*** are carried out to determine whether the abilities and physical status of a person with a disability can match the physical demand characteristics of the job so that the worker can return to his or her old job or apply for a particular new job. Under the ADA, a "formal job analysis" is not required because it may not be job specific and may not adequately identify the essential functions of a particular job. To meet the ADA criteria, a job analysis must focus on the purpose of the job and how essential the actual job function is in achieving this purpose. Factors determining the essentiality of a task or function include its frequency, the amount of time required to perform the task, and the consequences if it is not performed (i.e., does removal of that task or function fundamentally change the job or make the position nonexistent?). Job analysis should preferably be carried out at the worksite or, if that is not feasible, it may be simulated (e.g., in work hardening centers). Data collection for job analysis in the workplace and the clinic can either be expert-based (i.e., rated by expert observers) or incumbent-based (i.e., rated by the workers themselves).

I. **Surveys** are screening methods used to determine whether the workplace, job, individual worker, or working situation contributes significantly to the job stress. Once these problems are identified, surveys can be used to recommend work interventions to reduce the problem or further objective studies (e.g., quantifying a worker's performance on the job and the physiological cost of that performance). Survey questionnaires may include objects handled (weight, size, shape, surface texture, presence or absence of handles); amount and frequency of physical tasks such as lifting, pushing, pulling, climbing, stooping, and squatting; positions and postures that must be utilized to successfully perform the job; tools used (handle size, weight, vibration, position of use); layout of worksite (e.g., a desk or table with appropriate height, width, length, and presence of space underneath; height of workbench; and arrangement of tools utilized); amount of lighting present (type and intensity of lighting, windows); temperature of the facility; amount of noise present (e.g., are hearing protectors available and used if excess noise is present?); cleanliness of floor surface (e.g., spills, greasy spots, clutter, and obstacles present on floor that could lead to stumbles and falls); and general ambiance of the facility (e.g., pleasant, relaxed, clean, organized, and orderly or hurried, hostile, and hectic jobs).

II. **Time activity analyses**

- **Job activity analysis** is similar to a job description. It is used to estimate the whole job and define its overall physical workload demands to establish the need for a recovery time that will bring the job demands within the worker's capacities.
- **Work task analysis** consists of a detailed recording of the pattern of activities over the shift, the distribution of heavy and light physical work, the time required to perform a task (used to assess time pressure), and the frequency of occurrence for more demanding activities. It is used to identify the tasks that are most likely to exceed the worker's capacities.
- **Work cycle analysis** measures the time to complete a task and is expressed in minutes. It is used to identify the variability in performance of a task and the potential fatigue factors (i.e., time to complete a task usually increases during a shift when fatigue is occurring).
- **Methods–time measurement (MTM)** is a technique in which work is broken down into elemental tasks such as "move, grasp, turn". It is used for evaluating individual efficiency of motion, especially on highly repetitive jobs (e.g., how long a highly repetitive task should take or how it can be modified to reduce the time required). It can also be used for setting production standards in some plants and for identifying where new methods can increase productivity. Because it is too finely divided, it is unable to make an accurate estimate of the energy demands and physiological stresses on the worker; therefore, it is less useful than work task or work cycle analysis for characterizing job demands.

III. **Motion analyses** are used to analyze complex, repetitive motions in industry (i.e., the frequency, degrees of rotation, duration, positions or postures, and dexterity or coordination requirements of a task); to determine the efficiency of motion and the effectiveness of training; and to investigate movements that might contribute to joint irritation. They include goniometry (e.g., electrogoniometers; see Chapter 2.5, section I.B.4) and photometric or video-based motion analysis systems (see Chapter 2.5, section I.E).

IV. **Biomechanical analyses** include the use of force transducers (dynamometers and cable tensiometers; see Chapter 2.5, section II.D), force plates (to study ground reaction force that resists the feet during standing, walking, and running, and which can be used to study the dynamic aspects of industrial tasks when a worker is standing, walking, or lifting), electromyography (EMG), accelerometers (to help determine limb vibration), and motion analysis systems. These devices can be used to follow the motion of the limb during task performance; to identify the maximum torque in the most active muscles; to determine the time of contraction for each muscle group and derive the recovery time (to assess work endurance); to define resistance force and the direction of force; to determine the exact position of the joint around which the muscles are active; and to determine if there are any postural changes. Some applications of biomechanical analyses include assessment of back stress during manual lifting activities (e.g., by measuring reach, forces and torques, and load weight and dimensions; see Chapter 2.5, section III); evaluation of the effects of different body postures during seated and standing work; determination of the effects of vibration or cumulative stress on the joints; and for setting work speed according to the time of contraction and the derived recovery time.

V. **Cardiovascular and metabolic measurements of job demands**

- **Heart or pulse rate** is the most convenient measure of the physiological cost of work, for example, the time required for the heart rate to return to a pre-exercise level can be used to evaluate work stress and individual fitness levels. Heart or pulse rate can be measured by palpation (radial pulse, carotid pulse), radiotelemetry, or continuous electrocardiogram.
- **Blood pressure** is not commonly used because its measurement requires that the work be stopped during the measurement period. The blood pressure can be used to evaluate the stress of postural static work, which may show very high blood pressure changes with minimal heart rate changes.
- **Minute ventilation** measures the volume of gas breathed out per minute to determine the respiratory demand of work. The expired volume is measured by breathing through a spirometer, which mechanically determines the volume per breath (tidal volume) and accumulates the volume measurement over several breaths (respiratory rate) for a fixed time period, such as 1 minute. To collect the expired air, the worker must wear a partial face mask or a mouthpiece and nose clip, which can become a problem when communication and good visual control are needed on the job. Minute ventilation is usually measured in conjunction with measurement of oxygen consumption and carbon dioxide production. During sample taking, the worker must be in a steady state (i.e., the ventilation rate is not changing frequently) to reflect an average of all of the activities performed during the time of the sample.
  - **Oxygen consumption** in the lungs is determined by measuring the amount of air exchanged per minute (minute ventilation) and determining the amount of oxygen in the inspired and expired air. The difference between the amount of oxygen breathed in and the amount breathed out is the measure of the amount consumed. In reporting the oxygen consumption values for a job or task, one should include the average demands over the shift, the working demands over the shift weighted for the amount of time spent in each activity, and the peak demands.
  - **Carbon dioxide production** is estimated by measuring the minute ventilation and the amount of carbon dioxide in the expired air. It is very reliable if the work sustains a steady state for at least 5 minutes so adequate amounts of expired air sample can be collected.

b. ***Situational assessments*** involve placing a worker into a realistic work situation and systematically altering variables, such as physical demands or stress factors, to ascertain the worker's performance under each circumstance (e.g., how will a worker's performance be affected by increasing the distance a load must be transported?).

c. ***Psychometric instruments*** include numerous pencil-and-paper as well as apparatus instruments used for measuring vocational interests, general intelligence, achievement, aptitude, personality, and other related psychological issues. These tests are commonly used in chronic pain patients who are unable to return to their former job duties. They can be used to delineate the individual's response to pain and stress (e.g., depression, coping strategies, and self-image of pain and disability), to identify the patient's interpersonal and vocational strengths and weaknesses, and to determine the best method to motivate the patient to succeed in the rehabilitation program. Most of these tests are described in Chapter 2.9 and in Chapter 5.10, section IV).

I. **Vocational interest tests** are designed to identify broad categories of work with characteristics that an individual would find suitable. Examples include: Wide Range Interest-Opinion Test (WRIOT); California Occupational

Preference Survey (COPS); Strong-Campbell test; Work Values Inventory; and Kuder Occupational Interest Survey.

II. **General aptitude tests** are useful in vocational counseling for placement in work settings or training programs. Examples include: Differential Aptitude Tests (DAT); General Aptitude Test Battery (GATB); and Oral Directions Test (ODT). The GATB has been standardized for more than 450 different occupations, especially in unskilled and semi-skilled areas, and it is useful for individuals with limited transferable skills.

III. **Specific aptitude tests** are used for further evaluation of specific aptitudes recognized to be important in particular vocations. Examples include: Bennett Mechanical Comprehension Test; Revised Minnesota Paper Form Board Test; Minnesota Clerical Test; Computer Operator Aptitude Battery; Computer Programmer Aptitude Battery; MacQuarrie Test for Mechanical Ability; General Clerical Test; and SRA Tests of Clerical Aptitude.

IV. **General intelligence tests** (see Chapter 2.9, section II) include: Wechsler Adult Intelligence Scale, III (WAIS-III); Stanford-Binet Intelligence Test, fifth edition (SB5); Peabody Picture Vocabulary; and California Test of Mental Maturity. In some cases, memory assessments may be used to provide a memory quotient.

V. **Achievement tests** (see Chapter 2.9, section III) are used to determine past learning performance. Examples include: Wide Range Achievement Test-3 (WRAT-3); Woodcock-Johnson III Psycho-Educational Battery (WJ-III) Tests of Achievement; Adult Basic Learning (ABLE); and Peabody Individual Achievement Test-Revised (PIAT-R).

VI. **Personality inventories** (see Chapter 2.9, section I) that assess major personality characteristics related to personal and social adjustment can help to determine an individual's suitability for adapting to particular work environments. Examples include: Minnesota Multiphasic Personality Inventory-2 (MMPI-2); Millon Clinical Multiaxial Inventory III (MCMI-III); Millon Behavioral Health Inventory (MBHI); the Neuroticism, Extroversion, and Openness Personality Inventory-Revised (NEO-PI-R); Strong Interest Inventory (SII), Sixteen Personality Factors Questionnaire (16PF), and the Edwards Personal Preference Schedule (EPPS).

VII. **Tests for depression** (see Chapter 2.9, section VII) include the Beck Depression Inventory (BDI) and the Zung Self-Rating Depression Scale.

VIII. **Multidimensional pain questionnaires** (see Chapter 5.10, section IV.C.2.b) include the McGill–Melzack Pain Questionnaire (MPQ), the West Haven–Yale Multidimensional Pain Inventory (WHYMPI), and the Emory University Pain Estimate Chart.

IX. **Functional status or life-style impact scales** (see Chapter 5.10, section IV.D.1) include the Sickness Impact Profile (SIP) and Activity Diaries.

X. **Tests of general psychopathology in chronic pain patients** (see Chapter 5.10, section IV.D.2) include the Symptom Checklist 90-revised (SCL-90R) and the Millon Behavioral Health Inventory (MBHI).

XI. **Other psychological tests** include the Back Stress Indices Determination and the Symptom Magnification Testing.

d. ***Work samples*** are the primary technique of work evaluation used to assess an individual's vocational aptitude, worker characteristics, and vocational interests. They consist of a well-defined work activity involving tasks, materials, and tools that are identical or similar to those in an actual job or cluster of jobs. In addition to the systems described below, other work sample series include Singer Vocational Evaluation System, the Philadelphia Jewish Employment and Vocational Service Work Sample Battery, the Talent Assessment Program, the Key Functions Assessment, the Work Recovery Systems, the Isernhagen Work Systems, Blankenships, and ARCON, ERGASYS.

I. **Testing, Orientation, and Work Evaluation in Rehabilitation (TOWER) system** is the oldest complete work evaluation system originally developed and normed for people with physical disabilities. It is useful for thorough evaluation in limited areas and may take up to 3 weeks to complete. It is not commonly used because it has not been normed for the industry, and its applications are limited to jobs that relate to the TOWER work samples and do not relate to *Dictionary of Occupational Titles* classifications.

II. **Work Evaluation Systems Technology (WEST)** series of work samples commonly used in RTW programs include the WEST 2A-Whole Body Range of Motion Work Sample, the WEST 3-Comprehensive Weight System, WEST 4A-Upper Extremity Strength and Fatigue Tolerance Work Sample, and WEST 7-Bus Bench. They all include norms for healthy male college students or MTMs identified by the *Dictionary of Occupational Titles.*

III. **Valpar Component Work Samples (VCWS)** is the most widely used work assessment tool in the United States. It consists of subtests to measure those worker characteristics that have been found to be basic indicators of success within numerous job families. They are keyed to the worker traits listed in the *Dictionary of Occupational Titles* and include MTMs and norms derived from various groups of employed workers and special disability groups. There are at least 20 VCWS, the most popular of which include Small Tools (measures the person's ability to understand and work with small mechanical tools for repair of small appliances or for jewelry making), Upper Extremity Range of Motion (measures upper torso work tolerance), Multilevel Sorting (measures a person's ability to make decisions while performing tasks requiring physical manipulation and visual discrimination of colors, numbers, letters, and a combination of these), Simulated Assembly (measures a person's ability to do a task requiring repetitive physical manipulation and bilateral use of the upper limbs), Whole Body Range of Motion (measures the agility of a person's gross body movements as they relate to the functional ability to perform job tasks), and Dynamic Physical Capacities (composed of 28 individual tasks, such as lifting, climbing, stooping, and balancing, which are similar to those of a shipping and receiving clerk or parts order clerk).

IV. **Baltimore Therapeutic Equipment (BTE) Work Simulator II** is a computerized system that quantifies work output by measuring repetitive upper limb motions against measurable resistance over a specified amount of time. The BTE system consists of interchangeable attachments, which simulate the physical demands of most jobs, such as gripping, pinching, lifting, carrying, and reaching. It can be used to estimate work tolerance, cardiac stress, and pulmonary stress, and to provide feedback for work hardening tasks.

VI. Work rehabilitation

Rehabilitation for work benefits the workers by making them learn ways to safely and productively do their job; by building their strength, flexibility and endurance; by hastening their return to gainful employment; by returning them to productive roles with family and coworkers; by helping them gain confidence in their physical ability to do the job; and by lessening their chances of a repeat or new injury. For the employer, work rehabilitation has the following benefits: reduction in direct costs, facilitation of claim settlement, increase in successful RTW attempts, improvement in employee job satisfaction, and regaining productive use of an injured employee. Case managers should ideally be involved in work rehabilitation (especially in chronic cases) to ensure that the worker does not get "lost in the system". Specifically, the case manager assesses job availability with the current employer or in another company and investigates the existence of light-duty alternatives or other jobs to which the patient's skills can be transferred. He or she also communicates with the insurer to be sure that prompt coverage is provided for the necessary diagnostic, therapeutic, and rehabilitative efforts and to be certain that the insurer fully understands the proposed program, expected outcome, and time frames. Communication with the worker is critical, thereby preventing any misunderstandings about diagnosis, treatment plans, and RTW options. The case manager also monitors attendance by the injured worker at appropriate therapy sessions; and helps ensure compliance if nonattendance occurs. RTW options should preferably be the same job with the same employer or even with a different employer. If this is not possible, then a more extensive vocational training program may be needed for a different job, preferably with the same employer.

A. **ACUTE (EARLY) INTERVENTIONS** include first-aid measures, as well as appropriate acute and postacute care. The goals of acute intervention are accurate diagnosis and appropriate treatment to facilitate the worker's safe return to work as soon as possible. The worker should be seen promptly after the injury and followed up closely at short intervals (daily if necessary) so he or she does not "get lost in the system". In the acute stage, about 80–85% of workers generally experience improvement and return to productive work. If symptoms (e.g., pain, stiffness, or weakness) persist longer than expected into the subacute phase, the treatment effort should be intensified to prevent chronicity (see section VI.A.2). In the subacute phase, the patient may need a structured and regularly scheduled therapy program focused around reconditioning (similar to the work conditioning program in section VI.B.1).

1. **Acute management** is generally directed toward the symptomatic treatment of pain (which is a major complaint in the acute phase) and other accompanying symptoms (e.g., sleep disorders). The acute management is described in Chapter 5.10. Often the **PRICE** (i.e., **P**rotection, **R**elative rest, **I**ce, **C**ompression, and **E**levation) treatment approach can be initially helpful. Studies have shown that rest should be limited in duration (e.g., 1–2 days of complete bed rest with bathroom privileges for patients with acute back pain). When resting, patients with acute back pain should lie in the supine or side-lying position with bent hips and knees, and if they need to be upright they should avoid full sitting, which is 40% more stressful on the back than standing (instead, the patient should stand or semi-sit on the back of a chair or on a high stool). Appropriate physical modalities (see Chapter 4.1) such as heat, cold, transcutaneous electrical nerve stimulation units, massage, and gentle stretching may be used with or without non-narcotic analgesics and/or anti-inflammatory agents (e.g., nonsteroidal anti-inflammatory drugs or steroids; all described in Chapter 4.8, sections I.A.3 and III respectively). Muscle relaxants and narcotics may also be helpful in the acute phase. Tricyclic antidepressants (see Chapter 4.8, section V.A) may be used to improve the accompanying sleep disorder and may also help reduce pain (probably by increasing pain threshold). Active exercises (e.g., mobility, resistance, or aerobic exercises – all described in Chapter 4.2, sections I to III) may be started as early as the third day postinjury to prevent deconditioning. Splints (e.g., wrist splints for patients with carpal tunnel syndrome, lumbosacral corsets for back pain patients, or cervical orthosis for neck pain patients) may be used temporarily. As acute symptoms subside, use of medications, physical modalities, and splints should be decreased, but active exercises should increase.
2. **Preventive measures** must be initiated in the acute or subacute phase to prevent future recurrences. Instead of symptomatic treatment, preventive measures should be directed towards the underlying factors (e.g., poor physical conditioning, unhealthy life-style, poor posture and body mechanics, and poor working

conditions), which led to the injury in the first place. Patients must be taught about the underlying causes as well as the anatomy and pathomechanics of musculoskeletal injuries. Patient education may be given individually or in groups (e.g., Back School or Neck School). See Chapter 5.10, section VI.A for discussion of patient education techniques.

a. ***Early return to work*** (e.g., "light duty" or a modified job) is encouraged as long as the medical outcome is not compromised and no further tissue damage occurs. This helps prevent both physical and mental deconditioning.

b. ***Healthy life-style*** includes appropriate treatment for drug and alcohol abuse, cessation of smoking, proper nutrition (for weight loss if needed), regular conditioning exercises (i.e., mobility, resistance, and aerobic exercises – all described in Chapter 4.2), and relaxation exercises (described in Chapter 4.2, section VI).

c. ***Proper body mechanics***

I. **Postural awareness** can be trained through exercises (e.g., using McKenzie's "slouch-overcorrect" procedure or nontraditional techniques such as the Alexander technique or the Feldenkrais method) and patient education. The neck or back should be maintained either in a neutral (normal lordosis) or slightly extended position. A lumbar roll is useful in maintaining normal lumbar lordosis. Excessive forward bending and rotation of the neck or back should be avoided (because they increase spinal load and can overstretch the ligaments making them prone to injury). Workers who sit and do repetitive, monotonous, or static workload should be taught to take a stand-and-stretch moment (also called mini-break or pause gymnastics) every 20–30 minutes. This is not a break or rest period, but simply a means of getting the worker out of the chair to perform 2–3 minutes of gentle movements (see sample exercise program in Table 5.11-2) designed to loosen the muscles, break up the constrained posture, and improve blood flow and tendon lubrication in the affected areas.

II. **Proper lifting and carrying techniques** include the following practical points:

- Avoid excessive forward bending (because forward bending, even slightly, increases the back stress by 50%) by standing close to object and bending the knees even to pick up light objects or to reach for objects close to the ground (e.g., garage door handle located near the ground).
- Avoid trunk twisting, instead use the feet to pivot.
- Use the strong lower limb muscles for lifting (i.e., knee and hip extensors).
- Maintain normal lumbar lordosis.
- Use wide stance for balance and support.
- Use low loads. If heavy (e.g., 25 lb or 11.5 kg is considered heavy), get help from another person or use a mechanical lifting device.
- Pace the lift so it is sufficiently slow and deliberate to allow for the use of good body mechanics.
- Mentally lift (i.e., mentally plan and review the lifting or carrying techniques prior to carrying it out).
- Emphasize the lowering of the carried object as well as its lifting.
- Get a firm grasp on the object.
- Keep the load close to the body (especially moving objects such as babies or pets).
- Use symmetrical upper body motions to carry or move objects (e.g., use knapsack or two grocery bags instead of one).
- Put the shoulder strap of the bag on the opposite shoulder to even out the load.

Table 5.11-2 An example of a stand-and-stretch (or mini-break) program for people who sit

The following program takes 3 minutes to complete (each exercise is performed for 20 seconds).

1. Inhale slowly through your nose and gently exhale through your lips.
2. Drop your ear toward your shoulder and repeat on the other side.
3. Make circles with your shoulders by shrugging them up to your ears, pulling them back, and dropping them down.
4. Rotate your ankles in a circle to pump blood back up to your heart.
5. Place your hands on your pelvis and practice increasing and reducing the curve of your low back.
6. Drop your head down to your knees and rub the muscles on your back.
7. Place hands on your seat on either side of your hips. Push down and attempt to lift your weight off the chair.
8. When standing, support your low back with your hands and gently arch backwards.
9. Stand with your back flat against a wall and gently slide down the wall, 4 or 5 inches, bending your knees. Count to 3 and stand tall. If no wall is available, walk on site.
10. Sit up straight! Pull your head back while tucking your chin in.

Reprinted with permission of the Back School and Neck School programs of the Occupational and Industrial Orthopedic Center, Hospital for Joint Diseases-Orthopedic Institute, New York, NY.

- Push instead of pull (use firm grasp on load; keep a wide stance by putting one foot in front of the other; stay down low; and shift weight in the legs as needed).
- Use a wheeled cart (with wheels sufficiently maintained and large enough to allow smooth movement and to easily clear obstacles such as irregularities in the workplace floor).

d. ***Ergonomic intervention*** refers to human factors designed to fit or accommodate the workplace to the individual and to enhance worker comfort, safety, and productivity.

I. **Workplace redesign** includes modification in the workspace design (see Chapter 4.5, section II.B.2.e for barrier-free architectural design) or tools and equipment. The traditional workplace in the United States is based on anthropometric measurements of selected men or women in the Air Force and is inappropriate for the increasing number of women in the workforce today (especially minority women with different anthropometric measurements). Ideally, the furniture should be fully adjustable for use in multiple tasks. If the company cannot afford new furniture, modifications may be made, such as elevating the chair and providing footstools if the work surface is too high; elevating the work surface with blocks if it is too low; using pillows or lumbar rolls if chairs are too deep; or wrapping arm rests in foam if they are too short or too widely separated.

- **Visibility distance**, which is the distance needed between the eye and the work object (e.g., computer screen or book), should be about 12 inches or adjusted to the worker's focal distance (if wearing glasses) to prevent leaning forward to see. While holding the head upright and looking straight ahead, the eye should focus a little below the horizontal top of the book or screen to prevent head extension. Workers are discouraged from wearing bifocals to prevent the backward tilting of the head.

- **Lighting** must be sufficient to see well, and there should be no blinding reflections.
- **Work surface** should have the same height as the level of the elbow. The traditional work surface height of 29–31 inches (74–79 cm) for a 5′10″ (1.79 m) man is inappropriate for a 5′1″ (1.57 m) female who needs a surface height of 23–25 inches (58–63 cm). Everything on the work surface should be arranged so that it is within easy reach and, if tilt is needed, the surface (not the person's head) should be tilted.
- **Keyboards and peripherals** (e.g., mouse and trackball) should be positioned so that the worker can type with shoulders relaxed, elbows comfortably at the side of the body, and bent at a 90° angle or slightly more open. The worker should also be provided with a wrist rest for the keyboard and a separate one for the mouse or trackball. Ideally, the wrist rest should have a foam core, a smooth surface (e.g., felt, or, for multiusers, vinyl) and rounded edges. It should extend under the keyboards so that it is weighted down, and it should be about 4 inches deep by 1–1.5 inches thick (10 cm by 2.5–3.8 cm; i.e., deep enough to comfortably support the wrist during use of all keys including the space bar and thick enough so that the wrist of the user is not extended or flexed in use). It should also be placed at the edge of the work surface to eliminate ulnar pressure from the sharp edge of the desk. Adjustable forearm support (clamped on the work surface edge and articulated for full movement of the forearms) may also be used.
- **Chairs** should have a back support below the shoulder blades, a well-designed lumbar support (detachable or adjustable lumbar rolls or pillows may be used), swivel and rollers (to avoid twisting the spine), arm rests for support, and adjustable seat height. The seat height should allow the feet to rest comfortably flat on the floor or footrest with hips and knees bent at about 90°. The seat edge should be rounded and the seat depth should be three-quarters of leg length. A high sit–stand stool on which the worker can lean back against a semi-sit surface is useful if the worker has a high work surface and needs to frequently stand.
- **Phone adaptations** are described in Chapter 4.5, section II.A.4.d. For those involved in heavy phone work, a headset is effective in preventing neck and upper back problems associated with trying to hold the phone between the neck and shoulder while using the hands for a different task.
- **Tool adaptations** include grip modification (e.g., covering tool handles with caulking or thermophylic plastic to make them larger, softer, and rougher to reduce the force of grip and wrist deviation or covering mouse or trackballs with a piece of sponge to provide a custom grip and to reduce the finger flexion needed to depress the buttons) and toolweight modification to increase functional efficiency.

II. **Administrative changes** include rotation of job assignments (e.g., by cross-training), staggered breaks, encouraging breaks away from work area, regular supervised stand-and-stretch mini-breaks (see Table 5.11-2), varying of work tasks (to reduce repetitiveness), lowering production rates (e.g., slow down typing rates), allowing only limited overtime, training employees on safe and efficient use of equipment (e.g., keying with forearms and wrists relaxed), and proper pre-employment selection.

B. CHRONIC INTERVENTION is indicated in a small percentage of workers (about 10%) who still have pain complaints and physical disabilities that prevent return to work after the completion of acute and subacute care. It is well recognized that the longer workers are off the job (whether measured as time since date of injury or last date worked), the more difficult it becomes to return them to work (regardless of the type of impairment). In chronic cases (i.e., more than 3–6 months consecutively out of work), the initial injury is often resolved, but because of prolonged inactivity and sedentary life-style, the worker may develop chronic weakness and deconditioning as well as inflexibility and poor endurance. In addition, the worker may also be psychologically deconditioned. They also tend to smoke more, drink more, and take more medications than they were taking prior to the injury. Other characteristics of chronicity include patient's negative perception of disability, disability claims for compensation, subjective complaints that are disproportionate to objective signs, symptom magnification (see section V.B.3), lack of motivation to recover, and negative attitude to work return.

1. **Work conditioning** is a RTW program consisting of progressive structured reconditioning, which is recommended for a patient with an uncomplicated injury but whose physical limitations preclude return to work. It is typically provided as a unidisciplinary or bidisciplinary (i.e., occupational or physical therapy, or both) program that uses exercise, aerobic conditioning, education, and limited work tasks to restore an individual's systemic and neuromusculoskeletal function (strength, endurance, movement, flexibility, and motor control). The treatment focus is on active rehabilitation and physical restoration rather than passive modalities and medications. Work conditioning is usually tailored to the specific needs of the job (determined by worksite visit, if possible; see section V.D.2.a), e.g. emphasizing upper torso exercises for jobs requiring upper torso functions. It can usually be made acceptable to the worker if it is presented as a sports medicine model of treatment (e.g., using the analogy of an injured athlete who initially requires a period of rest after an acute injury, after which the athlete has to return to the training room to restore fitness before returning to competition). The work conditioning program usually consists of half-day sessions given three to five times per week for a relatively short period of time (e.g., 3–6 weeks) with periodic reassessment of the worker's fitness level and work capacity. When the worker is sufficiently conditioned to perform light duties, the worker is usually returned to the job, and arrangements are made to continue the conditioning program until the worker has maximally improved or has met the requirements for returning to the original job.
2. **Work hardening** (also called work simulation, work readiness training, or work rehabilitation) is a work-oriented, highly structured, individualized program that uses the interdisciplinary approach to provide a transition for the deconditioned, disabled worker to return him or her to work-ready status through progressively strenuous work (real or simulated) or work-related activities. Unlike work conditioning, which is limited to the physical components of flexibility, strength, coordination, and endurance for RTW, work hardening is more comprehensive because it also integrates behavioral and vocational components of the RTW process. Work hardening is recommended for workers who have been off work for protracted periods of time (e.g., longer than 3–6 months) and whose injury and physical limitations are complicated by more severe deconditioning as well as by psychosocial factors that interfere with ability to return to work. The interdisciplinary team members (i.e., physician, physical therapist, occupational therapist, psychologist, vocational specialist, social worker, ergonomist, and industrial engineer) must have a complete understanding of the worker's job and work conditions. Since 1988 (updated in 1992), the guidelines from the Commission of Accreditation for Rehabilitation Facilities (CARF) have ensured the quality of work-hardening programs for structure and content.

   The work-hardening process includes job analysis (see section V.D.2.a), establishing a work-tolerance baseline (e.g., medical history, worker interview, job description with critical work demands, pain assessment, physical assessment, lifting and carrying ability, pushing and pulling, stooping and bending, kneeling and crawling, sitting and standing, and work-task simulation), and an individualized work-hardening plan with the goal of maximizing the patient's functional improvement while simultaneously providing it in a safe environment. Other goals are increasing physical tolerance identified as deficient for critical work demands, attaining optimal work tolerance and ability, increasing proficiency with work adaptations or assistive devices, reducing fear and increasing confidence for resumption of productive work, developing problem-solving skills for self-management at the worksite, facilitating appropriate worker behaviors (e.g., timeliness, attendance, and dress), maximizing cognitive and psychosocial functioning, and identifying problems that may require placement in an alternative job.

Although physical modalities and medications may be used to help reduce pain perception and increase work tolerance, active exercise remains the single most important approach for the greatest number of patients. Aside from continuing to emphasize generalized conditioning (similar to that provided by the work-conditioning program), work hardening also incorporates job-specific work-task simulation activities (e.g., if the job requires the patient to lift boxes, then box lifting is incorporated into the program), which can be graded in difficulty or length of time involved. A typical program initially trains the patient to develop endurance for remaining in static positions, including sitting and standing postures, while performing activities. As the patient's tolerance improves, additional work-type activities (e.g., lifting, carrying, bending, kneeling, or climbing – depending on the patient's work requirements) are added. Examples of work-hardening modalities include a balance monitor that provides feedback on weight bearing and symmetry of posture; a multiworkstation, which simulates construction jobs; a truck or a car simulator with a computerized video road screen to simulate and measure the driving process; a computerized pneumatic lift to simulate the lifting process; an upper-limb work simulator (e.g., BTE) to simulate various upper-limb work tasks (including reaching overhead and manipulating tools); and a lower-limb simulator (e.g., foot controls). Most of these modalities are homemade, although many are commercially available.

Work-hardening programs also try to simulate actual working conditions (e.g., the worker is required to clock in and out daily; breaks are scheduled; and warehouse or other "work-like" settings are used, instead of a medical clinic or hospital, to minimize the worker's perception of illness and sickness). Patients also maintain an activity log to develop a sense of responsibility for their own rehabilitation and pain control. Another integral part of the program is education in proper use of the body to avoid reinjury, proper pacing on the job, relaxation (e.g., biofeedback, hypnosis, and progressive muscle relaxation techniques), stress management skills, assertiveness, interpersonal skills to facilitate conflict avoidance and resolution, and maintaining a healthy life-style. Education can be provided through discussion, demonstration, active participation, and audiovisual aids. It may be given individually or in a group setting (e.g., Back or Neck School).

A typical schedule for work hardening is usually 5 days per week (4 or 8 h/day) for up to 6–12 weeks. Treatment time is gradually increased to equal the person's premorbid work schedule. The cost of these programs is relatively high, but well-organized programs often have favorable success rates. Work hardening is most effective in patients who are motivated to return to work, have jobs available, and are free of overwhelming psychological or secondary gain issues, which can undermine progress. Return-to-work rates, obtained from individual programs that carefully select their clients, range from 50–60% to 85–88%. The RTW rate decreases as the length of disability (whether measured as time since date of injury or last date worked) increases. The chance of returning to work after 6 months of disability is about 50%. By 1 year, it decreases to about 25%;

and by 2 years, almost no patient returns to work even with exhaustive rehabilitation measures.

3. **Vocational training** is considered if the injured worker does not have the option of returning to his or her former job because of inability to physically meet the job demands despite work conditioning or work hardening; poor worker–job match, which would increase the risk of reinjury; lack of desire on the worker's part to return to the former job; or lack of willingness on the former employer's part to accept the worker back on the job. Vocational training refers to the actual training program the worker has to undergo to learn the chosen trade or profession. It involves an interdisciplinary team effort coordinated by the vocational counselor.

   The vocational counselor should be familiar with job options in the geographic area and be able to assist the individual with formulating a reasonable plan in finding a suitable vocation and training program. After medical clearance by a physician, the patient is given vocational testing (e.g., vocational interest inventories, achievement testing, aptitude testing, and assessment of the ability to perform work activities) and psychological testing to determine aptitude for specific vocations and for various levels of vocational or educational training (e.g., vocational school, junior college, and college). If the patient does not have a job after training, the vocational counselor can assist with job or volunteer work placements. The vocational counselor may also coach the prospective worker on filling out a job application, preparing a resumé, dressing for and conducting oneself at a job interview as well as on the job, dealing with authority figures and coworkers effectively, dealing with stress or conflict in the work situation, and managing finances. For prospective workers with physical impairments (e.g., head injuries or spinal cord injuries), the physical and occupational therapists as well as the ergonomist, industrial engineer, or employer can help formulate specific job and workplace adaptations or modifications.

4. **Chronic pain center treatment program** is an interdisciplinary team approach that focuses on behavioral modification, exercise for reactivation, stress reduction, and pain management. It is recommended as the last resort for workers with chronic pain whose primary nociceptive insult may no longer account for the greater part of the patient's disability and who are resistant to the above methods. Drug (e.g., narcotic) detoxification (e.g., using "pain cocktail" described in Chapter 5.10, section VI.E.3) may be necessary and antidepressant medications may be used for sleep and for pain modification. Psychologic counseling may be needed for the patient and family (to help them understand and adjust to the patient's behavior). Because most of these patients will not return to their previous employment, alternative vocational strategies (e.g., vocational training as in section VI.B.3) should be incorporated in the program.

Further reading

Burt CM: Work evaluation and work hardening. In Pedretti LW, Early MB, editors: *Occupational therapy practice skills for physical dysfunction*, ed 5, St Louis, 2001, Mosby, pp. 226–236.

Chaffin DB, Andersson GBJ, Martin BJ: *Occupational biomechanics*, ed 3, New York, 1999, Wiley-Interscience.

Cocchiarella L, Andersson GBJ, editors: *American Medical Association: guides to the evaluation of permanent impairment*, ed 5, Chicago, 2001, American Medical Association.

Commission on Accreditation of Rehabilitation Facilities (CARF): *Guidelines for work hardening programs*, Chicago, 1988, CARF.

Commission on Accreditation of Rehabilitation Facilities (CARF): *Standards manual for organizations serving people with disabilities*, Tucson, AZ, 1992, CARF.

Demeter SL, Andersson GBJ, editors: *American Medical Association: disability evaluation*, ed 2, St Louis, 2003, Mosby.

Eastman Kodak Company: *Kodak's ergonomic design for people at work*, ed 2, Hoboken, NJ, 2004, John Wiley & Sons.

Herrington TM, Morse LH, editors: *Occupational injuries: evaluation, management, and prevention*, St Louis, 1995, Mosby-Year Book.

Jacobs K: Preparing for return to work. In Trombly CA, Radomski MV, editors: *Occupational therapy for physical dysfunction*, ed 4, Philadelphia, 1995, Williams & Wilkins, pp. 329–349.

Matheson LN, Ogden L, Violette K, *et al.*: Work hardening: occupational therapy in industrial rehabilitation. *Am J Occup Ther* 39(5):314–321, 1985.

National Institute for Occupational Safety and Health (NIOSH): *Applications manual for the revised NIOSH lifting equation*, DHHS (NIOSH) Publication No. 94-110. Cincinnati, OH, 1994, US Department of Health and Human Services.

Scheer SJ, Weinstein SM: Industrial rehabilitation medicine. 1. An overview. *Arch Phys Med Rehabil* 73:S356–S359, 1992.

Scheer SJ, Mital A: Ergonomics. *Arch Phys Med Rehabil* 78:S36–S45, 1997.

Schuchmann JA: Occupational rehabilitation. In Braddom RL, editor: *Physical medicine and rehabilitation*, ed 2, Philadelphia, 2000, WB Saunders, pp. 984–1004.

Smith P: American with Disabilities Act: accommodating persons with disabilities. In Pedretti LW, Early MB, editors: *Occupational therapy practice skills for physical dysfunction*, ed 5, St Louis, 2001, Mosby, pp. 237–248.

US Department of Labor Bureau of Labor Statistics data on injuries, illnesses, and fatalities. Available at: *http://data.bls.gov*. Accessed August 8, 2004.

United States Department of Labor Employment and Training Administration: *Dictionary of occupational titles*, vol II, ed 4, revised, Washington, DC, 1991, US Government Printing Office.

Waddell G, McCulloch JA, Kummel E, Verner RM: Nonorganic physical signs in low-back pain. *Spine* 5:117–125, 1980.

Weinstein SM, Scheer SJ: Industrial rehabilitation medicine. 2. Assessment of the problem, pathology, and risk factors for disability. *Arch Phys Med Rehabil* 73:S360–S365, 1992.

Williams CT, Reno VP, Burton Jr JF, *et al.*: *Workers' compensation: benefits, coverage, and costs, 2001*, Washington, DC, 2003, National Academy of Social Insurance.

CHAPTER 5.12
Chronic pulmonary problems

Chronic pulmonary diseases can be classified into those primarily causing oxygenation impairment [e.g., chronic obstructive pulmonary disease (COPD)], those causing primarily ventilatory impairment (e.g., chronic restrictive pulmonary disease, extrapulmonary cause), and those causing both. Patients with chronic pulmonary diseases tend to avoid activities for fear of causing pulmonary discomfort (e.g., dyspnea). This sedentariness leads to deconditioning, which makes physical exertion even more unpleasant, hence leading to a slow and insidious, but steady, downward spiral in physical capability. The purpose of pulmonary rehabilitation is to halt this downward spiral. Ideally, the pulmonary rehabilitation program should involve an interdisciplinary team, which, aside from the patient and the patient's support system, consists of physicians, physical therapists, occupational therapists, nurses, respiratory care practitioners (formerly called respiratory therapists), cardiopulmonary technologists, exercise physiologists, dietitians or nutritionists, speech–language pathologists, social workers, psychologists, vocational counselors, durable medical equipment suppliers, and other allied health professionals.

The general goals of pulmonary rehabilitation are to at least stabilize or possibly reverse both the physical and psychopathological aspects of the pulmonary disease, and to help the patient return to the highest possible functional capacity despite the pulmonary disease. Specific goals include measures to support or improve cardiopulmonary function as well as prevent and treat complications; foster compliance with medical regimens; reduce the number of exacerbations, emergency room visits, and hospitalizations; educate the patient to confront the disease realistically; prepare the patient to take responsibility for his or her rehabilitation and well-being; optimize psychosocial functioning and coping mechanisms; and return the patient to a more active, productive, and emotionally satisfying life.

According to the 1997 American College of Chest Physicians (ACCP) and American Association of Cardiovascular and Pulmonary Rehabilitation (AACVPR) Pulmonary Rehabilitation Guidelines Panel, pulmonary rehabilitation has the following documented benefits in COPD patients: reduced number of hospitalizations and number of days of hospitalization; reduced symptoms of dyspnea; improved health-related quality of life; and, possibly, increased survival. Patients with chronic pulmonary diseases may have a superimposed acute pulmonary disease (e.g., upper respiratory tract infection, common cold, or pneumonia). In acute pulmonary disease, treatment generally includes appropriate medications (e.g., antibiotics and bronchodilators) and a program of breathing exercises (to expand the lungs and increase breathing efficiency), secretion removal techniques (to enhance gas exchange), and general conditioning exercises (to maintain functional capacity).

According to the American Thoracic Society (ATS, 1999), pulmonary rehabilitation is indicated for patients with chronic respiratory impairment who, despite optimal medical management, are dyspneic, have reduced exercise tolerance, or experience a restriction in activities. The need for pulmonary rehabilitation should be dictated by the symptoms, disability, and handicap, not the severity of physiologic impairment of the lungs (thus, there are no specific pulmonary function criteria that can be used to indicate the need for pulmonary rehabilitation). This chapter gives an overview of pulmonary rehabilitation as it pertains only to chronic pulmonary problems encountered in the PM&R setting.

I. Epidemiology

In 1998, COPD and allied conditions were the fourth leading cause of death and the fourth largest cause of major activity limitation (including loss of work days and premature retirement because of disability) in the United States. The incidence of COPD has doubled since 1970, and the prevalence has been increasing. In patients with traumatic tetraplegia and neuromuscular disorders, the most common cause of premature death is respiratory insufficiency.

II. Pulmonary evaluation

A. HISTORY

1. **Chief complaint**. Dyspnea (most common symptom of individuals with chronic pulmonary disease; see Table 5.12-1 for dyspnea grading), cough, sputum production, wheezing, fatigue, orthopnea, decreased exercise tolerance, morning headache, excessive drowsiness (with particular attention to symptom frequency), precipitating factors (such as infection, allergy, and humidity), relieving factors, complicating factors, rate of progression, and past treatments.
2. **Past and present occupational history**. Exposures to toxins and irritants.
3. **Functional history**. Effect of pulmonary disease on self-care and on vocational and avocational activities.
4. **Allergy and medication history**. Prolonged use of corticosteroids can potentially cause osteoporosis.

Table 5.12-1 Questionnaire for grading dyspnea

Dyspnea grade	Question*
I	"Are you ever troubled by breathlessness, other than on strenuous exertion?"
II	"Are you short of breath when hurrying on level ground or walking up a slight hill?"
III	"Do you have to walk slower than most people on level ground? Do you have to stop after a mile or so (or after 15 minutes) when you walk on level ground at your own pace?"
IV	"Do you have to stop for breath after walking about 100 yards (or after a few minutes) on level ground?"
V	"Are you too breathless to leave the house or breathless after undressing?"

**An affirmative answer to one of the questions establishes a patient's grade.*
From: Nishimura K, Izumi T, Tsukino M, et al.: *Dyspnea is a better predictor of 5-year survival than airway obstruction in patients with COPD.* Chest *121:1434–1440, 2002, with permission.*

5. **Personal history**. Smoking, alcohol consumption, and recreational or habitual drug use.
6. **Social history**. Home situation and architectural barriers, psychosocial history, and support system.
7. **Family history**. α-Antitrypsin deficiency, which predisposes the patient to emphysema.

B. **PHYSICAL EXAMINATION** is generally directed to the pulmonary (and cardiac) systems. Observe the patient's breathing rate (e.g., tachypnea), breathing pattern (e.g., shallow; abdominal; chest; pursed lip; paradoxical, i.e., inward motion of abdomen with inspiration; and respiratory alternans, i.e., alternating movements of the rib cage and abdomen are pathognomonic of diaphragmatic fatigue), chest shape (e.g., barrel-chested), posture (e.g., kyphosis, scoliosis, or forward-leaning posture described in section IV.B.4), respiratory muscle aids (e.g., ventilators), signs of advanced lung disease [e.g., use of accessory muscle activity during quiet breathing, jugular venous distention because of cor pulmonale, cyanosis (e.g., perioral and periorbital sites), clubbing, and dependent edema]; and capacity to clear secretions (e.g., cough). Auscultate the lungs (for decreased breath sounds, crackles or rales, wheezing, rhonchi) and heart (for tachycardia, arrhythmia, increased intensity of the pulmonic second sound). Check vital signs including temperature, blood pressure, height (which has a direct relationship with lung volumes), and weight (weight increase may be due to dependent edema or to generalized edema or anasarca secondary to right heart failure; unexplained loss may be due to carcinoma or other systemic disease). Also assess cognitive function, health status, emotional and mood state, and nutritional status (disturbances in body weight, body composition, and changes in eating habits are common in patients with advanced COPD).

C. **DIAGNOSTIC AND MONITORING TESTS**

1. **Radiographic tests** include chest radiographs (described in Chapter 5.13, section III.C.1), computed tomography scans, and magnetic resonance imaging scans to image the chest and the intrathoracic structures (to help identify tumors, infections, cardiovascular changes, lung parenchymal changes, etc.). They must be correlated with the clinical findings and may need to be done serially for follow-up.
2. **Cardiac tests** include electrocardiogram (ECG) (described in Chapter 5.13, section III.C.2a) and echocardiogram (described in Chapter 5.13, section III.C.2.b) to rule out cardiac dysfunctions, which may contribute to pulmonary problems.
3. **Laboratory tests**

a. ***Blood tests,*** such as complete blood count (hemoglobin and hematocrit), serum electrolytes, serum protein electrophoresis (for α_1-antitrypsin), and serum prealbumin or albumin (to determine nutritional status).

b. ***Sputum examination*** (microscopy, Gram stain, culture and sensitivity, cytology) to help diagnose specific infections and malignant conditions.

c. ***Blood gas monitoring*** includes arterial blood gas (ABG) (see Chapter 2.6, section IV.A), capillary blood gas monitoring, transcutaneous or pulse oximetry (see Chapter 2.6, section IV.B), and capnography (end-tidal CO_2 monitoring). Although ABG testing is more accurate than other methods, obtaining the arterial sample may be difficult in about 25% of patients [if the patient either hyperventilates or hypoventilates during ABG sampling (because of anxiety or pain), the ABG result may not reflect the patient's actual pulmonary condition]. The invasive ABG sampling is usually unnecessary in stable patients without intrinsic pulmonary disease. Daytime ABG for confirming suspicions of nocturnal hypoventilation may be misleading (as it may be normal) in patients with severe paralytic respiratory insufficiency (but no intrinsic lung disease). In these patients, pulse oximetry and capnography, both of which are noninvasive methods, are useful for continuous overnight monitoring of their blood gases. Pulse oximetry and capnography are also useful for monitoring the patient's blood gases during exercise.

d. ***Pulmonary function tests (PFTs)*** are fully described in Chapter 2.6. They include tests of ventilation (i.e., lung volumes and flow rate), pulmonary mechanics (airway resistance and lung compliance), lung diffusion capacity, and blood gases (see section II.C.3.c). In the PM&R setting, they are primarily used to differentiate between obstructive and restrictive pulmonary disorders and to estimate the severity and progression of a disease. They are usually carried out with the patient seated; however, in patients with chronic alveolar hypoventilation (CAH), PFTs should also be done in the supine position. For functional classification of pulmonary impairment or disability based on PFT, see Table 5.12-2.

e. ***Integrated cardiopulmonary (CP) exercise tolerance tests*** are fully described in Chapter 2.7, section II. They are used to assess cardiovascular and pulmonary parameters during exercise in patients with an established pulmonary diagnosis to determine a safe and individualized prescription of exercise or activity (e.g., intensity of exercise or activity or need for O_2 supplementation during exercise or activity). They include the cardiopulmonary graded exercise tolerance tests (CP-GXTT) (see Chapter 2.7, section II.A) using treadmill or bicycle ergometers for 6–12 minutes and the timed-walking test (see section

Table 5.12-2 Impairment classification for respiratory disorders, using pulmonary function and exercise test results

Parameters	CLASS 1 (0% impairment of the whole person)	CLASS 2† (10–25% impairment of the whole person)	CLASS 3† (26–50% impairment of the whole person)	CLASS 4 (51–100% impairment of the whole person)
FVC	≥80% Pr **and**	60–79% Pr **or**	51–59% Pr **or**	≤50% Pr **or**
FEV_1	≥80% Pr **and**	60–79% Pr **or**	41–59% Pr **or**	≤40% Pr **or**
FEV_1/FVC*	≥0.70 **and**			
D_{LCO}	≥70% Pr **or**	60–69% Pr **or**	41–59% Pr **or**	≤40% Pr **or**
VO_2max‡	>25 **or**	20–25	15–20	<15
METs‡	>7.1	5.7–7.1	4.3–5.7	<4.3
Comment	Must meet all the PFT criteria	Must meet only one PFT criterion	Must meet only one PFT criterion	Must meet only one PFT criterion

% Pr, per cent of predicted value; FVC, forced vital capacity; FEV_1, forced expiratory volume in 1 second; D_{LCO}, lung diffusion capacity using carbon monoxide.

** The ratio FEV_1/FVC is expressed as an absolute number (rather than as % Pr which can be confusing).*

† In classes 2 and 3, if the FVC, FEV_1, and FEV_1/FVC ratio are normal and the D_{LCO} is between 41% and 79%, then an exercise test is required.

‡ VO_2max (see Chapter 2.7, section II.A) = maximum volume of oxygen consumption [expressed in mL O_2/min/kg; can be converted into metabolic equivalents (METs) by dividing VO_2max with 3.5, since 1 MET = 3.5 mL of O_2 consumed/kg/min].

Data adapted from: Cocchiarella L, Andersson GBJ, editors: American Medical Association: Guides to the evaluation of permanent impairment, *ed 5, Chicago, 2001, American Medical Association, p. 107; American Thoracic Society: Evaluation of impairment/disability secondary to respiratory disease.* Am Rev Respir Dis *133:1206, 1986.*

VI.B.1.a; Chapter 2.7, section II.C), which involves the patient walking as far as possible in 12 minutes (may be modified to 6 or even 2 or 3 minutes for some patients).

f. ***Special pulmonary studies*** may occasionally be performed. They include

I. **Comprehensive sleep study**, which uses oral, nasal, or oronasal masks to detect airflow; chest wall monitoring to detect respiratory efforts; pulse oximetry to document desaturation; electroencephalogram (EEG) and electro-oculogram (EOG) to monitor the stages of sleep; ECG to detect hypoxia-induced arrhythmias; and chin electromyography (EMG). This is indicated only in COPD patients suspected of having sleep apnea/hypopnea syndrome (SAHS) or in those who have cor pulmonale or polycythemia and whose daytime arterial oxygen tension (PaO_2) is above 60 mmHg. In these patients (who are already hypoxemic when awake), overnight monitoring using only oximetry and capnography may be difficult to interpret.

II. **Airway reactivity tests** such as the bronchoprovocation test using methacholine inhalation to detect asthma.

III. Classification by etiology

A. CHRONIC OBSTRUCTIVE PULMONARY DISEASE, including emphysema, chronic bronchitis, bronchiectasis, asthma, and cystic fibrosis, is characterized by air trapping, increased flow work or energy expended in moving air, and normal or increased compliance. Pulmonary function test patterns (summarized in Table 2.6-2) generally show a decreased ratio of forced expiratory volume in 1 second to forced vital capacity (FEV_1/FVC), as well as low $FEF_{25-75\%}$, (i.e., the forced expiratory flow rate at 25–75% of the FVC). During maximal voluntary ventilation, the respiratory baseline gradually rises (as a result of air trapping) as ventilation progresses. The FEV_1 in COPD decreases by 45–75 mL per year, which is three times the normal rate of decline caused by aging. When the FEV_1 is less than 1500 mL, exertional dyspnea often occurs. In COPD patients with FEV_1 less than 750 mL, 30% die within 1 year and 50% within 3 years.

B. CHRONIC RESTRICTIVE PULMONARY DISEASES are characterized by reduction in the following PFT parameters (summarized in Table 2.6-2): total lung capacity (TLC), vital capacity (VC), residual volume (RV), expiratory reserve volume (ERV), functional residual capacity, minute ventilation, and compliance. Because air flow rates remain normal, however, the FEV_1/FVC ratio remains normal or may be increased. There is also increased elastic workload (i.e., energy consumed in stretching the elastic tissues of the lung) for which the patient compensates by producing rapid, shallow breathing. Unless the lungs are expanded by effective deep insufflations, these shallow breaths can eventually lead to atelectasis and hypoxia.

In addition, chronic restrictive pulmonary diseases often progress to CAH, which may be defined by the presence of chronic hypercapnia. Common symptoms of CAH include fatigue, dyspnea, headaches (morning or continuous), loss of concentration and memory, anxiety, personality changes (e.g., depression and irritability), sleep disturbances (e.g., daytime drowsiness, difficulty falling asleep, frequent awakening at night with shortness of breath, violent nightmares, difficulty awaking in the morning), and difficulty in managing airway secretions (especially with weak oropharyngeal and abdominal muscles). Sequelae of CAH include pulmonary problems (e.g., atelectasis, pneumonia, pulmonary scarring, decreased lung compliance, impaired ventilation/perfusion ratio, and pulmonary hypertension); cardiovascular problems (e.g., cor pulmonale, arrhythmia, systemic hypertension, and polycythemia); psychosocial problems (e.g., because of hypersomnolence, loss of concentration, anxiety, and irritability); and muscle aches and stiffness. The greater the severity of the CAH, the greater the risk of acute respiratory failure (which can be triggered by innocuous respiratory tract insults, fatigue, or stress). Chronic restrictive pulmonary diseases that can cause CAH can be classified into the following five categories:

1. **Neuromuscular causes** (the most common cause of neuromuscular respiratory failure in the United States is Guillain–Barré syndrome).

a. ***Suprasegmental CNS nuclei and pathways including upper motor neuron disease*** causing central alveolar hypoventilation syndrome because of idiopathic causes (Ondine's curse), brain disorders (Arnold–Chiari malformation, stroke, extrapyramidal disorders), spinal cord disorders (e.g., cervical or upper thoracic spinal cord injury, thoracic myelomeningocele, and syringomyelia), or both brain and spinal cord disorder (e.g., multiple sclerosis).

b. ***Combined upper and lower motor neuron disease,*** such as amyotrophic lateral sclerosis and progressive bulbar palsy.

c. ***Lower motor neuron disease*** involving the anterior horn cells (e.g., poliomyelitis, postpolio syndrome, and spinal muscular atrophies), peripheral nerves [e.g., Guillain–Barré syndrome, phrenic neuropathies, idiopathic or postsurgical diaphragm paralysis, polyneuropathies (because of toxic, metabolic, or infectious causes)], or neuromuscular junction (e.g., myasthenia gravis, Lambert–Eaton myasthenic syndrome, botulism, and organophosphate poisoning).

2. **Myopathic etiologies,** such as muscular dystrophies with dystrophinopathies (i.e., Duchenne's or Becker's), other muscular dystrophies (i.e., facioscapulohumeral, limb-girdle, and myotonic dystrophy), polymyositis, and congenital and metabolic myopathies.
3. **Chest wall and diaphragmatic defects,** such as kyphoscoliosis, ankylosing spondylitis, post-thoracotomy, and diaphragmatic hernia.
4. **Sleep disordered breathing,** which may be caused by SAHS or obesity.
5. **Primary pulmonary disorders,** for example tracheomalacia, bronchiectasis, chronic bronchitis, bronchopulmonary dysplasia, emphysema, cystic fibrosis, interstitial lung disease, adult respiratory distress syndrome, and chronic aspiration.

IV. Noninvasive management (see Table 5.12-3)

A. MEDICAL MODALITIES

1. General medical care

a. ***Cessation of smoking*** is the most important preventive component in the care of patients with chronic pulmonary diseases. Studies showed that cessation of smoking can decrease the excessive rate of decline in lung function associated with smoking. Smoke cessation techniques include the cognitive approach (e.g., information, books, articles, and physician's orders), propaganda (e.g., posters, brochures, and mass media messages), drugs (e.g., nicotine gum, patch, or nasal spray; buproprion), aversion–satiation (e.g., rapid smoking, imagination, smoky air in face or mouth, or electric shock), affective approach (e.g., fear), therapy programs (e.g., hypnosis, psychotherapy, smoking cessation clinics, and individual or group therapy), behavior modification (e.g., desensitization, role-playing, self-monitoring, sensory deprivation, and gradual reduction), and others (e.g., acupuncture, meditation, relaxation, and exercise). Resources on cessation of smoking are available from the American Lung Association (61 Broadway,

Table 5.12-3 Management options of chronic obstructive and restrictive pulmonary diseases

Classification	Management options
Obstructive	**Medical**: Medications (e.g., bronchodilator, pulmonary vaccines); nutrition therapy; hydration, cessation of smoking; patient education (avoid extremes of humidity and temperature, excessive fatigue, crowded areas) **Respiratory**: O_2 supplement to maintain $SaO_2 > 90\%$ (include home and/or long-term use); may consider nocturnal noninvasive intermittent positive pressure ventilation (IPPV) **PT/OT**: Controlled breathing techniques or CBT (e.g., diaphragmatic breathing; incentive spirometer; pursed lip breathing; paced breathing; ventilatory muscle training such as inspiratory resistive loading); secretion mobilization and airway clearance techniques; postural-relief techniques; abdominal strengthening exercises; general conditioning exercises [aerobic; extremity range-of-motion (ROM) and strengthening; avoid excessive fatigue]; energy and work conservation (including assistive and adaptive devices, and home modification); may combine CBT with biofeedback and relaxation techniques **Invasive**: Tracheal intubation **Others**: Psychosocial interventions; vocational counseling
Restrictive	**Medical**: Medications [e.g., vaccines (flu and bacterial); judicious use of antiviral agents (e.g., amantadine) or antibiotics; avoid sedatives and other drugs]; hydration; patient education (avoid obesity, heavy meals, extremes of humidity and temperature, excessive fatigue, crowded areas), cessation of smoking **Respiratory**: Mechanical ventilation (e.g., home ventilator; noninvasive IPPV; body ventilators); airway clearance management (consider *Mechanical In-Exsufflator*); use O_2 with caution; management of sleep disordered breathing **PT/OT**: CBT (e.g., diaphragmatic breathing; glossopharyngeal breathing; incentive spirometer; paced breathing; ventilatory muscle training such as inspiratory resistive loading); secretion mobilization and airway clearance techniques; abdominal strengthening exercises; may use abdominal binder; general conditioning exercises (e.g., extremity ROM and strengthening; avoid fatigue); postural-relief techniques; energy and work conservation (including assistive and adaptive devices, and home modification); may combine CBT with biofeedback and relaxation techniques **Invasive**: Tracheal intubation; diaphragmatic pacing **Others**: Psychosocial interventions, vocational counseling

6th Floor, New York, NY 10006; tel. (212) 315-8700; 1-800-LUNGUSA; website: *http://www.lungusa.org*); American Cancer Society (1599 Clifton Road, Atlanta, GA 30329; tel.1-800-ACS-2345; website: *http://www.cancer.org*); National Cancer Institute, 6116 Executive Boulevard, Bethesda, MD 20892; tel.1-800-4-CANCER website: *http://www.cancer.gov*; and Stanford Health Promotion Resource Center, 211 Quarry Road, Ground Floor, Stanford, CA 94305, tel. (650) 723-7049; website: *http://hprc.stanford.edu*.

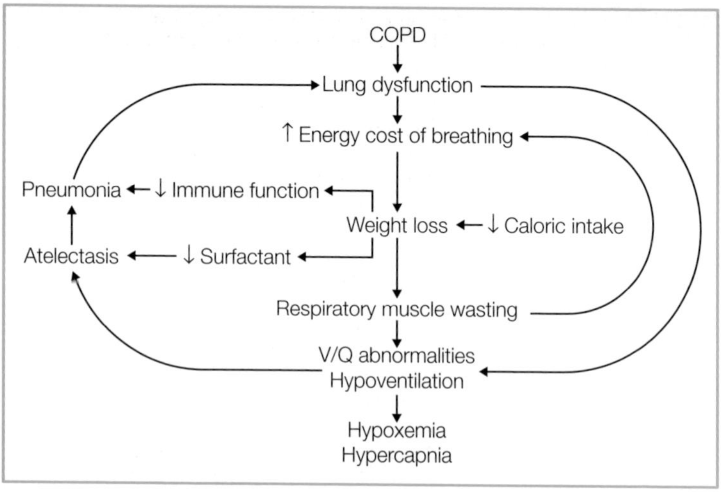

Figure 5.12-1 The vicious cycle whereby weight loss in patients with chronic obstructive pulmonary disease (COPD) leads to hypoxemia and hypercapnia. ↑, increased; ↓, decreased; V/Q, ventilation/perfusion. (Adapted from: Axen KV: Nutrition in chronic obstructive pulmonary disease. In Haas F, Axen K, editors: *Pulmonary therapy and rehabilitation. Principles and practice*, ed 2, Baltimore, 1991, Williams & Wilkins, p. 97.)

b. ***Nutritional therapy*** is essential for patients with chronic pulmonary disease whose body weight is low (especially those with COPD or on mechanical ventilation) because low body weight is associated with increased morbidity and mortality in COPD patients. Improving nutritional status increases endurance for activities of daily living (ADLs) and ambulation, reduces dyspnea, and increases subjective well-being; however, the resting ABGs usually remain unchanged. Also, the role of nutritional therapy in improving long-term outcomes outside the controlled hospital environment remains unclear. Nonetheless, nutritional support for patients with low body weight is recommended because of the above benefits in addition to improvement in respiratory function, immune function, skeletal muscle mass, and strength.

The two main reasons for weight loss in patients with chronic pulmonary disease are increased energy expenditure for breathing even at rest (thus increasing daily caloric need) and decreased caloric intake because of dyspnea while eating (especially large meals) caused by the need to breath-hold during swallowing. Other reasons for weight loss include the side-effects of prescribed medications (e.g., bronchodilators); decreased food intake, because eating limits whatever lung excursion is still possible in a diaphragm already depressed due to lung overexpansion (moreover, the depressed diaphragm is weakened by its position and is at a mechanical disadvantage, thus making excursion against a full stomach even more difficult); and concomitant reduced sense of taste and smell, as well as feelings of depression (thus causing loss of appetite and further weight loss). The vicious cycle whereby weight loss in COPD patients leads to hypoxemia and hypercapnia is shown in Fig. 5.12-1. Table 5.12-4 shows the general recommendations on feeding strategies to improve caloric intake for different pulmonary-related complaints of COPD patients.

Energy expenditure should be determined by indirect calorimetry. If this is unavailable, a practical method of calculating basal energy expenditure (BEE) uses the Harris–Benedict formula and then applies the correction factors for patients with COPD (see Chapter 5.6, section VII.B). Based on the BEE, the

Table 5.12-4 General recommendations on feeding strategies to improve caloric intake for different pulmonary-related complaints of COPD patients

Complaint	Estimated frequency*	General recommendations on feeding strategies
Early satiety	87%	1. Eat high-calorie foods first. 2. Limit liquid consumption during meal; sip liquids 1 hour after meals. 3. Eat cold food first as this can give less of a sense of fullness than hot foods.
Bloating	80%	1. Treat shortness of breath early to prevent air swallowing. 2. Eat smaller, more frequent meals. 3. Avoid rushed meals. 4. Avoid gas-forming foods (different for each patient).
Dyspnea	73%	1. Rest before meals. 2. Use bronchodilators before meals. 3. Use secretion clearance strategies if indicated. 4. Eat more slowly. 5. Use pursed-lip breathing between bites. 6. Use tripod position for meals. 7. Have readily prepared meals available for periods of increased shortness of breath. 8. Evaluate for meal desaturation; refer for O_2 evaluation if needed.
Anorexia	73%	1. Eat high-calorie food first. 2. Have favorite foods available. 3. Try more frequent meals and snacks throughout the day. 4. Instruct patients to push themselves to eat. 5. Add margarine, butter, mayonnaise, sauces, and gravies to diet to add calories.
Fatigue	60%	1. Rest before meals. 2. Have readily prepared meals available for periods of increased fatigue or illness. 3. Have patient try to eat larger meals when he or she is less tired.
Constipation	50%	1. Incorporate exercise as tolerated. 2. Instruct patient in high-fiber foods and adequate fluids. 3. Refer to Chapter 5.8, section VI.B for constipation management.
Dental problems	30%	1. Instruct patient to eat soft, high-calorie foods. 2. Refer to dental services as appropriate.

**Estimated frequency based on a survey of 19 malnourished COPD patients.*
Adapted from: Donahoe M, Rogers RM: Nutritional assessment and support in chronic obstructive pulmonary disease. Clin Chest Med *11:499, 1990*

caloric needs for the patient can be calculated and the patient can be given appropriate nutritional supplements to attain their ideal body weight (IBW). The cut-off weight for determining undernutrition in patients with chronic pulmonary disease is less than 90% IBW although values as low as below 70–85% IBW may be justifiable because: (a) the percentage IBW does not give information about body composition (i.e., lean vs. adipose tissue), hence a weight of 90% IBW may reflect athletic fitness if the low weight is because of loss of adipose tissue; (b) there is generally no associated biochemical or clinical sign of undernutrition at 90% IBW; and (c) the value used for calculating % IBW (i.e., the midpoint of the weight range for a given category) tends to overestimate the lower end of the weight range.

In general, appropriate intakes of fish, fat, and especially fresh fruits and vegetables, should be encouraged in patients with chronic pulmonary disease. Vitamin/mineral supplements should be considered in those unable to consume adequate nutrients from food. The use of supplements of omega-3 fatty acids and high-dose antioxidants is controversial. Moderate physical activity should be done regularly to maintain or improve muscle mass and tone, functional ability, and appetite.

As with other patients, protein usually makes up 20% of the total caloric requirement. Protein supplementation can also be given at 1.7 g/kg of body weight to promote nitrogen retention and physiologic improvement. The distribution of calories among fat and carbohydrate remains controversial. Dietary fat has a respiratory quotient (RQ) of 0.7 compared to 1.0 for carbohydrates. The RQ (see Chapter 2.7, section II.A) is the ratio of the carbon dioxide produced to the oxygen consumed, thus dietary fat produces lower levels of carbon dioxide per kilocalorie of energy expended than carbohydrate, making it more efficient as a source of fuel than carbohydrate. Studies have shown that the intake of relatively higher dietary fat is preferred in hypercapnic patients (e.g., severe COPD or acute respiratory failure requiring mechanical ventilator support) in whom a high-carbohydrate diet (particularly those providing an excess of calories to promote weight gain) may lead to further retention of carbon dioxide. However, this does not connote excessively high fatty intake, but rather the intermediate caloric distribution of about 45% carbohydrate and 35% fat (in addition to the 20% protein and recommended daily allowances of vitamins and minerals). In acute respiratory failure, a fat emulsion (e.g., Pulmocare) may be used not only to reduce carbon dioxide production but to provide a volume-concentrated source of calories in the fluid-restricted patient.

c. ***Patient education*** is a central component of pulmonary rehabilitation. Education classes (for both the patient and the family or support system) are generally conducted in a class format and may include the following topics: anatomy and physiology of the lung; pathophysiology of lung disease; the goal of treatment; symptom assessment and knowledge about when to seek medical treatment; diet and nutrition; smoking cessation; airway management; breathing training strategies; medication regimens (including drug action, side-effects, administration with inhaler technique, and self-care algorithms); energy conservation and work simplification techniques; benefits of exercise; exercise (including exercise conditioning programs) and safety guidelines; respiratory and chest therapy techniques; strategies for managing dyspnea; avoidance of environmental irritants (e.g., dust and chemicals); safe use of oxygen; the use and cleaning of respiratory therapy equipment; end of life planning; psychological factors (coping, anxiety, panic control), stress management; travel, leisure, and sexuality, including safe techniques for intimacy (see Supplemental references; see also Table 5.13-2 for sexual counseling of patients with concomitant cardiac problems). The amount of time allotted to each topic varies considerably across programs. In addition to lectures, the education component often includes printed handouts, demonstrations, and active coaching. Based on the few available studies, the 1997 ACCP/AACVPR Pulmonary Rehabilitation Guidelines Panel concluded that education outside the context of a multicomponent pulmonary rehabilitation program that includes exercise training may not be sufficient to improve the well-being of patients with COPD. For discussion on patient education techniques, see Chapter 5.10, section VI.A.

2. **Pharmacotherapy**. Because pulmonary drugs are primarily prescribed by pulmonologists, this section provides only an overview of the pulmonary drug as it

relates to patients undergoing pulmonary rehabilitation. The administration routes of some pulmonary drugs include inhalation routes [e.g., through nebulizers, metered-dose inhalers (MDIs) or dry-powder inhalers (DPIs)] and oral and parenteral routes. The advantages of the inhalation route over the oral and parenteral routes include a lower dose requirement and fewer side-effects; however, drugs given via the inhalation route have a shorter duration of action and must be given more frequently.

The most commonly used inhalation method is the MDI (e.g., for delivery of β-adrenergic, anticholinergic, steroid, and mast-cell-stabilizing drugs) because of its portability, relatively high lung deposition (10–15%), and low cost. The formerly recommended MDI technique in which the mouth is closed over the MDI mouthpiece has been shown to be ineffective as it results in greater deposition of aerosols in the mouth and throat rather than in the lung parenchyma; therefore, the following open-mouth technique is currently recommended by the American College of Chest Physicians:

- Shake the inhaler to mix the medication with the propellant (e.g., freon).
- Breathe out completely to end of a normal breath (i.e., to functional residual capacity).
- Open the mouth wide and hold canister in the upright position 2–4 cm from mouth, aiming the inhaler towards the mouth. In some patients (e.g., elderly or neurologic patients) spacers or aerosol reservoirs (which hold the MDI) may be used to decrease the proximal deposition of large particles.
- Depress the top of the MDI canister while breathing in deeply and slowly over a period of 5–6 seconds (to total lung capacity).
- Close the mouth and hold the breath for about 10 seconds.
- For each additional puff ordered, wait for at least 1–2 minutes between actuations.

The DPI, which appears to be equivalent to a properly used MDI, may cause heavy oropharyngeal deposition and clumping of particles in high-humidity environments. There are only a limited number of medications available through DPI [e.g., spin-inhaler for delivery of cromolyn sodium (Intal) and rotacaps for delivery of Ventolin]. Nebulizers (e.g., jet nebulizer and ultrasonic nebulizer) can deliver larger volumes and higher doses than MDIs; however, they are bulky, expensive, and subject to bacterial contamination. The nebulizer, therefore, is only used for patients who cannot use inhalers (e.g., because of cognitive or motor deficits) or who do not obtain relief of bronchospasm with inhalers (e.g., those with advanced COPD).

a. ***Bronchodilators*** are considered the first-line treatment for COPD.

I. **Sympathomimetic drugs**, in particular β_2-adrenergic agonists, cause the activation of adenyl cyclase, which catalyzes the conversion of adenosine triphosphate (ATP) to cyclic adenosine monophosphate (cAMP). Increased intracellular levels of cAMP, in turn, cause bronchodilation, increased mucus clearance, pulmonary artery dilation, and a decrease in antigen-induced release of mediators from basophils and mast cells. There are also nonpulmonary effects such as skeletal muscle tremors and some direct cardiac stimulation. Sympathomimetics are indicated for the relief of acute or chronic bronchospasm and in the prevention of exercise-induced bronchospasm. They are contraindicated in patients with hypersensitivity to any component of the drug or cardiac arrhythmias associated with tachycardia.

- **Catecholamines** are first-generation β_2-adrenergic agonists; however, they are nonspecific as they also stimulate α-adrenergic and β_1-adrenergic receptors, thus causing unwanted effects because of positive chronotropy and inotropy of the heart (e.g., palpitations, tachycardia, and hypertension) and hyperglycemia and hypokalemia. They generally have a short duration of action (only 1–2 hours) and can lead to the development of tolerance in some patients. Examples include **racemic epinephrine (Vaponefrin, MIcroNefrin), isoproterenol (Isuprel, Medihaler-Iso), isoetharine (Bronkosol; Bronkometer)**, and **bitolterol (Tornalate)**. Epinephrine is a potent stimulator of α- and β-adrenergic receptors. Isoproterenol has mostly β-adrenergic effect but is equally potent on both β_1 and β_2 receptors. Isoetharine has a more selective β_2 effect but is a less potent bronchodilator than isoproterenol. Bitolterol is a pro-drug that is inactive until it is cleaved in the lung by esterase to produce its active form, colterol. Because esterase levels are higher in the lung than in the heart, bitolterol has fewer cardiac side-effects. Bitolterol is also slowly hydrolyzed and has a sustained duration of up to 8 hours.

- **Resorcinols** are second-generation β_2-adrenergic agonists. They are more selective β_2-adrenergic agonists, more active orally, and have a longer duration of action (about 4–6 hours) than catecholamines. They include **metaproterenol (Alupent; Metaprel)**, and **terbutaline (Brethaire, Brethine, Bricanyl)**. Terbutaline is more β_2-specific than metaproterenol.
- **Saligenins** are third-generation β_2-adrenergic agonists. They show more β_2-specificity than the other sympathomimetic drugs, are active orally, and have a duration of action of 4–6 hours or longer. They include **albuterol (Proventil, Ventolin, Volmax), pirbuterol (Maxair), salmeterol (Serevent)**, and **levalbuterol (Xopenex)**. Pirbuterol has less potent bronchodilator effects than albuterol. Salmeterol, which was approved by the Food ad Drug Administration (FDA) in 1994, has a duration of action of up to 12 hours and is more potent than albuterol. Its only drawback is its slower onset of action than albuterol; hence, salbuterol is not indicated for rapid relief of acute bronchospasm. Levalbuterol is the first drug in a new subclass of inhaled β_2-adrenergic agonists. It is a more potent dilator than albuterol, with fewer side-effects. Like albuterol, its onset of action is about 15 minutes after administration (reaching peak effect in 30–60 minutes). Unlike albuterol, which lasts 4–6 hours, levalbuterol can last for 3–8 hours.

II. **Anticholinergic bronchodilators** compete with acetylcholine for receptors at the parasympathetic postganglionic effector cell junctions. Acetylcholine, which stimulates guanyl cyclase to produce cyclic guanosine monophosphate (cGMP), can cause both bronchial smooth muscle contraction and mast cell degranulation; therefore, anticholinergic agents, which decrease the intracellular level of cGMP, result in bronchodilation (this effect is independent from the actions of sympathomimetic drugs). In contrast to sympathomimetic drugs, which primarily affect the smaller distal airways, the anticholinergics primarily affect the larger central airways. Anticholinergics, which do not cause drug resistance, may be more effective when used on a long-term basis than β-adrenergic drugs.

Atropine sulfate, which is the prototypical parasympatholytic is not commonly used as a bronchodilator because of its many side-effects. The preferred anticholinergic bronchodilator is an inhaled form of ipratropium bromide (**Atrovent**), which is a derivative of atropine. Ipratropium acts locally as it is poorly absorbed from the bronchial mucosa and generally has fewer side-effects than atropine (common side-effects of atropine include dry mouth, tachycardia, blurred vision, and urinary retention). It reaches its peak effect in 1–2 hours and is thus not indicated for the initial treatment of acute bronchospasm. It is contraindicated in patients with allergy to atropine or other components of Atrovent (e.g., soya lecithin found in peanuts and soybeans) and is to be used with caution in patients with narrow-angle glaucoma, prostatic hypertrophy, tachycardia, and unstable cardiovascular status (e.g., myocardial ischemia and acute hemorrhage). Ipratropium bromide is available with albuterol in a single MDI canister as **Combivent** for patients responsive to both anticholinergic and sympathomimetic drugs.

A new anticholinergic bronchodilator, tiotropium bromide inhalation powder (**Spiriva**) was recently approved by the United States FDA for the long-term, once-daily, maintenance treatment of bronchospasms associated with COPD, including chronic bronchitis and emphysema. It should not be used for the initial treatment of acute episodes of bronchospasm (i.e., rescue therapy). It is administered using a special breath-activated DPI called HandiHaler®. It has similar side-effects and contraindications to ipratropium bromide.

III. **Methylxanthines** are traditionally believed to cause bronchodilation through phosphodiesterase inhibition, thus leading to increased intracellular levels of cAMP. Other proposed mechanisms include competitive antagonism at adenosine receptors, reduction in the uptake or metabolism of catecholamines, interference with the uptake and storage of calcium, and inhibition of prostaglandin synthesis. Aside from bronchodilation, they also stimulate breathing, enhance ciliary function, inhibit the release of histamine, vasodilate pulmonary vessels and decrease pulmonary hypertension, improve diaphragmatic contractility, and cause other nonpulmonary effects (e.g., vasodilate coronary artery blood vessels, vasoconstrict cerebral blood vessels, promote diuresis, stimulate the central nervous system and skeletal muscles, increase secretion of gastric acid, and relax uterine smooth muscle).

The methylxanthines most selective in their smooth muscle activity are theophylline (**Theo-Dur, Theolair, Theobid, Theoclear, Throchron, Uni-Dur, Aerolate, Quibron, Elixophyllin, Slo-phyllin, Slo-Bid, Respbid, Sustaire**) and its salts, aminophylline (**Mudrane**) and dyphylline (**Lufyllin, Dilor, Dyline**). Aminophylline is 75–85% less active than theophylline. A blood level of 10–20 mg/dL of theophylline is considered therapeutic, although many patients show mild bronchodilation with subtherapeutic levels of 5–10 mg/dL. Theophylline blood levels can be increased by many drugs (e.g., erythromycin, ciprofloxacin, flu vaccine, cimetidine, calcium-channel blockers, nonselective β-blockers, corticosteroids, isoniazid, allopurinol, and oral contraceptives) and conditions (e.g., pneumonia, congestive heart failure, liver disease, renal disease, shock, and diets high in caffeine). Some drugs that may decrease theophylline blood levels include β-adrenergic agonists, rifampin, phenytoin, and barbiturates. Loop diuretics and isoniazid may either increase or decrease theophylline blood levels. As a result of its absorption characteristics and potential side-effects, theophylline is contraindicated in patients with unstable blood pressure, gastrointestinal bleeding, hepatic failure, hyperthyroidism, nausea, history of seizures, tachyarrhythmias, extreme tremulousness, peptic ulcer, or vomiting.

Other methylxanthines such as caffeine (a central nervous system stimulant found in coffee, tea, cola, and cocoa) and theobromine (found in chocolates) are not approved for use as bronchodilators.

b. ***Glucocorticoids*** (discussed in Chapter 4.8, section III), which have bronchodilatory as well as potent anti-inflammatory effects, are used in pulmonary patients to treat primarily asthma and other pulmonary diseases (e.g., COPD, sarcoidosis). Steroids may be given intravenously [e.g., **hydrocortisone (Cortef; Solu-Cortef), methylprednisolone (Solu-Medrol)**], orally (e.g., **prednisone**), via a respiratory inhalant [e.g., **beclomethasone dipropionate (Beclovent; Vanceril), dexamethasone (Decadron Phosphate Respihaler), triamcinolone acetonide (Azmacort), flunisolide (AeroBid), fluticasone (Flovent), budenoside turbuhaler (Pulmicort)**], or through intranasal sprays [e.g., **beclomethasone (Vancenase Nasal Inhaler, Beconase Inhalation), dexamethasone (Decadron Phosphate Turbinaire), triamcinolone (Nasacort), flunisolide (Nasalide), fluticasone propionate (Flonase), budesonide (Rhinocort)** and **mometasone furoate (Nasonex)**].

c. ***Antiasthmatic agents***
   I. **Mast cell membrane stabilizers** act by stabilizing mast cells, thus inhibiting the release of inflammatory mediators. They include cromolyn sodium (also called **disodium cromoglycate, e.g., Intal, Gastrocrom, Nasalcrom), nedocromil sodium (Tilade)**, and the experimental drug, **ketotifen (Zaditen)**. These drugs are used to decrease the frequency and intensity of asthmatic attacks in both allergic and nonallergic asthma, to treat and prevent allergic rhinitis, and to prevent exercise-induced bronchospasm. Because they are not bronchodilators and have delayed onsets of action (4–6 weeks), they should not be used to reverse acute bronchospasm.
   II. **Leukotriene modifiers** are a new group of antiasthmatic agents that inhibit the leukotriene mediator cascade that leads to airway inflammation. They include **zileuton (Zyflo), zafirlukast (Accolate)**, and **montelukast (Singulair)**. They are considered as alternatives to low-dose inhaled steroids, cromolyn, or nedocromil in patients with mild to persistent asthma. They are used for long-term control, not acute treatment of asthma.

d. ***Mucokinetic agents*** alter the composition and volume of airway secretions to promote mobilization and removal of these airway secretions. The most important mucolytic agent is water. Adequate hydration (2–4 L/day) is essential for easier expectoration of mucus; however, patients should not be overhydrated as this may cause pulmonary edema in those with congestive heart failure or renal failure. Other mucokinetic agents (mostly in inhaled form) include **acetylcysteine (Mucomyst, Mucosol), sodium bicarbonate, hydrating agents** (iso-, hyper-, or hypotonic saline), **recombinant human deoxyribonuclease (Pulmozyne)**, and **propylene glycol**. The effectiveness of acetylcysteine in patients with COPD or asthma is controversial as it may also cause bronchospasm. If used at all, acetylcysteine should be limited to only a few doses and should be accompanied by bronchodilators.

e. ***Cough and cold preparations*** do not cure the cold or lessen its duration, but are used to modify or relieve the symptoms (e.g., nasal congestion, headache, fever, general malaise, cough, and rhinorrhea) of cold or allergy. They can be given singly or in combination with each other or with other chemicals (e.g., analgesics, anticholinergic agents, preservatives, caffeine, and alcohol). When using combination preparations, the benefits of each ingredient must be considered. Many cough and cold preparations are available over-the-counter and have high potential for abuse.
   I. **Antitussives** are used to suppress an ineffective, dry, hacking, nonproductive cough or in patients who cannot get enough rest because of excessive coughing. They can be given locally (e.g., topical anesthetics such as **lidocaine**) through an endotracheal or tracheostomy tube, or they can be given systemically using either narcotic (primarily **codeine**; see Chapter 4.8, section I.B.1.a.2) or non-narcotic preparations **[dextromethorphan** (e.g., **Robitussin DM, Drixoral, Vicks Formula 44), diphenhydramine** (e.g., **Tusstat, Benylin Cough**), and **benzonatate** (e.g., **Tessalon Perles**)]. Systemic antitussives act centrally by suppressing the cough reflex located at the medullary cough center.

II. **Expectorants** are used to relieve dry, nonproductive coughs by increasing the amount of fluid (i.e., mucus production) in the respiratory tract, therefore making the cough more productive. These include **guaifenesin** (e.g., **Robitussin, Humibid, Organidin), iodine products** (e.g., **potassium iodide, SSKI), ammonium chloride**, and **terpin hydrate**. Patients must be adequately hydrated for the expectorant to have maximal efficacy.

III. **Nasal decongestants** are sympathomimetic amines with primary α-adrenergic actions used to relieve nasal congestion and edema via local vasoconstriction of blood vessels in patients with upper respiratory allergies and the common cold. Nasal decongestants are to be used only on a limited basis (3–5 days) as prolonged use may result in rebound congestion upon drug discontinuation. Examples include **pseudoephedrine** (e.g., **Sudafed, Actifed), phenylephrine** (e.g., **Neo-Synephrine), ephedrine** (e.g., **Vicks Vatronol)**, and **oxymetazoline** (e.g., **Allerest 12-hour Nasal)**.

IV. **Antihistamines** reduce inflammation and allergic reactions by competitively antagonizing histamine at the H_1 receptor rather than binding to histamine to deactivate it. Most antihistamines also have anticholinergic, antipruritic, sedative, and antiemetic effects. The first-generation antihistamines include **alkylamines [chlorpheniramine** (e.g., **Chlor-Trimeton), dexchlorpheniramine** (e.g., **Poladex)], brompheniramine** (e.g., **Bromfed, Dimetane, Dallergy, Rondec, Lodrane, Poly-Histine CS**, and **Respahist), triprolidine** (e.g., **Actifed Cold)], ethanolamines** [i.e., **diphenhydramine** (e.g., **Benadryl), clemastine** (e.g., **Tavist)**, and **doxylamine** (e.g., **Nyquil, Unisom)], ethylenediamines** [i.e., **tripelennamine** (e.g., **PBZ)** and **pyrilamine** (e.g., **Triaminic, Codimal, Poly-Histine Elixir, Atrohist)], phenothiazines** [i.e., **prometazine** (e.g., **Phenergan, Prometh)], and piperidine** [i.e., **cyproheptadine** (e.g., **Periactin), azatadine** (e.g., **Trinalin)**, and **phenindamine** (e.g., **Nolahist)]**. They are short-acting and sedating. In contrast, the second-generation antihistamines, which include **fexofenadine (Allegra), terfenadine (Seldane), astemizole (Hismanal), loratadine (Claritin)**, and **cetirizine (Zyrtec)** are long-acting and are nonsedating. Terfenadine can cause QT-interval prolongation and ventricular arrhythmias and has been replaced by the safer fexofenadine.

f. ***Pulmonary vaccines*** are generally recommended for patients with chronic pulmonary diseases to prevent major respiratory tract infections, which can trigger respiratory failure.

I. **Pneumococcal vaccines (Pneumovax 23; Pnu-Immune 23)** contain purified capsular polysaccharide antigens of up to 23 of the most prevalent types of *Streptococcus pneumoniae* (pneumococci) which are responsible for approximately 90% of serious community-acquired pneumococcal diseases. The vaccine's popular name, "pneumonia vaccine", is misleading because pneumococci are responsible not only for pneumonia but for other infections also, such as meningitis and otitis media. The vaccine is effective only against the named types of pneumococci and is generally given once in a lifetime (with no booster dose) to individuals over 2 years old. It is injected intramuscularly (or subcutaneously) at a single dose of 0.5 mL and may be given concomitantly with the influenza virus vaccine (see below) injected at a different site. Aside from local muscle soreness, some patients may develop a low-grade fever and mild myalgia for about 24 hours. Although rare, there are reports of high fever, arthralgia, and anaphylaxis.

II. **Influenza virus vaccines** or **"flu shots"** (e.g., **FluShield, Fluvirin, Fluzone**) are prepared from extraembryonic fluids of chicken eggs infected with influenza virus. The infected fluid is then inactivated (hence it becomes noninfectious and cannot cause influenza), concentrated, and highly purified to create a surface antigen vaccine against types A and B strains of influenza. The formula is updated yearly to contain new strains which have developed since the previous year. It is contraindicated in patients with (a) allergy to hen's egg, chicken, or egg products; (b) allergy to any components of the vaccine, including thimerosal; (c) any signs of active infection; and (d) past history of Guillain–Barré syndrome. The vaccine is administered intramuscularly every year, ideally in the fall (before December) when influenza activity sharply increases, to individuals over 6 months old. The recommended dose for individuals over 3 years is 0.5 mL. Aside from local muscle soreness, the major but inconsequential side-effects of the influenza vaccine are fever, malaise, and myalgia, especially in patients who have not taken the flu vaccine previously. These symptoms usually appear in 6–12 hours and persist for 1 or 2 days.

g. ***Other pulmonary drugs*** include **diuretics** to reduce fluid overload (e.g., in cor pulmonale), **surface-active agent (ethanol)** to decrease surface tension of respiratory secretions (e.g., in fulminant pulmonary edema), and **anti-infective agents** to reduce mucus and improve ABGs in patients with pulmonary infection, especially in those with limited respiratory reserve. Ideally, anti-infective therapy should be directed by cultures. In pulmonary patients with viral infection, antibiotics are frequently prescribed because of the patient's increased susceptibility to secondary bacterial invasion resulting from altered immunity.

3. **Home oxygen therapy** is based on medical consensus and follows the guidelines established by Medicare for its reimbursement in the United States. Home oxygen is indicated for

- Exercise or activity use if the hemoglobin saturation (SaO_2) is equal to or less than 88%, or the arterial oxygen tension (PaO_2) is equal to or less than 55 mmHg with the exercise or activity for which oxygen is prescribed, or if there is demonstration of increased exercise tolerance or endurance with oxygen in conjunction with a rehabilitation program.
- Nocturnal use if SaO_2 is less than or equal to 88% or PaO_2 is less than or equal to 55 mmHg during sleep with evidence of cor pulmonale, erythrocytosis, or other physical or mental impairment attributable to nocturnal hypoxemia, or if sleep-related hypoxemia is corrected or improved by oxygen supplementation.
- Intermittent or stand-by oxygen if SaO_2 is less than or equal to 88% or PaO_2 is less than or equal to 55 mmHg in association with acute bronchospasm, heart failure, or other cardiopulmonary disease in a patient who is subject to frequent changes in clinical stability.
- Long-term oxygen therapy (LTOT) for continuous (24 hours/day) use if SaO_2 is less than or equal to 88% or PaO_2 is less than or equal to 55 mmHg when breathing room air as documented by two ABGs drawn at rest in the seated position in outpatients in stable condition receiving optimal medical therapy (if home oxygen is prescribed for an inpatient, the ABGs must be repeated 1–3 months after discharge when the patient has recovered from the acute illness and is receiving optimum therapy for any remaining chronic respiratory disease). However, because some patients with PaO_2 above 55 mmHg can have evidence of hypoxic organ dysfunction, the following criteria may also be used: PaO_2 less than or equal to 59 mmHg and evidence of at least one of the following: pulmonary hypertension (P wave greater than 3 mm in leads II, III, or aVF), cor pulmonale (dependent edema), or erythrocytosis (hematocrit above 56%).

When home oxygen is prescribed, the FiO_2 (fraction of inspired O_2) and oxygen flow rate should be titrated to the minimum needed to achieve adequate tissue oxygenation as confirmed by ABG to determine an increase in PaO_2 by

Table 5.12-5 Advantages and disadvantages of common modes of O_2 supply

Oxygen supply	Advantages	Disadvantages
1. Compressed gas cylinders	100% O_2 up to high flow rates; inexpensive; reliable; relatively portable; no power needed; for intermittent use (e.g., for sleep or exercise)	High pressure; unsafe to transfill at home; bulky; needs frequent deliveries from vendors
2. Liquid O_2 systems	100% O_2 at all flow rates; excellent portability; smaller storage volume; generally lighter; no power needed; for active patients or those who need high liter flows	Low pressure; can transfill from larger tanks; can freeze (may cause frostbite at connections and if spilled); settings can be inaccurate; evaporates if not used; expensive except for patients on >3 L/min rate
3. Molecular sieve O_2 concentrators	90–93% O_2 up to flow rates of about 3 L/min; least expensive for patients who stay home	Not portable; needs power from wall electrical outlet; needs back-up system; high maintenance; provides only flow rate of <2–3 L/min
4. Membrane-separator O_2 enrichers	Low maintenance (only filter needs to be changed); well humidified; ideal for transtracheal O_2 therapy	Low O_2 concentration (45%)

5 mmHg or to above 60 mmHg, or by using pulse oximetry to determine an increase in SaO_2 above 90%. To reduce the incidence of pulmonary oxygen toxicity (e.g., diffuse alveolar damage), an oxygen concentration of below 40–50% and oxygen pressure of 90–110 mmHg should be used. The oxygen flow should be increased over the resting requirement by 1 L/min during sleep or by 0.5 L/min during air travel. The advantages and disadvantages of different modes of oxygen supply and delivery are shown in Tables 5.12-5 and 5.12.6 respectively.

The use of home oxygen in COPD patients, when indicated, decreases reactive pulmonary hypertension, polycythemia, perception of effort during exercise, and hospitalizations, as well as improving cognitive function and prolonging life. In hypoxemic COPD patients, these potential benefits of home oxygen outweigh the risks of pulmonary oxygen toxicity (seen in 50% of COPD patients receiving LTOT for 7–60 months). In normoxemic COPD patients, the use of LTOT (to improve exercise performance or to treat dyspnea) remains controversial. In general oxygen should not be prescribed for prophylactic use or for "as needed" use at home (unless the patient meets the criteria described above).

The use of home oxygen may also be beneficial in patients with other chronic pulmonary diseases such as severe restrictive lung disease (e.g., kyphoscoliosis), cystic fibrosis, or pulmonary fibrosis (e.g., interstitial pneumonitis); however, the benefit is not as well documented as for COPD patients. In general, home oxygen is more harmful than beneficial in patients with chronic respiratory failure, especially those who are chronic carbon dioxide retainers (e.g., because of paralytic restrictive pulmonary diseases). These hypercapneic patients rely on the central hypoxic ventilatory drive; and oxygen supplementation may suppress ventilatory drive thus leading to more carbon dioxide retention and to respiratory arrest. In these patients, mechanical ventilation (see below) is recommended along with or instead of oxygen supplementation.

4. **Mechanical ventilation** (whether daytime or night-time) is mainly used in patients with CAH (as a result of various chronic restrictive pulmonary diseases;

Table 5.12-6 Advantages and disadvantages of common modes of O_2 delivery

Oxygen delivery	Advantages	Disadvantages
Continuous mode		
1. Nasal cannulae or prongs	Inexpensive; relatively comfortable; patient can eat, talk, sleep, expectorate; no CO_2 rebreathing; FiO_2 independent of nose or mouth breathers; FiO_2 delivered is 22–40% at 0.5–6.0 L/min*; the slower the inspiratory flow the higher the FiO_2	Less efficient than face mask; FiO_2 elevation is modest even at high flow rates; may cause mucosal drying and dermatitis unless well humidified
2. Face mask	Efficient delivery of air (if mask is tight) at wide range of FiO_2; air is humidified (except in the Venturi mask†, where gas is not completely humidified)	Less comfortable; awkward eating, talking, expectorating; not reliable when FiO_2 of <35% is needed; partial rebreathing of CO_2
3. Transtracheal	Cosmetic; lighter equipment; improved mobility; better oxygenation; reduced O_2 flow requirement; reduced inspiratory work; better sense of taste; good patient compliance	Invasive (needs mini-tracheostomy, e.g., with 16-gauge angiocatheter); needs humidification; causes complications (e.g., mucus balls; subcutaneous emphysema; cough; local infection; dislodged catheter; reinsertion failure)
Non-continuous mode:‡		
1. Reservoir O_2-conserving device§	Can be used with nasal cannulae; least expensive; simple; reliable	Unsightly; obtrusive; needs frequent replacement of filter; low compliance; decreased effectiveness in mouth breathers
2. Pulsed delivery¶	Most efficacious	Subject to mechanical failure

** Each liter per minute of oxygen flow adds about 3–4% to the FiO_2. A rough approximation is that a flow of 1 L/min of O_2 increases the FiO_2 to 24%, 2 L/min to 28%, and 3 L/min to 32%. These small increases are usually sufficient to increase the arterial oxygen content to acceptable clinical levels.*

† Venturi mask mixes O_2 with room air, creating high-flow enriched oxygen of a settable concentration. It provides an accurate and constant FiO_2. Typical FiO_2 delivery settings are 24, 28, 31, 35, and 40% oxygen. The Venturi mask is often used when there is concern about CO_2 retention.

‡ Maximizes O_2 delivery at the beginning of inspiration (because at the latter phase of inspiration, the O_2 enters the dead space and is wasted). The reduced O_2 flow requirement can reduce size and weight of O_2 equipment as well as potentially reduce cost of LTOT.

§ Uses a storage bag (e.g., in nonrebreathing or partial-rebreathing reservoir mask) with an internal diaphragm and a reservoir of about 20 mL which fills with O_2 during expiration. On inspiration, the diaphragm collapses, thus providing a volume of O_2 at the beginning of inspiration.

¶ Can deliver fixed or variable volume of O_2 at the end of expiration and the beginning of inspiration; uses thermistor detectors or pressure-sensors to detect chest wall motion; rapid, shallow breathing can cause continuous activation without O_2 conservation.

see section III.B) either as a life support system (e.g., high cervical spinal cord injury patients with respiratory muscle paralysis and patients with respiratory failure) or as an elective therapy (e.g., patients with progressive chronic respiratory insufficiency in an attempt to prevent acute respiratory failure, to preserve function, and possibly to increase survival). In general, the decision to initiate mechanical ventilation is based on the clinical assessment, that is, presence of apnea, tachypnea of over 40 breaths/min, and respiratory failure that cannot be adequately corrected by any other means. Other less reliable parameters (because they cannot distinguish between acute and chronic respiratory insufficiency) include ABG parameters, that is, PaO_2 less than 55 mmHg despite high-flow oxygen or $PaCO_2$ above 50 mmHg and PFT parameters (if patient is able to perform PFT) of vital capacity less than 15 mL/kg, inspiratory force less than –25 cmH_2O, and FEV_1 less than 10 mL/kg.

Indications for the elective use of chronic nocturnal mechanical ventilation in patients with CAH have not been clearly established. Factors to be considered include the rate of progression of the primary disease process, age, PFT results, ABG level (especially decreased PaO_2 and increased PCO_2) taken when awake and when asleep, sleep disordered breathing, acute respiratory compromise, or "fatigue" from intercurrent respiratory tract infections, and cognitive function, motivation, and cooperation. Noninvasive monitoring of nocturnal sleep blood gases (e.g., pulse oximetry or capnography) should be carried out at least once a year in patients whose supine VC is below 40–50% of predicted normal, especially in those patients with rapidly evolving conditions and loss of VC. More frequent nocturnal monitoring (every 3–12 months unless VC has increased) should be carried out in the presence of progressive paralytic restrictive pulmonary disease with a sudden drop in VC, a VC of less than 1000 mL or below 25–35% of predicted normal; a VC significantly lower in supine than sitting; or in any patients with symptoms or signs of CAH. Nocturnal ventilatory support is indicated in symptomatic patients with a VC less than 50% of predicted normal, mean SaO_2 below 95% for at least 1 hour during sleep, and maximum PCO_2 over 50 mmHg, and in nonsymptomatic patients with PCO_2 above 50 mmHg and mean SaO_2 below 95% during much of the night.

Mechanical ventilation (e.g., using oral or nasal intermittent positive-pressure airway ventilators, or using negative pressure body ventilators; see descriptions below) have been used at night in hypercapnic COPD patients to provide "rest" of "fatigued" respiratory muscles. However, this is controversial. Recent evidence suggests that the principal cause of hypercapnia in COPD patients with respiratory failure is weakness, not fatigue. The nocturnal use of mechanical ventilation in these patients, therefore, is actually to support weak respiratory muscles rather than to provide "rest" therapy as previously postulated. Reports on the benefits of nocturnal mechanical ventilation in COPD patients have been unpredictable and inconsistent. They include improvement in daytime blood gases, increased vital capacity, increased respiratory muscle strength and endurance (with increased 12-minute walking distance, functional activities, and quality of life), as well as decreased dyspnea and decreased need for hospitalizations. These potential benefits outweigh the potential adverse effects (e.g., air trapping) of nocturnal mechanical ventilation in COPD patients with any combination of the following: maximal inspiratory force below 50 cmH_2O, FEV_1 less than 25% of predicted normal, $PaCO_2$ over 45 mmHg, chronic tachypnea (over 30/min), or chest and abdomen dyssynchrony (i.e., paradoxical breathing).

When mechanical ventilation is applied to the body, a positive pressure pushes the diaphragm cephalad to cause expiration, while a negative extrathoracic pressure on the chest wall and abdomen causes inspiration. The opposite occurs when mechanical ventilation is directly applied to the airway, that is, positive airway pressure causes inspiration by pushing air into the lungs, and negative airway pressure causes expiration. The following sections discuss both positive- and negative-pressure mechanical ventilations applied to the body as well as positive-pressure airway mechanical ventilation. Negative-pressure airway mechanical ventilation, which is mainly used for exsufflation in airway clearance, is discussed in section IV.B.1.b.3. Major complications of mechanical ventilation include pulmonary barotrauma (e.g., pneumomediastinum, pneumothorax, and emphysema), pulmonary thromboemboli, gastrointestinal bleeding, dysrhythmias, accumulation of large amounts of secretions, and others (e.g., nosocomial infections, laryngotracheal injury, malnutrition, hypophosphatemia, and oxygen toxicity).

a. ***Positive-pressure airway ventilation*** can be intermittent, continuous, or bilevel. In the PM&R setting, the intermittent positive-pressure (airway) ventilation (IPPV) is the most common method used for noninvasive ventilatory support. Occasionally, a continuous positive-pressure mechanical ventilation [i.e., using continuous positive airway pressure (CPAP)] may be used to provide a "pneumatic splint" to maintain airway patency in patients with sleep disordered breathing (e.g., obstructive sleep apneas) or in nonintubated patients with rapidly reversible respiratory failure (for 24–48 hours). It must be noted that CPAP, which never provides positive pressure ventilation because it is not cycled, can provide easier breathing by increasing the FRC and thereby opening the airways. Noninvasive CPAP can be provided via a tight-fitting CPAP mask. The CPAP is inadequate and poorly tolerated in patients with restricted pulmonary volumes and CAH. Instead, a bilevel positive airway pressure (BiPAP), which is more effective and comfortable, or an IPPV is preferred in treating the sleep disordered breathing in these patients. A BiPAP has independently varying inspiratory positive airway pressures (IPAP) and expiratory positive airway pressures (EPAP). The greater the IPAP/EPAP difference (i.e., span), the greater the inspiratory muscle support. To ensure adequate ventilation, BiPAP spans of at least 20 cmH_2O are often needed. The BiPAP can be applied via a face or nasal mask through a home ventilator unit (e.g., Respironic BiPAP unit).

I. **Types**

- **Volume-preset airway ventilators** deliver a preset volume of air with each breath; thus maintaining constant ventilation by the minute despite changes in compliance or resistance (e.g., as a result of secretions) of the respiratory system. Volume-preset ventilators are the initial ventilators used in emergency situations (e.g., acute respiratory failure) and are the ventilator of choice for home use in adults. Examples of popular home-care ventilator units used for IPPV include Aequitron LP-6, LP-6 plus, and LP-10; Lifecare PLV-100 and 102; Respironics PLV-102b; Puritan–Bennett Achieva; and Intermed Bear 33. Most home-care airway ventilators are powered by 12-volt, direct current, automotive-type batteries (rather than deep-drain golf-cart type-batteries), are portable, and have alarm, monitors, and oxygen-enrichment capability. They are usually prescribed with a battery-powered suction machine, a manual resuscitator, and a back-up ventilator and power generator. For comparative evaluation of home-ventilator units, refer to the latest report of *Health Devices* (e.g., issue 21(8):1–289, 1992), published by Emergency Care Research Institute (ECRI), or to the standards published by the American Society of Testing and Materials (ASTM), e.g., ASTM: *Minimum standard specifications for electrically powered home care portable ventilators. Part I: positive pressure ventilators,* Philadelphia, 1991, ASTM, D1246-91.
- **Pressure-preset airway ventilators** deliver air until a preset amount of pressure is reached (to prevent excessive airway pressures); thus, the tidal volume varies with airway resistance. Although adults prefer using pressure-preset ventilators (because they could easily compensate for leakage), they are seldom prescribed for home use by adults because most volume-preset ventilators can be set to mimic a pressure-preset ventilator. Pressure-preset ventilators may be used by children who have large or variable leak around the tracheostomy tube or who need tidal volumes below 200 mL (because most

volume-preset ventilators are not reliable in delivering less than 200 mL of tidal volume). All of the above examples of volume-preset, home-care airway ventilators (except the Intermed Bear 33) have pressure-preset capabilities.

II. **Routes**

- **Invasive routes** include intubation and tracheostomy (see section V).
- **Noninvasive routes** are usually used for IPPV for elective long-term ventilatory support in patients with CAH. They are generally more convenient and provide good alternatives to invasive IPPV routes. Noninvasive IPPV is also more convenient and often more effective than the noninvasive negative-pressure body ventilators (NPBVs) (discussed in section IV.A.4.b.3) because, in at least 30% of patients, NPBV may cause significant nocturnal oxygen desaturation because of upper airway collapse. Noninvasive IPPV for long-term care can be provided using portable home-care ventilator units with pressure limits (the criteria for prescription of home ventilator units are given in section IV.A.4.a.4.b). An IPPV is contraindicated in patients with pneumothorax, bullous lung disease, asthma, recent esophageal or gastric surgery, cardiac dysfunction, or in an uncooperative patient.
  - **Nasal IPPV (NIPPV)** is the most popular and practical route for elective long-term nocturnal ventilatory support. It can also be used for elective long-term daytime ventilatory support in patients who cannot use oral IPPV (OIPPV) because of an inability to turn the neck and grab the mouthpiece for OIPPV or in patients with no significant ventilator-free time [i.e., the maximum period of time tolerated off ventilator support without resorting to glossopharyngeal breathing (GPB)]. A commercially available CPAP mask is generally used for NIPPV because it is simple to use, inexpensive, and durable. However, if the CPAP mask is not comfortable or produces air leaks (especially at NIPPV airflow pressures above 15 cmH_2O), a custom-molded nasal interface may be constructed (e.g., using acrylic materials or using the Lifecare SEFAM Mask assembly kit consisting of silicone putties, elastic straps, and small plastic housings) to increase comfort and decrease insulation leakage.
  - **Oral IPPV** is ideal for elective long-term daytime ventilatory support and can be as effective as a tracheostomy IPPV. It may also be used for elective long-term nocturnal ventilatory support if NIPPV is inadequate. Because OIPPV is safe, effective, and associated with few complications, it can also be used to convert patients from a tracheostomy to a noninvasive aid and can also be used in weaning a patient from ventilatory support. For daytime OIPPV, a mouthpiece is either kept in the patient's mouth or fixed near the mouth, adjacent to the powered-wheelchair controls (e.g., Sip-and-Puff, tongue, or chin controls; see Chapter 4.7, section III.B.2), so the patient can easily grab it up to six to eight times a minute for full ventilatory support. The commercially available mouthpiece is simple, inexpensive, and permits the patient to use a mouthstick, to eat, and, if the patient can do GPB (see section IV.B.2.a), to talk with a more normal rate, rhythm, and volume. For nocturnal OIPPV, a lip-seal retention flange (or bite-plate retention) is recommended to retain the mouthpiece and to prevent leakage from the mouth. For additional comfort and relief of orthodontic pressure, a soft, flexible scuba mouthpiece or a custom-molded acrylic mouthpiece may be used. In patients with excessive nasal leakage, cotton pledgets (for plugging the nose) or a nose clip may be used.
  - **Strapless oral–nasal interface IPPV (SONI-IPPV)** is indicated for the patient who cannot use a strap-retained interface or if NIPPV and OIPPV are inadequate or uncomfortable. A SONI consists of a custom-molded acrylic bite-plate with metal clasps for retention to the teeth. The bite-plate is then

fixed to an extraoral mask shell, which is connected through a hose to the ventilator. The air-tight extraoral mask may be open to both the nose and mouth, allowing concurrent nasal and mouth IPPV. If not needed, the SONI can be pushed out by tongue movement alone. Because the bite-plate is crucial to its construction, a SONI cannot be fitted in patients with inadequate or unstable dentition.

III. Modes of assisted ventilation

- **Assist/control ventilation or assisted mechanical ventilation** (AMV) allows the patient to trigger a ventilator-delivered breath (at a preset tidal volume) by initiating a minimal inspiratory effort. If the patient's inspiratory effort falls below a preset rate, the ventilator ensures a minimal minute ventilation at a preselected rate and tidal volume. The AMV is the recommended mode for home ventilator units because it allows the patient to interact with the ventilator thus minimizing discomfort and allowing for an increase in minute ventilation in response to changes in physiologic demands. The sensitivity of the patient-triggering mechanism should be set (usually at an inspiratory effort of 2–3 cm) so as to avoid unintentional machine ventilation (which can lead to hyperventilation, hypocapnia, and respiratory alkalosis) but should allow for patient-triggered breaths without excessive effort (or without "fighting the ventilator") especially during sleep to ensure adequate support of the ventilatory muscles.
- **Intermittent mandatory ventilation (IMV)** delivers a preset rate and tidal volume of air to guarantee a minimum ventilator-delivered minute ventilation, but also allows the patient to breathe spontaneously without triggering the ventilator. It should be tried in patients who are "fighting the ventilator" in the AMV mode or in patients whose cardiac output is reduced during positive pressure ventilation (e.g., because of hypovolemia) because it results in less reduction of cardiac output. It is also useful for treating patients with some capacity for spontaneous breathing (e.g., those with COPD or sleep apnea) because it helps maintain respiratory muscle tone. It can be used for expediting weaning (i.e., by reducing the IMV rate, the patient gradually assumes the bulk of the breathing work). In IMV, the work of breathing as well as oxygen consumption are increased (when compared to AMV), thus making it deleterious to patients with myocardial insufficiency. Moreover, IMV should not be used by patients with depressed respiratory drive or impaired neurologic status. A form of IMV that is synchronized with the patient's spontaneous inspiratory effort is called the synchronized IMV (SIMV). The SIMV prevents the stacking of mandatory breaths on spontaneous breaths. In home ventilator units (unlike the bedside consoles) there is no demand flow or continuous flow of gas, hence IMV/SIMV is not recommended because of the marked increase in breathing workload.
- **Controlled mechanical ventilation** (CMV) has a preset tidal volume and rate and does not allow the patient to breathe spontaneously (this can be uncomfortable). It is seldom used except in unconscious and apneic patients.

IV. Prescription guidelines

- **Ventilator setting.** Initially a volume-preset ventilator is used with the following parameters: tidal volume of 10–15 mL/kg (ideal body weight is preferred); respiratory rate of 12 machine-delivered breaths per minute (depending on the desired $PaCO_2$ or pH; i.e., to decrease $PaCO_2$, the rate should be increased); and an oxygen concentration (FiO_2) of 100% (unless with evidence that lower FiO_2 will provide adequate oxygenation; the goal is to reduce the FiO_2 to a nontoxic level of below 40–50%). The choice for mode of assist is discussed above. The ABGs should be obtained 15–30 minutes after initiating mechanical ventilation and periodically thereafter to adjust the ventilator settings. If arterial oxygenation is inadequate (e.g., PaO_2 less than 60 mmHg; SaO_2 below 90%) despite FiO_2 being above 50%, use positive end-expiratory pressure (PEEP) to prevent the closure of edematous small airways. The initial PEEP setting is 5 cmH_2O, which can be increased by 2–5 cmH_2O to maintain PaO_2 above 60 mmHg or SaO_2 above 90%. Subsequent ventilator settings are adjusted so that the lowest FiO_2 is used to maintain PaO_2 over 60 mmHg (SaO_2 over 90% in patients with normal pH) and the optimal minute ventilation (tidal volume × rate) is used to normalize the pH and $PaCO_2$.

- **Criteria for home ventilation**
  - **Clinical stability**, that is, no significant sustained dyspnea or severe dyspnea or tachypnea; acceptable ABG with PaO_2 at least 60 mmHg using FiO_2 less than or equal to 40%; psychosocial stability; no life-threatening cardiac dysfunction or arrhythmias; no anticipated readmission to hospital for more than 1 month; ability to clear secretions (by oneself or with assistive devices or techniques); presence of gag or cough reflex; no significant aspiration, and no endotracheal tube (tracheostomy is acceptable for home ventilator).
  - **Physiological stability**, that is, no acute infections; optimal acid–base and metabolic status; other organs are stable; stable time on and off the ventilator; stable lung impedance (i.e., resistance and compliance); and the following ventilator parameters: FiO_2 stable and below 40%, PEEP less than 10 cmH_2O, and IMV not in use.
  - **Commitment from the patient as well as the caregiver** (who must ensure that the ventilator unit as well as the IPPV route are properly adjusted, especially during the night).

V. **Weaning guidelines**

- **Criteria for ventilator weaning** include improved clinical status (i.e., the patient is alert and is hemodynamically stable); adequate oxygenation (PaO_2 over 60 mmHg on FiO_2 below 40–50%); pH 7.33–7.48, with acceptable $PaCO_2$; respiratory rate at or below 25/min (may be at or below 30 for COPD patients); vital capacity at least 10 mL/kg; tidal volume at least 5 mL/kg; resting minute ventilation less than 10 L/min, with ability to double the resting minute ventilation by maximum voluntary effort; maximum inspiratory pressure more negative than –25 cmH_2O; PEEP less than 5 cmH_2O; and spontaneous ventilation via T-tube (or other continuous airflow circuit tube, with or without CPAP) for 1–4 hours with acceptable blood gases, without marked increases in respiratory rate or heart rate, or with a change in general status. The above criteria are only guidelines. Some patients (e.g., those with COPD) can be weaned despite failure to meet these criteria.
- **Ventilator-weaning techniques** involve the progressive withdrawal of ventilator support, that is a progressive increase in ventilator-free time. Various ventilator-weaning protocols have been described, such as those that use or gradually reduce IMV, SIMV, AMV, positive-pressure support ventilation (PSV), CPAP, or PEEP. Following strict protocols (with strict time schedules), however, may cause unnecessary anxiety in the patient. A simple and effective method that decreases patient anxiety by allowing the patient to follow his or her own weaning schedule is by using the OIPPV, that is, the patient is given access to a mouthpiece so that he or she may take an assisted breath only when needed to prevent dyspnea and to maintain SaO_2 above 90% (e.g., monitored via pulse oximetry). In this method, other modes of ventilator assistance (e.g., IMV, SIMV, PEEP, and PSV) can be turned off, and as the patient becomes more capable of independent ventilation, he or she takes

fewer assisted breaths; thus, effectively weaning without an imposed schedule or any complicated protocols.

- **Criteria for termination of weaning** include a rise or fall in systolic blood pressure of at least 20 mmHg or a rise or fall in diastolic blood pressure of at least 10 mmHg; an increase in respiratory rate of at least 10/min, or a respiratory rate above 30/min; change in pulse rate of at least 20/min, or a pulse rate of at least 120/min or 20% greater than baseline; or when any of the following occur: onset of cardiac arrhythmias, a decrease in tidal volume, an increase in $PaCO_2$, and signs of increased work of breathing such as labored breathing, use of accessory muscles, or fatigue.
- **Reasons for failure to wean** include excessive airway secretions, incompletely treated pulmonary infection, bronchospasm, depressed cardiac output, respiratory muscle weakness, hypophosphatemia and nutritional deficiency, drug toxicity (e.g., excessive central nervous system depression from sedatives), significant acid–base disturbances, and hypothyroidism. All these problems are reversible and must be treated before reattempting weaning.

b. ***Body ventilation*** is another noninvasive technique used for ventilatory support in patients with CAH. It can be administered through either positive- or negative-pressure body ventilators.

1. **Positive-pressure body ventilators** promote expiration by assisting the cephalad movement of the diaphragm through positive pressure on the abdomen. As the pressure is removed and the diaphragm returns to its resting position, passive inspiration occurs (to which the patient can add his or her own tidal volume through inspiratory effort, if the patient has any).

- **Intermittent abdominal-pressure ventilator (IAPV)** (e.g., **Pneumobelt, Exsufflation Belt**) consists of a rubber air sac contained in an abdominal corset, which can be intermittently inflated to move the diaphragm cephalad, causing a forced expiration. The rubber air sac is connected by tubing to a portable ventilator, which provides positive pressure to inflate the air sac (not the lungs). The IAPV may be worn beneath the patient's outer clothing (for better cosmesis), but it must fit snugly over the abdomen from the xiphoid process to just above the pelvic arch. When the IAPV sac is deflated, the abdominal contents and diaphragm fall to the resting position, and inspiration occurs passively (which can be supplemented by active forms of inspiration). The usual IAPV cycle is 40% inspiration and 60% expiration.

  The IAPV is the most cosmetic and convenient mode of assisted ventilation in wheelchair-bound patients with no significant ventilator-free time (i.e., less than 1 hour). It can be used as an elective long-term noninvasive alternative to ventilatory aids if NIPPV, OIPPV, and SONI-IPPV are inadequate or uncomfortable. Its use is only effective, however, in the daytime because the patient must be in a sitting position (a trunk angle of 75° from horizontal is optimal, although 45° may be adequate in most cases). The patient also should not have significant scoliosis or be extremely obese. The IAPV can deliver a tidal volume from 250 to 500 mL (with reports of up to 1200 mL) and these volumes can be augmented by diaphragm action (when present) as well as by the use of GPB (see section IV.B.2.a). Although the IAPV has been used for daytime support by patients who receive tracheostomy IPPV overnight, its greatest benefit is derived when it is used in conjunction with the noninvasive nocturnal NIPPV or OIPPV. IAPV frees the mouth for the mouthstick and other activities.
- **Rocking bed with head down** (see section IV.A.4.b.2.a).
- **External oscillation ventilator set at *positive* pressure** (see section IV.A.4.b.2.b).

II. **Negative- and positive-pressure body ventilator**

- **Rocking bed.** This tilts the patient through a 15° or 30°, head-down position to a 30°, head-up position at an adjustable rate of 8 to 34 tilts per minute. When the head of the bed is up, negative pressure is produced to assist inspiration by using gravity to pull the diaphragm caudad; however, when the head is down, positive pressure is produced to assist expiration by the cephalad movement of the abdominal viscera, which pushes the diaphragm cephalad. In patients of relatively normal body weight and with some abdominal girth, the rocking motion of the bed assists in establishing tidal volumes of 250–400 mL. It is best for patients who have diaphragm paralysis and some accessory muscle use and who do not have primary pulmonary disease (i.e., those with good pulmonary compliance). The rocking motion produces a more physiologic type of breathing, aids circulation (thus preventing venous stasis and pressure ulcers), and assists in bowel motility and in the clearance of bronchial secretions. It is easy to use without the need for any restricting appliances, and it allows free access to the patient; however, it is one of the least effective ventilatory aids and is heavy, bulky, not portable, and rarely helpful in ventilating patients with poor chest wall or lung compliance. Although the bed has a break at the knee to prevent sliding, there are reports of patients falling from the bed. Moreover, although movement occurs only in one plane, some patients may complain of motion sickness.

  The rocking bed is not usually used simultaneously with another form of ventilation (OIPPV or NIPPV). However, it can be set up to have synchronous timing with these other ventilators, if it does not provide sufficient ventilation by itself. The other forms of ventilation are generally used when the patient either has stopped the bed for nursing care or is out of the bed in a wheelchair. The rocking bed provides extremely effective angle (head down) for postural drainage of the lung bases, and if the patient is prone, of the posterior segments.

- **External oscillation ventilator (Hayek Oscillator)** is a new type of ventilator, which consists of a lightweight flexible chest enclosure (cuirass) and an external computerized oscillating ventilator. The oscillating ventilator uses negative and positive pressures to generate a pressure change between the cuirass and the chest wall. The negative pressure causes the chest wall to expand and pulls air into the lungs thus producing inspiration. Positive pressure compresses the chest wall and forces air out to produce expiration. The oscillating ventilator provides full control over the whole respiratory cycle, because both inspiratory and expiratory phases are active and not reliant on passive recoil of the chest. While inspiratory pressure is always negative, expiratory pressure can be made positive, zero (atmospheric), or negative. This means that the ventilation cycle can commence above, at, or below functional residual capacity. The oscillating ventilator can also be used for secretion clearance by increasing the frequency of the oscillations (up to 999) per minute. It can be used for normal and abnormal lungs (including lungs with poor compliance) and has the same disadvantage as cuirass (see section IV.A.4.b.3.b).

III. **Negative-pressure body ventilators (NPBV)** promote inspiration by creating an intermittent negative extrathoracic (subatmospheric) pressure in the chest wall and abdomen. These are mainly used for nocturnal ventilatory support (except for the cuirass ventilators, which can also be used in the daytime in a sitting position), because they are not as convenient or as effective in providing long-term ventilation as the other noninvasive methods (e.g., NIPPV or OIPPV). Most NPBVs are not flexible in that they do not have mechanisms for aborting the development of negative pressure once the unit activates the inspiratory phase, regardless of what the patient desires (thus causing patient discomfort). In general, they are cumbersome and require the assistance of another person to apply or assemble the external device. Patients using NPBV also have difficulty in getting out of bed in the middle of the night or sleeping in any position but supine, are unable to sleep with their significant other, are unable to travel, and frequently complain of being cold during therapy because the negative pressure causes air to be drawn across the patient's chest during inspiration.

The NPBVs are contraindicated in patients with upper airway obstruction because they enhance the development of negative intrathoracic pressure (because the assisted breaths are not initiated by the patient), which increases the frequency and severity of upper airway collapse and obstruction to airflow during sleep (in these patients concurrent CPAP may be required). There are reports that associate NPBV with significant obstructive apneas and oxyhemoglobin desaturations during sleep (thus causing fatigue and other symptoms of ventilatory insufficiency, especially in patients using little or no daytime ventilatory aids) and with recurrent aspiration. The NPBVs should also not be used when there are excessive airway secretions (because of difficulty in the use of mechanical exsufflation or manually assisted airway secretion clearance techniques) or in other cases in which lung compliance or airway resistance is expected to vary extensively throughout the period of assisted ventilation.

- **Tank or "Drinker" ventilators** (e.g., **Emerson Iron Lung, Porta-lung**) enclose the entire body of the patient (sealed from neck down) in a chamber that produces intermittent subatmospheric pressure by a motor-driven bellow (Iron Lung) or by a separate negative-pressure generator (Porta-lung). They are reliable NPBVs with 100% efficiency as compared to a cuirass because there is no counterpressure on parts of the trunk when negative pressure is being produced in the tank. They are indicated for the management of patients with acute respiratory failure; for ventilatory support in otherwise hard to ventilate patients with decreased pulmonary compliance or significant scoliosis; and for temporary ventilatory aid in patients with acute upper respiratory tract infections who otherwise use NIPPV or OIPPV (because they free the nose and mouth for clearing secretions). General disadvantages of tank ventilators include difficulty in comfortable fitting of some patients with severe skeletal deformities or with an indwelling tracheostomy; claustrophobic reactions in some patients; and, although patients may be turned while inside the tank, other routine nursing or medical care requires that the patient be pulled out (or the chamber opened) and be given alternative ventilatory supports (preferably OIPPV or GPB). The Iron Lung is heavy (over 300 lb or 136 kg), immobile, requires assistance to enter or exit, and costly; while the Porta-lung also requires assistance to enter or exit but is lighter (about 110 lb or 50 kg) and can be portable.
- **Cuirass (or chest-shell) ventilators** (e.g., **Turtle Shell**) consist of an easy-to-don firm shell (which covers the anterior chest and abdomen) and a negative-pressure ventilator unit (which creates the subatmospheric pressure under the shell). They have only 45% efficiency compared to tank ventilators but are adequate for most patients provided that there is no complete respiratory paralysis or impairment of pulmonary compliance, apnea, intrinsic lung disease, severe back deformity, or morbid obesity. The cuirass ventilators are the only NPBV that can also be used for daytime ventilatory support in the seated position (although the IAPV, OIPPV, or NIPPV are invariably preferred). Because of their simplicity and convenience (functional

patient can enter and exit without assistance), the cuirass ventilators are the method of choice for providing temporary ventilatory support when converting a patient from tracheostomy- or intubation-IPPV to OIPPV or NIPPV (e.g., while waiting for the tracheostomy sites to close, which usually takes 2 or more days; or during extubation for patients being converted from IPPV through endotracheal intubation). The customized chest cuirass is better tolerated and provides less air leak than those mass-produced. In insensate patients, the cuirass ventilator may cause pressure ulcers especially at the area anterior to the axilla.

- **Wrap ventilators** (e.g., **Poncho; Pneumosuit**) consist of a firm plastic grid or frame (covering the thorax and abdomen) and are covered by a windproof wrap made of various materials (e.g., Gortex which is cooler, more flexible, and more comfortable but more expensive than plastic or cloth) in several styles (e.g., Poncho, which covers chest, part of arms, and torso to midhip, or a one-piece Pneumosuit). The wrap is sealed around the patient's wrists, neck, and abdomen or lower limbs depending on the style. As with cuirass ventilators, a negative-pressure ventilator unit is used to create the subatmospheric pressure under the grid and wrap; however, they provide greater volumes and are more efficient than cuirass ventilators. Wrap ventilators have about 60% efficiency compared to tank ventilators when carefully placed and correctly used. They are excellent for patients with difficult fit (e.g., patients with scoliosis but not for markedly obese patients) or with sensory deficits; however, they are time-consuming to don, are difficult to access for nursing or medical care of the body, and also make turning the patient difficult. As with other NPBVs, they are only used for nocturnal assisted ventilation.
- **Rocking bed with head *up*** (see section IV.A.4.b.2.a).
- **External oscillation ventilator set at *negative* pressure** (see section IV.A.4.b.2.b).

B. PULMONARY REHABILITATION MODALITIES

1. **Secretion removal techniques** consist of secretion mobilization followed by airway-clearance techniques. Their benefits include reduced work of breathing, increased ventilation and gas exchange capabilities, prevention of infection and atelectasis, and improved performance of exercise and ADL.

a. ***Secretion mobilization techniques*** usually involve the use of percussion, shaking, or vibration to loosen and mobilize secretions in a patient placed in specific positions for postural drainage. To be effective, they must be followed by airway-clearance techniques. An inhaled bronchodilator may be used 10–20 minutes prior to secretion mobilization to facilitate secretion movement. The patient should also be adequately hydrated by daily fluid intake. The use of inhaled moisture from a nebulizer or humidifier is mainly beneficial to patients with a tracheostomy because of loss of upper respiratory tract humidification. Secretion mobilization techniques are generally indicated for pulmonary conditions with more than 30 mL of secretions per day (e.g., cystic fibrosis, chronic bronchitis, bronchiectasis, and possibly asthma), aspirations, and atelectasis. Despite wide acceptance, there are no controlled studies that show that they shorten hospital stays, decrease the number of exacerbations, or reduce morbidity or mortality. They do not seem to be beneficial in treating pneumonia or viral bronchiolitis or as a routine postoperative measure. In acutely ill patients, they can cause hypoxemia and oxyhemoglobin desaturation.

I. **Postural drainage** involves the use of nine distinct gravity-assisted positions to improve the mobilization of secretions from individual lung lobes and segments. In general, the affected lung segment is positioned uppermost for drainage as well as for oxygenation. A commonly used position is the head-down (or Trendelenburg) posture with the patient either supine or prone and in varying degrees of trunk rotation or side-lying. The head-down angle of drainage is usually between 10° and 45° (except when the upper lobes are drained, which is accomplished by having the patient sit up or lie flat). Studies show that COPD patients are able to tolerate up to a 25° head-down tilt. Precautions for the head-down position include circulatory problems (e.g., pulmonary edema, congestive heart failure, and hypertension), abdominal problems (e.g., obesity, abdominal distention, hiatal hernia, nausea, and recent food consumption), and dyspnea. For the side-lying position, precautions include axillofemoral bypass graft and musculoskeletal pain (e.g., recent rib fracture) that could be aggravated by the position. In postural drainage, care must be taken to ensure that drainage from the uppermost part of the diseased lung does not spill into and compromise the dependent "good" lung. Postural drainage is best done after awakening in the morning (because of secretion accumulation at night) and 1–2 hours after meals (to avoid gastroesophageal reflux).

II. **Percussion (clapping)** is applied throughout the entire respiratory cycle by rhythmically striking the thoracic cage with cupped hands or by using a mechanical percussor to loosen airway secretions from bronchial walls. It is delivered at a frequency of about 5 Hz for 1–5 minutes (or longer) over the chest area that is draining. In patients with sensitive skin (e.g., elderly patients), a thin towel may be draped over the percussed zone. Precautions of percussion include circulatory problems [e.g., coagulation disorders, a platelet count below 50 000 mm^3 ($<50 \times 10^9$ L), and anticoagulation therapy] and musculoskeletal problems (e.g., fractured ribs, flail chest, degenerative bone disease, severe osteoporosis, or other fragile bone disorders). Contraindications include cardiovascular instability or failure, hemoptysis, increased intracranial or intraocular pressure, or aortic aneurysm.

III. **Shaking** is the application of a downward pressure type of bouncing maneuver (at 2 Hz) to a specific area on the thorax (corresponding to the underlying involved lung segment) throughout the expiratory phase of breathing. It is commonly used following percussion. It has the same precautions and contraindications as percussion.

IV. **Vibration** is a gentler modification of shaking applied manually to specific areas of the thorax during expiration. A vibrator may also be used with a frequency of 10–15 Hz and applied throughout the respiratory cycle. Because vibration uses little or no pressure to the thorax, it may be used when percussion and shaking are contraindicated. The use of expensive vibrating modalities (e.g., vibrating vests, air vibration under chest shells, or high-frequency oscillators) has not been shown to be significantly effective to justify their costs. However, in patients requiring chest vibration several times a day (e.g., cystic fibrosis or advanced bronchiectasis), their initial high cost may be worthwhile because they provide vibration with ease and their application is not labor intensive and does not require skilled personnel.

b. ***Airway-clearance techniques*** depend on intact mucociliary clearance mechanisms and the generation of optimal peak cough expiratory flow (PCEF) rates of more than 5–6 L/s. The mucociliary clearance mechanisms (i.e., ciliary and alveolar macrophage activities) are incapacitated by intubation and tracheostomy tubes as well as during infections, while PCEF is decreased in patients with pulmonary restrictive disease, ventilator assistance, oropharyngeal muscle weakness, abdominal muscle weakness, or intubation/tracheostomy tube (because of inability to close the glottis to generate expiratory pressures). Although airway suctioning can clear secretions from the upper airways, it does not help clear or mobilize the deeper secretions. Moreover, suction can cause potential complications (see below). Techniques to increase PCEF (i.e., cough maneuvers and their variations) are more effective than airway suctioning. In patients with COPD, the most effective mechanical aid for clearing the airway is the use of mechanical insufflator–exsufflators.

I. **Cough maneuvers** are the most common and easiest means of clearing the larger upper and central airways. They must be controlled to prevent dynamic airway collapse, bronchospasm, syncope, chest wall pain, and dyspnea. The sequence of cough involves deep inspiration, glottic closure, thoracoabdominal pressure generation, and glottic opening and expulsion. The glottis closure and the increased intrathoracic pressure can collapse the small airways in some patients with COPD, thus trapping the air behind the closed airway and making the cough ineffective (in these patients, the huffing techniques described below are recommended).

- **Controlled cough** is a timed, deliberate, coordinated forceful expiration used to mobilize the mucus without causing airway collapse. It is most effective when done in an upright or seated position in patients with a PCEF of at least 5–6 L/s, a maximum insufflation capacity (MIC) over 500 mL, and excessive airway secretion production (e.g., more than 30 mL/day). During the cough, a transient expiratory air velocity as high as 200–250 m/s can be created in the central airways to provide a shearing force to expel mucus that adheres to airway walls. The upright patient inhales deeply, holds the breath for several seconds (to close the glottis), contracts the abdominal muscles (i.e., "bears down" to create an increased intrathoracic pressure of 50–200 mmHg), then opens the glottis and forcefully and rapidly expels the air while contracting the abdominal muscles and leaning slightly forward. Two or three coughs are carried out with open mouth without taking another breath. The patient then takes a slow deep inhalation and repeats the whole procedure two or three times, then rests and breathes normally for several minutes before repeating the controlled coughing.
- **Tracheal cough stimulation** is used for patients who are unable to cough on command (e.g., after stroke or head trauma). A quick inward and downward pressure on the trachea (applied by placing the clinician's finger or thumb just above the suprasternal notch) is used to elicit the cough reflex.
- **Active-assistive cough** is used in patients with ineffective cough (i.e., PCEF of less than 6 L/s) as a result of weak or paralyzed abdominal muscles (e.g., because of cervical tetraplegia). If the patient's vital capacity is below 1200–1500 mL, a deep mechanical insufflation may be provided, followed by active-assistive cough to provide a PCEF of 5–7 L/s. Active-assistive coughing may be inadequate during severe upper respiratory tract infections or in patients with scoliosis or impaired function of the glottis (i.e., MIC of less than 500 mL). In these patients, the mechanical insufflator–exsufflator (described below) is recommended.
  - **Manually assisted cough** involves the use of the clinician's (or assisting person's) arm or heel of the hand to apply forces at various sites of the trunk in synchrony with the patient's expiratory or coughing effort. The pressure may be applied at the navel pushing up against the diaphragm while the patient is side-lying (i.e., Heimlich-type assist or abdominal thrust assist); the costophrenic angles of the rib cage with the patient assuming any position (i.e., costophrenic assist); the upper and lower anterior chest while the patient lies on one side or in a three-quarter supine position (i.e., anterior chest compression assist); or in a counterrotational stretch direction of chest expansion applied to the patient's shoulder and pelvis during inspiration followed by reversing the pressure direction to compress the thorax on all planes to facilitate forceful expulsion (i.e., counterrotation assist).

- **Self-assisted cough** is more advanced and involves more active participation from the patient. The patient assumes or is physically assisted into one of the following positions: prone-on-elbows, long-sitting, short-sitting (e.g., on bedside), hands-and-knees, or standing. The patient is then taught to extend the head and trunk during maximal inspiration followed by flexion of the head and trunk during cough.

- **Electrically stimulated cough** has been used for patients with paralyzed or weak abdominal muscles (e.g., spinal cord injury above the mid-thoracic level) by timing the stimulation of the abdominal muscles with expiration; however, this method needs further study.

II. **Huffing** is similar to controlled coughing except that the glottis remains open. The patient inhales deeply and immediately expels the air out by contracting the abdominal muscles and saying, "Ha, ha, ha". Huffing does not increase the intrathoracic pressure (as in coughing), hence the collapsible airway walls (e.g., in COPD patients) are stabilized, thus making expiration and secretion removal more effective in these patients.

- **Forced expiratory technique (FET)** is a form of huffing used for "milking" the secretions from the more peripheral airways that coughing may not affect. The patient is first taught to expand the lower chest (i.e., diaphragmatic breathing, with or without percussion and shaking), then to inhale a normal amount of air (resting tidal volume) followed by abdominal contractions to produce one or two forced exhalations starting at mid-lung volume and continuing to a low lung volume. This is followed by expectoration or a controlled cough at high lung volume to clear mucus from the central airways and then by a period of diaphragmatic breathing. The advantages for FET include less fatigue, less likelihood of bronchospasm, and less dynamic airway collapse (because of reduced transpulmonary pressures). The FET can be used in patients with COPD (including cystic fibrosis and asthma).
- **Positive expiratory pressure (PEP) technique** may be used prior to huffing. The patient exhales down to the functional residual capacity through a face mask or a mouthpiece (including a nose clip) with a one-way valve (to which variable expiratory resistance is applied) to achieve a PEP of 10–20 cmH_2O (as measured by a pressure manometer in mid-exhalation), for five to 15 breaths. This is followed by a few short, quick huffs and spontaneous coughs as needed. The use of PEP can theoretically limit the dynamic expiratory airway closure while also increasing lung volume and directing air distal to and behind airway secretions so that these secretions can be more easily expelled.

III. **Mechanical insufflation–exsufflation technique (e.g., Emerson CoughAssist® Mechanical In-Exsufflator (MI-E) Cough Machine)** is highly effective in removing airway secretions in patients with chronic restrictive pulmonary disease. It provides a deep inspiration (by positive-pressure insufflation) either through a mask or through the tracheal tube (tracheostomy or endotracheal) followed rapidly by a controlled suction (by negative-pressure exsufflation) of secretions into the mouth, mask, or tracheal tube where it can easily be suctioned. The sudden drop of insufflation pressure to exsufflation pressure (usually about 80 cmH_2O) occurs in less than 0.1 second and is sustained for 1.5–3 seconds to create a PCEF of 7–11 L/s. The duration of negative-pressure exsufflation is significantly longer than those produced by all other forms of airway clearance. The technique is easy, comfortable, and has no reported complications. Because it effectively clears secretions and mucus plugs, it also increases pulmonary volumes and normalizes SaO_2. It is effective even in patients with severe URIs, scoliosis, impaired function of the glottis, or dysphagia. It also allows earlier ventilator weaning of intubated or tracheostomized patients, as well as continued ventilatory support without a tracheostomy.

IV. **Suctioning** may be performed through the mouth or nose but is facilitated by an endotracheal tube (ET) or tracheostomy tube (TT). When suctioning the TT (or ET) in the hospital setting, a sterile technique is mandatory; while for suctioning (of TT) outside the hospital, a clean technique (using clean reusable suction catheters) is usually employed. Suctioning should be performed in conjunction with other airway-clearance techniques or when the other techniques fail to remove secretions adequately. Suctioning must be done judiciously as it may lead to complications including hypoxemia, brady- or tachycardia, hypo- or hypertension, increased intracranial pressure, atelectasis, tracheal damage, or nosocomial infections. Suctioning can also irritate the airway membranes and exacerbate secretion problems as well as causing airway edema and wheezing.

2. **Controlled-breathing techniques** are generally used to improve PFT parameters, reduce dyspnea, reduce the work of breathing, and improve ventilatory muscle function. These techniques also facilitate relaxation (see Chapter 4.2, section VI) and are indicated in patients with obstructive or restrictive pulmonary problems. Patients are usually instructed to inspire nasally (to ensure a slow, even inspiration, and prevent mouth drying) and to exhale orally (to provide the least resistance to air flow). Controlled-breathing techniques can be classified by the intended specific goals as follows:

a. ***Controlled-breathing techniques to improve PFT parameters,*** i.e., to increase lung volume, redistribute ventilation, maintain or restore functional residual capacity, and improve gas exchange.

I. **Diaphragmatic breathing** involves retraining the patient to use the diaphragm while relaxing abdominal muscles during inspiration (i.e., the abdomen rises while the chest wall remains stationary). It is first taught to the patient in a semi-Fowler's (semi-reclined sitting) position, then progressed to sitting, standing, walking, stair-climbing, and other activities. It may be synchronized with range-of-motion exercises of the upper limbs (e.g., shoulder elevation on inspiration) to promote lung expansion. Theoretically, the use of the diaphragm (the principal and most efficient muscle of inspiration) can make breathing more efficient with decreased oxygen cost. However, studies done in COPD patients have shown that it tends to increase rather than decrease the level of dyspnea because of overall chest wall motion asynchrony, abdominal paradox, reduced mechanical efficiency of the chest wall, and increased work of breathing with this maneuver without improvement in the distribution of ventilation to the lung bases. Thus the American Thoracic Society (1999) does not recommend its routine use in COPD patients. It may, however, be taught to non-COPD patients during pulmonary rehabilitation.

II. **Segmental breathing** is aimed at hypoventilated segments of the lungs in patients with pleuritic pain and splinting (e.g., because of surgery or trauma) as well as segmental atelectasis. Prior to segmental breathing, any airway obstruction must be cleared (e.g., mucus plugs must be removed by secretion removal techniques described above; bronchogenic tumors must be resected). The patient is asked to inspire against the resistance of the clinician's hand(s) placed at the thorax over the area of hypoventilation. As the clinician feels the local expansion of the thorax, the hand resistance is released to allow full inhalation.

III. **Sustained maximal inspiration (or incentive spirometer technique)** involves slow inspiration through the nose or pursed lips. When maximal inspiration is reached, it is held for 3 seconds before passively exhaling the volume. It is used in acute situations for patients with post-traumatic pain, postoperative pain, or acute lobar collapse. An incentive spirometer may be used to provide visual feedback of the volume of inspired air.

IV. **Glossopharyngeal breathing (GPB) or frog breathing**, which can technically be considered an IPPV, is a technique used by patients with chronic restrictive pulmonary disease in which the patient takes a deep (maximum) breath, and then uses the pistoning action of the tongue and pharyngeal muscle to project boluses of air past the glottis into the lungs. The lips, soft palate, and vocal cords open and close in rhythm during each pistoning stroke. In one breath, the patient usually performs six to eight (or up to 65) boluses or gulps, with each gulp consisting of 30 to 150 mL (usually 60–100 mL) of air. For GPB to be effective, the patient must have intact oropharyngeal muscle strength and should not be tracheostomized (even if the tracheostomy tube is plugged, gulped air can still leak around the tube and out of the tracheostomy site). Glossopharyngeal breathing enables the patient (even those with little or no vital capacity) to breathe without mechanical ventilation (up to 4 or more hours if the lungs are normal; otherwise, GPB may only be tolerated for minutes). This ventilator-free time is important when switching between different types of noninvasive aids and for security in case of ventilator failure. The GPB can also improve the volume of the voice (some patients may be able to shout for help), improve the flow and rhythm of speech, provide the deep breath needed for an effective assisted cough, help prevent microatelectasis, and improve or maintain pulmonary compliance. If during GPB, the SaO_2 falls to 85–90% or less, the patient typically complains of fatigue and requires mechanical ventilatory assistance.

b. ***Controlled-breathing techniques*** to reduce dyspnea and the work of breathing.

I. **Pursed lip breathing (PLB)** is used to reduce dyspnea and the work of breathing in patients with chronic airflow obstruction (e.g., COPD) by preventing air trapping caused by the collapse of small airways. The patient inhales through the nose for several seconds with the mouth closed, then exhales slowly for 4–6 seconds through pursed lips (i.e., a whistling or kissing position). During PLB, there should be no expiratory airflow through the nose and the patient usually bends forward slightly. The abdominal muscles are usually relaxed but may be contracted judiciously to increase the exhaled volume (making sure not to increase intrathoracic pressure as this might produce airway collapse). To prolong the expiration phase, the clinician may apply gentle pressure on the patient's abdomen. Pursed lip breathing, together with diaphragmatic breathing, is used during and following an exercise or activity that can induce tachypnea leading to dyspnea. Additional effects of PLB include reduced respiratory rate, increased tidal volume, maintenance of minute ventilation while decreas-ing the work of breathing, improved gas mixing at rest, and facilitation of relaxation.

II. **Paced breathing** is a process in which the patient breaks down an activity (that might otherwise be unattainable because of dyspnea) into small attainable tasks, then uses PLB and rest periods to complete each task at a comfortable tempo until the whole activity is completed without dyspnea and fatigue. For example, to climb one flight of stairs, the patient inhales at rest, then on exhalation (using PLB) the patient ascends one or two steps at a time and stops to rest until full recovery. The patient repeats this process until the whole flight is ascended without dyspnea.

c. ***Controlled breathing technique to improve ventilatory muscle functions*** (i.e., to increase the strength, endurance, and efficiency of ventilatory muscles).

The strength and endurance of the ventilatory skeletal muscles can be improved by general aerobic exercise alone as well as by using controlled breathing for ventilatory muscle training. Recent studies have shown that the exercise-induced improvement in ventilatory muscle function appears to be mode-specific, that is, endurance training improves the ability to increase sustained hyperpnea, whereas pure strength training improves inspiratory pressures. There are currently, however, no definitive data on the long-term benefits of ventilatory muscle training, the effect on functional activities, or criteria for patient selection or which ventilatory muscle training protocol to use.

I. **Inspiratory resistance training (IRT)**. According to the 1997 ACCP/AACVPR Pulmonary Rehabilitation Guidelines Panel, there is no scientific evidence to support the routine use of IRT as an essential component of pulmonary rehabilitation. However, IRT may be considered in selected patients with COPD who have decreased respiratory muscle strength and who remain dyspneic despite optimal therapy.

- **Inspiratory resistive loading** can be attained by using an inspiratory muscle trainer (IMT), which loads the inspiratory muscles by having the patient inhale through inspiratory orifices of progressively decreasing diameter (and to exhale without resistance). The initial aperture opening is determined by using 30–40% of the maximum inspiratory pressure (MIP) or by selecting the smallest aperture the patient can tolerate for a 10-minute exercise period. The training is carried out at a rate of 10–20 breaths/minute for 15–30 minutes, once or twice per day. After attaining a duration of 30 minutes, the exercise intensity is progressed by narrowing the aperture. For endurance training, use either a lower percentage of MIP or the aperture opening that would allow a longer exercise duration. The IMTs are indicated in stable patients with chronic restrictive pulmonary disease (i.e., with decreased compliance, decreased intrathoracic volume, or decreased strength of the respiratory muscle caused by long-term ventilatory support) and COPD (i.e., with resistance to airflow or alteration in length–tension relationship of ventilatory muscles in a barrel chest). The use of IMTs has been shown to improve strength, endurance, and functional capacity (i.e., ability to do ADLs).
- **Inspiratory threshold loading** can be attained by using a threshold loading device that permits inspiration only after reaching a threshold mouth pressure (set by means of a weighted plunger or by adjusting the tension of a spring-loaded valve). Unlike IMTs, the threshold loading device produces inspiratory resistance without relying on inspiratory flow rates. Inspiratory threshold loading improves ventilatory strength and endurance but not functional capacity.

II. **Voluntary isocapnic hyperpnea** uses prolonged periods of hyperpnea to provide low tension and a high level of repetitive activity for the diaphragm and other inspiratory muscles, thus leading to improved endurance. The patient is asked to maintain as high a level of minute ventilation as possible (breathing frequency is usually between 30 and 60 breaths per minute) for periods of 10–15 minutes usually twice daily. Voluntary isocapnic hyperpnea has been shown to improve endurance but not functional capacity. However, training systems for voluntary isocapnic hyperpnea are not generally portable and require monitoring so that patients need to train at a medical facility.

3. Abdominal muscle exercise and support

a. ***Abdominal strengthening exercises*** may be performed to help improve airway clearance (e.g., by increasing coughing force). These include partial sit-up exercises and possibly the use of neuromuscular electrical stimulation in innervated muscles (see Chapter 4.1, section V.B.3).

b. ***Abdominal binders*** may be used to enhance the expiratory phase of breathing in patients with weak abdominal muscles (e.g., high thoracic and cervical spinal cord injuries). However, they must not be so tight as to restrict inspiration. In COPD patients, abdominal binders should not be used because they impede breathing.

4. **Postural relief techniques** involve the use of appropriate positioning to reduce dyspnea by optimizing aeration, improving perfusion, and/or maximizing ventilation–perfusion ratios. Patients with COPD frequently lean forward at the waist (about 20–45° from the vertical) and bear weight on the elbows for support with the arms and shoulders (usually elevated) in a locked position. If seated, the patient supports himself or herself by bracing the elbows or hands on the knees or on a table. When ambulating, a rolling walker or bilateral canes may be used to allow forward leaning. The forward-leaning position has been shown to decrease dyspnea and to increase exercise tolerance. The physiologic basis for dyspnea relief in the forward-leaning posture is probably the result of the improved length–tension status of the diaphragm making it more efficient. In some COPD patients with low, flat, and overly shortened diaphragms, the head-down (Trendelenberg) position at 10° to 20° tilt may facilitate diaphragm movement, thus decreasing dyspnea. In general, a flat, supine position is poorly tolerated by most pulmonary patients.

5. **General reconditioning exercises** are used to improve functional capacity. According to the 1997 ACCP/AACVPR Pulmonary Rehabilitation Guidelines Panel, training of the lower extremities and upper extremities should be included in rehabilitation programs for patients with COPD. All exercises must emphasize proper breathing techniques, proper body mechanics, and must include adequate warm-up and cool-down periods. In patients with neuromuscular diseases, exercises should not be performed to the point of fatigue. All patients must be given an appropriate home exercise program and instructed to keep a log of their exercise. Patients must be followed at a regular interval to ensure that they are doing the exercises properly and with appropriate progression. Patients must maintain a regular exercise regime, or they will lose any gains made from the exercise.

a. ***Lower-extremity endurance training,*** i.e., low- to moderate-impact aerobic (cardiopulmonary) endurance exercises (described in Chapter 4.2, section III.A) of the muscles of ambulation, includes treadmill walking, ground-based walking, stair climbing, calisthenics, stationary bicycle, and pool activities. To date, the optimal specific exercise prescription guidelines for lower-extremity training have not been defined with certainty. Although lower-extremity exercises do not improve measures of lung function, they can improve the functional capabilities for ambulation. If possible, a graded-exercise tolerance test (see Chapter 2.7, section II.A), a PFT (see Chapter 2.6), and an ABG should be done prior to starting the exercise program. Graded-exercise tolerance tests may be used to determine the mode, intensity, duration, and frequency of lower-extremity training. A 10% decrease in FEV_1 or $FEF_{25-75\%}$ indicates the need for pre-exercise bronchodilator therapy. Supplemental oxygen (see section IV.A.3) is needed if there is a decrease in PaO_2 of more than 20 mmHg or if the PaO_2 is less than 55 mmHg during exercise.

b. ***Upper extremity training***

I. **Aerobic (cardiopulmonary) endurance exercises** (described in Chapter 4.2, section III.A) of the upper extremities include: arm ergometry (start at approximately 50 rpm without resistance, then gradually increase resistance at 5-week intervals until 20–30 minutes of exercise are tolerated); and repetitive lifting of free weights (or dowels, or elastic bands) up to shoulder level (start with the lowest resistance, then increase as tolerated until

20–30 minutes of exercise). The exercise response is monitored in terms of arm fatigue and dyspnea.

II. **Strengthening exercises** (described in Chapter 4.2, section II) of the arms involve low-repetition of weight-lifting (ranging from 50 to 85% of one-repetition maximum; see Chapter 4.2, section II.B.2.a.1) to increase peripheral upper-extremity muscle strength. Although there was no concomitant increase in maximal endurance exercise capacity, there was a measured improvement in quality of life.

6. **Relaxation techniques** (see Chapter 4.2, section VI)
7. **Energy conservation techniques** can lower the energy expenditure and the oxygen consumption of an activity, thus allowing patients with pulmonary problems to perform essential ADLs (without dyspnea or fatigue) independently or with the least amount of assistance. Energy conservation techniques involve the use of assistive and adaptive devices (see Chapter 4.5, section I.B.3), activity planning and preparation (i.e., scheduling, organizing, and prioritizing of tasks or choosing the "best breathing" time), paced breathing (see section IV.B.2.b.2), efficient breathing techniques (see section IV.B.2 on breathing exercises for relaxation and reduction of the work of breathing). Specific energy conservation and work simplification techniques used in pulmonary rehabilitation are described by Rashbaum and Whyte (see Further reading section).
8. **Psychosocial and behavioral interventions** may be recommended for appropriate chronic pulmonary patients with concomitant psychological (e.g., depression, anxiety) and/or psychosocial (e.g., low self-esteem, poor social relations, marital conflict) problems. According to the 1997 ACCP/AACVPR Pulmonary Rehabilitation Guidelines Panel, evidence to date does not support the benefits of short-term psychosocial interventions as single therapeutic modalities, but longer term interventions may be beneficial components of comprehensive pulmonary rehabilitation programs for COPD patients.
9. **Vocational measures** may be needed for appropriate patients to help them cope with vocational issues related to their chronic pulmonary problems.

V. Invasive management

Invasive management is used only if noninvasive methods fails or are inadequate.

A. TRACHEAL INTUBATION can be attained by either using an ET or TT. The indication for tracheal intubation or tracheostomy is acute respiratory failure (PaO_2 below 55 mmHg or $PaCO_2$ above 50 mmHg) as a result of acute pulmonary disease, intrinsic lung disease, or obstructive or restrictive respiratory disease that necessitate:

- Supplemental oxygen for which noninvasive mechanical ventilation is inadequate or not possible because of poor access to oral or nasal routes (e.g., facial fractures, osteogenesis imperfecta, inadequate bite for mouthpiece entry, or presence of nasogastric tube; or upper airway obstruction) or for other reasons (e.g., mental incompetence, obtundation, uncooperativeness, substance abuse, heavy sedative or narcotic use, uncontrollable seizures, or oropharyngeal muscle weakness)
- Ongoing aggressive management of respiratory tract secretions (e.g., as a result of PCEF less than 3 L/s or an MIC of less than 500 mL) for which a mechanical exsufflation device may be contraindicated or unavailable, and there is unreliable access to effective assisted coughing.

In the PM&R setting, most patients with CAH who require 24-hour/day ventilatory support do not need or desire tracheal intubation (using ET or TT) because of the availability of effective, safer, more comfortable, and cheaper noninvasive mechanical ventilation methods (see section IV.A.4.a.2.b). Irrespective of the extent of the ventilatory failure, a tracheostomized (or intubated) patient receiving pulmonary rehabilitation should, as soon as medically indicated, be weaned off the TT (or ET) and, if needed, be considered for noninvasive mechanical ventilation.

The guidelines for ventilator setting and ventilator weaning of intubated or tracheostomized patients are the same as those used for patients on noninvasive mechanical ventilation (see sections IV.A.4.a.4.a and IV.A.4.a.5). Suctioning is described in section IV.B.1.b.5. In intubated or tracheostomized patients, cuff care is important to avoid tracheal ischemia. A high-volume, low-pressure cuff should be used to seal the airway with minimal pressure against the tracheal wall, that is, cuff pressure maintained below capillary filling pressure (below 25 mmHg) as monitored every 8 hours with a manometer (e.g., a sphygmomanometer may be used with an adapter). The use of periodic cuff deflation is not recommended as it is inadequate in reducing tracheal trauma.

1. **Endotracheal tube** is usually applied in an emergency setting via the direct laryngoscopic technique for orotracheal placement. The preferred ET size is no. 8 (i.e., with 8-mm internal diameter) or larger to reduce airway resistance and the work of breathing in acute respiratory failure as well as to facilitate suctioning. The ET may be extubated if the patient can tolerate unassisted spontaneous breathing for 30–90 minutes (for example, through a T-tube or other continuous airflow circuit tube). Prolonged T-tube breathing may cause fatigue, especially if the ET size is small.
2. **Tracheostomy tube** should be considered if the ET cannot be successfully extubated after 2 weeks (or earlier than 2 weeks if a prolonged intubation period is anticipated). If weaning from mechanical ventilation is imminent, however, TT may be postponed safely for up to 4 weeks. To use a TT, a tracheostomy must first be created via a tracheotomy (i.e., a surgical incision in the trachea). A new tracheostomy site usually takes at least 72 hours to mature. If the TT is dislodged during this period, the TT should not be reinserted blindly as this may lead to malposition of the TT in the pretracheal space or elsewhere outside the trachea. The responsible surgical service should, therefore, be consulted; however, if the TT is dislodged after the initial 72-hour period (i.e., when the tracheostomy site has most likely matured into a well-formed track from the skin to the trachea), the TT can easily be reinserted and, if needed, position confirmed through radiograph.

   The early major complications of a tracheostomy include mediastinal or subcutaneous emphysema, postoperative bleeding, pneumomediastinum, pneumothorax, tube displacement, and aspiration, while the late major complications include nosocomial pneumonia, tracheal stenosis, tracheoinnominate fistula (i.e., between trachea and innominate artery), tracheomalacia (i.e., erosion or thinning of the tracheal wall), tracheoesophageal fistula, swallowing dysfunction (see Chapter 5.6, section VI.A for management of dysphagia in tracheostomized patients), and stomal infection. Tracheomalacia is highly suspected if the ratio of cuff size to tracheal size (C/T ratio) is more than 1.5. The C/T ratio (determined by radiogram) should ideally be less than or equal to 1. If the C/T ratio is above 1.5, the cuff should be inflated at a different site, by using a TT with a different length (e.g., Portex extra-long TT) or by inflating the second cuff of a double-cuffed TT or using an ET and cutting it to a different length.

   All TTs have a cannula or shaft (some have a single shaft, whereas others have an outer and inner shaft) and a neck plate (or neck flange), which rests on the neck between the clavicles. The neck plate contains small holes on the outer edge, which are used to secure the tracheostomy ties. Unlike the ET, the tip of the TT is not beveled but is straight cut to maximize air flow and prevent occlusion of the tip by the tracheal wall. Most adult TTs contain an inner cannula, although some do not (e.g., Bivona Fome-cuff and some other Portex tubes). The inner cannula can be removed from the outer cannula (e.g., every 8 hours) for cleaning of crusted secretions that may occlude the airway (e.g., in patients who are not suctioned frequently); while the outer cannula is left in place (to keep the tracheostomy stoma open) and can be changed every 6 weeks or more frequently. The outer cannula on most tubes or the inner cannula in some tubes has a 15-mm adapter for direct connection to the ventilator unit or manual resuscitator (e.g., AMBU bag). Because the TT completely bypasses the upper airway, the inspired air must be warmed and humidified. The more effective water reservoir-type humidifier (e.g., Fisher–Paykel Humidifier) is preferred by patients with increased secretions over the heat–moisture exchange humidifier (e.g., Artificial Nose); however, the Artificial Nose is more portable.

a. ***Size.*** The length of a TT is usually 2–6 inches (5–15 cm), with the exception of the Portex TT, which is available in an extra-long size. In general, the shorter the tube, the smaller the internal diameter (ID) unless the TT is customized by using an ET, which can be cut into any desired length. The ID of the TT ranges from 5 to 11 mm; while the outer diameter (OD) ranges from 7 to 15.3 mm. In most tubes, the ID is about 3 mm smaller than the OD. The ID size (usually printed on the TT neck flange) determines the TT size. The TT size for Jackson metal TT and Shiley double-cannula TT uses the Jackson equivalent number, that is, a no. 6 tube is equal to a 7.0 mm ID. This can be confusing, hence the ID size should be used instead of the TT size. If the TT size is used, it can be converted to OD size (in mm) by adding 4. The OD (in mm) size can then be multiplied by 3 to obtain the French size.

b. ***Types***

I. **Metal TT vs. plastic TT**

- **Metal TTs** (e.g., Jackson, Hollinger) are cuffless, reusable tubes made of durable stainless steel or silver. Although a latex cuff can be placed, it is not recommended as it may slip. Compared to plastic TTs, metal TTs cause less local tissue reaction, may be left in place for longer periods, and may be less costly in prolonged use than most plastic tubes. They are used to keep the tracheostomy stoma patent in spontaneously breathing patients until the tracheostomy is no longer needed.
- **Plastic TTs** (e.g., Shiley, Portex, Bivona) are disposable tubes most of which are made of polyvinyl chloride (PVC), whereas some are made of nylon, silicone, or Teflon. The rigidity of the PVC ranges from hard to soft, and it is available in either single or double cannulae, with or without a cuff.

II. **Cuff-inflated TT vs. uncuffed TT**

- **Cuff-inflated TTs** are used to provide an adequate seal to protect the lower airway from aspiration (e.g., patients who are unconscious or when eating or drinking especially in patients with dysphagia) and to ensure adequate ventilation to the lungs and prevent air leaking upward through the upper airway (e.g., when using CPAP or in patients with poor laryngeal control). Cuff inflation does not guarantee complete safety from aspiration (see discussion in Chapter 5.6, section III.C.1.a.2.b), and it does not allow the patient to speak. Most modern cuff-inflated TTs have high-volume/low-pressure balloon cuffs (see section V.A for monitoring guidelines) which evenly distribute the intracuff pressure on the tracheal mucosa, thus minimizing the complications of tracheal lesions. The lowest volume and pressure required for maintaining an adequate cuff seal are used. The Bivona Fome-cuff TT uses self-inflating foam (instead of a balloon), which does not require cuff pressure monitoring; however, it may not seal well (e.g., in patients using PEEP) and may require more frequent tube changes.

- **Uncuffed TTs** allow some patients to talk while receiving mechanical ventilation; however, to assure adequate ventilation, the exhaled tidal volume and ABGs should be checked regularly. It may be used right after a tracheostomy when there is loose fit of the TT on the stoma (thus allowing considerable leakage) or to prevent subcutaneous emphysema. An uncuffed TT should not be used in patients known to aspirate.

III. Fenestrated TT vs. nonfenestrated TT

- **Fenestrated TTs** have a straw-sized hole cut into the outer cannula of a cuffed or cuffless TT (e.g., Portex or Shiley cuffed TT with precut fenestration), thus allowing increased flow to the upper airway so the patient can speak (as well as breathe and cough) while the TT is uncuffed, the inner cannula is removed, and the TT is plugged and disconnected from the mechanical ventilation. If the patient needs mechanical ventilation, the inner cannula (which has no fenestration) is reinserted to occlude the fenestration of the outer cannula. The fenestrations should lie within the lumen of the trachea (this can be checked by direct vision with a flashlight) and should not touch the tracheal wall (otherwise granulation tissue can form into and around the holes, thus causing obstruction or bleeding, i.e., when the TT is pulled out). The fenestrated TT should only be used if the patient can breathe spontaneously for 2 hours or more without the need of mechanical ventilation and can swallow without aspiration when the TT is uncuffed (aspiration can be evaluated by performing a swallowing test using blue food coloring as described in Chapter 5.6, section III.C.1.a.2). It also allows the patient to breathe through the mouth.
- **Nonfenestrated TTs** are used if the patient needs continuous mechanical ventilation (i.e., is unable to have more than 2 hours of ventilator-free time) or is unable to protect the airway when swallowing. If the patient wants to talk, a one-way talking valve (e.g., Passy–Muir Speaking Valve; see next section) may be used, or the TT size can be decreased, or its cuff can be deflated to allow air leakage.

IV. Talking tubes vs. speaking valves. Both of these specialized tubes allow a patient to speak. As discussed above, other nonspecialized tubes may be used for speaking by allowing air leakage into the larynx (e.g., uncuffed tubes, cuff-deflated fenestrated or unfenestrated tubes, or use of smaller TT size). The use of tracheal buttons or plugs (see below) may also divert air to the larynx for speaking. For nonspeaking communication options, see Chapter 5.5, section IV.B.2.

- **Talking tracheostomy tubes (pneumatic speaking tubes)** are indicated for alert and motivated patients who need an inflated cuff for ventilation and who have intact vocal cords and the ability to mouth words. They are specialized TTs capable of supplying pressurized gas mixtures (at a flow rate of 1.5–10 L/min) through a cannula that travels through the wall of the talking tube, then enters the trachea through small holes above the inflated tube cuff so the patient can use the larynx to speak while the cuff is inflated (thus leaving mechanical ventilation undisturbed). The quality of speech is altered (e.g., lower pitch, coarser, or whisper-like) and patients need to speak in short sentences (because constant flow through the vocal cords can cause the voice to fade away). Also, the patient needs a fair amount of manual dexterity and minimal strength to occlude the external port to initiate flow of gas through the vocal cord (if needed, the occlusion of the external port may be done by the person with whom the patient is speaking through the patient's use of an eye blink or similar signal). Talking TTs should not be used within the first 5–7 days after tracheostomy because the pressurized gas may flow retrograde through the tracheostoma around the tube and cause subcutaneous emphysema. Talking TTs may not work if there are secretions or granulation tissue above the cuff, which may occlude the exit port for the gas. They are available as single-lumen cannula cuffed tubes (e.g., Portex "Talk" tube, Bivona Fome-cuff with sideport airway connector), which are easier for the patient to learn to use and less likely to become occluded, or as a double-lumen cannula cuffed tube (e.g., Communi-trach; Pitt Trach Speaking Tube).

- **One-way speaking valves** (e.g., Passy–Muir Speaking Valve, Olympic Trach-talk) are made of plastic and can be fitted on any TT with a 15-mm adapter. The valve opens on inspiration, bypassing upper airway pathology, thus making it easier to inspire; then on expiration, the valve closes and forces the air through the vocal cords, thus allowing vocalization (as well as helping to blow out any food residue in the trachea; see Chapter 5.6, section VI.A). They are used either in mechanically ventilated patients (with the cuff deflated) or in tracheostomized patients who can spontaneously breathe but cannot tolerate tracheal plugs or buttons. The Passy–Muir Speaking Valve is most frequently used because of its simple-to-use one-piece design. In contrast, the multipiece Olympic Trach-talk has a spring-loaded one-way valve attached to a T-piece. Speaking valves should only be used when the patient is awake and medically stable, able to manage his or her secretions effectively and not aspirate, has no severe tracheal or laryngeal stenosis, and is able to tolerate cuff deflation.

V. **Tracheal buttons vs. tracheal plugs**. Both are used to keep the tracheostomy stoma patent during tracheostomy weaning when there is some doubt about the success of the weaning (i.e., in case suction is needed or the patient needs to be reattached to the ventilator) or when a planned surgical procedure may require tracheostomy and mechanical ventilation. It can also be used to allow the patient to speak (but unlike speaking valves, it does not allow inspiration). There are other reasons for placement of these tubes, such as easy access for suctioning the lower airway, sleep apnea (leaving the plug open during sleep), vocal cord paralysis, and in neurologic disorders, such as myasthenia gravis.

- **Tracheal buttons** extend only to the inner surface of the anterior tracheal wall without encroaching on the lumen (and, therefore, do not cause tracheal lumen obstruction). To ensure that the tip does not extend into the trachea, spacers or rings are inserted on the outside of the button. The Olympic button is made of rigid plastic (Teflon), while the Kistner button is made of flexible plastic. Proper size must be used, because if the button is too short the tracheostomy tract may granulate and occlude ventilation; if too long, the button may occlude the trachea (thus limiting ventilation and removal of secretions); and if the button diameter is too small, it can be dislodged at night, thus inadvertently allowing the stoma to shrink.
- **Tracheal plugs** or **decannulation cannulae** are specially fitted, short, closed-lumen cannulae, inserted into the outer cannula for plugging. They can easily be removed for suctioning or for reconnection to the mechanical ventilator.

c. ***Guidelines for TT decannulation***. In general, TT decannulation or removal is considered when the patient no longer needs mechanical ventilation (see section IV.A.4.a.5 for ventilator-weaning guidelines) and can adequately clear secretions from the airway. A patient with a cuffed TT is weaned to a cuffless TT by gradual cuff deflation. The patient should not have an increased propensity for pneumonia or aspiration (aspiration may be checked by a blue food coloring test; see Chapter 5.6, section III.C.1.a.2), should be adequately ventilated with the cuff deflated, and should be able to cough secretions out of the TT. The cuffless TT is then downsized to the next smaller size and checked for the above parameters. Once the TT is downsized to about 8 mm outer diameter (e.g., Shiley no. 4 or Portex no. 5.0 mm ID) and the patient does not need excessive suctioning, then the TT can be discontinued or a tracheal button or plug may be used temporarily (see section V.A.2.b.5).

After decannulation, the tracheostomy stoma is covered with a dry dressing or a dressing with petrolatum-impregnated gauze (Vaseline or Xeroform gauze) taped in place. The patient's voice may be raspy or gravelly for several days until the stoma closes completely and spontaneously. During this time the stoma is assessed and cleaned and its dressing is changed at least daily. Occasionally, the tracheostomy stoma does not heal and may require plastic surgery for closure.

B. DIAPHRAGMATIC PACING (ELECTROPHRENIC NERVE PACING) is a highly sophisticated form of portable mechanical ventilation that leaves the patient's face free for ADLs. It is indicated in patients who have central damage to the respiratory control centers or their pathways (in the brainstem and spinal cord); at least partially intact C3–C5 anterior horn cells, phrenic nerve, and diaphragm; and who are unable to use an OIPPV. Some of the common cases that can benefit from diaphragmatic pacing include idiopathic central hypoventilation syndrome or Ondine's curse; acquired central hypoventilation syndrome; and high spinal cord injury (i.e., C1–C2). The diaphragmatic pacemaker, which can be implanted by a simple operation (with brief hospitalization), consists of an electrode (implanted cervically onto phrenic nerve fibers) and radio receivers (implanted on the anterior chest wall).

An external radio transmitter (whose batteries last up to 2–3 weeks) produces impulses that are delivered via the external antenna loop taped to the skin over the implanted receiver site. The radio transmitter may be accessed via a telephone for remote assessment of stimulation effectiveness and diagnosis of technical problems. Simultaneous bilateral diaphragmatic pacing is more effective and is preferred. In some adults, unilateral pacing may be used, however it can lead to paradoxical diaphragm movement which results in marginal ventilation. Potential complications of diaphragmatic pacing include infection, sudden operational failure, and the need to retain a tracheostomy because of obstructive sleep apnea. Recent advances in technology have increased its reliability, and it has been used successfully by some patients for over 15 years.

C. OTHER SURGICAL TREATMENTS include intercostal nerve-to-phrenic nerve anastomosis with implantation of a pacing electrode for the recently denervated diaphragm; bilateral carotid body resection (BCBR) for the relief of severe dyspnea (BCBR can also remove the respiratory drive for breathing produced by O_2 desaturation); and lung/lung–heart transplant for end-stage lung disease of various causes.

VI. Outcome assessment

Assessment of outcome according to ATS (1999) is an important component of comprehensive pulmonary rehabilitation both for determining individual patient responses and for evaluating the overall effectiveness of the program. Minimal requirements include prerehabilitation and immediate postrehabilitation assessment of: dyspnea; exercise ability; health status; and activity levels (if this is not sufficiently evaluated by the health-status questionnaire). If feasible, follow-up measurements (e.g., at 6- and 12-months postrehabilitation) should be done. For commonly used outcome measures in pulmonary rehabilitation, refer to Table 5.12-7.

Table 5.12-7 Commonly used outcome measures in pulmonary rehabilitation

Outcome measures	Impairment	Disability	Handicap	Symptoms*
A. Exercise ability				
Incremental exercise tests	√			
Submaximal exercise tests	√			
Walking tests		√		
B. General health status				
Sickness Impact Profile (SIP)		√	√	
Quality of Well-Being Scale		√	√	
Medical Outcomes Study, Short Form 36		√	√	P
C. Respiratory-specific health status				
St George's Respiratory Questionnaire		√	√	D
Chronic Respiratory Disease Questionnaire		√		F
D. Respiratory-specific functional status				
Pulmonary Functional Status and Dyspnea Questionnaire or modified version		√	√	D
Pulmonary Functional Status Scale		√	√	D/F
E. Exertional dyspnea (during exercise testing)		√	√	
Visual analog scale rating				D/F/P
Category rating (Borg)				D/F/P
F. Overall dyspnea				
Medical Research Council Scale		√		
Baseline and Transitional Dyspnea Indexes		√		

**Symptoms independently evaluated from activities designated as follows: D = dyspnea; F = fatigue; P = pain.*
From: American Thoracic Society: Pulmonary Rehabilitation. Am J Resp Crit Care Med 1999: 159(5):1666–1682, Table 7, p. 1675, with permission.

A. **OUTCOME MEASURES OF IMPAIRMENT** assess the patient's ability to exercise.

1. **Incremental exercise test** on a stationary bicycle or treadmill involves increasing the work rate at regular intervals to maximal tolerance or to a heart rate of 85% of predicted maximum. Routine measurements include heart rate (HR), respiratory rate (RR), blood pressure (BP), electrocardiogram (ECG), and oxygen saturation. If available to the exercise laboratory, exhaled gases may be analyzed to determine or calculate minute ventilation, oxygen consumption, carbon dioxide production, anaerobic threshold, and dead space (see Chapter 2.7, section II.A). Although often symptom-limited in chronic lung disease, incremental exercise testing is reproducible and sensitive to improvements from pulmonary rehabilitation.
2. **Submaximal exercise test** using a stationary cycle or treadmill exercise testing at a constant fraction of the maximal work rate is frequently used to measure exercise endurance capacity in pulmonary rehabilitation (i.e., a longer exercise

time on the treadmill or cycle ergometer indicates greater exercise endurance). It is more effort-dependent than incremental exercise testing and is often quite responsive to pulmonary rehabilitation intervention, with postrehabilitation exercise endurance times considerably longer than corresponding prerehabilitation values.

B. OUTCOME MEASURES OF DISABILITY

1. **Walking tests** are field tests where distance walked is the outcome measured.

a. ***Timed walking test*** (see Chapter 2.7, section II.C) is simple to perform, well-tolerated, and relevant to many daily activities. The patient is instructed to walk as far as possible in a corridor or large room at his/her own pace within 12 minutes (this may be modified to 6 or even 2 or 3 minutes for some pulmonary patients). Routine measurements include HR, RR, BP, and walking time and distance. Additional measurements may include oxygen saturation, ECG, and perceived exertion. Timed walking tests correlate with peak exercise performance on graded exercise tests and self-reported data on functional status questionnaires. Patients with COPD show significant learning effects for the timed walk tests, especially when the tests are repeated over relatively short intervals. The minimal clinically meaningful increase in the 6-minute walking test is about 54 m.

b. ***The shuttle walking test*** is an externally paced measure of exercise capacity designed for COPD patients. The patient must walk up and down a 10-m distance (shuttle) at gradually increasing speeds. Walking speed, dictated by a beeping signal, is increased after every minute of walking by shortening the time between signals. The shuttle walking test differs from the timed walk test in two aspects. First, it is more a measure of exercise capacity than of endurance because of its incremental nature. Second, self-pacing (which is of considerable importance to the timed walk) is eliminated because the walking pace is externally dictated. The shuttle walk is reproducible, correlates well with maximum oxygen consumption during incremental treadmill exercise, and is highly responsive to therapeutic intervention.

2. **Dyspnea ratings** are used to evaluate the impact of exercise training on dyspnea.

a. ***Exertional dyspnea*** is directly rated during exercise testing, such as incremental treadmill exercise tests or timed walking tests.

I. **The Borg's rate of perceived exertion (RPE) scale** (see Chapter 4.2, section III.A.3) can be used to rate the level of dyspnea (by selecting a number corresponding to a verbal descriptor ranging from no breathlessness, i.e., zero, to maximal breathlessness) during exercise.

II. **The visual analog scale** or **VAS** (see Chapter 5.10, section IV.C.2.a.1) can be used to measure dyspnea by having the patient point along a horizontal or vertical line, which is 100 mm in length and anchored at either end with descriptors such as "greatest breathlessness" and "no breathlessness". The distance (mm) from the beginning of the line to the point noted by the patient represents the level of dyspnea.

b. ***Overall dyspnea*** can be assessed by determining its effects on ADLs. The instruments used include: the Medical Research Council (MRC) dyspnea questionnaire, the University of California San Diego Shortness of Breath Questionnaire (UCSD-SOBQ), the dyspnea component of the Chronic Respiratory Disease Questionnaire , the Baseline and Transitional Dyspnea Indexes (BDI and TDI), and the Pulmonary Functional Status and Dyspnea Questionnaire (PFSDQ) and its modified version (PFSDQ-M).

C. OUTCOME MEASURES OF HANDICAP AND DISABILITY listed below have the ability to discriminate between different levels of impaired health among patients. However, the respiratory-specific measures demonstrate greater sensitivity to change from baseline after pulmonary rehabilitation.

1. **General health status or general health-related quality of life** has more restricted measurement focus than quality of life (see Chapter 2.8, section IV for discussion of quality of life assessment). It pertains only to the domains of life insofar as they affect "health" (or are affected by "health"). They can be assessed by using the Quality of Well-Being Scale or general health questionnaires, such as the Sickness Impact Profile (see Chapter 2.8, section IV.B) and the Medical Outcomes Study Short Form-36 (SF-36) (see Chapter 2.8, section IV.A).
2. **Respiratory-specific health status** can be assessed using the Chronic Respiratory Disease Questionnaire (CRDQ) and the St George's Respiratory Questionnaire (SGRQ).
3. **Respiratory-specific functional status.** Functional status has four dimensions: capacity, performance, reserve, and capacity utilization. Functional capacity is what the patient is capable of doing, whereas functional performance is what the patient actually does on a day-to-day basis. The difference between functional capacity and functional performance is the functional reserve, which is called upon in time of need. Pulmonary rehabilitation can increase the functional reserve, allowing the patient greater ability to engage in ADLs. However, whether the patient takes advantage of this "reserve" is an individual choice, which may account for the variability in postrehabilitation performance of patients. Functional capacity utilization refers to how closely performance approaches the patient's functional capacity. In pulmonary disease, functional performance evaluation focuses on the patient's ability to perform ADLs. The questionnaires used successfully in pulmonary rehabilitation include Pulmonary Functional Status and Dyspnea Questionnaire (PFSDQ) and its modified version (PFSDQ-M), and the Pulmonary Function Status Scale (PFSS). They provide an estimate of the impact of pulmonary rehabilitation on various activities, recognizing that the results are limited by the patient's motivation, recall, and perception of improvement.

D. MEASURES OF PSYCHOLOGICAL STATUS OUTCOMES

1. **Cognitive function assessment** should be considered in patients with suspected memory problems since a limitation might impede rehabilitation efforts by interfering with the patient's ability to follow instructions or articulate his or her health status. Cognitive deficits can be evaluated using one of several easy to administer instruments such as the Mini-Mental State Examination (MMSE) or the Neurobehavioral Cognitive Status Examination (NCSE). These questionnaires screen for general factors such as memory, alertness, attention, orientation, and reasoning. Normative values for patients with COPD are available for the MMSE.
2. **Questionnaires relying primarily on cognitive changes** may be more appropriate for pulmonary patients. The following questionnaires are commonly used in pulmonary patients, but they vary in the degree to which they measure cognitive changes. Questionnaires commonly used to measure coping and mood include the Psychosocial Adjustment to Illness Scale-Self Report and the Profile of Mood States. Questionnaires more specific to symptoms of depression and/or anxiety include the Geriatric Depression Scale, the Center for Epidemiological Studies-Depression Scale, the Hospital Anxiety and Depression Scale, the Beck Depression Inventory (see Chapter 2.9, section VII.A), the Zung Self-Rating Depression Scale (see Chapter 2.9, section VII.B), and the Spielberger State-Trait Anxiety Inventory (see Chapter 2.9, section VII.C).

Further reading

Alba, AS: Concepts in pulmonary rehabilitation. In Braddom RL, editor: *Physical medicine and rehabilitation*, ed 2, Philadelphia, 2000, WB Saunders, pp. 687–701.

American Association of Cardiovascular and Pulmonary Rehabilitation (AACVPR): *Guidelines for pulmonary rehabilitation programs*, ed 2, Champaign, IL, 1998, Human Kinetics.

American College of Chest Physicians (ACCP) and American Association of Cardiovascular and Pulmonary Rehabilitation (AACVPR) Pulmonary Rehabilitation Guidelines Panel: Pulmonary rehabilitation. Joint ACCP/AACVPR evidence-based guidelines. *Chest* 112: 1363–96, 1997.

American Thoracic Society: Pulmonary rehabilitation. *Am J Resp Crit Care Med* 159: 1666–1682, 1999.

Bach JR: Pulmonary rehabilitation in neuromuscular disorders. *Sem Resp Med* 14(6):515–529, 1993.

Bach JR: Rehabilitation of the patient with respiratory dysfunction. In DeLisa JA, Gans BM, Walsh NE, *et al.*, editors: *Physical medicine and rehabilitation: principles and practice*, ed 4, Philadelphia, 2005, Lippincott, Williams & Wilkins, pp. 1843–1866.

Bach JR, Alba AS, Garrison SJ: Pulmonary rehabilitation. *Arch Phys Med Rehabil* 71 (suppl 4):S238–S243, 1990.

Brannon FJ, Foley MW, Starr JA, *et al.*: *Cardiopulmonary rehabilitation: basic theory and application*, ed 3, Philadelphia, 1998, FA Davis.

Casaburi R: Principles of exercise training. *Chest* 101 (Suppl 5):263S–267S, 1992.

Casaburi R, Petty TL: *Principles and practice in pulmonary rehabilitation*, Philadelphia, 1993, WB Saunders.

Colbert BJ, Mason BJ: *Integrated cardiopulmonary pharmacology*, Upper Saddle River, NJ, 2002, Prentice Hall.

Dettenmeier PA: *Pulmonary nursing care*, St Louis, 1991, Mosby-Year Book.

Fishman AP, editor: *Pulmonary rehabilitation*, New York, 1996, Marcel Dekker.

Haas F, Axen K, editors: *Pulmonary therapy and rehabilitation: principles and practice*, ed 2, Baltimore, 1991, Williams & Wilkins.

Harmon-Weiss S: *Chronic obstructive pulmonary disease. Nutrition management for older adults*, Washington, DC, 2002, Nutrition Screening Initiative (NSI).

Hodgkin J, Connors GL, Bell CW, editors: *Pulmonary rehabilitation: guidelines to success*, ed 3, Philadelphia, 2000, Lippincott, Williams & Wilkins.

Howder CL: *Cardiopulmonary pharmacology: a handbook for cardiopulmonary practitioners and other allied health personnel*, ed 2, Baltimore, 1996, Williams & Wilkins.

Levenson C: Breathing exercises. In Zadai C, editor: *Clinics in physical therapy: pulmonary management in physical therapy*, New York, 1992, Churchill Livingstone.

Massery M: Manual breathing and coughing aids. *Phys Med Rehabil Clin North Am* 7(2):407–422, 1996.

O'Donohue Jr WJ, editor: *Long-term oxygen therapy: scientific basis and clinical application*, New York, 1995, Marcel Dekker.

O'Donohue WJ, Giovannoni RM, Goldberg AF, *et al.*: Long-term mechanical ventilation: guidelines for management in the home and alternate community site. *Chest* 90 (suppl):1S–37S, 1986.

Rashbaum I, Whyte N: Occupational therapy in pulmonary rehabilitation: energy conservation and work simplification techniques. *Phys Med Rehabil Clin North Am* 7(2):325–340, 1996.

Rogers RM, Donahoe M: Nutrition in pulmonary rehabilitation. In Fishman AP, editor: *Pulmonary rehabilitation*, New York, 1996, Marcel Dekker, pp. 543–564.

Wilson DJ, Shepherd KE: Modern airway appliances and their long-term complications. In Roberts JT, editor: *Clinical management of the airway*, Philadelphia, 1994, WB Saunders.

Supplemental references

Eckert RC, Bartsch K, Dowell D, *et al.*: *Being close*, Denver, 1984, National Jewish Hospital/ National Asthma Center.

Hossler CJ, Cole SS: *Intimacy and chronic lung disease*, Ann Arbor, 1983, University of Michigan.

Kravetz HM: *A visit with Harry* (slide-tape program), Prescott, AZ, 1982, HM Kravetz.

Kravetz HM: *A visit with Helen* (slide-tape program), Prescott, AZ, 1982, HM Kravetz.

Kravetz HM, Weiss M, Meadows R: *Sexual counseling for the male pulmonary patient* (slide-tape program), Prescott, AZ, 1980, HM Kravetz.

Selecky PA: *Sexuality and chronic breathing problems*, Santa Ana, CA, 1989, American Lung Association of Orange County.

Shimberg EF: *Coping with COPD: understanding, treating, and living with chronic obstructive pulmonary disease*, New York: 2003, St Martin's Press.

CHAPTER 5.13
Cardiac problems

This chapter gives an overview of cardiac rehabilitation in patients with medical cardiac diagnoses [e.g., postmyocardial infarction, chronic stable angina, compensated congestive heart failure, coronary heart disease (CHD), and cardiac arrhythmias] and surgical cardiac diagnoses [e.g., postcoronary arterial bypass graft surgery (post-CABG), postcoronary angioplasty, postcardiac valvular surgery, and postcardiac transplantation]. The general goals of cardiac rehabilitation are to optimize the patient's physiologic, psychosocial, and vocational function, as well as to reduce the morbidity and mortality of cardiac diseases. The cardiac patient is given an educational program (e.g., life-style modification such as low-cholesterol diet, stress reduction, and smoking cessation) to reduce the risk factors for heart disease, as well as reconditioning exercises to improve safety and tolerance of daily activities (e.g., vocational, recreational, and sexual activities). The approach to cardiac rehabilitation is usually interdisciplinary, involving physicians, nurses, physical therapists, occupational therapists, exercise physiologists, nutritionists, psychologists (or psychiatrists), social workers, and vocational counselors. Cardiac rehabilitation services must include comprehensive long-term programs involving medical evaluation, exercise prescription, modification of CHD risk factors, education, counseling, and vocational programs.

I. Epidemiology

Cardiovascular disease, which is responsible for 29% of all deaths, is the leading cause of morbidity and mortality in the adult population in the United States (*National Vital Statistics Reports*). The major category of cardiovascular disease is CHD, which can clinically manifest as stable or unstable angina pectoris, myocardial infarction (MI), silent myocardial ischemia, or sudden death. Among working adults, CHD is a leading cause of premature, permanent disability. Another category of cardiovascular disease is congestive heart failure, which is increasing in prevalence and which in 1994 ranked as the first-listed discharge diagnosis in 874000 hospital discharges (alive or dead). In 2003, the cost related to CHD was estimated to exceed $351 billion. The death rate from CHD still remains high despite its decrease from 228.1 per 100000 population (in 1970) to 94.9 per 100000 (in 1994). This decline in mortality rate has been attributed to advances in medical treatment and technology, increase in exercise participation, and reductions in cigarette smoking and red meat consumption.

There are more than 13.5 million Americans with a history of MI or who have experienced angina pectoris. Every year, approximately 1.5 million Americans sustain an MI, of which nearly 500000 are fatal. The majority of patients (over 50%) with acute MI are over age 65, whereas about 45% are between age 40 and 65 and 5% are under age 40. The MI survivors (approximately 1 million Americans per year) are potential candidates for cardiac rehabilitation as are those with stable angina pectoris (more than 7 million Americans per year), post-CABG (309000 patients in 1993, 45% of whom were under age 65), and percutaneous transluminal coronary angioplasty (PTCA) and other transcatheter interventional procedures (362000 patients in 1993, 54% of whom were under age 65). Among these potential candidates, only

11–38% participate in cardiac rehabilitation programs, despite studies showing that cardiac rehabilitation can reduce the mortality and morbidity of CHD.

II. Coronary heart disease risk factors

A. MODIFIABLE CHD RISK FACTORS. Hypertension [blood pressure (BP) >140/90 mmHg or >130/80 for those with diabetes or chronic kidney disease], cigarette smoking, obesity (over 30% ideal body weight, especially those with abdominal fat pattern), habitually sedentary life-style, hypercholesterolemia (>200 mg/dL), high levels of low-density lipoprotein (LDL) cholesterol (>100 mg/dL), low levels of high-density lipoprotein (HDL) cholesterol (<40 mg/dL), hypertriglyceridemia (>150 mg/dL), hyperinsulinemia, diabetes mellitus, and "type A" behavior (this last is controversial because of problems in measuring "type A" behavior).

B. UNMODIFIABLE CHD RISK FACTORS. Advanced age (male at least 45; female at least 55 or prematurely menopausal without estrogen replacement therapy); male gender (rate of CHD is three to four times higher in men than women in the middle decades of life and roughly twice as high in the elderly); black race (because of higher rates of hypertension), family history of premature CHD (i.e., MI or sudden death before age 55 in a first-degree male relative or before age 65 in a first-degree female relative), past history of CHD, cardiac event, or abnormal ECG [e.g., left ventricular hypertrophy (LVH)]; and a past history of occlusive peripheral vascular disease (PVD) or cerebrovascular disease.

III. Cardiac evaluation

A. HISTORY

1. Chief complaint

a. ***Chest pain,*** that is typical anginal pain, which is described as tight, vise-like, aching, squeezing, burning, and pressing, is located at the substernal area but may also involve the left chest, arms, neck, or jaw; lasts 3–5 minutes or up to 15 minutes; is precipitated during exertion, emotional upset, cold weather, or exertion after meals; and is relieved within 3–5 minutes after rest or sublingual nitroglycerin.

b. ***Other chief complaints*** are dyspnea (usually exertional), orthopnea (often with paroxysmal nocturnal dyspnea), palpitation, syncope, fatigue, edema, dizziness or lightheadedness, nausea or vomiting, cyanosis, and pallor.

2. Past history, such as past cardiac event (e.g., MI) or abnormal electrocardiogram (ECG) (e.g., LVH), cardiovascular surgery or procedure (e.g., CABG, PTCA, or cardiac pacemaker insertion), congestive heart failure, hypertension, diabetes mellitus, occlusive PVD, cerebrovascular disease, pulmonary embolism, bacterial endocarditis, rheumatic fever, ankylosing spondylitis (associated with aortic valve disease or conduction defects), Down syndrome (associated cardiac abnormalities), myasthenia or other neuromuscular disease (associated with cardiomyopathy or conduction disease), and congenital heart defects.

3. Medication history, such as antianginals (nitrates, β-blockers, calcium-channel blockers), antiarrhythmics (sodium-channel blockers, β-blockers, potassium-channel blockers, calcium-channel blockers), antihypertensives (diuretics, β-blockers, angiotensin-converting enzyme inhibitors, angiotensin-receptor blocker, calcium-channel blockers, aldosterone antagonist), heart-failure treatment drugs (inotropics, diuretics, peripheral vasodilators), anticoagulants, antiplatelet agents, and antilipemic agents.

4. **Functional and occupational history**, such as the function and level of activity tolerance at present and prior to the cardiac event and level of activity required at home and at work.
5. **Personal history**, such as cigarette use, alcohol use, substance abuse, leisure activities, exercise history, diet history, personality type, and emotional adaptation to stress.
6. **Social history**, such as home situation, support system, architectural barriers, and financial condition.
7. **Family history**, such as premature MI or sudden death, hypercholesterolemia or hyperlipidemia, arrhythmias, hypertrophic cardiomyopathies, and Marfan's disease.

B. PHYSICAL EXAMINATION

1. **General**. Weight, height, skinfold measurement, body habitus, skin (pallor, diaphoresis, xanthelasma; if postsurgery, check incisional drainage, wound healing, as well as tubes and drains that limit mobility), arcus cornealis, facial appearance, anxiety, and gait.
2. **Vital signs**. Temperature, blood pressure (resting hypertension, orthostatic and symptomatic hypotension), pulse and heart rate and rhythm, and respiratory rate and pattern.
3. **Cardiovascular**

a. ***Inspection***. Jugular venous pulse and waveform, and cyanosis (e.g., perioral).

b. ***Palpation***. Precordium (point of maximal impulse, thrills, systolic heave), major arterial pulses (carotid, brachial, radial, femoral, popliteal, posterior tibial, and dorsalis pedis pulses), and peripheral dependent edema.

c. ***Auscultation***

I. **Heart sounds**: S1 (mitral and tricuspid valve closure; soft S1 is heard in mitral regurgitation, low-output states, and first-degree heart block; loud S1 is heard in mitral stenosis, high-output states, and short PR intervals), S2 (pulmonic and aortic valve closure), fixed S2 splitting with respiration (atrial septal defect), paradoxical S2 splitting during expiration (left bundle branch block, left ventricular failure, aortic stenosis), gallop sounds (S3 because of ventricular filling sounds, and S4 during atrial systole as a result of decreased ventricular compliance), ejection click (aortic or pulmonic valve opening), mid-systolic click (mitral valve prolapse), and opening snap (opening of mitral valve in mitral stenosis).

II. **Heart murmurs**. Systolic ejection murmurs (functional or innocent flow murmurs, aortic stenosis, pulmonic stenosis, idiopathic hypertrophic subaortic stenosis, atypical mitral regurgitation), pansystolic or holosystolic murmurs (mitral regurgitation, tricuspid regurgitation, ventricular septal defects), late systolic murmurs (mitral valve prolapse), immediate diastolic decrescendo murmurs (aortic regurgitation, pulmonic regurgitation), delayed diastolic murmurs (mitral stenosis, tricuspid stenosis), and continuous systolic and diastolic murmurs (arteriovenous fistula, patent ductus arteriosus).

III. **Pericardial rub** (pericarditis, acute MI).

4. **Pulmonary**. Breath sounds (decreased, crackles or rales, wheezes, ronchi).
5. **Neurologic and musculoskeletal**. Focal neurologic signs, altered mental status, joint range of motion, muscle strength, and endurance.

C. DIAGNOSTIC TESTS are needed to detect subclinical findings; however, they must be correlated with clinical findings, and, if needed, they must be performed serially for follow-up.

1. **Chest radiograph** is used to detect cardiac and pulmonary pathologies (e.g., cardiac enlargement, aortic calcification, pulmonary congestion, and pneumonia). A systematic approach to reading chest radiographs includes (a) soft tissues, bones, and thorax, (b) pulmonary vasculature and lungs, (c) size and contour of

the heart and individual chambers, (d) great vessels and mediastinal structures, (e) abnormal densities and lucencies, and (f) pleura and diaphragm.

2. **Cardiac tests**

a. ***Electrocardiography (ECG)*** is commonly used to identify structural changes (e.g., ventricular or atrial enlargement), ischemic changes (e.g., ST-T segment displacement), infarction (e.g., Q-wave or non-Q-wave), conduction abnormalities (e.g., bundle branch block and heart block), rhythm abnormalities (e.g., atrial fibrillation or flutter, premature atrial or ventricular contractions, and ventricular fibrillation), and metabolic abnormalities (e.g., hyperkalemia). It can also determine drug effects on the heart (e.g., digitalis or quinidine) and can be used to guide the exercise prescription. Table 5.13-1 shows a quick method of ECG interpretation.

b. ***Echocardiography*** **(or *cardiac ultrasound*;** see Chapter 2.2, section III.B)

   I. **Transthoracic echocardiography** is used to evaluate known or suspected CHD or MI (e.g., global or segmental wall motion abnormalities; assessment of left ventricular ejection fraction; and detection of ventricular aneurysm, mural thrombus, or right ventricular infarction), valvular heart disease [e.g., functional murmur vs. organic valvular abnormality, aortic valve stenosis vs. hypertrophic cardiomyopathy, specific causes of mitral regurgitation murmurs, prosthetic valve abnormalities, valvular vegetations (e.g., endocarditis), and ventricular function in valvular heart disease], pericardial disease (e.g., pericarditis, pericardial effusion, and cardiac tamponade), cardiomyopathy, congenital heart disease, and cardiac tumors. It may also be used in cardiac stress testings (see below).

   II. **Transesophageal echocardiography (TEE)** is particularly useful in the diagnosis of atrial pathology (thrombus, tumor, atrial septal defect, patent foramen ovale), mitral valve dysfunction (endocarditis, regurgitation), aortic pathology (dissection, abscess, endocarditis), and pulmonary artery pathology (thrombus).

3. **Laboratory tests**

a. ***Blood tests*** including complete blood count (hemoglobin and hematocrit); serum electrolytes, cardiac-specific troponins I or T [cTnI or cTnT are increased within 4–6 hours after onset of angina or MI, peak at about 24 hours, and stay elevated for 7–10 days; they are usually measured two or three times during a 12- to 16-hour period; a positive or negative qualitative troponin test takes 15 minutes to do and is used for rapid screening; the quantitative troponin test takes 45–90 minutes to do and is reported as: <0.5 ng/mL = normal; 0.5 to 2.0 ng/mL = unstable angina (may also be seen in chronic kidney failure); >2.0 ng/mL = significant MI]; serum creatine kinase (CK), especially the CK-MB isoenzyme (increased within 4–8 hours after the onset of MI then peaks between 8 and 24 hours, and returns to normal by 48–72 hours); serum lactate dehydrogenase (LDH) especially LD_1 isoenzymes (elevated from 48–96 hours after the onset of MI); and serum drug levels (e.g., digoxin, procainamide, and quinidine).

b. ***Cardiac stress tests***

   I. **Cardiovascular exercise tolerance testing (CV-ETT)** uses a treadmill or cycle ergometry (bicycle or arm crank) for cardiac diagnostic, prognostic, and functional purposes. In the PM&R setting, it is used primarily as the basis for prescribing an individualized and safe exercise program. Chapter 2.7, section I describes fully CV-ETT.

   II. **Echocardiographic stress testing** is usually carried out in conjunction with a treadmill or bicycle ergometer (or occasionally with a pharmacologic stress test; see below) to detect cardiac ischemia (i.e., left ventricular dyssynergia, regional wall motion abnormalities, and wall motion changes). The use of bicycle ergometry allows for continuous monitoring and the detection of

Table 5.13-1 Quick method of electrocardiogram (ECG) interpretation

ECG parameters	Normal	Comments
A. Measurement*		
1. Heart rate†	50–90 bpm‡	• Measure atrial and ventricular rates, if different; • <50 bpm = sinus bradycardia; • >90 bpm = sinus tachycardia; • Variable beat to beat rate = sinus arrhythmia
2. PR interval	0.12–0.20 seconds	• <0.12 = ventricular pre-excitation (e.g., Wolff–Parkinson–White syndrome); AV-junctional rhythm; • >0.2 = first-degree AV block
3. QRS duration	0.06–0.10 seconds	• >0.10 = BBB; nonspecific IVCD; ventricular tachycardia
4. QT interval	Depends on HR§	• Prolonged in: CHD; drug therapy (quinidine, procainamide, TCA); hypokalemia; stroke
5. QRS axis in frontal plane	+90° to −30°	• Deviated in: ventricular hypertrophy; fascicular blocks involving LBB
B. Rhythm and conduction analyses	Normal sinus rhythm	1. Abnormal-impulse (arrhythmia) analyses: a. Site of origin: atria, AV junction, ventricles b. Rate of occurrence: normal, slow, fast c. Response: regular; irregular d. Onset: premature (active), escape (passive) 2. Conduction-delay analyses: a. Site of delay: sinoatrial, intra-atrial, AV junction, intraventricular (left or right BBB); b. Direction of block: antegrade; retrograde; c. Degree of AV block: first degree; second degree [type I (Wenckebach); type II (Mobitz)]; third degree
C. Waveform description		
1. **P waves**: RAE (tall, peaked P waves in II, III, aVF); LAE (wide, notched P wave in frontal plane; increased negativity of P wave in V_1).		
2. **QRS complexes**: RVH (increased R-wave voltage in V_{1-2}; increased S-wave voltage in V_{5-6}); LVH (increased R-wave voltage in V_{5-6}; increased S-wave voltage in V_{1-2}); MI [increased T-wave amplitude and width; terminal position of T wave inverts as MI becomes evolved; ST-segment elevation (>2 mm); "pathologic" Q wave (i.e., >0.04 seconds wide; depth ~1/3 QRS amplitude).		
3. **Nonspecific ST-T wave changes**: myocardial ischemia or infarction; electrolyte abnormalities; drugs; ventricular hypertrophy; central nervous system disease		

bpm, beats per minute; AV, atrioventricular; BBB, bundle branch block; IVCD, intraventricular conduction disorder; CHD, coronary heart disease; TCA, tricyclic antidepressant; RAE or LAE, right or left atrial enlargement; RVH or LVH, right or left ventricular hypertrophy.

**In measuring ECG tracings, one big box = 0.2 seconds; one small box = 0.4 seconds.*

† For HR estimation (at a paper speed of 25 mm/s), each successive big box (between successive P waves or between successive QRS complexes) corresponds to 300, 150, 100, 75, 60, 50 bpm.

‡ The normal HR range of 50–90 bpm (based on actual data) is more clinically relevant than the traditional 60–100 bpm (See Spodick DH, Raju P, Bishop RL, et al.: *Operational definition of normal sinus heart rate.* Am J Cardiol *69:1245–1246, 1992).*

§ QT interval is <0.40 seconds at 70 bpm; for every 10 bpm increase in HR, the QT interval decreases by 0.02 seconds, and vice versa.

transient ischemic changes, while the use of treadmill testing is limited to scanning before and after exercise. Exercise echocardiography, which compares favorably with the results of ETT using ECG, is used when ECG-ETT is ambiguous or nondiagnostic, in women (because of a higher likelihood of a false-positive ECG test), and in those with abnormalities on the resting ECG.

III. **Radionuclide stress testing** uses thallium-201 or technetium-99m perfusion scintigraphy to assess myocardial perfusion and to detect ischemia in CHD (and also to detect acute MI). The imaging can be performed in conjunction with a treadmill or a bicycle ergometer test or with pharmacologic stress testing (see below). Radionuclide scintigraphy can image all patients regardless of habitus and has been shown to be more accurate than stress echocardiography alone or ECG alone; however, it is invasive (injection of a radioactive agent with a long half-life) and is expensive.

IV. **Pharmacologic stress testing** involves the injection of coronary artery vasodilators (e.g., dipyridamole and adenosine) or dobutamine (inotropic, chronotropic, and moderate coronary vasodilator) to induce cardiac stress for the diagnosis of CHD and for risk stratification. Coronary artery vasodilators cause a "cardiac steal" phenomenon in which normal arteries dilate (thus increasing blood flow), but diseased arteries (which are already dilated) are unable to dilate further (thus causing a relative "decrease" in blood flow). Pharmacologic stress testing is usually used in conjunction with ECG monitoring and either echocardiography or radionuclide perfusion scintigraphy. Although patients can be tested regardless of their ability to perform adequate levels of exercise, the usefulness of pharmacologic stress testing remains questionable for determining exercise prescription in cardiac rehabilitation. Pharmacologic stress testing, however, can provide information about ventricular function and the extent of myocardium that may become ischemic, thus they are useful in determining the level of risk stratification, as it relates to the exercise program.

V. **Isometric hand-grip stress test** is performed by having the patient squeeze a hand dynamometer at 25–75% of maximum hand strength for as long as tolerable to provide exercise stress. This technique, which has been used in older research publications, is generally not recommended for clinical use because it does not provoke ischemia as effectively as ETT and other stress testings.

c. ***Invasive cardiovascular diagnostic procedures***, such as cardiac catheterization (right and left side of the heart), coronary angiography, intracardiac electrophysiologic studies, and endomyocardial biopsy.

IV. Cardiac rehabilitation

Cardiac rehabilitation consists of four distinct, successive phases. Many clinicians, however, divide it into three phases by combining phases III and IV and calling it the "long-term" or "maintenance" cardiac rehabilitation phase. Each phase of cardiac rehabilitation has specific goals with educational or life-style modification components as well as an activity or exercise component, but differs with respect to location (inpatient, outpatient, or community), duration of the phase, amount of supervision, and intensity of activity.

A. PHASE I, the inpatient phase of cardiac rehabilitation, can be divided into Ia or acute phase (which generally involves 3 to 6 days of hospitalization) and Ib or long-term acute phase (which requires prolonged hospitalization because of secondary complications or other disabilities). Phase I is designed primarily for patients recovering from MI or CABGs. Other cardiac patients that may benefit from a phase I program include those with angioplasty (PTCA), valve surgery, cardiac transplantation, stable angina, and CHD risk factors. Phase I is started as soon as the patient's condition has stabilized, usually on the 2nd to 4th day after MI or after surgery. It is considered the initial point and cornerstone for all other phases in preparing the patient for return to an active and productive life-style.

The goals of phase I (i.e., Ia and Ib) are as follows:

- to prevent the sequelae of immobilization and assist the patient in tolerating self-care activities and household ambulation;
- to prepare the patient (and family) for a healthy life-style (i.e., by identifying and modifying the risk factors of CHD);
- to reduce psychologic and emotional disorders that accompany the cardiac diagnosis (anxiety and depression are the most common; they are usually self-limiting but may last more than 6 months in up to 30% of patients);
- to facilitate adjustment to the acute event and to the hospital environment; and
- to motivate the patient to make a long-term commitment to the cardiac rehabilitation program.

By the end of phase I, the cardiac patient should be able to perform self-care, activities of daily living, and household ambulation (except stair climbing); understand the benefits of exercise and be able to perform the prescribed exercises; understand and be able to take medications independently; adhere to the prescribed diet (e.g., low-fat diet); check the pulse rate; and identify cardiac symptoms. Phase I programs include:

1. **Education and risk-modification programs**. Patient education techniques are discussed in Chapter 5.10, section VI.A. Specific topics for the phase I educational program include orientation to cardiac rehabilitation, anatomy and physiology of the heart, disease and the healing process, recognition of angina and other cardiac symptoms, cardiovascular medications, pulse taking, benefits of physical activity and exercise, psychosocial adjustment to disability (for patient and family), and sexual counseling (see Table 5.13-2; see also Chapter 5.9). The patient is also taught to identify modifiable CHD risk factors and to take the following steps:

a. ***Hyperlipidemia control,*** that is, lowering of cholesterol to desirable levels to reduce risk for CHD. For a practical approach to lipid screening and treatment based on the 2001 National Cholesterol Education Program (NCEP) Expert Panel on Detection, Evaluation, and Treatment of High Blood Cholesterol in Adults (Adult Treatment Panel III or ATP III), refer to Fig. 5.13-1. The therapeutic life-style changes recommended by ATP III primarily consist of: dietary modification to primarily reduce intake of saturated fats and cholesterol and increase intake of viscous (soluble) fiber (see Table 5.13-3 for overall recommendation of dietary modification; see Supplemental references for books on low-fat diet programs and recipes; consider referral to registered dietitians or other qualified nutritionists); increased physical activity; and weight reduction to maintain body mass index (BMI) of 18.5–24.9 kg/m^2 (where BMI = weight in kg divided by the square of height in meters). For discussion about weight-loss programs, that is dietary change, exercise, behavior modification, life-style modification, drug treatment, weight-loss surgery, and combination therapies, refer to the articles by the 1998 Expert Panel on the Identification, Evaluation, and Treatment of Overweight and Obesity in Adults and the 1992 National Institute of Health Technology Assessment Conference Panel (see Further reading section).

Table 5.13-2 General sexual counseling for patients after a cardiac event (e.g., myocardial infarction or coronary artery bypass graft surgery)

Parameter	General sexual counseling
MET requirement	• The maximal activity during sexual intercourse approximates 4.7–5.5 METs for <30 seconds and ~3.5 METs during the pre- and postorgasmic periods.[1,2] • Noncoital activities (e.g., masturbation) have lower energy expenditures than coitus.[3]
Safe time of sexual resumption	• When patient is stable or asymptomatic; in general, If the patient can exercise at levels of 5–7 METs without symptoms, abnormal pulse rate, or changes in blood pressure or ECG.[1] • Time period is variable (usually within 3–6 weeks after cardiac event).
Tests for readiness to resume sexual activity	• Clinical test: two-flight stair-climbing test [i.e., 10 min of rapid walking at 120 paces/min or 3 miles/hour, followed by climbing two flights of stairs (about 22 steps with 17 cm height) in 10 seconds or at two steps/second];[4] or • Laboratory test: exercise tolerance test (see Chapter 2.7, section I) with maximum workload of at least 5–7 METs.
Benefits of exercise	• Exercise training can lessen the peak coital heart rate.[5]
Positions[6]	• Suggested positions: patient at the bottom; side-by-side, face-to-face, face-to-back; sitting on a chair with partner sitting on patient's lap. • Most patients do not make changes in patterns of foreplay or position adopted during coitus.
Precautions	• Avoid sexual activities in the following conditions (associated with sudden death during coitus)[7]: illicit sexual affairs; unfamiliar surroundings; after a large meal; or after high alcohol intake. • Also avoid sexual activities soon after physical or emotional stress.
Warning signs[6] that warrant a physician consultation	• Tachycardia and dyspnea/tachypnea that persist for 10–15 min after coitus; extreme fatigue persisting until the next day; arrhythmias; dizziness, lightheadedness or "blacking out"; chest pain during or after coitus; sexual dysfunction.

Data adapted from:
[1] *Hellerstein HK, Friedman EH: Sexual activity and the postcoronary patient.* Arch Intern Med *125:987–999, 1970.*
[2] *Douglas JE, Wilkes TD: Reconditioning cardiac patients.* Am Fam Physician *11(1):123–129, 1975.*
[3] *Bohlen JG, Held JP, Sanderson MO,* et al.: *Heart rate, rate-pressure product, and oxygen uptake during four sexual activities.* Arch Intern Med *144:1745–1748, 1984.*
[4] *Larson JL, McNaughton MW, Kennedy JW,* et al.: *Heart rate and blood pressure responses to sexual activity and a stair-climbing test.* Heart Lung *9:1025–1030, 1980.*
[5] *Stein RA: The effect of exercise training on heart rate during coitus in the post myocardial infarction patient.* Circulation *55:738–740, 1977.*
[6] *Papadopoulos C: Education and counseling of the patient and family: Sexual problems/interventions. In Wenger NK, Hellerstein HK, editors.:* Rehabilitation of the coronary patient, *ed 3, New York, 1992, Churchill Livingstone, pp. 473–481.*
[7] *Massie E, Rose EF, Rupp JC,* et al.: *Sudden death during coitus: Fact or fiction?* Med Aspects Hum Sex *3(6):22–26, 1969.*

If after 6 weeks, the therapeutic life-style changes fail to attain the LDL goal, the following drugs are considered: statins or HMG-CoA reductase inhibitors [lovastatin (Mevachol), pravastatin (Pravachol), simvastatin (Zocor)]; bile acid sequestrants or bile acid binding resins [cholestyramine (Questran, Cholybar), colestipol (Colestid)]; nicotinic acid (niacin); fibric acid derivatives [gemfibrozil

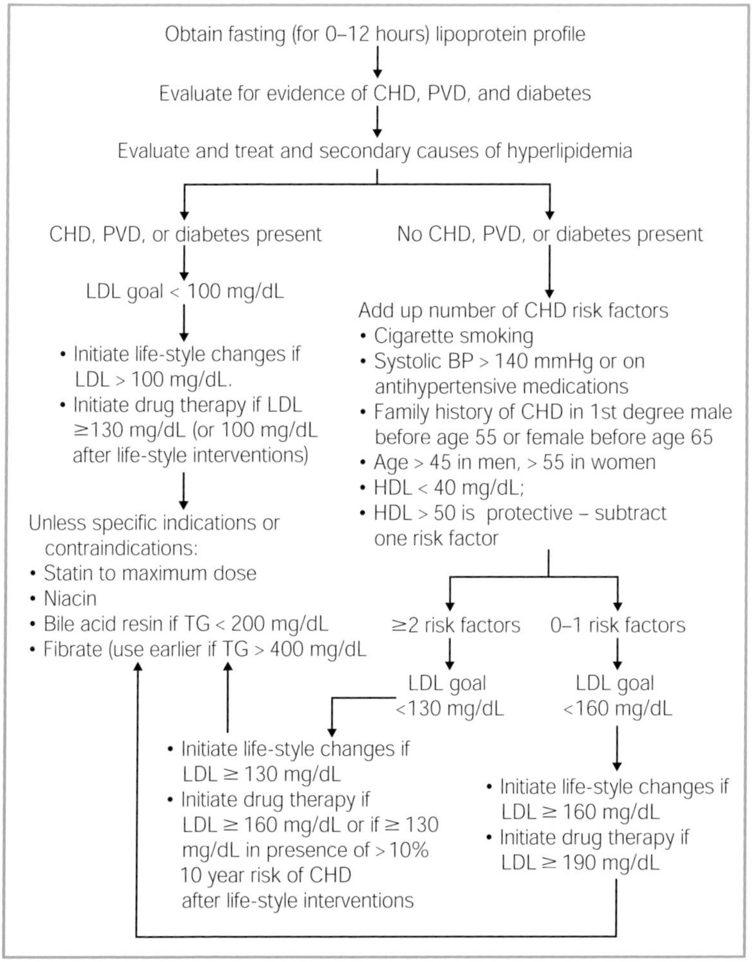
Obtain fasting (for 0–12 hours) lipoprotein profile
Evaluate for evidence of CHD, PVD, and diabetes
Evaluate and treat and secondary causes of hyperlipidemia
CHD, PVD, or diabetes present
No CHD, PVD, or diabetes present
LDL goal < 100 mg/dL
• Initiate life-style changes if LDL > 100 mg/dL.
• Initiate drug therapy if LDL ≥130 mg/dL (or 100 mg/dL after life-style interventions)
Unless specific indications or contraindications:
• Statin to maximum dose
• Niacin
• Bile acid resin if TG < 200 mg/dL
• Fibrate (use earlier if TG > 400 mg/dL
Add up number of CHD risk factors
• Cigarette smoking
• Systolic BP > 140 mmHg or on antihypertensive medications
• Family history of CHD in 1st degree male before age 55 or female before age 65
• Age > 45 in men, > 55 in women
• HDL < 40 mg/dL;
• HDL > 50 is protective – subtract one risk factor
≥2 risk factors
0–1 risk factors
LDL goal <130 mg/dL
LDL goal <160 mg/dL
• Initiate life-style changes if LDL ≥ 130 mg/dL
• Initiate drug therapy if LDL ≥ 160 mg/dL or if ≥ 130 mg/dL in presence of > 10% 10 year risk of CHD after life-style interventions
• Initiate life-style changes if LDL ≥ 160 mg/dL
• Initiate drug therapy if LDL ≥ 190 mg/dL

Figure 5.13-1 Practical approach to lipid screening and treatment based on the 2001 Adult Treatment Panel III recommendations. The lipoprotein profile screening is repeated every 6 weeks until goal is achieved, after which it should be monitored every 4–6 months to determine adherence to treatment. BP = blood pressure; CHD = coronary heart disease; HDL = high-density lipoprotein; LDL = low-density lipoprotein; PVD = peripheral vascular disease; TG = triglycerides. (From: Witztum JL, Steinberg D: The hyperlipoproteinemias. In Goldman L, Ausiello D, editors: *Cecil textbook of medicine*, vol 2, ed 22, Philadelphia, 2004, Saunders, p. 1265, with permission.)

(Lopid), clofibrate (Atromid-S)]; and antioxidants [probucol (Lorelco)]. The use of Metamucil (see Chapter 5.8, section VI.B.3.a.1) in counteracting the constipating effects of bile acid sequestrants also helps lower cholesterol. Other cholesterol-lowering agents under investigation include fish oils; vitamins A, C, and E; and estrogen replacement therapy.

b. ***Hypertension control***, that is lowering of BP to <140/90 mmHg (or <130/80 mmHg for those with diabetes or chronic kidney disease), to reduce cardiovascular, renal, and central nervous system morbidity and mortality associated with long-standing hypertension. Based on the 2003 JNC 7 (i.e., The Seventh

Table 5.13-3 Dietary modification for hyperlipidemia control based on the 2000 Dietary Guidelines for Americans

Nutrient	Recommended intake
Saturated fat*	<7% of total calories
Polyunsaturated fat	Up to 10% of total calories
Monosaturated fat	Up to 20% of total calories
Total fat	25–35% of total calories
Carbohydrates†	50–60% of total calories
Fiber	20–30 g/day
Protein	Approximately 15% of total calories
Cholesterol	<200 mg/day
Total calories‡	Balance energy intake and expenditure to maintain desirable body weight or prevent weight gain

*Trans *fatty acids, which can also raise low-density lipoprotein, should be kept at low intake.*
† Carbohydrates should be derived predominantly from foods rich in complex carbohydrates including grains, especially whole grains, fruits, and vegetables.
‡ Daily energy expenditure should include at least moderate physical activity (contributing approximately 200 kcal/day).
From: Expert Panel on the Detection, Evaluation, and Treatment of High Blood Cholesterol in Adults: Executive summary of the third report of the National Cholesterol Education Program (NCEP) Expert Panel on Detection, Evaluation, and Treatment of High Blood Cholesterol in Adults (Adult Treatment Panel III). JAMA *285(19):2490, 2001, with permission.*

Report of the Joint National Committee on Detection, Evaluation, and Treatment of High Blood Pressure), the following "stepped-care" approach is recommended:

Step 1. Life-style modification is encouraged in patients with normal systolic BP (i.e., SBP <120 mmHg) and normal diastolic BP (i.e., DBP <80 mmHg). In prehypertensive patients (SBP = 120–139 and DBP = 80–89), life-style should be modified without using antihypertensive drugs unless there are compelling indications (see Table 5.13-4). In all hypertensive patients, life-style modifications should be made throughout their life. They include:

- Weight reduction (see discussion under section IV.1.a.);
- Adoption of DASH or **D**ietary **A**pproaches to **S**top **H**ypertension eating plan which is rich in potassium and calcium (i.e., diet high in fruits, vegetables, and low-fat dairy products with a reduced content of saturated and total fat – see section IV.A.1.a);
- Reduction of daily sodium intake [i.e., less than 2.4 g sodium, which is approximately less than 6 g salt (sodium chloride) per day];
- Moderation of alcohol intake (i.e., patients suspected of alcohol abuse as identified by a "yes" response on the CAGE questionnaire, see Table 1.1-1, should be referred to programs for the treatment of alcoholism; patients with no alcohol abuse problems should limit daily alcohol intake to no more than two drinks per day or 1 oz of ethanol (e.g., 24 oz beer, 10 oz wine, or 3 oz 80-proof whiskey) in most men and no more than 1 drink per day in women and lighter-weight persons;
- Participation in a regular aerobic exercise program (see section IV.A.2.a), e.g., brisk walking 30 minutes per day, three to four times a week;
- Smoking cessation (see section IV.A.1.c);

Table 5.13-4 Individual drug classes recommended for hypertensive patients with compelling indications						
Compelling indications	**Diuretic**	**BB**	**ACEI**	**ARB**	**CCB**	**Aldo ANT**
Heart failure	√	√	√	√		√
Postmyocardial infarction		√	√			√
High coronary disease risk	√	√	√		√	
Diabetes	√	√	√	√	√	
Chronic kidney disease			√	√		
Recurrent stroke prevention	√		√			

Note: The compelling indication is managed in parallel with the blood pressure.
A thiazide diuretic is used as the initial therapy for most patients with hypertension.
Drug abbreviations: BB = β-blocker; ACEI = angiotensin-converting enzyme inhibitor; ARB = angiotensin-receptor blocker; CCB = calcium-channel blocker; Aldo ANT = aldosterone antagonist.
Adapted from: Chobanian AV (chair): JNC 7 Express: The seventh report of Joint National Committee on Prevention, Detection, Evaluation, and Treatment of High Blood Pressure, *US Department of Health and Human Services, May 2003, p.15.*

- Stress management (controversial; not recommended by the JNC 7 because of a lack of convincing data; see section IV.A.1.e).

Step 2. If blood pressure is >140/90 mmHg or >130/80 mmHg (in patients with diabetes or chronic kidney disease), continue life-style modification and add first-line drugs:

- For stage 1 hypertension (SBP = 140–159 or DBP = 90–99 mmHg) without compelling indications (as listed in Table 5.13-4), thiazide-type diuretics may be used for most. But in some, the following drugs may be considered: angiotensin-converting enzyme inhibitor (ACEI), angiotensin-receptor blocker (ARB), β-blocker (BB), calcium-channel blocker (CCB), or a combination of these.
- For stage 2 hypertension (SBP >160 or DBP >100 mmHg) without compelling indications (as listed on Table 5.13-4), a two-drug combination may be used for most (usually thiazide-type diuretic plus ACEI, or ARB, or BB, or CCB)
- For hypertensive patients with compelling indications refer to Table 5.13-4.

Step 3. If still not at the goal BP, continue life-style modification and optimize dosages or add additional drugs until the goal BP is achieved, or consider consulting with a hypertension specialist.

c. ***Smoking cessation*** (see techniques in Chapter 5.12, section IV.A.1.a) to reduce the risk of CHD by 50–70% in the primary prevention of CHD and to reduce up to 50% the risk of sudden death and fatal reinfarction in patients with MI (i.e., tertiary prevention). Smoking cessation is essential and must be emphasized in all patients undergoing cardiac rehabilitation.

d. ***Diabetes mellitus control,*** that is lowering of blood sugar to less than 140 mg/dL, to reduce the risk of cardiovascular disease (especially CHD), peripheral vascular disease, and cerebrovascular disease. Management includes nonpharmacologic (e.g., weight loss program if obese, dietary control, and exercise) and pharmacologic (e.g., oral hypoglycemics and insulin) treatment.

e. ***Stress management,*** that is relaxation techniques (see Chapter 4.2, section VI), biofeedback (see Chapter 4.1, section VI), and psychological techniques on coping with stress have been reported to reduce coronary morbidity and mortality, especially in patients with "type A" behavior. These beneficial effects, however, are controversial because of the difficulty in diagnosing "type A" behaviors. Recent studies seem to indicate that impatience and free-floating hostility (rather than ambition and competitive drive) are the key elements of a "type A" behavior pattern.

2. **Exercise**. The following cardiac patients may generally proceed with phase I exercises and activities: those with uncomplicated cardiac events, first-degree heart block, sinus bradycardia, and infrequent premature ventricular contractions (PVCs). Although significant improvements in cardiovascular fitness or other physical measurements are not expected during phase I, studies have shown that early physical activity reduces the complications of immobilization (i.e., by reducing venous thromboembolism, maintaining muscle tone, reducing orthostatic hypotension, and maintaining joint mobility).

Absolute contraindications for exercise training in cardiac patients include unstable angina, heart failure (acute, uncompensated), uncontrolled atrial or ventricular arrhythmias, uncontrolled sinus tachycardia (>120 beats/min), second- or third-degree atrioventricular block (without pacemaker), resting ST-segment displacement over 3 mm, resting BP above 200/110 mmHg, inappropriate asymptomatic postural or exertional BP responses, orthostatic BP drop >10 mmHg with symptoms, severe and symptomatic aortic stenosis (more than 50 mmHg gradient), hypertrophic obstructive cardiomyopathy, active pericarditis or myocarditis, idiopathic hypertrophic subaortic stenosis, dissecting aneurysm, severe pulmonary hypertension, recent embolism, acute or chronic thrombophlebitis, uncontrolled diabetes mellitus (resting blood glucose >400 mg/dL), and acute systemic illness (acute thyroiditis, hypo- or hyperkalemia, hypovolemia) or fever (above 100°F or 37.8°C).

Relative contraindications of exercise training in cardiac patients include resting BP over 180/100 mmHg, hypotension, inappropriate rise in BP during exercise, sinus tachycardia at rest (more than 120 beats/min), resting ST-segment depression over 2 mm, moderate aortic stenosis, ventricular aneurysm, compensated heart failure, pericarditis associated with CABG, excessive incisional drainage after CABG, new ECG change suggestive of new infarction, poorly controlled diabetes mellitus, symptomatic anemia (hematocrit less than 30%), significant emotional stress or psychological disorders, or neuromuscular, musculoskeletal, or orthopedic problems that would prohibit exercise.

a. ***Exercise programs*** include low metabolic demand exercises and activities that are performed for 5–10 minutes (progressing up to 20–30 minutes), two to four times daily. These activities require less than 4.0 METs (see Chapter 2.7, section I.A for discussion of METs or metabolic equivalents; see also Tables 4.2-3 and 4.2-4 for METs of different activities) and should generally not raise the patient's heart rate (HR) above 20 beats/min over the resting heart rate. At the beginning of phase I, the exercises emphasize range of motion (ROM), which is advanced through a series of active exercises (and, if tolerated, mild resistance exercises) in the supine, sitting, and upright positions. If the patient is confined to bed, leg and foot exercises (e.g., ankle pumps) are encouraged to reduce venous stasis. Passive or active-assistive ROM exercises may be necessary for some patients (e.g., those with severe myocardial damage, status postcardiac transplantation, or other compromising complications). Otherwise, as a result of the short duration of phase I, the patient is immediately advanced to active exercises and activities under close monitoring during and after the session (which may later be progressed to telemetric ECG monitoring of activities).

Exercise parameters monitored include pulse or HR, BP, ECG, and activity-induced symptoms. In general, HR monitoring is preferred as it is easier to monitor during exercise than auscultatory BP. The exercise or activity should be stopped if the patient develops any of the following signs and symptoms: angina, light-headedness, nausea, dyspnea, fatigue, pallor, cyanosis, ataxia, hypoxia, altered mental status, peripheral circulatory insufficiency (e.g., leg claudication); inappropriate bradycardia (drop in HR of more than 10 beats/min); activity-induced BP changes (e.g., >20 mmHg drop in SBP; SBP >220 mmHg or DBP > 110 mmHg); activity-induced ECG changes [e.g., ST displacement over 2–3 mm from rest, ventricular tachycardia, symptomatic supraventricular tachycardia, new-onset left bundle branch block, new-onset second- or third-degree atrioventricular block, R on T PVCs, and frequent multifocal PVCs (i.e., more than 30% of PVCs)].

As soon as tolerable, the patient is progressed to independent self-care and short-distance ambulation (in the corridor or on a treadmill) or bicycle ergometry. In general, the energy cost of almost all activities of daily living is less than 4 METs. Unless the patient is able to tolerate 5–7 METs (e.g., from exercise tolerance testing described in Chapter 2.7, section I.A), he or she should not climb stairs, which generally requires 5–7 METs. Patients who have CABG and PTCA have little or no permanent damage to the myocardium, hence they can generally be exercised more aggressively than those who have sustained an MI. For patients who are postcardiac transplantation, passive ROM exercises are initiated at extubation and performed twice a day. Borg's rating of perceived exertion (RPE) scale at an intensity of 11–13 in the original Borg's RPE scale (see Table 4.2-5; see also discussion of Borg's RPE scale in Chapter 4.2, section III.A.3) is recommended in cardiac transplant patients because cardiac denervation decreases the reliability of other parameters such as HR (i.e., HR does not increase until circulating catecholamines rise after 3–5 minutes of exercise and does not reach maximum levels predicted for the donor age).

b. ***Exercise testing.*** At the end of phase I or prior to starting phase II (i.e., from 3 days to 3 weeks after a cardiac event), a low-level exercise tolerance test (ETT; see Chapter 2.7, section I) is generally ordered. End-points for ETT are shown in Table 2.7-2. Other end-points that may be used in low-level exercise tolerance testing include attaining the following: increase in HR of 20–30 beats above resting HR; maximal heart rate of 120–140 beats/min; 70–75% age-estimated maximal HR; 4–6 METs, or, in patients on β-blockers, a Borg's RPE scale of "hard" (see Table 4.2-5). The ETT is used to stratify patients based on prognostic risks (see Table 5.13-5). Its specific goals are to assess the patient's progress, the adequacy of the current medical regimen, and the need for coronary revascularization; and to help determine the extent of ECG-monitoring needed during exercise and the appropriateness of progression to supervised phase II or to a home exercise program. Based on ETT, the prognoses of patients with MI are as follows (see also Fioretti *et al.*, 1984; Theroux *et al.*, 1976; Weld *et al.*, 1981; and Krone *et al.*, 1985).

- Patients with at least 1 mm of ST-segment depression, or who cannot achieve a peak workload of 4 METs, or cannot increase their SBP at least 30 mmHg (or at least to 110 mmHg) during the ETT are at increased risk for coronary mortality within the first year after MI. The abnormal BP response is probably a more sensitive predictor of mortality at 1 year than the maximal workload achieved or ischemic ST-segment changes.
- Patients with exercise-induced ST-segment depressions within 10–21 days after MI have a 2 to 20 times greater risk of having a subsequent coronary event than do patients without this ECG finding.
- Patients unable to achieve a peak workload of 4 METs during ETT by 3 weeks after MI are at significantly higher risk for recurrent MI, coronary death, cardiac arrest, or necessity for CABG at a 2-year follow-up than those capable of performing at least 4 METs of peak workload.

Table 5.13-5 Risk stratification criteria of cardiac patients for exercise participation

RISK CLASSIFICATION AND DESCRIPTORS
Lowest risk for exercise participation (all must be present for patient to remain at lowest risk) Absence of complex ventricular arrhythmias during exercise testing and recovery Absence of angina or other significant symptoms (e.g., unusual shortness of breath, lightheadedness, or dizziness during exercise testing and recovery) Presence of normal hemodynamics during exercise testing and recovery (i.e., appropriate increases and decreases in heart rate and systolic blood pressure (BP) with increasing workloads and recovery) Functional capacity ≥7 METs* **Nonexercise testing findings:** Rest ejection fraction ≥50% Uncomplicated myocardial infarction (MI) or revascularization procedure Absence of complicated ventricular arrhythmias at rest Absence of congestive heart failure (CHF) Absence of signs or symptoms of postevent/postprocedure ischemia Absence of clinical depression
Moderate risk for exercise participation (any of these findings places patient at moderate risk) Presence of angina or other significant symptoms [e.g., unusual shortness of breath, lightheadedness, or dizziness, occurring only at high levels of exertion (≥7 METs)] Mild to moderate level of silent ischemia during exercise testing or recovery (ST segment depression <2 mm from baseline) Functional capacity <5 METs* **Nonexercise testing findings:** Rest ejection fraction = 40–49%
High risk for exercise participation (any of these findings places a patient at high risk) Presence of complex ventricular arrhythmias during exercise testing and recovery Presence of angina or other significant symptoms [e.g., unusual shortness of breath, lightheadedness, or dizziness at low levels of exertion (<5 METs) or during recovery] High level of silent ischemia (ST-segment depression ≥2 mm from baseline) during exercise testing or recovery Presence of abnormal hemodynamics with exercise testing (i.e., chronotropic incompetence, or flat or decreasing systolic BP with increasing work loads) or recovery (i.e., severe postexercise hypotension) **Nonexercise testing findings:** Rest ejection fraction <40% Family history of cardiac arrest or sudden cardiac death Complex arrhythmias at rest Complicated MI or revascularization procedure Presence of CHF Presence of signs or symptoms of postevent/postprocedure ischemia Presence of clinical depression

**Note: If measured functional capacity is not available, this variable is not considered in the risk-stratification process.*
1 MET (metabolic equivalent) = 3.5 mL O_2/kg/min; EF = ejection fraction.
From: Williams MA: Exercise testing in cardiac rehabilitation: Exercise prescription and beyond. Cardiol Clin *19(3):418, 2001, with permission.*

B. PHASE II is a continuation of phase I and is usually conducted in an outpatient setting or towards the end of hospitalization. If the patient is discharged from the hospital, phase II should generally start within 2 weeks and last 8–12 weeks. Indications and contraindications to phase II are essentially the same as those for phase I. The goals of phase II are:

- to enhance cardiovascular function and physical work capacity (i.e., strength, endurance, and flexibility),

- to detect ECG changes (e.g., arrhythmias) during exercise,
- to teach the patient proper techniques of exercise and provide him or her with guidelines for long-term exercise,
- to establish healthy life-styles in the patient and family; and
- to enhance the patient's psychologic function and prepare him or her for a return to work and resumption of normal familial and social roles.

By the end of phase II, the cardiac patient should be able to perform the daily self-administered exercise program safely, have adequate knowledge of his or her disease and symptoms to pursue vocational, recreational, and sexual activities safely; sustain healthy habits (e.g., low-fat diet) to reduce CHD risks; and comply with medications and medical follow-up. Phase II programs include:

1. **Education and risk-modification programs.** These programs are a continuation and reinforcement of programs learned in phase I (see section IV.A.1) and are designed to help patients maintain a healthy life-style. Prepared education programs may be used (e.g., *An Active Partnership for the Health of Your Heart*, American Heart Association, 7272 Greenville Avenue, Dallas, TX 75231-4596, tel. 1-800-AHA-USA; *http://www.americanheart.org*).
2. **Exercise.** Depending on the ETT (see section IV.2.b) and the patient's risk stratification (see Table 5.13-5), the patient is given an individualized prescription of intensity, duration, frequency, and mode of activity. The exercise is supervised with either continuous or intermittent ECG monitoring (telemetry or hard-wired ECG). Phase II activities emphasize physical reconditioning and begin with dynamic–rhythmic or aerobic exercises (see Chapter 4.2, section III.A for discussion of aerobic exercises) at a level of 5 METs. The exercise involves both the upper- and lower-limb muscle groups because there is little crossover of adaptation between arm and leg exercises. Equipment used generally includes treadmills, bicycle ergometers, arm ergometers, wall pulleys, steps, rowing machines, vertical climbing devices, cross-county ski simulators, and light weights. The patient performs 5–10 minutes of exercise at each station with approximately 1 minute of rest between bouts. Each exercise session generally lasts 1 hour (including warm-up and cool-down periods) and is performed three times per week. The goal is to exercise within the target heart rate (described in Chapter 4.2, section III.A.1) for at least 20–30 minutes for training adaptation to occur. The exercise intensity is increased on a weekly basis as the patient's symptoms and physical conditioning permit, ultimately progressing to 8 METs before starting phase III.
3. **Return-to-work (RTW) program** (see also Chapter 5.11, section IV). Patients are prepared to return to their original job (or to a modified duty initially) or, in some cases, to an alternative job. In general, patients who can perform more than 7 METs of workload without any abnormal responses should be able to return to most jobs except heavy industrial work (see Table 5.11-1 for correlation of MET levels with the US Department of Labor classification of work). Studies show that in the United States, more than two-thirds (70–75%) of patients with MI return to work (usually within 2–3 months); however, only 30% of cardiac patients from low socioeconomic levels or with low educational achievement are able to return to work. Among those cardiac patients who initially return to work, about 20% drop out within 1 year.

C. PHASES III AND IV are considered the maintenance (long-term) phase of cardiac rehabilitation. The maintenance phase is important because if it is neglected, the benefits gained during the training phases (i.e., I and II) are lost within a few weeks. Low-risk patients who did not participate in phases I or II may participate in the maintenance phase. Phase III usually lasts from 6 to 24 months and generally includes clinical supervision and intermittent ECG monitoring (e.g., through real-time ECG transmission over the telephone for home-based exercise). Exercises may initially be performed in an outpatient setting, then progressed to a community or home setting. The goals of phase III are similar to those of phase II. Phase III is designed to provide a smooth transition from the structured, closely supervised, and monitored phase II program to one that is less monitored, supervised, and structured.

Phase IV, which is an extension of phase III, is a lifelong program, which generally does not include clinical supervision or ECG monitoring. The goals of phase IV are to continue in improving and maintaining fitness and a healthy life-style (to minimize cardiac disease morbidity and mortality). Other noncardiac patients (including healthy adults interested in enhancing physical fitness) may enter the phase IV program (even without going through phase III). A minimum of 2 weeks is generally needed to assess the patient's readiness for unsupervised and nonmonitored activities. The unsupervised patients may periodically need supervised exercise and ECG-monitored classes at the rehabilitation center to assess the patient's progress, to update the exercise program, and to evaluate the patient's clinical status. Phase III and IV programs include:

1. **Education and risk-modification programs.** These programs consist of review and reinforcement of topics learned in phases I and II (see sections IV.A.1 and IV.B.1) for patients who underwent the training phases. For patients who are directly entering phase III or IV, the education and risk-modification programs (discussed in phases I and II) are initiated.
2. **Exercise.** As with phase II, the results from the ETT are used to determine the intensity of phase III training. The exercises selected involve the muscle groups trained in phase II and should fit within the interests and life-style of the individual patient. As a result of training specificity, upper-limb exercises should also be prescribed in addition to the lower-limb exercises. The minimum requirement is to exercise at least three times per week for 30–60 minutes (with a regimen of 5–10 minutes warm-up, 20–30 minutes aerobic training, and 5–10 minutes cool-down). For those who have completed phase II, a target heart rate range (THRR) of 80% of maximum heart rate (MHR) is usually used, and the patient progresses gradually until 85% MHR when training adaptation is normal. However, for low-risk cardiac patients or healthy subjects who did not participate in phase II, a more conservative intensity is initially used (e.g., THRR at 70% of MHR attained in an ETT), which may progress at a more rapid rate (especially in healthy individuals depending on such factors as physical condition, age, musculoskeletal limitations) to 85–90% MHR (for healthy individuals and other select patients). The types of exercise include:

a. ***Aerobic endurance exercises.*** For full discussion of aerobic endurance exercises, see Chapter 4.2, section III.A. To help ensure long-term compliance, fun games and recreational sports may be used, preceded by a program of general conditioning and clinical assessment, including ECG monitoring with telemetry during actual play.

b. ***Resistance training*** (see Chapter 4.2, section II). The use of resistance exercises has been shown to be safe and beneficial for phase III and IV cardiac patients. Contraindications and termination criteria for resistive exercises are similar to those described in section IV.A.2 and those shown in Table 2.7-2 respectively. A popular form of resistive exercise is circuit weight training (CWT; see Chapter 4.2, section II.B.2.b) using resistive machines, which seem to be more beneficial than free weights. Specific benefits of circuit weight training include improvement in strength, lean body mass, flexibility, and cardiovascular endurance, and perhaps increase in bone mineral content (thus reducing the possibility of osteoporosis with aging). Circuit weight training also reduces the potential for musculoskeletal discomfort, is generally safe, and provides added fun and satisfaction.

Circuit weight training is usually performed after the aerobic phase (to ensure adequate warm-up and to decrease the risk of musculoskeletal injury), on alternate days, three times per week. All major muscle groups are exercised starting from large muscles then progressing to small muscles. The level of resistance (i.e., low-to-moderate or 30–60% of 10 repetition maximum) should allow the exercise sets to be completed comfortably (without straining) with 8–20 (usually 10–15) repetitions per station. Depending on the patient's fitness level and time allotted for circuit weight training, the number of sets varies from one to three and the number of stations varies from 5 to 18.

In the beginning, the patient should attempt one set of exercises then gradually build up to three sets. When the patient can easily complete 12 to 15 repetitions at a Borg's RPE of 12 to 13 (see Borg's RPE scale in Table 4.2-5), then resistance can be increased (depending upon the patient's time allotment for the session, fitness level, and fatigability). When lifting is involved, it must be done through the full arc (if possible) at the following speed: lift to a count of 2 and lower to a count of 4. Each CWT session should last from 20 to 30 minutes with rest intervals of 30–60 seconds between stations. In general, shorter rest intervals allow for greater improvement in cardiovascular endurance; while longer rest intervals provide for greater recovery of heart rate and blood pressure and less risk of cardiovascular complications.

c. ***Aquatic-exercise programs*** (see Chapter 4.2, section V). Water exercises (including swimming) are safe and are less stressful on bones and joints than land-based weight-bearing activities. Moreover, they can be performed in a horizontal position, thus enhancing venous return and augmenting stroke volume by reducing the effects of gravity. The cooling effect of water can also decrease the risk of heat overload. The recommended water temperature for cardiac patients ranges from 26 to 33°C (80–92°F). Most patients find the warmer temperature range more comfortable (especially those with peripheral vascular disease as heat causes vasodilation); however, the cooler temperature range is better for dissipation of heat.

Aquatic activities with varying intensities include water walking (with and without use of the arms), swimnastics, water aerobics, aqua stepping or step aerobics, swimming that incorporates a variety of strokes, and water games (e.g., volleyball). The exercise intensity is individually prescribed based on the ETT (see Chapter 2.7, section I). Although bicycle ergometer or treadmill tests may be used, an arm ergometer test is preferred if the aquatic program consists mainly of upper body work (e.g., swimming). The exercise frequency (three times per week) and intensity are similar to those for aerobic endurance exercises (see Chapter 4.2, section III.A). However, the THRR is preferred for estimating intensity, because the Borg RPE scale may be less accurate with water exercise, and there are limited data on the actual energy cost (METs) of water activities in cardiac patients.

Further reading

American Association of Cardiovascular and Pulmonary Rehabilitation (AACVPR): *Guidelines for cardiac rehabilitation and secondary prevention programs*, ed 4, Champaign, IL, 2004, Human Kinetics.

Bartels MN: Cardiac rehabilitation. In Grabois M, Garrison SJ, Hart KA, *et al.*, editors: *Physical medicine and rehabilitation: the complete approach*, Malden, MA, 2000, Blackwell Science, pp. 1435–1456.

Chobanian AV, Bakris GL, Black HR, *et al.*: The seventh report of the Joint National Committee on Prevention, Detection, Evaluation, and Treatment of High Blood Pressure: The JNC 7 report, *JAMA* 289(19):2560–2572, 2003.

Expert Panel on the Detection, Evaluation, and Treatment of High Blood Cholesterol in Adults: Executive summary of the third report of the National Cholesterol Education Program (NCEP)

Expert Panel on Detection, Evaluation, and Treatment of High Blood Cholesterol in Adults (Adult Treatment Panel III). *JAMA* 285(19):2486–2497, 2001.

Expert Panel on the Identification, Evaluation, and Treatment of Overweight and Obesity in Adults: Executive summary of the Clinical Guidelines on the Identification, Evaluation, and Treatment of Overweight and Obesity in Adults. *Arch Intern Med* 158:1855–1867, 1998.

Fardy PS, Yanowitz FG: *Cardiac rehabilitation, adult fitness, and exercise testing,* ed 3, Baltimore, 1995, Williams & Wilkins.

Fioretti P, Brower R, Simoons ML, *et al.*: Prediction of mortality in hospital survivors of myocardial infarction: comparison of predischarge exercise testing and radionuclide ventriculography at rest. *Br Heart J* 52:592–598, 1984.

Flores AM, Zohman LR: Rehabilitation of the cardiac patient. In DeLisa JA, Gans BM, editors: *Rehabilitation medicine: principles and practice,* ed 3, Philadelphia, 1998, Lippincott-Raven, pp. 1337–1357.

Halar EM, editor: Cardiac rehabilitation: Part 1. *Phys Med Rehabil Clin North Am* 6(1):1–223, 1995.

Krone RJ, Gillespie JA, Weld FM, *et al.*: Low-level exercise testing after myocardial infarction: usefulness in enhancing clinical risk stratification. *Circulation* 71:80–89, 1985.

Moldover JR, Bartels MN: Cardiac rehabilitation. In Braddom RL, editor: *Physical medicine and rehabilitation,* ed 2, Philadelphia, 2000, WB Saunders, pp. 665–686.

National Institute of Health Consensus Development Panel: Physical activity and cardiovascular health. *JAMA* 276(3):241–246, 1996.

National Institute of Health Technology Assessment Conference Panel: Methods for voluntary weight loss and control. *Arch Intern Med* 116:942–949, 1992.

Pashkow FJ, Dafoe WA, editors: *Clinical cardiac rehabilitation: a cardiologist's guide,* Philadelphia, 1999, Lippincott, Williams & Wilkins.

Pollock ML, Wilmore JH: *Exercise in health and disease: evaluation and prescription for prevention of rehabilitation,* ed 2, Philadelphia, 1990, WB Saunders.

Theroux P, Waters DD, Halphen C, *et al.*: Prognostic value of exercise testing soon after myocardial infarction. *N Engl J Med* 301(7):341–345, 1976.

United States National Vital Statistics Reports 52(9):9, 2003.

Weld FM, King-Lee C, Bigger JT, *et al.*: Risk stratification with low-level exercise testing 2 weeks after acute myocardial infarction. *Circulation* 64:306–314, 1981.

Wenger NK, Froelicher ES, Smith LK, *et al.*: *Cardiac rehabilitation: clinical practice guideline No. 17.* AHCPR Publication No. 96-0672, Rockville, MD, October 1995, Agency for Health Care Policy and Research and the National Heart, Lung, and Blood Institute, US Department of Health and Human Services.

Wenger NK, Hellerstein HK, editors: *Rehabilitation of the coronary patient,* ed 3, New York, 1992, Churchill Livingstone.

Supplemental references

Connor SL, Connor WE: *The new American diet,* New York, 1986, Simon & Schuster.

American Heart Association: *American Heart Association low-fat, low-cholesterol cookbook,* ed 3, New York, 2004, Clarkson-Potter.

Ornish D: *Dr Dean Ornish's program for reversing heart disease,* New York, 1996, Ivy (Ballantine) Books.

PART VI

PHYSICAL MEDICINE AND REHABILITATION: APPENDICES

Appendix A

Appendix A-1 Average ranges of motion for the cervical spine and upper limbs

Joint	Motion	AAOS	AMA
Cervical spine	Flexion	0 to 130–150°*	0–60°
	Extension	0 to 130–150°*	0–75°
	Lateral flexion	0 to 80–100°*	0–45°
	Rotation	0 to 155–180°*	0–80°
Shoulder	Flexion	0–180°	0–180°
	Hyperextension	0–60°	0–50°
	Abduction	0–180°	0–180°
	Adduction	Not measured	0–50°
	Medial rotation	0–70°, or thumb tip reaches T6–T10	0–90°
	Lateral rotation	0–90°	0–90°
Elbow	Flexion	0–150°	0–140°
Forearm	Pronation	0–75°	0–80°
	Supination	0–80°	0–80°
Wrist	Flexion	0–80°	0–60°
	Extension	0–60°	0–60°
	Radial deviation	0–20°	0–20°
	Ulnar deviation	0–30°	0–30°
Thumb			
Carpometacarpal	Palmar abduction	0–70°	Not measured
	Radial abduction	0–80°	0–50°
	Adduction (radial)	Not measured	0–8 cm†
	Opposition	Thumb tip to 5th base	0–8 cm‡
Metacarpophalangeal	Flexion	0–50°	0–60°
	Hyperextension	Not measured	0–40°
Interphalangeal (IP)	Flexion	0–80°	0–80°
	Hyperextension	Not measured	0–30°
Fingers			
Metacarpophalangeal	Flexion	0 to 86–105°	0–90°
	Hyperextension	0 to 18–23°	0–20°
Proximal IP	Flexion	0 to 102–108°	0–100°
	Hyperextension	0 to 6–9°	0–30°
Distal IP	Flexion	0 to 63–72°	0–70°
	Hyperextension	0–8°	0–30°

Data adapted from Greene WB, Heckman JD, editors: American Academy of Orthopaedic Surgeons (AAOS): The clinical measurement of joint motion, *Rosemont, IL, 1993, AAOS; and Cocchiarella L, Andersson GBJ, editors:* American Medical Association (AMA). Guides to the evaluation of permanent impairment, *ed 5, Chicago, 2001, AMA Press.*

** Represents total values of passive cervical range of motion (i.e., right + left rotation or lateral flexion; flexion + extension); also age-dependent.*

† Smallest possible distance from flexor crease of thumb interphalangeal joint to distal palmar crease of fifth metacarpophalangeal joint.

‡ Largest possible span from flexor crease of thumb interphalangeal joint to distal palmar crease of third metacarpal.

Appendix A-2 Average ranges of motion for the thoracolumbosacral spine and lower limbs

Joint	Motion	AAOS	AMA
Thoracic spine	Flexion*	NS	0–50°
	Rotation*	0–30°	0–30°
Lumbar or lumbosacral spine	Flexion*	0 to 45–65°	0 to ≥60°
	Extension*	0–27°	0–25°
	Lateral flexion*	0 to 19–38°	0–25°
	Rotation*	0–21°	NM
Hip	Flexion	0–120°	0–100°
	Hyperextension	0–20°	0–30°
	Abduction	0–40°	0–40°
	Adduction	0–30°	0–20°
	Medial rotation	0–45°	0–40°
	Lateral rotation	0–45°	0–50°
Knee	Flexion	0–140°	0–150°
Ankle and foot	Dorsiflexion	0–20°	0–20°
	Plantar flexion	0–50°	0–40°
	Inversion	0 to 28–37°	0–30°
	Eversion	0 to 21–28°	0–20°
Toes			
First metatarsophalangeal (MTP)	Flexion	NM	0–30°
	Extension	NM	0–50°
First interphalangeal (IP)	Flexion	NM	0–30°
	Extension	0°	0°
Second MTP	Flexion	NM	0–30°
	Extension	NM	0–40°
Third MTP	Flexion	NM	0–20°
	Extension	NM	0–30°
Fourth MTP	Flexion	NM	0–10°
	Extension	NM	0–20°
Fifth MTP	Flexion	NM	0–10°
	Extension	NM	0–10°
Second to fifth proximal and distal IP	Flexion/extension	NM	NM

Data adapted from: Greene WB, Heckman JD, editors: American Academy of Orthopaedic Surgeons (AAOS): The clinical measurement of joint motion. *Rosemont, IL, 1993, AAOS; and Cocchiarella L, Andersson GBJ, editors:* American Medical Association (AMA): Guides to the evaluation of permanent impairment, *ed 5, Chicago, 2001, AMA Press.*

** Measured by double inclinometer technique; NS = not specified; NM = not measured.*

Appendix A-3 Laboratory reference values (used at New York University Medical Center)

Common laboratory tests	Normal values (adult)
Biochemistry, blood	
Acid phosphatase	0.1–0.8 IU/L
Alanine aminotransferase	3–36 U/L
Albumin	4.0–5.0 g/dL
Aldolase	<6 U/L
Alkaline phosphatase	39–117 U/L
Alpha-1-antitrypsin	85–313 mg/dL
Ammonia	11.0–35.0 Umol/L
Amylase	20–220 U/L
Anion gap at K^+	9–18 mEq/L
Aspartate aminotransferase	7–37 U/L
B-12	200–900 pg/mL
Bilirubin	
direct	0–0.6 mg/dL
indirect	0.2–0.7 mg/dL
total	0.2–1.0 mg/dL
Blood urea nitrogen	10–20 mg/dL
Calcium	8.4–10.2 mg/dL
Carbon dioxide	21–29 mEq/L
Chloride	100–112 mEq/L
Cholesterol	
high-density lipoprotein	Male: 35–55 mg/dL Female: 45–65 mg/dL
low-density lipoprotein	65–175 mg/dL (calculated value)
total cholesterol	120–240 mg/dL
Creatine kinase	25–225 U/L
Creatinine	0.6–1.6 mg/dL
Folic acid (folate)	5–15 mg/mL
Gamma glutamyl transpeptidase	7.0–60.0 IU/L
Glucose (fasting and nonfasting)	70–110 mg/dL
Iron group	
iron	42–135 μg/dL
total iron binding capacity	280–400 μg/dL
saturation	11–46%
Lactic dehydrogenase	100–250 U/L
Magnesium	1.6–2.3 mg/dL
Osmolality	280–295 mosm/kg
Phosphorus, inorganic	2.7–4.5 mg/dL
Potassium	3.5–5.3 mEq/L
Prealbumin	17–42 mg/dL
Protein, total	6.0–8.0 g/dL
Sodium	136–148 mEq/L
Triglyceride*	30–160 mg/dL (30–50 years old); 30–190 mg/dL (>50 years old)
Troponin	<0.5 ng mL
Uric acid	2.5–7.0 mg/dL
Endocrine, blood	
Free thyroxine index	1.8–4.3
Thyroxine (T_4)	4.5–11.5 μg/dL
Triiodothyronine (T_3)	90–185 ng/dL
T_3 resin uptake	35–45%
Thyroglobulin RIA	≤25.0 ng/mL
Thyroid-binding globulin	11–36 μg/mL
Thyroid-stimulating hormone	0.2–4.8 mU/mL
Hematologic	
Complete blood count	
white blood cell	$4.0–12.0 \times 10^9$/L
red blood cell	male: $4.4–6.1 \times 10^{12}$/L female: $4.2–5.5 \times 10^{12}$/L

(Continued)

Appendix A-3 (*Continued*)

hemoglobin	male: 14–18 g/dL female: 12–16 g/dL
hematocrit	male: 41–51% female: 37–47%
reticulocyte count	0.5–1.5%
mean corpuscular volume	82–92 fL (femtoliters)
mean corpuscular hemoglobin (MCH)	27–31 pg/cell
MCH concentration	32–36%
red-cell distribution width	11.5–14.5%
platelets	130–400 × 10^9/L
Erythrocyte sedimentation rate	male: 0–10 mm/hr female: 0–20 mm/hr
Glycosylated hemoglobin	5.5–9.5%
Coagulation	
activated partial thromboplastin time	27–37 seconds
prothrombin time†	10.5–13.0 seconds
fibrinogen	150–380 mg%
Immunologic, blood	
Total hemolytic complement (CH_{50})	150–250 units/mL
Complement components	
Clq	11–22 mg/dL
C3	55–120 mg/dL
C4	20–50 mg/dL
Urinalysis	
pH	5.0–7.0
Specific gravity	1.001–1.030
Color, appearance	Yellow, clear
White blood cell	0–2
Red blood cell	0–2
Urobilinogen	0.2–1.0 eu/dL
Casts, bilirubin, blood	Negative
Protein, glucose, ketones	Negative
Nitrate, yeasts, bacteria	Negative
Crystals, epithelial cells	Variable

* *See also Chapter 5.13, sections II.A and IV.A.1.a, for undesirable and desirable levels, respectively.*

† *See Chapters 4.8 (VII.A.1) and 5.3 (IV.B.1.a and V.A.2) for therapeutic international normalized ratio (INR) levels.*

Appendix A-4

Reference values for motor nerve conduction studies (these values are to be used as guidelines as every laboratory should ideally collect its own set of reference values; also, the patient's unaffected limb may be used as a "normal" reference)

	Distal motor latency		Motor conduction velocity	
	Segment (distance from stimulating → pick-up electrode)	**Onset latency Mean ± 1 SD (range)**	**Segment (stimulating → pick-up electrode; using tape measure)**	**Mean ± 1 SD (range)**
Median[a]	Wrist mid-crease → APB (8 cm along nerve course)	3.7 ± 0.3 ms (3.2–4.2 ms)	Above elbow → wrist	56.7 ± 3.8 m/s (50–67.3 m/s)
Ulnar[b,c]	Wrist → ADQ (6.5–8 cm)	3.0 ± 0.4 ms (2.2–3.8 ms)	Above elbow → wrist (elbow flexed ~70°)	62.7 ± 5.5 m/s (52–74 m/s)
Radial (PIN)[d,e]	Forearm → EIP[i] (8 cm)	2.4 ± 0.5 ms	Above elbow → EIP[i]	61.6 ± 5.9 m/s (48–75 m/s)
Deep peroneal[f,g]	Ankle → EDB (8 cm)	3.8 ± 0.7 ms (2.3–5.9 ms)	Fibular head → ankle	49.9 ± 5.9 m/s (41.6–64.6 m/s)
			Popliteal area → ankle	51.1 ± 6.3 m/s (41.6–62.7 m/s)
Tibial[h]	Ankle → AH[j] (8 cm)	3.4 ± 0.5 ms	Popliteal area → ankle	54.9 ± 7.6 m/s

Data adapted from:

[a] *Melvin JL, Schuchmann JA, Lanese RR: Diagnostic specificity of motor and sensory nerve conduction variables in the carpal tunnel syndrome,* Arch Phys Med Rehabil *54:69–74, 1973.*

[b] *Eisen A: Early diagnosis of ulnar nerve palsy,* Neurology *24:256–262, 1974.*

[c] *Checkles NS, Russakov AD, Piero DL: Ulnar nerve conduction velocity: effect of elbow position on measurement,* Arch Phys Med Rehabil *52:362–365, 1971.*

[d] *Trojaborg W, Sindrup EH: Motor and sensory conduction in different segments of the radial nerve in normal subjects,* J Neurol Neurosurg Psychiatry *32:354–359, 1969.*

[e] *Jebsen RH: Motor conduction velocity in proximal and distal segments of the radial nerve,* Arch Phys Med Rehabil *47:597–602, 1966.*

[f] *Jimenez J, Easton JKM, Redford JB: Conduction studies of the anterior and posterior tibial nerves,* Arch Phys Med Rehabil *51:164–169, 1970.*

[g] *Checkles NS, Bailey JA, Johnson EW: Tape and caliper surface measurements in determination of peroneal nerve conduction velocity,* Arch Phys Med Rehabil *50:217–218, 1969.*

[h] *Fu R, DeLisa JA, Kraft GH: Motor nerve latencies through the tarsal tunnel in normal adult subjects: standard determinations corrected for temperature and distance,* Arch Phys Med Rehabil *61:243–248, 1980.*

[i] *Needle recording electrode is inserted at the EIP.*

[j] *Ankle → AH segment specifically tests distal motor latency of medial plantar branch of tibial nerve.*

ADQ = abductor digiti quinti; AH = abductor hallucis; APB = abductor pollicis brevis; EDB = extensor digitorum brevis; EIP = extensor indices propius; PIN = posterior interosseous nerve branch of radial nerve; SD = standard deviation; cm = centimeter; ms = millisecond; m/s = meters per second.

Appendix A-5 Reference values for sensory nerve conduction studies (these values are to be used as guidelines as every laboratory should ideally collect its own set of reference values; also, the patient's unaffected limb may be used as a "normal" reference)

	Distal segment		Distal latency		Amplitude
Sensory nerve	**Antidromic technique stimulating → recording electrode)**	**Distance (cm)**	**Onset latency Mean ± 1 SD**	**Peak latency Mean ±1 SD (range)**	**Mean ± 1 SD (range)**
Median[a,b]	Distal crease of wrist → 2nd or 3rd digit	14	2.4 ± 0.3 ms	3.0 ± 0.3 ms	41.6 ± 25 μV (10–90 μV)
Ulnar[a,c]	Wrist → 5th digit	14	2.4 ± 0.3 ms	3.0 ± 0.3 ms	(15–50 μV)
Superficial radial[d]	Forearm → 1st web space	10 12 14	1.8 ± 0.3 ms 2.1 ± 0.3 ms 2.4 ± 0.3 ms	2.3 ± 0.4 ms 2.6 ± 0.4 ms 2.9 ± 0.4 ms	31 ± 20 μV (13–60 μV)
Superficial peroneal[e]	Anterolateral leg → anteromedial area of lateral malleolus[g]	12		2.9 ± 0.3 ms	20.5 ± 6.1 μV
Sural[f]	Lower calf → area behind lateral malleolus[h]	14		3.5 ± 0.2 ms (3.0–4.0 ms)	(5–30 μV)

Data adapted from:

[a] Cohn TG, Wertsch JJ, Pasupuleti DV, et al.: *Nerve conduction studies: orthodromic vs. antidromic latencies,* Arch Phys Med Rehabil *71:579–582, 1990.*

[b] *Melvin JL, Schuchmann JA, Lanese RR: Diagnostic specificity of motor and sensory nerve conduction variables in the carpal tunnel syndrome,* Arch Phys Med Rehabil *54:69–74, 1973.*

[c] *Johnson EW, Melvin JL: Sensory conduction studies of median and ulnar nerves,* Arch Phys Med Rehabil *48:25–30, 1967.*

[d] *Mackenzie K, DeLisa JA: distal latency measurement of the superficial radial nerve in normal adult subjects;* Arch Phys Med Rehabil *62:31–34, 1981.*

[e] *Jabre JF: The superficial peroneal sensory nerve revisited, Arch Neurol 38:666–667, 1981.*

[f] *Schuchmann JA: Sural nerve conduction: a standardized technique,* Arch Phys Med Rehabil *58:166–168, 1977.*

[g] *Normal sensory conduction velocity of superficial peroneal nerve (specifically intermediate dorsal cutaneous branch) = 65.7 ± 3.7 m/sec.*

[h] *Normal sensory conduction velocity of sural nerve for 0–14 cm = 40.1 m/sec.*

SD = standard deviation; cm = centimeter; ms = millisecond; m/s = meters per second; μV = microvolt.

Appendix A-6

Reference values for F-wave studies (these values are to be used as guidelines as every laboratory should ideally collect its own set of reference values; also, the patient's unaffected limb may be used as a "normal" reference)

Motor nerve	Pick-up site	F-Latency[d] Mean ± 1 SD	M-Latency Mean ± 1 SD	F-Wave conduction velocity[e] (to and from SC) mean ± 1 SD	F-Ratio[f] Mean ± 1 SD
Median[a,b]	APB	Wr = 29.1 ± 2.3 ms El = 24.8 ± 2.0 ms Ax = 21.7 ± 2.8 ms	Wr = 3.5 ± 0.5 ms El = 7.8 ± 0.8 ms Ax = 11.3 ± 1.0 ms	Wr = 59.2 ± 3.9 m/s El = 62.2 ± 5.2 m/s Ax = 64.3 ± 6.4 m/s	El = 1.04 ± 0.09
Ulnar[a,b]	ADQ	Wr = 30.5 ± 3.0 ms bEl = 26.0 ± 2.0 ms aEl = 23.5 ± 2.0 ms Ax = 21.9 ± 1.9 ms	Wr = 2.9 ± 0.5 ms bEl = 6.7 ± 0.7 ms aEl = 9.2 ± 0.9 ms Ax = 11.2 ± 1.0 ms	Wr = 56.7 ± 2.9 m/s bEl = 58.2 ± 2.9 m/s aEl = 61.1 ± 5.4 m/s Ax = 63.1 ± 5.9 m/s	bEl = 1.40 ± 0.11
Peroneal[b,c]	EDB	An = 51.3 ± 4.7 ms Kn = 42.7 ± 4.0 ms	An = 4.5 ± 0.9 ms Kn = 12.9 ± 1.4 ms	An = 53.3 ± 3.8 m/s Kn = 56.3 ± 4.9 m/s	Kn = 1.11 ± 0.09
Tibial[b,c]	AH	An = 52.3 ± 4.3 ms Kn = 43.5 ± 3.4 ms	An = 4.1 ± 0.6 ms Kn = 12.9 ± 1.3 ms	An = 51.3 ± 2.9 m/s Kn = 54.4 ± 3.6 m/s	Kn = 1.17 ± 0.10

Data adapted from:

[a] *Kimura J: F-wave velocity in the central segment of the median and ulnar nerves: a study in normal subjects and in patients with Charcot-Marie-Tooth disease,* Neurology *24:539–546, 1974.*

[b] *Kimura J: F-wave determinations in nerve conduction studies. In Desmedt JE, editor: Motor control mechanisms in health and disease, New York, 1983, Raven Press, pp. 961–975.*

[c] *Kimura J, Bosch P, Linday GM: F-wave conduction velocity in the central segment of the peroneal and tibial nerves,* Arch Phys Med Rehabil *56:492–497, 1975.*

[d] *The F latency is the shortest onset latency after 10–20 F-wave stimulations.*

[e] *F-wave conduction velocity (m/sec) = (nerve distance in mm × 2)/(F latency in msec − M latency in msec − 1), where nerve distance is measured using a tape measure as follows: (a) for the median or ulnar nerve, measure from the stimulus site along the course of the nerve to the axilla (with arm abducted 90°), then around the back of the shoulder (posteriorly) to the C7 spinous process; (b) for the peroneal or tibial nerve, measure from the stimulus site along the course of the nerve to the greater trochanter of the femur then posteriorly to the lower border of the T12 spinous process.*

[f] *The F ratio refers to the ratio between proximal and distal segments of the nerve, with cathode stimulation at the volar crease of the elbow (for median nerve); 3 cm above the medial epicondyle (for ulnar nerve), just above the fibular head (for peroneal nerve), and in the popliteal fossa (for tibial nerve). The F-ratio formula is (F latency in msec − M latency in msec − 1)/(M latency in msec × 2). By using the F ratio, there is theoretically less potential for errors as it circumvents the need for measuring nerve length. However, F ratio assumes that various limbs of different length have the same proportion for the proximal and distal segments (bisected at either the elbow or knee).*

ADQ = abductor digiti quinti; AH = abductor hallucis; An = ankle; APB = abductor pollicis brevis; Ax = axilla; EDB = extensor digitorum brevis; El = elbow; Kn = knee; SC = spinal cord; SD = standard deviation; Wr = wrist; aEL = above elbow; bEL = below elbow; ms = millisecond; m/s = meters per second.

Appendix A-7 Reference values for motor nerve conduction studies (these values are to be used as guidelines as every laboratory should ideally collect its own set of reference values; also, the patient's unaffected limb may be used as a "normal" reference)

Distal motor latency			Motor conduction velocity	
Motor nerve	**Segment (Distance from stimulating? Pick-up electrode)**	**Onset latency mean ± 1 SD (Range)**	**Segment (Stimulating? Pick-up electrode; using tape measure)**	**Mean ± 1 SD (Range)**
Median	Wrist mid-crease → APB (8 cm along nerve course)	3.7 ± 0.3 ms (3.2–4.2 ms)	Above elbow → wrist	56.7 ± 3.8 m/s
Ulnar	Wrist → ADQ (6.5–8 cm)	3.0 ± 0.4 ms (2.2–3.8 ms)	Above elbow → wrist (elbow fixed ~ 70°)	62.7 ± 5.5 m/s (52–74 m/s)
Radial (PIN)	Forearm → EIP (8 cm)	2.4 ± 0.5 ms	Above elbow → EIP	61.6 ± 5.9 m/s (48–75 m/s)
Deep peroneal	Ankle → EDB (8 cm)	3.8 ± 0.7 ms (2.3–5.9 ms)	Fibular head → ankle Popliteal area → ankle	49.9 ± 5.9 m/s (41.6–64.6 m/s)
Tibial	Ankle → AH (8 cm)	3.4 ± 0.5 ms	Popliteal area → ankle	

ADQ, abductor digiti quinti; AH, abductor hallucis; EDB, extensor digitorum brevis; EIP, extensor indicis proprius.

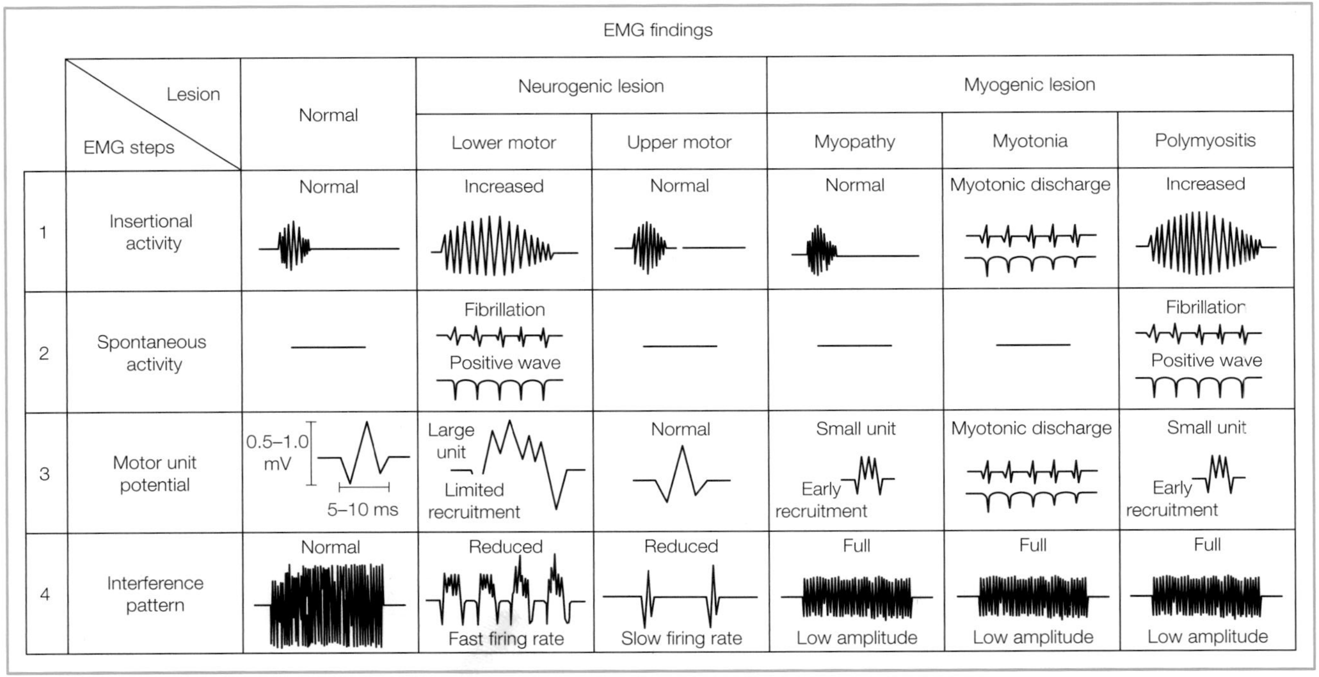

Appendix A-8 Summary of typical findings of needle electromyography in normal muscle and in neurogenic and myogenic lesions. (Redrawn from Kimura J. *Electrodiagnosis in diseases of nerve and muscle: principles and practice*, ed 2, Philadelphia, 1989, F.A. Davis, p. 252, with permission.)

Appendix B

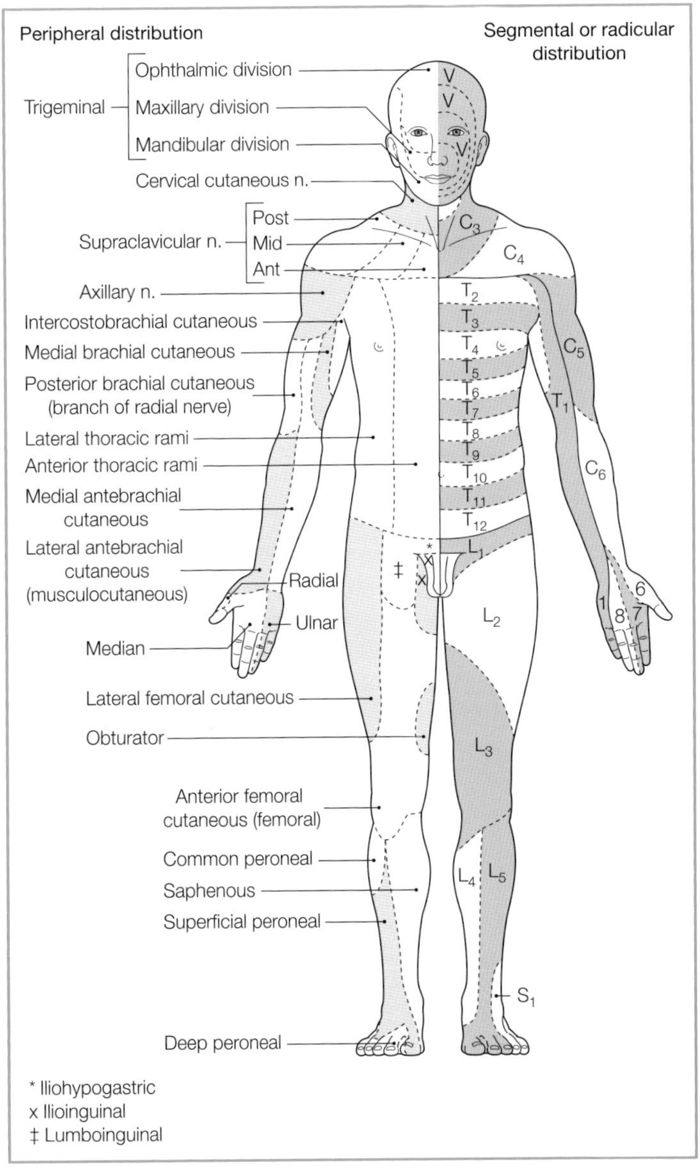

Appendix B-1 Sensory distribution of major peripheral nerves and dermatomes corresponding to spinal cord segments, anterior view. (Redrawn from: Chusid JG: *Correlative neuroanatomy and functional neurology*, ed 19, Los Altos, CA, 1985, Lange Medical Publications, p. 233, Copyright © 1985 Appleton & Lange, McGraw Hill Companies with permission.)

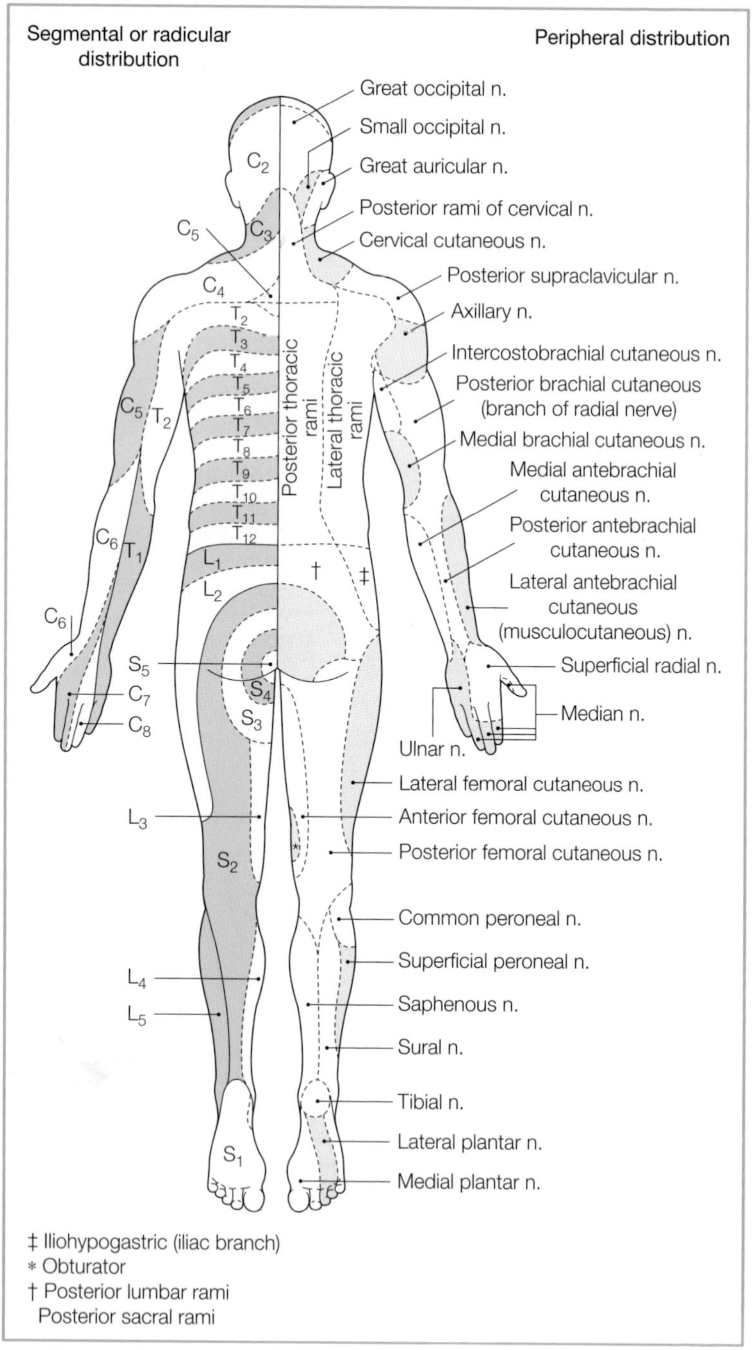

Appendix B-2 Sensory distribution of major peripheral nerves and dermatomes corresponding to spinal cord segments, posterior view. (Redrawn from: Chusid JG: *Correlative neuroanatomy and functional neurology*, ed 19, Los Altos, CA, 1985, Lange Medical Publications, p. 233, Copyright © 1985 Appleton & Lange, McGraw Hill Companies, with permission.)

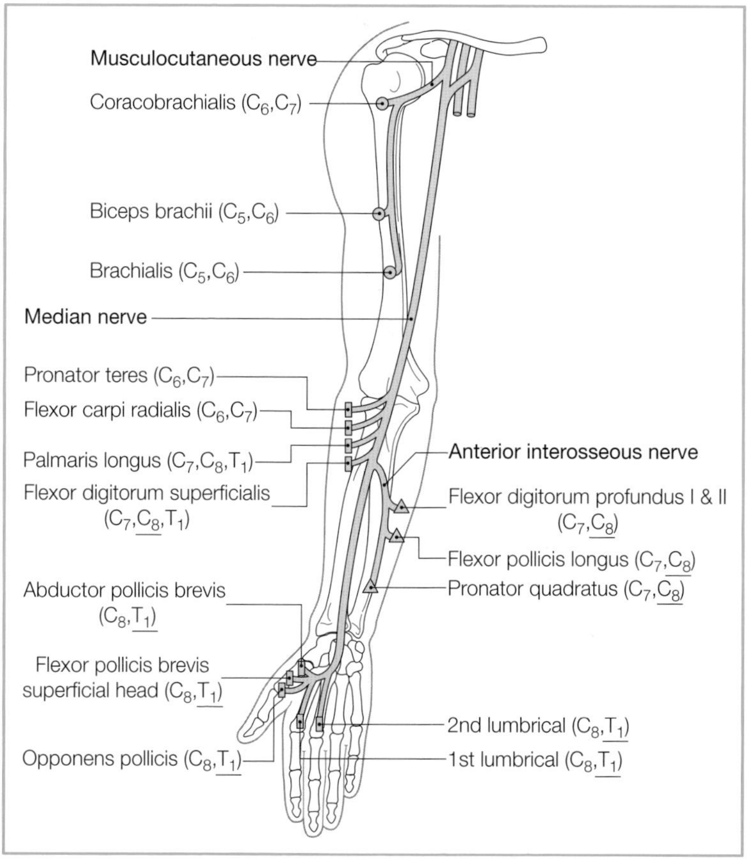

Appendix B-3a Diagram of motor innervation of the upper limb showing the branches of the musculocutaneous and median nerves. The predominant root supply is underlined. (Adapted from: *The guarantors of brain: aids to the examination of the peripheral nervous system,* East Sussex, England, 1986, Balliére Tindall.)

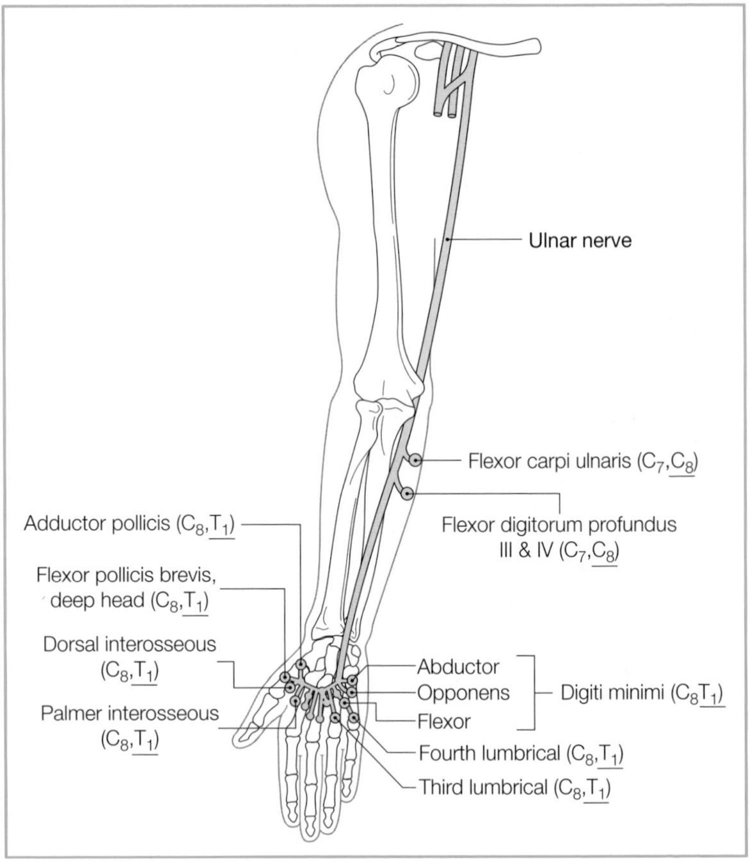

Appendix B-3b Diagram of motor innervation of the upper limb showing the branches of the ulnar nerve. The predominant root supply is underlined. (Adapted from: *The guarantors of brain: aids to the examination of the peripheral nervous system*, East Sussex, England, 1986, Balliére Tindall.)

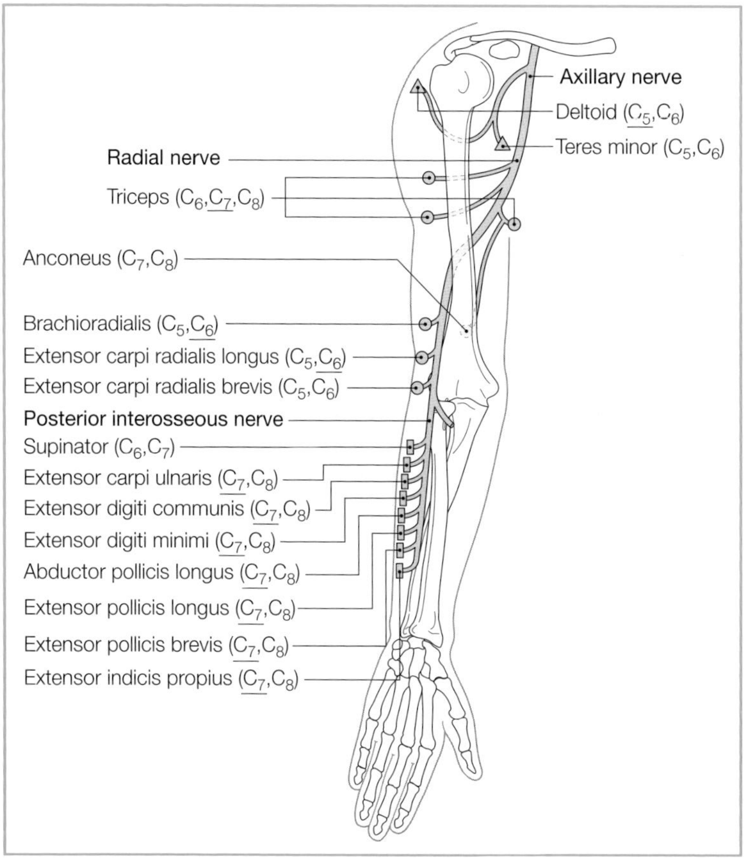

Appendix B-3c Diagram of motor innervation of the upper limb showing the branches of the axillary and radial nerves. The predominant root supply is underlined. (Adapted from: *The guarantors of brain: aids to the examination of the peripheral nervous system*, East Sussex, England, 1986, Balliére Tindall.)

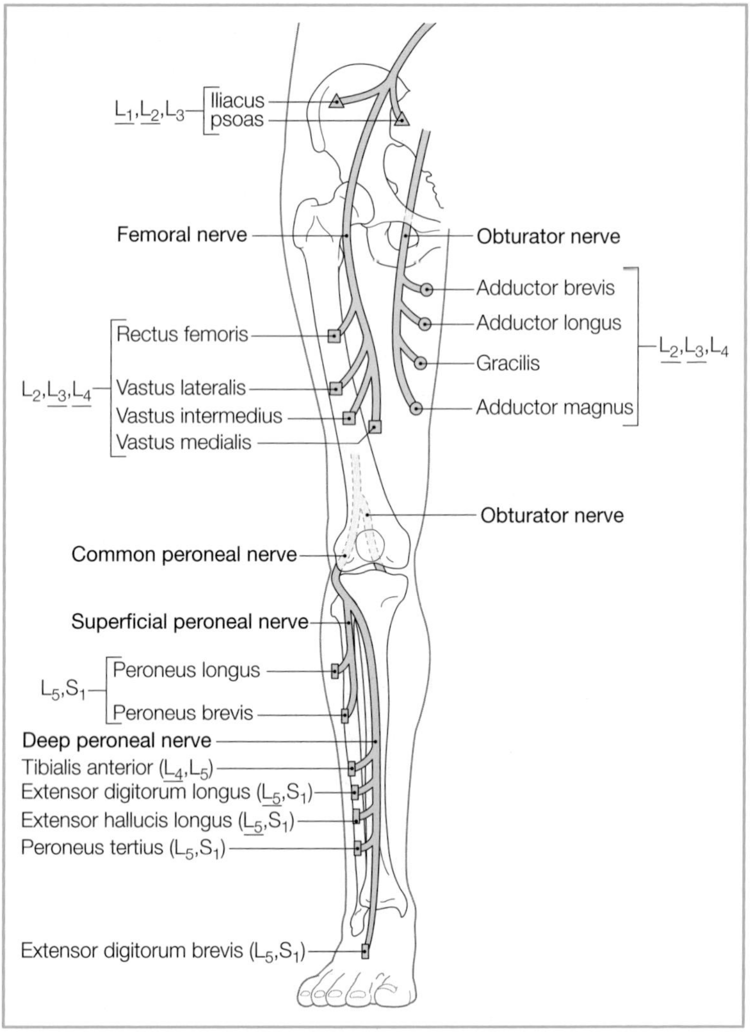

Appendix B-4a Diagram of motor innervation of the lower limb showing the branches of the femoral, obturator, and common peroneal nerves. The predominant root supply is underlined. (Adapted from: *The guarantors of brain: aids to the examination of the peripheral nervous system*, East Sussex, England, 1986, Balliére Tindall.)

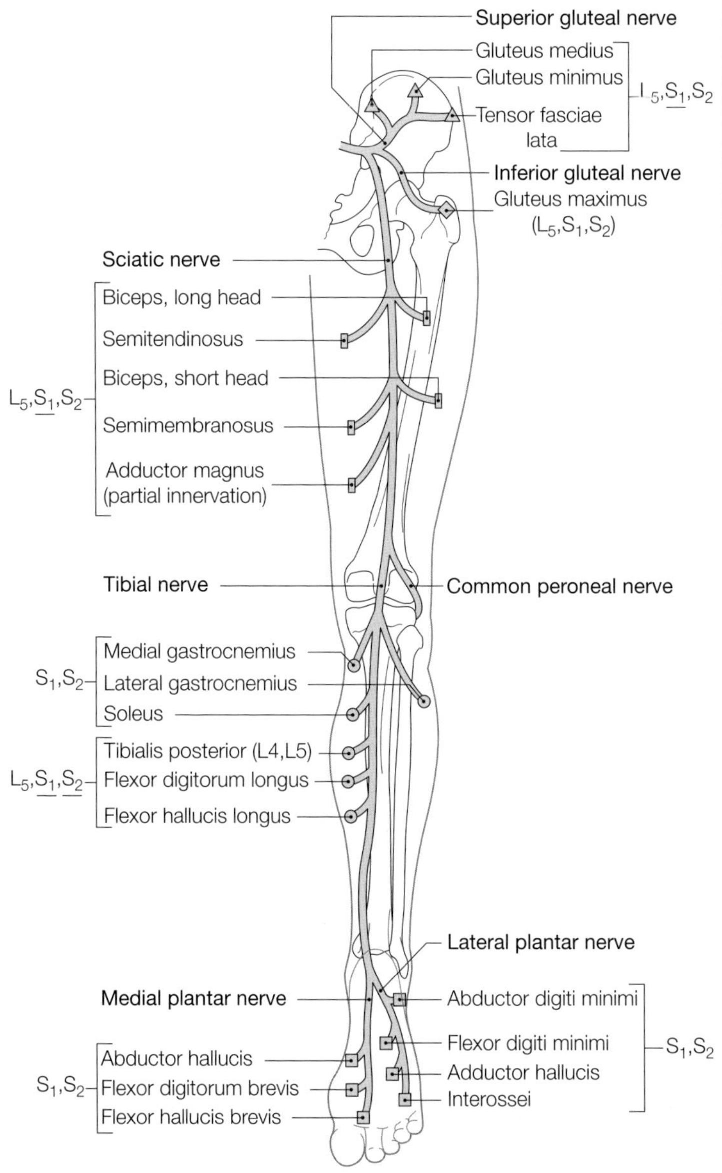

Appendix B-4b Diagram of motor innervation of the lower limb showing the branches of the gluteal, sciatic, and tibial nerves. The predominant root supply is underlined. (Adapted from: *The guarantors of brain: aids to the examination of the peripheral nervous system*, East Sussex, England, 1986, Balliére Tindall.)

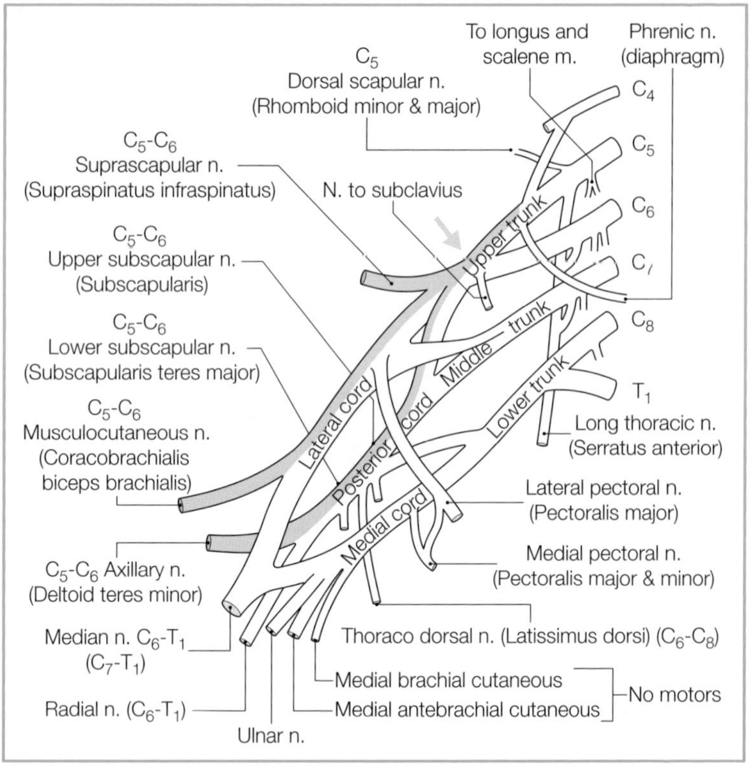

Appendix B-5 Diagram of the brachial plexus. The arrow indicates the Erb's point. Posterior nerves are shaded. (From: Torg JS, Shephard RJ: *Current therapy in sports medicine*, ed 3, St Louis, 1995, Mosby, p. 62; with permission.)

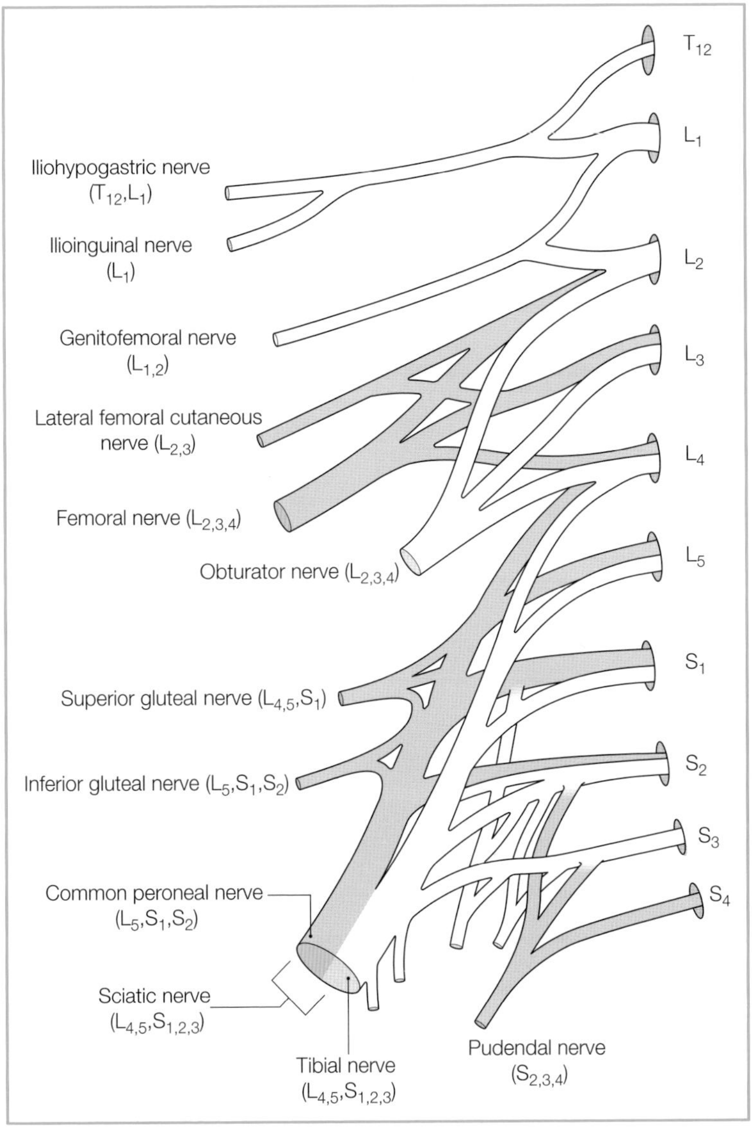

Appendix B-6 Diagram of the lumbosacral plexus; posterior nerves are shaded.

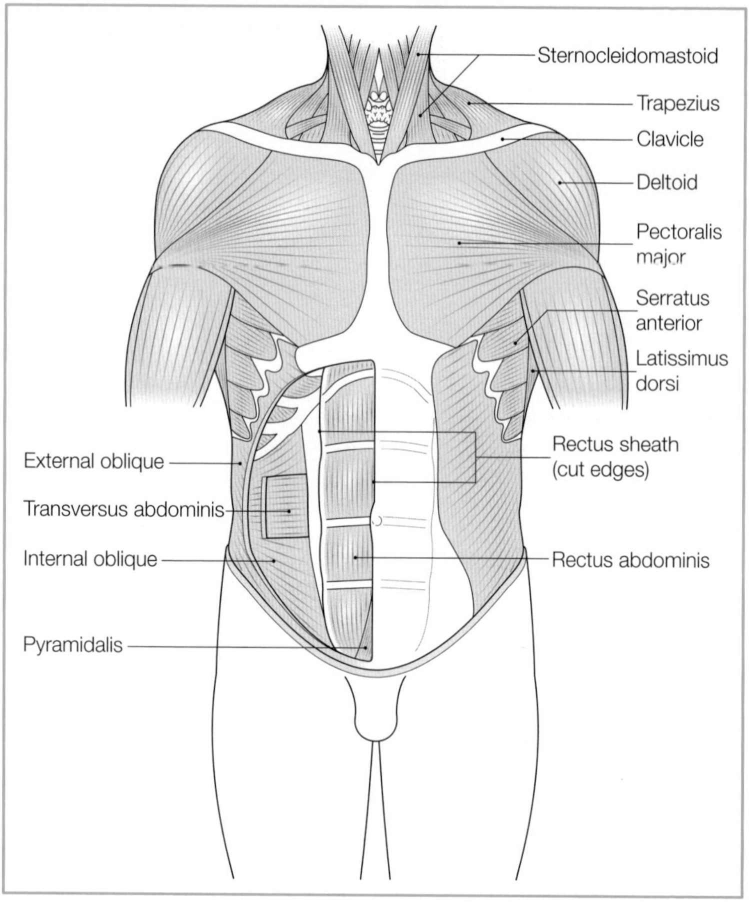

Appendix B-7 Superficial muscles of the trunk, anterior view. (From: Seidel HM, Ball JW, Dains JE, *et al.*: *Mosby's guide to physical examination*, ed 3, St Louis, 1995, Mosby, p. 650, with permission.)

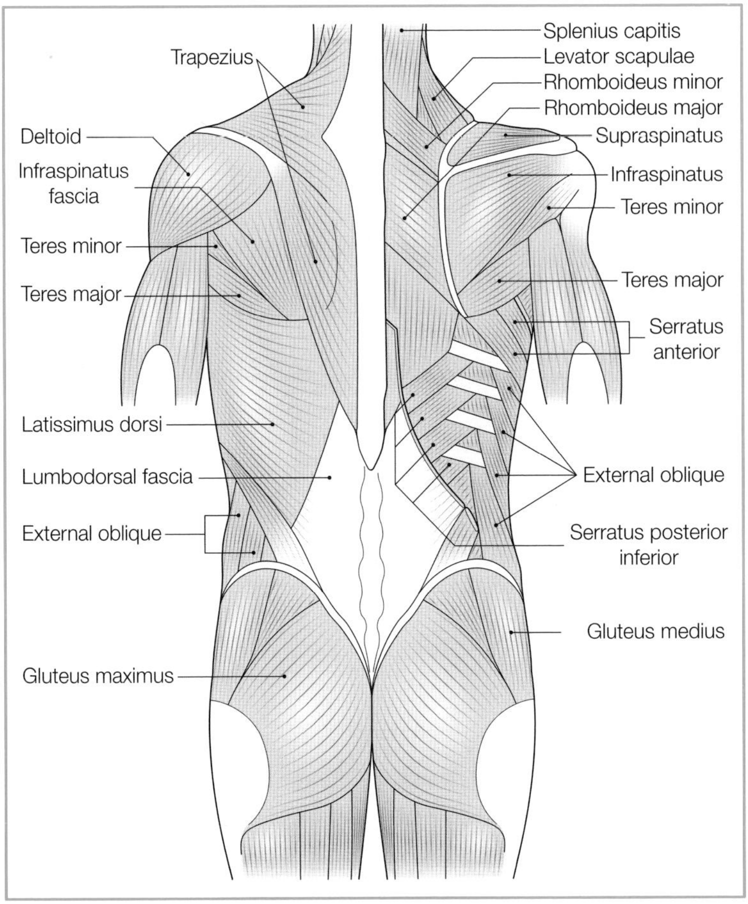

Appendix B-8 Superficial muscles of the trunk, posterior view. (Redrawn from: Seidel HM, Ball JW, Dains JE, *et al.*: *Mosby's guide to physical examination*, ed 3, St Louis, 1995, Mosby, p. 651, with permission.)

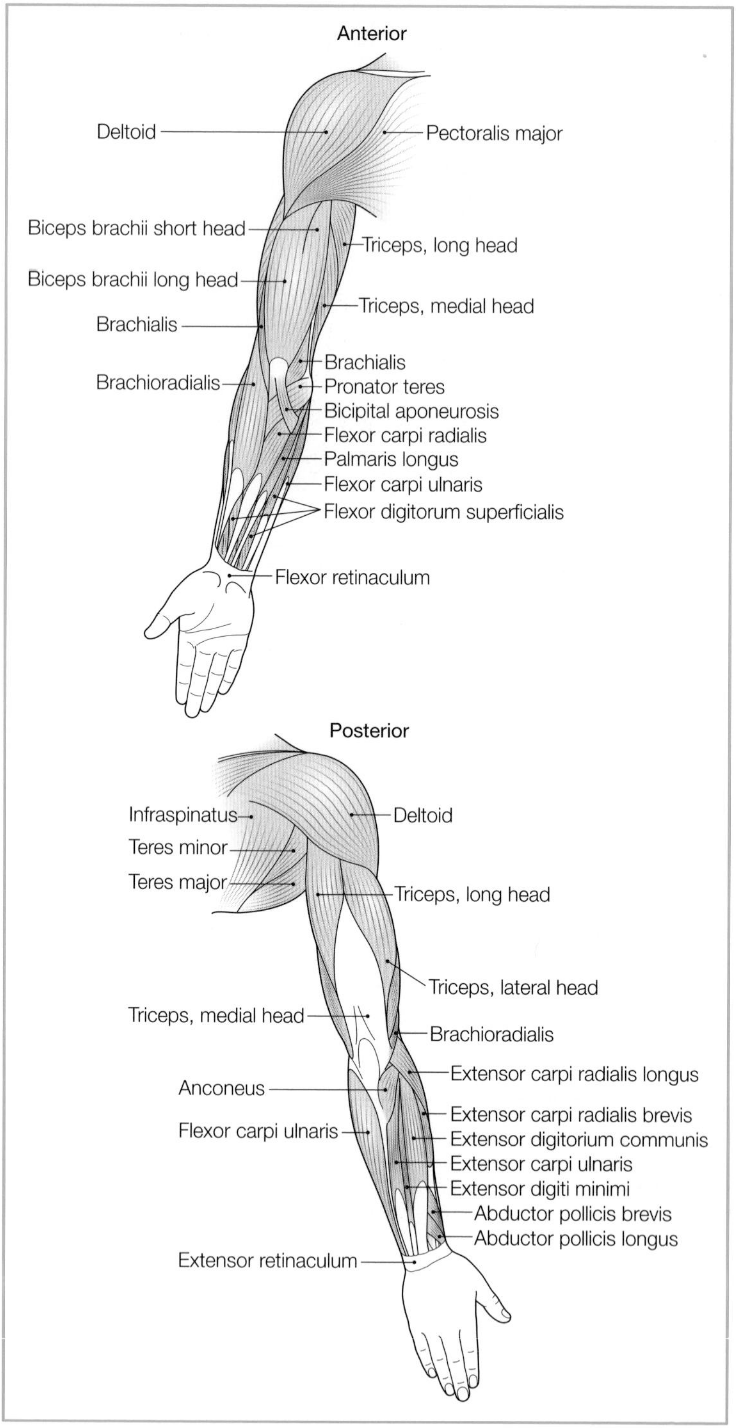

Appendix B-9 Muscles of the upper limbs. (Redrawn from: Seidel HM, Ball JW, Dains JE, *et al.*: *Mosby's guide to physical examination*, ed 3, St Louis, 1995, Mosby, p. 646, with permission.)

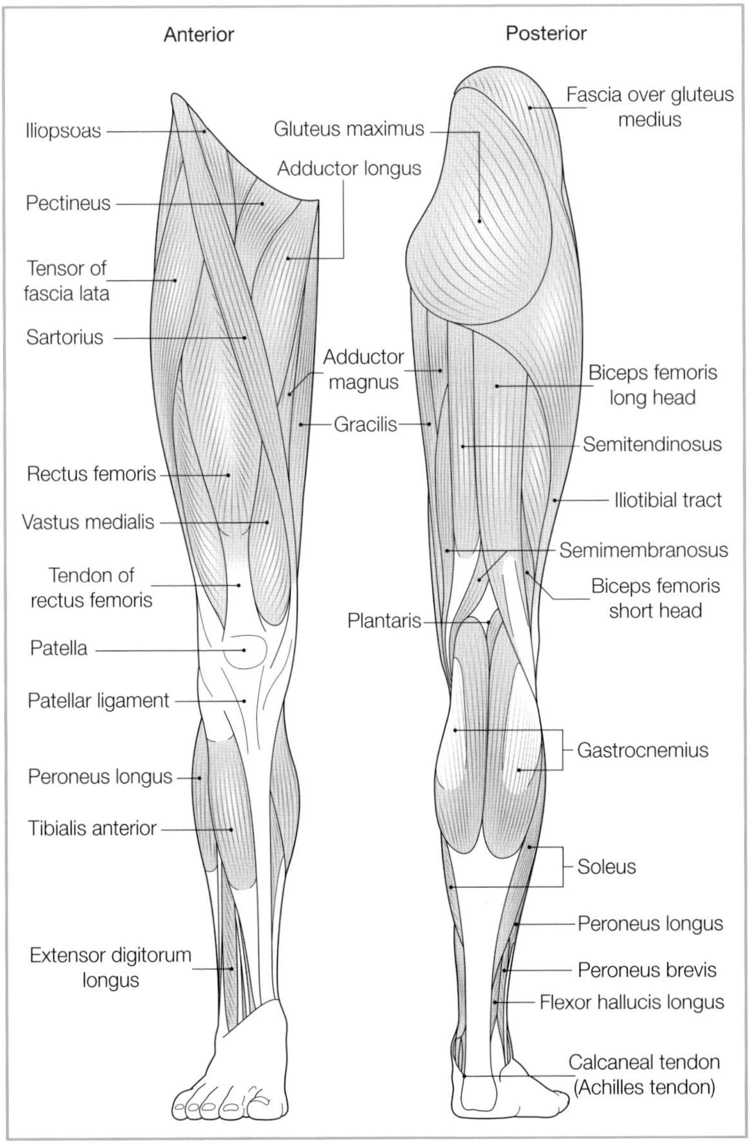

Appendix B-10 Muscles of the lower limbs. (Redrawn from: Seidel HM, Ball JW, Dains JE, *et al.*: *Mosby's guide to physical examination*, ed 3, St Louis, 1995, Mosby, p. 647, with permission.)

Appendix C

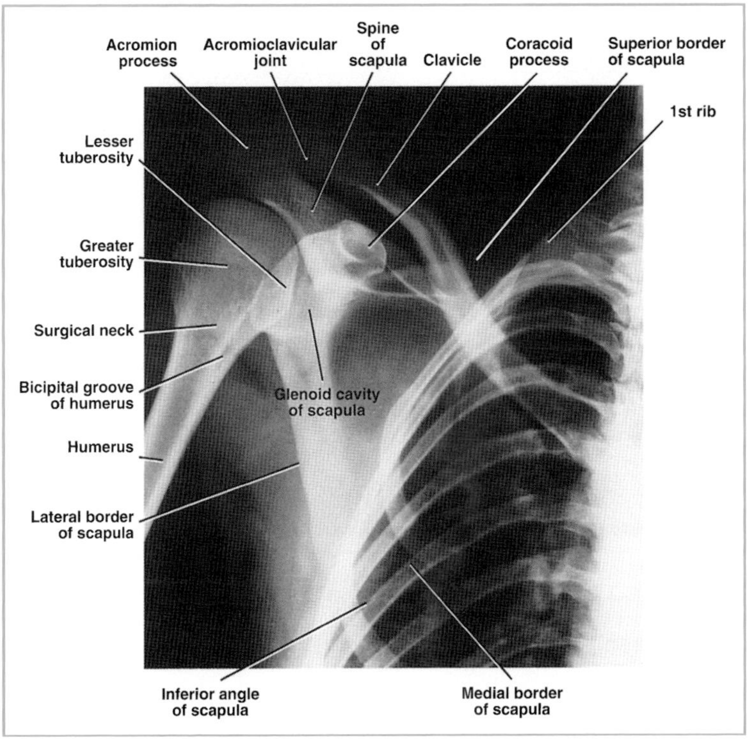

Appendix C-1 Anteroposterior radiograph of the shoulder joint with the humerus medially rotated. (From Snell R, Smith M: *Clinical anatomy for emergency medicine*, St Louis, 1993, Mosby, p. 590, with permission.)

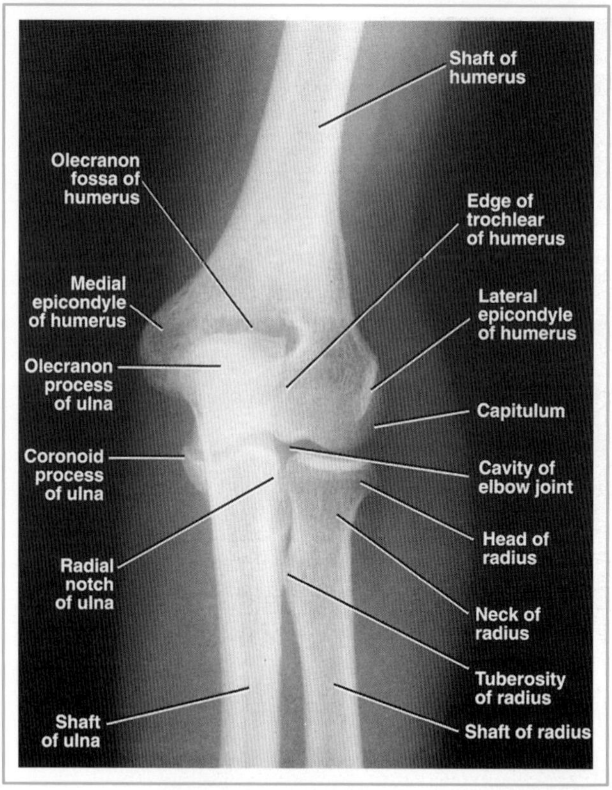

Appendix C-2 Anteroposterior radiograph of the elbow joint. (From: Snell R, Smith M: *Clinical anatomy for emergency medicine*, St Louis, 1993, Mosby, p. 592, with permission.)

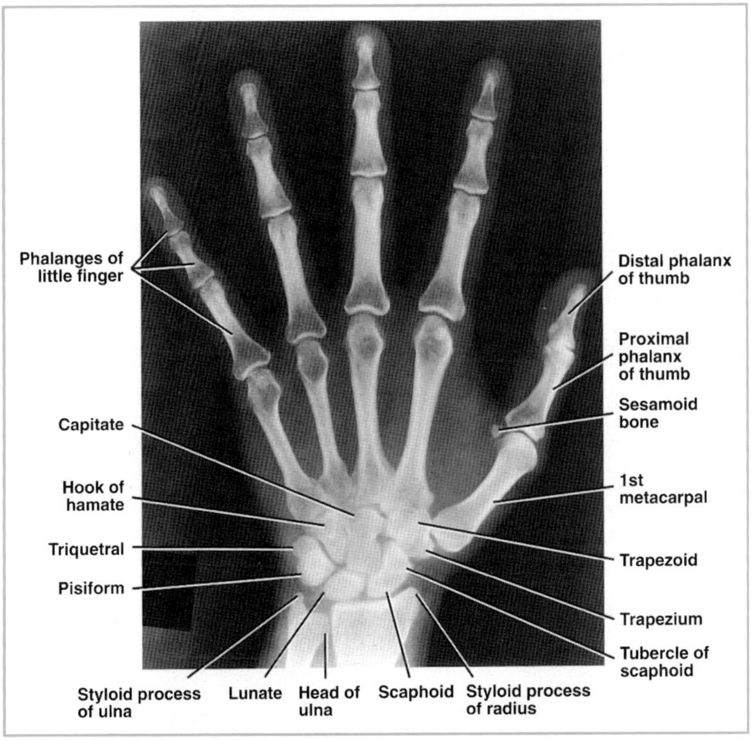

Appendix C-3 Posteroanterior radiograph of the wrist and hand with the forearm pronated. (From: Snell R, Smith M: *Clinical anatomy for emergency medicine*, St Louis, 1993, Mosby, p. 650, with permission.)

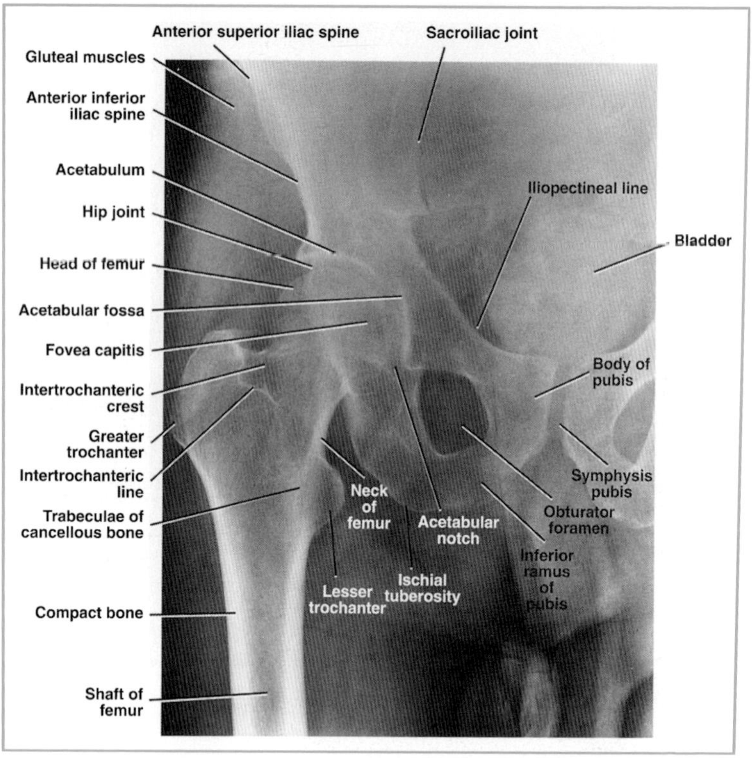

Appendix C-4 Anteroposterior radiograph of the hip joint and pelvis. (From: Snell R, Smith M: *Clinical anatomy for emergency medicine*, St Louis, 1993, Mosby, p. 703, with permission.)

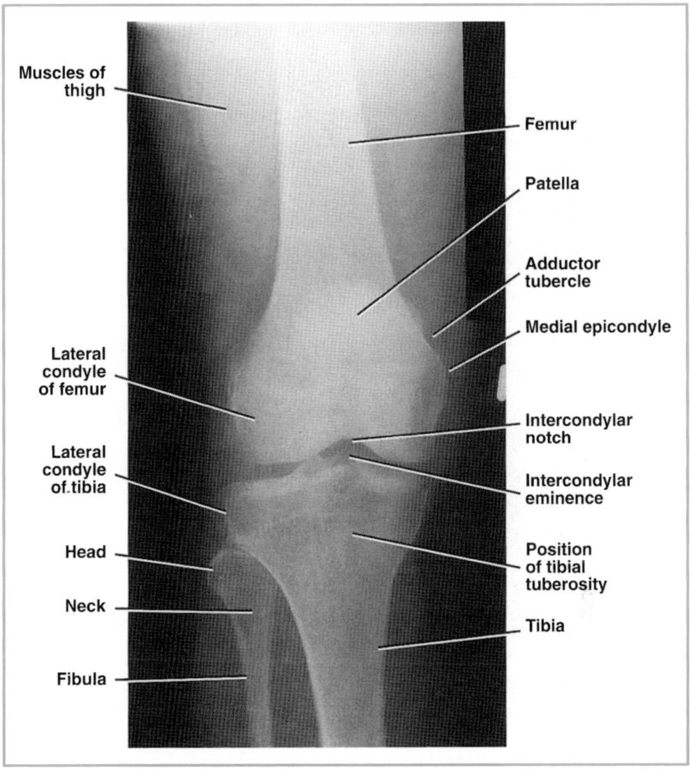

Appendix C-5 Anteroposterior radiograph of the knee joint. (From: Snell R, Smith M: *Clinical anatomy for emergency medicine*, St Louis, 1993, Mosby, p. 707, with permission.)

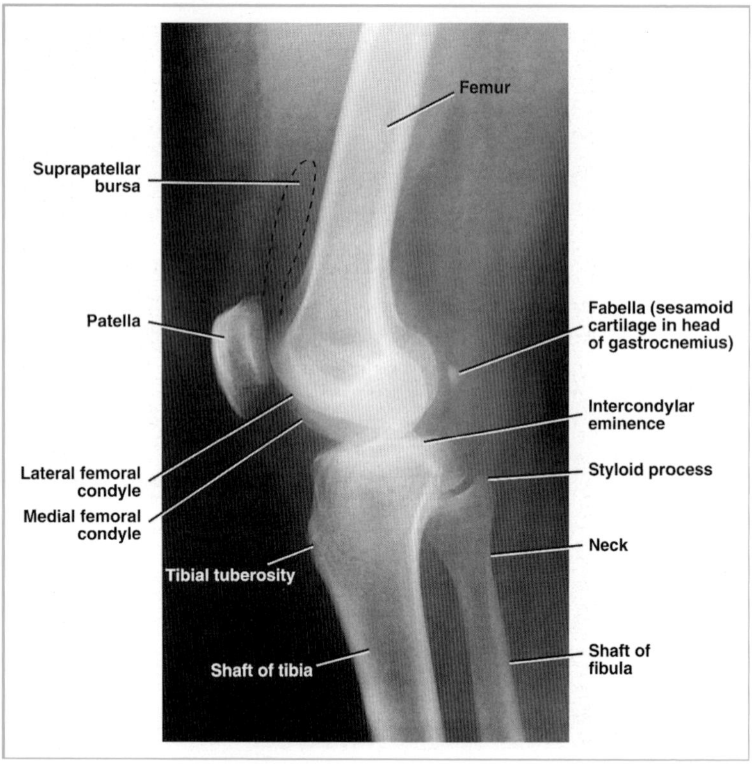

Appendix C-6 Lateral radiograph of the knee joint. (From: Snell R, Smith M: *Clinical anatomy for emergency medicine*, St Louis, 1993, Mosby, p. 708, with permission.)

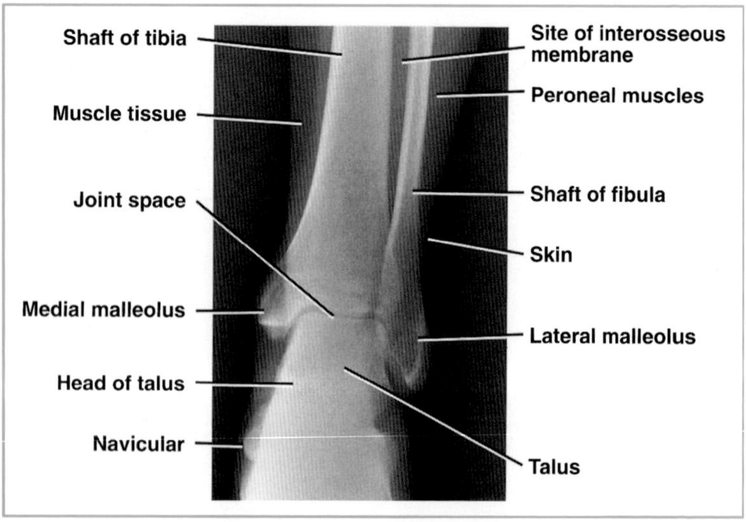

Appendix C-7 Anteroposterior radiograph of the ankle joint. (From: Snell R, Smith M: *Clinical anatomy for emergency medicine*, St Louis, 1993, Mosby, p. 711, with permission.)

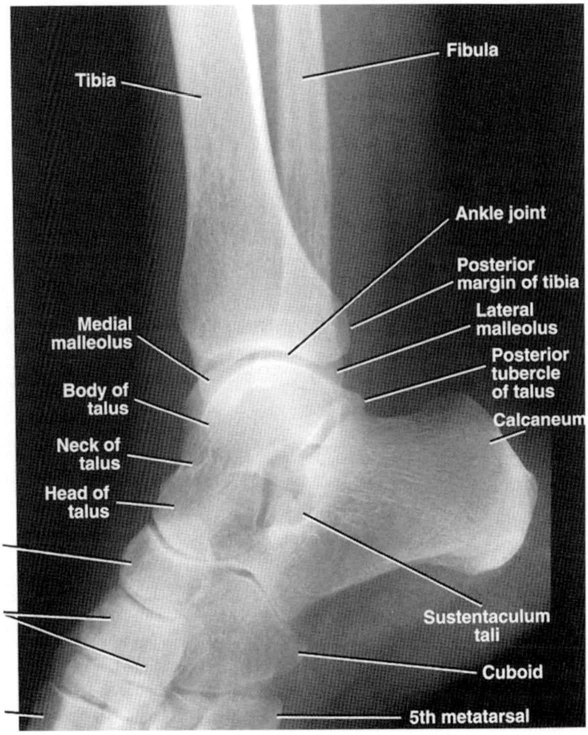

Appendix C-8 Lateral radiograph of the ankle joint. (From: Snell R, Smith M: *Clinical anatomy for emergency medicine*, St Louis, 1993, Mosby, p. 711, with permission.)

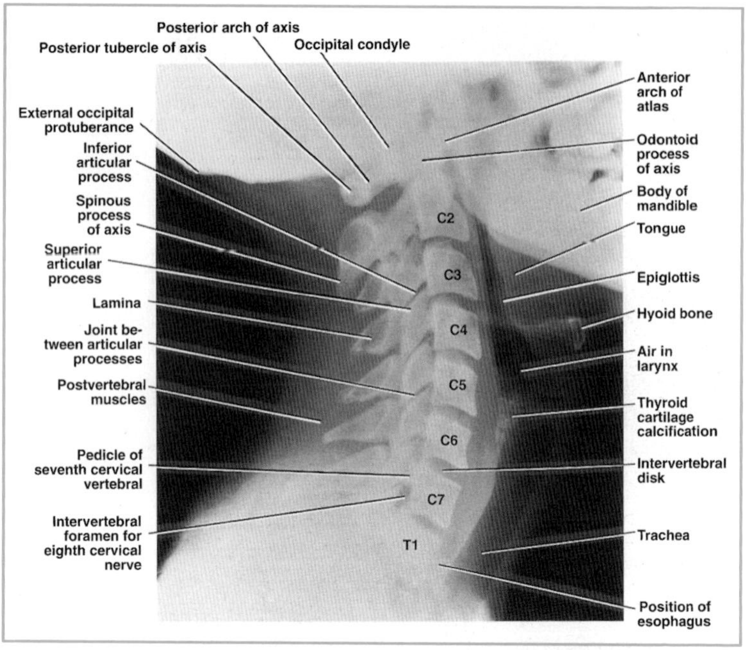

Appendix C-9 Lateral radiograph of the cervical spine. (From: Snell R, Smith M: *Clinical anatomy for emergency medicine*, St Louis, 1993, Mosby, p. 186, with permission.)

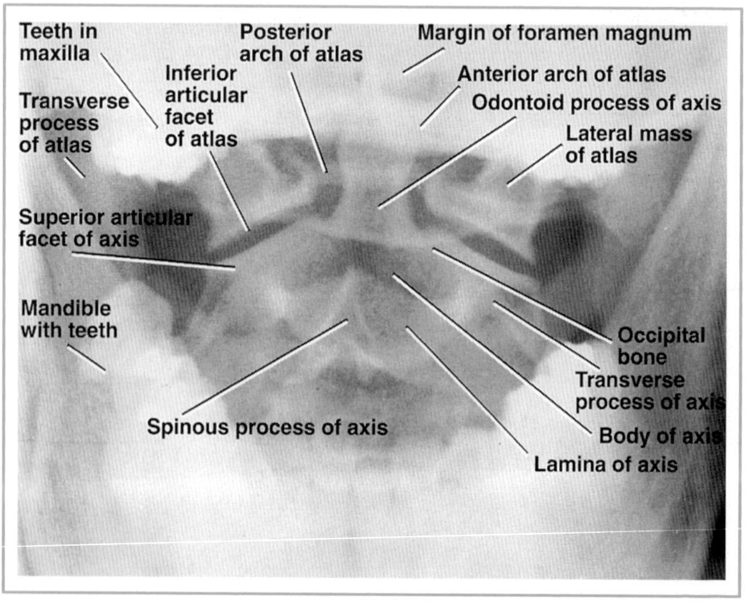

Appendix C-10 Anteroposterior radiograph of the upper cervical spine with the patient's mouth open to show the odontoid process. (From: Snell R, Smith M: *Clinical anatomy for emergency medicine*, St Louis, 1993, Mosby, p. 360, with permission.)

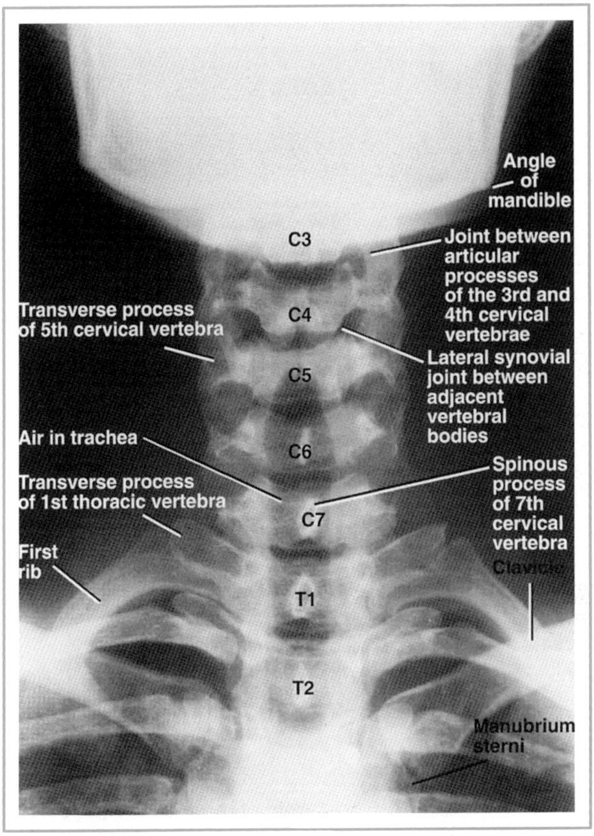

Appendix C-11 Anteroposterior radiograph of the cervical spine. (From: Snell R, Smith M: *Clinical anatomy for emergency medicine*, St Louis, 1993, Mosby, p. 360, with permission.)

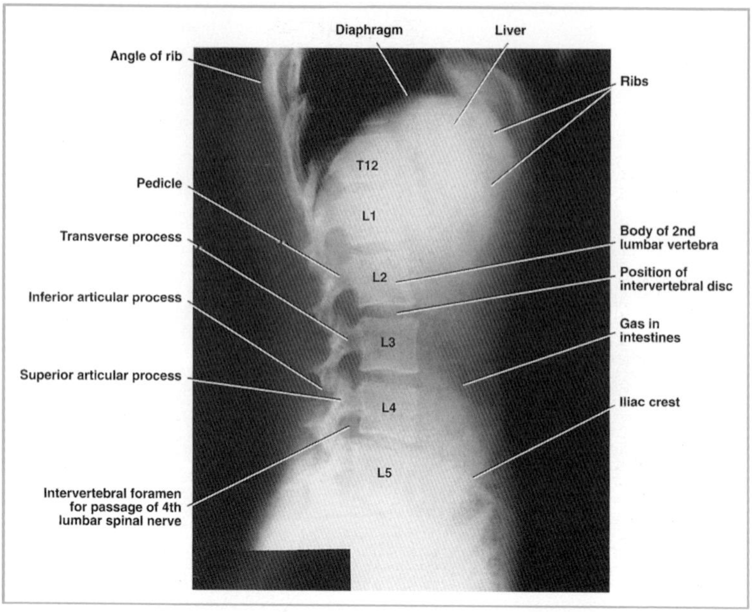

Appendix C-12 Lateral radiograph of thoracolumbar spine. (From Snell R, Smith M: *Clinical anatomy for emergency medicine*, St Louis, 1993, Mosby, p. 365, with permission.)

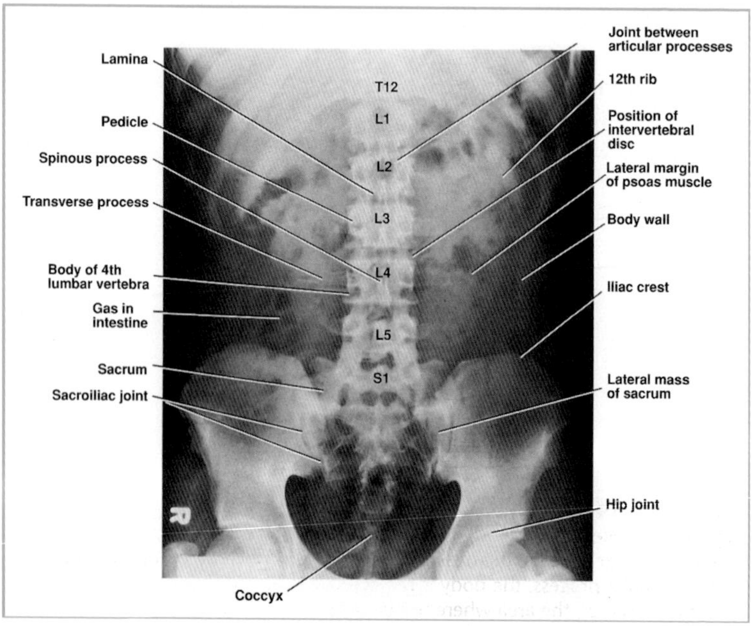

Appendix C-13 Anteroposterior radiograph of the lumbosacral and coccygeal spine. (From Snell R, Smith M: *Clinical anatomy for emergency medicine*, St Louis, 1993, Mosby, p. 364, with permission.)

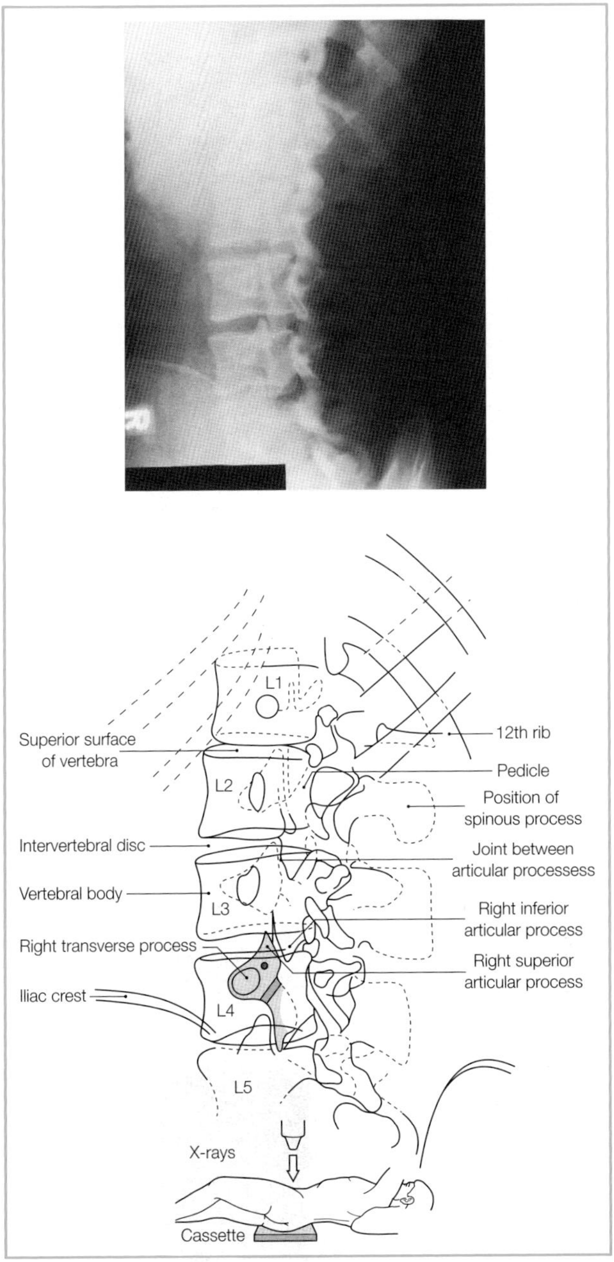

Appendix C-14 Oblique radiograph of the lumbar spine. The stippled "Scotty dog" appearance is seen on the fourth lumbar vertebra. The ear of the dog is the superior articular process, the nose is the ipsilateral pedicle, the front leg is the inferior articular process, the body is the contralateral pedicle, the neck is the pars interarticularis (i.e., the area where the pedicle, lamina, and articular processes all converge), and the presence of a "collar" on the dog's neck indicates a defective area of ossification or a traumatic break in the pars interarticularis, called spondylolysis. (From: Snell R, Smith M: *Clinical anatomy for emergency medicine*, St Louis, 1993, Mosby, p. 366–367, with permission.)

Appendix D

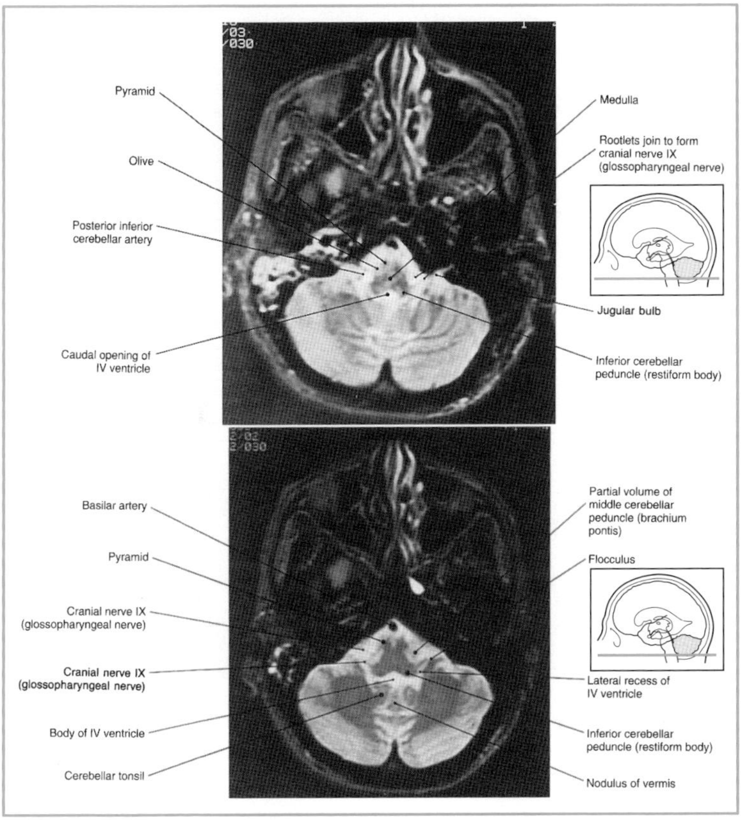

Appendix D-1 to D-10 Normal brain MRI, axial views: the following are consecutive T_2-weighted magnetic resonance images [with repetition time/echo time (TR/TE) of 2000/80 ms] of the adult brain in axial sections. (From: Hayman LA, Pfleger MJ, Pagani JJ, *et al.*: *Atlas of the adult brain*. In Hayman LA, Hinck VC, editors: *Clinical brain imaging: Normal structure and functional anatomy*, St Louis, 1992, Mosby, pp. 79–97, with permission.)

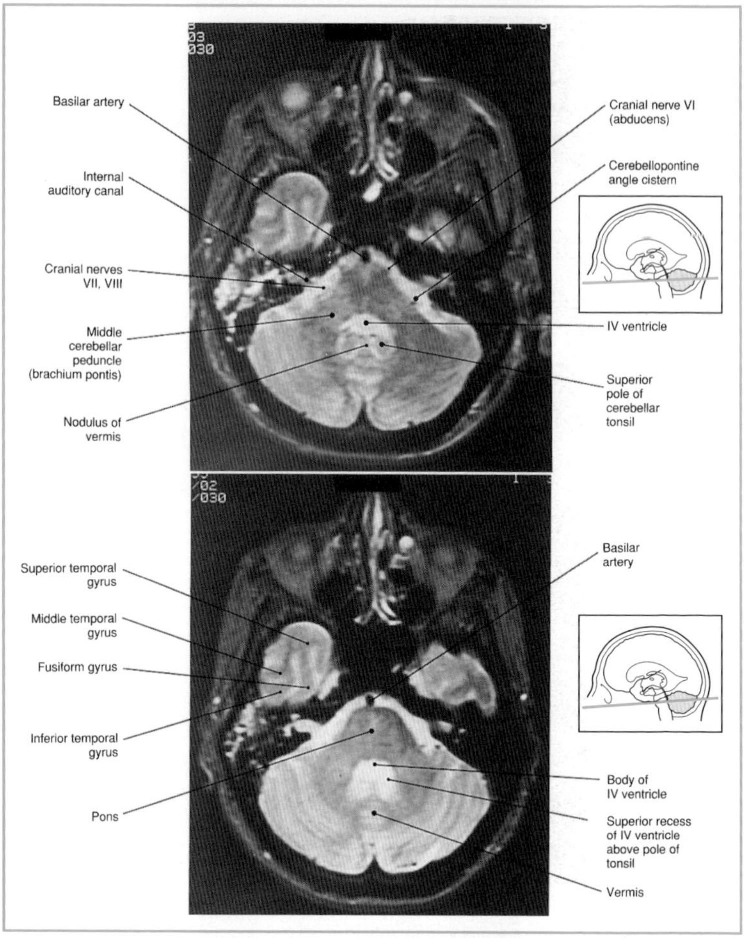
Basilar artery
Internal auditory canal
Cranial nerves VII, VIII
Middle cerebellar peduncle (brachium pontis)
Nodulus of vermis
Cranial nerve VI (abducens)
Cerebellopontine angle cistern
IV ventricle
Superior pole of cerebellar tonsil
Superior temporal gyrus
Middle temporal gyrus
Fusiform gyrus
Inferior temporal gyrus
Pons
Basilar artery
Body of IV ventricle
Superior recess of IV ventricle above pole of tonsil
Vermis

Appendix D-2

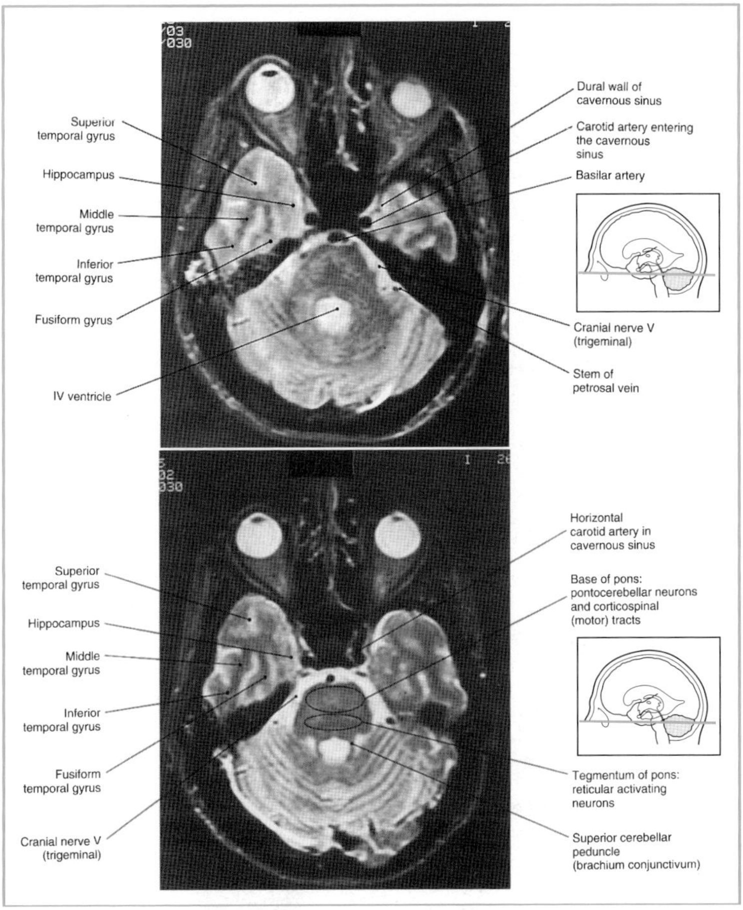

Superior temporal gyrus
Hippocampus
Middle temporal gyrus
Inferior temporal gyrus
Fusiform gyrus
IV ventricle
Dural wall of cavernous sinus
Carotid artery entering the cavernous sinus
Basilar artery
Cranial nerve V (trigeminal)
Stem of petrosal vein
Superior temporal gyrus
Hippocampus
Middle temporal gyrus
Inferior temporal gyrus
Fusiform temporal gyrus
Cranial nerve V (trigeminal)
Horizontal carotid artery in cavernous sinus
Base of pons: pontocerebellar neurons and corticospinal (motor) tracts
Tegmentum of pons: reticular activating neurons
Superior cerebellar peduncle (brachium conjunctivum)

Appendix D-3

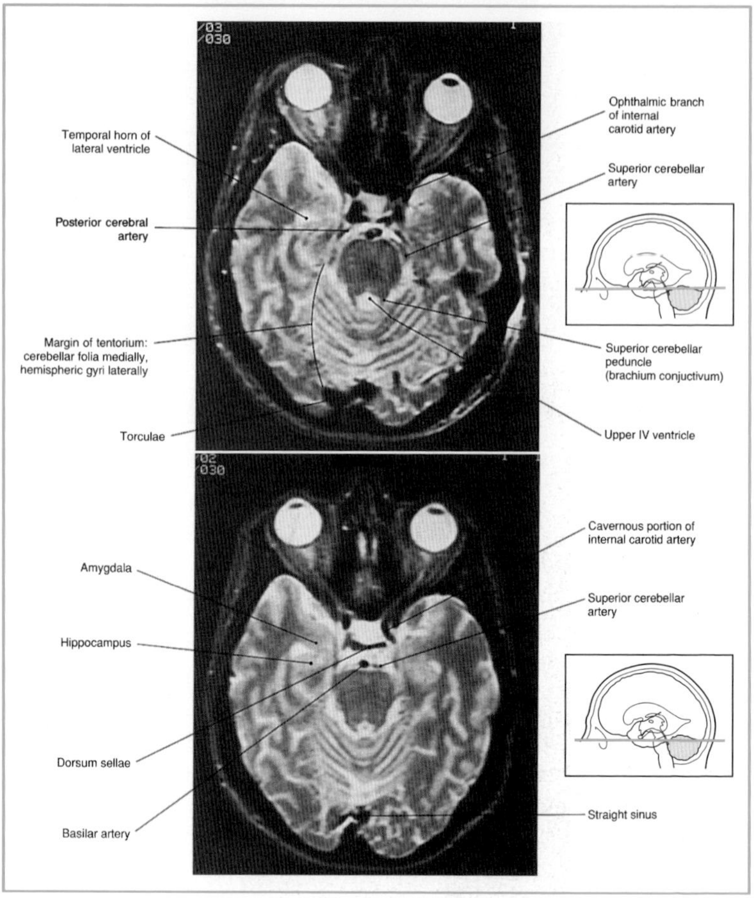
/03
/030
Temporal horn of lateral ventricle
Posterior cerebral artery
Margin of tentorium: cerebellar folia medially, hemispheric gyri laterally
Torculae
Ophthalmic branch of internal carotid artery
Superior cerebellar artery
Superior cerebellar peduncle (brachium conjuctivum)
Upper IV ventricle
/02
/030
Amygdala
Hippocampus
Dorsum sellae
Basilar artery
Cavernous portion of internal carotid artery
Superior cerebellar artery
Straight sinus

Appendix D-4

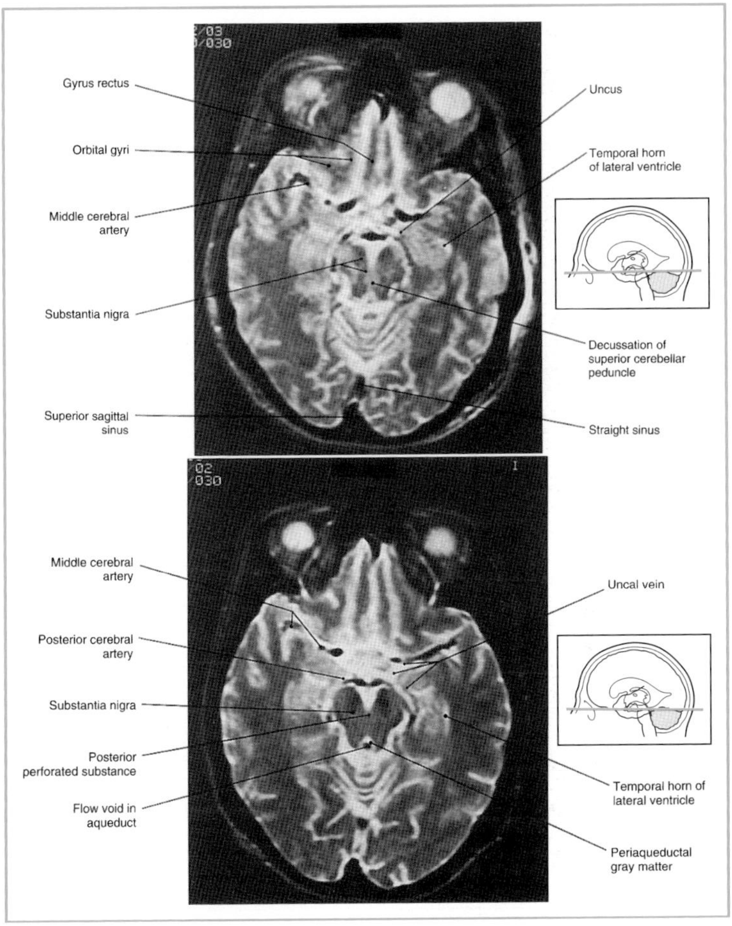

Gyrus rectus
Orbital gyri
Middle cerebral artery
Substantia nigra
Superior sagittal sinus
Uncus
Temporal horn of lateral ventricle
Decussation of superior cerebellar peduncle
Straight sinus
Middle cerebral artery
Posterior cerebral artery
Substantia nigra
Posterior perforated substance
Flow void in aqueduct
Uncal vein
Temporal horn of lateral ventricle
Periaqueductal gray matter

Appendix D-5

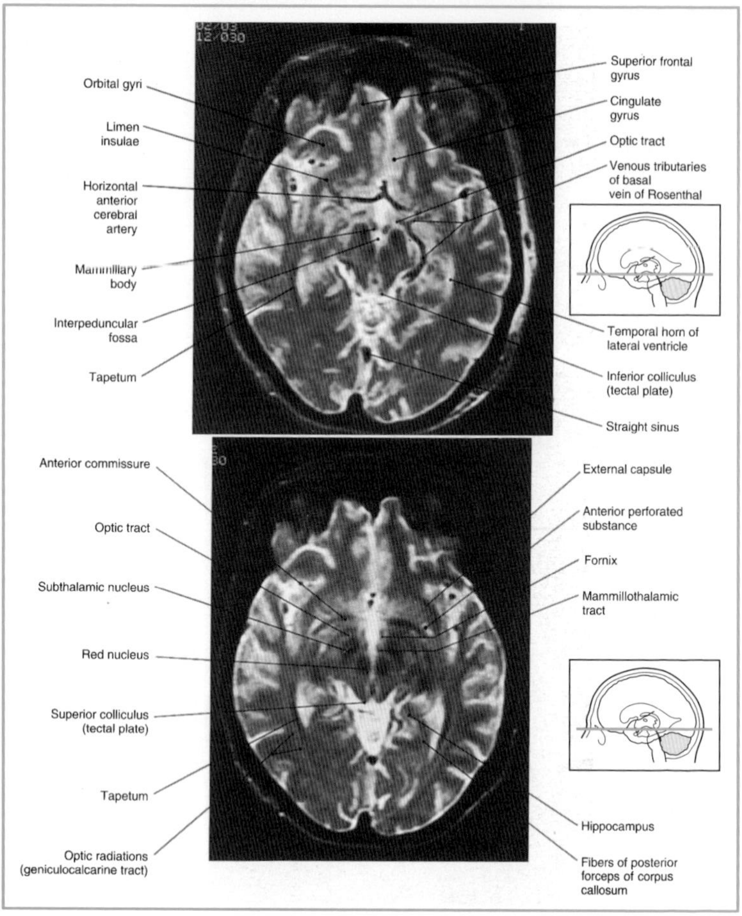
Orbital gyri
Limen insulae
Horizontal anterior cerebral artery
Mammillary body
Interpeduncular fossa
Tapetum
Superior frontal gyrus
Cingulate gyrus
Optic tract
Venous tributaries of basal vein of Rosenthal
Temporal horn of lateral ventricle
Inferior colliculus (tectal plate)
Straight sinus
Anterior commissure
Optic tract
Subthalamic nucleus
Red nucleus
Superior colliculus (tectal plate)
Tapetum
Optic radiations (geniculocalcarine tract)
External capsule
Anterior perforated substance
Fornix
Mammillothalamic tract
Hippocampus
Fibers of posterior forceps of corpus callosum

Appendix D-6

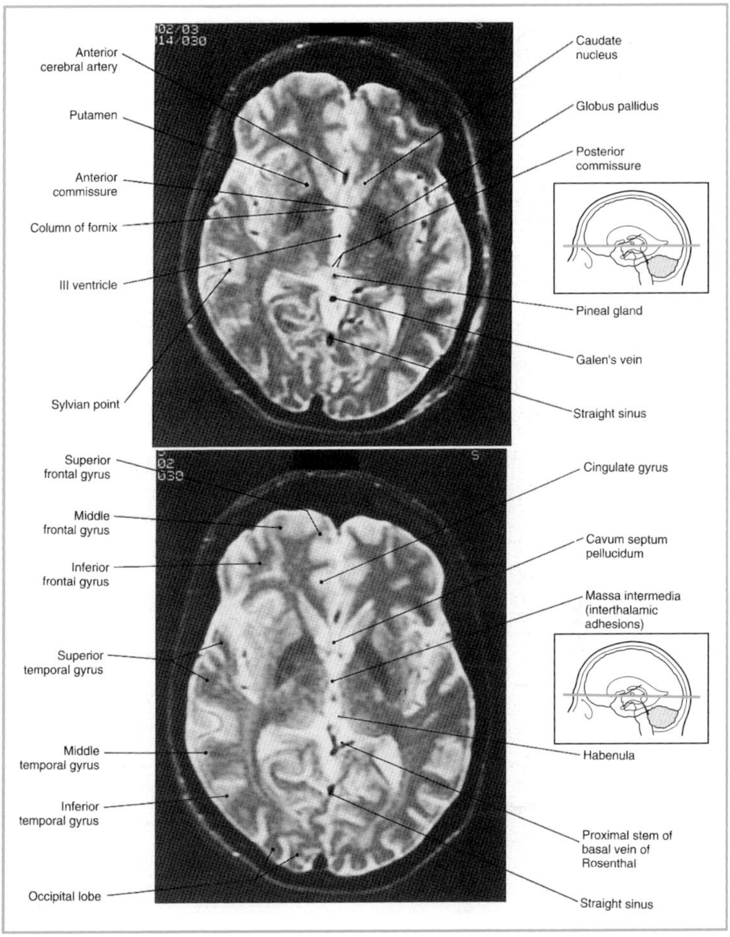
Anterior cerebral artery
Putamen
Anterior commissure
Column of fornix
III ventricle
Sylvian point
Caudate nucleus
Globus pallidus
Posterior commissure
Pineal gland
Galen's vein
Straight sinus
Superior frontal gyrus
Middle frontal gyrus
Inferior frontal gyrus
Superior temporal gyrus
Middle temporal gyrus
Inferior temporal gyrus
Occipital lobe
Cingulate gyrus
Cavum septum pellucidum
Massa intermedia (interthalamic adhesions)
Habenula
Proximal stem of basal vein of Rosenthal
Straight sinus

Appendix D-7

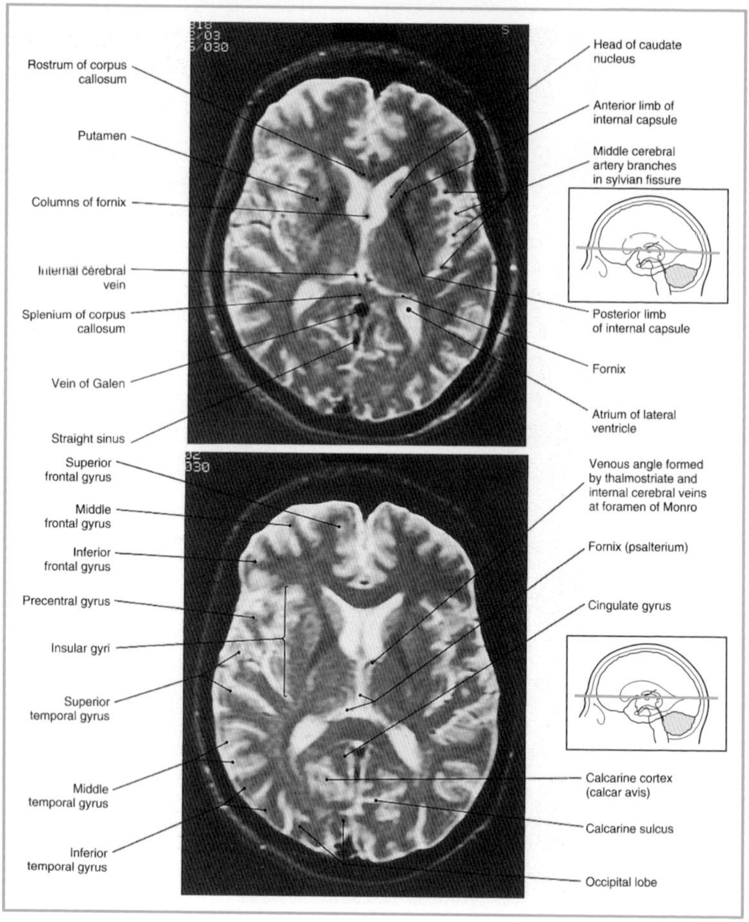
Rostrum of corpus callosum
Putamen
Columns of fornix
Internal cerebral vein
Splenium of corpus callosum
Vein of Galen
Straight sinus
Head of caudate nucleus
Anterior limb of internal capsule
Middle cerebral artery branches in sylvian fissure
Posterior limb of internal capsule
Fornix
Atrium of lateral ventricle
Superior frontal gyrus
Middle frontal gyrus
Inferior frontal gyrus
Precentral gyrus
Insular gyri
Superior temporal gyrus
Middle temporal gyrus
Inferior temporal gyrus
Venous angle formed by thalmostriate and internal cerebral veins at foramen of Monro
Fornix (psalterium)
Cingulate gyrus
Calcarine cortex (calcar avis)
Calcarine sulcus
Occipital lobe

Appendix D-8

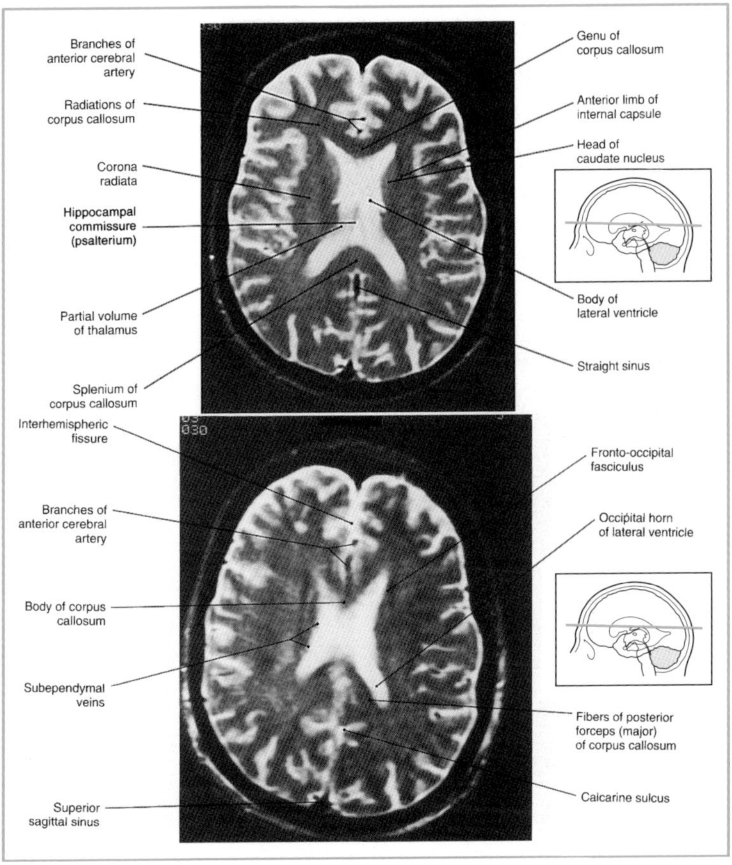
Branches of anterior cerebral artery
Radiations of corpus callosum
Corona radiata
Hippocampal commissure (psalterium)
Partial volume of thalamus
Splenium of corpus callosum
Genu of corpus callosum
Anterior limb of internal capsule
Head of caudate nucleus
Body of lateral ventricle
Straight sinus
Interhemispheric fissure
Branches of anterior cerebral artery
Body of corpus callosum
Subependymal veins
Superior sagittal sinus
Fronto-occipital fasciculus
Occipital horn of lateral ventricle
Fibers of posterior forceps (major) of corpus callosum
Calcarine sulcus

Appendix D-9

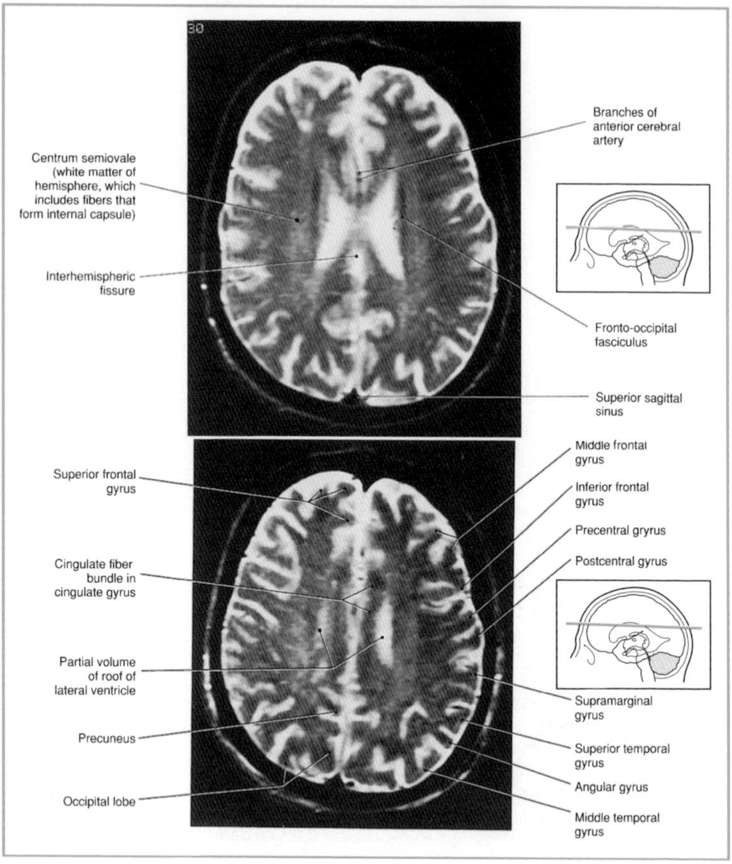
30
Branches of anterior cerebral artery
Centrum semiovale (white matter of hemisphere, which includes fibers that form internal capsule)
Interhemispheric fissure
Fronto-occipital fasciculus
Superior sagittal sinus
Middle frontal gyrus
Superior frontal gyrus
Inferior frontal gyrus
Precentral gryrus
Postcentral gyrus
Cingulate fiber bundle in cingulate gyrus
Partial volume of roof of lateral ventricle
Supramarginal gyrus
Precuneus
Superior temporal gyrus
Angular gyrus
Occipital lobe
Middle temporal gyrus

Appendix D-10

Appendix E

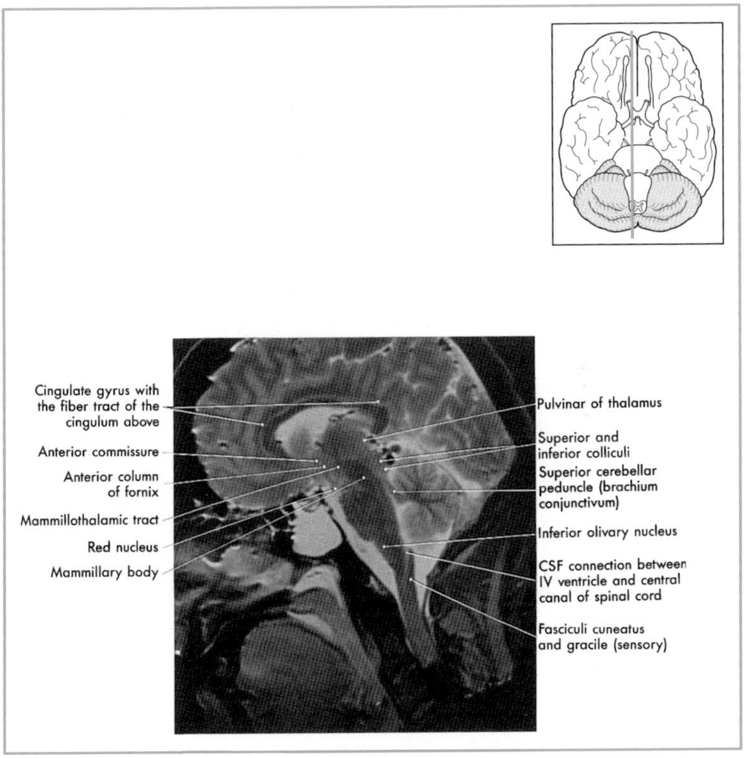

Appendix E-1 to E-7 Normal brain MRI (sagittal view). The following are consecutive T_2-weighted magnetic resonance images [with repetition time/echo time (TR/TE) of 2000/80 ms] of the adult brain in sagittal sections. (From: Hayman LA, Pfleger MJ, Pagani JJ, *et al.*: *Atlas of the adult brain.* In Hayman LA, Hinck VC, editors: *Clinical brain imaging: Normal structure and functional anatomy,* St Louis, 1992, Mosby, pp. 99–111, with permission.)

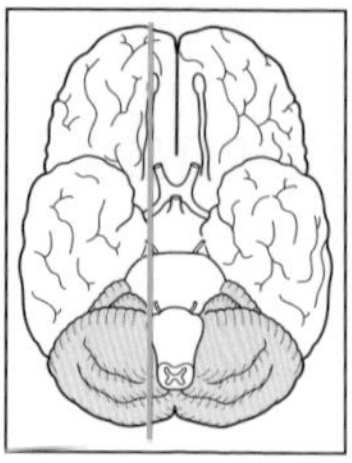

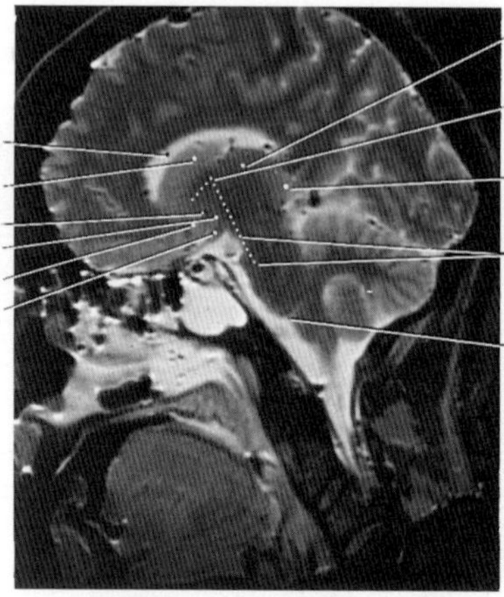
Frontal horn of the lateral ventricle
Head of the caudate
Anterior commissure
Putamen
Globus pallidus
Optic tract
Thalamus
Genu of internal capsule extends ventrally as anterior limb and dorsally as posterior limb
Pulvinar of thalamus
Posterior limb of internal capsule continues inferiorly through cerebral peduncle (crus cerebri) as pyramidal (corticospinal) tract
Foramen caecum separates base of pons from olive of medulla

Appendix E-2

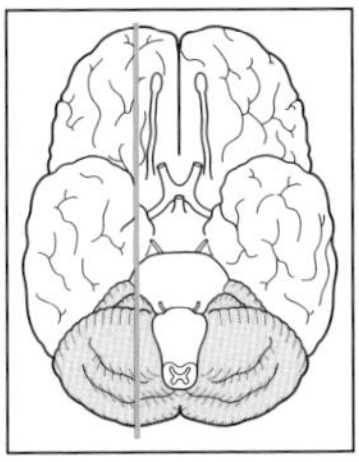

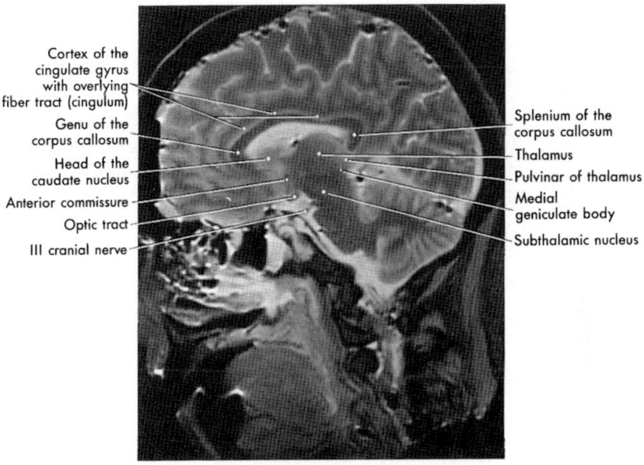
Cortex of the cingulate gyrus with overlying fiber tract (cingulum)
Genu of the corpus callosum
Head of the caudate nucleus
Anterior commissure
Optic tract
III cranial nerve
Splenium of the corpus callosum
Thalamus
Pulvinar of thalamus
Medial geniculate body
Subthalamic nucleus

Appendix E-3

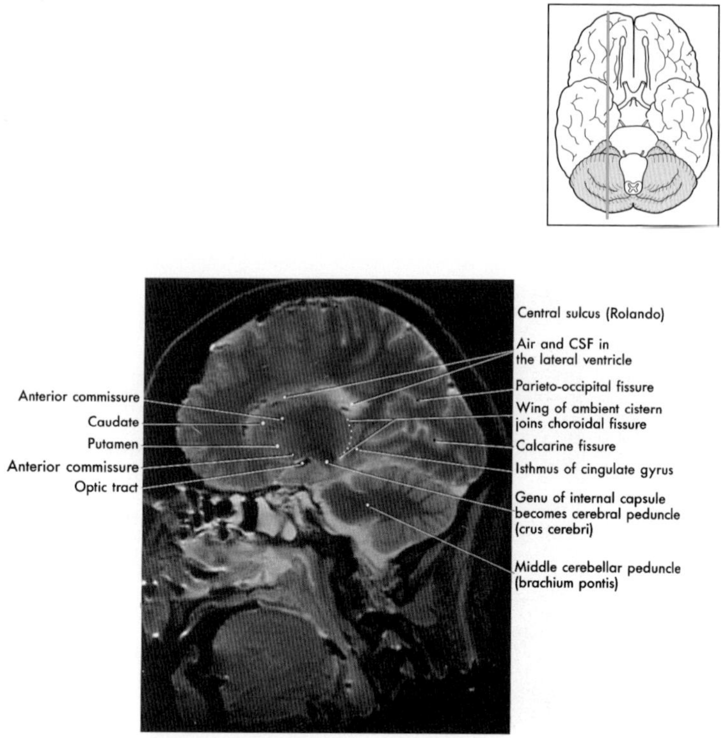
Central sulcus (Rolando)
Air and CSF in the lateral ventricle
Parieto-occipital fissure
Wing of ambient cistern joins choroidal fissure
Calcarine fissure
Isthmus of cingulate gyrus
Genu of internal capsule becomes cerebral peduncle (crus cerebri)
Middle cerebellar peduncle (brachium pontis)
Anterior commissure
Caudate
Putamen
Anterior commissure
Optic tract

Appendix E-4

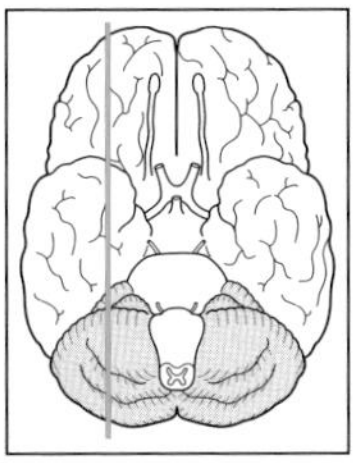

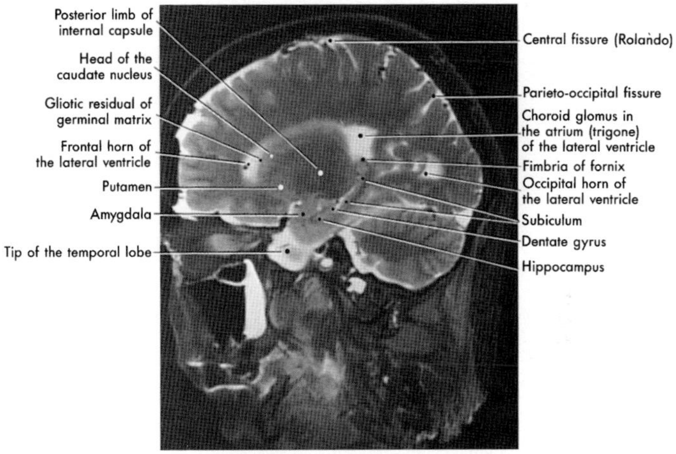
Posterior limb of internal capsule
Head of the caudate nucleus
Gliotic residual of germinal matrix
Frontal horn of the lateral ventricle
Putamen
Amygdala
Tip of the temporal lobe
Central fissure (Rolando)
Parieto-occipital fissure
Choroid glomus in the atrium (trigone) of the lateral ventricle
Fimbria of fornix
Occipital horn of the lateral ventricle
Subiculum
Dentate gyrus
Hippocampus

Appendix E-5

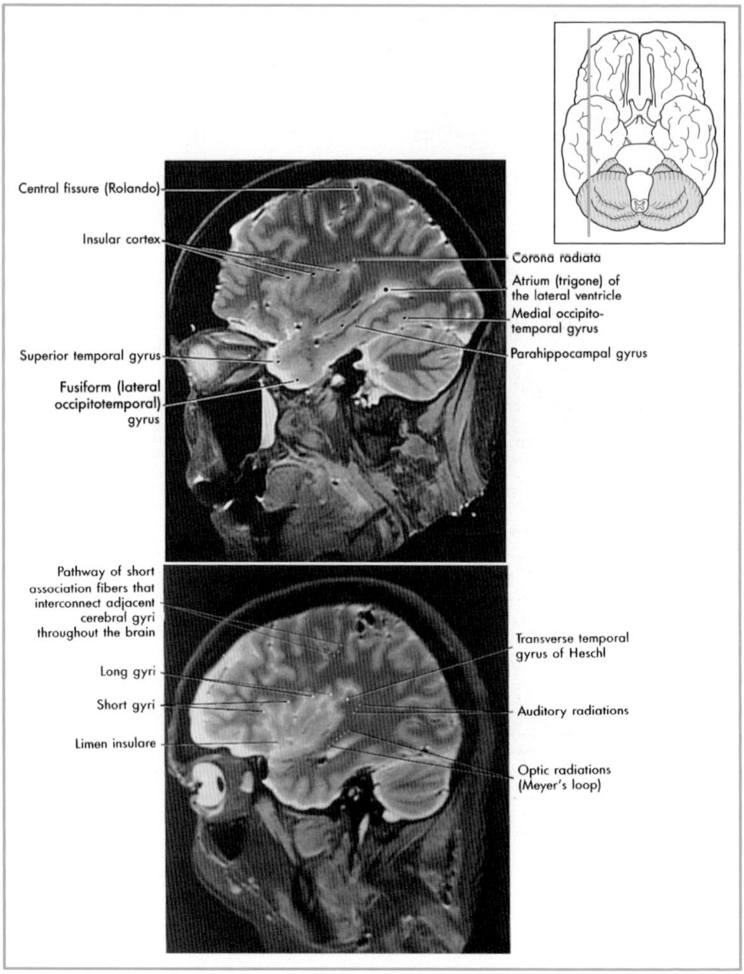
Central fissure (Rolando)
Insular cortex
Corona radiata
Atrium (trigone) of the lateral ventricle
Medial occipito-temporal gyrus
Parahippocampal gyrus
Superior temporal gyrus
Fusiform (lateral occipitotemporal) gyrus
Pathway of short association fibers that interconnect adjacent cerebral gyri throughout the brain
Transverse temporal gyrus of Heschl
Long gyri
Short gyri
Auditory radiations
Limen insulare
Optic radiations (Meyer's loop)

Appendix E-6

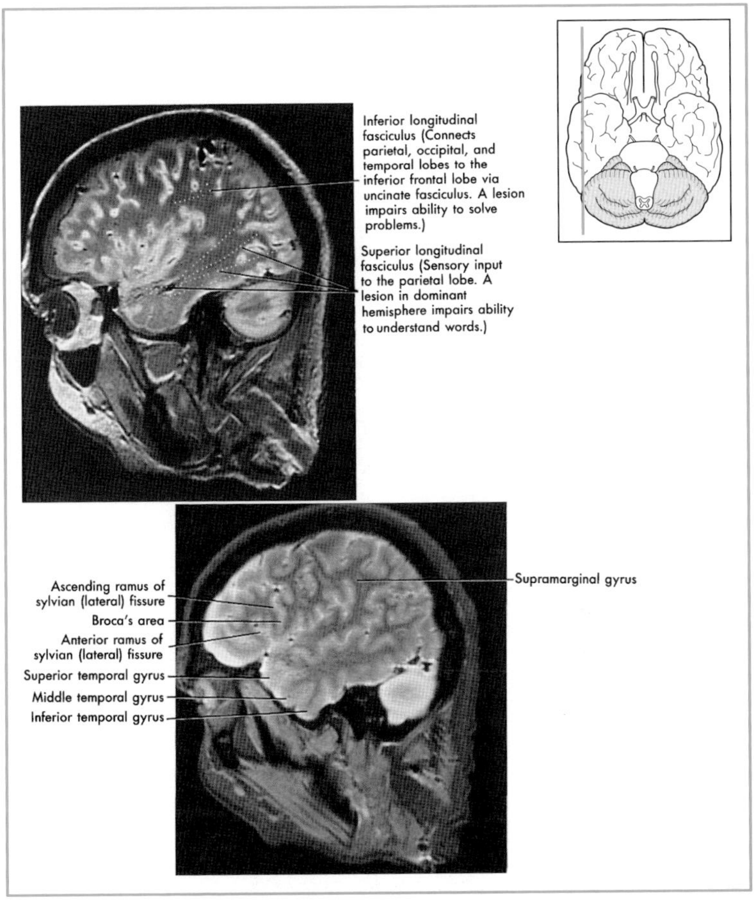
Inferior longitudinal fasciculus (Connects parietal, occipital, and temporal lobes to the inferior frontal lobe via uncinate fasciculus. A lesion impairs ability to solve problems.)
Superior longitudinal fasciculus (Sensory input to the parietal lobe. A lesion in dominant hemisphere impairs ability to understand words.)
Supramarginal gyrus
Ascending ramus of sylvian (lateral) fissure
Broca's area
Anterior ramus of sylvian (lateral) fissure
Superior temporal gyrus
Middle temporal gyrus
Inferior temporal gyrus

Appendix E-7

Appendix F

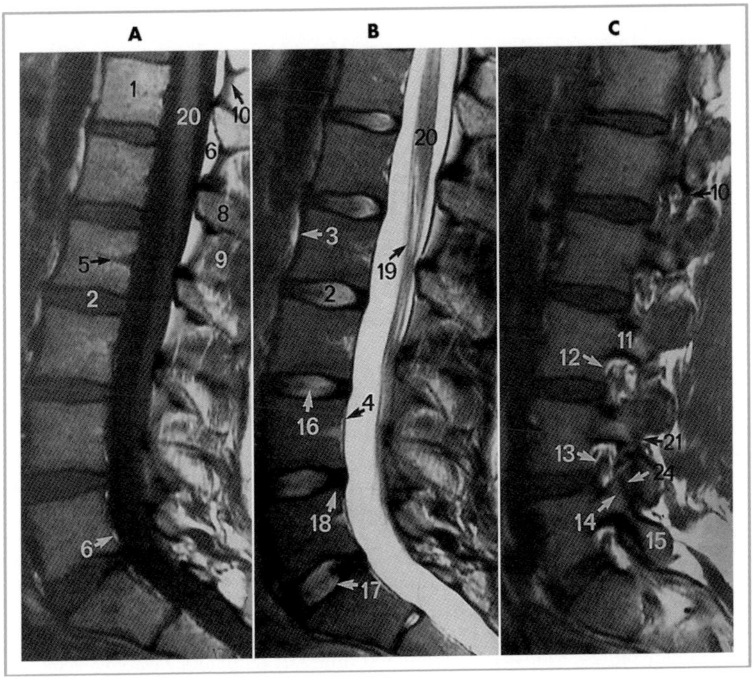

Appendix F-1 High-resolution magnetic resonance imaging of the sagittal section of the lumbar spine. (**A**) (T_1-weighted) and (**B**) (T_2-weighted) demonstrate normal midline anatomy. (**C**) is a T_1-weighted sagittal scan through the neural foramen showing the relationship of the soft tissues to the surrounding bone and intervertebral disk. 1, vertebral body; 2, intervertebral disk (nucleus pulposus); 3, anterior longitudinal ligament; 4, posterior longitudinal ligament; 5, basivertebral venous plexus; 6, epidural fat; 8, spinous processes; 9, interspinous ligament; 10, ligamentum flavum; 11, pedicle; 12, neural foramen with epidural fat and veins; 13, dorsal root ganglion; 14, superior articular facet; 15, inferior articular facet; 16, intranuclear cleft; 17, inner annular fibers of disk; 18, outer annular fibers of disk; 19, cauda equina; 20, conus medullaris; 21, pars interarticularis; 24, facet joint. (From: Osborne AG: *Diagnostic neuroradiology*, vol 1, St Louis, 1994, Mosby, p. 789, with permission.)

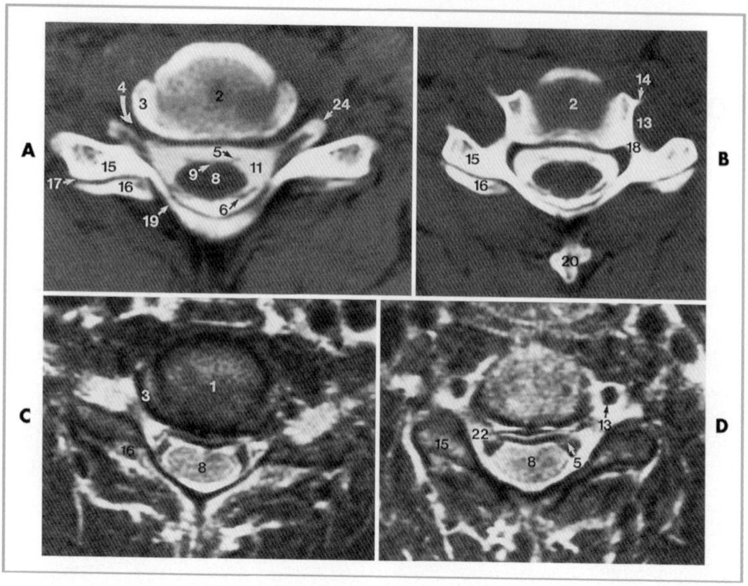

Appendix F-2 Multimodality imaging studies showing the axial anatomy of the spine. Axial computed tomography scans (**A** and **B**) with intrathecal contrast are shown at the level of the uncovertebral joint and neural foramina (**A**) and the pedicles (**B**). (**C**) and (**D**) are axial T_2-weighted magnetic resonance imaging scans which depict normal cervical spinal cord and soft tissue anatomy. Prominent areas of high-velocity signal loss from pulsatile cerebrospinal fluid flow are present. 1, vertebral body; 2, intervertebral disk (nucleus pulposus); 3, uncinate process; 4, neural foramen; 5, anterior roots; 6, posterior roots; 8, cervical spinal cord; 9, ventral medial fissure; 11, subarachnoid space; 13, vertebral artery in foramen transversarium; 14, transverse process; 15, superior articular facet; 16, inferior articular facet; 17, facet joint; 18, pedicle; 19, lamina; 20, spinous process; 22, epidural fat; 24, root sleeve. (From: Osborne AG: *Diagnostic neuroradiology*, vol 1, St Louis, 1994, Mosby, p. 796, with permission.)

Index

Note: page numbers in *italics* refer to figures, tables, and appendices.

Index